Praise for the
American Dietetic Association Complete Food and Nutrition Guide

". . . jam-packed with practical eating and food safety tips."

—USA Today

"It's always refreshing to find a nutritionist interested in good taste!"

—Julia Child, author, culinary expert, TV personality

"[A] remarkable reference."

—Graham Kerr

"[The book] may be the ultimate healthy-eating primer. How often can it be said of a book that it may extend your life?"

—Fitness magazine

". . . brimming with tips from baby food to eating for healthy aging."

—Shape magazine

"Duyff really covers nutrition and healthy eating from all angles . . . without overusing the 'd' word ['don't']."

—Tufts University Health & Nutrition Letter

"Intelligent advice about sensible eating."

—Washington Times

"Everything you ever wanted to know about everything you ever wanted to eat is in this guide."

—Food Management magazine

". . . a must for everyone's kitchen, from the teenager learning about food and nutrition to adults changing their eating styles."

—Cheri Svoboda, The Oregonian

". . . in short, it's a winner!"

—Washington Post

". . . set out so anyone, even those not nutritionally inclined, can open the book and find something interesting."

—Janice Denham, food editor, *St. Louis Journal* Publications

". . . covers everything from deciphering food labels to maintaining a family-friendly kitchen to changing dietary needs as we age."

—St. Louis Post-Dispatch

"An essential resource for consumers seeking to make healthy food choices, and nutrition professionals requiring a science-based reference tool."

—Susan Lerner Barr, M.S., R.D., contributing nutrition editor, *Self* magazine

". . . solid all-around guide to nutrition that's fun just to pick up and peruse . . . sure to become dog-eared over time."

—Environmental Nutrition

"Translates nutrition science into the everyday food advice people need to make healthy choices when grocery shopping, cooking dinner, or ordering from a restaurant menu."

—Carolyn O'Neil, MS, RD, award-winning television food journalist, former CNN nutrition news correspondent

". . . tackles most of the nutritional issues that concern Americans today . . . up-to-date and helpful."

—Seattle Times

"Readable and timely. . . . Duyff gives sound advice."

—Library Journal

"A wealth of practical information [to] refer to time and time again."

—Journal of Nutrition Education

"Excellent and thorough . . . Includes solid, science-based content on many nutrition topics, up-to-date healthy eating guidance, and ways to evaluate current nutrition research."

—Johanna Dwyer, DSc, RD, professor, School of Nutrition and Medicine, Tufts University, and director of Frances Stern Nutrition Center

American Dietetic Association
Complete Food and Nutrition Guide

2ND EDITION

Roberta Larson Duyff

MS, RD, FADA, CFCS

John Wiley & Sons, Inc.

About the ADA

The American Dietetic Association is the largest group of food and nutrition professionals in the world. As the advocate of the profession, the ADA serves the public by promoting optimal nutrition, health, and well-being.

For more information . . .

Visit the ADA's Web site at *http://www.eatright.org*. The American Dietetic Association's Web site offers nutrition information for consumers and health professionals, and the Find a Dietitian feature to locate a dietetics professional in your area. The ADA's Consumer Nutrition Information line, at (800) 366-1655, also provides referrals to local registered dietitians as well as recorded nutrition messages in English and Spanish.

This book is printed on acid-free paper. ∞

Copyright © 2002 by The American Dietetic Association. All rights reserved

Illustrations on part and chapter openers and on pages 298, 372, 374, and 392 copyright © 2002 by Jackie Aher.

Published by John Wiley & Sons, Inc., Hoboken, New Jersey
Published simultaneously in Canada

Design and production by Navta Associates, Inc.

No part of this publication may be reproduced, stored in a retrieval system, or transmitted in any form or by any means, electronic, mechanical, photocopying, recording, scanning, or otherwise, except as permitted under Section 107 or 108 of the 1976 United States Copyright Act, without either the prior written permission of the Publisher, or authorization through payment of the appropriate per-copy fee to the Copyright Clearance Center, 222 Rosewood Drive, Danvers, MA 01923, (978) 750-8400, fax (978) 750-4470, or on the web at www.copyright.com. Requests to the Publisher for permission should be addressed to the Permissions Department, John Wiley & Sons, Inc., 111 River Street, Hoboken, NJ 07030, (201)748-6011, fax (201) 748-6008, email: permcoordinator@wiley.com

Limit of Liability/Disclaimer of Warranty: While the publisher and author have used their best efforts in preparing this book, they make no representations or warranties with respect to the accuracy or completeness of the contents of this book and specifically disclaim any implied warranties of merchantability or fitness for a particular purpose. No warranty may be created or extended by sales representatives or written sales materials. The advice and strategies contained herein may not be suitable for your situation. You should consult with a professional where appropriate. Neither the publisher nor author shall be liable for any loss of profit or any other commercial damages, including but not limited to special, incidental, consequential, or other damages.

Readers are advised to seek the guidance of a licensed physician or healthcare professional before making changes in healthcare regimens, since each individual case or need may vary. This book is intended for informational purposes only and is not for use as an alternative to appropriate medical care. While every effort has been made to ensure that the information is the most current available, new research findings, being released with increasing frequency, may invalidate some data.

For general information about our other products and services, please contact our Customer Care Department within the United States at (800) 762-2974, outside the United States at (317) 572-3993 or fax (317) 572-4002.

Wiley also publishes its books in a variety of electronic formats. Some content that appears in print may not be available in electronic books.

ISBN 0-471-44144-9

Printed in the United States of America

10 9 8 7 6 5 4 3 2 1

Contents

PART I   Eat Smart, Live Well: It's About You!

PART II   Healthful Eating: The Basics

PART IV Food for Health: Every Age, Every Stage of Life

Foreword

Food nourishes us in many ways. Eating is one of life's pleasures. Food is tied to memories of our youth and to social occasions, celebrations, and other aspects of our culture. Food also fuels our bodies. What we eat is a controllable factor in keeping us as healthy and as fit as possible.

The fundamentals for fostering a healthy body remain constant. A well-balanced approach to eating and getting plenty of rest and physical activity are, and always have been, keys to good health. Research about nutrition and its impact on everything from childhood development to disease control and prevention, however, shows that our knowledge about the role of nutrition in a healthful lifestyle is continually evolving. Since the last published edition of this book, scientists have made exciting discoveries about nutrition and how much it can affect our overall health. We now know more about health-promoting substances in fruits, vegetables, and grain products called phytonutrients. We have expanded the way we look at vitamins and minerals. Consumers are increasingly turning to "alternative" medicine and therapies to treat or prevent disease. In addition, the impact of biotechnology on the food supply is changing the way we think about how our food is grown and processed.

All these important issues and more are discussed in the second edition of the *American Dietetic Association Complete Food and Nutrition Guide.* Written and reviewed by qualified nutrition practitioners—registered dietitians and dietetic technicians, registered—the book is scientifically based. But more than that, it is practical and easy to understand. Registered dietitians counsel people to attain optimal health by eating a variety of nutrient-rich foods with an emphasis on taste, quality, moderation, balance, and food safety.

In the second edition of the *American Dietetic Association Complete Food and Nutrition Guide,* Roberta Duyff shows you how to maximize your health while enjoying food. Her practical suggestions are backed up by the latest scientific evidence, as well as by her extensive experience as a registered dietitian. Best of all, the book can serve as a reference for your entire family's health—and it's right at your fingertips.

Enjoy the book and optimize your health.

Julie O'Sullivan Maillet, RD, PhD, FADA
President, American Dietetic Association

Acknowledgments

At every phase in developing the *American Dietetic Association Complete Food and Nutrition Guide,* I've been grateful and indebted to the many professionals, colleagues, and friends—in the fields of nutrition and dietetics, health, family and consumer sciences, food science, culinary arts, education, and communications—who have shared their knowledge, experience, and expertise throughout my career. I'm especially grateful to:

The American Dietetic Association, for the honor of writing this book on behalf of the association's more than seventy thousand members.

Betsy Hornick, editor and registered dietitian, on behalf of ADA Publications, for her nutrition expertise, editorial guidance, and commitment to excellence at every phase in the development of this book in both its first and second editions.

ADA staff: Diana Faulhaber, ADA director of book publishing, who offered constant support and encouragement for a consumer-focused, healthy-eating book; Sharon Denny and Lorri Fishman, ADA Knowledge Center, for their quick, enthusiastic help in preparing the manuscript; Saudia Muhammad and Alison Loviska, publications department, who helped with permissions; Anne Coghill, acquisitions editor, who began the second-edition process; Michael Weitz, ADA director of marketing, for the many promotional efforts for the book; Lori Ferme, ADA media relations manager, for ADA's publicity of the book; and to those who work with them.

ADA members—with expertise as either a *registered dietitian* or a *dietetic technician, registered*—who volunteered countless hours to review the manuscript for content accuracy, clarity, and comprehensiveness:

● To those who reviewed this entire edition: Sharon Denny, Lorri Fishman, and Lisa Kelly.

● To those who provided their unique expertise for portions of the book: Keith-Thomas Ayoob, Leila Beker, Felicia Busch, Maureen Callahan, Beverly Clevidence, Mildred Cody, Eleese Cunningham, Connie Diekman, Robert Earl, Deborah Fillman, Susan Finn, Julie Fulton, Molly Gee, Barbara Gollman, Dayle Hayes, Lenore Hodges, Edith Hogan, Sherri Hoyt, Barbara Ivens, Judith Jarvis, Cynthia Kupper, Linda McDonald, Elaine McLaughlin, Julie O'Sullivan Maillet, Wendy Marcason, Jacqueline Marcus, Mildred Mattfeldt-Beman, Libby Mills, Marlene Most, Tammie Otterstein, Linda Rhodes Pauly, Anne Piatek, Christine Polisena, Diane Quagliani, Christine Rosenbloom, Allison Sarubin Fragakis, Lana Shepek, and Joanne Slavin.

● To those who reviewed the first edition: Susan Borra, Mary Carey, Dayle Hayes, Marsha Hudnall, Nancy Schwartz, and Madeleine Sigman-Grant, as well as Julie Burns, Suzanne Havala, Sue Murvich, and Ann Semenske.

Sherri Hoyt, colleague and registered dietitian, for her contributions on food sensitivity, infant and child feeding, nutrition during pregnancy, and breast-feeding.

Registered dietitians and other food, nutrition, and health professionals who work in government agencies, the food industry, and educational institutions throughout the country, and who served as resources and experts.

Organizations who granted permission for the use of supporting illustrations and graphics.

Dietetic students for their careful fact checking: Sehr Jangda, Adrienne Kraemer, and Grace Lange.

The fine team of editors and staff at John Wiley & Sons, especially Kitt Allan, Kellam Ayres, Tanya Barone, Laura Cusack, Sabrina Eliasoph, Tom Miller, John Simko, and Elizabeth Zack, who handled the publication of this book; copyeditor William Drennan; the design team at Navta Associates; as well as the Chronimed Publishing team responsible for its first edition.

Other friends and family who reviewed the manuscript from their unique consumer and professional perspectives: Ann Hagan Brickman, Linda Carpenter, Julie Duyff, Phil Duyff, Patty Fletcher, Karen Marshall, Patricia McKissack, and Linda Valiga.

Edith Syrjala Eash, Diva Sanjur, and Hazel Spitze, who encouraged my early career as a registered dietitian and in nutrition education.

Anne Piatek, colleague and culinary dietitian, for encouraging me to write this book.

My family, especially my mother, Jeane Larson, and my friends, who shared their support, understanding, and encouragement for both editions.

My husband, Phil, who read every chapter for clarity and consumer friendliness . . . and who offered the sensitivity and loving support I needed to write this book.

Roberta Larson Duyff, MS, RD, FADA, CFCS
Author/Food Nutrition Consultant
Duyff Associates, St. Louis, Mo.

This book went to press prior to release of the 2002 Dietary Reference Intakes for macronutrients and fiber; recommendations for these dietary components reflect previous guidelines.

Unless otherwise noted, the nutrient and calorie data in this book were derived from:

- U.S. Department of Agriculture/Agricultural Research Service, *Nutrient Data Library, http://www.nal.usda.gov/fnic/foodcomp/*

- Jean A. T. Pennington, *Bowes & Church's Food Values of Portions Commonly Used,* 17th ed. (New York: J. B. Lippincott, 1998)

- Selected data from food manufacturers and fast-food chains

Introduction

The *American Dietetic Association Complete Food and Nutrition Guide* has been created for you as a practical, up-to-date resource for healthful eating. From cover to cover, you'll see how smart eating—combined with physical activity—promotes fitness. As important, you'll learn how healthful eating and taste go hand in hand!

To offer *solutions* for your everyday eating dilemmas, this book is filled with practical advice—whatever your lifestyle or needs. From weight control to heart-healthy eating . . . supermarket shopping to eating out . . . food safety to kitchen nutrition . . . vegetarian eating to sports nutrition, you'll find many tips for ease, convenience, and good taste. Look for today's "hot" food issues, too: phytonutrients, functional foods, dietary supplements, and food biotechnology, among others.

As your complete resource on nutrition, you can refer to this book again and again at every age and stage of your life—from choosing the healthiest baby food or feeding a child or teen, to dealing with unique nutrition needs in a woman's life or challenges of aging. It's also filled with advice for preventing, slowing, or dealing with heart disease, cancer, diabetes, and other common health problems. This book is meant for you, and for all those you care about . . . perhaps a child, spouse, companion, aging parent, or friend.

For your personal nutrition "checkup," you'll find opportunities to assess your own everyday food choices. Start in chapter 1 with "Looking for 'Healthy Solutions'?" to identify your personal eating challenges. For more information, each question refers you to in-depth answers throughout the book. In fact, in almost every chapter, "Your Nutrition Checkup" gives you a close-up look at your own food decisions.

Whenever nutrition makes the news (print, television, radio, or online), this book can help you judge the headlines and separate sound fact from fad. Its food and nutrition advice comes from the American Dietetic Association, the authority the United States turns to for food and nutrition advice, with more than eighty-five years of nutrition expertise and research.

With questions posed to nutrition experts—in part through the American Dietetic Association's Knowledge Center—thousands of consumers have helped shape the focus and content of the *American Dietetic Association Complete Food and Nutrition Guide*. We hope the answers to their food and nutrition questions will also answer many of yours!

Read, enjoy, be active, and eat healthy . . . for life!

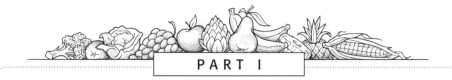

PART I

Eat Smart, Live Well
It's About You!

CHAPTER 1

Food Choices for Fitness

Your life is filled with choices! Every day you make thousands of choices, many related to food. Some seem trivial. Others are important. A few may even set the course of your life. But as insignificant as a single choice may seem, made over and over, it can have a major impact on your health—and your life!

This book is about choices—those you, your family, and your friends make every day about food, nutrition, and health. Within its pages, you'll find reliable nutrition information and sound advice, based on scientific evidence. It offers you practical ways to eat healthfully in almost any situation and at every phase of life. And it encourages you to enjoy the pleasures of food. After all, taste is the number one reason most people choose one food over another.

Most important, the practical tips and flexible guidelines on its pages help you choose nutritious, flavorful foods to match your own needs, preferences, and lifestyle—even as your life and family situation change. Eating for health is one of the wisest decisions you'll ever make!

Fitness: Your Overall Health!

What does being fit mean to you? Perhaps, being free of disease and other health problems? Or having plenty of energy, or a trim or muscular body, or the ability to finish a 10K run? Actually, "fitness" is far broader and more personal. It refers to your own *optimal health and overall well-being*. Fitness is your good health—at its very best.

Being fit defines every aspect of your health—not only your physical health, but your emotional and mental well-being, too. In fact, they're interconnected. Smart eating and active living are fundamental to all three. When you're fit, you have:

● Energy to do what's important to you and to be more productive

● Stamina and a positive outlook to handle the mental challenges and emotional ups and downs of everyday life, and to deal with stress

● Reduced risk for many health problems, including serious, often life-changing diseases, such as heart disease, cancer, diabetes, and osteoporosis

● The chance to look and feel your best

● Physical strength and endurance to protect yourself in case of an emergency

● A better chance for a higher quality of life, and perhaps a longer one, too

Fit Is Ageless

Fitness at every age and stage in life depends on healthful eating and active living. The sooner you make them your priorities, the better your health.

That, too, is what this book is all about—how to eat for health and stay physically active throughout the cycle of life, and enjoy great-tasting food along the way!

Good nutrition and regular physical activity are two lifestyle habits that promote fitness—but certainly not the only ones. To stay fit, make other lifestyle choices for good health, too: get adequate sleep, avoid smoking, manage stress, drink alcoholic beverages only in moderation (if you drink), wear your seat belt, observe good hygiene, get regular medical checkups, obtain adequate health care—to name a few.

Smart Eating: Fuel for Fitness

What does it take to be fit? You don't need special or costly foods, or fancy exercise equipment or health club membership. You don't need to give up your favorite foods, or set up a tedious system of eating rules or calorie counting. And you don't need to hit a specific weight on the bathroom scale.

You've heard the term "nutrition" all your life. The food-fitness connection is what it's all about. In a nutshell, nutrition is how food nourishes your body. And

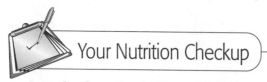

Your Nutrition Checkup

Ready for Healthier Eating?

Where do you fit on this "healthy eating" readiness test? Check one.

☐ *"My food choices are okay as they are."* Okay, but read on to find out why you might consider taking a few steps in the future to eat for better health (and perhaps move more, too).

☐ *"I'll change my eating habits sometime, but I can't make myself do it now."* Good initial thought. Check here for sensible, realistic ways to eat smarter (and move more)—but *now* rather than later. The sooner you start, the greater the benefits.

☐ *"I'm ready to eat smarter, starting now."* Good. Look through these chapters for small steps to healthful eating that you can take. As you achieve them, try a few more. Be active, too.

☐ *"I'm already a 'healthy eater.'"* Great, keep it up! Flip through this book for more practical ways to eat smart. In fact, get adventuresome with your eating. And take time for active living.

☐ *"Healthy eating and active living are second nature to me."* Excellent! Share the practical advice here and your own success with someone else!

being well nourished depends on getting enough of the nutrients your body needs—but not too much.

At every stage in life, healthful eating fuels fitness. Well-nourished infants, children, and teens grow, develop, and learn better. Good nutrition helps ensure a healthy pregnancy and successful breast-feeding. And healthful eating and active living help people at any age feel their best, work productively, and lower their risks for some diseases.

Today's understanding of nutrition is based on years of scientific study. Interest in food and health actually has a long history and was even recorded by the ancient Greeks. But it wasn't until the nineteenth century that the mysteries of nutrition began to be solved. Since then, scientists have been able to answer many nutrition questions. And research continues as scientists explore emerging questions about food, nutrients, phytonutrients, and their role in health.

Today we know that healthful eating dramatically lowers the risk for the main causes of disability and death in the United States: heart disease, certain cancers, diabetes, stroke, and osteoporosis. Good nutrition and regular physical activity also can lower risks for obesity, high blood pressure, and high blood cholesterol—all risk factors for serious disease.

Nutrition advice, with the consensus of today's nutrition experts, is supported by solid scientific evidence. So unlike the ancients, you have a valid basis for choosing food for health. It's up to you to apply nutrition principles and advice for your own well-being.

To make wise food choices, you need science-based nutrition information. What you know—and don't know—just may surprise you!

Smart Eating: Pleasure, Too!

Why do you choose one food over another? Besides the nutrition benefits, food is a source of pleasure, adventure, and great taste! It's no surprise that people entertain and celebrate with food, or look forward to a special dish.

Your own food choices reflect you and what's important to you: your culture, your surroundings, the people around you, your view of yourself, the foods available to you, your emotions, and certainly what you know about food and nutrition. To eat for health, you don't need to give up your food favorites. Simply learn how to fit them in. Good nutrition adds pleasure to eating—especially as you eat a greater variety of vegetables, fruits, grain products, and other nutrient-rich foods.

Throughout this book, you'll get plenty of guidance to do just that! You'll learn more about nutrition and fitness—and how you can eat the foods you like, even try new foods, in an eating plan that promotes your personal fitness.

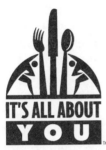

IT'S ALL ABOUT YOU ™

Make Healthy Choices That Fit Your Lifestyle
So You Can Do The Things You Want To Do.

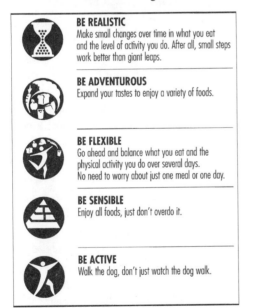

BE REALISTIC
Make small changes over time in what you eat and the level of activity you do. After all, small steps work better than giant leaps.

BE ADVENTUROUS
Expand your tastes to enjoy a variety of foods.

BE FLEXIBLE
Go ahead and balance what you eat and the physical activity you do over several days. No need to worry about just one meal or one day.

BE SENSIBLE
Enjoy all foods, just don't overdo it.

BE ACTIVE
Walk the dog, don't just watch the dog walk.

Source: The Dietary Guidelines Alliance, 1999; © Cattlemen's Beef Board and National Cattlemen's Beef Association.

What's Smart Eating? Guidelines for Americans

Healthful eating: it's one of your best personal investments! While your genes, age, surroundings, lifestyle, healthcare, and culture strongly influence your health,

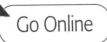 **Check Your "Eat Smart" Score!**

Go Online

Want a snapshot view of your food choices for the day? Score the quality of your day's meals and snacks online—and see how your food choices match up to the Dietary Guidelines for Americans and the Food Guide Pyramid. Using the U.S. Department of Agriculture's Interactive Healthy Eating Index (IHEI), go online to compare the types and amounts of food you consume with healthful eating advice from the Pyramid. This interactive Web site also shows how much total fat, saturated fat, cholesterol, and sodium your day's food choices contain. Use it for one day to get a quick look, or up to twenty days to check the quality of what you eat over time. Access it through *http://www.usda.gov/cnpp* to the Interactive Healthy Eating Index online.

what you eat and how much you move are key factors in your fitness equation.

What's the secret to healthful eating? It's no secret at all, just solid advice. In a nutshell, enjoy an overall approach to eating, with most of your energy, or calories, coming from grain products, vegetables, fruits, lower-fat milk products, lean meat, fish, poultry, and legumes. Consume less energy, or calories, from fats and sweets. Let's explore just what that means—and how to do it.

In ten statements, the Dietary Guidelines for Americans sum up the basics about eating and being active for health. Follow their advice, and promote your health for the long run, while reducing your risks for many health problems, including some leading causes of disability and death among Americans. By following the guidelines you may reduce risk factors (obesity, high blood pressure, and high blood cholesterol) that lead to chronic disease. And you may lower your chances for heart disease, some cancers, diabetes, stroke, and osteoporosis.

So if you're not following the Dietary Guidelines already, why not? And why not start now?

Developed by the U.S. Department of Agriculture and the U.S. Department of Health and Human Services, the Dietary Guidelines have been developed for you—in fact, for all healthy Americans ages two and over. Updated every five years, these guidelines offer the most current, science-based advice, based on the consensus of many nutrition experts.

The Dietary Guidelines are flexible, with plenty of room for you to eat what you enjoy *and* eat for health! They're sensible, too, recognizing that what you eat over several days, rather than for just one day, or one meal or snack, is what really counts!

The advice of the Dietary Guidelines is summed up with the ABCs for good health:

- *Aim for fitness . . .* with a healthy body weight and active living.
- *Build a healthy base* . . . with a variety of nutritious, health-promoting foods, kept safe to eat.
- *Choose sensibly . . .* without overdoing on fat, especially saturated fat; sugars; salt; and for adults who choose to drink them, alcoholic beverages.

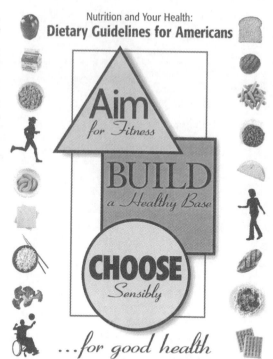

Nutrition and Your Health:
Dietary Guidelines for Americans

Aim *for Fitness*

BUILD *a Healthy Base*

CHOOSE *Sensibly*

. . . for good health

lems, among others. Did you know that premature death is linked to excess body weight as well? And that being overweight also can take a toll on emotional health?

Despite the known risks, overweight and obesity have become a national and global pandemic, and not just for adults. The typical American adult gains weight with every decade. The risk for and the actual incidence of overweight among children and teens are rising dramatically, too.

No matter what your age, aim for a healthy weight. For adult women, more than 35 inches around the waistline, and for men, more than 40 inches around the waistline are quick markers for excess abdominal fat and the potential risk for some health problems. What's your "measure" of fitness?

As an adult in a healthy weight range, set your goal on maintaining your present weight. However, if you're overweight, and especially if you already have one of these health problems, you're wise to trim down gradually. At the very least, manage your weight so you don't gain more. (Note: Being overweight is a problem when extra pounds come from excess body fat. Because strenuous workouts build muscle, extra weight from muscle isn't a problem.)

If children and teens can keep a healthy weight while they're growing, their chance of being overweight adults is lower. More active play, fewer sedentary activities (such as TV and video and computer games), and healthful eating are their best strategies to a healthy weight.

For children, teens, and adults of any age, a healthy weight is key to a long, healthy, and productive life. The smart way to achieve that goal? Eat mostly nutrient-rich foods such as vegetables, fruit, grain products, lean meats, and low-fat dairy foods, choose sensible food portions, and keep physically active. *For more about weight management and health, see chapter 2, "Your Healthy Weight."*

Aim for Fitness

When you focus on fitness, remember that two guidelines—aiming for a healthy weight and putting physical activity into your everyday life—pay off: helping you work productively, enjoy life, and feel your best. These same guidelines help children and teens thrive, develop, and succeed at school.

"Weight" for Health

Guideline 1: Aim for a healthy weight.

Are you at your healthy weight? Appearance or fitting into a clothes size are commonly cited reasons to maintain a healthy weight. Yet, even a few pounds of excess weight may be more risky to your health than you think. Research shows that overweight and obesity increase the risk factors for chronic disease, including high blood pressure and high blood cholesterol, and up the chances for developing serious health problems: heart disease, stroke, diabetes, certain types of cancer, arthritis, and breathing prob-

Move It: The Food-Activity Connection

Guideline 2: Be physically active each day.

Physical activity is essential for your health, yet most Americans don't get enough. For those reasons, being active every day is its own Dietary Guideline! Your healthy weight is one key reason for regular physical activity. But the benefits extend much farther. *See "Ten Reasons to Make the 'Right Moves'" later in this chapter.* Try to accumulate each day at least thirty minutes of moderate physical activity if you're an adult, and sixty minutes for children and teens. *For examples of moderate physical activity, see "Moderate Activity: What Is It?" below.*

Get active . . . stay active . . . or become even more active. Spread out your activity, or do it all at once; either way offers benefits. If you haven't been active,

Exercise Your Options

For more about the benefits of physical activity and about ways to be more physically active, check here:

- *For most healthy people, including those managing their body weight* . . . "Get Physical!" in chapter 2
- *For children* . . . "Get Up and Move, Turn Off the Tube!" in chapter 16
- *For teens* . . . "Move Your 'Bod'" in chapter 16
- *For older adults* . . . "Never Too Late for Exercise" in chapter 18
- *For travelers* . . . "When You're on the Road" in chapter 19
- *For athletes* . . . chapter 19, "Athlete's Guide: Winning Nutrition"

MODERATE ACTIVITY: WHAT IS IT?

If some activities use more energy than others, you may wonder: Just what does "moderate physical activity" really mean? It equates to the energy you need to walk 2 miles in 30 minutes.

Moderate physical activity uses about 150 calories a day, or about 1,000 calories a week. For that amount of energy expenditure, you might spend more time on less vigorous activities, such as brisk walking, or spend less time on more vigorous activities, such as running.

COMMON CHORES	DURATION	*Less Vigorous, More Time**	SPORTING ACTIVITIES	DURATION
Washing and waxing a car	45–60 min.	↑	Playing volleyball	45 min.
Washing windows or floors	15–60 min.		Playing touch football	30–45 min.
Gardening	30–45 min.		Walking 1¾ miles (20 min./mile)	35 min
Wheeling self in wheelchair	30–40 min.		Basketball (shooting baskets)	30 min.
Pushing a stroller 1½ miles	30 min.		Bicycling 5 miles	30 min.
Raking leaves	30 min.		Dancing fast (social)	30 min.
Walking 2 miles (15 min./mile)	30 min.		Water aerobics	30 min.
Shoveling snow	15 min.		Swimming laps	20 min.
Stairwalking	15 min.	↓	Basketball (playing a game)	15–20 min.
		More Vigorous, Less Time	Jumping rope	15 min.
			Running 1½ miles (15 min./mile)	15–20 min.

* Some activities can be performed at various intensities. The suggested durations correspond to the expected intensity of effort.

Source: Practical Guide to the Identification, Evaluation and Treatment of Overweight and Obesity in Adults (Bethesda, Md.: National Institutes of Health, 2001).

Ten Reasons to Make the "Right Moves"

Whether you're involved in sports or simply live an active lifestyle, physical activity pays big dividends. Physical activity is the "right move" for fitness—for almost everyone, not just for athletes. Consider just a few reasons why:

1. *Trimmer body.* If you're physically active, you'll have an easier time maintaining a healthy weight, or losing weight and keeping it off if you're overweight. *For more about the benefits of physical activity for weight management, see chapter 2, "Your Healthy Weight."*

2. *Less risk for health problems.* An active lifestyle—or a sports regimen—can help protect you from many ongoing health problems.

   Studies show that regular physical activity helps lower risk factors. For example, physical activity lowers total and LDL ("bad") cholesterol and triglyceride levels while boosting the HDL ("good") cholesterol level, controls blood pressure, and improves blood sugar levels. Your risks for heart disease, type 2 diabetes, and colon cancer also go down when you fit physical activity into your everyday living.

   Active living also may reduce or eliminate the need for medication to lower blood lipids, lower blood pressure, or manage diabetes.

3. *Stronger bones.* Regular, weight-bearing activities such as walking, running, weight lifting, cross-country skiing, and soccer help make your bones stronger. If you're past age thirty-five, weight-bearing exercise helps maintain your bone strength and reduce your chance of fractures.

4. *Stronger muscles.* Strength-training activities such as lifting weights at least two times a week keep your body strong for sports and everyday living.

When you're strong, it's easier to move, carry, and lift things. When you exercise your muscles, you also give your heart a workout. Remember, it's a muscle, too. A strong heart pumps blood and nutrients more easily through your 60,000 miles of blood vessels.

5. *More endurance.* You won't tire as easily when you're physically active. And you may have more stamina during the rest of the day, too.

6. *Better mental outlook.* Active people describe feelings of psychological well-being and self-esteem when they make active living a habit. It's a great way to reinforce that "can do" attitude.

7. *Stress relief and better sleep.* Research shows that physical activity helps your body relax and release emotional tension. That promotes longer, better-quality sleep, and you may fall asleep faster.

8. *Better coordination and flexibility.* Your body moves with greater ease and range of motion when you stay physically active.

9. *Injury protection.* When you're in shape, you more easily can catch yourself if you slip or trip . . . and can move away from impending danger more quickly.

10. *Feel younger longer.* Research suggests that physical activity slows some effects of aging. Active people have more strength and mobility, and fewer limitations.

For more about the benefits of physical activity, see "Active Play: Good Moves for Children" in chapter 16, and for older adults, "The Reasons Are Many" in chapter 18.

start gradually. Work up to longer, more intense activities for more benefits. As you plan, try to fit in physical activities that are especially beneficial:

● *For flexibility,* try stretching, yoga, and dancing.

● *For strength,* try weight-bearing activities (walking, tennis) for bone strength, and carrying groceries or weight lifting to build muscles.

● *For cardiovascular fitness,* try aerobic activities that increase your heart rate and breathing.

Have You Ever Wondered

. . . if you set a safe pace for physical activity? Take the "talk-sing test" to find out. If you can talk as you move, you're okay. If you're too breathless to talk, slow down. And if you can sing, step up your pace!

Unless you have a health problem, you probably can start moving more now! Talk to your healthcare provider first if you have an ongoing health problem—including heart disease, high blood pressure, diabetes, osteoporosis, arthritis, or obesity, if you're at high risk for heart disease, or if you're over age forty for men, or over age fifty for women.

Build a Healthy Base

Four more Dietary Guidelines establish your base for healthful eating. The familiar Food Guide Pyramid is an easy-to-use planning guide that helps you get the nutrients you need from food each day. Vegetables, fruits, and grains form the foundation of the Pyramid for good reason: you need plenty of them for good nutrition and health, and to reduce your health risks. In fact, try new foods from these groups in place of high-calorie, less nutritious foods you may be used to eating. And *always* keep your food safe—wherever, whatever you eat!

Food Variety—a Priority!

Guideline 3: Let the Pyramid guide your food choices.

If variety is the "spice of life," in your food choices variety is key to enjoying food and to good nutrition and health. Each day your body needs the nutrients and other healthful substances that a variety of food provides. Most foods and beverages have more than one nutrient. But no one food or food category has them all.

The Food Guide Pyramid is an easy guide for what to eat each day: *for variety,* so you get a range of nutrients, and *for adequacy,* so you get enough without overdoing on calories. In fact, it's flexible enough to fit any healthful way of eating and include any food, even occasional fats and sweets. The Pyramid recommends a range of servings, and identifies serving sizes. It acts as a guide for an appropriate amount of food for you.

The Food Guide Pyramid translates nutrient recommendations from the Dietary Reference Intakes (DRIs) and the Dietary Guidelines for Americans into practical advice for all healthy people, ages two years and over. *In chapter 10 learn how to use the Pyramid to plan meals and snacks.*

Grain Products, Fruits, and Vegetables—Enjoy!

Guideline 4: Choose a variety of grains daily, especially whole grains.

Guideline 5: Choose a variety of fruits and vegetables daily.

Grain products, fruits, and vegetables (including legumes)—you need more of these foods than others. Just check the serving recommendations in the Food Guide Pyramid.

Grain products belong at the base of the Pyramid; their complex carbohydrates should supply most of your food energy. These same foods also supply a unique array of vitamins, minerals, and

Food Guide Pyramid
A Guide to Daily Food Choices

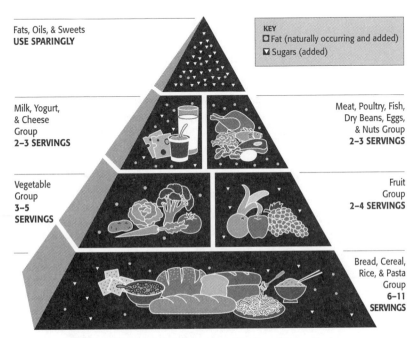

Fats, Oils, & Sweets
USE SPARINGLY

KEY
☐ Fat (naturally occurring and added)
☑ Sugars (added)

Milk, Yogurt, & Cheese Group
2–3 SERVINGS

Meat, Poultry, Fish, Dry Beans, Eggs, & Nuts Group
2–3 SERVINGS

Vegetable Group
3–5 SERVINGS

Fruit Group
2–4 SERVINGS

Bread, Cereal, Rice, & Pasta Group
6–11 SERVINGS

Source: U.S. Department of Agriculture/U.S. Department of Health and Human Services

other plant substances (called phytonutrients). Folic acid, a B vitamin in fortified grain products, is among them; folic acid protects against some birth defects, and perhaps lowers the risk for heart disease and cancer. Why the emphasis on whole grains? Besides fiber, whole grains contain other protective plant substances.

Despite their health benefits, many people don't consume enough fruits and vegetables. Yet they're the major source of several vitamins and minerals, a source of fiber—and phytonutrients with potential health-promoting qualities. Legumes also are high in protein. Because the nutrient and phytonutrient content of fruits and vegetables differs so much, variety is important.

Other benefits: unless you add sauces, dressings, and other high-fat ingredients, or use high-fat cooking methods such as frying, grain products, fruits, and vegetables are low in fat, too. Eating plenty of whole grains, fruits, and vegetables may help lower your risk for some health problems, including heart disease and certain types of cancer as well.

How might you eat more of these foods? "Redesign" your dinner plate. Mentally divide it into pie-shaped sections, filling about 75 percent with grain products, vegetables, and fruits.

For more about the vitamins and minerals in grain products, vegetables, and fruits, see chapter 4. For more about their fiber and complex carbohydrates, see chapters 5 and 6.

For Your Health and Safety's Sake

Guideline 6: Keep food safe to eat.

Healthful eating is about more than *what* you eat; it's also about *how* you keep whatever you eat safe. Foodborne illnesses, from even a small amount of food, strike millions of Americans each year, causing mild to severe, even life-threatening symptoms. The effects may last just a few hours or days, or for weeks, months, and years to come. Be aware that young children, older adults, pregnant women, and those with weakened immune systems or some chronic diseases are especially vulnerable.

Keeping food safe is up to you, not just the responsibility of farmers, food manufacturers, retailers, and restaurant workers. Many cases of foodborne illness

---

Variety, Balance, Moderation: Cornerstone of Healthy Eating

Food variety, along with balance and moderation, make eating enjoyable and healthful. You've heard these terms before. Just what do they mean?

● *Vary your food choices,* especially fruits, vegetables, and grain products, to consume nutrients and phytonutrients for health. Variety adds to food's enjoyment, too!

● *Balance your food choices over time* to get enough, but not too much, of each type of food and each nutrient.

● *Moderate how much you eat* to control food energy (calories) as well as fat, cholesterol, sugars, sodium, and alcoholic beverages (if you consume them).

How do you eat to get the variety, balance, and moderation that's best for your health? Just climb the Food Guide Pyramid to fitness!

---

could be avoided if consumers handle food properly as they choose, prepare, serve, and store food. *See chapter 12 for an in-depth look at foodborne illnesses and how you can keep your food safe and healthful.*

Choose Sensibly

Four more Dietary Guidelines help you choose foods sensibly to promote your health and lower your chances for some chronic health problems. With these guidelines you can fit any food into your day's meals and snacks as long as you don't overdo on fat (especially saturated fat), sugars, salt, and alcoholic drinks. Nutrition Facts on food labels can help you do that!

The "Lowdown" on Fats, Saturated Fats, and Cholesterol

Guideline 7: Choose a diet that is low in saturated fat and cholesterol and moderate in total fat.

Fat is a nutrient essential for health. Besides supplying energy, it contains essential fatty acids and carries some vitamins (A, D, E, and K) into your bloodstream. Yet, it's well known that too much fat, especially saturated fat, and too much cholesterol are linked to a higher risk for high blood cholesterol levels and heart disease. High-fat diets also increase the chances for some cancers.

Although many people consume less fat, saturated fat, and cholesterol than they did a decade ago, Americans on average still consume too much. A diet that's moderate in fat (no more than 30 percent of calories) and low in saturated fat (no more than 10 percent of calories) is the goal to strive for.

Cutting down on fat and saturated fat—but not cutting it out entirely—is a sensible way to eat for health. Among the strategies: learn to choose lean meat, fish, and poultry, and low-fat and fat-free foods; use low-fat cooking methods; eat plenty of grain products, vegetables, and fruits; and go easy on high-fat dressings, sauces, and spreads. Nutrition Facts on food labels can help you choose foods with less fat. *For more about fat and cholesterol in moderation in a healthful eating plan, see chapter 3, "Fat Facts."*

Sugars—a Moderate Issue

Guideline 8: Choose beverages and foods to moderate your intake of sugars.

In one form or another, sugars—a form of carbohydrate—are present in many foods you eat. Some are naturally occurring sugars, such as the sugars found in fruits and dairy foods. Others are added sugars, used for both flavor and function in a variety of foods during processing and preparation. Complex carbohydrates (starches) from grain products, vegetables, and fruits are broken down into sugars during digestion. To the human body, all sugars look and act alike, regardless of their source.

Carbohydrates, including sugars, are your body's main source of energy. So what's the main health issue? Foods with sugars or starches can promote tooth decay.

A second health issue: some foods and beverages with added sugars supply energy, or calories, but few nutrients. Consuming too many calories from these foods may contribute to weight gain or to eating fewer nutrient-rich foods from the Pyramid's five major food groups. For sugars, moderation is your guideline for consuming enough, but not overdoing, especially if your energy needs are low.

To help you choose beverages and foods to moderate sugars in your day's meals and snacks, read the Nutrition Facts on food labels. *For more about sugars in a healthful eating plan, see chapter 5, "Sweet Talk: Sugar and Other Sweeteners."*

Salt and Sodium—Moderation Again

Guideline 9: Choose and prepare foods with less salt.

Salt is a combination of two nutrients: sodium and chloride. Sodium itself is naturally present in many foods. As nutrients, sodium and chloride help your body regulate fluids and blood pressure. So why the guideline?

For many people, extra sodium passes right through the body. However, others have blood pressure that's sodium-sensitive; for them, high sodium intake, along with obesity, heredity, or getting older, contribute to high blood pressure. Choosing and preparing foods with less salt helps reduce their risk of high blood pressure. That's wise advice, even for healthy people, who may not know if their blood pressure is sodium-sensitive.

Another reason to go easy on sodium: eating less salt may decrease calcium loss from bone, and so help protect bones from the risks of osteoporosis and fractures.

The main source of sodium is food itself, not salt added at the table. To consume less salt and sodium, enjoy more fresh fruits and vegetables. Use herbs and spices as your main flavor enhancers. And use Nutrition Facts on food labels to identify and compare sodium in food, especially prepared food. *For more about salt and sodium in a healthful eating plan, see chapter 7, "Sodium: A Salty Subject."*

Alcoholic Beverages—Go Easy

Guideline 10: If you drink alcoholic beverages, do so in moderation.

Do you enjoy an occasional drink? If so, drink alcoholic beverages in moderation. That's no more than one drink a day for women and two for men. A drink is 12 ounces of beer, 5 ounces of wine, or 1.5 ounces of 80-proof distilled spirits. Any more can be risky.

On their own, alcoholic beverages offer calories but essentially no nutrients, so they don't nourish your body. Instead, if they substitute for nutritious food and beverages, the risk for malnutrition goes up. In excess, their alcohol can be harmful.

What are the risks? Too much alcohol may impair judgment, which can lead to accidents and injury. Drinking beyond moderation is linked to many health problems, including high blood pressure, stroke, heart disease, certain cancers, and diseases of the liver and pancreas. And it's linked to social problems, too, including violence and suicide. Drinking during pregnancy increases the chances of birth defects. And even one drink a day slightly increases a woman's risk for breast cancer. Another potential problem: over time some people become dependent on alcohol.

When should you avoid drinking? Before and while you drive, and whenever you may put yourself or others at risk. *Don't drink at all* if you can't control your drinking; if you're a child or a teen; if you plan to work with equipment that takes attention, skill, or coordination; or if you're taking medications that may interact with alcohol. Pregnant women and those trying to become pregnant shouldn't drink either.

Alcoholic beverages can make meals more enjoyable. Also, for men over age forty-five and women over fifty-five, moderate drinking may lower the risk for heart disease.

For more about alcoholic beverages and advice for consuming them, see "Alcoholic Beverages: In Moderation" in chapter 8.

Your Food Choices: The Inside Story

While you enjoy the sensual qualities of food—the mouth-watering appearance, aroma, texture, and flavor—your body relies on the life-sustaining functions that nutrients in food perform. Other food substances, including phytonutrients (or plant substances), appear to offer even more heath benefits beyond nourishment. What's inside your food? How do these substances promote health? And how much is enough, but not too much?

Nutrients—Classified Information

Your body can't make most nutrients from food, or produce energy, without several key nutrients. You need a varied, adequate supply of nutrients from food for your nourishment—and for life itself.

Whether a pizza, a chef's salad, milk, or chips, your food choices are digested, or broken down, into nutrients, then absorbed into your bloodstream and carried to every cell of your body. Most of the body's work takes place in cells, and food's nutrients are essential to your body's "do list."

Saying that foods are complex substances is an understatement! More than forty nutrients in food, classified into six groups, have specific and unique functions for nourishment. Their work is linked in partnerships for your good health.

Carbohydrates. As your body's main source of energy, or calories, carbohydrates belong in two groups: complex carbohydrates (or starches) and sugars. *Chapter 5, "Sweet Talk: Sugars and Other Sweeteners," explores carbohydrates.*

Fiber, another carbohydrate, aids digestion, promotes health, and offers protection from some diseases. Despite its role in health, fiber isn't a nutrient, because it is not digested and absorbed into the body. *See chapter 6, "Fiber: Your Body's Broom."*

Fats. Fats supply energy. They play a role in other physiological functions, too, such as nutrient transport, growth, and being part of many body cells. Fats are complex substances made of varying combinations of fatty acids. All fatty acids aren't the same. Some are more saturated (harder at room temperature); others, more unsaturated. Fatty acids that your body can't make are considered "essential." *You'll learn about fat and cholesterol (a fatlike substance) in chapter 3, "Fat Facts."*

Proteins. Proteins are sequenced combinations of amino acids that build, repair, and maintain all your

---

Have You Ever Wondered

. . . how the Dietary Guidelines for Americans compare with the American Heart Association (AHA) and the American Cancer Society (ACS) guidelines? All these dietary guidelines offer sound, science-based advice for health eating. Based on strong scientific evidence, they're consistent with each other. *See pages 543 and 553 for the AHA and the ACS guidelines.*

body tissues. Your body makes nonessential amino acids; others are considered "essential" from food because your body can't make them. Especially when carbohydrates and fat are in short supply, proteins provide energy. If they're broken down and used for energy, amino acids can't be used to maintain body tissue. *For more about amino acids, see chapter 20, "The Vegetarian Way."*

Vitamins. Vitamins work like spark plugs, triggering chemical reactions in body cells. Each vitamin regulates different body processes. Because their roles are so specific, one cannot replace another. *To learn more, see chapter 4, "Vitamins, Minerals, Phytonutrients: Variety on Your Plate."*

Minerals. Somewhat like vitamins do, minerals spark body processes. They, too, have unique job descriptions. *See chapter 4, "Vitamins, Minerals, Phytonutrients: Variety on Your Plate."*

Water. Water makes up 55 to 75 percent of your body weight—and it's a nutrient, too. It regulates body processes, helps regulate your body temperature, carries nutrients and other body chemicals to your cells, and carries waste products away. *For more about water and health, see chapter 8, "Fluids: Often Overlooked."*

Nutrients: How Much?

Everyone around you needs the same nutrients—just in different amounts. Why differences? For healthy people, age, gender, and body size are among the reasons. Children and teenagers, for example, need more of some nutrients for growth. Pregnancy and breastfeeding increase the need for some nutrients, too, and for food energy. Because their bodies are typically larger, men often need more of most nutrients than women do.

How much of each nutrient do you need? Dietary Reference Intakes (DRIs), established by the Food and Nutrition Board of the Institute of Medicine, National Academy of Sciences, include daily nutrient recommendations for healthy Americans based on age and gender. The DRIs include four types of recommendations:

● *Recommended Dietary Allowances (RDAs)* are recommended levels of nutrients that meet the needs of almost all healthy individuals in specific age and gender groups. Consider them as a goal.

● *Adequate Intakes (AIs)* are similar in meaning to RDAs. They're used as guidelines for some nutrients that don't have enough scientific evidence to set firm RDAs.

● *Tolerable Upper Intake Levels (ULs)* aren't recommended amounts. In fact, there's no scientific consensus for recommending nutrient levels higher than the RDAs to most healthy people. Instead, ULs represent the maximum intake that probably won't pose risks for health problems for almost all healthy people in a specific age and gender group. Why set limits? With the growing use of fortified foods and dietary supplements, especially in large doses, you're wise to recognize safe upper limits and so avoid adverse reactions.

● *Estimated Average Requirements (EARs)* are used professionally to assess groups of people, not individuals. When used with research, the EAR is the nutrient amount whereby half the population would have their nutrient needs met; the other half wouldn't.

Groups of experts regularly review the DRIs, using the most current research evidence, and update the dietary recommendations. *A listing of the DRIs appears in the Appendices.*

How do you use the DRIs? For the most part, you don't need to add up the numbers; it takes considerable effort to calculate the nutrients in all your food choices, then make an assessment with DRIs. If you choose to do that, remember, however, that the recommendations—RDAs and AIs—apply to your average nutrient intake over several days, not just one day and certainly not one meal.

DRIs are nutrient intake goals to strive for; they're also used by professionals to set standards for nutrition programs, food labeling, nutrition education guides, food fortification, and medical nutrition therapy. The Food Guide Pyramid and Nutrition Facts on food labels offer consumer-friendly ways to plan and assess the nutritional quality of your food choices.

More Than Nutrients: Foods' Functional Components

Food contains much more than nutrients! Science is beginning to uncover the benefits of other substances in food: phytonutrients (including fiber), omega fatty acids, conjugated linoleic acid, and pre- and probiotics, to name a few. Described as "functional," these substances do more than nourish you. They appear to promote your health and protect you from health risks related to many major health problems, including heart disease, some cancers, diabetes, and macular degeneration, among others.

At least for now, no DRIs exist for the functional components of food, except for fiber (released in 2002). And scientists don't yet fully understand their roles in health. However, within this book you'll get a glimpse of emerging knowledge about functional substances in food. And you're bound to hear more as new studies about functional substances in food unfold.

Solutions for Healthful Eating, Active Living

Almost any time is the perfect time to start taking control of your food choices, and to change your eating style if needed. The sooner you invest in your health, the greater the benefit!

If you're ready to eat smarter or move more, use these goal-setting steps to invest in your health and the health of your family, one easy step at a time:

Audit your food choices and lifestyle. Start by keeping track of what you eat or drink, along with how much, when, and why. For example, if you snack when you feel stressed or bored, or order fast foods with fries and soda when you need a quick meal, write that down. Use a food log to pinpoint eating behaviors you want to change. *See "Dear Diary . . ." in chapter 2 for tips on keeping a food log. Take the personal assessments in "Your Nutrition Checkup" throughout this book for a glimpse at what you do already.*

Set goals. Know what you want—perhaps a healthier weight or lower cholesterol levels. And be realistic. Change doesn't mean giving up a food you like. However, smaller portions, different ways of cooking, and being more physically active give you more "wiggle room" to occasionally enjoy foods with more calories.

Make a plan for change. Divide big goals, such as "I will eat better," into smaller, more specific goals, such as "I will eat more vegetables." List practical steps to achieve your goals. For example:

Goal: Eat less fat.

Steps: Use low-calorie salad dressing. Buy lean meat. Order a regular burger, not the deluxe size; skip the "special" sauce. Order a baked potato rather than fries, or share an order of fries.

Be patient. Make gradual changes. Change for the long run takes time, commitment, and encouragement. Most health goals (e.g., losing weight, lowering blood cholesterol levels) take a lifelong commitment. Stick with your plan, even if success takes several months or longer. And remember that small steps toward reaching a goal add up over time!

Monitor your progress. If you get off track, pick up where you left off, and start again. You can do it!

Seek help from a qualified health professional. A registered dietitian can help you on your journey to fitness.

Reward yourself. Change is hard work that deserves recognition. Pat yourself on the back with a bike ride, a walk with a friend, a new CD, or a new outfit. Feeling good is the best reward!

Reevaluate your plan every month or two. See how changes you've made fit with your goals. You may even tackle a new goal!

Looking for "Healthy Solutions"?

Looking for a practical approach to sound nutrition? Check here for sensible, easy solutions to eat for fitness. Some advice is meant for you; other advice may apply to family members or friends.

DO YOU ...	YES OR NO?	FOR "HEALTHY SOLUTIONS," CHECK HERE ...
Feel confused by nutrition news and advice?	☐ Yes ☐ No	*Chapter 24, "Well Informed?,"* to decipher today's and tomorrow's news about food and health. (This whole book translates what's known about nutrients, phytonutrients, and health to smart eating.)
Get frustrated trying to control your weight?	☐ Yes ☐ No	*Chapter 2, "Your Healthy Weight,"* to find a way to your healthy weight that works—and to sort through diets that don't.
Think you need to give up foods you enjoy to eat healthy?	☐ Yes ☐ No	*Chapter 10, "Planning to Eat Smart,"* to see how you can enjoy any food and still eat for your good health!
Feel life's just too hectic to eat healthy?	☐ Yes ☐ No	*Chapter 10, "Planning to Eat Smart,"* to find quick, healthful, easy meals and snacks when you're tight on time.
Feel overwhelmed by all the food choices in the supermarket?	☐ Yes ☐ No	*Chapter 9, "What's on Today's Table?,"* to keep updated on today's "new" foods (functional, health-positioned, organic, ethnic, others), food regulations, and food biotechnology. *Chapter 11, "Supermarket Smarts,"* to shop easily for taste, convenience—and good health.
Wonder if the "bug" you caught might be foodborne illness?	☐ Yes ☐ No	*Chapter 12, "The Safe Kitchen,"* for essential ways to keep your food safe for you to eat.
Think healthful cooking takes extra effort?	☐ Yes ☐ No	*Chapter 13, "Kitchen Nutrition,"* for simple ways to healthier food "prep"—for less fat, salt, and added sugars, and more fruits, vegetables, fiber, calcium, and more.
Think eating out a lot keeps you from eating right?	☐ Yes ☐ No	*Chapter 14, "Your Food Away from Home,"* to eat out (fast food, ethnic food, sit-down food) your way— and enjoy it, too!
Feel unsure if you're feeding your kids right?	☐ Yes ☐ No	*Chapter 15, "Off to a Healthy Start,"* for baby-feeding basics. *Chapter 16, "Food to Grow On,"* for strategies that work for helping your child or teen learn to eat right.

Looking for "Healthy Solutions"? *(continued)*

Do you ...	Yes or no?	For "Healthy Solutions," check here ...
Know that women have some special nutrition issues, but what?	☐ Yes ☐ No	*Chapter 17, "For Women Only,"* for sound eating advice for pregnancy, breast-feeding, and menopause.
Want to slow down the aging process?	☐ Yes ☐ No	*Chapter 18, "For Mature Adults: Healthful Eating!"* for smart eating if you're age "fifty plus" or if you're caring for someone that age. (Check this whole book, too.)
Want to "max out" your sports performance?	☐ Yes ☐ No	*Chapter 19, "Athlete's Guide: Winning Nutrition,"* for ways to eat for your physical best: before, during, and after a workout.
Feel uncertain about your own (or your teen's) approach to vegetarian eating?	☐ Yes ☐ No	*Chapter 20, "The Vegetarian Way,"* for practical advice, no matter what your approach to vegetarian eating.
Think you have a food allergy or other food sensitivity?	☐ Yes ☐ No	*Chapter 21, "Sensitive about Food,"* to deal with lactose intolerance, a food allergy, or other food sensitivities.
Need help to reduce your risks for—or to deal with—specific health problems?	☐ Yes ☐ No	*Chapter 22, "Smart Eating to Prevent and Treat Disease,"* for the healthy eating basics for common health problems—heart disease, diabetes, cancer, and osteoporosis, among others. (This book also is filled with tips!)
Think you need a nutrient or herbal supplement, but you're not sure what—*and if?*	☐ Yes ☐ No	*Chapter 23, "Supplements: Use and Abuse,"* to sort through smart advice and misinformation about supplements.

Every "yes" is one more reason to use this book as your healthy eating resource!

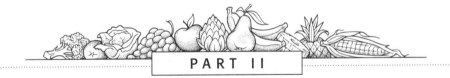

PART II

Healthful Eating
The Basics

CHAPTER 2

Your Healthy Weight

We often take it for granted, but good health is one of the most precious gifts of life. A healthy weight—maintained throughout life—helps you achieve good health in many ways: look your best, feel your best, and reduce your risk for many serious and ongoing diseases.

What is a healthy weight? It's the weight that's best for you—not necessarily the lowest weight you think you can be. A healthy weight actually is a range that's statistically related to good health. Being above or below that range increases the risk of health problems, or decreases the likelihood of good health.

The smart approach to your best weight is really no secret—only common sense. A healthful lifestyle, which includes regular physical activity with an eating pattern chosen for variety, balance, and moderation, makes all the difference. Maintaining a healthy weight throughout life is best for health. Does that mean you need to be "everyday perfect"? No. Just try to manage your weight by eating smart and living actively most of the time.

Body Basics: What's Your Healthy Weight?

The answer isn't as simple as stepping onto a bathroom scale, then comparing your weight to a chart. Your own healthy weight is one that's right for you. It may be quite different from someone else's weight,

even if he or she is the same height, gender, and age as you are.

What makes the difference? Your genetic makeup plays a role because it determines your height and the size and shape of your body frame. A genetic link to body fat also may exist. Of course, genetics isn't the only reason why weight differs from person to person. Your metabolic rate, the rate at which your body burns energy, makes a difference. So does your body composition. Muscle burns more calories than body fat does. Your level of physical activity and what you eat both play a role, too.

So what's your healthy weight? That depends. The right weight for you takes several things into account: (1) your Body Mass Index, or your weight in relation to your height; (2) the location and amount of body fat you have; and (3) your risks for weight-related problems such as diabetes or high blood pressure.

Body Mass Index: Fit or Fat?

Body Mass Index (BMI) is one "tool" for judging your body weight in relation to your height—and, at the same time, your risks for weight-related health problems. It doesn't directly measure body fat. For adults, there's no difference in BMI weight ranges for age; health risks appear to be the same, regardless of age. The same chart applies to men and women.

The generous BMI range of healthy weights allows for individual differences. Higher weights within the healthy range typically apply to people with more muscle and a larger frame, such as many men and some women. After all, muscle and bone weigh more than fat. Gaining or losing weight within these ranges isn't necessarily healthful for you.

People with a higher percentage of body fat tend to have a higher BMI than those who have a greater percentage of muscle. Carrying excess body fat puts you at greater risk for health problems such as heart disease, diabetes, and certain types of cancer. The higher your BMI, the greater your risk.

What's Your BMI?

Use the chart "Are You at a Healthy Weight?" to find out.

If you fit within the healthy weight range—BMI 18.5 to 24.9—that's good. Take steps to keep it there:

Right for You: Fit at Any Size

Healthy people come in many sizes and shapes: tall or short, stocky or lanky, muscular or not. These differences are a unique part of being human. For this reason, there's no such thing as a "perfect body," or an ideal body weight, shape, or size that everyone should strive for. The most important thing is being healthy, so you can enjoy a healthful lifestyle with the body you have.

Likewise, losing weight, or maintaining a healthy weight, is easier for some people than others—in spite of their commitment to healthful eating and physical activity. That, too, is part of what makes each of us unique.

Regardless of your size and shape, you can choose a healthful lifestyle—and so live a fuller, more productive life and reduce your risk for health problems:

● Assess your own health habits.

● Make choices for good health with yourself in mind.

● Enjoy a delicious, healthful eating style and fun, physical activity.

● Get regular physical checkups.

● Monitor your "numbers" (blood cholesterol, triglycerides, blood pressure, fasting blood sugar levels), and keep them within a healthy range. *See "Your Body's 'Maintenance' Program" on page 537 for normal levels.*

● Make your goal your personal healthy weight, not some unattainable goal!

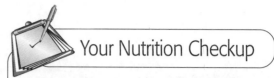

Your Nutrition Checkup

Are You at a Healthy Weight?

Figuring Your BMI. To calculate your exact BMI:

1. Multiply your weight in pounds by 0.45.
   For example: 132 pounds × 0.45 = 59.4

2. Multiply your height in inches by 0.025, then square the result.
   For example: 65 inches × 0.025 = 1.625
   1.625 × 1.625 = 2.64

3. For your Body Mass Index:
   Divide your answer in step 1 by the answer in step 2.
   For example: 59.4 ÷ 2.64 = 22.5 BMI

   An easier way to calculate your BMI: check out one of these Web sites, for example:

● Partnership for Healthy Weight Management: *www.consumer.gov/weightloss/bmi.htm*

● National Heart, Lung, and Blood Institute: *www.nhlbisupport.com/bmi/bmicalc.htm*

---

move more and eat fewer calories if your BMI starts to creep up. Be aware: some people fit within the healthy weight range but still have excess body fat and little muscle. Read on to *"Body Weight, Body Fat?"*

What if your weight puts you above a BMI of 25? For most people, that's less healthy—unless the extra weight is muscle, not fat. Try to avoid more weight gain. The higher your weight is above the healthy range, the greater your risk for weight-related health problems.

What if your weight falls below "healthy"? Again, that may be okay for you, but it also may suggest a health problem. A BMI under 18.5 may increase the risk for menstrual irregularity, infertility, and osteoporosis. It also may be an early symptom of a health problem or an eating disorder. Check with your health professional if you lose weight suddenly or for unexpected reasons.

Like other measures, use the BMI *only* as a guideline. For people who have lost muscle mass, including some elderly people, even a BMI within the "healthy weight" range may not be healthy. Muscular people who are healthy and fit may have a BMI above the healthy range. Consult your doctor about the BMI

ARE YOU AT A HEALTHY WEIGHT?

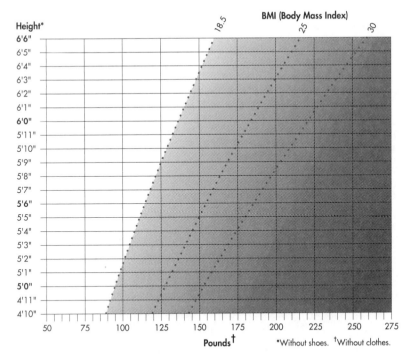

BMI measures weight in relation to height. The BMI ranges shown above are for adults. They are not exact ranges of healthy and unhealthy weights. However, they show that health risk increases at higher levels of overweight and obesity. Even within the healthy BMI range, weight gains can carry health risks for adults.

Directions: Find your weight on the bottom of the graph. Go straight up from that point until you come to the line that matches your height. Then look to find your weight group.

Healthy Weight BMI from 18.5 up to 25 refers to healthy weight.

Overweight BMI from 25 up to 30 refers to overweight.

Obese BMI 30 or higher refers to obesity. Obese persons are also overweight.

Source: Report of the Dietary Guidelines Advisory Committee on the Dietary Guidelines for Americans, 2000, page 3.

that's healthy for you. Remember that looking at your BMI alone doesn't determine whether your weight is healthy. The location and amount of body fat you carry, and your weight-related risk factors, including your family history of health problems, count, too.

Note: This BMI chart is meant for adults, not for growing children or teens. *See the Appendices for the growth charts with Body Mass Index for Age percentiles for boys and for girls two to twenty years.* Pediatric charts take individual growth patterns into account.

Body Weight, Body Fat?

Your body composition (how much of your weight is body fat), not necessarily where you fit on any chart, is an important part of evaluating your weight. In fact,

the location and amount of body fat may predict your weight-related health risk more than body weight alone. For example, a person's weight may fit right within the healthy range on a BMI chart, but he or she still may carry too much body fat. Conversely, a muscular person may seem to be overweight according to charts, but may not be overfat. Why? Muscle weighs more than fat.

How can you determine how much of your weight is body fat (often referred to as percent body fat)? Short of expensive tests such as underwater weighing, getting an exact measure isn't easy, and it's especially hard to figure it out on your own. A health or fitness professional might use a skinfold caliper to measure the fat layer on several parts of your body, such as your arm, midriff, and thigh. New electronic scales and other devices also can measure body fat percentages.

Remember, your weight on a scale by itself can't tell you if you're carrying too much fat and how your weight is distributed. And perhaps most importantly, body weight shouldn't dictate how you feel about yourself.

Here are some other ways to judge how you are doing in terms of body fat and health.

Of Apples and Pears

Stand in front of a full-length mirror, preferably nude. How do you look? Be your own judge. Are you shaped like an apple or a pear? For health, being an "apple" can be riskier than being a "pear."

Where your body stores fat is a clue to your healthy weight. Abdominal or upper body fat (applelike shape) increases the risk for some health problems such as diabetes, high cholesterol levels, early heart disease, and high blood pressure, even when the BMI falls within a healthy range. In contrast, excess weight carried below the waist in the hips, buttocks, and thighs (pearlike shape) doesn't appear to be as risky for most health problems. However, it may increase your risk for varicose veins and orthopedic problems.

For the most part, being an "apple" or a "pear" is an inherited tendency for those who gain weight. In other words, fat distribution is partially influenced by genes. However, smoking and drinking too many alcoholic beverages also seem to increase fat carried in the stomach area; as a result, they increase the risk of weight-related health problems. Conversely, vigorous exercise can help to reduce stomach fat, helping to decrease these health risks.

Waist Whys. Health risks go up as your waist size increases. That's especially true if your waist measures more than 35 inches for a woman or more than 40 inches for a man. So a simple tape measure is another tool for assessing your abdominal fat. Stand, and measure your waist just above your hipbone. (Hint: Relax, and breathe out. Don't cinch in the tape measure or pull in your stomach!)

What Are Your Health Risks?

Have you ever finished a physical exam feeling that your weight was within a healthy range, only to have your doctor suggest that you lose—or perhaps gain—a few pounds? For some physical conditions, such as high blood pressure, diabetes, high blood cholesterol,

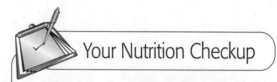
Your Nutrition Checkup

Are You at Risk for Chronic Disease?

The more of these risk factors you have, the more likely you are to benefit from weight loss if you're overweight or obese.

☐ Do you have a personal or family history of heart disease?

☐ Are you a male older than forty-five years or a post-menopausal female?

☐ Do you smoke cigarettes?

☐ Do you have a sedentary lifestyle?

☐ Has your doctor told you that you have:

    ☐ High blood pressure?

    ☐ Abnormal blood lipids (high LDL cholesterol, low HDL cholesterol, high triglycerides?)

    ☐ Diabetes?

Source: U.S. Department of Agriculture and U.S. Department of Health and Human Services, *Nutrition and Your Health: Dietary Guidelines for Americans* (2000).

For more about these risk factors, see chapter 22, "Smart Eating to Prevent and Treat Disease."

or arthritis, your physician may advise weight loss even though you appear to have a healthy weight.

See "Are You at Risk for Chronic Disease?" above. The higher your BMI and waist measurement and the more weight-related risk factors you have, the more likely you are to benefit from losing a few pounds.

A doctor may advise some weight gain for other reasons, perhaps to replace weight loss and aid recovery after a prolonged illness or surgery, or to help withstand some medical treatments, perhaps cancer treatment. *For benefits of a healthy weight for women's health, see "Every Age and Stage of Life: Why a Healthy Weight?" in chapter 17.*

RISK OF ASSOCIATED DISEASE ACCORDING TO BMI AND WAIST SIZE

BMI		WAIST LESS THAN OR EQUAL TO 40 IN. (MEN) OR 35 IN. (WOMEN)	WAIST GREATER THAN 40 IN. (MEN) OR 35 IN. (WOMEN)
18.5 or less	Underweight	–	N/A
18.5–24.9	Normal	–	N/A
25.0–29.9	Overweight	Increased	High
30.0–34.9	Obese	High	Very high
35.0–39.9	Obese	Very high	Very high
40 or greater	Extremely obese	Extremely high	Extremely high

Source: Partnership for Healthy Weight Management (2001).

Energy Basics: Calorie Math

You can't touch them or see them. Food supplies them, but they're not nutrients. Your body burns them to keep you alive—and moving. What are they? They're calories! To understand how to achieve and maintain a healthy weight, you need to start with the calorie basics.

A Measure of Energy

Calories actually are units of energy. Back in science class, you probably learned the technical definition: One calorie is the amount of energy needed to raise the temperature of 1 gram of water by 1 degree Celsius. In the world of nutrition and health, the term "calorie" refers to the amount of energy in food and the amount of energy the body uses.

In food, calories are energy locked inside three groups of nutrients: carbohydrates, fats, and proteins. These nutrients are released from food during digestion, then absorbed into the bloodstream and converted to glucose, or blood sugar.

In your body, the food energy in glucose finally gets released into trillions of body cells, where it's used to power all your body's work—from your heartbeat, to push-ups, to the smile that spreads across your face. Energy from food you don't need right away can be stored as body fat or perhaps as glycogen, a storage form of carbohydrate. If your body doesn't use them, they just "hang around" as stored energy for later use.

Food Power

Read food labels or check a calorie counter. You'll see that most foods supply calories, or energy—some more than others. What accounts for the differences?

Three nutrient categories—carbohydrates, proteins, and fats—and alcohol supply energy, or calories, in food. Gram for gram, fat and alcohol supply more than either carbohydrate or protein do.

SOURCE OF ENERGY	CALORIES PER GRAM
Fats	9
Alcohol	7
Carbohydrates	4
Proteins	4

Three nutrient categories don't provide calories: vitamins, minerals, and water; neither do cholesterol and fiber.

As a rule of thumb, foods that are watery, watery-crisp (rather than greasy-crisp), or fibrous tend to have fewer calories than foods that are more fatty or greasy. (Remember, water is calorie-free.) For example, celery, which has more water and fiber than French fries, also has fewer calories.

How Many Calories for You?

Your body's need for energy, or fuel, never stops. Every minute of every day, your body needs a constant supply of energy to stay alive and to function well.

How much? Energy needs vary from person to person. Even your own energy needs change at different ages and stages of life. Your age, basal metabolic rate, body size and composition, physical condition, and activity level all contribute to how much energy you need.

Powering your body can be compared to fueling your car. Both your car and your body need a source of energy just to keep idling. When you move, your body—like your car—burns more fuel, and uses even more to go faster and farther. Some bodies—and some cars—are more fuel-efficient than others. That is, they use less energy to do the same amount of work. Age, size, shape, gender, physical condition, and even the type of "fuel" affect fuel efficiency. *"How Does Your Body Use Energy?" on page 26 shows the proportion of energy used for each role in your body.*

Your Basic Energy Needs

Energy for basal metabolism (basic needs) is energy your body burns on "idle." In scientific terms, basal metabolic rate (BMR) is the level of energy needed to keep involuntary body processes going. These include pumping your heart, breathing, generating body heat, perspiring to keep cool, transmitting messages to your brain, and producing thousands of body chemicals.

When we think of calories, energy burned through physical activity often comes to mind. Yet, for most people, basal metabolism represents about 60 percent of the body's energy needs!

How Does Your Body Use Energy?

If you're like most people, here's how your body uses the energy it "burns" each day:

Basic energy needs (basal metabolism)	60%
Physical activity	30%
Digestion of food and absorption of nutrients	10%
Energy use for the day	*100%*

The simple "rule of ten" offers a quick, easy estimate of how much energy your body uses for basal metabolism daily. Figure on 10 calories per pound of body weight for women, and 11 calories per pound for men, to meet routine energy demands. Here's an example:

Consider an active 130-pound female. She would burn about 1,300 calories (130 pounds × 10 calories per pound) per day for basal metabolism and about 2,200 calories total per day. (That's 60 percent of total calories for her basic energy needs.) Now calculate for yourself: About how much energy might your body require for your basic needs?

Why can one person consume more calories day after day and never gain a pound? For another person of the same age, height, and activity level, weight control is a constant challenge. The "rule of ten (or eleven)" doesn't allow for individual differences in basal metabolic rate (BMR). Age, gender, genetics, and body composition and size, among other factors, affect basic energy needs. Although you don't need to know your BMR to achieve and maintain a healthy weight, that may be useful information for some people, perhaps athletes in training. Health or fitness professionals can determine that for you. *Worth noting:* A handheld palm device is available that individuals can use to measure their metabolic rate at rest.

Age Factor. Young people—from infancy through adolescence—need more calories per pound than adults do for growing bone, muscle, and other tissues. During infancy, energy needs are higher per pound of body weight than at any other time in life. And just watch a growing teenager eat; you know that energy needs are high during adolescence! (The "rule of ten" isn't meant for kids—especially not infants.)

By adulthood, food energy (calorie) needs—and BMR—start to decline: 2 percent for each decade. For example, a woman who needs about 2,200 calories per day for her total energy needs at age twenty-five might need 2 percent less, or 2,156 calories per day, at age thirty-five. She may need another 2 percent less by age forty-five, and so on.

Why the decline in BMR? Body composition and hormones change with age. And with less physical activity, muscle mass decreases; body fat takes its place. Because body fat burns less energy than muscle, fewer calories are needed to maintain body weight, and the basal metabolic rate goes down. (As an aside, regular physical activity can help keep energy needs up.)

If you continue to follow your teenage eating habits—and live a less active lifestyle—the extra pounds that creep on with age should come as no surprise! Unused calories get stored as body fat.

Family Matters. Genetic makeup and inherited body build account for some differences in basal metabolic rate—differences you can't change! (Families tend to pass on food habits to one another, too, which also may account for similarities in body weight.)

Body Size, Shape, and Composition. Consider the impact on BMR and energy needs:

● A heavy, full-size car usually burns more fuel per mile than a small, sleek sports car. Likewise, the more you weigh, the more calories you burn. Body size makes a difference. It takes somewhat more effort to move if you weigh 170 pounds compared to 120. That's one reason why men, who often weigh more, use more calories than women.

● A lean, muscular body has a higher metabolic rate than a softly rounded body with more fat tissue. Why? Ounce for ounce, muscle burns more energy than body fat does. So the higher your proportion of muscle to fat, the more calories you need to maintain your weight. A softly rounded body type has a greater tendency to store body fat then a lean, sinewy body.

Tip: Stay physically active to maintain your muscle mass—and give your BMR a boost.

● A tall, thin body also has more surface area than a short body, and as a result, more heat loss; the net result—more calories burned (higher BMR) to maintain normal body temperature.

Gender Gap. The ratio of muscle to fat differs with gender, accounting for differences in basal metabolic rate. Up to age ten or so, energy needs for boys and girls are about the same, but then puberty triggers change. When boys start developing more muscle, they need more calories; their added height and size demand more energy, too.

By adulthood, men usually have less body fat and 10 to 20 percent more muscle than women of the same age and weight. That's one reason why men's basic energy needs are higher. In contrast, women's bodies naturally keep body fat stores in reserve for pregnancy and breast-feeding.

During pregnancy and breast-feeding, a woman's energy needs go up. To meet the energy demands of a full-term pregnancy, women need about 300 extra calories a day—or about 80,000 extra calories over nine months. To breast-feed her baby, a woman needs about 500 extra calories a day during the time she's breast-feeding.

Hot—or Cold? Outside temperature affects internal energy production. On chilly days, your BMR "burns" a little higher to keep you warm during prolonged exposure to cold. Shivering and moving to keep warm use energy, too. And in hot temperatures, your body's air conditioning system burns a bit more energy—for example, as you perspire to cool down.

The Diet Factor. Do you think that skipping meals or following a very-low-calorie eating plan offers a weight-loss edge? Think again. Severe calorie restriction actually can make your body more energy efficient and cause the rate at which your body burns energy from food to slow down! You then require fewer calories to perform the same body processes. This slowdown in metabolic rate is your body's strategy for survival.

An Exercise Perk. Depending on the length and intensity of exercise, a physical workout can boost your BMR for several hours afterward.

Physical Activity: An Energy Burner

Movement of any kind—a blink of your eye, a wave of your hand, or a jog around the block—uses energy. In fact, about 30 percent of your body's energy intake is used to power physical activity! But at best, that estimate is imprecise because activity levels differ so much. Very active people need more calories, using up about 40 percent of their total energy for physical activity.

Common sense says that some physical activities burn more energy than others. The amount of energy used to power physical activity actually depends on three things: the type of activity, its intensity, and how long you do it. Suppose you walk with a friend of the same age and body size. The one who pumps his or her arms and takes an extra lap around the block burns more energy. *The chart "Burning Calories with Activity" on page 28 shows how much energy—or how many calories—get used for common, nonstop activities.*

The Food Connection

Eating itself actually burns calories. Digesting food and absorbing nutrients use about 10 percent of your day's energy expenditure—about 180 calories if you consume 1,800 calories daily. But don't count on these processes to burn up all the energy in anything you eat!

Energy in Balance

There's nothing magical about controlling weight. To maintain weight, "energy in" must balance "energy out." In other words, your calorie intake must equal the calories your body burns. To lose or gain, just tip the energy balance.

● *For weight loss,* you need to consume fewer calories than you burn each day. Do that by either cutting back on calories or by moving more. Better yet, do both.

● *If you need to gain weight,* tip the balance in the other direction: consume more calories than your body uses.

What's the bottom line? Be aware that no matter what their source—carbohydrates, fats, or proteins—your body stores most excess calories you consume as body fat.

BURNING CALORIES WITH ACTIVITY

CALORIES BURNED PER HOUR, BY BODY WEIGHT			CALORIES BURNED PER HOUR, BY BODY WEIGHT		
ACTIVITY	120 LBS.	170 LBS.	ACTIVITY	120 LBS.	170 LBS.
Aerobic dance	330	460	Racquetball	385	540
Archery	190	270	Reading	70	100
Basketball	330	460	Rowing, stationary	385	540
Bicycling (<10mph)	220	310	Running, 10 mph	880	1,230
Bowling	165	230	Sitting (watching TV)	55	75
Calisthenics	250	345	Sitting (writing, typing)	100	140
Driving a car	110	155	Skating, roller	385	540
Eating	80	115	Skiing, cross-country	440	615
Food preparation	135	190	Skiing, downhill	385	540
Gardening	275	385	Sleeping	50	70
Golf (walking)	250	345	Soccer	385	540
Hiking	330	460	Swimming, leisure	330	460
Horseback riding	220	310	Tennis	385	540
Housework	135	190	Walking, brisk	220	310
Jogging	385	540	Weight training	165	230
Mowing lawn	300	425			

Source: "Compendium of Physical Activities: Classification of Energy Costs of Human Physical Activities," *Medicine and Science in Sports and Exercise* 25 (1993): 71-80.

Calorie Myths

Over the years, calorie myths of all kinds have developed. Do any of these unfounded notions sound familiar?

Myth: Margarine has fewer calories than butter.

Fact: Regular stick margarine and stick butter contain the same number of calories—about 36 per teaspoon. For a spread with fewer calories, try jelly or jam with 16 calories per teaspoon, or whipped butter or whipped margarine, about 26 calories per teaspoon.

Myth: A rich, fudgy brownie, before bedtime, is more fattening than the same brownie eaten at lunchtime.

Fact: What you eat, not when, makes the difference. No matter when they're eaten, calories seem to have the same effect in the body. Too many can add up to extra body fat. Timing has no direct effect on how your body uses the calories. Evidence does suggest that eating regular meals, especially breakfast, helps to reduce fat intake and minimize impulsive snacking, which can add up to excess calories over the course of a day.

Myth: Potatoes and bread are fattening.

Fact: By themselves, they're not high in calories—88 calories for a medium (4-ounce) potato and 70 calories for an average-size slice of bread. Both potatoes and bread are great sources of complex carbohydrates. However, high-fat toppings or spreads can add up to excess calories. Consider the calories in one tablespoon: sour cream (about 30 calories), butter or margarine (about 100 calories), and regular mayonnaise (about 100 calories).

Myth: Excess carbohydrates, not fats, cause weight gain.

Fact: Excess carbohydrates are no more fattening than excess calories from any source: fats, carbohydrates, and proteins. Despite claims of "low-carb" weight loss regimens, a high-carbohydrate diet doesn't promote body fat storage by enhancing insulin resistance. Excess calories from any source are stored as body fat.

Weighing the Risks

Overweight and obesity are epidemic in the United States. According to the Centers for Disease Control and Prevention, 61 percent of American adults are overweight or obese (with a BMI of 25 or above)—up significantly, just in the past decade. Young people are increasingly overweight, too! An estimated 20 percent of children in the United States are overweight or obese, according to the USDA Symposium on Childhood Obesity.

Gaining, or Losing, 1 Pound

One pound of body fat equals about 3,500 calories. Therefore, losing 1 pound requires a 3,500-calorie deficit. The opposite is true for weight gain. The following scenarios describe how an average person might gain or lose weight.

● To gain 1 pound: *If you added 250 calories* from an extra sandwich, fruit salad, or a bag of chips to your normal eating plan every day—without boosting your activity level—how long might it take *to gain 1 pound?*

   3,500 calories = 1 pound of body fat

   3,500 calories ÷ 250 calories per day = *14 days, or 2 weeks*

● To lose 1 pound: *If you burned 100 extra calories* by walking about 30 minutes during your lunch hour 5 days a week—without boosting your calorie intake—when would that *pound come off?*

   100 calories per day × 5 days = 500 calories per week

   500 calories per week × 7 weeks = 3,500 total calories burned

   3,500 calories = 1 pound of body fat

Have You Ever Wondered

. . . if my weight problem is really a thyroid problem? Maybe—but before you blame your thyroid, check with your doctor, who may order a test to find out. *Hypothyroidism,* when the thyroid doesn't produce enough thyroid hormone, is the most common form of thyroid disease; one symptom is weight gain. On the flip side, an overactive thyroid causes *hyper*thyroidism; one symptom is weight loss. *See chapter 22, page 545, with a "Have You Ever Wondered" question about thyroid disease and high blood cholesterol.*

According to the Institute of Medicine, obesity is defined as an excess of body fat, whereas overweight refers to an excess of body weight that includes fat, bone, and muscle. Globally, a BMI of 25 to 29.9 for adults is considered overweight; a BMI of 30 or more, obese.

The causes of overweight? Energy imbalance: more calories consumed than used. Today's inactive lifestyles contribute heavily to weight problems. For example, studies link excessive television viewing to the incidence of obesity. Today's technology, including computers, video games, and work-saving devices, play a role, too!

The causes of obesity are more complex than energy imbalance. Other psychological, social, and lifestyle factors add to the complex reasons for individual problems of obesity.

Because it runs in families, genetics may play a role—especially if the conditions are right. For example, people who inherit a sluggish metabolism are more likely to have a weight problem. A child's surroundings and upbringing are factors, too. With one obese parent, the chances of being overweight are 40 percent; that doubles when both parents are obese.

What about being too thin? The reasons for being underweight are as complex and unique as being overweight. Genetics may be a factor here, too. As with obesity, thinness tends to run in families. Some people may inherit a speedy metabolism. For many reasons, the appetite center of the brain may not signal hunger, so people may feel full even when they're not. Other psychological, physical, economic, social, and lifestyle factors also may get in the way of eating well. *See "Too Thin—a Problem?" later in this chapter.*

Overweight and Obesity: Hazards to Health

Sometime spend an hour or so carrying around a 5- or 10-pound bag of sugar or flour, or a heavy phone book. Tiring? That's the extra burden on your body and heart when you carry extra pounds of body fat. The more excess body fat you have, the greater that burden. Every body system—including the lungs, the heart, and the skeleton—has to work harder just to move.

Many health problems, *noted in the chart "Risky Business" on page 31,* are linked to overweight and obesity. That's why the Dietary Guidelines for Americans advises: *Aim for a healthy weight.* In other words, achieve and maintain your healthy weight—or at least avoid further weight gain. *Chapter 22 explores the links between overweight and obesity, and cardiovascular health, some cancers, and diabetes.*

Your "Weigh": Figuring Your Energy Needs

How much energy does your body need in a day? For a rough guesstimate, do the following "energy math."

1. *Figure your basic energy needs (BMR).* Multiply your healthy weight (in pounds) by 10 for women and by 11 for men. If you see from your BMI that you're overweight, use the average weight within the healthy weight range given for your height in "Are You at Your Healthy Weight?" earlier in this chapter.

   weight × ____ (either 10 or 11) = ____ calories for basic needs

2. *Figure your energy needs for physical activity.* Check the activity level that matches your lifestyle for most days of the week:

   ____ Sedentary: mainly sitting, driving a car, lying down, sleeping, standing, reading, typing, or other low-intensity activities

   ____ Light activity (for no more than 2 hours daily): light exercise such as light housework, grocery shopping, walking leisurely

   ____ Moderate activity: moderate exercise such as heavy housework, gardening, dancing, or brisk walking (and very little sitting)

   ____ Very active: active physical sports, or in a labor-intensive job such as construction work or ditch digging

   Multiply your basic energy needs by the percent that matches your activity level: sedentary, 20%; light activity, 30%; moderate activity, 40%; or very active, 50%.

   ____ calories for basic needs

   × ____% for activity level

   = ____ calories for physical activity

3. *Figure energy for digestion and absorbing nutrients.* Add your calories for basic needs and calories for physical activity, then multiply the total by 10%.

   (____ calories for basic needs + ____ calories for physical activity) × 10% =

   ____ calories for digestion and absorbing nutrients

4. Add up your total energy needs by adding calories for each purpose.

   + calories for basic needs

   + calories for physical activity

   + calories for digestion and absorbing nutrients

   = ____ calories for your total energy needs

   As an example, consider this 40-year-old female, who works at a desk and walks during her lunch hour. She weighs 125 pounds, which is healthy for her height.

   Basic energy needs: 125 pounds × 10 = 1,250 calories

   Energy for physical activity: 1,250 calories × 0.30 = 375 calories

   Energy for digestion and absorbing nutrients: (1,250 + 375 calories) × 0.10 = 162.5 calories

   Total energy needs: 1,250 calories + 375 calories + 162.5 calories = *1,787.5 calories*

RISKY BUSINESS

OVERWEIGHT AND OBESITY: KNOWN RISK FACTORS FOR . . .

- Diabetes
- Heart disease
- Stroke
- High blood pressure
- Gallbladder disease
- Osteoarthritis (degeneration of the cartilage and bone in joints)
- Sleep apnea and other breathing problems
- Some forms of cancer (uterine, breast, colorectal, kidney, gallbladder)

OBESITY: ASSOCIATED WITH . . .

- High blood cholesterol
- Complications of pregnancy
- Menstrual irregularities
- Excess body and facial hair
- Stress incontinence (urine leakage cause by weak muscles in the pelvic area)
- Psychological disorders such as depression
- Increased surgical risk

Source: National Institute of Diabetes and Digestive and Kidney Diseases/National Institutes of Health, *Statistics Related to Overweight and Obesity* (2000).

Obesity can lead to a cycle of inactivity. Often extra body weight makes physical activity more tiring— even for everyday activities such as walking up stairs or through a mall. Inactivity can lead to more weight gain, more muscle loss, and other health problems. Obesity can have an emotional price tag, too, if a negative body image leads to poor self-esteem and social isolation.

Now consider the upside: the health benefits of trimming down. If you're overweight, reducing even 10 to 20 pounds of excess body weight may be enough to improve your health and your quality of life. Even this small weight shift can help lower the risk factors for many chronic diseases: lower blood pressure, total and LDL blood cholesterol levels, triglyceride levels, and blood sugar. In addition, HDL cholesterol levels may go up. *To learn about total, LDL, and HDL cholesterol and triglycerides, see the "'Fat' Dictionary" in chapter 3.*

Obesity and Kids: A Heavy Burden

America's youth are getting fatter! Today 13 percent of children (six to eleven years) and 14 percent of teens (twelve to nineteen years) are considered obese, according to the Centers for Disease Control and Prevention. The effects can last a lifetime. Inactivity also is on the rise, contributing significantly to the prevalence of overweight and obesity.

Although obese children don't automatically become obese adults, there's reason for concern. Eating and activity patterns for life often are established during childhood. For these children, the risk for being overweight as teens and adults is higher. According to some studies, those who are overweight as teens have a greater chance for ongoing health problems such as diabetes as adults. What's more, weight problems affect self-image, and as a result, self-esteem. How children feel about themselves can affect almost every aspect of their lives now—and on into their adult years.

Weight-loss programs for adults are not meant for children or teens. Young people need enough calories and nutrients for their growth and development. Often increased physical activity, rather than cutting calories, is enough to help overweight children achieve a healthful weight. Before devising a plan to help your child or teenager lose weight, talk to your doctor or registered dietitian (RD).

For more about healthy food choices and lifestyles for children and teens, see chapter 16, "Food to Grow On." There you'll also find guidelines for helping young people reach and maintain a healthy weight; *see "Weighty Problems for Children—Overweight" and "If Your Child or Teen Has a Weight Problem . . ."*

Weight Management: Strategies That Work!

The key to managing your weight throughout your life? A positive "can do" attitude and the right kind of motivation! If you're trying to lose weight to fit into a

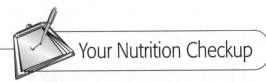

Weight-Loss Readiness Test

Are you ready to lose weight? Your attitude affects your ability to succeed. Take this readiness quiz to see if you're mentally ready before you begin. Mark each statement as "true" or "false." Be honest with yourself! The answers should reflect the way you really think—not how you'd like to be!

1. I have thought a lot about my eating habits and physical activities, and I know what I might change.

2. I know that I need to make permanent, not temporary, changes in my eating and activity patterns.

3. I will feel successful only if I lose a lot of weight.

4. I know that it's best if I lose weight slowly.

5. I'm thinking about losing weight now because I really want to, not because someone else thinks I should.

6. I think losing weight would solve other problems in my life.

7. I am willing and able to increase my regular physical activity.

8. I can lose weight successfully if I have no slipups.

9. I am willing to commit time and effort each week to organize and plan my food and activity choices.

10. Once I lose a few pounds but reach a plateau (I can't seem to lose more), I usually lose the motivation to keep going toward my weight goal.

11. I want to start a weight loss program, even though my life is unusually stressful right now.

Now Score Yourself

Look at your answers for items 1, 2, 4, 5, 7, and 9. Score "1" if you answered "true" and "0" if you answered "false." For items 3, 6, 8, 10, and 11, score "0" for each "true" answer and "1" for each false answer.

No one score indicates if you're ready to start losing weight. But the higher your total score, the more likely you'll be successful.

If you scored 8 or higher, you probably have good reasons to lose weight now. And you know some of the steps that can help you succeed.

If you scored 5 to 7 points, you may need to reevaluate your reasons for losing weight and the strategies you'd follow.

If you scored 4 or less, now may not be the right time for you to lose weight. You may be successful initially, but you may not be able to sustain the effort to reach or maintain your weight goal. Reconsider your reasons and approach.

Interpret Your Score

Your answer can clue you in on some stumbling blocks to your weight management success. Any item you scored as "0" suggests a misconception about weight loss, or a problem area for you. So let's look at each item a bit more closely.

1. You can't change what you don't understand, and that includes your eating habits and activity pattern. Keep records for a week to pinpoint when, what, why, and how much you eat—as well as patterns and obstacles to regular physical activity.

2. You may be able to lose weight in the short run with drastic or highly restrictive changes in your eating habits or activity pattern. But they may be hard to live with permanently. Your food and activity plans should be healthful ones you can enjoy and sustain.

3. Many people fantasize about reaching a weight goal that's unrealistically low. If that sounds like you, rethink your meaning of success. A reasonable goal takes body type into consideration—and sets smaller, achievable "mile markers" along the way.

4. If you equate success with fast weight loss, you'll have problems keeping weight off. This "quick fix" attitude can backfire when you face the challenges of weight maintenance. The best and healthiest approach is to lose weight slowly while learning strategies to keep weight off permanently.

5. To be successful, the desire for and commitment to weight loss must come from you—not your best friend or a family member. People who lose weight, then keep it off, take responsibility for their weight goals and choose their own approach.

6. Being overweight may contribute to some social problems, but it's rarely the single cause. While body image and self-esteem are strongly linked, thinking you can solve all your problems by losing weight isn't realistic. And it may set you up for disappointment.

7. A habit of regular, moderate physical activity is a key factor to successfully losing weight—and keeping it off. For weight control, physical activity doesn't need to be strenuous to be effective. Any moderate physical activity that you enjoy and will do regularly counts.

8. Most people don't expect perfection in their daily lives, yet they often feel they must stick to a weight-loss program perfectly. Perfection at weight loss isn't realistic. Rather than viewing lapses as catastrophes, see them as opportunities to find what triggers your problems and develop strategies for the future.

Source: American Dietetic Association.

9. To successfully lose weight, you must take time to assess your problem areas, then develop the approach that's best for you. Success requires planning, commitment, and time.

10. First of all, a plateau in an ongoing weight-loss program is perfectly normal, so don't give up too soon! Before you lose your motivation, think about any past efforts that have failed, then identify strategies that can help you overcome those hurdles.

11. Weight loss itself can be a source of stress, so if you're already under stress, you may find a weight-loss program somewhat difficult to implement right now. Try to resolve other stressors in your life before starting your weight-loss effort.

---

bathing suit before vacation, or to look good for your school reunion, or because your spouse is nagging you to drop a belt size, your commitment and efforts are likely to fizzle out over time. Internal motivators—health, increased energy, self-esteem, feeling in control—increase your chances for lifelong success.

If you're at your healthy weight, these strategies for weight management are meant for you, too. *A word of caution:* If your weight problem is excessive—too much or too little—or if you have health problems, talk to your doctor before you get started. Children, pregnant women, and people over age sixty-five shouldn't attempt weight loss without advice from their health professional.

Ready? Set . . . Go for It!

Whether your objective is weight loss, weight gain, or weight maintenance, lifelong success depends on some new ways of thinking.

● Make health, not appearance, your weight-management priority. Strive for your best weight for health. That's not necessarily the lowest weight you could be—or what you consider your "ideal" number.

● For weight loss gain, follow these tactics for weight management: (1) healthful eating, (2) regular physical activity, and (3) acceptance of the weight you can achieve through a healthy lifestyle.

● Set realistic, attainable goals—for you! Start with your current weight or your lifestyle, not where you want to be. The challenge of trimming 5 pounds at a time may seem more doable than losing 25 or more pounds.

● Focus on a healthy lifestyle—for a lifetime—not on "dieting." Dieting alone is often a short-term tactic without long-term results. The concept of "dieting" carries a lot of negative baggage: guilt, "shoulds," and "can't haves." For most people, "dieting" results in failure.

● Focus your strategies: action-oriented and specific. Perhaps you'll walk for 15 minutes each day during your lunch break, or you'll drink milk rather than a milk shake with your fast-food lunch.

● Tailor your strategies to your schedule, your budget, your family situation, and your personal needs, to name a few. Experts have found that two out of three people who were successful at weight control personalized their efforts to fit their lifestyles. *See "Check It Out!" later in this chapter.*

● Think long-term and act gradually. It's true that fasting and starvation-type diets can peel off pounds, but most of the weight that's lost quickly is only water loss! Grueling exercise regimens may tone the body, but for most people, these tactics aren't realistic ways to live—and they may not be healthful, either.

Weight Cycling–the "Yo-Yo" Problem

Have you gained and lost the same 10, 20, or even 30 pounds over and over again? The cycle of repeatedly losing and regaining weight can make weight management more difficult in the long run. Lost weight that repeatedly comes back may lead to feelings of frustration, failure, and poor self-esteem. According to some studies, weight cycling may even increase the risk for ongoing health problems such as heart disease and some forms of cancer.

Weight cycling often comes from quick-fix diets, weight-loss gimmicks, and other risky strategies. Without physical activity, each time the dieter sheds a few pounds, he or she loses lean body mass, along with body fat. Because the approach for weight loss is short-lived, pounds quickly return. Without exercise, those regained pounds are mostly body fat, which burns less energy than muscle. As the cycle repeats itself, the dieter needs fewer and fewer calories to maintain weight, and it gets harder and harder to lose weight. The cycle of "failure, success, failure" makes it psychologically harder to try again, too.

If repeated "ups and downs" of dieting describe your weight problem, shift your approach to one of lifetime weight management. Break the cycle with long-term approaches rather than short-term results. Make gradual and permanent changes in the way you eat, your activity level, and your lifestyle. It's the only way to be healthy—for life.

Instead of trying quick fixes, plan for a gradual weight shift of ½ to 1 pound a week. That's safe and healthy. With any more weight loss, you may be exercising too much or eating too little.

If you need to lose weight, losing about 10 percent of your weight over 6 months is safe; that's 20 pounds in 6 months (26 weeks) for someone who weighs 200 pounds. Remember: Your extra pounds didn't creep on overnight. They don't disappear that way either!

● Be realistic with your self-talk. Skip the absolutes—"always," "never," and "must" in your tactics. "I'll never eat another french fry." "I must swim twenty laps every other day." Get rid of "shoulds," too. "I should get up early and walk."

● Cut yourself some slack. Nobody's perfect. Allow for occasional slipups in your eating strategies, without feeling guilty.

● Plan to indulge sensibly. By planning for "treats" and "splurges" you may be more successful in the long run.

● Expect success. Reaching life's goals is often a self-fulfilling prophecy. Positive self-talk and an enthusiastic approach to weight management can set you up for success!

Get Physical!

Move it to lose it! Physical activity has been cited as the most powerful tool for weight management. A physically active lifestyle offers many rewards—from heart health to strong bones to stress relief, plus many other benefits. Yet many people don't get enough. *See "Moderate Activity: What Is It?" in chapter 1.*

Think of the impact of the personal computer. Back in the days of the manual typewriter, a typist, on average, burned 15 more calories an hour than someone doing the same work today on a computer. For

Put Action in Your Lifestyle!

Like sound eating habits, regular physical activity is part of a healthful lifestyle. Apply the same principles—variety, balance, and moderation—to both your food choices and your physical activities. Always check with your healthcare provider before beginning any rigorous physical activity program.

● *Variety.* Enjoy many different activities to move different muscles, including your heart: perhaps power walking for your heart and leg muscles, gardening for arm muscles, and sit-ups for abdominal muscles.

● *Balance.* Because different activities have different benefits, balance your physical activity pattern. For overall fitness, choose activities that build cardiovascular endurance (aerobic activities), muscular strength, bone strength, and flexibility.

● *Moderation.* Move enough to keep fit, without overdoing. You don't need a heavy workout. At least thirty minutes of moderate physical activity most and preferably all days of the week will do. Once you achieve this goal, consider moving more to help keep your body fit.

someone who does word processing for four hours a day, that adds up to 60 calories a day, or 300 calories over a five-day workweek. When you add up all the energy savings—from escalators and moving sidewalks, to cars and motorbikes, to home appliances and electric garage door openers—you can see that inactivity has become a way of life and why weight control has become an everyday challenge. The more you sit, the less energy you need, and the more likely you are to gain weight!

The Active Edge

Study after study shows that people who keep physically active are more successful at losing—and keeping off—extra pounds of body fat. In fact, physical activity appears to be the key to maintaining a healthy weight. Here are eight reasons why. Regular, moderate physical activity:

● *Burns energy.* The longer, more frequently, and more vigorously you move, the more energy you

---

Twenty Everyday Ways to Get Moving

Do you find it difficult to fit thirty minutes of physical activity into your life every day? It may be easier than you think—even with a busy lifestyle. These everyday activities can count toward your day's total if they're done with moderate intensity—and most take only a little extra time.

1. Wake up thirty minutes earlier, and take a brisk walk to start your day. Need someone to get you going? Schedule your walk with your spouse or a neighbor.

2. Forget the drive-through car wash. Wash the car yourself. Bonus: You'll save money at the same time.

3. Take stairs instead of the elevator or escalator. Walking up stairs is a great heart exerciser, calorie burner, and muscle builder!

4. Park at the far end of the parking lot for a longer walk. Get off the bus a stop ahead, then walk the rest of the way to your destination. Walk your kids to and from school.

5. Are you a computer user—on and off the job? Give yourself at least five minutes off for every hour or two of computer time: walk to the water fountain, or go up and down a few flights of stairs.

6. Walk around your building—outside or inside—during your lunch or coffee break. You'll burn energy rather than being tempted to nibble on a snack.

7. Get a dog, and walk together. No dog? Then borrow a neighbor's dog or push a baby stroller.

8. Play actively with your kids, grandkids, or pets. Some dogs like to play with a Frisbee as much as kids do!

9. Before and after dinner, walk—and talk—with your family. To burn more energy if you have an infant, use a baby carrier on your back rather than pushing a stroller.

10. Do some backyard gardening. (*Bonus:* Grow fresh vegetables and herbs if you can.) In the fall, rake leaves.

11. Ride your bike (the kind you pedal) to work or to a friend's home—if it's safe to do. Walk to do nearby errands, such as grocery shopping for small things or going to the post office.

12. While you watch television, do household chores or projects: mop the kitchen floor or refinish a piece of furniture. Avoid the "couch potato" syndrome.

13. Catch up with your around-the-house work: wash the windows, vacuum or shampoo the carpet, clean the garage or basement, sweep the sidewalk.

14. Use the exercise equipment you already own. Do two things at one time: ride your stationary bicycle while you read the morning paper or a newsmagazine. Watch the morning news while you work out on your rowing machine.

15. Push your lawn mower instead of using the power-assisted drive. Skip the snow blower; shovel the snow by hand if you're fit.

16. Make homemade bread. Knead the dough by hand, not with a bread machine or a food processor.

17. Use a rest room or pay phone at the other end of the building so you get an opportunity to walk.

18. Plan an active family vacation or a weekend outing. Rather than sit on a beach, go canoeing, hiking, or snow skiing.

19. "Walk your talk!" If you like to chat on the phone, buy a portable one so you don't need to sit still. (Use hand weights while talking on the phone.)

20. Rent an exercise video rather than a movie. And work out with the video as a leisure time activity.

burn. When you burn more than you consume, your body uses its energy stores, and you lose weight. Just adding thirty minutes of brisk walking to your day makes a difference!

● *Helps you keep muscle and lose body fat.* Without physical activity, you tend to lose lean body tissue along with body fat.

● *Builds lean body mass.* Even when you're not moving, lean body mass requires more energy to maintain than fat tissue.

● *Speeds up your basal metabolic rate*—for up to twelve hours, even after you stop. You'll burn more energy even at rest.

● *May suppress appetite a bit.* In fact, people who get regular physical activity often eat less than those who don't.

● *Helps relieve stress.* Remember: Stress may lead to nibbling on more food and consuming more calories than your body needs.

● *Creates a "trimmer" mind-set.* As some people get more physically active, they opt for foods with less fat, fewer calories, and more complex carbohydrates. The reason? It just seems to "feel good."

● *"Looks good" on you.* A firm, lean body from physical activity looks trimmer than one that's flabby with more body fat, even at the same weight. Think of your body as a "package" of lean tissue and body fat; muscles take less space than body fat. Although looks aren't the only reason for being physically active, they're a great side effect!

What if you need to *gain* weight? Because the benefits go beyond weight control, everyone needs to get moving. There's no need to cut back on physical activity unless a person's physical activity pattern is excessive—or if a physician advises a slower pace.

Weight control is just one reason to keep physically active. *For other benefits, see "Ten Reasons to Make the 'Right Moves'" in chapter 1.*

Simply Living an Active Lifestyle

To benefit from active living, you don't need to be an exercise fanatic with strenuous daily workouts. Step aerobics at a fitness club, kick boxing, or thirty minutes on an exercise bike every day may not be right for you. That's okay; any kind of moderate, consistent physical activity can do the job. In fact, any activity you enjoy and stay with can be the right one for you. If it's enjoyable, you're more likely to stick with it.

To manage your weight—and get other health benefits—try to fit thirty minutes or more of moderate activity into your daily life. Do it all at once, or spread it out: for example, ten minutes of brisk walking during your lunch hour, fifteen minutes of leisure bike riding, and five minutes of sidewalk sweeping at home. If you haven't been physically active, then build up gradually. Even a little more physical activity can make a difference.

Remember: *the energy expenditure of physical activity goes up in three ways.* The *longer,* the *more frequent,* and the *more intense* your activity, the more energy you burn. Regardless, choose physical activities that you enjoy and can stick with for the rest of your life.

Even though some weight-loss regimens make "spot-reducing" promises, your body can't get rid of fat in just the problem places. As you exercise and burn more calories than you consume, your body draws energy from all its fat stores, including the problem spots. If you keep on moving, fat will eventually disappear in all the right places.

When You Want to Lose

Eating to control weight and eating for good health are one and the same. One simple food plan—based on the Food Guide Pyramid—can accomplish both objectives. To tip the energy balance for weight loss or gain, or to keep it level, simply adjust your food choices and the number of servings you consume within each of the five major groups of the Food Guide Pyramid. *For more about following these guidelines, see "The Food Guide Pyramid: Your Healthful Eating Guide" in chapter 10.*

Remember: one pound of body fat contains 3,500 calories worth of stored energy. For weight loss, create a 3,500-calorie deficit for each pound you want to lose. Experts suggest striving for a 250- to 500-calorie deficit per day to lose weight at the safe rate of about ½ to 1 pound per week. Do that by cutting back on what you eat or being more physically active—or better yet, by doing both.

To trim energy intake, should you count calories or count fat grams? Perhaps neither one. Just eating smarter might be enough: cut back to smaller portions; eat fewer high-fat, sugary snacks; choose mostly lean and low-fat foods; and enjoy more fruits and vegetables and fewer higher-calorie foods.

Counting calories to manage weight takes effort. If you choose to do this, get a calorie counter that lists calories in many foods, or try a computer program that makes the task easier.

Count fat grams? That, too, can be time-consuming. You might keep track of fat grams to learn the fat content of foods. After all, fat does provide more than twice the calories per gram than carbohydrate or protein. If you moderate the fat you consume, you'll likely cut back on calories. But keep in mind: "low-fat" doesn't always mean "low-calorie." Some "low-fat" and "fat-free" foods, such as desserts and muffins, have more sugars and as many calories as their counterparts. *See "Low-'Cal' and Low-Fat: Not the Same!" on page 39.* Remember: the total calories (not fat grams) you consume and burn through physical activity determine your body weight.

Not every food you eat needs to be low in calories. The idea is to balance high-calorie foods with low-calorie foods over the course of a day—or even a few days—so your total calorie intake is less than what you use.

How many calories? To get *enough of the nutrients* your body needs, eat *at least 1,600 calories a day.* That's easier to do wisely if you choose mostly lean and low-fat foods. Children and teenagers especially need adequate calories and nutrients for growth, as well as for normal body function and physical activity.

Try these calorie-cutting, healthful eating strategies:

● Follow the advice of the Food Guide Pyramid. For each of the five food groups, eat the servings recommended for the lower end of the serving range. With mostly lean and low-fat foods, that's about 1,600 calories.

● Watch your portion sizes. Even calories in low-fat foods can tip your energy balance toward weight gain when portions are bigger than you need.

Get Portion Savvy

"It's not too big. It's not too small. It's just right!" As a weight management strategy, keep tabs on portion sizes to, in turn, manage the number of calories you consume. Even low-fat foods—for example, pasta, rice, beans, or potatoes—can add up to a hefty calorie count when portions get big.

How portion savvy are you? Without using a measuring cup, try pouring one cup of dry cereal—or scooping a half cup of ice cream—into a bowl. Now check the size with a measuring cup. Chances are, you've overestimated. Most people do. That's why many people quite innocently overdo their calorie intake.

The Food Guide Pyramid offers standard serving sizes as part of its guideline for healthy eating. Use measuring cups and spoons, and perhaps a kitchen scale to compare your helpings with Pyramid serving sizes or the serving sizes listed on the Nutrition Facts of food labels.

Need specific strategies to be more portion savvy? Check here for "how-tos":

● Size up your servings—see chapter 10.

● Be aware of portion distortion—see chapter 10.

● Control restaurant portions—see chapter 14.

● When you shop, cook, and eat out, cut back on fat in your food choices. Switching from high- to low-fat foods may be enough to make a difference if the calorie content in the food is less. Read Nutrition Facts on foods labels to find out.

● Fill up on fruits, vegetables, and whole grains. Being high in fiber and usually low in calories, they can help satisfy you faster. *Bonus:* They may take more time to chew—so you eat less!

● Learn how to eat what you like! No one food by itself can make you fat. You'll more likely stick to your eating plan if you don't deprive yourself. Just eat small amounts of higher-calorie food. *For tips on taming food cravings, see "Eat What You Crave!" later in this chapter.*

Check It Out!

Ready to start a weight control plan? To make sure the approach is healthful and effective, ask yourself a few questions before you begin. Does the program include:

- A variety of foods from all five major groups in the Food Guide Pyramid?
- Appealing foods you will enjoy eating for the rest of your life, not just a few weeks or months?
- Foods that are available at the supermarket where you usually shop?
- The chance to eat your favorite foods—in fact, any foods?
- Eating strategies that fit your lifestyle and budget?
- An adequate amount of nutrients and energy—from at least the minimum number of servings from the Food Guide Pyramid?
- Enough regular physical activity?

If you *cannot* answer "yes" to all these questions, chances are this weight-loss program won't bring long-term success because you may not stick to it. Success is possible only when you make healthful, permanent changes in your eating and physical activity habits.

- Use the Nutrition Facts on food labels to compare calories in different foods. The amount for one serving is on the label. A serving isn't necessarily the whole package! Check the front of the label, too, where you may find nutrition claims for foods with fewer calories. What do the label terms mean? *Check "Label Lingo: Calories" on page 39.*

- Go easy on wine, beer, and other alcoholic drinks: no more than one drink a day for women and two for men. Alcohol supplies calories—7 calories per gram. A 12-ounce beer contains about 150 calories, and a 5-ounce glass of white wine has 100 calories. Downing a six-pack of beer on a hot summer day can add up to a whopping 900 calories, and splitting a 1-liter bottle of wine can supply 325 calories or more; excessive amounts aren't healthful, either. Drinking alcoholic beverages also can stimulate your appetite, so you may eat more.

- Snack smart. It's easy to think about meals yet forget about snacks. Choose snacks wisely by the calories and nutrients they supply. Practice the art of calorie balancing so you can enjoy some higher-fat snacks, such as chocolate bars, nuts, ice cream, or chips. Just eat them less often, in small amounts. And balance them with lower-calorie, lower-fat snacks—pretzels, bread sticks, raisins, fruit, or raw vegetables—the next time.

- Ask a registered dietitian for more guidance on choosing healthful foods for weight loss.

Need specific calorie-cutting strategies? Check here for "how-tos":

- Take control of calories in alcoholic drinks—see chapter 8.
- Snack smart for fewer calories—see chapter 10.
- Get "calorie-wise" as you shop—see chapter 11.
- Cut calories by trimming fat in food "prep"—see chapter 13.
- Eat out with calorie savvy—see chapter 14.

Slimming Habits

Look at your eating habits. Do you snack on high-calorie foods at work because everyone else does? Do you eat fast so you can get on quickly with your day? Are you a stand-up diner?

- Rethink your old ways of eating—and identify those habits that promote weight gain. Consider what, when, why, where, and how you eat. Then, if you need to, make some changes for a more healthful eating style.

- Plan meals and snacks ahead. Haphazard eating often becomes high-calorie eating. Pack low-calorie snacks, such as raw vegetables, to eat at work when others snack on candy, doughnuts, or chips.

- Shop on a full stomach to help avoid the temptation to buy extra goodies or to nibble on free samples. Write out your shopping list when you're not hungry.

- Stick to a regular eating schedule. (There's no hard-and-fast rule about eating three meals a day.)

Label Lingo

Calories

Nutrition Facts on the food label list the calories in a single serving. In addition, "calorie lingo" on the package can alert you to lower-calorie food products as you search supermarket displays.

LABEL TERM	MEANS
Calorie-free	Less than 5 calories
Low-calorie	40 calories or less
Reduced or fewer calories	At least 25% fewer calories*
Light or lite	One-third fewer calories or 50% less fat*; if more than half the calories are from fat, fat content must be reduced by 50% or more
Low-calorie meals	120 calories or less per 100 grams
Light meal	"Low-fat" or "low-calorie" meal

*As compared with a standard serving size of the traditional food

Studies show that missed meals can lead to impulsive snacking and overeating and may lower the rate at which your body burns energy.

● Eat from plates, not from packages. When you nibble chips or crackers from a package or snack on ice cream from the carton, you don't know how much you've eaten. It may be more, much more, than you think!

● Serve foods right on the dinner plate, not in serving bowls and platters on the table. You'll likely eat less. Use smaller bowls and dinner plates so small portions look like more. *See "Get Portion Savvy" earlier in this chapter for more tips on portion control.*

● Eat slowly. Savor the flavor of each bite. After all, it takes about twenty minutes for your stomach to signal your brain that you're full—which curbs your urge for a second helping. Slow down by putting down your fork between bites. Eat with chopsticks if they slow you down. Sip, rather than gulp, beverages. Swallow before filling your fork again.

● Forget the "clean-plate club." You don't need to eat everything on your plate if you're satisfied already.

● Sit down to eat. Focus on your food, rather than nibbling, while you do other things. That way you know that you've eaten.

● Make eating the only event—and enjoy it. Eating unconsciously while you watch television, read, or drive may lead to eating more than you think.

● Choose foods that take more time to eat. For example, peeling and eating an orange takes longer than drinking a glass of orange juice.

● Stop eating when you leave the table. Avoid the urge to nibble on leftovers as you clear the table and clean up.

LOW-"CAL" AND LOW-FAT: NOT THE SAME!

Read the label! Compare the calories. Being fat-free doesn't make a food calorie-free. A fat-free or reduced-fat product may have as many (even more) calories per serving than regular products.

Fig cookie (1)
Fat-free	51 calories
Regular	56 calories

Vanilla frozen yogurt (1/2 cup)
Nonfat	100 calories
Regular	104 calories

Caramel topping (2 tablespoons)
Fat-free	103 calories
Homemade with butter	103 calories

Peanut butter (2 tablespoons)
Reduced-fat	187 calories
Regular	191 calories

Cereal bar (1.3 ounce)
Low-fat	130 calories
Regular	140 calories

Source: National Institutes of Health, *Practical Guide to the Identification, Evaluation, and Treatment of Overweight and Obesity in Adults* (2001).

- When you get the urge to nibble (especially if you're not hungry), do something else. Jog, call a friend, walk the dog, or step out into your garden.

- Be aware of the influence of others. You don't need to eat that cake, muffin, or bagel in the break room just because your officemate brought it to work.

Eating Triggers

You have all the best intentions. Then something triggers your desire to eat—even though you're not hungry. Instead of looking inside the refrigerator or diving into a bowl of snacks, get in touch with the emotions and situations that trigger your eating. Learn to differentiate between physical hunger and other, emotionally-driven hungers. Find an appropriate diversion.

Dear Diary . . .

Help yourself to weight control by keeping tabs on what you eat. Research shows that people who keep a food and activity diary are often more successful at weight management than those who don't.

There's nothing complicated about keeping a record. Use any kind of notebook as your diary, or buy a day-to-day food and activity diary for handwritten records. If you carry your laptop computer everywhere, keep your records there. Or get a hand-held palm monitoring device with software to log these data and carry with you.

For the record, keep track of the amounts and kinds of foods and beverages you eat every day. To get a handle on any eating "triggers," write your mood and rate your hunger level each time you eat. Put down the time and place, too. List the amount of time you spend in physical activity, along with what you do. Keep your food and activity record for at least a week or two. Then review it to get a closer look at your eating and physical activity habits.

Most people can spot problem areas easily: perhaps the high-fat snack every afternoon at 3:00 P.M., or the nighttime snacks eaten in front of the television. Keeping records offers one way to identify areas you might need to change. It also can help you focus on your weight goals—and think twice before indulging in a high-fat snack when you're not hungry.

Emotional Overeating: Take Control!

To relax, quell anger, or overcome depression or loneliness, mood-triggered eating may feel good—at first. But eating to cope with emotions can lead to more negative feelings (guilt, lack of personal control, and poor self-esteem) and perhaps to a cycle of mood-triggered eating. Any excessive calorie intake can promote weight gain. As important, using food to satisfy emotions may distract you from handling serious issues in your life.

On the plus side, learning to control mood-triggered eating promotes feelings of personal power and self-esteem!

Learn to deal with emotions in a positive, more appropriate way. Address the real problems. Resolve your moods with positive self-talk or a brief change of scenery. Compared with nibbling, physical activity—perhaps a brisk walk, a bike ride, or a tennis game—often does the trick!

- Do you eat when you're bored or stressed? Find some other options. Make a list of fun activities: enjoy your garden, play with the dog, go shopping, call a friend, surf the Internet, or play with your kids. Post your list on the refrigerator. When you're bored or upset, pick one of these activities instead of eating. *See "Emotional Overeating: Take Control!" above.*

- Be aware of social situations that trigger eating—such as parties, entertaining friends, dating, talking around the coffeepot at work, and happy-hour business meetings. Then create your own ways to avoid overeating.

- Remember: out of sight, out of mind. If the sight of candy, chips, and other high-calorie foods lures you, store them in an inconvenient place. Better yet, don't keep them around. Instead stock up on fruit, raw vegetables, and other foods with fewer calories.

- Accomplished something special? Reward yourself, but not with food. Treat yourself to a massage or a day spa. Buy something new to wear, read, or entertain you. Go to a play, concert, or sports event. Indulge yourself by calling your friends. Don't make success your trigger for eating.

● Watch out for seasonal triggers: perhaps nibbling while watching fall and winter sports on television, "cooling off" in hot weather with a few beers or an extra-large soft drink, or eating and entertaining during the holidays. Or eat smaller portions or different foods if only eating will do. If you're not sure what triggers your eating, keep a food diary for a week or two. *"Dear Diary . . ." on page 40 offers some tips for doing so.*

Party "Tid-bites"

Celebrate! Food is one of the pleasures of parties, holiday festivities, and other social gatherings at every time of year. Just because you're trying to eat healthfully doesn't mean you need to avoid celebrations or accept a few extra party pounds. Any foods—even traditional holiday fare—can fit into a healthful eating plan for the calorie-conscious. The secret is moderation and balance.

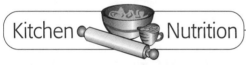

Kitchen Nutrition

Celebration Meals Go Lean!

Celebration menus—or almost any meal—may be modified to lower the calories and the fat content. Often the differences go almost unnoticed. Compare this traditional menu with its leaner version. *Then see chapter 13 for tips on trimming calories and fat in food preparation.*

ORIGINAL MENU	LEANER MENU
3½ oz. roasted turkey with skin	3½ oz. skinless, roasted turkey
½ cup stuffing	½ cup wild rice pilaf
½ cup broccoli with 2 tbsp. hollandaise sauce	½ cup broccoli with lemon juice
½ cup cranberry relish	¼ cup cranberry relish
1 medium crescent roll	1 whole-grain roll
1 slice pecan pie	1 slice pumpkin pie
Total calories: 1,140	*Total calories:* 735
Total fat: 50 g	*Total fat:* 20 g

Whether a stand-up event or a sit-down dinner, these party tips can help you hold the line:

● Be realistic. Trying to lose weight during the holidays may be a self-defeating goal. Instead strive to maintain your weight.

● Balance party eating with other meals. Eat small, lower-calorie meals during the day so you can enjoy celebration foods, too—without overdoing your energy intake for the day.

● Take the edge off your hunger before a party. Eat a small, low-fat snack such as fruit or a bagel. Feeling hungry can sabotage even the strongest willpower!

● When you arrive at a party, avoid rushing to the food. Greet people you know—conversation is calorie-free! Get a beverage, and settle into the festivities before eating. You may eat less.

● Ask for sparkling water and a lime twist rather than wine, champagne, or a mixed drink. Sparkling water doesn't supply calories.

● Move your socializing away from the buffet table. When conversations take your attention away from food, unconscious nibbling becomes too easy.

● Make just one trip to the party buffet. And be selective. Choose only the foods you really want to eat, and keep portions small. Often just a taste satisfies a craving or curiosity.

● Opt for lower-calorie party foods. Perhaps enjoy raw vegetables with a small dollop of dip, just enough to coat the end of the vegetable. Try boiled shrimp or scallops with cocktail sauce or lemon. Go easy on fried appetizers and cheese cubes.

● If you're bringing a dish, make it healthfully delicious—and low-calorie, too. That way, you'll know there's something with fewer calories you can munch on. Perhaps bring raw vegetables with a yogurt or cottage cheese dip, or bring a platter of juicy, fresh fruit.

● Enjoying a sit-down dinner party? Make your first helping small—especially if your host or hostess expects you to take seconds. The total amount may be about the same as your normal-size portions.

● Forget the all-or-nothing mind-set. Depriving yourself of special holiday foods, or feeling guilty

Noodlin' over "Carb" Headlines?

Can "carbs" make you fat—as some headlines suggest? The Dietary Guidelines for Americans and the Food Guide Pyramid recommend an eating pattern with plenty of complex carbohydrates from foods such as breads, cereals, rice, pasta, fruits, vegetables, and legumes (beans).

Limited research notes that carbohydrate-rich foods may cause weight gain in "insulin-resistant" people. For these individuals, it's speculated, the body reacts to sugars and starches by overproducing insulin—and so causing too much starch to be stored as fat. However, most of us don't gain weight on a high-carbohydrate diet, unless it provides excess calories. The real culprits for weight are inactivity, high-fat eating, and uncontrolled portion sizes from any source of food, including bread, pasta, and other grain products. See "Insulin Resistance Syndrome, or 'Syndrome X'" in chapter 22.

when you do enjoy them, isn't a healthful eating strategy. And deprivation and guilt certainly are not part of the holiday spirit!

● When you're entertaining, make over your menus with fewer calories and fat. Your guests probably won't detect the difference. Be sensitive to any guests with weight goals in mind, too. *For a dinner makeover, see "Kitchen Nutrition: Celebration Meals Go Lean!" earlier in this chapter.*

● Have fun! Sharing food is part of many celebrations. Enjoying a traditional holiday meal and party foods with family and friends doesn't need to destroy healthful food habits you've nurtured all year long.

Motivation Boosters

With weight control as part of your lifestyle, healthful eating and physical activity become second nature. When you need a boost to stay on track, try this!

● Make lifestyle changes with a friend or a family member! A partner increases the enjoyment factor of physical activity and healthful eating.

● Enlist support. Family and friends can help you keep on track. Those who have the support of family members, particularly a spouse, more likely manage their weight successfully. Watch out for

those who attempt to sabotage your efforts. If it's right for you, join a support group.

● Track your progress—but not too often. Avoid the urge to step onto the scale every day. Once a week is often enough. Since weight fluctuates from day to day due to fluid loss and retention, you may not get a true picture if you weigh yourself too frequently.

● Remember that for women, weight gain from water retention may be a normal part of a monthly menstrual cycle. Usually that passes in a few days.

Have You Ever Wondered

. . . why it seemed easy to lose weight in your teens and twenties . . . and why it's so hard now? There could be several reasons why it seems harder as an adult—a less active lifestyle, different eating habits, or changes in your body. Metabolism slows during each decade of your adult years.

Many past attempts at dieting may complicate the picture. Low-calorie diets help you shed fat and some muscle tissue. But when you regain weight, you tend to regain it as fat. Because fat tissue requires fewer calories to maintain than muscle does, you need to cut calories even more. The remedy? Move more. Physical activity burns fat and can build muscle, making weight loss easier. Increased physical activity can boost the rate at which your body uses energy for your basic energy needs.

. . . if your stomach shrinks when you eat less? No, your body doesn't work that way. Although your stomach can expand to accommodate a large intake of food, it doesn't stretch out indefinitely. As food passes to your intestines, the stomach goes back to its normal size. When you cut back on calories, your stomach keeps its normal size, even if your appetite isn't as big.

. . . if every person's body has a unique set point, or a preset weight, that it tries to return to? That's a theory with no conclusive evidence. Even if a set point exists, it's probably a range that can be set a little lower with more physical activity and food choices with fewer calories and fat. Or for someone who's too thin, eating a few extra calories may help adjust the set point a bit higher.

● Celebrate any success. Weight loss doesn't need to be an all-or-nothing venture. If you've been carrying around excess pounds, even small changes can make a difference in your health and reduce your risk for disease.

● Enjoy how good your healthy weight feels. Reward yourself with a new garment, a bouquet of flowers, a new CD, or a special outing. Still, there's no greater motivation than knowing you're in control and caring for yourself!

Too Thin—a Problem?

Maybe. Being too thin can be a health risk, especially if being underweight results from undereating. An eating pattern with too few calories may not supply enough of the nutrients a person needs to keep his or her body running normally. Children who undereat may not get enough nutrients or energy for growth and development either. A lack of food energy may cause fatigue, irritability, and lack of concentration. And those with a poor diet may have trouble warding off infections.

For normal-weight people, a layer of body fat just under the skin helps protect the body from cold. But very thin people have only a very thin fat layer, so they lack insulation to keep them warm. That becomes an increasing problem for the thin, frail elderly, especially if they don't have adequate heating in their homes.

If you lose weight suddenly and don't know the cause, talk to your doctor. This may be an early symptom of other health problems.

When You Want to Gain

There's plenty written about weight loss; that's because it's a common problem. However, under some circumstances, people may need to gain weight. For some people weight gain is as hard as weight loss is for others!

The obvious approach for weight gain is this—consume more energy than your body burns. For every pound of body weight you gain, you need to consume 3,500 calories more than your body burns. As with weight loss, do so in a healthful way. *Note:* The suggestions indicated here are not meant for people with eating disorders, whose weight problems are complex and often life-threatening.

● Follow the guidelines of the Food Guide Pyramid—and eat more servings from the five major food groups. Go for the higher end of the serving ranges. Trying to gain weight by overdoing foods from the Pyramid tip and other high-fat foods isn't a healthful answer, even for someone who's thin!

● Stick to the guideline: no more than 30 percent calories from fat *(see chapter 3),* unless your doctor advises more. Controlling fat in your eating is good for your heart and your whole body, not just your weight.

● Choose some foods with concentrated calories. That way you won't need to increase the volume of food too much. Try dried fruits or fruits canned in heavy syrup, instead of fresh fruits. Fortify soups, casseroles, and fluid milk with dry milk powder. Enjoy some higher-calorie condiments, such as a dollop of sour cream on a baked potato. Garnish salads with olives, avocados, nuts, and cheese, which have more calories.

● Eat more frequently—five to six small meals a day—if your appetite is small. For example, eat breakfast at 7:00 A.M. and again at 10:00 A.M. Eating two or three large meals during the day may be too much to handle at one time.

● Drink fluids thirty minutes before and after meals—not with meals. By limiting beverages at mealtime, you'll have more room for food.

● Focus on nutrient-rich foods and beverages. Don't fill up on low- and no-calorie foods or drinks, such as diet sodas or hard candies. Rather than coffee, tea, and water, drink juice, milk, and milkshakes.

● Enjoy a snack before bedtime.

● Stimulate your appetite if you just don't feel like eating. *See the following section, "No Appetite?," for ideas.*

● Use the Nutrition Facts on the food label to choose nutrient-rich foods, which also supply the calories you need. *See chapter 11 for more on label reading.*

● Try adding a commercial liquid meal replacement, or make your own shake or smoothie if you can't get enough calories from your regular meals and snacks. Check with your healthcare provider or registered dietitian for guidance.

● Ask a registered dietitian for more guidance on choosing healthful foods for weight gain. *See chapter 24, "Well-Informed?," for tips on finding a qualified nutrition expert in your area.*

● Stay physically active—good for muscle building and feeling energetic. It also may help stimulate appetite!

Source: Adapted from Gail Farmer, *Pass the Calories, Please!* (Chicago: The American Dietetic Association, 1994). Used with permission.

No Appetite?

People lose their appetite for all kinds of reasons: illness, pain, fatigue, depression, stress, medication, disease, or a combination of these.

If that happens, the appetite control center of your brain might be affected, signaling that you're not hungry even when you should be. You may lose your appetite and tolerance for food when you're sick—even though you need nourishment to get well. Or emotional stress may affect your desire for and ability to handle food.

Cope with a loss of appetite. Eat by the clock rather than by hunger. It may be easier to consume all the calories you need. Take advantage of the "up" times. When you feel well and your appetite is good, eat and enjoy! And try these ideas for stimulating your appetite:

● Add some pizzazz to your foods! Colorful foods, appealing texture, and an appetizing aroma are helpful aids to increasing food intake.

● Become involved in food selection and preparation.

● Drink a glass of beer or wine before meals. This often gives your appetite a jump start. But check with your doctor first.

● Eat meals with friends. The pleasure of being with others may be an appetite booster.

● Fill the house with enticing food aromas such as freshly baked bread, cake, or cookies.

● Keep favorite foods on hand for meals and snacks. You may eat more when food is readily available.

● Make mealtimes pleasant. A relaxed and attractive setting with soft music or flowers on the table may perk up your appetite.

● Try eating your meal away from the dining room table, such as picnic style in the living room or at a candlelit table in front of the fireplace. Sometimes a change of place helps.

● Plan for longer mealtimes. Don't schedule activities close to meals.

● Walk before meals. A short walk often helps stimulate an appetite.

● Stay away from unpleasant or unsettling topics of conversation at mealtimes, especially if stress is a problem for you.

Source: Adapted from Gail Farmer, *Pass the Calories, Please!* (Chicago: The American Dietetic Association, 1994). Used with permission.

Disordered Eating: Problems, Signs, and Help

Several million Americans suffer from disordered eating. Between 5 and 20 percent will die from medical complications as a result. Eating disorders—anorexia nervosa, bulimia, and binge eating disorder—are actually distorted eating habits often related to emotional problems. Anorexia typically results in low body weight; it's linked to menstrual irregularity, osteoporosis in women, and greater risk of early death in women and men. Bulimia may or may not be linked to low body weight. And binge eating disorder, probably the most common eating disorder, typically results in overweight and often in repeated weight gain and loss. All require qualified medical care, including psychological or psychiatric, and nutrition counseling.

Anorexia and Bulimia: What Are They?

Anorexia nervosa is sometimes called the "starvation sickness." Obsessed with food, weight, and thinness, people suffering from anorexia deny their hunger and refuse to eat—even after extreme weight loss. As they consume too few calories for their basic needs, their bodies slowly waste away. By starving themselves, people with anorexia don't get the nutrients they need for normal bodily functions.

Bulimia nervosa is marked by binge eating and purging (self-induced vomiting). The person gorges, usually on high-calorie foods, and then intentionally vomits or uses laxatives or diuretics. A diuretic increases urine production. The consequences are serious: dehydration, organ damage, internal bleeding from the stress of vomiting, tooth decay from acids in vomit, and in some cases, death. Many people with these eating disorders alternate between anorexia and bulimia. Reports indicate that 60 percent of people who have dieted extensively or starved themselves resort to bingeing, and then purging to keep their weight off.

When does an eating disorder start? Generally it begins with an ordinary weight-loss diet, begun either just before or after a major life change or trauma. However, there's no clear understanding of the exact causes.

We do know, however, that eating disorders are more than food problems. The person's whole life—schoolwork or career, family life, day-to-day patterns, emotions, growth, overall health—gets wrapped up in the eating issues.

Who's at Risk for Anorexia and Bulimia?

People of almost any age and either gender may develop an eating disorder. However, some groups of people are more at risk than others.

- Females clearly are the most susceptible. In fact, approximately 95 percent of all people with anorexia are women.
- Adolescents are at particular risk. Estimates indicate that as many as 1 of every 250 teenage girls will develop at least some symptoms of anorexia.
- Athletes such as dancers and gymnasts, who must control their weight, are susceptible.
- Eating disorders are being increasingly identified in males, as well as in adults and even in children as young as eight, nine, and ten years old.

Anorexia and Bulimia: The Warning Signs

Eating disorders produce warning signs. If you or someone you know shows any combination of these symptoms, be concerned!

People with anorexia may:

- Eat tiny portions, refuse to eat, and deny they are hungry.
- Show abnormal weight loss—as much as 15 percent or more of body weight—or a large weight loss in a short time.
- Act hyperactive, depressed, moody, or insecure.
- Have an intense fear of being fat.
- See themselves as fat, wanting to lose more weight, even when they are very thin.
- Exercise excessively and compulsively.
- Suffer from constipation or irregular menstrual periods.
- Develop fine, downy hair on their arms and face.
- Complain of nausea or bloating after eating normal amounts of food.
- Binge-eat, then purge, perhaps by vomiting or using laxatives or diuretics.

People with bulimia may:

- Eat mainly in private.
- Disappear after eating—often to the bathroom.
- Show great fluctuations in weight, and may be of normal weight or be overweight.
- Feel out of control when eating.
- Eat enormous meals but not gain weight.
- Feel ashamed and depressed after gorging.

Three Things to Know about Disordered Eating

Experts aren't certain about the exact causes of disordered eating. But they do agree on these key points:

1. **Food itself is not the primary problem.** Instead, eating patterns are symptoms of serious distress.

2. **Early detection is crucial.** The sooner the person gets help, the better the chance for permanent recovery.

3. **Help is available.** Team treatment, including medical and dental care, psychotherapy, nutrition education, and family counseling, provides the best results.

● Have swollen parotid glands. The parotid glands, located near the ears, are one type of salivary glands.

● Experience irregular menstrual periods.

● Binge-eat, then purge.

● Abuse alcohol or drugs.

● Become dependent on laxatives, diuretics, emetics, or diet pills to lose weight. Emetics such as syrup of ipecac induce vomiting.

● Develop dental problems caused by acid from vomiting. Acids eat away at tooth enamel.

Binge Eating Disorder: A More Common Problem

Binge eating disorder (BED), different from occasional overindulging, is the uncontrollable eating of large amounts of food in a short time. Unlike bulimia, a person with BED usually doesn't purge, fast, abuse diuretics or laxatives, or overexercise. Estimates suggest that 2 percent (as many as 4 million) of Americans have this disorder—and many of them are obese or overweight.

The concerns are physical, psychological, and social. Large amounts of food eaten by binge eaters are typically high in fats and sugars, and may lack sufficient vitamins and minerals. With the likelihood of overweight and obesity comes an increased risk for serious health problems, including diabetes, heart disease, high blood pressure, gallbladder disease, and some cancers. Binge eating often results in depression, embarrassment, and social isolation; those with the disorder are often upset by both the problem and their inability to control their eating.

Although the cause of BED isn't clear, there's a link to depression and other negative emotions. Among the areas of research: the effect of brain chemicals and metabolism, and whether depression is a cause or a result of binge eating disorder.

Who's at Risk for Binge Eating Disorder?

Although many people with BED are overweight or obese (often severely obese), even normal-weight people have this disorder. More women than men deal with BED, but it's the most common eating disorder among men.

BED: The Warning Signs

Being overstuffed after an exceptional meal isn't necessarily a warning sign. Instead, people with binge eating disorder typically have several characteristics; they:

● Feel out of control when eating.

● Eat unusually large amounts of food.

● Eat very fast.

● Eat until they feel uncomfortable.

● Eat a lot, even when they aren't hungry.

● Feel embarrassed about the amount of food they eat, so eat alone.

● Feel disgusted, depressed, or guilty about overeating.

What to Do

If you suspect a friend or a family member has anorexia, bulimia, or binge eating disorder, don't wait until a severe weight problem or a serious medical problem proves you are right. There's plenty you can do before that happens:

● *Act to get help.* Speak to the person about your concern. Enlist assistance from family and friends. Talk to medical professionals, a social worker, or the school nurse or counselor if the person is a student. Call your local mental health association. A registered dietitian also can give you an expert perspective on eating disorders. *See chapter 24, "Well Informed?," to locate a registered dietitian in your area.*

As an aside: People with disordered eating may encourage disordered eating among others; today that problem has spread through the use of Web sites with private chat rooms.

For people with BED, a weight-loss diet alone may not be successful. Losing weight and keeping it off may be harder (for physical and emotional reasons) than for people without an eating disorder. Normal-weight people with binge eating disorder shouldn't be on a weight-loss diet.

The best treatment for disordered eating combines medical, psychological, and nutrition counseling. Participation in self-help groups for the patient, as well as group counseling for family members, are important parts of treatment.

● *Expect resistance.* A person with anorexia usually doesn't believe that he or she needs assistance or is in any danger. Someone with bulimia or BED may acknowledge the problem but still refuse to seek help. But the faster he or she gets help, the greater the chances for recovery.

● *Prepare for long-term treatment.* Recovery may take several months to several years. Symptoms and attitudes related to eating disorders rarely disappear quickly. Treatment includes helping people achieve an appropriate weight. Family support groups are particularly effective in helping relatives of people with disordered eating survive the long ordeal.

● *For more guidance, see "More Weighty Problems for Children—Fear of Weight Gain" and "Mainly for Girls . . . Pressure to Be Thin" in chapter 16.*

"Diets" That Don't Work!

Every year Americans spend billions of dollars on the weight-loss industry—often for diet plans, diet books, services, and gimmicks that don't work! The lure of quick, easy weight loss is hard to resist, especially for those unwilling to make a commitment to lifelong behavioral change. Although the diets are ineffective in the long run, weight-loss hopefuls willingly give the next craze a chance. The result? Perhaps temporary results. But overall, wasted money, weight regained, a feeling of failure, and perhaps damage to health.

The next craze is often a past craze that's simply

QUICK CHECK: DOES THIS DIET WORK?

Probably not—and certainly not in the long run—if a popular diet promotes . . .

- Miracle foods or diet magic
- Little or no physical activity
- Odd food quantities
- Quick weight loss
- Rigid menus
- Specific food combinations

Source: Adapted from Wheat Foods Council, *The Truth about Fad Diets.* 1999. Educational information provided by the Wheat Foods Council, 1999.

---

resurfaced with a new name, a new twist, yet still no sound science to back up the claims. Fad diets typically rely on nonscientific, unproved claims, personal stories, testimonials, or poorly controlled studies. Not surprisingly, many people feel confusion and diet fatigue as they sort through the contradictory popular approaches to weight loss. Sound familiar? For those who try one fad diet after another, weight cycling becomes a common and frustrating problem. *See "Weight Cycling—The 'Yo-Yo' Problem" earlier in this chapter.*

"Magical, One-Food" Diets

The "grapefruit diet," the "all-you-can-eat fruit diet," the "rice diet," "the cabbage soup diet," "the no dairy foods diet"! There's a weight-loss diet for almost every taste.

The facts are . . . Often touted to help melt fat away, no single-food or single-food-group diet has any special ability to do that. These diets don't work for several reasons. They lack variety. They don't provide adequate amounts of all the nutrients and protective phytonutrients the body needs for health, especially when some foods are off-limits. With unlimited quantities of "magical foods," the dieter runs the risk of overeating the foods featured on the so-called diet plan. Any weight loss—and lower calorie intake—comes from eliminating entire groups of other foods, not to any "magic" from any single food or food group.

The bottom line is that no super food can reverse weight gain resulting from inactivity and overeating. Eliminating a food or food category doesn't work either. Also, because these diets don't teach new eating habits, people usually don't stick with them!

High-Protein, Low-"Carb" Diets

Recent headlines and best-selling books promote protein as a new solution to weight loss and fitness. Carbohydrates—complex carbohydrates and/or sugars—are often falsely accused as the culprits. In fact, these diet plans aren't new. They've been around with different names for years.

The facts are . . . Simply because these diets are lower in calories, they may promote loss—if you stick with them. However, a high-protein diet doesn't build muscle and burn fat, as some people think. Only regular physical activity and training build muscle strength and burn calories stored in body fat. Most Americans consume more than enough protein.

Because these weight loss plans are common today, research is under way looking at low to moderate carbohydrate diets for weight loss. They may be appropriate for some people, perhaps those with insulin resistance. Stay tuned. *See "Insulin Resistance Syndrome, or 'Syndrome X'" in chapter 22.*

For most people, there are concerns related to a high-protein, low-carbohydrate eating approach to weight loss:

● These diets do promote rapid weight lost—at first. Their diuretic effect promotes loss of water weight, not body fat, however. The psychological lift offers a false sense of success that's quickly gone when water weight returns.

● Depending on the protein-rich foods consumed, a high-protein, low-"carb" diet may be high in total fat, saturated fat, and cholesterol. Inconsistent with sound nutrition advice, this weight loss regimen over time can increase the risk for heart disease and perhaps some forms of cancer.

● Excessive protein may leach some calcium from bones, according to emerging research, adding to the risk for osteoporosis.

● A diet that restricts complex carbohydrates is often low in fiber. The possible result? Constipation and other gastrointestinal disorders. A low-fiber diet isn't consistent with overall guidelines for health.

● Very-high-protein diets also can strain the liver and the kidneys as the body breaks down protein.

● A condition called ketosis (increased blood ketones from incomplete fat breakdown) can result with these regimens. Ketosis suppresses hunger and thus contributes to lower calorie intake. Some popular diets claim that ketosis hastens weight loss. In truth, muscle also breaks down due to a lack of carbohydrate for energy. In addition, ketosis can cause weakness, nausea, dehydration, light-headedness, and irritability. It can be fatal to people with diabetes, and during pregnancy may cause birth defects or fetal death.

High-Fiber, Low-Calorie Diets

The flip side of the high-protein craze may be the high-fiber approach to dieting. It's true that most of us need more fiber to promote good health. Twenty to 35 grams of fiber daily are recommended. Too much—perhaps resulting from fiber supplements—may be too much of a good thing!

The facts are . . . As a component of food, fiber isn't absorbed by the body; therefore it doesn't contribute calories. That's why high-fiber foods such as whole grains, vegetables, legumes, and fruits—usually lower in calories—are included in weight-loss diets. Their high-fiber content makes these diets quite filling, so you might eat less overall.

Very-high-fiber diets also may come up short on protein foods. An excessively high-fiber diet can cause constipation and dehydration if extra fluids aren't consumed.

Bulk fillers, which are high in fiber, aren't advised. They reduce hunger by first absorbing liquid, then swelling up in the stomach. These products can be harmful when they obstruct the digestive tract. *See "Supplement Watch: About Fiber Pills and Powders . . ." in chapter 6.*

Moderation of dietary fiber, as part of an overall healthful diet, is a smarter approach to weight loss. Adding fiber to a healthful weight-loss plan—one that doesn't go below 1,600 calories per day—is a smart idea!

Very-Low-Calorie Liquid Diets

Very-low-calorie liquid formulas have been developed for short-term use under the supervision of a physician. To help some obese people, they serve a purpose for short-term weight loss—if there's also a commitment to new eating and active living habits. Used as a liquid diet without other foods, they're very low in calories, providing just 400 to 800 calories a day.

Several years ago these formulas were changed after deaths were attributed to their use. Newer formulas have more vitamins, minerals, and high-quality protein.

The facts are . . . Without medical supervision and nutrition education, liquid diets don't teach new ways of eating. Since people usually don't stay with them, there's usually no long-term weight loss. They also may result in fatigue, constipation, nausea, diarrhea, or hair loss. For people with some health problems such as insulin-dependent diabetes or kidney disease, a very-low-calorie liquid diet can be harmful.

A very-low-calorie diet is different from over-the-counter meal replacements (typically in liquid form) that may substitute for a meal. Although these products may be low in calories, they don't provide the full range of vitamins, minerals, fiber, phytonutrients, and other functional benefits supplied by the great-tasting variety of food.

Fasting

Fasting has been touted as a tactic for jump-starting weight loss. Does it work?

The facts are . . . As with very-low-calorie diets, fasting deprives the body of energy and nutrients needed for normal functions. Any rapid weight loss is mostly water and muscle loss. Fasting also may cause fatigue and dizziness, with less energy for physical activity. And it feeds the cycle of "yo-yo" dieting.

As an aside, there's a misconception that fasting "cleans out" the system, removing toxic wastes. To the contrary, body chemicals called ketones build up in the body when carbohydrates aren't available for energy. Ketosis puts a burden on the kidneys; as noted earlier in this chapter, ketones that accumulate can be harmful to health.

Gimmicks, Gadgets, and Other "Miracles"

Promoters advertise the "great wonders of the weight-loss world"—weight-loss patches, electric muscle stimulators, spirulina (a species of blue-green algae), starch and fat blockers, creams that melt fat away, ephedra, and many, many others. Some sound almost amusing. *Chapter 23 addresses some supplements promoted for weight loss.*

The facts are . . . All these products have been offered for sale and purport to promote weight loss. Yet none proves effective. Some even may be harmful. And they're all a waste of money!

For instance, the popular press often advertises massages and other therapies for getting rid of "cellulite." But there's nothing unique about dimpled fat on thighs and hips. Cellulite is simply normal body fat under the skin that looks lumpy when the fat layer gets thick, allowing connective, fibrous-looking tissue that holds fat in place to show. The lumpy look can lessen or disappear with normal weight loss.

You've also probably seen weight-loss programs based on sweating off extra weight. Sweating in a sauna—or wearing a rubber belt or nylon clothes that make you perspire during exercise—may cause weight loss. However, the pounds that disappear come from water loss, not body fat. As soon as you drink or eat, weight returns.

Instead of helping to achieve a healthful weight goal, "sweating off" pounds may damage health through dehydration. *See chapter 8, "Fluids: Often Overlooked," for more about dehydration and the body's need for water.*

Eat What You Crave!

If the sight of certain foods puts your mind into a tailspin, you may need to readjust your approach to eating. An overly restrictive diet may "feed" a food craving—and set you up to overindulge!

The jury is still out on the true cause of food cravings. It may be physiological, psychological, or both. We don't yet know if food cravings are linked to a need to resupply the body with nutrients it lacks, or if cravings are reinforced by positive emotional and social links to certain foods.

Studies suggest that avoiding certain foods altogether often makes them irresistible. The result? Giving in to a food craving, and perhaps overeating. Then guilt creeps in, and people try to resist those foods once again, only to overindulge and feel guilty again.

What's a better approach? Eat a small portion of any food you enjoy—even if it's higher in fat or calories. Even when you're trying to shed pounds, you can enjoy high-calorie foods as long as your eating plan is varied, balanced, and moderate. As another option, try to satisfy your palate with a low-fat, low-calorie version.

Need more strategies for sensible and effective weight management? Check here for "how tos":

● Help your child or teen keep a healthy weight—see chapter 16.

● Encourage your kids to move more and sit less—see chapter 16.

● Stay physically active in your later years— see chapter 18.

● Gain, maintain, or lose weight as an older adult—see chapter 18.

When You Need Help . . .

If you have weight problems of any kind or more questions about controlling your own weight, it's okay to seek outside advice and help. But be wary. Not every weight-loss "professional" is qualified to give the help you need. Steer clear of weight-loss programs and products that offer claims for quick fixes. They often promise far more than they can deliver.

First and foremost, choose a program that suits your personality and lifestyle. In addition, find a program with a maintenance plan that includes physical activity, and counseling that focuses on realistic behavioral changes. In the end, you supply your own motivation, but the plan must promote your good health. Above all, choose a plan you can live with. *See the checklist in the following section, "Questions to Ask . . . About Diet Programs," to judge a weight management plan.*

If you need help finding a weight-control program, talk with a registered dietitian, who is trained to help you figure out what kind of weight-management system will fit your lifestyle. *For more help in finding a qualified nutrition professional and for reliable information about nutrition and health, see chapter 24, "Well Informed?"*

Questions to Ask . . . about Diet Programs

Millions of Americans participate in organized weight-loss programs each year. Today the Internet even provides this service. Many of these programs are run by qualified medical and nutrition experts who can effectively help their clients lose weight and keep it off permanently. However, others make overblown claims and tout products that are ineffective and costly, and their staff may not have appropriate credentials. Before you sign on the dotted line, ask questions such as these:

● What is the approach, and what are the goals of the program?

● What are the health risks?

● How will you assess my health status before recommending the program? Many programs recommend a medical checkup before starting.

● Will the program include instruction, guidance, and skill building to help me learn to eat in a more healthful way for the long term? How?

● Will the program include guidance on physical activity for a lifetime? How?

● What data can you show me that prove your program works? What has been written about the program's success besides individual testimonials?

● Do customers keep off the weight after they leave the diet program? Ask for results over two to five years. The Federal Trade Commission requires weight-loss companies to back up their claims.

● What are the costs for membership, weekly fees, food, supplements, maintenance, and counseling? What's the payment schedule? Are any costs covered under health insurance? Do you give refunds if I drop out?

Spotting a Fraud

Does it sound too good to be true? Then it probably is! Be wary. Over the years, promoters of fraudulent weight-loss schemes have laced their claims with words and phrases such as these:

Ancient	Exotic
Balances hormones	Fast
Banish fat	Guaranteed
Breakthrough	Magical
Cure	Miraculous
Discovered in Europe	Mysterious
Easy	New discovery
Effortless	Quick
Enzymatic process	Secret

● Will you monitor my success at three- to six-month intervals, then modify the program if needed?

● Do you have a maintenance program? Is it part of the package, or does it cost extra?

● What kind of professional support is provided? What are the credentials and experiences of these professionals? (Detailed information should be available on request.)

● What are the program's requirements? Are there special menus or foods, counseling visits, or exercise plans?

For more guidance on evaluating a weight-control plan, see "Check It Out!" earlier in this chapter.

Have You Ever Wondered

. . . if food combining can help you lose weight? Forget this claim! It's just one more case of wishful thinking. No scientific evidence suggests that combining certain foods or eating them in careful sequence aids weight loss. And no food combinations cause food to either turn to body fat or produce toxins.

. . . if over-the-counter diet pills help with weight loss? Over-the-counter diet pills, or appetite suppressants, work by curbing the appetite, but usually just for a few weeks. Some have unpleasant side effects and some can be addictive, with potential damage to the heart and the nervous system. They may be prescribed to help a person start a lifelong program for weight management, but they're not a substitute for adopting healthful eating habits over the long term. They should never be taken for very long—and only under a doctor's supervision.

. . . if obesity can be controlled with medication? For some people, medication may be prescribed—under a doctor's care—as part of an obesity treatment program. Such medication isn't effective for everyone, and can have potential side effects. The U.S. Food and Drug Administration has approved two kinds. Sibutramine is an appetite suppressant that seems to work with natural hormones (norepinephrine and serotonin) in the brain; however, it may increase blood pressure and induce an abnormally rapid heartbeat. Orlistat reduces the absorption of dietary fat; however, it may reduce the absorption of some fat-soluble vitamins, too. Research continues on these and other medications.

. . . if surgery and liposuction are options for weight loss? Not for most people. Gastric bypass surgery, done by shortening the small intestine or by making the stomach smaller, does promote weight loss. However, because the side effects can be harmful, doctors rarely advise surgery—and then only as a final resort in life-threatening situations when other approaches haven't worked. Liposuction, the surgical removal of fat tissue from various body areas, is often only a short-term solution. If eating and exercise habits remain the same, it's likely that the weight will be regained.

. . . what to do when your weight seems to hit a plateau? Be patient. Plateaus are a normal part of weight loss. Your body requires fewer calories to function as you lose weight. Allow time to readjust. Gradually adding more activity may help nudge you off the weight-loss plateau.

. . . if you should join a support group to lose weight? Perhaps, but that's an individual matter. Weight-loss organizations and support groups often educate participants as they offer psychological support. And many, but not all, are coordinated by qualified nutrition experts. The section, *"Questions to Ask . . . about Diet Programs,"* can help you judge. For some people, peer support offers motivation, especially if they pay to attend the program. There's a downside, however. Without a weight maintenance program, many people gain weight again when they're no longer in the group.

. . . if "cyberdieting" works? Logging on to the Internet may offer support for weight loss. Some people like the anonymity; others like personalized help with feedback at home. Some research suggests that well-designed, interactive programs are effective—at least in the short term. The challenge is finding a site that offers sound guidance and privacy of personal data, rather than one that's mostly in business to sell products. There's another potential problem. Face-to-face weight loss counseling with a registered dietitian addresses other issues—related health problems, personal lifestyles, and food preferences, among others—that may affect your weight loss success; cyberdieting may not. *See "Nutrition in Cyberspace" in chapter 24.*

CHAPTER 3

Fat Facts

Fat is a hot topic! For more than a decade, health issues related to fat and cholesterol have captured consumer attention. Health experts advise lowering the total fat, especially saturated fat, and cholesterol in our food choices. Media stories continually report new research linking various types of fat, cholesterol, and health. Cookbooks and magazine articles tout low-fat recipes. The food industry has launched many fat-modified products: "reduced-fat," "fat-free," and now "with omega-3s," and "trans fat-free." Not surprisingly, many people are making a "change of plate" by buying and preparing foods in a lean and flavorful way.

While other nutrition-related concerns have emerged, attention to fat likely will be around for some time. Evidence is clear that a high-fat diet is linked to many chronic health problems, among them cardiovascular disease, some types of cancer, diabetes, and obesity. As science reveals more, it's also becoming quite clear that the links between the different types of fat and health are more complex than we once thought.

Aging baby boomers are being forced to face the "fat facts of life." And people of all ages recognize that cutting back to a moderate fat intake—and going easy on "sat fats"—will promote their good health in the long run. In fact, the government's Dietary Guidelines for Americans advises: *Choose a diet that is low in saturated fat and cholesterol and moderate in total fat.*

Americans already have cut down on their total fat intake. On average, people consume about 33 percent of their calories from total fat. While this figure reflects a downward trend, there's still room to improve.

Fats Matter

Suppose your doctor said, "You need to get your serum cholesterol level down. Your triglycerides are borderline high. And cut the fat, especially the saturated fat, in your diet." Just what would this mean to you? And what would you do? To understand the role of fats in food, health, and chronic disease, we need to start with the basics.

Fat: A Nutrient for Health

With all the attention on fat today, you may be surprised to learn that fats have some positive benefits. Fat is a nutrient necessary for your health. In moderate amounts, fats perform a full workload of bodily functions. You actually can't live without them! That's why a fat-free diet isn't a healthful goal. There's more to healthful eating than simply cutting back on fats. In fact, the type of fat you eat may be just as important as the total amount of fat in your diet. Evidence suggests that the various types of fats in foods have different effects on health; some fats may even offer health-protective benefits. So just how does fat help keep you healthy?

Fats: Essential Work

For one, fats work as partners in your body, supporting the work of other nutrients. Just as sugar dissolves in water, so some vitamins dissolve in fat. That's how vitamins A, D, E, and K, as well as carotenoids, are carried in food and into your bloodstream. Without fats these fat-soluble vitamins cannot fully nourish your body.

Certain fats are considered essential, specifically two fatty acids—linoleic acid and alpha-linolenic acid—which your body can't make. (Fatty acids are the building blocks of fat.) For children to grow normally and for adults and children to maintain healthy skin, food choices must supply linoleic acid. For children, alpha-linolenic acid is important, too. Alpha-linolenic acid converts to omega-3 fatty acids, which keep your brain and nervous system functioning normally. You may know some omega-3s by their nicknames: EPA (eicosapentaenoic acid) and DHA (docosahexaenoic acid). Linoleic acid is an omega-6 fatty acid. *See "Eat Your Omega-3s and -6s" on page 56.*

Have You Ever Wondered

... if "low-fat" is "low-calorie," too? Not necessarily. It's true that fat itself is a concentrated source of energy, or calories. However, cutting back on foods high in fat may not trim calories if too many carbohydrate-rich foods take their place. Note that the calorie content of the "regular" and "low-fat" version of a food may be similar because carbohydrate-containing ingredients often are added to help replace flavor that's lost when fat is removed. To find out, read the Nutrition Facts on the food label for packaged foods. Even if the calories are less, go easy on your portion size of low-fat or fat-free foods. Eating a whole box of fat-free cookies isn't a "low-calorie" experience!

... if a reduced-fat food is always "low-fat"? Not necessarily. It just may have less fat (at least 25 percent less) than its full-fat counterpart. Check the Nutrition Facts on food labels to find out. *See "Label Lingo" later in this chapter to know what the terms mean.*

FISH: HOW MUCH OMEGA-3?

RAW FISH, ABOUT 3½ OUNCES (100 GRAMS)	OMEGA-3S (GRAMS)	TOTAL FAT (GRAMS)
Fatty fish		
Sardines in sardine oil	3.3	15.5
Atlantic mackerel	2.5	13.9
Atlantic herring	1.6	9.0
Chinook salmon	1.4	10.4
Anchovy	1.4	4.8
Atlantic salmon	1.2	5.4
Less fatty fish		
Tuna	0.5	2.5
Brook trout	0.4	2.7
Catfish	0.3	4.3
Shrimp	0.3	1.1
Flounder	0.2	1.0

Source: Adapted from S.L. Conner and W.E. Conner, "Are Fish Oils Beneficial in the Prevention and Treatment of Coronary Artery Disease?," *American Journal of Clinical Nutrition* 66 (1997): 1020S–1031S.

Both linoleic acid and alpha-linolenic acid are widely available in food: for example, linoleic acid from vegetable oils and poultry fat, and alpha-linolenic acid from soy oil, nuts, and seeds. If your food choices are varied, getting enough of these fatty acids is easy. EPA and DHA are naturally part of some foods, especially fatty fish and fish oils. *See "Fish: How Much Omega-3?"*

A "Power Source"

Like carbohydrates and proteins, fats supply energy, or calories, to power your physical activity and the many body processes that keep you alive. (Remember, a calorie is defined as a unit of energy.) Fats are a concentrated energy source, supplying 9 calories for each fat gram. To compare, carbohydrates and proteins provide less than half that amount—just 4 calories per gram. Although your body uses fat for energy, it's not the body's preferred fuel source. And often fat isn't used for energy.

If you consume more energy from fat than your body needs, your body saves the extra in your body's fatty tissues, mostly in fat cells. Body fat also is known as adipose tissue. When you need an extra energy supply, your body can draw on this stored fat. Other body cells and blood plasma have some fat, too.

Fat for Satiety

A little fat in food adds more than flavor to your meal. It also helps satisfy your hunger by making you feel full after eating. Why? Because fats take longer to leave your stomach than either carbohydrates or proteins do. If you eat a very-low-fat meal, you may feel hungry again within an hour or two.

Body Fat: Its Role

A certain amount of body fat serves several functions: to cushion and position your body organs, to protect your bones from injury, and to form a fat layer under your skin. This fat layer offers insulation, helping you stay warm on a cold winter day. And the soft fat pads on your buttocks and the palms of your hands protect your bones from bumps, bangs, and jolts. Fat that's stored around your organs isn't accessed for energy.

Why Foods Contain Fat

Fat offers sensory qualities that make food taste good. As an ingredient in food, fat carries flavor. It also gives a smooth, creamy texture to foods such as ice cream and peanut butter. When foods such as cake or a brownie seem to melt in your mouth, that's just what's happening—the fat is melting! And from meat to baked foods, fat makes many foods moist and tender, or brown and crispy.

But can you cut the fat in a recipe? To a certain extent, yes. The recipe still may work if you use less. But eliminating fat altogether may not give the result you expect. As a recipe ingredient, fat gives food many desirable qualities:

In baked foods. Fat tenderizes; adds moisture; holds in air so baked foods are light; and affects the shape, for example, in cookies. With too little fat, baked goods might be tough or dry, or they may not rise properly.

In sauces. Fat keeps sauces from curdling and forms part of an emulsion. An emulsion is a mixture of two substances, such as fat and water, that stay together instead of separating, as they normally would.

In other cooked foods. Fat helps conduct heat as food cooks—for example, when food is sautéed (cooked quickly in a small amount of fat) or fried.

In cooked meat, poultry, and fish. Fat seals in moisture as foods are basted, or brushed with liquid during cooking. Sometimes the surface gets dry if it isn't basted.

For foods cooked in a pan. Fat lubricates the pan so food won't stick.

In all kinds of food. Fat helps carry flavor and nutrients, provides texture (mouth feel), and adds satiety value.

Your "Fat Tooth"

Have a craving for rich chocolates or desserts? Your "fat tooth," not your "sweet tooth," may account for that urge to indulge. In this world of high-fat foods, a preference for high-fat foods may be culturally conditioned. Research suggests that it's learned early, when infants and young children learn through experience that fat is associated with satiety (reduction of feelings of hunger).

A smooth, creamy milk shake; a flaky, tender pastry; and a juicy steak: the appeal of high-fat foods may come from qualities that fat imparts. Or perhaps the appeal stems from on-again, off-again dieting. Some studies say that dieting may amplify a fat craving, or more likely, the craving for sweetened fat like that found in many rich desserts.

No matter what the reason for a "fat tooth," you can overcome, or at least manage, your preference for fatty foods:

- Fool your tastebuds. Get a smooth, creamy consistency with low-fat and fat-free ingredients: low-fat yogurt as a base for savory dips; thick, puréed fruit as a dessert sauce; and creamy buttermilk as a base for milk shakes.

- Indulge a "fat tooth." Share a rich dessert with someone else to cut your fat grams and calories in half.

- Recondition your eating style by gradually shifting to a lower-fat diet.

Sorting the Fats

"Lipids," "fats," "cholesterol," "fatty acids," "triglycerides," "lipoproteins," "hydrogenated," "omega-3s," "trans fatty acids"—the dictionary of fat terms seems endless and often confusing. Some describe fats in the body; others apply to fats in food; and some, to fats in both. Just what do all these terms really mean?

Actually, there's no one kind of fat. The term "lipids" refers to all kinds of fatty substances, including fats and cholesterol. A common quality among lipids is that they don't dissolve in water.

"Fat" Dictionary

Lipid. Scientific term that refers to all fats, cholesterol, and other fatlike substances; lipids do not dissolve in water.

Lipoproteins. Protein-coated packages that carry lipids, including cholesterol, in the bloodstream. Without the protein coating, lipids cannot travel through the bloodstream.

Cholesterol. Waxy, fatlike substance found in foods of animal origin and in every body cell. It's essential for cell building.

> *Blood (serum) cholesterol.* Cholesterol that travels in the bloodstream. The body manufactures most of its blood cholesterol; some is also absorbed from foods you eat.

> *Dietary cholesterol.* Cholesterol in food, found only in foods of animal origin, and never in foods from plant sources, even if they contain fat.

> *HDL blood cholesterol ("good" cholesterol).* Cholesterol carried by high-density lipoproteins (HDLs). HDLs carry cholesterol and other blood lipids away from body cells to the liver so they can be broken down and excreted. HDLs—with a higher ratio of protein to cholesterol—are made in the liver in response to physical activity and some foods. Food doesn't have them.

> *LDL blood cholesterol ("bad" cholesterol).* Cholesterol carried by low-density lipoproteins (LDLs). LDLs circulate to body cells, carrying cholesterol and other lipids, where they may be used. LDL cholesterol may form deposits on artery and other blood vessel walls. LDLs—with a higher ratio of cholesterol to protein—are also manufactured in the liver. They are only in the body, not in food.

Fats. Group of compounds made of glycerol and fatty acids. Fats are one of three main nutrient groups in food that supply energy; the others are carbohydrates and proteins. Fats also can be stored in the body.

Adipose tissue. Scientific term for body fat.

Dietary fat. Fat in food.

Triglycerides. Scientific name for the common form of fat found in both the body and in foods. Most body fat is stored in the form of triglycerides; triglycerides also circulate in the blood. Triglycerides, made of three fatty acids and glycerol, act like saturated fat: they trigger the liver to make more cholesterol so levels of total and LDL cholesterol rise.

Fatty acids. Basic units of fat molecules arranged as chains of carbon, hydrogen, and oxygen. Fats are mixtures of about sixteen different fatty acids, categorized by their structure. Each has its own unique physiological effect in your body.

> *Monounsaturated fatty acids.* Fatty acids missing one hydrogen pair on their chemical chain. They trigger less total or LDL cholesterol, and more HDL cholesterol, production. Canola, nut, and olive oils are high in monounsaturated fatty acids.

> *Polyunsaturated fatty acids.* Fatty acids missing two or more hydrogen pairs on their chemical chains. They also trigger lower total blood cholesterol, as well as lower LDL and HDL cholesterol, production. Corn, safflower, soybean, sesame, and sunflower oils are high in polyunsaturated fatty acids. Fatty acids in seafood are mainly polyunsaturated, too.

> *Saturated fatty acids.* Fatty acids that have all the hydrogen they can hold on their chemical chains. They trigger the liver to make more total and LDL cholesterol. In food, they come mainly from animal-based foods such as meat, poultry, butter, whole milk, and whole milk products, and from coconut, palm, and palm kernel oils.

Functional Nutrition: Eat Your Omega-3s and -6s

No doubt about it: seafood can be good for your health. Overall, it has less total fat and less saturated fat than meat and poultry. For this reason, eating fish regularly may help lower your blood cholesterol levels. Moreover, seafood supplies several vitamins and minerals. Recently there's been interest in the functional food benefits provided by the omega-3 fatty acid content of fish.

Omega-3 fatty acids—polyunsaturated fatty acids of a somewhat different structure—are found mostly in seafood, especially higher-fat, cold-water varieties such as mackerel, albacore tuna, salmon, sardines, Atlantic herring, swordfish, and lake trout. Flaxseed oil, soybean oil, and canola oil, as well as nuts and seeds, supply omega-3s, too. Nuts supply alpha-linolenic acid, which converts to omega-3s. And some eggs have more omega-3s if the chicken feed supplied it.

Research suggests that omega-3s may help thin blood and prevent blood platelets from clotting and sticking to artery walls. That, in turn, may help lower the risk for blocked blood vessels and heart attacks. Omega-3s may help prevent arteries from hardening, lower levels of triglycerides, and modestly reduce blood pressure levels. What's not clear is how much omega-3 fatty acids we need, how often, and their effect on heart disease.

Even if scientific evidence eventually understands the link, omega-3 fatty acids by themselves aren't a magic remedy for heart disease—and you can't simply add them to your meals and snacks to get the potential benefits. But combined with eating less saturated fat, they may have a protective effect. Researchers are exploring other links between omega-3 fatty acids and health: eye health, rheumatoid arthritis, and immunity. Stay tuned!

To enjoy nutritional and omega-3s' benefits from seafood, make fish a regular part of your eating style; try to eat seafood, including fatty fish, two or three times a week. And try using foods with omega-3s in place of foods with more saturated fats.

Although fish oil supplements contain omega-3 fatty acids, they're not advised as a substitute for fish—or as a dietary supplement for most people. Popping a fish oil capsule won't undo the effects of an otherwise high-fat diet. The safety, effectiveness, and proper dosage for fish oil supplements haven't been determined. Instead, enjoy fish for its nutritional benefits, flavor—and variety in your eating style.

What about omega-6s (the polyunsaturated fatty acids in vegetable oils)? They, too, may reduce the risk of cardiovascular disease by lowering total and LDL-cholesterol blood levels; however, they also may lower HDL levels.

Another fatty acid—conjugated linoleic acid (CLA)—may offer functional benefits, too. CLAs are found in dairy foods and some meat products (beef, lamb). Research is exploring a potential link to decreased risk for certain cancers and a role in improved body composition. Very little human research has yet been done.

Omega-3 fatty acids. Fatty acids that are highly polyunsaturated. They may help reduce blood clotting in the arteries and protect from hardening of the arteries. Mostly they come from seafood, especially fatty fish such as albacore tuna, mackerel, and salmon, as well as nuts, and soy, canola, and flaxseed oils.

Omega-6 fatty acids. Another group of polyunsaturated fatty acids. They, too, may help promote heart health by lowering total and LDL cholesterol. Vegetable oils—soybean, corn, safflower—are good sources.

Trans fatty acids. One type of fatty acid, formed during the process of hydrogenation. Although they're found naturally in some foods, most trans fatty acids in the diet come from hydrogenated fats. In the body, they act like saturated fats and tend to raise blood cholesterol levels.

Hydrogenated fats. Unsaturated fats that are processed to make them stable and solid at room temperature—for example in many packaged foods (such as crackers and cookies) and stick margarine. Hydrogen is added to their chemical makeup and makes them firmer and more saturated while extending their shelf life.

Fats and Oils: How do they Compare?

- Saturated Fat %
- Polyunsaturated Fat %
- Monounsaturated Fat %

	Saturated Fat %	Polyunsaturated Fat %	Monounsaturated Fat %
CANOLA OIL	6	32	62
MID OLEIC SUNFLOWER OIL	9	26	65
SAFFLOWER OIL	9	78	13
FLAXSEED OIL	10	32	62
SUNFLOWER OIL	12	69	19
CORN OIL	13	59	28
PEANUT OIL	14	32	50
SOYBEAN OIL	15	61	24
OLIVE OIL	17	11	72
COTTONSEED OIL	26	55	20
LARD	42	10	48
BEEF FAT	46	4	47
PALM OIL	50	10	40
BUTTERFAT	63	3	31
COCONUT OIL	92	2	6

Fats: Not Created Equal

Whether solid or liquid, the fats that we consume are made up of fatty acids and glycerol. Most fats in food are referred to as triglycerides. When digested, they're broken down into fatty acids and glycerol. In turn, the body uses them to form other lipids, which are used for a variety of bodily functions. When fat is stored in your body, it's in the form of a triglyceride.

In scientific terms, fatty acids are chains of carbon, hydrogen, and oxygen. They may be saturated or unsaturated. The term "saturation" refers to how many hydrogen atoms link to each carbon in the chain.

- When carbon atoms have as many hydrogens attached as possible on the chain, a fatty acid is *saturated.*

- When hydrogen atoms are missing, the fatty acid is *unsaturated.* A polyunsaturated fatty acid has two or more missing hydrogen pairs; a monounsaturated fatty acid is missing only one hydrogen pair on its chemical chain.

Now let's apply this to food. What, for example, makes margarine different from vegetable oil? The fatty acid content. All fats are mixtures of fatty acids: saturated, polyunsaturated, and monounsaturated. The proportion and differences in fatty acid content account for their varying characteristics—for example, liquid oil as compared with firm margarine. Their degree of saturation also has a significant role in how fatty acids from food affect health.

- Fats made mostly of saturated fatty acids usually are solid at room temperature. Animal-based foods and tropical vegetable oils (coconut, palm kernel, and palm) contain mainly saturated fatty acids. In general, harder and more stable fats are more saturated. They include butter, stick margarine, shortening, and the fat in cheese and meat.

- By contrast, fats that contain mostly polyunsaturated fatty acids usually are liquid at room temperature. Safflower, sunflower, corn, and soybean oils contain the highest amounts of polyunsaturated fats.

- Foods with mostly monounsaturated fatty acids are liquid at room temperature. They're found in some vegetable oils, such as canola, olive, and peanut oils.

"Fats and Oils: How do they Compare?" above shows the proportions of various fatty acids in fats and oils.

Besides fats and oils, the proportion of fatty acids varies in other fat-containing foods. For example, seafood and meat both have saturated and unsaturated

At a Glance: How Dietary Fat Affects Blood Lipids

Type of Fatty Acids	Effects of Blood Lipids
Saturated	↑ total cholesterol, ↑ LDL cholesterol
Polyunsaturated	↓ total cholesterol, ↓ LDL cholesterol, ↓ HDL cholesterol*
Monounsaturated	↓ total cholesterol, ↓ LDL cholesterol, may ↑ HDL cholesterol*
Omega-3	↓ triglycerides, ↓ total cholesterol*
Trans	↑ total cholesterol, ↑ LDL cholesterol, may ↓ HDL cholesterol

*Unsaturated fatty acids may have a beneficial effect if they replace saturated fats, but not if they're simply added, making the diet higher in fat.

fatty acids. However, seafood has a higher proportion of polyunsaturated fatty acids; meat, more saturated fatty acids.

About Trans Fats

Processing can change the structure of fat, making it more saturated. The process is called hydrogenation because missing hydrogen is added to fatty acid chains in their chemical makeup. As a result, oils become semisolid and more stable at room temperature. Usually hydrogenation is partial, making fat 5 to 60 percent saturated. The result: trans fatty acids.

The term "trans" simply describes the chemical makeup of a fatty acid. Although beef, pork, lamb, butter, and milk have small amounts of trans fatty acids, most trans fatty acids come from hydrogenated oil.

As an example, stick margarine is made by hydrogenating vegetable oil. All margarines are made from vegetable oil. In stick margarine, the fatty acids are more hydrogenated, with a higher proportion of saturated fatty acids, making it more firm than soft margarine that's sold in tubs or as "squeeze" margarine. Tub and squeeze margarines contain more water, and sometimes have air whipped in so they may be lower in fat and calories. Butter-margarine blends may be even firmer than stick margarine; the saturated fatty acids in butter help keep the product firm.

If more "sat fats" are formed, why hydrogenate the oil? This process gives desirable qualities to food. For example, because hydrogenated fats are more stable, they extend the shelf life of foods such as crackers and margarine. For that reason, these foods don't develop a rancid flavor and odor as quickly. Hydrogenating the oil in peanut butter gives a creamy consistency; oil stays mixed in and doesn't rise to the top. And stick margarine and vegetable shortening remain firm at room temperature when their oil is partially hydrogenated. In the fast-food industry, many foods are fried with these fats.

Why the concern about trans fats? Trans fatty acids act like saturated fats, potentially raising LDL blood cholesterol levels and decreasing HDL cholesterol. That, in turn, may increase the risk for fatty deposits on blood vessel walls and heart attacks. Trans fatty acids supply only about 2 to 4 percent of total calories in the American diet, compared with about 12 per-

Have You Ever Wondered

. . . what trans-free spreads are? They're usually margarine-type products processed with little or no trans fatty acids. Their formulas differ and may contain fat replacers. Look for trans fat claims on food labels.

. . . if melting a fat such as butter, stick margarine, or lard makes it less saturated? While unsaturated fats are liquid at room temperature, simply heating and melting doesn't change saturated fatty acids to unsaturated fatty acids. As soon as lard, margarine, or butter is cooled to room temperature, it's solid again.

. . . what stearic acid is? It's another saturated fat, found in animal products and some plant foods, under scientific study. Research suggests that its effect may be neutral, neither raising nor lowering blood cholesterol levels. For now, there's not enough evidence to offer advice—but enough to suggest that even saturated fats work in different ways.

. . . what shortening really is? It's simply another term that refers to fat. Solid at room temperature, shortening is vegetable oil (often hydrogenated soybean or cottonseed oil, palm oil, or coconut oil) sometimes combined with animal fat. Their being high in "trans fats" and perhaps "sat fats," go easy on shortening or foods made with shortening.

cent from saturated fat. Still, it's wise to be prudent, especially if you have high cholesterol levels already. You don't need trans fats for normal health.

How can you be a wise consumer and cut back on trans fats? Check food labels and go easy on foods with "partially hydrogenated vegetable oil": stick margarine, vegetable shortening, and many prepared foods, cakes, cookies, crackers, snack foods, and commercially fried foods, including fried fast foods. Look for "trans fatty acid" claims (perhaps "no trans fatty acids") on some food labels.

Fat: More Than Meets the Eye!

Visible or not, almost all foods contain fat in varying amounts. Some are very high in fat; others have just trace amounts.

The fat content of some foods is obvious: for example, in butter, oil, and margarine. Even in certain cuts of meat and poultry with the skin on, fat is easy to see—and easy to trim off.

In most foods, however, clues to a food's fat content appear on food labels. The Nutrition Facts panel tells how much per serving. Salad dressings, many baked foods, chips, crackers, chocolate, nuts, avocados, sauces, meat, poultry, fish, cheese, dairy products, and egg yolks, for example, all contain varying amounts of fat. Obviously, fried foods contain more fat than those that are baked or steamed.

Which foods supply the most fat in the typical American diet?

● On average, most fat in the American diet comes directly from fats and oils, as well as salad dressings, candy, gravies, and sauces.

● Animal-based foods provide varying amounts of fat, as well as saturated fat. With lean and fat-modified products on the market, check the Nutrition Facts on food labels to know how much.

● With only a few exceptions (avocados and olives), fruits and vegetables don't supply much fat

Have You Ever Wondered?

... if olive oil has fewer calories and less fat than butter? Because liquid oils are concentrated, and solid fats may contain other ingredients besides fat, oils generally contain slightly more fat and calories than equal amounts of solid fat. Per tablespoon, olive oil contains about 14 grams of fat and 120 calories compared to butter, with about 12 grams of fat and 100 calories. The main difference is in the types of fatty acids. Olive oil has a higher proportion of monounsaturated fatty acids, which may be healthier; butter has more saturated fatty acids.

... which has more saturated fat: butter or margarine? Although margarine has more trans fats than butter, it still has less saturated fat. Another way to compare is to look at the total of saturated fats plus trans fat. One tablespoon of butter has about 7.5 grams of saturated plus trans fats; the same amount of some stick margarine has about 4.5 grams of saturated plus trans fats. The amount of total fat is comparable—12 grams per tablespoon.

naturally. That's true for most grain products, too—unless it's added during food preparation or processing. French fries, fried okra, croissants, and hush puppies are all higher-fat choices.

About Fat Replacers . . .

Today's supermarkets sell options! Foods made with fat replacers can help you consume less fat if they really replace full-fat products in your food choices. These foods have much of the taste, texture, and appearance of their higher-fat counterparts. Besides being lower in fat, they're usually, but not always, lower in saturated fat, cholesterol, and calories as well.

Fat gives unique characteristics to food, so when fat is removed from a "recipe," perhaps to make a low-fat cookie, many characteristics of the food change, too. Fat replacers often give these foods a familiar texture, appearance, and taste.

Food manufacturers use different types of fat replacers: carbohydrate-based, protein-based, and fat-based. Most contribute calories, although less than fat does. Because no fat replacer acts exactly like fat, most reduced-fat and fat-free products contain a mixture of fat replacers. From a food safety standpoint, both scientific research and their review by the U.S. Food and Drug Administration (FDA) recognize fat replacers as safe.

Carbohydrate-Based Fat Replacers

Modified starches, dextrins, cellulose, gums, and other carbohydrate ingredients work by combining with water to provide texture, appearance, and mouth feel that are similar to fat. Fat-free salad dressings, for example, contain carbohydrate-based substitutes. The calories in carbohydrate-based replacers range from almost nothing to 4 calories per gram. The difference is that some, such as modified starches and dextrins, are digested; others, such as cellulose and other fibers, aren't digested, so they provide no energy. Most of these fat replacers can withstand some heat; however, they can't be used for frying.

Puréed prunes (dried plums) and applesauce sometimes are used as fat replacers in baked foods. They're an easy fat substitute you can try yourself. Prunes and applesauce add bulk, flavor, and nutrition.

Primer: Fat, Saturated Fat, and Cholesterol in Food

	Total Fat (g)	Saturated Fatty Acids (g)	Cholesterol (mg)	Calories
Breads, Cereals, Rice, Pasta				
Bread, 1 slice				
White	1	Trace	Trace	70
Whole-wheat	1	Trace	0	65
Bagel, with egg, 1	1	Trace	14	155
Biscuit, 1 medium	3	1	2	105
Roll, dinner, 1	2	Trace	0	85
Croissant, 1 medium	12	7	62	230
Muffin, 1 large	6	2	44	185
Pancake, 1 medium	3	1	26	90
Waffle, 1 medium	5	2	39	205
Doughnut, yeast, 1	14	5	21	245
Danish pastry, 1 (2 oz.)	13	4	49	240
Oatmeal, cooked, ½ cup	1	Trace	0	70
Shredded wheat, 1 large biscuit	Trace	Trace	0	85
Granola, ⅓ cup	10	2	0	180
Rice, white, cooked, ½ cup	Trace	Trace	0	110
Fried rice (with egg and vegetables), ½ cup	6	1	21	120
Cookie, 1 medium				
Oatmeal	3	1	5	60
Chocolate chip	4	1	6	70
Cake, devil's food, frosted, ¹⁄₁₂ of 8-inch	16	5	32	405
Milk, Yogurt, Cheese				
Milk, 1 cup				
Whole	8	5	33	150
2% reduced-fat	5	3	18	120
1% low-fat	3	2	10	100
Fat-free	Trace	Trace	4	85
Yogurt, 1 cup				
Nonfat plain	Trace	Trace	4	135
Low-fat plain	4	2	15	155
Low-fat fruit flavored	3	2	10	250
Cottage cheese, ½ cup				
Creamed	5	3	16	110
1% low-fat	1	1	5	82
Cheese, 1 oz.				
Natural Cheddar	9	6	29	115
Mozzarella, part fat-free	5	3	16	110
Process American	9	6	27	105
Vanilla ice cream, ½ cup	7	4	27	135
Vanilla ice milk, ½ cup	3	2	9	90
Frozen yogurt, ½ cup	2	1	8	105

	Total Fat (g)	Saturated Fatty Acids (g)	Cholesterol (mg)	Calories
Vegetables				
Potatoes				
Boiled, ½ cup	Trace	Trace	0	65
Potato salad, ½ cup	8	1	50	135
French fries, 10 strips	8	3	0	160
Au gratin, ½ cup	9	4	19	175
Chips, 1 oz.	10	3	0	150
Cabbage, ½ cup				
Cooked	Trace	Trace	0	15
Creamy coleslaw	11	2	6	125
Celery and carrot sticks, 8	Trace	0	0	10
Stir-fried vegetables, ½ cup	Trace	Trace	0	45
Meats, Poultry, Fish, Beans, Eggs, and Nuts				
Beef				
Lean cut (eye of round), roasted, 3 oz.				
Lean and fat	11	4	61	195
Lean only	4	2	59	145
Fattier cut (chuck blade), braised, 3 oz.				
Lean and fat	22	9	88	295
Lean only	11	4	90	215
Ground, cooked, 3 oz. patty				
Regular	17	7	76	245
Lean	16	6	73	230
Extra lean	14	5	71	215
Pork center loin, roasted, 3 oz.				
Lean and fat	11	4	68	180
Lean	8	3	67	150
Beef liver, braised, 3 oz.	4	2	331	135
Chicken, light and dark meat, roasted, 3 oz.				
With skin	12	3	74	200
Without skin	6	2	75	160
Halibut fillets, baked, 3 oz.	1	Trace	49	95
Tuna, canned, 3 oz.				
In oil	7	1	25	170
In water	1	Trace	25	115
Crabs, hard-shell, steamed, 2 medium	2	Trace	95	95
Shrimp, steamed or boiled, 8 extra large	2	Trace	160	110
Frankfurters, 2 (3 oz.)	27	10	47	300
Dry beans, cooked, ½ cup	Trace	Trace	0	110
Peanut butter, 2 tbsp.	16	3	0	190
Sunflower seeds, 2 tbsp.	10	1	0	105
Egg, large, cooked, 1	5	2	213	75
Yolk	5	2	213	60
White	0	0	0	15

PRIMER: FAT, SATURATED FAT, AND CHOLESTEROL IN FOOD *(continued)*

	TOTAL FAT (G)	SATURATED FATTY ACIDS (G)	CHOLESTEROL (MG)	CALORIES
Fruits				
Apple, 1 medium	Trace	Trace	0	80
Avocado, ½ medium	15	2	0	160
Banana, 1 medium	1	Trace	0	105
Olives, 5 large				
Green	3	Trace	0	25
Ripe	3	Trace	0	30
Orange, 1 medium	Trace	Trace	0	60
Peach, 1 medium	Trace	Trace	0	20
Strawberries, 5 berries	1	Trace	0	20
Mixed fruit cup with cream dressing, ½ cup	3	2	9	80
Fats, Oils, Sweets				
Butter, 1 tbsp.	12	7	31	100
Butter-margarine blend, 1 tbsp.	12	5	16	100
Margarine, 1 tbsp.				
Soft	12	2	0	100
Stick	12	2	0	100
Liquid (squeezable)	12	2	0	100
Diet	6	1	0	50
Vegetable oil (corn), 1 tbsp.	14	2	0	120
Hydrogenated vegetable shortening, 1 tbsp.	13	3	0	115
Salad dressing, 1 tbsp.				
Mayonnaise (regular)	12	2	7	100
Mayonnaise, reduced-calorie	5	1	5	50
Mayonnaise-type	7	1	4	70
Mayonnaise-type, reduced-calorie	4	1	4	45
Italian	7	1	0	70
Italian, low-calorie	1	Trace	1	15
Cream, 1 tbsp.				
Sour	3	2	6	30
Light (table)	3	2	10	30
Nondairy, frozen	1	Trace	0	20
Cream cheese, 1 tbsp.	5	3	16	50
Pie, apple, ⅛ of 9-inch	22	5	0	455
Cheesecake, 1/12 of 9-inch	25	10	86	405
Sherbet, ½ cup	2	1	7	135
Milk chocolate bar, 1 oz.	9	5	6	145

Source: Human Nutrition Information Service/U.S. Department of Agriculture, "Choose a Diet Low in Fat, Saturated Fat, and Cholesterol," *Home and Garden Bulletin* 253-4 (July 1993).

Protein-Based Fat Replacers

Made with protein from egg whites or fat-free milk, these fat replacers provide a creamy sensation and improve appearance and texture when fat is removed. Low-fat cheese made with a protein-based substitute gives an appearance and texture that come close to full-fat cheese. Most protein-based replacers aren't used in foods prepared at high temperatures. That's because the protein coagulates, and they no longer function in ways similar to fat.

Protein-based replacers contribute 1 to 4 calories per gram, compared with 9 calories per fat gram. What accounts for the calorie range? These replacers may be blended with ingredients such as cellulose that can't be digested. Protein-based replacers also provide small amounts of amino acids.

Fat-Based Replacers

These are made with fats that have been chemically altered. They provide few or no calories as compared to fat because the body is unable to fully absorb the fatty acids. They may be used in baked foods, some fried foods, cake mixes, frosting, and dairy foods.

Olestra is a calorie-free fat replacer made from vegetable oils and sugar. It contributes no calories because it passes through the body without being digested and absorbed. Olestra provides the characteristics of fat in cooking, especially for frying and snack foods. Olean is the brand name for olestra that you'll see on food labels. Because olestra isn't digested, some vitamins carried by fat aren't fully absorbed. For this reason, fat-soluble vitamins are added to foods made with olestra. For some people, consuming foods with olestra may be linked to digestive discomfort.

Salatrim is another fat-based replacer used in baked goods, dairy products, and confection-type products. It provides calories, but only 5 calories per gram (as compared to 9 calories per gram in fat) because it is only partially absorbed in the body.

FAT REPLACERS: ONE WAY TO LOWER FAT AND CALORIES

Fat-modified foods can make a difference in the calories and fat of a meal. Foods with fat replacers may have more carbohydrates; that's why the percent of fat reduction may be higher than the percent of calorie reduction.

You probably wouldn't make all these substitutions in this chart. Even if you do, you still need to be sensible. Portion size counts.

	CALORIES	FAT (GRAMS)
Regular Lunch		
2 slices bread	130	2
1 oz. American cheese	105	9
2 oz. bologna	180	17
1 tbsp. mayonnaise	100	11
Banana	105	0
2 chocolate cookies (30 g)	140	6
Total	760	45
Lunch with Fat-Modified Foods		
2 slices bread	130	2
l oz. reduced-fat cheese product	75	4
2 oz. fat-free bologna	40	0
1 tbsp. low-fat mayonnaise/dressing	25	1
Banana	105	0
2 reduced-fat chocolate cookies (30 g)	120	3
Total	495	10

Source: Adapted from International Food Information Council Foundation, *Food Insight Media Guide on Food Safety & Nutrition* (2002–2004). Reprinted with permission of the International Food Information Council Foundation.

What Foods Contain Fat Replacers?

If you scan the supermarket shelves you see low-fat or fat-free versions of full-fat foods: margarine, salad dressing, mayonnaise, cheese, sour cream, ice cream, cookies, baked foods, and candy, to name a few. They're made by replacing some or all of the fat with fat replacers.

To some degree, fat replacers supply calories, so the energy contributed by fat-modified foods may or

. . . what a label stating "98% fat-free" means? You might think this means that only 2% of the total calories come from fat. Actually, the percent is referring to weight and not calories. So "98% fat-free" means that 2% of the weight of the total serving comes from fat. By law, when manufacturers use a "% fat-free" on a label, the amount of total fat must be below 3 grams of fat per serving. This amount is quite low, but may be more than you'd think when reading the "% fat-free" claim.

may not be less than the original food. For the calories and fat per serving, check the Nutrition Facts panel on the food label. And go easy. Less fat is no license to overeat!

The bottom line: fat replacers can be a safe and effective option for making meals and snacks appealing—and at the same time, control the fat and energy in your food choices. With these ingredients, the variety of reduced-fat, low-fat, and fat-free products offers you even more ways to moderate fats in your food choices.

Cholesterol: Different from Fat

To clear up a common misperception, cholesterol is a fatlike substance, but it's not a fat itself. Cholesterol has a different structure from fat and performs different functions in the human body. Some functions promote health; some don't. Because fat and cholesterol often appear together in foods of animal origin, and because their roles in health are so intertwined, they're easily mixed up.

Like fat, cholesterol often gets a "bad rap," yet it's part of every body cell and of some hormones, including sex hormones such as estrogen. As part of a body chemical called bile, it helps the body digest and absorb fat, too. With the help of sunlight, a form of cholesterol in your skin can change to vitamin D, a nutrient essential for bone building. However, too much cholesterol in the bloodstream is linked to heart disease.

Blood vs. Dietary Cholesterol

Confused about cholesterol? You're not alone! Actually, the term itself refers to two different types. Blood, or serum, cholesterol circulates in the bloodstream. Dietary cholesterol comes from food.

Functional Nutrition: Stanol- and Sterol-Based Ingredients

New cholesterol-lowering spreads contain unique, functional ingredients: plant stanol esters or plant sterol esters. These ingredients are naturally present in small amounts in vegetables and plant oils. In fact, the average person consumes about 250 milligrams of plant stanols and sterols daily from many plant-based foods.

Butterlike spreads that contain plant sterol or stanol esters are promoted for their ability to lower LDL blood cholesterol by up to 14 percent; they don't affect HDLs. For a significant cholesterol-lowering effect, the health claim states that you need to consume two servings of a spread that contains plant stanol or sterol esters daily—with meals—as part of an eating plan that's low in saturated fat and cholesterol. Read the package label for the serving size.

These spreads offer cholesterol-lowering benefits to anyone. Research shows that people with elevated cholesterol levels benefit most. In fact, the 2001 National Cholesterol Education Program of the National Institutes of Health recommends the addition of 2 grams per day of stanols or sterols as part of the dietary management for high blood cholesterol levels. People on statin drug therapy can use these spreads for additional cholesterol-lowering as part of their healthful eating regimen.

Currently two brands of these spreads are sold: Take Control, which contains plant sterol esters, and Benecol, which contains plant stanol esters. Spreads with these unique dietary ingredients cost more to produce than regular spreads.

Use them in food preparation, not only as a spread. Benecol regular spread (with plant stanol esters) can be used in cooking and baking without changing the flavor of food. Use it like any other margarine, substituting it equally for the fat, oil, or shortening in a recipe. A spread that contains plant sterols (Take Control) isn't recommended for baking or frying.

Have You Ever Wondered

. . . if adding olive oil and canola oil to your eating approach is healthful? Sure—if you take saturated fats away, too. Olive and canola oils are both high in monounsaturated fatty acids and low in saturated fatty acids. Monounsaturated fatty acids in foods may help lower blood cholesterol levels more than polyunsaturated fatty acids do. However, simply adding olive or canola oils to an already high-fat diet is not the point. These oils are still 100 percent fat, with 120 calories per tablespoon. The goal for health is to use oils high in monounsaturated fatty acids instead of other fats and oils.

. . . what's the source of canola oil? It comes from the canola plant, developed from its close relation the rapeseed plant, using traditional methods of plant breeding. Extracted from canola seeds, canola oil is very low in saturated fat, yet a great source of mono- and polyunsaturated fats.

Canola oil differs from rapeseed oil (consumed in Europe and Asia) in a significant way. Canola oil is extremely low in erucic acid. While erucic acid has not been shown to affect human health, it has been linked to cardiac abnormalities in experimental animals. The U.S. Food and Drug Administration deems canola oil as safe for use in food.

. . . if cholesterol supplies calories? Although cholesterol is often confused with fat, cholesterol is not a source of energy, or calories, so eating too much can't make you fat. Unlike fats, carbohydrates, and proteins, cholesterol isn't broken down, so the body cannot derive any energy from it.

While many factors affect blood cholesterol levels, the cholesterol that circulates in your body comes from two sources:

● *Your body produces cholesterol*—enough for your needs. Your liver makes most of it, but every body cell can make cholesterol, too. In fact, when the body makes too much, the risk for heart disease goes up. Unlike adults, infants and young children's bodies don't produce enough cholesterol, so for children under age two, it's important that their food choices supply cholesterol.

● *Cholesterol also comes from foods and beverages of animal origin:* eggs, meat, poultry, fish, and dairy foods. Animals produce cholesterol, but plants don't. A diet high in cholesterol is one factor that elevates blood cholesterol levels for some people. That's why moderation is advised. Dietary cholesterol doesn't automatically become blood cholesterol. The total fat, especially saturated fat and trans fats, in your food choices has a more significant effect on blood cholesterol levels than dietary cholesterol alone does.

The "Good" and the "Bad"

Have you ever wondered what the terms "good" cholesterol and "bad" cholesterol really mean? They actually refer to cholesterol carried in your blood by two types of lipoproteins, and not to cholesterol in food.

Because cholesterol doesn't mix with water, it can't be carried alone in your bloodstream. Instead, it's combined in "packages" with fats and proteins. These packages, called lipoproteins, carry cholesterol both to and from your body cells.

The nicknames "good" and "bad" cholesterol relate to risk factors for heart disease. High levels of HDL, or "good," cholesterol are linked to *lower* heart disease risk; high levels of LDL, or "bad," cholesterol, to *higher* heart disease risk. Think "high" for health and "low" for less healthy. Your total blood cholesterol count consists of both HDL and LDL cholesterol.

Although HDL and LDL cholesterol aren't found in food, your food choices do influence LDL levels. If you lower the saturated fat and cholesterol in your diet, you'll likely bring down LDL blood cholesterol levels. And if you're physically active, you'll likely lower your LDL cholesterol and keep your HDL blood cholesterol higher. What you eat and how active you are are just two of many factors that affect LDL, HDL, and total blood cholesterol levels. *To learn more, refer to "HDLs and LDLs: The Ups and the Downs" on page 540.*

Cholesterol: In What Foods?

What foods contain cholesterol? Only foods of animal origin. Egg yolks and organ meats are especially high in cholesterol. And in varying amounts, meat, poultry, seafood, dairy products, and animal fats such as butter or lard all supply cholesterol, too. Cholesterol is not found in vegetable oils, margarine, egg whites, or in plant-based foods such as grains, fruits, vegetables, beans, and peas.

As mentioned before, cholesterol and saturated fatty acids often occur together in animal-based foods. That's why they sometimes get confused. Sirloin steak, butter, and Cheddar cheese, for example, all contain both saturated fatty acids and cholesterol. On the other hand, shellfish and organ meats are high in cholesterol, yet they're low in saturated fatty acids.

In foods of animal origin, both lean and fatty tissues contain cholesterol. That's why some low-fat foods, such as squid and shrimp, can be relatively high in cholesterol. The sauce or butter they're dipped in can boost their cholesterol content, too.

Even though some plant-based foods (margarine, vegetable oil, nuts, and seeds) are high in fat or saturated fat, they have no cholesterol, even margarines made with trans fats. Although nuts have no cholesterol, they derive 80 to 89 percent of their calories from fat.

So why do some vegetable dishes and grain-based baked goods contain cholesterol? It's the added ingredients: egg yolks, cheese, milk, meat, poultry, butter, or lard. Some common examples are refried beans made with lard, greens cooked with bacon, and muffins made with butter and egg yolks. The amount of cholesterol per serving varies with the recipe.

When shopping, if you spot a food that's labeled "no cholesterol" or "cholesterol-free," it cannot have any more than 2 grams of saturated fat. However, you'll want to read the rest of the food label to find out about the total fat content; it may not be low in fat.

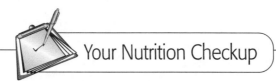

Your Nutrition Checkup

Fat and Cholesterol Audit

What's the fat and cholesterol quotient of your eating style? For each section, check one box in each column that matches your usual food choices over the course of a day or several days. Choosing from every column is okay. That's part of making trade-offs! Remember, your overall fat intake over time is what counts—not each individual choice.

COLUMN 1 (3 POINTS)	COLUMN 2 (2 POINTS)	COLUMN 3 (1 POINT)
☐ Reasonable portions, totaling 5 to 7 oz. of meat, poultry, or fish per day	☐ Some reasonable portions and some bigger portions, totaling somewhat more than 7 oz. of meat, poultry, or fish per day	☐ Big portions of meat, poultry, and fish, totaling much more than 7 oz. per day
☐ Low-fat and fat-free milk dairy products	☐ Both low-fat and whole-milk dairy products, and some higher-fat products, such as cheese	☐ Whole-milk dairy products and higher-fat products, such as cheese
☐ Variety of lean meat, skinless poultry, and fish	☐ Some lean and some higher-fat meat and poultry	☐ High-fat meat, such as juicy steak or high-fat sausage, or poultry with skin on

COLUMN 1 (3 POINTS)	COLUMN 2 (2 POINTS)	COLUMN 3 (1 POINT)
☐ Broiled, grilled, or roasted foods such as meat, poultry, and fish, and steamed, boiled, or baked vegetables	☐ Some broiled, grilled, or roasted foods, and others that are fried	☐ Mostly fried or sautéed meat, poultry, fish, and vegetables
☐ Little or no gravy or creamy, high-fat sauces	☐ Some gravy or high-fat sauces	☐ Plenty of gravy and/or high-fat sauces
☐ Low-fat salad dressing or small amount (1 tbsp per serving) of regular salad dressing	☐ Some regular salad dressing	☐ Liberal use of regular salad dressing
☐ Fruit, frozen yogurt, and other low-fat desserts and snacks	☐ Some low-fat desserts and snacks, and some with more fat, such as regular ice cream, cake, and cookies	☐ Plenty of high-fat desserts and snacks
☐ Small amounts of stick margarine, butter, or high-fat spread or toppings on breads or vegetables—or none at all	☐ Mostly just small amounts of stick margarine, butter, or other high-fat spreads or toppings on breads or vegetables	☐ Liberal amounts of stick margarine, butter, or other high-fat spreads or toppings on bread or vegetables
☐ Bagels, bread, tortillas, and other low-fat breads	☐ Some low-fat breads and some higher-fat breads such as croissants, muffins, and doughnuts	☐ Mostly higher-fat breads
☐ An egg yolk or less a day	☐ Usually an egg yolk or less a day, but sometimes more	☐ 2 or 3 egg yolk breakfasts, almost daily
Column 1 subtotal _____	*Column 2 subtotal* _____	*Column 3 subtotal* _____

Now for the totals . . .

Your score: _____. Depending on which column you checked, each box is worth 3, 2, or 1 point(s).

If you scored . . .

20 to 30 points—You've taken a low-fat eating style to heart!

16 to 19 points—You've got the idea of moderation. Yet you still have room to trim fat and cholesterol in your food choices a bit more. Read on!

10 to 15 points—For your good health, you're wise to rethink your overall eating style for less fat and cholesterol. Read on for simple, practical tips!

Too Much of a Good Thing?

Today, many Americans are concerned about the amount of fat in their diets. Rightly so. On average, Americans consume more than they need. Although our fat intake is dropping, it's still higher than the guideline set by health experts: no more than 30 percent of total calories from fat in your total diet. Most of us also eat too much saturated fat. *See "What's Your Upper Limit on Fat and Saturated Fat?" later in this chapter.*

High-fat, especially high-saturated-fat, eating is

linked to higher blood cholesterol levels and a greater chance for heart disease. There's more reason for caution: eating a high-fat diet also increases the risk for some types of cancer and obesity. For this reason, the Dietary Guidelines for Americans advise: *Choose a diet that is low in saturated fat and cholesterol and moderate in total fat.* Cutting back on fat and cholesterol may account partly for a slight, recent decline in death rates from heart disease.

Weight control is a good reason to go easy on fat, since high-fat foods are often high in calories, too. Whether they're saturated or unsaturated, calories from fat are all alike. Every fat gram supplies 9 calories, or more than twice the amount provided by 1 gram of carbohydrate or protein. And excess calories, whether from fat, carbohydrate, or protein, are stored in the body as fat. Remember: the total amount of calories eaten, not just the calories from fat, is the issue in weight management. *Check "Primer: Fat, Saturated Fat, and Cholesterol in Food" earlier in this chapter to compare the calories in several higher-fat foods.*

For more about the effects of fat, saturated fat, and cholesterol on heart disease and cancer, see "Your Healthy Heart" and "Cancer Connection" in chapter 22.

Fat and Cholesterol: Know Your Limits

How much fat and cholesterol is enough? For fat, the advice depends on your overall energy needs. By now, the guideline for fat intake is well known: for healthy Americans after age two, consume no more than 30 percent of total calories from fat. No matter what your energy intake, the cholesterol guideline for healthy individuals remains the same: 300 milligrams or less per day.

Here's how the "no more than 30 percent" guideline is divided:

- 7 to 10 percent of total calories from saturated fats

- 10 to 15 percent from monounsaturated fats

- about 10 percent from polyunsaturated fats.

Of the other 70 or more percent of calories, 55 to 60 percent should come from carbohydrates, mostly

---

Fat Math

The recommended advice: no more than 30 percent of your calories from total fat, with less than 10 percent from saturated fat. How many fat grams is that? That depends on your energy needs. Here's how to make those calculations if you consumed 2,000 calories a day:

To figure 30-percent calories from total fat per day . . .
30% (or 0.30) × 2,000 calories = 600 calories from total fat

To figure total fat grams per day . . .
600 calories from total fat ÷ 9 calories per gram of fat = 66.66 or 67 grams of total fat per day

To figure 10 percent calories from saturated fat per day . . .
10% (or 0.10) × 2,000 calories = 200 calories from saturated fat*

To figure grams of saturated fat per day . . .
200 calories from unsaturated fat ÷ 9 calories = 22 grams of saturated fat (of the 67 grams total fat) per day*

*To calculate monounsaturated fats or polyunsaturated fats, use this same equation. The guidelines are: 10 to 15 percent of total calories from monounsaturated fats, and about 10 percent from polyunsaturated fats. Remember: total fat *equals* saturated fats plus monounsaturated fats *plus* polyunsaturated fats.

---

complex carbohydrates from foods such as bread, cereal, rice, and pasta; the remainder, from protein.

To clear up any confusion, the "no more than 30 percent" guideline for total fat and "7 to 10 percent" guideline for saturated fat apply to your total diet, *not* to a single food or a single meal. And the percent of calories you consume from fat—over several days—impacts your health. So don't worry or feel guilty if you occasionally eat more. Just make it up by eating less on other days.

In real numbers, how much is 30 percent calories from total fat—and 10 percent calories from "sat fat"? The specific amount depends on a person's energy needs. And that depends on age, gender, body size, and activity level. *To figure your own fat budget, see the example in "Fat Math" above.* You also can check the bottom of the Nutrition Facts panel on many food

What's Your Upper Limit on Fat and Saturated Fat?

IF YOU EAT THIS MANY CALORIES A DAY . . .	YOUR CALORIES FROM FAT WOULD BE NO MORE THAN . . .	YOUR DAILY SATURATED FAT INTAKE SHOULD BE NO MORE THAN . . .	YOUR DAILY FAT INTAKE SHOULD BE NO MORE THAN . . .
1,600	480	18 g	53 g
2,000	600	20 g*	65 g*
2,200	660	24 g	73 g
2,500	750	25 g*	80 g*
2,800	840	31 g	93 g

*Percent Daily Values on Nutrition Facts labels are based on a 2,000-calorie diet. Values for 2,000 and 2,500 calories are rounded to the nearest 5 grams to be consistent with the Nutrition Facts panel.

Source: Adapted from *Dietary Guidelines for Americans* (2000).

labels. For a 2,000- and a 2,500-calorie diet, it shows how many fat grams equal the "less than 30 percent" guideline.

To guesstimate how many calories you need to maintain your current weight, see "Your 'Weigh': Figuring Your Energy Needs" in chapter 2.

Trim Fat in Your Eating Style

Do you consume too many calories from fat? From a health standpoint, you'd probably benefit by cutting back!

Cutting back from 33 or 40 percent calories from fat to 30 percent doesn't need to be a huge change in your eating pattern. Even small changes add up. Often eating a smaller portion of a high-fat dessert, switching to lean meat and low-fat or nonfat dairy products, and eating broiled rather than fried foods are enough to make a daily difference. As an added benefit, cutting back on high-fat foods may leave room to enjoy more carbohydrate-rich foods—if calories remain the same.

Keep in mind that you can reduce fat, including saturated fat, from your food choices in many ways. You don't need to use them all. To start, try a few strategies listed here. Once you've mastered them, try a few more. Here's how:

For Less Total Fat . . .

● Know where fat comes from. You can't cut back unless you know the sources of fat. *See "Primer: Fat, Saturated Fat, and Cholesterol in Food" earlier in this chapter.*

Check the Nutrition Facts on food labels for how much fat, including saturated fat, and cholesterol a single serving contains. You could tally up how much fat you ate per day, using the labels. But that would be time-consuming. So instead consider the following tips! *To learn how to best use the Nutrition Facts panel, see "Get All the Facts!" in chapter 11.*

● Look for nutrient content claims on the label, perhaps "low-fat" or "lean." As you shop, use these clues to help guide your food purchases. *To learn what these claims mean, see "Label Lingo: Fats and Cholesterol" later in this chapter.*

● Think positive! Use the Food Guide Pyramid guidelines to fit in all the foods you enjoy. A healthful diet—without too much fat or cholesterol—contains enough, but not too much of foods from the five food groups: (1) grain products; (2) fruits; (3) vegetables; (4) lean meat, skinless poultry, fish, cooked beans and peas (legumes), moderate amounts of eggs and nuts; and (5) mostly low-fat and fat-free dairy foods.

● Choose lean meat (beef, veal, and/or pork) and skinless poultry. Loin and round cuts of meat have less fat. Trim visible fat from meat and poultry, too. Lean meat isn't the same as fat-free; it just has less fat.

Lean meat contains cholesterol in both the fat and in lean muscle tissue. Trimming the fat and buying lean cuts reduce the cholesterol in meat but won't make it cholesterol-free.

● Make your meals "fishy." Enjoy seafood two or three times a week, prepared a low-fat way. Go for fattier fish, such as salmon, occasionally to get the potential omega-3 benefits.

● Eat "five a day" fruits and vegetables. Besides being low in fat, fruits and veggies fill you up and help curb your appetite for higher-fat foods. Soluble fiber in some fruits, vegetables, and grain products also has a cholesterol-lowering effect. *To think about the variety of tasty fruits and vegetables in today's supermarkets, see "Garden of Eatin': Less Common Vegetables" and "Fresh Ideas: Uncommon Fruit" in chapter 9.*

● Go for grains! Choose lower-fat grain products— pasta, rice, breakfast cereal, bagels, tortillas, pita, and other lower-fat breads; include those with soluble fiber, such as oats. Go easy on doughnuts, sweet rolls, higher-fat muffins, cakes, and cookies. Consume more of your food energy from carbohydrate-rich foods and less from fat!

● Choose mostly low-fat or fat-free dairy products. The bone-building nutrients in low-fat and whole-milk products are about the same.

● Go easy on fats and oils. That includes vegetable oils, butter, margarine, lard, cream cheese, and bacon used in cooking, as well as high-fat salad dressings, sauces, and many candies. Add flavor to food with herbs and seasonings rather than high-fat sauces. Interestingly, while butter is an animal fat and margarine is a vegetable fat, their fat content is the same: about 12 fat grams and 100 calories per tablespoon.

● Consider today's reduced-fat, low-fat, and fat-free foods on supermarket shelves: for example, fat-free salad dressing, low-fat snacks, trans-free spreads, and low-fat ice cream. Remember: many lower-fat processed foods have the same or more total calories than their traditional counterparts. Read the Nutrition Facts on the food label to compare.

● Balance higher-fat food choices with lower-fat foods to stay within your fat budget—and still enjoy moderate amounts of higher-fat foods.

● Watch your "snack fats." Smart snacks fill in missing nutrient gaps, help control hunger, and can provide an energy boost between meals. But some popular snack foods are higher in fat, perhaps saturated fat, than you may realize. *See "Check Out the Difference: Snacks with More and with Less Fat!" on this page for nutritious snack options.*

CHECK OUT THE DIFFERENCE: SNACKS WITH MORE AND WITH LESS FAT!

SNACKS	FAT (GRAMS)	CALORIES
Apple (1 medium)	0	80
Spiced applesauce (½ cup)	0	95
Apple pie (⅛)	20	410
Banana (1)	0	105
Milk chocolate bar (1½ oz.)	13	225
Broccoli, raw (½ cup)	0	10
Chocolate chip cookie 2¼-in. (1)	4	80
Carrot (1 medium)	0	30
Carrot cake (1/12 of 9-in.)	11	240
Orange (1)	0	60
Corn chips (1 oz.)	10	155
Strawberries (½ cup)	0	20
French fries (10)	9	170
Salsa (¼ cup)	0	20
Sour cream dip (¼ cup)	8	100
Saltines (10 crackers, or 1 oz.)	4	130
Potato chips (1 ounce)	10	150
Frozen yogurt (½ cup)	4	115
Ice cream, regular (½ cup)	7	135
Angel food cake (1/12 of cake)	0	75
Pound cake (1/16 of loaf cake)	13	230
Gingersnaps (4) (1 oz.)	3	120
Butter cookies 2-in. (6) (1 oz.)	6	140
Bagel 3½-in. (1)		
With 2 tbsp. jam	1	290
With 2 tbsp. part skim ricotta cheese	4	240
With 2 tbsp. cream cheese	11	195
Doughnut (1 glazed/sugared)	10	190

● Defat your cooking style without losing flavor. For example, broil, bake, boil, steam, stir-fry, or microwave foods, rather than fry.

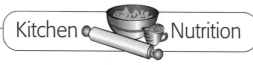

Kitchen Nutrition

Yogurt Cheese

Create this "fat replacer" in your kitchen. Yogurt cheese makes a thick spread for crackers or bagels; a creamy dip or salad dressing; a flavorful topper on baked potatoes and tacos; or a rich-tasting cheesecake or cream soup. Best of all, it's low in fat and high in calcium.

- Line a strainer with cheesecloth (double thickness) or a paper coffee filter. Or use a strainer specially designed for making yogurt cheese. Place the strainer over a deep bowl.

- Spoon gelatin-free yogurt into the strainer and cover. (Check the label to find out if it contains gelatin. Yogurt may be plain-, vanilla-, lemon-, coffee-, or fruit-flavored; however, this doesn't work with fat-free yogurt.) Refrigerate. Allow the liquid whey to drain into the bowl for two to twenty-four hours, depending on how firm you want the "cheese" to be. Drained for twenty-four hours, 32 ounces of yogurt will yield about 1½ cups of yogurt cheese.

- To flavor, blend 1½ cups of plain yogurt cheese with one of these combinations:

  - ⅔ cup apricot preserves and 3 tablespoons chopped almonds or walnuts

  - ¼ cup crumbled blue cheese, 1½ cups grated apple or pear, and 1 teaspoon sugar

  - 3 ounces salmon, 2 tablespoons chopped green onion, and 1 tablespoon chopped parsley

  - 3 tablespoons herb blend, 1 teaspoon garlic, and pepper (to taste)

For more low-fat cooking tips, see chapter 13, "Kitchen Nutrition."

Source: St. Louis District Dairy Council.

- Add flavor with herbs and spices instead of high-fat flavorings or sauces. Rub mixtures of seasonings on tender cuts of meat before cooking for wonderful blends of flavors. Use low-fat or fat-free marinades to tenderize and add flavor to lean cuts of meat.

- When you can, substitute foods and ingredients high in unsaturated fatty acids for those high in saturated fatty acids. *The chart "Easy Substitutions to Cut Fat and/or Cholesterol" in chapter 13 offers a list of easy ways.*

- Watch your portion size. The amount of fat and cholesterol in your food choices depends on both what you eat and how much. Extra-large portions of higher-fat foods provide extra-large amounts of fat.

- Make beans the "main event" at meals occasionally. Meals with cooked dry beans as the main protein source have several cholesterol-lowering qualities. *Usually* bean dishes are lower in total fat, saturated fat, and cholesterol—yet higher in complex carbohydrates and fiber—than dishes made with meat or cheese.

- Order "lean" when you order out. In a fast-food or table-service restaurant, look for menu clues that suggest less fat, such as "grilled" or "broiled." Ask questions about how food is prepared. And go easy on foods that are fried, breaded, or prepared with rich sauces or gravy.

Need more lean and low-fat strategies for healthful eating? Check here for "how-tos":

- Shop for foods with less fat and cholesterol—see chapter 11.

- Trim fat in your kitchen without giving up flavor—see chapter 13.

- Cut back on fat in restaurant orders—and enjoy food, too—see chapter 14.

- Enjoy a vegetarian approach to low-fat eating—see chapter 20.

- Handle fats, "sat fats," and cholesterol to manage heart disease and other chronic diseases—see chapter 22.

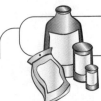

Label Lingo

Fats and Cholesterol

Check food labels for clues about fat and cholesterol. On the front of the package you may find nutrient content claims.

LABEL TERM . . .	MEANS . . .
For Fat Content . . .	
Fat-free	Less than 0.5 gram fat per serving
Low-fat	3 grams or less of fat per serving
Reduced or less fat	At least 25% less fat* per serving
Light	1/3 fewer calories or 50% less fat* per serving
____ % fat-free	The food meets the definition of "low-fat" or "fat-free" if stated as 100% fat-free
Light meal	"Low-fat" (at least 50% less fat per serving*) or "low-calorie" meal (at least 1/3 fewer calories per serving*)
Low-fat meal	3 grams or less fat per 100 grams, and 30 percent or less calories from fat
For Saturated Fat Content . . .	
Saturated-fat-free	Less than 0.5 gram saturated fat and less than 0.5 gram trans fatty acids per serving
Low saturated fat	1 gram or less saturated fat per serving and no more than 15% of calories from saturated fat

LABEL TERM . .	MEANS . . .
Reduced or less saturated fat	At least 25% less saturated fat*
For Cholesterol Content . . .	
Cholesterol-free	Less than 2 milligrams cholesterol and 2 grams or less of saturated fat per serving
Low cholesterol	20 milligrams or less cholesterol and 2 grams or less of saturated fat per serving
Reduced or less cholesterol	At least 25% less cholesterol* and 2 grams or less of saturated fat per serving
For Fat, Saturated Fat, and Cholesterol Content . . .	
Lean†	Less than 10 grams total fat, 4.5 grams or less saturated fat, and 95 milligrams cholesterol per 3-ounce serving and per 100 grams
Extra lean†	Less than 5 grams total fat, 2 grams saturated fat, and 95 milligrams cholesterol per 3-ounce serving and per 100 grams

*As compared with a standard serving size of the traditional food

†On packaged seafood or game meat, cooked meat, or cooked poultry

For Less Saturated Fat . . .

● Limit solid fats such as butter, stick margarine, lard, and partially hydrogenated shortenings; when you can, use vegetable oils instead. Liquid vegetable oils have less saturated fatty acids and more unsaturated fatty acids than fats that are firm at room temperature. Go easy on animal fats, too, since they're more saturated. For example, choose soft tub or squeeze (liquid) margarine in place of stick margarine or butter. And try polyunsaturated or monounsaturated oil in recipes calling for melted shortening or butter. *Check "Lean Tips . . . for Baked Goods" in chapter 13 for making substitutions with vegetable oil in baked goods.*

● Cut back on total fat. You'll likely reduce saturated fats—and trans fats, too. Tip: if you eat less "sat fat," you'll have some leeway for plant-based foods with unsaturated fat. That doesn't mean overdoing on total fat or calories, however.

● Check the Nutrition Facts on food labels for the saturated fat in one serving; choose foods with less. Check the ingredient list, too. If any of these ingredients is among the first several listed, the food is likely higher in saturated fat: butter, partially hydrogenated vegetable oil, coconut oil, palm oil, palm kernel oil, cocoa butter, meat fat, lard, egg yolks, whole milk solids, cream, or cheese.

For Less Cholesterol . . .

● Go easy on egg yolks to keep under the 300-milligram limit for cholesterol in your day's food choices. That includes the eggs in prepared foods such as bread,

cakes, and pancakes. Remember, the yolk has all the cholesterol—about 215 milligrams in the yolk from a large egg. An egg white has no cholesterol. Tip: substitute two egg whites for one whole egg in baked goods, or use an egg substitute.

● Go easy on organ meats such as liver. Even though they're nutritious, they're high in cholesterol.

● Look for leaner meat, fish, poultry, and low-fat dairy foods. You won't eliminate all the cholesterol, but you'll trim away some cholesterol along with less fat.

● Check food labels to find foods that are low in cholesterol or cholesterol-free. *See "Label Lingo: Fats and Cholesterol" on page 72.*

Have You Ever Wondered

. . . if coconut milk is high in fat? One cup of canned coconut milk (made by combining grated coconut meat and coconut water) contains 445 calories and 48 fat grams (of which 43 fat grams are saturated). Coconut water, or liquid, drained from a fresh coconut—without any grated coconut meat—has just 46 calories and less than 1 fat gram per cup. Just ¼ cup of dried, sweetened coconut has 87 calories and 6 fat grams.

. . . if salmon is lower in fat than chicken? Salmon has about 185 calories and 9 fat grams per 3-ounce cooked portion compared with 190 calories and 9 fat grams in the same portion of roasted, light-meat chicken with the skin on. Skinless, this same portion of chicken contains about 150 calories and 3 fat grams. The potential benefits of salmon: more omega-3 fatty acids.

. . . if air-popped popcorn is always low in fat? Not always. If you buy it ready-made, check the Nutrition Facts for the fat and saturated fat content. Although the package may say "air-popped," oil may be added after

popping as a flavoring. For microwave popcorn, check the label to see if oil is added—and how much and what kind. And what about the bucket of popcorn you buy in malls or movie theaters? It's usually loaded with fat; satisfy your appetite with the small-size order.

. . . if ghee is a good substitute for butter? Commonly used in the cuisine of India, ghee is clarified butter. It's been heated, then strained to remove milk solids so the fat is slightly concentrated—with more fat and calories per teaspoon. Why clarify butter? Without the milk solids, it can be heated to a higher temperature without burning.

. . . how the fat in feta cheese compares with that in other cheeses? It's somewhat lower—but not much. An ounce of feta cheese has 6 grams of fat, which includes 4 grams of saturated fat. By comparison, 1 ounce of Cheddar cheese has 9 total fat grams, including 6 grams of saturated fat. With their intense pungent flavors, however, smaller amounts of stronger cheeses such as feta, Parmesan, and blue cheese go a long way in delivering flavor.

CHAPTER 4

Vitamins, Minerals, and Phytonutrients

Variety on Your Plate!

Vitamins, minerals, and phytonutrients: your body needs them—*perhaps more of them*—for your good health. That's positive nutrition! Just how much do you need for optimal health, not just enough to avoid a deficiency? What foods are your best sources? And how do these food substances keep you fit?

Although headlines may seem confounding, there's plenty that's well known about the roles of vitamins, minerals, and phytonutrients (plant substances) in health. Over the past century, research has unlocked puzzles related to widespread deficiencies. Today's nutrition breakthroughs focus less on cures and more on the roles of nutrients, phytonutrients, and other food substances in health promotion and in protection from cancer, heart disease, and osteoporosis, to name a few health problems.

- *Today,* more than forty nutrients, including vitamins and minerals, have been identified in food. Their functions, the amount you need at different stages of your life, and their food sources are better understood.

- *Today,* we know more about the balance of vitamins and minerals—and the variety of foods—that allow the body to absorb and use them most efficiently. In other words, we're discovering what's enough, but not too much, for our unique, individual needs.

- *Today,* science is exploring a new frontier: substances in food, including phytonutrients, that offer health benefits beyond basic nourishment.

The bottom line? A variety of food (not a cabinetful of supplements)—with plenty of vitamins, minerals, and phytonutrients—is part of your ticket to good health!

Vitamins and Minerals: Team Players!

Vitamins and minerals are key to every process that takes place in your body. They don't work alone, but instead in close partnership with other nutrients to make every body process happen normally: from helping carbohydrates, proteins, and fats produce energy, to assisting with protein synthesis (the creation of new proteins), to building your healthy bones, to helping you think about the words on this page.

- Vitamins are complex substances that work as regulators. Often they act as coenzymes, or partners, with enzymes, the proteins that cause reactions to take place in your body.

- Minerals are part of many cells, including (but not only) the hard parts: bone, teeth, and nails. Minerals also are part of enzymes and may trigger your body's enzymatic reactions.

Compared with carbohydrates, proteins, and fats, your body needs vitamins and minerals in only small amounts, so they're called *micro*nutrients. Don't let these small amounts fool you, however. Vitamins and minerals don't supply energy directly. But they do regulate many processes that produce energy—and do a whole lot more!

Read on to explore the many vitamins and minerals we know most about: their varied, yet integrated roles in health; recommended intakes (for most, but not all); and food sources. *The Appendices give specific recommendations—Dietary Reference Intakes (DRIs)—for vitamins and minerals, for people of all ages.* Within this chapter, you'll also get a broader look at vitamins A and C, calcium, and iron, which often appear on the Nutrition Facts of food labels. *For more about vitamins and mineral supplements, see "Vitamin and Mineral Supplements (Selected): Claims, Benefits, Risks" in chapter 23.*

Vitamins: The Basics

Vitamins belong in two groups: water-soluble and fat-soluble. The category describes an important quality—how they are carried in food and transported in your body.

As their name implies, water-soluble vitamins (B-complex vitamins and vitamin C) dissolve in water. They're carried in your bloodstream. For the most part,

---

Click Here!

How do your favorite foods stack up for vitamins and minerals? Other nutrients? Calories? All these facts are within your easy reach; just check the Nutrition Facts on a food package. *For the nutrient database from the U.S. Department of Agriculture, http://www.nal.usda.gov/fnic/foodcomp is the appropriate Web site.*

---

water-soluble vitamins aren't stored in your body—at least not in significant amounts. Instead, your body uses what it needs, then excretes the extra amount through urine. Since they aren't stored, you need a regular supply of water-soluble vitamins from your food choices.

How much do you need? Enough, but not too much. Even though you excrete excess amounts of water-soluble vitamins, moderation is still the best approach. For example, taking large doses of vitamin C from a dietary supplement may create extra work for your kidneys, causing kidney stones, as well as diarrhea. Likewise, too much niacin, vitamin B_6, folate, or pantothenic acid also may be harmful. Read on to learn why.

You've probably guessed that fat-soluble vitamins (vitamins A, D, E, and K) dissolve in fat. That's how they're carried into your bloodstream and throughout your body—attached to body chemicals made with lipids, or fat. And that's one reason why you need only moderate amounts of fat in your food choices.

Your body can store fat-soluble vitamins in body fat, so consuming too much of any fat-soluble vitamins for too long—usually from vitamin pills or other dietary supplements—can be harmful. Vitamins A and D, for example, can build up to toxic levels. High intakes of vitamins E and K usually aren't linked to symptoms of toxicity. *For more about dietary supplements, see chapter 23.*

Alphabet Soup: What Are DRIs?

Dietary Reference Intakes (DRIs). Daily nutrient recommendations—expressed as RDAs or AIs—based on age and gender; set at levels to decrease the risk of chronic disease through nutrition

Recommended Dietary Allowances (RDAs). Recommended daily levels of nutrients to meet the needs of almost all healthy individuals in a specific age and gender group; used when there's scientific consensus for a firm nutrient recommendation

Adequate Intakes (AIs). Similar to RDAs, and used for nutrients that lack sufficient scientific evidence to determine a firm RDA

Tolerable Upper Intake Level (UL). Not a recommendation; maximum intake that most likely won't pose risks for health problems for almost all healthy people in that age and gender group

Source: Institute of Medicine, National Academy of Sciences.

Daily Values (DVs) for nutrients aren't DRIs, although they are based on RDA values from the past. DVs are used for food labeling.

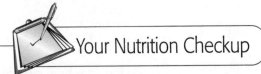

Your Nutrition Checkup

Can You Count Up to "Five a Day"?

Fruits and vegetables are among your body's best sources of many (but not all) vitamins and minerals—and phytonutrients, including fiber. Fruits and vegetables are rich sources of carotenoids (which form vitamin A), vitamin C, folate, and potassium; *for examples, see the chart "Produce Package" in chapter 10.* And even though they're filling, most are naturally low in calories and fat.

That's why the Dietary Guidelines for Americans advise you to enjoy a variety of fruits and vegetables in your daily food choices: eat five servings a day. Better yet, eat more—but at least two servings of fruits and three servings of vegetables a day!

● Try to eat at least one carotene-rich choice daily.

● Eat at least one vitamin C-rich choice daily.

● Eat plenty of high-fiber choices.

Now take a moment to consider what you ate yesterday. How many fruit and vegetable servings did you consume? Were they good sources of carotenoids (vitamin A) and vitamin C? If so, make a check to show which one.

	HOW MANY?		CHECK FOR	
	VEGETABLES	FRUITS	CAROTENOIDS	VITAMIN C
At breakfast?	_____	_____	_____	_____
At lunch?	_____	_____	_____	_____
For snacks?	_____	_____	_____	_____
At dinner?	_____	_____	_____	_____
For dessert?	_____	_____	_____	_____
Subtotals	_____	_____	_____	_____

Now repeat this exercise for today, then for two more days . . . and keep track. Answer "yes" or "no." Did you consume . . .

	DAY 1	DAY 2	DAY 3
At least five servings of vegetables and fruits?	_____	_____	_____
A source of carotenoids?	_____	_____	_____
A source of vitamin C?	_____	_____	_____

If most of your answers are "yes," you get the nutrient benefits of plenty of fruits and vegetables.

If you mostly answered "no," *check out the ideas in chapter 13 for fitting more fruits and vegetables in.*

On the Label

Without looking, do you know which vitamins and minerals appear on food labels? The four required on the Nutrition Facts need your special attention: vitamins A and C, calcium, and iron. Consume enough of these nutrients to reduce your risk for some common health problems. Other nutrients may appear on the label: some voluntarily, others required if these nutrients are added.

Be aware: Daily Values (DVs) for nutrients, used with food labeling, may differ from today's DRIs. DVs for nutrients are based on previous RDAs. *See "% Daily Values: What Are They Based On?" in the appendices.*

Nutrition Facts
Serving Size 1 cup (248g)
Servings Per Container 4

Amount Per Serving

Calories 150   Calories from Fat 35

% Daily Value*

Total Fat 4g	**6%**
Saturated Fat 2.5g	**12%**
Cholesterol 20mg	**7%**
Sodium 170mg	**7%**
Total Carbohydrate 17g	**6%**
Dietary Fiber 0g	**0%**
Sugars 17g	
Protein 13g	

Vitamin A 4%	•	Vitamin C 6%
Calcium 40%	•	Iron 0%

Percent Daily Values are based on a 2,000 calorie diet. Your daily values may be higher or lower depending on your calorie needs:

		Calories:	2,000	2,500
Total Fat	Less than		65g	80g
Sat Fat	Less than		20g	25g
Cholesterol	Less than		300mg	300mg
Sodium	Less than		2,400mg	2,400mg
Total Carbohydrate			300g	375g
Dietary Fiber			25g	30g

Calories per gram:
Fat 9 • Carbohydrate 4 • Protein 4

Read on to find out how vitamins keep you healthy: their functions, effects of getting too little or too much, Dietary Reference Intakes (DRIs), and their food sources. *Note:* On the following pages, the amounts of vitamins in food have been rounded.

Fat-Soluble Vitamins

Vitamin A (and Carotenoids)

See also "Carotenoids: 'Color' Your Food Healthy" in this chapter.

What it does:

● Promotes normal vision, and helps your eyes see normally in the dark, helping adjust to the lower level of light.

Vitamin-Rich Cures

Nutrition history is full of fascinating stories of nutrient-deficiency diseases that confounded doctors of the past.

● The scourge of *scurvy,* which plagued seafarers several hundred years ago, was finally cured by stocking ships with lemons, oranges, and limes; hence, British sailors were called "limeys." Scurvy is caused by a deficiency of vitamin C, a nutrient that citrus fruits provide in abundance.

● *Night blindness,* often caused by a deficiency of vitamin A, was known in ancient Egypt. The recommended cure of the day: eating ox or rooster livers. Today it's well known that liver contains more vitamin A than many other foods.

● Giving children cod liver oil to prevent *rickets* was practiced in the nineteenth century. But not until 1922, when vitamin D was discovered, did scientists know what substance in cod liver oil gave protection.

● *Beriberi,* a deficiency of thiamin, was noted in Asia as polished, or white, rice became more popular than unrefined, or brown, rice. The cure was discovered accidentally when chickens with symptoms of beriberi ate the part of rice that was discarded after polishing. It contained the vitamin-rich germ. Today the process of enrichment adds thiamin and other B vitamins back to polished rice; today rice is fortified with folic acid, too.

● Promotes the growth and health of cells and tissues throughout your body; important for reproduction and development of the embryo

● Protects you from infections by keeping skin and tissues in your mouth, stomach, intestines, and respiratory, genital, and urinary tracts healthy.

● Works as an antioxidant in the form of carotenoids, and may reduce your risk for certain cancers and other diseases of aging.

Carotenoids (which form vitamin A) are thought to have health benefits beyond being precursors for vitamin A; *these potential health benefits are addressed later in this chapter.*

If you don't get enough: Night blindness; other eye problems; dry, scaly skin; problems with reproduction; and poor growth are symptoms of a significant deficiency. The deficiency disease from too little vitamin A is called xerophthalmia.

If you consume excess amounts: Because it's stored in your body, large intakes of vitamin A, taken over time, can be quite harmful: headaches, dry and scaly skin, liver damage, bone and joint pain, vomiting or appetite loss, abnormal bone growth, nerve damage, and birth defects. Almost always, these symptoms result from high intakes of vitamin A from dietary supplements, not from food. Beta carotene from fruits and vegetables is okay! The Tolerable Upper Intake Limit is 2,800 micrograms of Retinal Activity Equivalent (RAE) daily for ages fourteen to eighteen, and 3,000 micrograms daily during adulthood. (Retinol, beta carotene, and other provitamin A carotenoids determine RAE.)

How much you need: From age fourteen on, the RDA is 900 micrograms RAE of vitamin A for males and 700 micrograms RAE for females. During pregnancy, the recommendation is 770 micrograms per day, and during breast-feeding, 1,200 micrograms RAE daily.

Note: The 2001 RDAs measure vitamin A in Retinol Activity Equivalents (RAEs), reflecting retinol and carotenoid units. You might see vitamin A expressed in other ways: International Units (IU)—used for food labels and dietary supplements, or as Retinol Equivalents (RE)—used in the 1989 RDAs and many nutrient databases.

Here's how to convert Retinol Equivalents to Retinol Activity Equivalents. For vitamin A derived from:

● Animal-based foods or supplements   1 RE = 1 RAE

● Plant-based foods   1 RE divided by 2 = 1 RAE

Where it's mostly found: The body gets vitamin A in two ways:

● In animal sources of foods, vitamin A, in the form of retinol, is completely made (or preformed). Vitamin A comes from liver, fish oil, eggs, milk fortified with vitamin A, and other vitamin A–fortified foods.

● Carotenoids, such as alpha carotene and beta carotene, come from foods of plant origin. Certain carotenoids are modified to form vitamin A (referred to as "provitamin A carotenoids") in your body. Carotenoids are found in red, yellow, orange, and many dark-green leafy vegetables. Plant sources of carotenoids are especially important to those who eat few animal-based foods.

Do you get most or all of your beta carotene (which turns to vitamin A) from fruits and vegetables? If so, you may need to eat more of them! According to the 2001 DRI report from the Institute of Medicine, the conversion of carotenoids to vitamin A was overestimated in the past. In fact, it takes twice the amount of carotene-rich foods to meet the body's vitamin A needs as once thought.

See the following "Vitamin A and Carotenoids: Good Picks" for a list of good sources and amounts.

Vitamin D

See also "Vitamin D: The Sunshine Vitamin" in chapter 18.

What it does:

● Promotes the absorption of two minerals—calcium and phosphorus—and regulates how much calcium remains in your blood.

● Helps deposit these minerals in bones and teeth, making them stronger and healthier.

If you don't get enough: In your older years, you may have greater loss of bone mass (osteoporosis), and

---

Vitamin A and Carotenoids: Good Picks

Besides supplying essential carotenoids, enjoy at least one serving of carotene-rich fruit or vegetables daily for the antioxidant power, too! Vitamin A content is given below in two ways: in approximate Retinol Equivalents (currently used in many nutrient databases) and in approximate Retinol Activity Equivalents (used with 2001 RDAs for vitamin A).

FOOD	RETINOL EQUIVALENTS (RE)* (APPROXIMATE)	RETINOL ACTIVITY EQUIVALENTS (RAE)* (APPROXIMATE)	FOOD	RETINOL EQUIVALENTS (RE)* (APPROXIMATE)	RETINOL ACTIVITY EQUIVALENTS (RAE)* (APPROXIMATE)
Beef liver, cooked (3 oz.)	9,085	9,085	Egg, large (1)	95	95
Sweet potato, mashed (½ cup)	2,800	1,400	Milk, whole (1 cup)	75	75
Carrot (1 medium)	2,025	1,015	Tomato, medium, raw (1)	75	35
Kale, boiled (½ cup)	480	240	Broccoli, raw (½ cup)	70	35
Mango, medium (½)	405	200	Green bell pepper, raw (½ cup)	30	15
Turnip greens, cooked (½ cup)	395	200	Collards, frozen, boiled (½ cup)	30	15
Spinach, raw (1 cup)	375	185	Orange, medium (1)	30	15
Papaya, medium (½)	305	150			
Red bell pepper, raw (½ cup)	285	140			
Apricot (3)	275	135			
Cantaloupe (½ cup)	260	130			
Milk, fat-free (1 cup)	150	150			
Romaine lettuce (1 cup)	145	70			

Many fortified foods, including breakfast cereals, supply vitamin A, too. Read the Nutrition Facts on food labels to see how much.

*The % Daily Values—used on food labels and many dietary supplements—are based in International Units (IUs) for vitamin A.

your risk of softening of the bones (osteomalacia) increases. Children with a significant vitamin D deficiency may develop rickets, or defective bone growth. Fortifying milk with vitamin D has virtually wiped out rickets in the United States. Rickets may, however, become a problem again if juice or soft drinks are consumed regularly in place of milk.

If you consume excess amounts: Because it's stored in your body, too much vitamin D can be toxic, possibly leading to kidney stones or damage, weak muscles and bones, excessive bleeding, and other problems. An overdose usually comes from dietary supplements, not food—and not from overexposure to sunlight. For that reason, an upper limit, or Tolerable Upper Intake Level (ULs), of 2,000 International Units (IU), or 50 micrograms, per day for people ages one and over was set as part of the Dietary Reference Intakes (DRIs).

How much you need: From birth through age fifty, the recommendation for an Adequate Intake (AI) has been set at 5 micrograms cholecalciferol (which is the form of vitamin D in an animal-based food) or 200 International Units (IU) daily, with no increased need during pregnancy or breast-feeding. One microgram cholecalciferol = 40 IU vitamin D. To maintain healthy bones, the guideline for vitamin D goes up to 10 micrograms, or 400 IU, daily for adults over age fifty. Over seventy years, the guideline increases to 15 micrograms, or 600 IU, per day.

Vitamin D from plant-based foods is in a different form.

Where it's mostly found: Known as the "sunshine vitamin," your body can make vitamin D after sunlight, or ultraviolet light, hits your skin. That's no excuse for overexposure to sun from sunbathing. To get enough, it takes only twenty to forty minutes of sun, three times a week, on your hands, arms, and face without sunscreen. Darker skin needs more sun exposure; lighter skin, less.

As a precaution (especially during the winter), for people who don't get outdoors much, and for older people whose skin is less efficient at converting sun exposure to vitamin D, milk is fortified with vitamin D. Cheese, eggs, some fish (sardines and salmon), and fortified breakfast cereals and margarine also contain small amounts of vitamin D.

Food	Vitamin D (International Units)
Salmon with bones, canned (3 oz.)	190–535
Milk, most types (1 cup)	100
Cornflakes (1 cup)	40
Egg, large (1)	25
Margarine (1 tsp.)	20

Vitamin E

See also "Vitamin E: One Main Mission" later in this chapter.

What it does:

● Works as an antioxidant, preventing the oxidation of LDL cholesterol, and perhaps lowering the risk for heart disease and stroke. Its antioxidant activity also may help reduce the risk of other health problems, such as some types of cancer.

● As an antioxidant, protects essential fatty acids and vitamin A. *See "Antioxidant Vitamins: A Closer Look" later in this chapter to learn how antioxidants seem to work.*

If you don't get enough: Most Americans consume enough vitamin E to meet recommendations, according to the Institute of Medicine (2000). Because it's so abundant in food, a deficiency of vitamin E is rare. The two exceptions are premature, very-low-birth-weight infants and people with poor fat absorption, cystic fibrosis, or some other chronic health problems. In these cases, the nervous system can be affected. Because vegetable oils are good sources of vitamin E, people on low-fat diets might not get enough.

If you consume excess amounts: Eating plenty of vitamin E-rich foods doesn't appear to be a problem. However, taking large doses of vitamin E as a dietary supplement appears to have no benefits—and isn't recommended. Too much may increase the risk of bleeding, may impair vitamin K action, and may increase the effect of anticoagulant medication.

That's why a Tolerable Upper Intake Level (UL) has been set: 800 milligrams daily for teens ages fourteen to eighteen; 1,000 milligrams of alpha-tocopherol daily for adults ages 19 and over. If you take a supplement, 1,000 milligrams equal about 1,500 IU of natural vitamin E or 1,100 IU of dl-alpha-tocopherol synthetic vitamin E.

How much you need: The RDA guideline for males and females age 14 and over is 15 milligrams of alpha-tocopherol each day. Children need less, depending on their age. During pregnancy, women still need 15 milligrams daily; during breast-feeding the recommendation goes up to 19 milligrams daily.

Note: Vitamin E is a group of substances called tocopherols with different potencies. Alpha-tocopherol is its most potent form. On food and supplement labels, the amount is given in International Units (IU) of alpha-tocopherol, not in milligrams.

To make the conversion, 15 milligrams of alpha-tocopherol (the RDA for adults) equal:

- About 22 IU of d-alpha-tocopherol ("natural" vitamin E in some supplements)

- About 33 IU of dl-alpha-tocopherol (a synthetic form in fortified foods and some supplements)

The "natural" form of vitamin E is more fully used than the synthetic form. That's why there's a difference in the conversion factor.

Where it's mostly found: The best sources of vitamin E are vegetable oils—for example, soybean, corn, cottonseed, and safflower. That includes margarine, salad dressing, and other foods made from oil. Nuts (especially almonds and hazelnuts), seeds (especially sunflower seeds), and wheat germ—all high in oil—are good sources, too. Green, leafy vegetables provide smaller amounts.

Food	VITAMIN E (MG ALPHA-TOCOPHEROL)
Sunflower seeds (1 oz.)	14
Almonds, dried (1 oz. or 24 nuts)	7
Hazelnuts, dried (1 oz.)	7
Wheat germ (¼ cup)	5
Peanut butter (2 tbsp.)	3
Corn oil (1 tbsp.)	3
Spinach, raw (1 cup)	1
Pecans, dried (1 oz. or 31 large nuts)	1

Have You Ever Wondered?

. . . if hair analysis is a valid way to diagnose a vitamin or mineral deficiency? Except to detect poisonous elements such as lead or arsenic, hair analysis isn't a valid way to check your nutritional status. Why? Hair grows slowly; the condition of hair strands differs along their length. Chemicals used to clean and treat hair affect its composition. Differences in age and gender also affect the quality of hair. Too often, those who promote hair analysis for nutrition reasons are also trying to promote dietary supplements. Buyer, beware!

. . . if vitamin E in skin moisturizers gets rid of wrinkles? Vitamins, amino acids, cocoa butter, or other nutrients in skin creams and cosmetics can't remove or prevent aging skin. The only possible exception is Retin-A, sold by prescription, which may slow the process. However, there's no research on its long-term effects. Protecting your skin from damage caused by ultraviolet light (sunshine) is the most important way you can slow the process of wrinkling. And moisturizing your skin daily with skin cream, preferably one containing a sun block of SPF 15 or more, will help, too.

Vitamin K

What it does:

- Makes proteins that cause your blood to coagulate, or clot, when you're bleeding. That way, bleeding stops.

- Helps your body make some other body proteins for your blood, bones, and kidneys.

If you don't get enough: Blood doesn't coagulate normally. Except for rare health problems, a deficiency of vitamin K is very unlikely. Prolonged use of antibiotics could be a problem, since they destroy some bacteria in your intestines that produce vitamin K.

If you consume excess amounts: No symptoms have been observed, but moderation is still the best approach. People taking blood-thinning drugs, or anticoagulants, need to eat foods with vitamin K in moderation. Too much can make blood clot faster. No Tolerable Upper Intake Level (UL) is established.

How much you need: The Adequate Intake (AI) advises 75 micrograms daily for teens ages fourteen to eighteen. During adulthood the intake goes up: 120

micrograms daily for men and 90 micrograms daily for women. Neither pregnancy nor breast-feeding increases the recommendation. To make sure infants have enough, newborns typically receive a shot of vitamin K.

Where it's mostly found: Like vitamin D, your body can produce vitamin K on its own—this time from certain bacteria in your intestines.

The best food sources are green, leafy vegetables such as spinach and broccoli. However, a variety of foods provide smaller amounts: milk and other dairy foods, meat, eggs, cereal, fruits, and other vegetables.

FOOD	VITAMIN K (MCG)
Spinach, raw (1 cup)	150
Broccoli, raw (½ cup)	60
Egg, large (1)	25
Wheat bran (1 oz.)	25
Wheat germ (1 oz.)	10
Milk (1 cup)	10
Strawberries (½ cup)	10
Orange, medium (1)	5

Water-Soluble Vitamins

Thiamin (vitamin B₁)

What it does:

● Helps produce energy from carbohydrates in all the cells of your body.

If you don't get enough: Because most people consume many grain products, a thiamin deficiency is rare in the United States today, with one exception: chronic alcoholics. Symptoms include fatigue, weak muscles, and nerve damage. Before refined grains were enriched with thiamin, a deficiency was common, sometimes resulting in a disease called beriberi, which affects mainly the cardiovascular and nervous systems.

If you consume excess amounts: Your body excretes any excess amount you may consume. Contrary to popular claims, extra amounts have no energy-boosting effect.

How much you need: The RDA for thiamin is tied to your energy needs: 1.2 milligrams daily for males age fourteen through adulthood. For females, the recom-

mendation is 1.0 milligram daily from ages fourteen through eighteen and 1.1 milligrams daily from age nineteen on. During pregnancy and breast-feeding, the amount recommended goes up to 1.4 milligrams daily.

Where it's mostly found: Whole-grain and enriched grain products such as bread, rice, pasta, tortillas, and fortified cereals provide much of the thiamin we eat. Enrichment adds back nutrients, including many B vitamins, lost when grains are refined. Pork, liver, and other organ meats provide significant amounts, too.

FOOD	THIAMIN (MG)
Pork, lean, broiled (3 oz.)	0.8
Beef liver, braised (3 oz.)	0.2
Enriched corn tortilla (1)	0.2
Enriched rice, cooked (½ cup)	0.2
Whole-grain bread (1 slice)	0.1

Riboflavin (vitamin B₂)

What it does:

● Helps produce energy in all cells of your body.

● Helps change the amino acid called tryptophan in your food into niacin. (Protein is made of many different amino acids.)

If you don't get enough: Except for people who are severely malnourished, a deficiency isn't likely. Deficiency symptoms include eye disorders (including cataracts); dry and flaky skin; and a sore, red tongue.

Have You Ever Wondered ?

... *what B complex vitamins are?* They're a "vitamin family" with related roles in health: thiamin (vitamin B₁), riboflavin (vitamin B₂), niacin, vitamin B₆, folate, vitamin B₁₂, biotin, and pantothenic acid. Besides their varied, unique body functions, most B vitamins help your body produce energy within its trillions of cells.

... *how cooking affects the vitamin content of foods?* Water-soluble vitamins are destroyed more easily by food preparation, processing, and storage than fat-soluble vitamins are. *For food handling tips to retain vitamins, see "Simple Ways to Keep Vitamins in Food" in chapter 13.*

Contrary to popular myth, riboflavin deficiency doesn't cause hair loss.

If you consume excess amounts: No reports suggest problems from consuming too much.

How much you need: Like thiamin, the RDA for riboflavin is tied to your energy needs. Adult men need 1.3 milligrams daily and adult women need 1.1 milligrams daily. During pregnancy, the recommendation is 1.4 milligrams; during breast-feeding, the amount goes up to 1.6 milligrams daily.

Where it's mostly found: Milk and other dairy foods are major sources of riboflavin. Some organ meats—liver, kidney, and heart—are excellent sources. Enriched bread and other grain products; eggs; meat; green, leafy vegetables; and nuts supply smaller amounts. Because ultraviolet light, such as sunlight, destroys riboflavin, milk is packed in opaque plastic or cardboard containers, not clear glass.

FOOD	RIBOFLAVIN (MG)
Beef liver, braised (3 oz.)	3.5
Yogurt, fat-free with dry milk solids (1 cup)	0.4
Milk, fat-free (1 cup)	0.4
Enriched corn tortilla (1)	0.2
Egg, large (1)	0.2
Whole-grain bread (1 slice)	0.1

Niacin

What it does:

● Helps your body use sugars and fatty acids.

● Helps enzymes function normally in your body.

● Helps produce energy in all the cells of your body.

If you don't get enough: For people who consume adequate amounts of protein-rich foods, a niacin deficiency isn't likely. Pellagra is caused by a significant niacin deficiency. Symptoms include diarrhea, mental disorientation, and skin problems.

If you consume excess amounts: Consuming excessive amounts, likely from a dietary supplement, may cause flushed skin, rashes, or liver damage. The Tolerable Upper Intake Level (UL) is 35 milligrams daily for adults, and 30 milligrams daily for teens ages fourteen to eighteen. Self-prescribing large doses of niacin to lower blood cholesterol may lead to adverse effects—and may not give cholesterol-lowering benefits. If your doctor prescribes niacin, be sure to take it in the recommended dosage.

How much you need: Niacin recommendations are given in NE, or niacin equivalents. That's because it comes from two sources: niacin itself and from the amino acid called tryptophan, part of which converts to niacin.

Like thiamin and riboflavin, the recommendation is tied to energy needs. The advice for adult males is 16 milligrams NE daily, and for adult females, 14 milligrams NE daily. During pregnancy, 18 milligrams NE is advised; during breast-feeding, 17 milligrams NE daily.

Where it's mostly found: Foods high in protein are typically good sources of niacin: poultry, fish, beef, peanut butter, and legumes. Niacin is also added to many enriched and fortified grain products.

FOOD	NIACIN (MG NE)
Turkey breast, roasted, without skin (3 oz.)	6.0
Peanut butter (2 tbsp.)	4.0
Codfish, cooked (3 oz.)	2.0
Enriched corn tortilla (1)	1.5
Enriched spaghetti, cooked (½ cup)	1.0
Black-eyed peas, frozen, cooked (½ cup)	0.5
Lima beans, boiled (½ cup)	0.5
Yogurt, fat-free with dry milk solids (1 cup)	0.5

Pyridoxine (vitamin B$_6$)

What it does:

● Helps your body make nonessential amino acids, or protein components, which are then used to make body cells.

● Helps turn the amino acid called tryptophan into two important body substances: niacin and serotonin (a messenger in your brain).

● Helps produce other body chemicals, including insulin, hemoglobin, and antibodies that fight infection.

If you don't get enough: A deficiency can cause mental convulsions among infants; depression; nausea; or greasy, flaky skin. For infants, breast milk and properly prepared infant formulas contain enough.

If you consume excess amounts: Large doses, taken over time, can cause nerve damage. The Tolerable Upper Intake Level (UL) is 100 milligrams daily for adults and 80 milligrams daily for teens ages fourteen to eighteen.

How much you need: The RDA is 1.3 milligrams daily for adult males and females through age fifty. After age fifty, the RDA increases to 1.7 milligrams daily for males and 1.5 milligrams for females. The amount increases to 1.9 milligrams daily during pregnancy and 2.0 milligrams daily during breast-feeding.

Where it's mostly found: Chicken, fish, pork, liver, and kidney are the best sources. Whole grains, nuts, and legumes also supply reasonable amounts.

FOOD	PYRIDOXINE (MG)
Chicken, light meat, skinless, roasted (3 oz.)	0.5
Pork, loin, roasted (3 oz.)	0.5
Peanut butter (2 tbsp.)	0.1
Black beans, boiled (½ cup)	0.1
Whole-wheat spaghetti, cooked (½ cup)	0.1
Almonds (1 oz.)	<0.1

Folate (folic acid or folacin)

What it does:

● Plays an essential role in making new body cells by helping to produce DNA and RNA, the cell's master plan for cell reproduction.

● Works with vitamin B_{12} to form hemoglobin in red blood cells.

● May help protect against heart disease.

● Helps lower the risk of delivering a baby with neural tube defects such as spina bifida.

● Helps control plasma homocysteine levels, a substance associated with increased risk of cardiovascular disease.

If you don't get enough: A deficiency affects normal cell division and protein synthesis, especially impairing growth. Anemia, caused by malformed blood cells that can't carry as much oxygen, may result from a folate deficiency.

Pregnant women who don't get enough folate, especially during the first trimester, have a greater risk of delivering a baby with neural tube defects such as spina bifida. (The neural tube in an embryo becomes the spinal cord and brain.) To reduce risk, all women of childbearing age should consume adequate amounts. *See "Before Pregnancy" in chapter 17.*

If you consume excess amounts: Consuming too much can mask a vitamin B_{12} deficiency and may interfere with certain medications. Taking excess amounts as a dietary supplement offers no known benefits. For adults, the Tolerable Upper Intake Level (UL) is 1,000 micrograms daily of folic acid, the form of folate in fortified foods and supplements. For teens ages fourteen to eighteen, it's 800 micrograms daily.

Have You Ever Wondered

. . . about the difference between the terms "enriched" and "fortified"? Both terms indicate that nutrients—usually vitamins or minerals—were added to make a food more nutritious. *Enriched* means adding back nutrients that were lost during food processing. For example, B vitamins, lost when wheat is refined, are added back to white flour. *Fortified* means adding nutrients that weren't present originally. For example, milk is fortified with vitamin D, a nutrient that helps your body absorb milk's calcium and phosphorus. According to a recent law, most enriched grain products are now fortified with folic acid to reduce the incidence of certain birth defects.

. . . if microwave cooking destroys vitamins? Even if you cook foods properly, some water-soluble vitamins, such as B vitamins and vitamin C, can be destroyed. For several reasons, more vitamins are retained with microwave cooking than with most other methods: very short cooking time, covered cooking, and little or no cooking water.

How much you need: For folate, the RDA for males from age fourteen through adulthood is 400 micrograms daily. Folate can come from foods with naturally occurring folate, as well as from foods fortified with folic acid and from supplements.

As added protection against neural tube defects, women capable of becoming pregnant (fourteen to fifty years) should get 400 micrograms of folic acid daily from fortified foods, vitamin supplements, or a combination of the two, in addition to the folate found naturally in certain foods. Pregnancy increases the recommended amount to 600 micrograms daily; during breast-feeding, 500 micrograms are advised.

Where it's mostly found: Orange juice, lentils, dried beans, spinach, broccoli, peanuts, and avocados are among the good sources of naturally occurring folate. Enriched grain products—such as most breads, flour, crackers, corn grits, cornmeal, farina, rice, macaroni, and noodles—must be fortified with folic acid. Folic acid is the form of folate in fortified foods and supplements. Some breakfast cereals are fully fortified at 400 micrograms per serving—100 percent of the daily recommendation for many people. Unenriched grain products, such as some imported pastas, may not be fortified with folic acid. To be sure, check the Nutrition Facts on the label of grain products to see if folic acid has been added and how much.

FOOD	FOLATE (MCG)
Breakfast cereals, fortified with folic acid (¾–1 cup)	100–400
Spinach, boiled (½ cup)	130
Navy beans, boiled (½ cup)	125
Orange juice (1 cup)	110
Wheat germ (¼ cup)	80
Avocado (½)	55
Pasta, fortified with folic acid, cooked (½ cup)	50
Rice, fortified with folic acid, cooked (½ cup)	45
Bread, fortified with folic acid (1 slice)	40
Romaine lettuce, shredded (½ cup)	40
Peanuts, dried (1 oz.)	40
Milk, fat-free (1 cup)	15

Vitamin B_{12} (cobalamin)

See "Vitamin B_{12}: A Challenge for Vegans" in chapter 20.

What it does:

● Works closely with folate to make red blood cells.

● Serves as a vital part of many body chemicals and so occurs in every body cell.

● Helps your body use fatty acids and some amino acids.

If you don't get enough: A deficiency may result in anemia, fatigue, nerve damage, a smooth tongue, or very sensitive skin. A deficiency of vitamin B_{12} can be masked—and even progress—if extra folic acid is taken to treat or prevent anemia.

For either genetic or medical reasons, some people develop a deficiency—pernicious anemia—because they can't absorb vitamin B_{12}. They're missing a body chemical called intrinsic factor that comes from their stomach lining. This problem can be medically treated with injections of vitamin B_{12}.

Strict vegetarians, who eat no animal products, and the infants of vegan mothers are at risk for developing a vitamin B_{12} deficiency. This could cause severe anemia and irreversible nerve damage. The elderly also are at risk. Including foods fortified with vitamin B_{12} or dietary supplements can prevent vitamin B_{12} deficiency.

If you consume excess amounts: No symptoms are known, but taking extra vitamin B_{12} to boost energy has no basis in science.

How much you need: The RDA is 2.4 micrograms daily for adults. The recommendation increases to 2.6 micrograms daily during pregnancy and 2.8 micrograms daily during breast-feeding.

Where it's mostly found: Vitamin B_{12} comes from animal products—meat, fish, poultry, eggs, milk, and other dairy foods. Some fortified foods may contain it, too.

FOOD	VITAMIN B_{12} (MCG)
Salmon, cooked (3 oz.)	3.0
Beef tenderloin lean, broiled (3 oz.)	2.2

Food	
Yogurt, fat-free with dry milk solids (1 cup)	1.4
Shrimp, cooked (3 oz.)	1.3
Milk (1 cup)	0.9
Egg, large (1)	0.5
Chicken, light meat, skinless, roasted (3 oz.)	0.3

Biotin

What it does:

● Helps your body produce energy in your cells.

● Helps metabolize (or use) proteins, fats, and carbohydrates from food.

If you don't get enough: That's rarely a problem for healthy people who eat a healthful diet because the body also produces biotin from intestinal bacteria. In rare cases of deficiency, these symptoms may appear: heart abnormalities, appetite loss, fatigue, depression, or dry skin.

If you consume excess amounts: There are no reported effects of consuming excess amounts.

How much you need: The Adequate Intake (AI) for biotin is 30 micrograms daily for adult males and females, including during pregnancy. The AI increases to 35 micrograms daily during breast-feeding.

Where it's mostly found: Biotin is found in a wide variety of foods. Eggs, liver, yeast breads, and cereals are among the best sources.

Food	Biotin (mcg)
Egg, large (1)	10
Wheat germ (¼ cup)	6
Oatmeal, cooked (½ cup)	5
Shredded wheat cereal (1½ oz.)	4
Pancakes (three 4-in.)	3

Pantothenic Acid

What it does:

● Helps your body cells produce energy.

● Helps metabolize (or use) proteins, fats, and carbohydrates from food.

If you don't get enough: That's rarely a problem for healthy people who eat a healthful diet.

If you consume excess amounts: The only apparent effects are occasional diarrhea and water retention.

How much you need: The Adequate Intake (AI) for pantothenic acid is 5 milligrams daily for teens ages fourteen to eighteen and for adults. During pregnancy and breast-feeding, the AI increases to 6 and 7 milligrams, respectively.

Where it's mostly found: Pantothenic acid is widely available in food. Meat, poultry, fish, whole-grain cereals, and legumes are among the better sources. Milk, vegetables, and fruits also contain varying amounts.

Food	Pantothenic Acid (mg)
Salmon, cooked (3 oz.)	1.3
Chicken, light meat, skinless, roasted (3 oz.)	0.9
Yogurt, whole milk (1 cup)	0.9
Sweet potato, mashed, cooked (½ cup)	0.9
Milk, fat-free (1 cup)	0.8
Corn, boiled (½ cup)	0.7
Egg, large (1)	0.6
Ham, lean (3 oz.)	0.4
Whole-wheat macaroni, cooked (½ cup)	0.3
Kidney beans, cooked (½ cup)	0.2

Choline

What it does: Choline, a vitaminlike substance, plays a role in many body processes.

● Promotes the transport of fats and helps make substances that form cell membranes.

● Helps make acetylcholine, which is a neurotransmitter in your body needed for many functions, including muscle control and memory storage.

● Plays a role in liver function and reproductive health.

If you don't get enough: No clear cases of deficiencies in humans have been identified, but choline status may depend on consuming enough folate. Since scientific data are insufficient, it's not known if choline is essential in the diet; if so, how much is needed; and the effects of a deficiency.

If you consume excess amounts: The Tolerable Upper Intake Level (UL) for adults is 3.5 grams of choline daily; for teens ages fourteen to eighteen, 3.0 grams daily.

How much you need: There is no RDA for choline. However, Adequate Intake (AI) levels were set in 1998: 550 milligrams daily for males ages fourteen and older; 400 milligrams daily for girls ages fourteen to eighteen; and 425 milligrams daily for women. During pregnancy and breast-feeding, the AI increases to 450 milligrams and 550 milligrams, respectively.

Where it's mostly found: Choline, a natural food component, is widely distributed in food. Meat, liver, eggs, soybeans, and peanuts are especially good sources. Since the U.S. Food and Drug Administration has authorized nutrient content claims on food labels for choline, you may find new choline-fortified products.

FOOD	CHOLINE (MG)
Beef liver (3 oz.)	455
Egg, large (1)	345
Beef steak (3 oz.)	60
Peanuts (1 oz.)	30
Milk, whole (1 cup)	10

Vitamin C (ascorbic acid)

See "Vitamin C: More Jobs than You Think!" later in this chapter.

What it does:

- Helps produce collagen, a connective tissue that holds muscles, bones, and other tissues together.

- Helps keep capillary walls and blood vessels firm, and so protects you from bruising.

- Helps your body absorb iron and folate from plant sources of food.

- Helps keep your gums healthy.

- Helps heal any cuts and wounds.

- Protects you from infection by stimulating the formation of antibodies and so boosting immunity.

- Works as an antioxidant to inhibit damage to body cells.

If you don't get enough: Eventually, a severe deficiency of vitamin C leads to scurvy, a disease that causes loose teeth, excessive bleeding, and swollen gums. Wounds may not heal properly either. Because vitamin C-rich foods are widely available, scurvy is rare in the United States today.

If you consume an excess amount: Because vitamin C is water-soluble, your body excretes the excess; high levels of vitamin C in urine can mask the results of tests for diabetes. Very large doses may cause kidney stones and/or diarrhea, and for those with iron overload, excessive vitamin C (which enhances iron absorption) can make the problem worse. But the effects of taking large amounts for a long time isn't known. A Tolerable Upper Intake Level (UL) for vitamin C has been set: 2,000 milligrams daily for adults; 1,800 milligrams daily for teens ages fourteen to eighteen.

How much you need: The RDA for females and males ages fourteen to eighteen is 65 milligrams and 75 milligrams of vitamin C daily, respectively. Adult males need 90 milligrams daily; adult females, 75 milligrams of vitamin C daily for everyday needs (about the amount in ¾ cup of orange juice). Women need somewhat more during pregnancy (80 to 85 milligrams) and breast-feeding (115 to 120 milligrams).

For people who smoke, the RDA for vitamin C is *increased* by 35 milligrams daily to help counteract the oxidative damage from nicotine.

Have You Ever Wondered

. . . if bleeding gums mean you're not getting enough vitamin C? It's not likely unless you have a severe deficiency. Most cases of bleeding gums come from poor oral hygiene. Brushing and flossing regularly help keep your gums healthy. *For more about healthy gums, see chapter 22, page 575.*

Vitamin C: More than Citrus

Citrus fruits—oranges, grapefruits, tangerines—are well-known sources of vitamin C. Yet many other fruits and vegetables are excellent sources, too. Enjoy at least one serving of vitamin C-rich foods daily.

Food	Vitamin C (mg)
Guava, medium (1)	165
Red bell pepper (½ cup)	95
Papaya, medium (½)	95
Orange juice, from frozen concentrate (¾ cup)	75
Orange, medium (1)	60
Broccoli, boiled (½ cup)	60
Green bell pepper (½ cup)	45
Kohlrabi, boiled (½ cup)	45
Strawberries (½ cup)	45
Grapefruit, white (½)	40
Cantaloupe (½ cup)	35
Tomato juice (¾ cup)	35
Mango, medium (½)	30
Tangerine, medium (1)	25
Potato, baked with skin (1)	25
Cabbage, raw (½ cup)	25
Tomato, medium, raw (1)	25
Collard greens, frozen, boiled (½ cup)	25
Spinach, raw (1 cup)	15

Some fruit drinks and other processed foods are fortified with vitamin C. Check the Nutrition Facts on the label for the amount per serving. And remember, if you rely only on fortified foods as your vitamin C source, you may miss out on other nutrients and compounds present in foods with naturally occurring vitamin C.

Where it's mostly found: Vitamin C mainly comes from plant sources of food. All citrus fruits, including oranges, grapefruits, and tangerines, are good sources. And many other fruits and vegetables, including berries; melons; peppers; many green, dark leafy vegetables; potatoes; and tomatoes supply significant amounts, too. *See the sidebar "Vitamin C: More than Citrus" above for a list of good sources and amounts.*

Antioxidant Vitamins: A Closer Look

You've probably read the headlines "Antioxidants Promote Health!" or "Antioxidants Prevent Aging." A quick trip through the supermarket shows that many food manufacturers are fortifying food with beta carotene (which forms vitamin A in the body), vitamin C, and vitamin E, as well as selenium (a mineral).

Just what are antioxidants? They're dietary substances, including a handful of nutrients, that significantly slow or prevent the oxidative (damage from oxygen) process and so prevent or repair damage to your body cells. They may also improve immune function and perhaps lower risk for infection and cancer. What makes them unique? What foods supply them naturally? How might they work in your body? And how may antioxidants promote health and reduce the risk of chronic, or ongoing, diseases? Since antioxidants research is new, there's no conclusive evidence yet on their role in health. However, *"Rounding Up Free Radicals" later in this chapter explains how antioxidants appear to work.*

Carotenoids: "Color" Your Food Healthy

Imagine a beautiful autumn day. Leaves of red, orange, and yellow rustle in the branches overhead. The colors of the season belong to carotenoids, or plant pigments that generally are red, orange, and deep yellow.

The array of colors in fruits and vegetables also comes from carotenoids. The clues to their presence are obvious in the vibrant palette of produce in your supermarket. It's no surprise that apricots, cantaloupes, mangoes, carrots, red and yellow peppers, and sweet potatoes, for example, all contain carotene. Broccoli, kale, romaine lettuce, and spinach have carotene, too—even though they're dark green! The orange-yellow color of their carotene gets hidden by the chlorophyll in the leaves. *"Vitamin A and Carotenoids: Good Picks" earlier in this chapter lists good food sources and amounts.*

Beta carotene is the carotenoid most familiar to us. Actually, the plant world has more than six hundred known carotenoids. Of those, only a few have been analyzed in fruits and vegetables: alpha carotene, beta carotene, beta cryptoxanthin, gamma carotene, lycopene, lutein, and zeaxanthin; even then, the data are limited.

Beta carotene and other carotenoids perform many functions in your overall health. You have just read about their role as a precursor to vitamin A; *also see "Vitamins: The Basics" earlier in this chapter.* Carotenoids also play a functional role in health— many antioxidants potentially offer protection from some diseases and degenerative changes that accompany aging.

For foods high in beta carotene and other carotenoids, try to choose red, orange, deep-yellow, and some dark-green leafy vegetables every day. Be aware that color is a clue, not an assurance, that fruits and vegetables are good sources of beta carotene. For example, despite their color, neither corn nor snow peas have much beta carotene—but they do supply other nutrients.

No Dietary Reference Intakes (no RDA, AI, or UL) specifically for carotenoids have been established yet except as precursors to vitamin A. Be cautious; consuming too much of them from dietary supplements may have an adverse effect. *See "Vitamin/Mineral Supplements: Benefits and Risks" in chapter 23.*

Vitamin C: More Jobs than You Think!

Over the years, vitamin C, also known as ascorbic acid, developed celebrity status with claims that it can prevent or cure the common cold. Although those claims have been overblown, an adequate intake of vitamin C does play an important role in fighting infection. For colds, extra vitamin C may have a mild antihistamine effect, perhaps shortening the duration of a cold and making the symptoms more mild. However, scientific evidence doesn't justify taking large

---

Have You Ever Wondered

. . . if beta carotene supplements offer protection for smokers? No research supports any benefit. More importantly, a large study of smokers indicated that beta carotene supplements may be harmful to smokers. Smokers who used supplemental beta carotene had a higher incidence of lung cancer than those who didn't. For nonsmokers, it's still unknown whether higher intakes of beta carotene offer benefits. Unless your doctor prescribes a supplement for a vitamin A deficiency, skip carotenoid supplements!

---

doses of vitamin C regularly to boost immunity. For those who choose to take vitamin C for colds, research suggests that the placebo effect may be responsible for more benefits than taking extra vitamin C.

Here's what we do know: vitamin C is a water-soluble vitamin with many functions in health. Among them, vitamin C helps form the connective tissue that holds the many parts of your body together. It keeps capillaries healthy so you don't bruise easily, and your gums healthy so they don't bleed.

Vitamin C works in partnership with iron, too, helping the body to absorb iron from plant sources of food. *See "Iron in Foods: Heme vs. Nonheme" later in this chapter.* In fact, an adequate daily supply of vitamin C in your food choices can increase the absorption of nonheme iron (mostly from plant sources) by as much as two to four times. For those who get most of their iron from plant sources of food, including vegetarians, vitamin C is of special importance.

Of newer interest, as an antioxidant, vitamin C may protect your body in much the same way that beta carotene and vitamin E do. However, vitamin C attacks free radicals in body fluids, not in fat tissue. Preliminary research is exploring a link to reduced risk of cataracts and cancer protection; no evidence exists to advise consuming more than the RDA for vitamin C.

Because vitamin C isn't stored in the body, you're wise to consume a vitamin C-rich food daily. *"Vitamin C: More than Citrus" earlier in this chapter lists several good sources.* If you habitually consume a vitamin C-rich fruit or juice with breakfast, you probably consume enough.

Vitamin E: One Main Mission

For years, vitamin E has been surrounded by pseudo-scientific myths. It's been misguidedly acclaimed as a cure for almost all that ails you: for example, improving sexual prowess, curing infertility, preventing aging, curing heart disease and cancer, and improving athletic performance, to name just a few. The benefits of vitamin E don't extend this far, but it does appear to play a broad role in promoting your health.

The main role of vitamin E—a fat-soluble vitamin—appears to be as an antioxidant. It may help prevent the oxidation of LDL, or "bad," cholesterol, which contributes to plaque buildup in the arteries; although the jury's still out, that may help reduce the risk for heart disease and stroke. Vitamin E also may help protect from cell damage that can lead ultimately to health problems such as cancer. Vitamin E appears to work hand in hand with other antioxidants such as vitamin C and selenium to protect you from some chronic diseases.

Vitamin E is actually a group of substances called tocopherols, all with different potencies. For this reason they're often measured as milligrams of alpha-tocopherol equivalents.

Where do you get vitamin E? Vitamin E is found most abundantly in vegetable oils, salad dressings, margarine, and other processed foods made with vegetable oils. Vitamin E also is in wheat germ, whole-grain products, seeds, nuts (especially hazelnuts and almonds), and peanut butter. In addition, vitamin E is added to processed foods as a preservative. (*Note:* Heating vegetable oils to high temperatures, as in frying, destroys vitamin E.)

In vegetable oils, nuts, and seeds, vitamin E protects their unsaturated fats from oxidation. Typically, foods high in unsaturated fats also are good sources of vitamin E.

Rounding Up Free Radicals

Just how do antioxidant vitamins work? First let's look closely inside the body to learn more about oxygen. To produce energy, every cell in your body needs a constant supply of oxygen. For this reason, oxygen is basic to life.

There's another side to the oxygen story. When body cells burn oxygen, they form free radicals, or oxygen by-products; a free radical is an unstable molecule with a missing electron. These free radicals can damage body cells and tissues, as well as the DNA, which is your body's master plan for reproducing cells. Environmental factors such as cigarette smoke and ultraviolet light also cause free radicals to form in your body.

Damage caused by oxidation is quite familiar: for example, the quick browning on a cut apple or pear, and rancidity in oils. However, if you dip your apple or pear in orange juice, which has vitamin C, it stays white. And if vitamin E is added as a preservative to vegetable oil, it doesn't turn rancid as fast.

In your body, the process is similar. Free radicals cause oxidation, or cell damage, as they "steal" an electron from body cells to become stable. Over time, that may lead to cell dysfunction and contribute to the onset of health problems such as cancer, artery and heart disease, cataracts, age-related macular degeneration, diabetes, and some deterioration that goes with aging. Antioxidants in your body counteract the action of free radicals.

Three antioxidant vitamins appear to neutralize free radicals: beta carotene and other carotenoids, vitamin C, and vitamin E. Some enzymes that have trace minerals—selenium, copper, zinc, and manganese—and some phytonutrients act as antioxidants, too. As scavengers, antioxidant vitamins mop up free radicals by donating an electron of their own. The result? Antioxidants may control free radicals or convert them to harmless waste products that get eliminated before they do damage. Antioxidants even may help undo some of the damage already done to body cells.

Each antioxidant has its own biological job description. Being water-soluble, vitamin C removes free radicals from fluids inside and outside of body cells. Beta carotene and vitamin E, because they're fat-soluble, are present in lipids and fat tissues in your body. Antioxidants seem to complement each other. Because they work together, an excess or a deficiency of one may inhibit the benefits of other antioxidants.

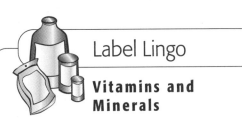

Label Lingo

Vitamins and Minerals

The lingo on the front of many food packages describes the amount of vitamins or minerals found in a single serving. For specific amounts of the nutrients described, check the Nutrition Facts on the label.

High, Rich in, Excellent source of means 20% or more of the Daily Value.*

Good source, Contains, Provides means 10 to 19% of the Daily Value.*

More, Enriched, Fortified, Added means 10% or more of the Daily Value.*

*As compared with a standard serving size of the traditional food

Be aware that scientific evidence can't promise that antioxidant nutrients provide a "safety shield" from chronic disease. Their role and potential interactions in reducing the risk of certain chronic diseases are among the many unknowns. And we don't know the potentially adverse affects of ongoing, high intakes of these nutrients from supplements either. Still, a varied diet—that follows the Food Guide Pyramid—with plenty of antioxidant-containing fruits, vegetables, and whole grains is still smart eating!

A "Garden" of Antioxidants

Where should your antioxidant vitamins come from? An eating style with plenty of fruits and vegetables (at least five servings a day) is undisputed as the wisest approach to good health. Eating plenty of whole-grain foods (at least three servings daily), as well as nuts, containing vitamin E provides them, too.

Many foods on supermarket shelves are fortified with antioxidant vitamins: C, E, and beta carotene. While these foods may not supply enough of the antioxidant vitamins for their possible protective benefits, they're often good sources of these essential nutrients. For carotenoids and vitamin C, fruits and vegetables still are the best sources, as they contain other phytonutrients that may help prevent health problems such as some cancers and heart disease.

Antioxidants in Supplements

Even if a little is good, a lot may not be better. So far no research proves that taking beta carotene, vitamin C or E, or other antioxidant supplements will prevent disease.

To date, scientists haven't pinpointed which antioxidants offer specific benefits, how much would be enough—or how many years you'd need to take them. And they don't know enough about side effects that might appear from taking supplemental antioxidants over long periods of time. Moreover, the mix of

Fruits and Vegetables: A Look at Their Antioxidant Potential

A food's health-promoting benefits likely come from many antioxidants, not just a single antioxidant nutrient or food substance. With this in mind, a scientific scoring method—the ORAC (oxygen radical absorbency capacity) score—has been created to estimate the overall antioxidant potential of fruits and vegetables. The higher the ORAC score, the greater the antioxidant potential.

FRUIT (RAW)	ORAC UNITS	VEGETABLES (RAW)	ORAC UNITS
Dried plums (prunes) (4)	1,939	Kale (1 cup)	1,186
Blueberrries (½ cup)	1,740	Beets (½ cup)	571
Blackberries (½ cup)	1,466	Red bell peppers (½ cup)	533
Strawberries (½ cup)	1,170	Brussels sprouts (½ cup)	431
Raisins (¼ cup)	1,026	Corn (½ cup)	420
Raspberries (½ cup)	756	Spinach (1 cup)	378
Oranges (½ cup sections)	675	Onions (½ cup)	360
Plums (1)	626	Broccoli florets (½ cup)	320
Red grapes (½ cup)	591	Eggplant (½ cup)	320
Cherries (½ cup)	516	Alfalfa sprouts (½ cup)	149

Sources: USDA Agricultural Research Service, *Food and Nutrition Research Briefs* (April 1999). Calculated to serving sizes, J. Walsh, "The Growing Allure of Antioxidants," *Environmental Nutrition* (January 2000).

Remember: The ORAC score offers a scientific method for looking at food in a new way. No guidelines exist to suggest how many ORAC units you need. *Be aware:* A high ORAC value doesn't mean a food performs better as an antioxidant source; the bioavailability of these antioxidants isn't known, either.

antioxidants in food, not just one or two from supplements, may offer positive and powerful antioxidant action.

Other antioxidant issues need research, too. For one, high doses from antioxidant supplements may be harmful, perhaps by working as pro-oxidants that promote, rather than neutralize, oxidation. Second, not all free radicals are harmful. Some offer protection by attacking harmful bacteria or cancer cells in the body. Very high intakes of antioxidants may destroy or hinder these protective free radicals.

Until more is known, continue to enjoy the wide variety of fruits, vegetables, and grain products with their many naturally occurring antioxidants. And avoid high doses in supplements. *For more about dietary supplements, see chapter 23.*

Minerals–Not "Heavy Metal"

The term "minerals" may conjure up thoughts of rocks. But to your body, minerals are another group of essential nutrients, needed to both regulate body processes and give your body structure.

Like vitamins, minerals help trigger, or regulate, a myriad of processes that continually take place in your body, so they are essential to your life. For example, they regulate fluid balance, muscle contractions, and nerve impulses.

Even though they make up only a small percentage—about 4 percent—of your weight, minerals also help give your body structure. They not only give structure to bones and teeth, but muscles, blood, and other body tissue all contain minerals, too.

Unlike vitamins, minerals are inorganic. Minerals can't be destroyed by heat or other food-handling processes. In fact, if you've ever completely burned food, perhaps while cooking over a fire, the little bit of ash left over is its mineral content.

You might think of minerals in two categories— major minerals and trace minerals—depending on how much you need. Regardless of amount, they're all essential.

● *Major minerals:* Major minerals are needed in greater amounts than trace minerals are—more than 250 milligrams are recommended daily for each one. Calcium, phosphorus, and magnesium fit in this cate-

gory, along with three electrolytes—sodium, chloride, and potassium.

Electrolytes, grouped together because their work is interrelated, regulate body fluids in and out of every cell. Electrolytes also transmit nerve, or electrical, impulses. *To learn more about electrolytes, see "Sodium: You Need Some!" in chapter 7.*

● *Trace minerals:* Your body needs just small amounts—fewer than 20 milligrams daily—for each of the trace minerals, or trace elements: chromium, copper, fluoride, iodine, iron, manganese, molybdenum, selenium, and zinc. Recommended Dietary Allowances have been set for only some: copper, iodine, iron, molybdenum, selenium, and zinc. Until science learns more, others are presented in DRI Charts as Adequate Intake Levels (AIs).

Nutrition experts have reviewed research on other trace elements: arsenic, boron, nickel, silicon, and vanadium. They don't appear to have a role in human health. However, Tolerable Upper Intake Levels (UL) have been set for some: boron (20 milligrams a day), nickel (1.0 milligram a day), and vanadium (1.8 milligrams a day) for adult levels.

All minerals are absorbed in your intestines, then transported and stored in your body in different ways. Some pass directly into your bloodstream, where they're carried to cells; any excess passes out of the body through urine. Others attach to proteins and become part of your body structure; because they're stored, excess amounts can be harmful if the levels consumed are too high for too long.

Read on for a summary of how minerals keep you healthy: their functions, effects of getting too little or too much, Dietary Reference Intakes, and sources.

Note: On the following pages, the amounts of minerals in foods have been rounded.

Major Minerals

Calcium

See "Calcium: A Closer Look" later in this chapter.

What it does:

- Builds bones, both in length and strength, becoming part of bone tissue.

- Helps your bones remain strong by slowing the rate of bone loss as you age.

- Helps your muscles contract and your heart beat.

- Plays a role in normal nerve function.

- Helps your blood clot if you're bleeding.

If you don't get enough: For children, not getting enough calcium may interfere with growth; a severe deficiency may keep children from reaching their potential adult height. Even a mild deficiency over a lifetime can affect bone density and bone loss, increasing the risk for osteoporosis, or brittle bone disease. *See "Bone Up on Calcium" later in this chapter.*

If you consume excess amounts: Unless the doses are very large (more than 2,500 milligrams daily), adverse effects for adults are unlikely. Very large doses over a prolonged period of time may cause kidney stones and poor kidney function, and may affect the absorption of other minerals such as iron, magnesium, and zinc. These problems could occur from consuming too much through a calcium supplement, not from milk or other calcium-rich foods. The Tolerable Upper Intake Level (UL) from the Dietary Reference Intakes

is set at 2,500 milligrams daily from age one on through adulthood.

How much you need: For ages nine through eighteen, the Adequate Intake (AI) is 1,300 milligrams daily. As an adult through age fifty, the AI is 1,000 milligrams of calcium daily. After that, the recommendation goes back up, to 1,200 milligrams of calcium daily for both men and women to help maintain bone mass. Calcium recommendations for women who are pregnant or breast-feeding are the same as for other women in their respective age group.

To reduce the risks of osteoporosis, many nutrition experts believe that even more calcium is better for your bones, so the National Institutes of Health Consensus Panel on Osteoporosis advises an optimal calcium intake that's higher than the AI—1,500 milligrams calcium daily for postmenopausal women not on estrogen and for adults over age sixty-five.

Where it's mostly found: Milk and other dairy foods such as yogurt and most cheeses are the best sources of calcium. In addition, some dark-green leafy vegetables (kale, broccoli, bok choy), fish with edible bones, calcium-fortified soy milk, and tofu made with calcium sulfate also supply significant amounts. *See "Counting Up Calcium" later in this chapter for a list of good sources and amounts.*

Phosphorus

What it does:

- Helps generate energy in every cell of your body.

- Acts as the main regulator of energy metabolism in your body's organs.

- Is a major component of bones and teeth, second only to calcium.

- Serves as part of DNA and RNA, which are your body's master plan for cell growth and repair.

If you don't get enough: A deficiency is quite rare, except for small, premature babies who consume only breast milk, or for people who take an antacid with aluminum hydroxide for a long time. In those rare cases, the symptoms include bone loss, weakness, loss of appetite, and pain.

If you consume excess amounts: An excess amount may lower the level of calcium in the blood—a problem if calcium intake is low. As a result, bone loss may increase. Besides that, consuming too much phosphorus doesn't appear to be a problem in the United States. The Tolerable Upper Intake Level (UL) for phosphorus is 4,000 milligrams a day for people ages nine through seventy; after age seventy, it's 3,000 milligrams of phosphorus daily. For pregnancy, the level drops slightly, to 3,500 milligrams of phosphorus daily.

How much you need: The RDA for phosphorus is 1,250 milligrams daily for ages nine through eighteen, then decreases to 700 milligrams daily for adults of all ages. Scientific evidence shows that people need less than previously thought.

Where it's mostly found: Almost all foods contain phosphorus. Protein-rich foods—milk, meat, poultry, fish, and eggs—contain the most. Legumes and nuts are good sources as well. Even bread and other baked foods have some. You'll also find phosphorus in colas and pepper-type soft drinks.

FOOD	PHOSPHORUS (MG)
Milk, whole (1 cup)	230
Perch, cooked (3 oz.)	220
Cheddar cheese (1 oz.)	145
Lean ground beef, cooked (3 oz.)	140
Kidney beans, cooked (½ cup)	125
Tofu (½ cup)	120
Peanut butter (2 tbsp.)	105
Egg, large (1)	90
Cola (12 oz.)	45

Magnesium

What it does:

● Serves as an important part of more than three hundred body enzymes. Enzymes are body chemicals that regulate all kinds of bodily functions, including producing energy, making body protein, and muscle contractions.

● Helps maintain body cells in nerves and muscles, and signals muscles to relax and contract.

● Serves as a component of bones.

If you don't get enough: A deficiency is rare except in diseases where the body doesn't absorb magnesium

properly. Then symptoms might include irregular heartbeat, nausea, weakness, and/or mental derangement.

If you consume an excess amount: Consuming too much magnesium from food probably won't do any harm—unless it can't be excreted properly due to kidney disease. The Tolerable Upper Intake Level is 350 milligrams a day; this amount is less than the RDA because it represents only the amount of magnesium in supplements or drugs.

How much you need: The RDA for teenage boys is 410 milligrams of magnesium daily to age eighteen; for teenage girls, 360 milligrams daily. The RDA for adult males is 400 milligrams daily through age thirty, then 420 milligrams daily after that. For females, the recommendation is 310 milligrams daily through age thirty, then 320 milligrams daily after age thirty. Neither pregnancy nor breast-feeding increases the need for magnesium.

Where it's mostly found: Magnesium is found in varying amounts in all kinds of foods. The best sources are legumes, nuts, and whole grains. Green vegetables are good sources, too.

FOOD	MAGNESIUM (MG)
Spinach, boiled (½ cup)	80
Peanut butter (2 tbsp.)	50
Pecans, dried (1 oz.)	50
Black-eyed peas, boiled (½ cup)	45
Lima beans, boiled (½ cup)	40
Whole-wheat bread (1 slice)	25
Parsnips, boiled (½ cup)	25
Whole-wheat spaghetti, cooked (½ cup)	20

Major Minerals: Electrolytes

Chloride

What it does:

● Helps regulate fluids in and out of body cells.

● As a component of stomach acid, helps with the digestion of your food and the absorption of nutrients.

● Helps transmit nerve impulses, or signals.

If you don't get enough: Because salt is such a common part of the diet, a deficiency of chloride isn't likely if you're healthy. Chloride loss goes along with sodium loss; they're replenished together. Their deficiency symptoms are similar, too.

If you consume excess amounts: For people who are sensitive, there may be a link to high blood pressure, but more study is needed.

How much you need: There's no RDA for chloride. However, most healthy people can satisfy their chloride needs with a minimum of 750 milligrams daily. Higher amounts don't appear to have any extra benefits.

Where it's mostly found: Salt is made of sodium and chloride, so salt and salty foods are the main sources of chloride. As a point of reference, ¼ teaspoon of salt contains 750 milligrams of chloride.

Potassium

See "Potassium: Another Reason for 'Five a Day'" in chapter 7.

What it does:

- Helps regulate fluids and mineral balance in and out of body cells.
- Helps maintain your normal blood pressure.
- Helps transmit nerve impulses, or signals.
- Helps your muscles contract.

If you don't get enough: For healthy people, a potassium deficiency is rare. But when vomiting, diarrhea, or laxative use goes on for too long, the body may lose excess amounts. Kidney problems also may cause severe loss. The deficiency symptoms caused by these problems include muscle cramps, weakness, appetite loss, nausea, and fatigue. You may need a potassium supplement if you're taking medication for high blood pressure. Talk to your doctor.

If you consume excess amounts: Harmful effects from consuming too much are rare because excess amounts usually are excreted. If an excess can't be excreted, it can cause heart problems. People with kidney problems may not be able to get rid of excess potassium and may be advised to limit potassium-containing foods and to avoid using potassium chloride as a salt substitute.

How much you need: There is no RDA for potassium, but the minimum amount suggested for adults is 2,000 milligrams a day; some experts suggest more, about 3,500 milligrams per day, to help protect against high blood pressure.

Where it's mostly found: Potassium is found in a wide range of foods, especially fruits, many vegetables, and fresh meat, poultry, and fish. Less processed foods tend to have more potassium.

FOOD	POTASSIUM (MG)
Banana, medium (1)	450
Milk, whole (1 cup)	370
Haddock, cooked (3 oz.)	340
Tomato, raw (1)	275
Turkey, light and dark meat, roasted, skinless (3 oz.)	260
Orange, medium (1)	235
Okra, boiled (½ cup)	190
Bell pepper (½ cup)	90

Sodium

See chapter 7, "Sodium: A Salty Subject."

What it does:

- Helps regulate the movement of body fluids in and out of your body cells.
- Helps your muscles, including your heart, relax.
- Helps transmit nerve impulses, or signals.
- Helps regulate your blood pressure.

If you don't get enough: Unless you've experienced diarrhea or vomiting for a long time, or you have kidney problems, a sodium deficiency isn't likely. But if that happens, symptoms might include nausea, dizziness, and muscle cramps.

If you consume an excess amount: For healthy people, excess sodium is excreted, but some kidney diseases interfere with sodium excretion, causing fluid retention and swelling. For people who are sodium-sensitive, a diet high in sodium can promote high blood pressure.

How much you need: As with the other electrolytes, there is no RDA for sodium. However, the minimum amount considered safe and adequate is 500 milligrams daily for healthy adults, which is much less than most people consume. The Daily Value used for food labeling is 2,400 milligrams of sodium.

Where it's mostly found: Processed foods account for about 80 percent of the sodium in food. The rest comes from table salt and the small amount that occurs naturally in food. As a point of reference, $\frac{1}{4}$ teaspoon of salt contains 500 milligrams of sodium.

FOOD	SODIUM (MG)
Beef bologna (1 oz.)	310
Cheddar cheese (1 oz.)	175
Whole-wheat bread (1 slice)	160
Milk, whole (1 cup)	120

The Nutrition Facts on food labels tell how much sodium comes from a single serving of food. *See "Get All the Facts!" in chapter 11 to learn how to read sodium information on the food label.*

Trace Minerals

Chromium

What it does:

- Works with insulin to help your body use glucose, or blood sugar. *See "Sugar: What Is It?" in chapter 5 to learn more about glucose.*

If you don't get enough: Because chromium works closely with insulin, a deficiency can look like diabetes. *See "Diabetes: A Growing Health Concern" in chapter 22 for more about diabetes.*

If you consume excess amounts: Consuming harmful amounts from dietary sources is highly unlikely.

How much you need: There is no RDA for chromium; however, a level of Adequate Intake (AI) has been set: 35 micrograms per day for males ages fourteen to fifty, and 30 micrograms per day from age fifty-one on. For females, 24 micrograms daily from ages fourteen to eighteen; 25 micrograms daily from ages nineteen through fifty; and 20 micrograms daily from age fifty-

one on. During pregnancy, the AI level is an additional 5 micrograms daily higher; during breast-feeding, an additional 20 micrograms..

Where it's mostly found: Meat, eggs, whole-grain products, and cheese are all good sources.

FOOD	CHROMIUM (MCG)
Shredded wheat cereal (2 oz.)	65
Peas (1 cup)	60
Cheese, American (1 oz.)	48
Liver, braised (3 oz.)	42
Egg, large (1)	26

Copper

What it does:

- Helps your body make hemoglobin, needed to carry oxygen in red blood cells.
- Serves as a part of many body enzymes.
- Helps your body develop connective tissue, myelin, and melanin.
- Helps your body produce energy in the cells.

If you don't get enough: A deficiency rarely comes from a lack of copper in the diet, but instead from genetic problems or from consuming too much zinc. As another cause, excess zinc from dietary supplements can hinder copper absorption.

If you consume excess amounts: Harmful effects of copper from dietary sources are extremely rare in the United States. The Tolerable Upper Intake Level (UL) is 8,000 micrograms daily for teens ages fourteen to eighteen, and 10,000 micrograms daily for adults.

How much you need: The RDA for copper is set at 890 micrograms per day for teens ages fourteen to eighteen, and 900 micrograms daily for adults. During pregnancy the level is 1,000 micrograms daily; during breast-feeding it's 1,300 micrograms daily.

Where it's mostly found: Organ meats, especially liver; seafood; nuts; and seeds are the best sources of copper. Cooking in copper pots also increases the copper content of foods.

FOOD	COPPER (MCG)
Beef liver, braised (3 oz.)	3,860
Clams, cooked (3 oz.)	580
Sunflower seeds, dry roasted (1 oz.)	520
Peanuts, dry roasted (1 oz.)	190
Mushrooms, canned (½ cup)	180

Fluoride

See "The Fluoride Connection" in chapter 8.

What it does:

● Helps harden tooth enamel and so helps protect your teeth from decay.

● May offer some protection from osteoporosis, or brittle bone disease, by helping to strengthen bones.

If you don't get enough: Tooth enamel may be weak.

If you consume excess amounts: With excessive fluoride, teeth become mottled, or marked with brown stains, although teeth are healthy in every other way. Be aware that these stains may have other causes as well. The Tolerable Upper Intake Level (UL) is 2.2 milligrams of fluoride daily for children ages four through eight; from age nine through adulthood, the UL is 10 milligrams of fluoride daily.

How much you need: An Adequate Intake (AI) for fluoride has been set. AI levels for children are as follows: ages four to eight, 1 milligram of fluoride daily, and ages nine to thirteen, 2 milligrams of fluoride daily. For teens the AI is set at 3 milligrams of fluoride daily. For adults, the guideline is 4 milligrams of fluoride daily for males and 3 milligrams daily for females. There are no increased needs during pregnancy or breast-feeding. A fluoride supplement may be prescribed during infancy. *See "Vitamin and Mineral Supplements for Breast-Fed Babies" in chapter 15.*

Where it's mostly found: Fluoride is not widely available in food. Two significant sources are tea, especially if it's made with fluoridated water, and fish with edible bones, such as canned salmon.

The primary means for obtaining fluoride is drinking and cooking with fluoridated (fluoride added) water. Many municipal water supplies are fluoridated; however, most bottled waters are not. Some types of cooking utensils, such as Teflon with its fluoride-containing polymer, also can increase the fluoride content of food. The content of fluoride in food varies widely and is affected by the environment in which the food originated.

Iodine:

What it does:

● Serves as part of thyroid hormones such as thyroxin, which regulate the rate at which your body uses energy.

If you don't get enough: With an iodine deficiency, the body can't make enough thyroxin. As a result, the rate at which the body burns energy slows down, and weight gain may become a problem. Goiter, an enlarged thyroid gland, is the deficiency disease often caused by a lack of iodine. With the use of iodized salt, goiter rarely is caused by an iodine deficiency.

If you consume excess amounts: Goiter also can be induced when people consume high levels of iodine—but not at levels consumed in the United States. Too much also can result in irregular heartbeat and confusion. The Tolerable Upper Intake Level (UL) is 900 micrograms daily for teens ages fourteen to eighteen, and 1,100 micrograms daily during adulthood.

How much you need: The RDA for iodine is 150 micrograms daily for adults. During pregnancy, the recommendation goes up to 220 micrograms; during breast-feeding, 290 micrograms daily.

Where it's mostly found: Iodine is found naturally in saltwater fish. Foods grown near coastal areas also contain iodine, but many people don't have access to these foods. For this reason, salt is iodized, assuring an adequate amount of iodine in the food supply, even if you consume only modest amounts of salt. One-half teaspoon of iodized salt provides almost enough iodine to reach the RDA for a day.

FOOD	IODINE (MCG)
Table salt, iodized (¼ tsp.)	100
Cod, cooked (3 oz.)	87
Potato, cooked (1 medium)	7
Spinach, cooked (½ cup)	5
Almonds (1 oz.)	4

Iron

See "Iron: A Closer Look" later in this chapter.

What it does:

● Serves as an essential part of hemoglobin, which carries oxygen in your blood from your lungs to every body cell, and other enzymes.

● Helps in brain development.

● Supports a healthy immune system.

If you don't get enough: Although there may be other causes, an iron deficiency can lead to anemia, along with fatigue and infections. Among women with regular menstrual loss, iron deficiency is more common. In fact, in the United States, iron deficiency is the most common nutrient deficiency.

If you consume excess amounts: Iron can build up to dangerous levels for people with a rare genetic problem called hemochromatosis, whereby the body absorbs and stores too much iron. That excess can cause an enlarged liver, bronze skin pigmentation, and diabetes, as well as pancreatic, liver, cardiac, and other organ damage. Ten times more common in men, symptoms of hemochromatosis usually begin to appear in adulthood, often in the thirties.

Taking adult iron supplements can be dangerous for children. Children should get immediate medical attention if they take an overdose of iron supplements. The Tolerable Upper Intake Level (UL) is 45 milligrams of iron per day for ages fourteen and over.

How much you need: The RDA for teen males ages fourteen to eighteen is 11 milligrams of iron daily; for adult men it's 8 milligrams daily. For teen females to age eighteen, 15 milligrams of iron daily; for females ages nineteen to fifty, 18 milligrams are recommended daily. From age fifty-one on, women need about 8 milligrams of iron daily.

During pregnancy the recommendation goes up to 27 milligrams daily; during breast-feeding, the RDA is 10 milligrams daily for females age eighteen and younger and 9 milligrams daily for females ages nineteen and over.

Where it's mostly found: Iron comes from foods of both animal (heme iron) and plant (nonheme) sources. It's much better absorbed from heme iron and when vitamin C is consumed with nonheme iron at the same meal. *See "Counting Up Iron" later in this chapter for a list of good sources and amounts.*

Manganese

What it does:

● Serves as part of many enzymes.

● Helps in bone formation.

● Helps in the metabolism of energy-producing nutrients.

If you don't get enough: The chances of not getting enough are very low, since manganese is so widely distributed in the food supply.

If you consume excess amounts: Consuming harmful levels from food is very rare, too. The Tolerable Upper Intake Level (UL) is set at 9 milligrams daily for teens ages fourteen to eighteen, and at 11 milligrams daily during adulthood.

How much you need: There is no RDA for manganese. However, the AI is set at 2.2 milligrams and 1.6 milligrams daily for males and females ages fourteen to eighteen, respectively. For adults the AI is 2.3 milligrams daily for males and 1.8 milligrams daily for females. During pregnancy (teens and adults), the AI is 2.0 milligrams daily; during breast-feeding, 2.6 milligrams daily.

Where it's mostly found: Whole-grain products are the best sources of manganese, along with some fruits and vegetables. Tea also is a good source.

Whole Grains: For Goodness Sake

Why the advice to make three of your daily Grains Group servings whole grain? Whole-grain foods are rich in complex carbohydrates and fiber and low in fat. Beyond that, they're important sources of antioxidant nutrients, including vitamin E and selenium. Whole grains supply minerals such as zinc, copper, and iron, and vitamin B_6. And they're sources of some disease-fighting phytonutrients such as lignans and flavonoids.

"What Is a Whole Grain?" in chapter 6 explains where the nutrients and fiber come from within the grain. In that chapter, also see "Fiber's 'Benefit Package': A Closer Look," and "Which Bread Is Whole Grain?" Check "Today's Grains" in chapter 9 for descriptions of lesser used whole grains.

FOOD	MANGANESE (MG)
Pineapple, raw (½ cup)	1.3
Whole-wheat spaghetti, cooked (½ cup)	1
Whole-wheat bread (1 slice)	0.6
Tea, instant powder (1 tsp.)	0.5
Lentils, boiled (½ cup)	0.5
Kale, boiled (½ cup)	0.3
Strawberries (½ cup)	0.2

Molybdenum

What it does:

- Works with riboflavin to incorporate the iron stored in the body into hemoglobin for making red blood cells.

- Is part of many body enzymes.

If you don't get enough: With a normal diet, there's no need to worry about a deficiency. A deficiency of the enzymes made with molybdenum affects the nervous system, and in extreme cases may result in death.

If you consume excess amounts: Too much may have reproductive effects, but harmful levels are quite uncommon. The Tolerable Upper Intake Level (UL) is 1,700 micrograms daily during the years fourteen to eighteen, and 2,000 micrograms daily during adulthood.

How much you need: The RDA for molybdenum is 43 micrograms daily during the years fourteen to eighteen, and 45 micrograms daily during adulthood. During pregnancy and breast-feeding, the RDA level goes up to 50 micrograms daily for teen and adult women.

Where it's mostly found: Molybdenum is found mostly in milk, legumes, liver, breads, and grain products. The amount consumed in a typical eating pattern appears adequate. Little is known about the actual amounts in foods.

Selenium

What it does:

- Works as an antioxidant with vitamin E, to protect cells from damage that may lead to heart disease, and perhaps cancer and other health problems.

- Aids cell growth.

- Boosts immune function.

If you don't get enough: The general signs of a deficiency in humans aren't clear, but it may affect the heart muscle.

If you consume excess amounts: A normal diet with a variety of foods generally provides moderate levels of selenium. Very high levels from dietary supplements can be quite harmful. The Tolerable Upper Intake Level is set at 400 milligrams daily for people ages fourteen and over.

How much you need: The RDA is 55 micrograms daily for people ages fourteen and over. During pregnancy the recommendation remains the same, 55 micrograms daily; during breast-feeding it goes up to 70 micrograms daily.

Where it's mostly found: The richest sources are seafood, liver, and kidney, as well as other meats. Grain products and seeds contain selenium, but the amount depends on the selenium content of the soil in which they're grown. Fruits and vegetables generally don't have much.

FOOD	SELENIUM (MCG)
Chicken, light meat, skinless (3 oz.)	26
Brown rice, cooked (½ cup)	13
Egg, large (1)	12
Whole-wheat bread (1 slice)	11
Peanuts (¼ cup)	3

Zinc

What it does:

- Promotes cell reproduction and tissue growth and repair. Adequate zinc intake is essential for growth.

- Associated with more than two hundred enzymes.

- Helps your body use carbohydrates, proteins, and fats.

If you don't get enough: A deficiency during childhood can impair growth, and during pregnancy can cause birth defects. Other symptoms include appetite loss, skin changes, and reduced resistance to infections.

If you consume excess amounts: Too much zinc from dietary supplements can have harmful side effects, including impaired copper absorption. The Tolerable Upper Intake Level (UL) for zinc is 34 milligrams daily for teens ages fourteen to eighteen, and 40 milligrams daily for adults.

How much you need: The RDA for males is 11 milligrams daily for ages fourteen on. For females it's 9 milligrams daily for teens ages fourteen to eighteen, and 8 milligrams daily during adulthood. During pregnancy the recommendation increases to 13 milligrams daily for teens, and 11 milligrams daily for adults; during breast-feeding, 14 milligrams and 12 milligrams daily, respectively.

Where it's mostly found: Good sources of zinc include foods of animal origin, including meat, seafood, and liver. Eggs and milk supply zinc in smaller amounts. Whole-grain products, wheat germ, black-eyed peas,

Your Nutrition Checkup

Yesterday . . . Did You Consume Enough Calcium?

Food	No. of Servings	Calcium Quality Points	Score	Food	No. of Servings	Calcium Quality Points	Score
8 oz. milk (any type)	____	× 3 =	____	1 cup cooked greens (mustard, dandelion, beet)	____	1	____
8 oz. yogurt	____	3	____	1 cup cooked soybeans	____	1	____
3½ oz. sardines	____	3	____	1 cup cooked acorn squash or butternut squash	____	1	____
½ cup ricotta cheese	____	3	____				
10 oz. milkshake	____	3	____	1 cup tofu (treated with calcium sulfate)	____	1	____
2 slices processed cheese	____	3	____	1 packet instant oatmeal	____	1	____
8 oz. high-calcium orange juice	____	3	____	1 sourdough English muffin	____	1	____
8 oz. calcium-fortified soy milk*	____	3	____	½ cup softserve vanilla ice milk	____	1	____
1 oz. hard cheese	____	2	____	½ cup chocolate, vanilla, tapioca, or rice pudding	____	1	____
⅓ cup grated cheese	____	2	____	1 slice medium cheese pizza	____	1	____
1 cup black-eyed peas	____	2	____	1 medium cheeseburger	____	1	____
2 tbsp. blackstrap molasses	____	2	____	*Total calcium score*			____
3 oz. canned salmon with bones	____	2	____			× 100	
1 cup frozen yogurt	____	2	____	Approximate milligrams of calcium			____
1 cup cottage cheese	____	1	____				
1 cup baked beans	____	1	____				
1 cup cooked broccoli, kale, or bok choy	____	1	____	*Fortified at about 500 milligrams calcium per 8 ounces			

Source: Adapted from C. Pierre, *Calcium in Your Life,* American Dietetic Association's Nutrition Now Series (New York: John Wiley & Sons, 1997). This material is used by permission of John Wiley & Sons.

and fermented soybean paste (miso) also contain zinc, but in a form that's less available to the body.

FOOD	ZINC (MG)
Beef, ground lean (3 oz.)	4.5
Wheat germ (¼ cup)	3.6
Crab, canned (3 oz.)	3.5
Wheat bran (½ cup)	2
Sunflower seeds (1 oz.)	1.5
Black-eyed peas, frozen, boiled (½ cup)	1
Almonds (1 oz.)	1
Milk, whole (1 cup)	1
Tofu, raw (½ cup)	1
Peanut butter (2 tbsp.)	0.9
Tuna, canned, packed in water (3 oz.)	0.7
Egg, large (1)	0.5
Whole-wheat bread (1 slice)	0.5

Calcium: A Closer Look

The human body contains more calcium than any other mineral. For an average 130-pound adult, about 1,200 grams—almost 3 pounds—of the body is calcium. Your body composition, of course, depends on the size of your body frame; the density of your bones; and, if you're older, how much bone you've lost through aging.

Of that amount, about 99 percent of your body's calcium is in your bones. The remaining 1 percent is in your other body fluids and cells. Calcium is as important to you as an adult as it was during your childhood. The reasons really aren't that different.

Bone Up on Calcium

Most of us mentally connect the growing years with the need for calcium. That's true, but "boning up" is actually a lifelong process—starting at the moment of conception. During the childhood and teen years, bones grow long and wide. In fact, 40 percent or more of the body's bone mass is formed during adolescence. By age twenty or so, that phase of bone building is complete. But the period of building toward peak bone mass continues until the early thirties. Bones become stronger and more dense as more calcium becomes part of the bone matrix.

Your bones are in a constant state of change. Because bones are living tissue, calcium gets deposited and withdrawn daily from your skeleton, much like money in a bank, in a process called remodeling. As small amounts are withdrawn, they're used for other body functions; at the same time, calcium is deposited in bones. To keep your bones strong and to reduce bone loss, you need to make regular calcium deposits to replace the losses—and even build up a little "nest egg" of calcium for when your food choices come up short.

Calcium doesn't work alone. It works in partnership with other nutrients, including phosphorus and vitamin D. Vitamin D helps absorb and deposit calcium in bones and teeth, making them stronger. Phosphorus also is an important part of the structure of bone.

If you don't consume enough calcium—or if your body doesn't adequately absorb it (perhaps because you're short on vitamin D)—your body may withdraw more calcium from bones than you deposit. You need calcium, for example, for muscle contraction and your heartbeat, too. This process gradually depletes bone, leaving a void in places where calcium otherwise would be deposited, eventually making bones more porous and fragile. *See "Which Bone Is Healthy?" in chapter 22 to compare healthy bone with osteoporotic bone.*

After age thirty or so, bones slowly lose minerals that give them strength. That's a natural part of the aging process. Whatever calcium a woman has "banked" in her skeleton will be the amount in her bones when she enters menopause. Even then, consuming enough calcium can help women retain their bone density and lower the risk for osteoporosis later.

During the childbearing years, the hormone estrogen appears to protect bones, keeping them strong. But with the onset of menopause, bone loss speeds up for women as estrogen levels go down. If women achieve their peak bone mass as younger adults, their risk for osteoporosis, or brittle bone disease, later in life is reduced. Their bones are strong enough before menopause to offer protection.

For older adults (ages fifty-one and over), calcium

remains important for bone health as well as for protection from high blood pressure and cancer. It's not too late to get the benefits from consuming more calcium, even if you're starting now.

An adequate calcium intake is one important factor in building healthy bones. Adequate exercise is another. Regular, weight-bearing physical activities such as walking, strength-training, dancing, kickboxing, and tennis stimulate bone formation. These types of activities trigger nerve impulses that, in turn, activate body chemicals to deposit calcium in bones.

Women—and men, too: You can build bone until about age thirty. After that, you can only slow the bone loss that comes with aging. Follow these tips:

● Consume adequate amounts of calcium—at every age and stage of life!

● Be careful about weight loss; eating plans that severely restrict food often restrict calcium, too. If you're concerned about calories or fat, choose fat-free or low-fat milk and still get the bone-building benefits of milk.

● Participate regularly—at least three times weekly—in weight-bearing activities.

● Avoid smoking and an excessive intake of alcohol; both interfere with bone health.

For more about calcium during the bone-building adolescent years, see "Calcium: A Growing Issue" in chapter 16. And to review the many factors that relate to osteoporosis, see "Osteoporosis: Reduce the Risks" in chapter 22.

More than Bone Health!

Looking for ways to stay healthy? Bone-building benefits are just one reason to make calcium a smart-eating priority! Like other nutrients, calcium is well known for "multitasking."

Daily "Chores." Although used in just a small amount, calcium helps your muscles contract, your heart beat, your blood clot, and your nervous system send messages. These functions are vital to your health.

More Protection. A growing body of research supports a functional benefit for calcium-rich foods. Calcium appears to play an important role in promoting health and protecting you from several health risks that begin to appear in midlife. If you're already consuming

enough calcium for bone health, the benefits may multiply!

● Calcium helps your blood pressure. The good news: research shows that a low-fat diet with low-fat dairy foods, fruits, and vegetables may help reduce your risk for hypertension (high blood pressure). Already hypertensive? Consuming adequate calcium may help bring your blood pressure level down. *Read about the DASH (Dietary Approaches to Stop Hypertension) diet and the calcium link in chapter 22.* Remember, lowering your blood pressure reduces the risk of heart disease and stroke, too.

● Are you at risk for colon cancer, perhaps with a history of polyps? Although the research isn't conclusive, calcium-rich or low-fat dairy foods appear to offer

Have You Ever Wondered

... if calcium supplements or calcium-fortified foods can substitute for dairy foods? For most people, fortified foods and supplements are meant to supplement, not replace, foods with naturally occurring calcium.

Although they may fill the calcium gap, supplements and calcium-fortified foods (such as juice, cereal, pasta, and rice) don't supply all the other health-promoting nutrients and food substances found in dairy foods. Besides calcium, Milk Group foods are key sources of protein, vitamins A, B$_2$ (riboflavin), B$_{12}$, and D (if fortified) and the minerals phosphorus, potassium, magnesium, and zinc. Beyond that, dairy foods offer substances with potential functional benefits: conjugated linoleic acid (CLA), sphingolipid, and butyric acid, which may help protect you from some cancers and other health conditions. *For more about CLA, see "Functional Nutrition: Eat Your Omega-3s and -6s" in chapter 3.*

You can overdo calcium if you regularly consume calcium-fortified juice and/or calcium-fortified breakfast cereal—and take a calcium supplement as "insurance." What's the downside? Too much calcium, most likely from fortified foods and supplements, may limit the absorption of iron and zinc, two minerals that often come up short for many Americans.

... if eggs count as a calcium-rich dairy food? Although they're typically sold in the dairy case, eggs aren't a dairy food! Since you don't eat the shell (your body can't use that form of calcium), eggs supply very little calcium.

some protection from abnormal cell growth in the colon—more protection than calcium supplements offer.

● Although research has just begun, calcium or dairy foods may reduce the risk of other health problems: kidney stones, premenstrual syndrome, polycystic ovary syndrome, breast cancer, lead toxicity, and obesity. Stay tuned—and consume enough calcium!

Calcium: When You Need More . . .

For people of every age, food choices can supply an adequate amount of calcium. However, as an extra

---

Counting Up Calcium

Dairy foods supply 73 percent of all the calcium available in the U.S. food supply. Besides providing calcium, they supply protein, vitamin D (if fortified), and phosphorus, which together help the body absorb and deposit calcium in bones, Dairy foods also are important sources of vitamin A, riboflavin, vitamin B_{12}, magnesium, and potassium.

Other foods also supply calcium. Some dark-green leafy vegetables and fish with edible bones provide significant amounts. Many processed foods such as soy milk, tofu, orange juice, and breakfast cereal may be fortified with calcium.

Green, leafy vegetables and grain products supply some calcium. However, some vegetables such as spinach contain oxalates; grains may contain phytates. Both bind with some minerals, including calcium, magnesium, and iron, partially blocking their absorption. Caffeine can interfere with calcium absorption, too.

FOOD	CALCIUM (MG)	FOOD	CALCIUM (MG)
Yogurt, plain, nonfat (1 cup)	450	Sardines with edible bones (1 oz.)	90
Tofu, regular (processed with calcium*) (½ cup)	435	Dried figs (3)	90
		Ice cream (½ cup)	85
Yogurt, plain, low-fat (1 cup)	415	Cottage cheese (½ cup)	75
Yogurt, fruit (1 cup)	315	Tempeh (½ cup)	75
Milk, fat-free (1 cup)	300	Okra (½ cup)	75
Milk, 2% (1 cup)	295	Parmesan cheese (1 tbsp.)	70
Milk, whole (1 cup)	290	Milk chocolate bar (1 oz.)	70
Chocolate milk, 1% (1 cup)	285	Mustard greens (½ cup)	50
Chocolate milk, 2% (1 cup)	285	Orange (1)	50
Swiss cheese (1 oz.)	270	Kale (½ cup)	45
Calcium-fortified soy milk (8 oz.)	250–300	Broccoli (½ cup)	45
Calcium-fortified orange juice (¾ cup)	225	Anchovies with edible bones (5)	45
Cheese pizza† (⅛ of 15-in. pizza)	220	Tortillas (made from lime-processed corn*)	40
Cheddar cheese (1 oz.)	205	Pinto beans (½ cup)	40
Salmon, canned with edible bones (3 oz.)	205	Rutabaga (½ cup)	40
Mozzarella cheese, part skim (1 oz.)	185	Chinese cabbage, raw (½ cup)	30
Macaroni and cheese† (½ cup)	180	Cream cheese (2 tbsp.)	25
Blackstrap molasses (1 tbsp.)	170	Tuna, canned (3 oz.)	10
Pudding (½ cup)	150	Lettuce greens (½ cup)	10
Tofu, raw (processed without calcium*) (½ cup)	130		
Frozen yogurt (½ cup)	105	*Read the labels.	
Turnip greens (½ cup)	100	†The amount of calcium may vary, depending on the ingredients.	

safeguard, many doctors also recommend calcium supplements, especially for menopausal and post-menopausal women to help slow bone loss that comes with hormonal changes. Many women simply don't consume enough calcium.

If you're advised to take calcium supplements, use them to your best advantage to fill the calcium gap—and not as a substitute for calcium-rich foods. *See "Calcium Supplements: A Bone Builder" in chapter 23 for ways to get the most benefit.*

Calci-Yumm: How to Eat More!

Need more calcium in your food choices? Give your meal and snack choices a calcium boost in these easy ways:

● Make it a habit! Eat two to three servings—or more—of foods from the Milk, Yogurt, and Cheese Group each day. Include fruity yogurt with breakfast and a refreshing glass of milk for lunch or dinner for two easy servings. Three cups of milk, regardless of whether it's whole, fat-free, or flavored, supply about 900 milligrams of calcium.

● Reach for milk—during your "coffee break." If there's no place to buy a carton of milk, bring it from home. Refrigerate milk for a day at work in a small water bottle. Some experts say that just choosing milk at snacktime could make a big impact toward reducing the risk for osteoporosis.

● Give goat milk a try. One cup supplies about 325 milligrams of calcium, slightly more than 1 cup of cow milk. The fat content varies, so you need to check the Nutrition Facts on the label. Look for low-fat goat milk that's fortified with vitamins A and D.

● For the "new taste" of milk, try flavored milk—blueberry, banana, peanut butter—or yogurt-fruit drinks. Or make your own fruity drinks by blending milk or yogurt with fruit and ice in a blender or food processor.

● Enjoy calcium-rich snacks: frozen yogurt, ice milk, cheese with crackers, plain yogurt, pudding, milk, or calcium-fortified juice. *For a calcium-rich, low-fat dip or cracker spread, see "Kitchen Nutrition: Yogurt Cheese" in chapter 3.*

● At a coffee bar, order latte (steamed milk with espresso coffee) or cappuccino. Lower the calories and hold the fat by asking for fat-free milk. For more flavor, sprinkle on a little cinnamon or nutmeg. While caffeine can interfere with calcium absorption, this effect is readily offset by consuming the amount of steamed milk typically added to latte or cappuccino.

● Lighten up with milk. Add milk to your coffee or tea (milk tea), rather than drinking it black. Milk has more calcium than powdered nondairy creamer.

● Choose vegetables and fruits with more calcium: dark-green leafy greens such as kale and mustard, collard, and turnip greens; broccoli, dried beans, and bok choy are good sources of calcium. Other nondairy options include dried figs and calcium-fortified fruit juices.

● Drink calcium-fortified soy milk (from the carton or blended in smoothies) and use it in cooking, especially if you choose to avoid milk.

● Say "cheese" when you make or order sandwiches.

● Choose canned fish with edible bones: salmon, sardines, and anchovies. Mix salmon in salads, casseroles, pasta dishes, salmon cakes, and other mixed dishes.

● Add tofu (soybean curd) made with calcium to salads, casseroles, chili, stir-fries, smoothies, and other dishes.

● Boost the calcium in your food preparation. Make soups, chowders, and hot cereal with milk. Top salads, soups, and stews with shredded cheese. Mix dry milk powder into meat loaf and casseroles. Make vegetable dips with plain yogurt, calcium-fortified tofu, or cottage cheese. Add bok choy, broccoli, or kale to soups, casseroles, and other mixed dishes. *For more ways to add calcium-rich foods in food preparation, see "Calcium Boosters" in chapter 13.*

● Look for calcium-rich foods in the grocery store. Check the Nutrition Facts on food labels, listing the calcium in a single serving. The amount is given as the % Daily Value, which approximates the percentage of your day's calcium need supplied by one serving of that food.

● Try high-calcium milk. If milk is fortified with extra calcium, you'll find the amount per serving (perhaps 500 milligrams in one cup of milk) listed in the Nutrition Facts on the label.

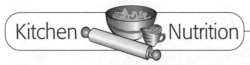

Kitchen Nutrition: Milk Plus

You say you're not a milk drinker? Just whisk one or two ingredients, such as those below, with one cup of milk—cold or hot, fat-free or whole—and give it a refreshing new flavor! (And enjoy the added benefits of 300 milligrams of calcium from a cup of milk.)

- ½ cup of fresh or frozen puréed berries: strawberries, raspberries, blackberries, or blueberries
- 2 tablespoons of fruit juice concentrate and ½ teaspoon of flavor extract
- ¼ teaspoon of almond, anise, hazelnut, maple, or vanilla extract. Or try a flavored oil, perhaps cinnamon or peppermint: use 2 drops of flavored oil in place of ¼ teaspoon of extract.
- 1 puréed banana or peach, with ½ teaspoon of honey
- ½ cup of cranberry juice cocktail and a small scoop of low-fat vanilla ice cream
- 1 tablespoon of creamy peanut butter and 2 tablespoons of chocolate syrup

You'll find many calcium-rich foods in the dairy case of the supermarket: for example, milk, yogurt, and cheese. However, descriptions on food labels can help you identify other foods that are good calcium sources. Look for "calcium-rich," "good source of calcium," and "more calcium." *See "Label Lingo: Vitamins and Minerals" earlier in this chapter to see what these descriptions mean.*

Note: If you frequently have gas, cramping, and bloating after consuming milk and milk products, you may be lactose intolerant. *For more on this condition and how to include calcium-rich foods in your meals and snacks, see "Lactose Intolerance: A Matter of Degree" in chapter 21.*

Iron: A Closer Look

Iron: it's a mineral that's widely available in food. You need it in small amounts to keep healthy. Yet, iron deficiency is a common nutrition problem everywhere in the world. Iron deficiency often leads to anemia and its symptoms: fatigue, weakness, and poor health, all interfering with a person's physical ability to perform at full potential.

Iron: Its Mission

Although iron has many biological functions, its main job is to carry oxygen in the hemoglobin of red blood cells. In fact, about two-thirds of your body's iron is in hemoglobin. Hemoglobin takes oxygen to your body cells, where it's used to produce energy. Iron in red blood cells also helps take away carbon dioxide, a by-product of energy production. Red blood cells have a "life span" of about four months. After that, some of their iron gets recycled; either it's stored or used immediately to make new red blood cells. This recycling action helps protect you from iron deficiency.

What happens when you don't consume enough iron—or when the iron stored in your body gets too low? Red blood cells can't carry as much oxygen, likely making you feel tired, perhaps weak, and less able to perform at your peak efficiency. These are among the symptoms of anemia. Be aware, however, that anemia has several causes—not just iron deficiency. *For more, see "Anemia: More than One Cause" in chapter 22.*

As part of its job description, iron also helps protect you from infections as part of an enzyme in your immune system. Iron helps change beta carotene to vitamin A, helps produce collagen (which holds tissues of your body together), and helps make body proteins (amino acids), among its other tasks.

How much iron do you need to consume? Your body is highly adaptive, absorbing more iron when its iron stores are low, and less when they're higher. Regardless, the Recommended Dietary Allowances (RDA) are set to meet the needs of the broad population.

Iron needs are highest during periods of rapid growth: childhood, adolescence, childbearing years for women, and pregnancy. Prior to menopause, women need enough iron to replace losses from menstrual flow. Iron needs also go up to support increases of blood volume during pregnancy. Not surprisingly, iron-deficiency anemia is most common among people at these ages and stages of life, too, when the dietary need for iron is highest. In fact, it's hard to get enough without taking an iron supplement.

With menopause, iron needs drop. That's the time to *stop* taking an iron supplement, especially for women at risk for hemochromatosis, a genetic disorder that results in high levels of stored iron in the body. Iron-rich foods can supply as much as most postmenopausal women need. *See the earlier discussion of iron in this chapter for a brief explanation of hemochromatosis.*

Iron in Foods: Heme vs. Nonheme

If iron is abundant, why don't many of us "pump enough iron" from food? Iron comes from a wide variety of foods—of both animal and plant origin. Most of the iron from meat, poultry, and fish is heme iron. That name comes from the way it's carried in food—as part of the hemoglobin and myoglobin (similar to hemoglobin in humans) in animal tissue. Foods of plant origin contain only nonheme iron. And egg yolks have mostly nonheme iron.

The deep-red color of animal muscle comes from hemoglobin. The darker the color, the higher the content of heme iron. For example, beef liver, which is redder than roast beef, has more iron. And dark turkey meat has more heme iron than the light meat.

What makes this difference nutritionally significant? First, consider that iron in food isn't absorbed efficiently. Much of the iron you consume never gets absorbed into your bloodstream. (Fortunately, the RDAs take this fact into account.) The amount of iron your body absorbs depends on several factors: among them, how much iron you consume and in what form (heme or nonheme); other nutrients in the meal or snack that can enhance or hinder its absorption; and

---

COUNTING UP IRON

This chart shows the amount of total iron in food. But remember, iron from most animal sources (heme iron) usually is better absorbed than iron from plant sources of food (nonheme iron).

To help reduce iron-deficiency anemia, many foods on today's supermarket shelves are enriched or fortified with iron: iron-enriched flour (also used in baked goods and pasta) and iron-fortified breakfast cereals.

FOOD	IRON (MG)	FOOD	IRON (MG)
Sources of Mostly Heme Iron		*Sources of Nonheme Iron (continued)*	
Beef liver, braised (3 oz.)	5.8	Lima beans, cooked (½ cup)	2.2
Lean sirloin, broiled (3 oz.)	2.9	Enriched rice, cooked (½ cup)	1.4
Lean ground beef, broiled (3 oz.)	1.8	Pretzels (1 oz.)	1.2
Skinless chicken, roasted		Raisins, seedless (⅓ cup)	1.0
dark meat (3 oz.)	1.1	Dried plums (prunes) (5)	1.0
Skinless chicken, roasted		Whole-wheat bread (1 slice)	0.9
white meat (3 oz.)	0.9	Green beans, cooked (½ cup)	0.8
Pork, lean, roasted (3 oz.)	0.9	White bread made with	
Salmon, canned with bone (3 oz.)	0.7	enriched flour (1 slice)	0.8
		Egg yolk, large (1)	0.6
Sources of Nonheme Iron		Peanut butter, chunky (2 tbsp.)	0.6
Fortified breakfast cereal (1 cup)*	4.5–18	Apricots, dried (3)	0.5
Pumpkin seeds (1 oz.)	4.2	Zucchini, cooked (½ cup)	0.3
Blackstrap molasses (1 tbsp.)	3.5	Cranberry juice drink (¾ cup)	0.3
Soybean nuts (½ cup)	3.5	Unenriched rice, cooked (½ cup)	0.2
Bran (½ cup)	3.0	Grapes (½ cup)	0.1
Spinach, boiled (½ cup)	3.2	Egg white, large (1)	<0.1
Red kidney beans, cooked (½ cup)	2.6		
Prune juice (¾ cup)	2.3	*The amount varies. Read the Nutrition Facts on food labels.	

how much iron your body has stored already. In fact, the bioavailability of iron in a mixed U.S. diet (animal- and plant-based foods) is about 18 percent; in a vegetarian diet, about 10 percent.

Heme iron is absorbed into your body more readily than nonheme iron. Depending on how much you already have stored, 15 to 35 percent of heme iron gets absorbed. That's good news.

Nonheme iron is a different story. Only 2 to 20 percent of nonheme iron gets absorbed. Even though foods with nonheme iron often contain more iron than those with heme iron, you may get less than you think. Again, there's good news. You can enhance your body's ability to absorb nonheme iron. Consuming vitamin C and foods such as meat with heme iron aids nonheme iron absorption.

On the reverse side, some phytonutrients—oxalic acid in spinach and chocolate; phytic acid in wheat bran and legumes; tannins in coffee and tea; and polyphenols in coffee—seem to inhibit nonheme iron

Iron: The Power of Partnership

To help your body absorb more iron, pair foods like these at your meals and snacks. Meat, poultry, fish (all three with heme iron), and vitamin C-rich foods help release more nonheme iron from foods of plant origin and egg yolks.

ABSORPTION ENHANCERS	NONHEME IRON SOURCES
Sirloin strips	With spinach salad
Barbecued beef	With refried beans and tortillas
Ground beef	With a whole-grain roll
Pork	With bean soup
Chicken	With brown rice
Ham	With scrambled eggs
Grapefruit	With bran cereal
Strawberries	With oatmeal
Red bell pepper	With whole-grain pasta
Papaya	With whole-wheat toast
Orange	With a peanut butter sandwich on whole-wheat bread

Source: Adapted from National Cattlemen's Beef Association, *Iron in Human Nutrition* (Chicago, 1998).

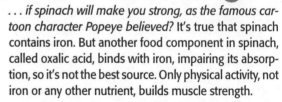

Have You Ever Wondered

. . . if spinach will make you strong, as the famous cartoon character Popeye believed? It's true that spinach contains iron. But another food component in spinach, called oxalic acid, binds with iron, impairing its absorption, so it's not the best source. Only physical activity, not iron or any other nutrient, builds muscle strength.

. . . if cooking in an iron skillet improves the iron content of food? It does. Before the days of aluminum and stainless steel cookware, great-great-grandma unknowingly supplemented her family's diet with iron from her iron pots and pans. If you have cast iron cookware, you can get the benefits, too. Foods with acids such as tomato juice, citrus juice, and vinegar help dissolve small amounts of iron from the pot into the cooking liquids—especially good for foods that simmer and stew for a while.

. . . if you need more iron if you seem tired all the time? Maybe—or maybe you need more sleep, less stress, or perhaps more physical activity to increase your stamina! Fatigue is a symptom of anemia, however. Check with your physician for a blood test. *See "Anemia: 'Tired Blood'" in chapter 22 for more about anemia and blood testing.*

absorption. But again, consuming vitamin C and iron from meat, fish, and poultry at the same time helps overcome these "inhibitors."

These quick nutrition tips can help your body better absorb iron (nonheme) from foods of plant origin and from egg yolks:

● Enjoy a vitamin C-rich food—such as an orange, cantaloupe, green pepper, or broccoli—right along with it; for example, you get more iron from a peanut butter sandwich on whole-wheat bread if you eat it with a glass of orange juice. This is especially important for vegetarians, who get most of their iron from plant sources. Add a little meat, poultry, or fish (with heme iron) to foods of plant origin and egg yolks; for example, include some ground beef in a pot of chili, or sliced lean ham in an egg omelette. The presence of heme iron boosts the absorption of nonheme iron.

● Drink coffee or tea between meals—not with meals.

● Cook in an iron skillet.

For more combinations, see "Iron: The Power of Partnership" on page 106.

Making the most of the iron in your food choices shows the power of nutrient partnerships—and underscores the reasons for enjoying a variety of food!

Need more strategies to boost your vitamin and mineral quotient? Check here for "how-tos":

- Explore new-to-you fruits, vegetables, and grain products—see chapter 9.

- Plan a day's food choices that deliver enough vitamins and minerals and plenty of phytonutrients—see chapter 10.

- Scout for nutrient-rich, phytonutrient-rich foods when you shop—see chapter 11.

- Lock vitamins in and boost calcium, too, when you prepare food—see chapter 13.

- Enjoy the flavors and get the benefits of "five a day" fruits and vegetables—see chapters 13 and 14.

- Use nutrient supplements wisely—see chapter 23.

Phytonutrients—a "Crop" for Good Health

Besides nutrients, plant-based foods (legumes, vegetables, fruits, whole grains, nuts, seeds, and teas as well as herbs and spices) have another "crop" of naturally occurring compounds with potential health benefits. Collectively they're called phytonutrients, meaning plant chemicals. "Phyto" means plant. Think *fight* for "phytos," since they appear to promote health by sparking body processes that fight, or slow, the development of some diseases.

Why have phytonutrients captured our attention? Because of their potential for health promotion! Today consumers are more interested in positive nutrition and self-care: adding (not avoiding) foods that may enhance fitness, boost immunity, slow aging, and prevent or slow the chance for chronic disease. Sound like you? Research on phytonutrients is the new frontier in nutrition, as exciting today as vitamin discoveries were a hundred years ago!

Phytonutrients: What Role in Health?

As public interest in phytonutrients soars, science is exploring their functional benefits. In fact, consumer and media interest is ahead of scientific evidence. Functional benefits are those that extend beyond the role of food's nutrients in promoting your health. In fact, the benefits are all about positive nutrition: what you can eat, *not* what you can't!

Phytonutrients are bioactive compounds in food that promote your health by helping to slow the aging process or reducing the risk for many diseases. Since the early 1980s, research has intensified in investigating how phytonutrients protect against some cancers, heart disease, stroke, high blood pressure, cataracts, osteoporosis, urinary tract infections, and other chronic health conditions.

These are among the ways that phytonutrients might work: serve as antioxidants, enhance immunity, change estrogen metabolism, enhance communication among body cells, cause cancer cells to die, detoxify carcinogens, and repair damage to DNA that's caused by smoking and other toxins. Yet the benefits and actions of phytonutrients are still uncertain. Do they work independently, together, with nutrients and fiber, or do their actions add up? Stay tuned!

"Phytos": In a Class of Their Own

Neither vitamins nor minerals, phytonutrients are substances that plants produce naturally to protect themselves against viruses, bacteria, and fungi, as well as insects, drought, and even the sun. Beyond that, they provide the color, aroma, and flavor that give food so much sensual appeal. Of the thousands of phytonutrients, more than two thousand are plant pigments that put a rainbow of colors on your plate! *See "Paint Your Plate with Color!" in chapter 13.*

Like nutrients, phytonutrients are grouped according to their biochemical characteristics and probable protective functions. Only a few hundred have yet been studied. What we know today is merely the "appetizer."

Research has revealed a few things. Most fruits and vegetables contain phytonutrients. Different plant-based foods supply different kinds and amounts; some have a remarkable variety. An orange, for example, has more than 170 different phytonutrients! In any fruit or vegetable, these substances appear to work together with nutrients and fiber for your good health.

For phytonutrients, food databases are limited to just a few hundred foods, with only a few key carotenoids and phytoestrogens. A database for flavonoids is being developed. No Dietary Reference Intakes exist for them yet. Here's a quick look at several phytonutrient categories:

Terpenes. Carotenoids, limonoids, and saponins are subgroups of terpenes, a large class of phytonutrients that work as potent antioxidants. The hundreds of carotenoids, often grouped by color, may decrease the risk of heart disease, stroke, blindness, and some cancers—and may help slow the aging process, improve respiratory function, and reduce problems associated with diabetes. *See "Carotenoids: 'Color' Your Food Healthy" earlier in this chapter.*

Phenols. This family group, which includes polyphenols (including flavonoids), offers protection from oxidative damage. Sometimes called bioflavonoids, more than eight hundred flavonoids work as antioxi-

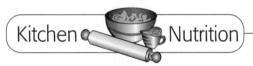

Boosting Phytonutrient Benefits

Research suggests that what you do in the kitchen can make a difference in food's phytonutrients benefits. For example:

- Cooking or food processing may enhance the body's ability to use (bioavailability) some phytonutrients. Carotenoids (including lycopene) are one example. In addition, dietary fat may enhance the absorption of carotenoids; dietary fiber impedes it.

- Heat damages anthocyanins, which are flavonoids. On the flip side, the anthocyanin content may increase in fresh fruit if it's stored for a few days.

- Flaxseed needs to be crushed or ground to get the benefits.

- For the most benefit from tea's polyphenols, brew each cup fresh (preferably in water that's not hard) and drink it soon. Three to five minutes of brewing for one tea bag brings out 80 percent of the catechins, which are flavonoids.

- Chop garlic for about fifteen minutes before heating to allow allyl sulfides to fully develop.

Functional Nutrition: More to Learn!

Phytonutrients aren't the only food substances with functional benefits. Check here to learn more:

- *"Prebiotics and Probiotics: What Are They?"* in this chapter.

- *"Eat Your Omega-3s and -6s"* in chapter 3.

- *"Stanol- and Sterol-Based Ingredients"* in chapter 3.

- *"Polyols: Sugar Replacers,"* about sugar alcohols, in chapter 5.

- *"Fiber: Your Body's Broom,"* chapter 6.

- *"Teatime: Health Benefits?"* in chapter 8.

- *"Functional Foods: A New Wave"* in chapter 9.

- *"A Toast to Heart Health"* in chapter 22.

- *"Functional Foods for Heart Health!"* in chapter 22.

- *"Functional Foods: How Much for Benefits?"* in chapter 22.

dants with many potentially protective health benefits; for example, some appear to promote cardiovascular health by helping to make blood cells less "sticky." Isoflavones, anthocyanins, and catechins are subgroups of flavonoids; some isoflavones are phytoestrogens—weak, nonsteroid estrogens. Lignans, other phenolic substances, are also phytoestrogens.

Phytosterols. Sometimes referred to as "plant cholesterol" because of their structural similarity, phytosterols are fatlike substances in plants. Phytosterols offer protection from heart disease by helping to decrease the absorption of dietary cholesterol from animal-based foods.

Thiols (organosulfuric compounds). Thiols are plant substances that contain sulfur naturally. Their food sources are easy to identify because of their pungent aroma. Some of these compounds you might hear about include glucosinolates, indoles, dithiolthiones, and isothiocyanates in cruciferous vegetables, and allyl sulfides in foods such as garlic and onions.

Organic Acids and Polysaccharides. These substances include organic acids such as oxalic acid, phytic acid, and tannins, which bind with iron and make it less available to your body. Yet they may have benefits, too; see the following chart. Caffeic and ferulic acids fit

FUNCTIONAL NUTRITION: A QUICK LOOK AT KEY PHYTONUTRIENTS

A HANDFUL OF PHYTONUTRIENTS*	WHAT THEY APPEAR TO DO	WHERE THEY'RE FOUND (SOME FOOD SOURCES)
Allyl Sulfides Allyl methyl trisulfide Diallyl sulfide	● May help lower LDL cholesterol ● May help maintain a healthy immune system ● May help control hypertension ● May reduce the risk of certain cancers	● Onions, garlic, leeks, chives, scallions
Carotenoids Beta carotene	● As an antioxidant, neutralize free radicals that may cause cell damage ● May help slow the aging process ● May reduce the risk of some cancers ● May improve lung function ● May reduce problems related to type 2 diabetes	● *Yellow-orange fruits and vegetables* such as apricots, cantaloupes, papayas, carrots, pumpkins, sweet potatoes, winter squash ● *Green vegetables* such as broccoli, spinach, kale
Lutein	● Contribute to maintaining healthy vision ● May reduce the risk of cataracts and macular degeneration ● May reduce the risk of some cancers	● *Green vegetables* such as kale, spinach, collard greens, Swiss chard, Romaine lettuce, broccoli, Brussels sprouts ● Kiwi fruit ● Egg yolks
Lycopene	● Reduce risk of prostate cancer ● May reduce risk for heart disease	● *Most red fruits and vegetables* such as tomatoes, tomato products, pink grapefruit, guava, watermelon (The red pigment in red peppers is from keto carotenoids, not lycopene.)
Zeaxanthin	● Contribute to maintaining healthy vision ● May help prevent macular degeneration	● Corn, spinach, winter squash, green vegetables, citrus fruits. (Eggs have a small amount of zeaxanthin, too.)
Flavonoids Anthocyanins (cyanidin, delphinidin, malvidin)	● As an antioxidant, neutralize free radicals ● May help reduce cancer risk ● May help prevent urinary tract infections	● Blueberries, blackberries, cranberries, cherries, strawberries, kiwifruit, plums, red grapes, red cabbage, eggplant (skin)
Catechins	● As an antioxidant, neutralize free radicals ● May help reduce risk for cancers of the stomach, skin, and esophagus	● Tea (black, oolong, or green), wine

FUNCTIONAL NUTRITION: A QUICK LOOK AT KEY PHYTONUTRIENTS *(continued)*

A HANDFUL OF PHYTONUTRIENTS*	WHAT THEY APPEAR TO DO	WHERE THEY'RE FOUND (SOME FOOD SOURCES)
Flavanones (hesperetin, naringenin)	● May help protect against heart disease	● Citrus fruit
Isoflavones(daidzein, genestein, glycitein)	● May reduce menopause symptoms such as hot flashes ● May offer protection from breast and prostate cancers ● May protect bone health after menopause	● Soybeans, soy-based foods
Quercetin	● Works as a potent antioxidant ● May reduce the growth and spread of cancer cells	● Onions ● Wine ● Tea ● Many vegetables
Resveratrol	● As an antioxidant, may help reduce the risk of heart disease ● Support normal cardiovascular health ● May help reduce the risk of cancer, blood clots, stroke	● Red grapes, red grape juice, red wine ● Peanuts
Tangeritin	● May protect against some cancers	● Citrus fruit
Glucosinolates† Sulphoraphane (†change to indoles and isothiocyanates when chewed or cooked)	● As antioxidants, neutralize free radicals ● May reduce the risk of some cancers ● May aid in detoxifying some carcinogens	● Cruciferous vegetables such as bok choy, broccoli, broccoli sprouts, cabbage, cauliflower, collard greens, kale, turnips, turnip greens
Lignan *Limonoids*	● As phytoestrogens, may protect against some cancers ● As antioxidants, may protect against heart disease by helping to lower LDL cholesterol, total cholesterol, and tryglycerides	● Flaxseed (not flaxseed oil unless some hull remains), rye, wheat bran, oatmeal, barley ● Vegetables ● Citrus fruits (rinds, edible white membranes)
Organic Acids Caffeic acid	● Has antioxidant action	● Fruits, including citrus
Ferulic acid	● May reduce the risk of heart disease, eye disease, other degenerative disease	● Vegetables
Ellagic acid	● May reduce the risk of some cancers ● May lower cholesterol levels	● Berries, red grapes, kiwifruit

A HANDFUL OF PHYTONUTRIENTS*	WHAT THEY APPEAR TO DO	WHERE THEY'RE FOUND (SOME FOOD SOURCES)
Phytic acid	● May reduce cancer risk ● May help control blood sugar, cholesterol, and triglycerides	● Cereal grains ● Nuts, seeds
Tannins	● May improve urinary tract health ● May reduce risk of CVD	● Cranberries, cranberry products, cocoa, chocolate
Oligosaccharides	● May improve gastrointestinal health	● Jerusalem artichokes, shallots, onion powder
Phytosterols Beta-sitosterol Campesterol Stigmasterol	● Support normal cholesterol levels ● Lower blood cholesterol levels by inhibiting cholesterol absorption	● Corn, soy, wheat, wood oils ● Modified margarine products
Saponins	● May lower LDL cholesterol ● Contains anticancer enzymes	● Soybeans, soy-containing foods, other legumes

*Fiber, another phytonutrient, is addressed in chapter 6.

Source: Adapted from: International Food Information Council (2001). Reprinted with permission of the International Food Information Council Foundation.

in this phytonutrient family, too. Oligosaccharides, made of many simple sugars, are yet another category of phytonutrients that work as prebiotics.

Bottom line: Already there's overwhelming evidence for the health benefits of plant-based foods: fruits; vegetables; legumes (including soy); nuts; seeds; and grains, especially whole grains. Research shows that you *lower the odds* for some cancers, heart disease, and other health problems by *eating more* fruits, vegetables, and grains.

Count on a variety of foods, not dietary supplements, to reap the benefits of the many phytonutrients from all kinds of plant-based foods. Supplements with just one or a few phytonutrients haven't been shown to be either effective or safe.

Functional Nutrition
Prebiotics and Probiotics: What Are They?

As other functional components of foods, prebiotics and probiotics may promote healthy bacteria, or microflora, in your intestines—and perhaps improve your health. *Prebiotics* stimulate or help activate bacteria growth; *probiotics* are the live cultures, or bacteria, themselves.

● *Prebiotics* are nondigestible substances such as oligosaccharides (indigestible carbohydrate) in food that promote the growth of normal, healthful bacteria that are already in your colon. Other substances in food, such as dietary fiber, starch, and sugar alcohols, may work as prebiotics, too.

● *Probiotics* are active cultures, such as some strains of lactic acid bacteria, or foods that contain them, that help reintroduce or change bacteria in the intestine. *Lactobacilli* and *Bifidobacteria* in yogurt with live cultures and other fermented dairy foods have probiotic cultures.

● Early research suggests that probiotic cultures may help keep your immune system healthy and help maintain the "good" bacteria in your intestine. Probiotics also may help reduce the risk of some health problems—for example, shorten the duration of diarrhea, reduce the symptoms of lactose intolerance, promote a healthy immune system, and decrease the risk of some cancers and high cholesterol levels.

CHAPTER 5

Sweet Talk
Sugar and Other Sweeteners

Were you born with a "sweet tooth"? Probably, yes. Studies show that newborns respond to sweet tastes quicker than to other tastes: bitter, sour, or salty. Sweetness adds to the pleasure of eating!

From one source or another, sweet flavors are recorded throughout culinary history. In the earliest times, hunter-gatherer societies enjoyed the sweetness of berries and other fruit. Perhaps, say some experts, sweetness indicated that the food was safe for them to eat. As far back as the Stone Age, primitive drawings show that humans collected honey. Biblical writings and ancient Greek manuscripts tell us that honey was the main sweetener three thousand years ago—and it remained so in the Western world until colonial times. Honey also was used by the Aztecs and the Mayans, and much farther north, maple syrup was used to sweeten food.

Although its origins aren't clear, sugarcane appears as early as 1200 B.C. An early epic describes a banquet of sweet things with "canes to chew" from the land of sugar, or Gur, known today as Bengal. Through trade and conquest, sugar found its way to Europe. But it remained very expensive and mainly medicinal until the 1500s. Then sugar changed population patterns, the world economy, and the course of history. With slave labor, sugar could be produced in the West Indies—and quickly took the place of honey as the Western world's primary sweetener in food and beverages.

Sugars: The Sweet Basics

Two categories of sweeteners flavor food: nutritive and nonnutritive. Traditional sweeteners—sugars and polyols (sugar alcohols)—are nutritive sweeteners, which nourish your body by supplying energy, and are measured by calories. Intense sweeteners, such as aspartame and saccharin, are many times sweeter than sugar. However, because they supply few if any calories, they're considered nonnutritive. In many prepared foods a blend of sweeteners is used, which gives the sweetness level that many people enjoy without too much energy, or calories.

Sugar: What Is It?

Along with starch and fiber, sugars belong to a nutrient category called carbohydrates. Carbohydrates—sugars and starches—are your body's main source of fuel. Some sugars occur in foods naturally. Others are added. Regardless of whether sugars are added or occur naturally, your body really can't tell the difference. Read on to learn why.

Carbohydrates' "Short Form"

Most often, when people hear the word "sugar," they think of table sugar. However, table sugar is just one of several sugars referred to as simple carbohydrates. Starches and fiber are structurally more complex. That's why they're called complex carbohydrates.

Have You Ever Wondered

. . . if honey or brown sugar is more nutritious than white sugar? That's a common misperception. Honey is a mixture of sugars (fructose, glucose, sucrose, and other sugars) formed from nectar by bees. Ounce for ounce, the nutrient content of honey and white (or table) sugar is about the same. Why a slight difference? A teaspoon of honey weighs slightly more than a teaspoon of white sugar, so it has somewhat more calories and carbohydrates: a teaspoon of white sugar has about 15 calories and 4 grams of carbohydrates; a teaspoon of honey, about 21 calories and 4.5 grams of "carbs."

Honey is sweeter than white sugar, so less is needed to sweeten foods. Brown sugar is merely sugar crystals flavored with molasses. From a nutritional standpoint, it has 16 calories and 4 grams of carbohydrates per teaspoon—about the same amounts as white sugar. No sugars contain vitamins, minerals, or fiber.

. . . what refined sugar is? Refined sugar is most simply described as sugar separated either from the stalk of sugarcane or from the beet root of sugar beet. The sugar-containing juice of the plant is extracted, then processed into dried sugar crystals. It's sold as granulated or white sugar. Molasses is the thick syrup that's left after sugar beet or sugarcane is processed for table sugar.

. . . what raw sugar really is? Raw sugar comes from processing sugarcane. It's a coarse, granulated solid sugar left when clarified sugarcane juice evaporates. Because of its impurities, you can't buy 100 percent raw sugar. You can, however, buy turbinado sugar. Even though it may be referred to as raw sugar, turbinado sugar is more like refined sugar. Turbinado sugar is raw sugar that's been refined in a centrifuge under sanitary conditions. It has a light tan color. Nutritionally speaking, its calorie and carbohydrate content are the same as refined, or table sugar. So-called natural sugars—raw sugar, date sugar, honey, maple syrup—aren't nutritionally better than other sugars.

Whether simple or complex, all carbohydrates are made of the same three elements: carbon, hydrogen, and oxygen. The name "carbohydrate" actually comes from its chemical makeup. "Carbo-" means carbon; "-hydrate" means water, or H_2O. To make different types of carbohydrates, these elements first are arranged in single units. Sugars are made of just one or two units; starches and fiber have many more.

In scientific language, sugars are either monosaccharides, with one sugar unit, or disaccharides, with two sugar units. ("Mono-" means one, "di-" means two, and "-saccharide" means sugar.) The three types of monosaccharides are fructose, galactose, and glucose. When two join together chemically, they become disaccharides:

Sucrose = glucose + fructose

Lactose = glucose + galactose

Maltose = glucose + glucose

Sucrose is another name for table sugar, but this same sugar is found naturally in some fruits and vegetables, too. Lactose is the naturally occurring sugar in milk, while fructose is the sugar in fruit and in honey.

The ingredient lists on food labels show all kinds of sweeteners. Some are simply other words for sugar: for example, words ending in "-ose."

Other nutritive sweeteners you'll find on food labels include:

Brown sugar	High-fructose corn syrup (HFCS)
Cane sugar	
Confectioner's sugar	Honey
Corn sweeteners	Invert sugar
Corn syrup	Malt
Crystallized cane sugar	Maple syrup
Dextrin	Molasses
Evaporated cane juice	Raw sugar
Fruit juice concentrate	Turbinado sugar

Made of Many Sugars

Starches and fiber have something in common; they're both polysaccharides. "Poly-" means many. If you concluded that both starches and fiber are composed of many sugar units, you're absolutely right! They're just longer chains of sugars. Starch comes from foods of plant origin such as rice, pasta, potatoes, beans, and grain products.

If starch is made of sugars, why doesn't it taste sweet? The size of the molecules makes the difference. Starch molecules are bigger. Unlike sugars, starch molecules don't fit on the receptors of your taste buds.

But keep a starchy cracker in your mouth for a while. Once digestive enzymes in saliva break down its starch into sugar, it starts to taste sweet because the sugar molecules are small enough to be tasted.

Another polysaccharide, called glycogen, is the form of carbohydrate that's stored in your body. Stored glycogen is of special interest to athletes involved in endurance sports. *For more about energy for athletic performance, see "Energy to Burn" in chapter 19.*

From Complex to Simple . . .

From complex to simple! In a nutshell, that's what happens to carbohydrates during digestion. Before they can be absorbed from your digestive tract into your bloodstream, complex carbohydrates from starches are broken down to the simplest sugars: glucose, galactose, and fructose. Then, in your bloodstream, single sugars move into your body cells, where they're converted to energy. Except for fiber, all carbohydrates—sugars and starches—break down to single sugars during digestion. Your body doesn't distinguish what foods they came from.

Because they're single sugars already, monosaccharides, such as the fructose in fruits, can be absorbed just as they are. That's not the case for disaccharides: sucrose, lactose, and maltose. Digestive enzymes break them down. Some people don't produce enough of an enzyme called lactase, so they have trouble digesting the disaccharide lactose, or milk sugar. *See "Lactose Intolerance: A Matter of Degree" in chapter 21.*

Only fiber, another polysaccharide, remains somewhat intact in the body. Many animals can digest fiber. However, human digestive enzymes can't break down fiber into units that are small enough for absorption, so fiber can't be an energy source. That very quality makes fiber uniquely qualified to promote your health in other ways. *See chapter 6, "Fiber: Your Body's Broom."*

Carbohydrates: Your "Power" Source

Carbohydrates are your body's main energy source, powering everything from jogging to breathing, to thinking, and even to digesting food. Actually, glucose is the main form of carbohydrate used for energy.

Fructose: A Sweeter Message

Is fructose any more healthful than sucrose, or table sugar? Surprisingly, no. All sugars nourish your body in the same way. Fructose and sucrose are just different sugars, and both types are simple carbohydrate. In fact, your body eventually breaks down sucrose into fructose and glucose.

Fructose is found naturally in fruit. But it's also added to certain foods, either as crystalline fructose or as high-fructose corn syrup (HFCS). Crystalline fructose is made from cornstarch, and looks and tastes much like sucrose. HFCS is a combination of fructose and dextrose, a sugar that comes from corn. Currently it's one of the most commonly consumed sweeteners in the United States.

Like any sugar, crystalline fructose and HFCS supply 4 calories per gram. They're both 1 1/2 times sweeter than table sugar, so a slightly smaller amount gives the same level of sweetness.

You might find crystalline fructose on the ingredient list of baked foods, frozen foods, beverages, and tabletop sweeteners. HFCS is used in nondiet soft drinks, fruit drinks, salad dressings, pickle products, ketchup, baked foods, tabletop syrups, fruits, candies, gums, and desserts.

Because it circulates in your bloodstream, glucose is often called blood sugar. It's carried to every body cell, each with its own "powerhouse" for producing energy.

Carbohydrates, absorbed from your digestive tract, cause blood sugar (glucose) levels to rise. Insulin helps glucose enter your cells, where it is used for energy production.

Your body doesn't turn all of its blood sugar into energy at the same time. As blood sugar levels rise above normal, insulin (a hormone from your pancreas) signals your liver, muscles, and other cells to store the extra. Some gets stored in the muscles and liver as glycogen, a storage form of carbohydrate. Some glucose also may be converted to body fat—if you consume more calories than your body needs.

When blood sugar levels drop below normal, another hormone, called glucagon, triggers the conversion of glycogen to glucose. That's how blood sugar levels stay within normal range between meals. Once glucose is back in your bloodstream, it's again ready to fuel your body cells.

Just a Spoonful of Sugar . . .

1 tsp. fructose	12 calories
1 tsp. honey	21 calories
1 tsp. high fructose corn syrup	18 calories
1 tsp. jelly	17 calories
1 tsp. brown sugar	16 calories
1 tsp. table sugar	15 calories

"Carbs" should be your main energy source, even though your body also derives energy from fat and protein in food. Rather than provide energy, let your body use protein for jobs that only protein can do: building and repairing your body tissues. If your energy intake is less than what your body needs and if your limited glycogen stores are used up, your body proteins are broken down and used as an energy source. Also unhealthy, in a low-"carb," high-fat diet, fat is used for energy; however, in the process, potentially harmful ketones can build up in the blood.

Whether from sugar or starch, 1 gram of carbohydrate fuels your body with the same amount of energy: 4 calories for each gram. By comparison, protein also supplies 4 calories per gram, while fat supplies more: 9 calories per gram. For health's sake, make foods with complex carbohydrates, or starch, your body's main energy source. Usually these same foods are loaded with vitamins, minerals, and perhaps fiber, too. An added bonus: many starchy foods are low in fat.

Foods with complex carbohydrates form the foundation of a healthful way of eating. Enjoy six to eleven servings of bread, cereal, pasta, and rice daily. Many vegetables are good sources of complex carbohydrates, too; eat three to five servings of veggies daily. *See chapter 10 to learn how you can fit these foods in.*

Your Smile: Sugar and Oral Health

Imagine the wide smile that comes with those popular words "Look, Mom, no cavities!" Today, 50 percent of America's children have cavity-free teeth, and the number is climbing. Good dental care, along with the widespread use of fluoride toothpaste, fluoride rinses, sealants, and fluoridated water, are making smiles healthier than ever.

Just what causes cavities—and how can you and your family protect your teeth? For years we've connected tooth decay to eating sugary foods. But whether you get cavities depends on many factors—and certainly not diet alone! Heredity, as well as the makeup and flow of saliva, are factors. Although part of the equation, sugar itself isn't the culprit it was once thought to be.

Plaque Attack!

The cavity-producing process starts when bacteria in your mouth mix with carbohydrates—both sugars and starches—to make acids. Bacteria are found in dental plaque, an invisible film that forms in your mouth and clings to the surfaces of your teeth and along your gumline.

Acids, produced by bacteria in the mouth, can eat away tooth enamel, causing tooth decay, also known as dental caries. Every time you eat sugars and starches, acids begin to bathe your teeth. The cavity-producing action continues for twenty to forty minutes after you eat something starchy or sugary.

These two "equations" offer a quick summary of the action that takes place in your mouth when bacteria in plaque mix with carbohydrate in food:

plaque + carbohydrate = acid

acid + tooth enamel = potential tooth decay

Have You Ever Wondered

. . . if presweetened cereals are more cavity-promoting than unsweetened cereals? There's really no difference. Carbohydrates in both starches and sugars "nourish" bacteria that promote decay. Whether or not they're presweetened, their cavity factor depends on how long cereals stick between teeth or in the crevices in molars. The total content of carbohydrates really makes no difference in a food's potential to cause cavities.

Although not a dental health issue, presweetened cereals often have more calories per serving—but perhaps no more than your own spoonful of sugar sprinkled on unsweetened cereal.

A Sticky Issue

Hard candy offers no more threat to your teeth than pasta does. Surprised? Any food that contains carbohydrates—pasta, bread, rice, chips, fruit, even milk, as well as cake, cookies, and candy—can "feed" the bacteria in plaque.

Table sugar, or sucrose, isn't the only sugar that plays a role in oral health. Any sugar—whether it's added or naturally occurring—could promote cavities. Fructose in fruit, and lactose in milk, for example, also cause bacteria to produce plaque acids. So fruit juice-sweetened cookies have the same cavity potential as cookies made with table sugar.

Among young children, baby-bottle tooth decay is caused when teeth or gums are exposed to milk, breast milk, formula, fruit juice, or another sweet drink for extended periods of time. This happens most often when babies fall asleep sucking on a bottle or fall asleep frequently while breast-feeding. *For more on baby-bottle tooth decay, see "Caring for Baby Teeth" in chapter 15.*

Do some foods promote cavities more than others? There's no definitive list that ranks the cavity-forming potential of food. However, two factors that make a difference include how often you eat (or how often carbohydrate comes in contact with your teeth) and how long it stays on your teeth.

Frequency. The more often you eat carbohydrate foods, especially between meals, the more likely acid will attack teeth. Sucking hard candy or cough drops, nibbling chips, or slowly sipping a sweetened drink all afternoon nourish bacteria and bathe teeth with plaque acids the whole time! The action continues for twenty to forty minutes after you finish each candy, nibble each chip, or drink each sip of the soft drink.

Type of Food. Because some foods stick to your teeth, plaque acids continue their action long after you stop eating or drinking. The word "sticky" may conjure up thoughts of caramels. Yet caramels dissolve and leave your mouth faster than bread or chips that stick between your teeth or in the pits of your molars. It may take hours for the food particles to finally leave your mouth. The faster food dissolves and leaves your mouth, the less chance it has to produce plaque acid. For example, sticky dried fruit, granola bars, and

Keep Teeth and Gums Healthy

- Enjoy a balanced variety of foods from the five groups of the Food Guide Pyramid. An adequate supply of nutrients is essential for healthy teeth and gums.

- Go easy on between-meals snacks. When you do snack, try to eat the snack at one time rather than over a longer period.

- Brush twice a day. Floss or use an interdental cleaner between your teeth daily. Use a fluoride mouth rinse. For some people, an interdental cleaner, made of soft rubber, can help clean the food particles and plaque between teeth; ask your dentist if it's right for you. Brushing too often may be abrasive to your tooth enamel.

- Brush with fluoride toothpaste that has the American Dental Association Seal of Acceptance. The optimal amount of fluoride from toothpaste comes from brushing twice a day, not any more often.

- Have regular dental checkups, which include a thorough cleaning.

- Talk to your dentist about sealants, which protect against decay in the pits and fissures of your teeth. (They're not just for kids.)

- For infants, avoid the urge to pacify your baby with a bottle of juice, formula, or milk. If you choose to use a bottle as a pacifier, fill it with water only.

- For children, talk to your dentist, doctor, or pediatric nurse about what amount of fluoride your child should have. If you live in a community that doesn't have an optimal amount of fluoride in the water, supplements may be recommended.

raisins may stay on your teeth longer than a soft drink or a hot fudge sundae does.

Will a box of raisins or a bunch of grapes be more cavity-promoting than a single raisin or a single grape? Eaten at one time, portion size makes no difference. Any amount of carbohydrate gets the decay process going. It's the frequency of snacking that seems to have a bigger impact on cavity formation than the size of the snack.

Brushing and flossing after eating remove the "decay duo": plaque and food particles. Swishing water around your mouth after meals and snacks may help rinse away food particles and sugars, but it won't remove plaque bacteria.

"Carbs"—Not the Only Link to Oral Health

Carbohydrates aren't the only nutrition factor linked to oral health. Some nutrients make teeth stronger. And some foods are even described as "anticavity" foods.

For children, an overall nutritious diet promotes healthy teeth, making them stronger and more resistant to cavities. Several nutrients are especially important, including calcium, phosphorus, and vitamin D. These nutrients also build the jawbone, which helps keep teeth in place. For adults, calcium intake has little effect on keeping teeth healthy, but these same nutrients continue to be important for keeping the jawbone strong.

Tooth loss, common among the elderly, may be linked to gum, or periodontal, disease. Constant infection causes the bone structure of the jaw to gradually deteriorate. *See "Keep Smiling: Prevent Gum Disease" in chapter 22.*

Before fluoridation of water was a common practice, tooth decay was much more prevalent. Now, adding fluoride—to drinking water, toothpaste, and mouth rinses—has become one of the most effective ways to prevent cavities. Fluoride makes the structure of teeth stronger by helping to add minerals back to microscopic cavities on the surface of tooth enamel. *To read about fluoridated water, see "The Fluoride Connection" in chapter 8.*

Get your juices flowing! Your body produces up to one quart of saliva a day—especially if you drink enough fluids. That's good news, because saliva helps protect your teeth from decay. By clearing carbohydrates from your mouth faster, saliva helps to reduce the time that plaque acids can form. Minerals in saliva—calcium, phosphorus, and fluoride—may have a protective effect, too.

Smile, and say cheese! Some aged cheeses—for example, sharp Cheddar, Monterey Jack, and Swiss—also may help protect your teeth from cavities. By increasing saliva flow, they lower acid levels. Like the milk it's made from, cheese also contains calcium and phosphorus, which may help remineralize tooth enamel.

Snack for a Healthy Smile

Keep your smile healthy! For everyone, especially children, smart snacking can lead to good oral health.

- Overcome the urge to snack frequently. Bacteria in plaque produce acids that can damage teeth for twenty to forty minutes after each exposure to carbohydrates in snacks.

- Choose snacks wisely for a well-balanced eating plan. Eat fresh vegetables, fruits (such as apples), plain yogurt, cheese, milk, and popcorn.

- Even though sugars from hard candy, cough drops, and lollipops may leave your mouth faster than snacks that stick between your teeth, go easy on sugary snacks that dissolve slowly in your mouth. Sucking on foods bathes your teeth in sugar for a while. Slowly sipping a sweetened beverage or a nondiet soft drink has the same effect.

- Brush as soon as you can after snacking. This removes plaque and so stops the cavity-producing action of bacteria. Or at least rinse your mouth with water to get rid of food particles.

Sugar Myths

Other than their role in tooth decay, sugars have no direct relationship to any health problem. After careful review of scientific studies, that's the conclusion of nutrition and health experts. Yet sugar myths are still widespread. Here's the real scoop on four common misconceptions about sugar.

Linked to Hyperactivity?

Following an afternoon of sweet snacks, friends, and active play, kids may be "all wired up." But don't blame the candy, cupcakes, or sweet drinks for a "sugar high." Sugar has been wrongly accused as a cause of hyperactivity or attention deficit-hyperactive disorder (ADHD). Even though no scientific evidence supports any link between the intake of sugars and hyperactivity, many parents and other caregivers seem reluctant to put this notion aside.

The causes of nervous, aggressive, and impulsive behavior and a short attention span aren't completely understood. But experts advise adults to take stock of a child's overall environment. The excitement of a party or a special event, such as trick-or-treating or a visit to Santa—and not the sweet snacks that go with the fun—may be the reason for unruly behavior. To the contrary, some studies suggest that sugars may have a calming effect, but there's still more to be learned; a body chemical called serotonin produced in and released from the brain may be a factor.

Causes Diabetes?

Again, the answer is no. Sugars don't cause diabetes. Even though the scientific community debunked this myth almost twenty-five years ago, the misperception persists.

In diabetes, the body can't use sugar normally. The causes are complex and still not fully known. Genetics certainly play a role, but illness, being overweight, or simply getting older also may trigger diabetes; being overweight seems to be a key factor in the growing diabetes epidemic.

While food choices don't cause diabetes, diet is part of the strategy for managing diabetes—along with physical activity and perhaps medication. To control blood sugar levels, people with diabetes manage the overall carbohydrates, proteins, and fats in their meals and snacks.

In the past, people with diabetes were warned to avoid or strictly limit sugar in their food choices. But today, experts recognize that refined sugars, naturally occurring sugars, and starches have similar effects on blood sugar levels. For people with diabetes, the amount of carbohydrates, not the source, is the issue. In fact, blood sugar levels after a meal or a snack are linked to many factors, including how the food is prepared, the meal size, how much fat was eaten, the other foods in the whole meal or snack, the absorption rate of the sugars (digested from sugars and starches)—and certainly a person's health status.

According to current advice from the American Diabetes Association, moderate amounts of sugar can be part of a well-balanced diabetic diet. For people with diabetes, a registered dietitian can help plan and monitor their diet. *For more on diabetes, as well as insulin resistance, see "Diabetes: A Growing Health Concern" in chapter 22.*

Have You Ever Wondered

. . . if eating sugar or a carbohydrate-rich diet causes an insulin reaction that results in weight gain? No, although some popular diet book gurus may say so. Consuming carbohydrate-rich foods doesn't cause insulin resistance; excessive calories do. People who are overweight and sedentary may have symptoms of insulin resistance, a condition often diminished with moderate physical activity and weight loss. *See "Insulin Resitance Syndrome, or 'Syndrome X'" in chapter 22.*

. . . if "carbs" affect your mood? No consistent research supports this notion. As serotonin, a body brain chemical, breaks down, it may help relieve stress. Although carbohydrates may help replenish the body's serotonin, no conclusive research suggests a calming effect. So does a bowl of ice cream or a mug of hot chocolate give you a feeling of comfort or calm? If so, perhaps it's really a link to pleasant memories.

Triggers Hypoglycemia?

It's highly unlikely. Yet many people explain away anxiety, headaches, and chronic fatigue as hypoglycemia caused by eating foods with sugar. Often self-diagnosed, hypoglycemic disorders are quite rare.

Hypoglycemia, or low blood sugar, is actually a condition, not a disease. Between meals, blood sugar levels naturally drop—but remain fairly constant between 60 and 110 milligrams per deciliter (mg/dL) among healthy people. A signal for hypoglycemia is when levels drop below about 40 mg/dL. When blood sugars fall below normal levels, there's not enough glucose immediately available for cells to produce energy. That can cause several symptoms, including sweating, rapid heartbeat, trembling, and hunger.

Among people with diabetes, hypoglycemia is caused by taking too much insulin, by exercising too much, or by not eating enough. In most other cases, low blood sugar is linked to other serious medical problems, such as liver disease or a tumor of the pancreas.

In rare cases, a disorder called reactive hypoglycemia occurs. As a rebound effect, the body secretes too much insulin after a large meal. The result is a drop in blood sugar well below normal, and symptoms such as shakiness, sweating, rapid heartbeat, and trembling may occur—but not until about two to four hours after eating. These symptoms are not to be confused with extreme hunger, which is characterized by gradually increased stomach rumbling, headache, and feelings of weakness—usually occurring six to eight hours after a meal.

If you think you're among those rare cases and that you have symptoms of reactive hypoglycemia, pay attention to how you feel two to four hours after eating. Then talk to your physician about a medical checkup and testing your blood glucose level while you're experiencing symptoms.

Also be cautious of so-called health clinics that diagnose "sugar-induced hypoglycemia" and offer treatment with costly remedies.

Makes You Fat?

Another no. Eating too many calories, not just sugars, causes your body to produce extra pounds of body fat. That includes too many calories from any source—carbohydrates, fats, or proteins. Actually, excess calories from fat turn into body fat first, before extra calories from carbohydrates do. Sugar itself isn't the villain. Instead, being overweight results from a complex interaction of genetics, environment, inactivity, and overall food choices.

Contrary to what some popular diet gurus say, sugar won't cause your body to make or store fat. It's true that insulin levels rise when "carbs" are absorbed. That's normal. Insulin regulates energy storage, allowing your body to move blood glucose elsewhere, perhaps to your cells for energy production or to your muscles or liver for storage. Once accomplished, insulin and glucose levels drop to normal if you're healthy. Glucose is only converted to body fat if you consume more calories than your body needs.

Eliminating foods with sugars and starches isn't the answer to weight loss either. The idea surrounding this myth probably relates to the "glycemic index (GI)," which rates foods by their ability to raise blood glucose levels. (From a scientific standpoint, this concept is quite complex. Among the issues, the GI of a single food is irrelevant in a mixed diet; we don't know what happens when foods of differing GIs are eaten at the same time.) There's no evidence that eliminating foods with a higher GI, such as baked potatoes,

carrots, cornflakes, or whole-grain bread, promotes weight loss; these same foods may offer phytonutrient benefits.

Do people with weight problems have a "sweeter tooth"? And do they consume more sugars than normal-weight individuals? No evidence says so. In fact, they may eat less sugar—but perhaps more fat. For those who are calorie-conscious, including some sweet flavors may help to make a low-calorie diet more appealing. So just because many people like sweet tastes doesn't mean that eating sugary foods will lead to overindulgence. And eating sweets won't stimulate the appetite for more!

To keep your weight healthy, you're wise to control all calories, including those from sugars, in your food choices. Sugary foods—for example, sweet, rich desserts and snacks—can supply more calories than you need. Those extra calories may come from fats, as well as carbohydrates. A "fat tooth" rather than a "sweet tooth" may be why some people overindulge. To maintain your weight ("no gain, no loss") when you're cutting back on fat, replace lost calories with energy from complex carbohydrates. Choose more foods from the lower part of the Food Guide Pyramid. If you're really physically active, sugars can help supply the extra energy you need.

How Much Carbohydrate?

Experts advise consuming about 55 to 60 percent of your total daily calories from carbohydrates, mostly complex carbohydrates, and no more than 30 percent of calories from fat. In a 2,000-calorie-a-day diet, that's 1,100 calories or more from carbohydrates.

To reach this guideline, most Americans need to boost their carbohydrate intake and lower their fat

Have You Ever Wondered

... if a "sugar-free" food is also "calorie-free"? Not necessarily, so don't let the term confuse you. A sugar-free food may not contain sugar but may contain calories from other carbohydrates, fats, and proteins. To find the calories and total sugars in one serving of any packaged food, read the Nutrition Facts on the food label.

intake. On average, Americans consume about 50 percent of their calories from carbohydrate and 33 percent from fat. Protein supplies about 15 percent, and alcohol the remaining 2 percent.

If experts recommend consuming less fat and more "carbs," why do the Dietary Guidelines advise: *Choose beverages and foods to moderate your intake of sugars?* There are two reasons.

First, sugars contribute energy, or calories, yet no other nutrients. Some foods high in sugar supply food energy and few other nutrients and, for some people, may take the place of more nutritious foods and the vitamins and minerals they provide. To compare, foods with complex carbohydrates usually have less fat but more vitamins, minerals, and fiber.

Second, both sugars and starches in foods can promote tooth decay, especially when eaten frequently as snacks. When you're really active, you may need extra calories for energy. If you've eaten a varied and balanced diet that meets the recommendations of the Food Guide Pyramid, sugars can supply some of that extra energy.

Sugars in Your Food

Natural or added, sugars are found in all kinds of food. Seventy-five years ago, homemakers baked with sugars and honey, prepared jellies and jams with sugars, and flavored homemade baked beans with molasses or sorghum molasses. In one recipe or another, about two-thirds of the sugars added to food came from domestic kitchens. Only about one-third were added during commercial food processing. Today those numbers are reversed as more and more households depend on convenience foods rather than home cooking.

No matter what their source, moderate amounts of sugars are part of healthful eating, especially since they're naturally part of many foods and an essential ingredient in others.

Where Do Sugars Come From?

Fruits and vegetables, milk and bread, ketchup and salad dressing, candies and soft drinks—all kinds of foods get flavor, texture, and bulk from sugars. Some sugars occur naturally; others are added during food processing.

Sugar naturally occurs in fruits and vegetables. Through photosynthesis, plants transform the sun's energy into carbohydrates as food for their own growth. Plants have the unique ability to change their carbohydrates. As fruit matures, its carbohydrates shift from starch to sugars, making fruit much sweeter and more appealing. By contrast, many vegetables—among them peas, carrots, and corn—are sweetest when they're young. As they mature, their sugars change to starches. What's the "chef's" lesson? Look for young, fresh vegetables—and serve them at their peak. In other words, don't store them too long. Serve fruits when they're ripe; you may need to allow ripening time after you buy them.

Milk, too, derives some of its pleasing flavor from lactose, its own naturally occurring sugar. Milk isn't perceived as a sweet beverage, however. Lactose is only one-sixth as sweet as sucrose.

Through food processing, sugars—mainly sucrose and fructose—also are added to many prepared foods. Although many plants supply sugars, sugarcane and sugar beets are key sources. Sugarcane grows in the subtropics; sugar beets, in temperate climates. Sucrose comes from both. Fructose, a sugar that occurs naturally in fruit, also takes a significant share of the sweetener market.

Don't forget your own kitchen. In one form or another, you're likely adding sugar as you prepare food: white and brown sugar, corn syrup, molasses, and honey, as well as jam, jelly, and syrup.

Although many nutritious foods contain sugars, regular soft drinks (soda or pop), candies, and other sweet snacks often contain them, too. The Food Guide Pyramid—your guide to healthful eating—shows the food groups that supply added sugars. But it doesn't show sugars that occur naturally.

There's nothing wrong with adding sugars to food or choosing sweetened foods. In fact, they may add appeal to nutritious foods you otherwise avoid. The health issue comes when high-sugar, low-nutrient foods crowd out more nutritious options—for example, when soft drinks, rather than milk or fruit juice, frequently accompany a meal. Following the recommendations from the Food Guide Pyramid is your first priority; then add sweets.

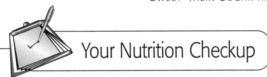

Your Nutrition Checkup

Sweet and Nutrient-Dense, Too?

Here's your chance to check your "sweet" choices. Are they packed with nutrients, too? Or do they provide mostly calories and few nutrients? Check the space that describes what choices you make!

Do You . . .	ALWAYS	MOSTLY	SOMETIMES	NEVER
☐ Reach for fruit as a snack, rather than candy?	___	___	___	___
☐ Drink juice—or milk—with lunch or dinner, rather than soft drinks?	___	___	___	___
☐ Top your cereal with fruit instead of—or along with—sugar?	___	___	___	___
☐ Sweeten waffles, pancakes, or French toast with fruit, rather than just syrup?	___	___	___	___
☐ Top ice cream with fruit, not just chocolate or caramel syrup?	___	___	___	___
☐ Order juice or milk with a fast-food meal or snacks, such as a burger meal?	___	___	___	___
☐ Choose fruit for dessert, not a rich, high-calorie dessert?	___	___	___	___
☐ Go for the smaller rather than the bigger slice of pie or cake?	___	___	___	___
☐ Snack on two or three cookies with milk, rather than simply down five or six cookies?	___	___	___	___
☐ Make hot cocoa with milk, not just water?	___	___	___	___

Now rate your choices.

Total the points in each column. For each answer, give yourself:

　　4 points for "always"

　　3 points for "mostly"

　　2 points for "sometimes"

　　1 point for "never"

If you scored . . .

30 or above. Your "sweet" choices are mostly high in nutrients, too. In fact, enjoy a bit of sugar now and then to add pleasure to eating.

20 to 29. If your overall diet is balanced and you're not overspending your calorie budget, your preference for sweets is probably okay.

10 to 19. Your "sweet tooth" may be crowding out nutritious foods. Check them out and consider some sweet options from the food groups, not just the Pyramid tip. You'll find great ideas in this chapter!

Sugars: More than Sweeteners

The sweetness of sugars is the attribute that gets attention. Yet sugars contribute far more than a pleasing flavor to recipes and processed foods. From the standpoint of kitchen chemistry, sugars work as multipurpose ingredients, fulfilling functions that you may not even think about:

In yeast breads . . . sugars are "food" for yeast, allowing the dough to rise. Yeast doesn't consume all the sugar, however. The rest adds flavor and contributes to the aroma and delicate-brown color of the crust.

In cakes . . . sugars contribute to the bulk, tenderness, smooth crumb texture, and lightly browned surface. In cakes that have air whipped in, such as angel food cake and sponge cake, sugars help hold the form.

Added Sugars: What Foods?

Do you eat a lot of these foods? If so, try to cut back. These foods are the most common sources of added sugars in the American diet.

- Soft drinks (not diet or sugar-free)
- Cakes, cookies, pies
- Fruitades and drinks such as fruit punch and lemonade
- Dairy desserts such as ice cream
- Candy

Source: Nutrition and Your Health, Dietary Guidelines for Americans, 5th ed. (Washington, D.C.: U.S. Department of Agriculture and U.S. Department of Health and Human Services, 2000).

In cookies . . . as sugars and shortening are creamed together, sugars help bring air into the dough. Sugars also contribute to the light-brown color, crisp texture, and even to the "cracked" surface of sugar cookies and gingersnaps.

In canned jams, jellies, and preserves . . . sugars help inhibit the growth of molds and yeast by tying up the water that these microorganisms need to multiply. For this reason, sugars act as preservatives.

In candy . . . sugars contribute to the texture—for example, the smoothness of hard candy and the creaminess of fudge. And as they cook, turning from white to yellow to brown, sugars develop a unique, tasty flavor.

In all kinds of food . . . sugars add to the flavor, aroma, texture, color, and body of food.

What happens if you cut back on sugar in recipes? That depends. In some recipes there's little difference—except for taste. In others, you'll notice a difference in volume, texture, color, and aroma. And in jams, jellies, and preserves, mold will grow quickly, even if they're refrigerated.

Sugars: In Healthful Eating

Sugars, in moderation, are part of healthful eating. By adding taste, aroma, texture, color, and body to all kinds of foods, sugars—naturally occurring or added—can make a variety of foods more appealing.

If your energy needs are low, go easy on the amount of sugars you consume, as well as the amount of fat. And consume mostly nutrient-dense foods. Those are foods that provide other nutrients, too—not just sugars or fats.

- Get your "carbs" mostly from starchy foods. Pasta, rice, bread, other grain products, legumes, potatoes, and other starchy vegetables are great sources of complex carbohydrates. Because they usually supply vitamins, minerals, and perhaps fiber, they're considered nutrient-dense.

- Enjoy the sweet flavor of fruit and fruit juice—and reap the nutritional benefits! Fruit gets its sweet flavor from fructose. At the same time, fruit supplies vitamins A or C, or both—and folate, potassium, and fiber, as well as other nutrients and phytonutrients. Some fruits are sour or bitter, not sweet. Cranberries

Label Lingo

Sugars

Nutrition Facts on food labels give the amount of sugars and total carbohydrates in one serving of a food product. And nutrient content claims give quick descriptions. Look for these terms as you walk the supermarket aisles:

LABEL TERM . . .	MEANS. . .
Calorie-free	Less than 5 calories
Sugar-free	Less than 0.5 gram sugars per serving
Reduced sugar or less sugar	At least 25% less* sugar or sugars per serving
No added sugars, without added sugar, no sugar	No sugars added during processing or packing including ingredients that contain sugar such as juice or dry fruit
Low sugar	(May not be used as a claim on food labels)

*As compared with a standard serving size of the traditional food.

Fruit Snacks: Sweet and Nutritious

Next time you have a craving for a sweet snack, reach for fruit! Besides satisfying a taste for sweets, fruit is packed with nutrients: vitamins A or C, or both—and folate, potassium, fiber, and phytonutrients, too!

Fruit pops. Freeze puréed fruit (mango, papaya, or apricot) or juice in ice cube trays or paper cups with wooden sticks.

Fruit mix. Mix up a zipper-top bag of dried fruits of your choice: apple slices, apricots, blueberries, cherries, cranberries, pear slices, and raisins, among others. (Hint: Brush your teeth—or rinse your mouth with water—after nibbling because dried fruit sticks to teeth!)

Frozen chips. Slice bananas into thin rounds. Spread them flat on a baking pan; cover. Freeze and serve frozen as a fun snack. (*Hint:* The same technique works for seedless grapes or berries.)

Frugurt. Top a rainbow of cut-up fruit with low-fat yogurt. (Hint: It looks pretty in a clear glass or a plastic cup.)

and limes are two examples. Sugars may be added to make these nutritious fruits or their juices more enjoyable.

● Drink water often. Enjoy milk, too. Soft drinks shouldn't replace calcium-rich beverages you need for healthy bones.

● Check food labels for sugar facts. To eat sugars in moderation, know their sources. Almost all food labels carry a Nutrition Facts panel, which lists the amount of calories, total carbohydrate, and sugars per serving. The sugars content is just part of the total carbohydrate. You'll find sugars in all kinds of foods, including milk, fruit, and grain products. Check for other nutrients, too, and for foods that provide plenty of nutrients along with sugars.

● If you're curious about a food's "recipe," look for sugars on the ingredient list of a food label. Even if you don't see the word "sugar," it may be added to food and drinks. Words such as "maltose," "dextrin," "corn syrup," and "molasses" are terms for sugar. And terms ending in "-ose" are sugars, also.

If sugar appears as the first or second ingredient or if several sugars are listed, check the Nutrition Facts panel on a food label. It tells if a food or a drink is high or low in sugars, total carbohydrates, and other nutrients. Sugars that occur naturally in foods, such as in fruit and milk, aren't listed on the ingredient list.

● Know the meaning of label language. You may find words such as "sugar-free" or "no sugar added" on flavored yogurt, canned fruit, breakfast cereal, or other foods. As you shop, read the label language, then check the Nutrition Facts panel for specific information.

● For healthy teeth, snack smart on foods with sugars and starchy foods—but not too often. *For more about healthful snacking, see "That Snack Attack!" in chapter 10.*

● Watching calories? Moderate sugars in your food preparation. *For tips, see "Sugar Savers" in chapter 13.*

● Make sugar trade-offs. Balance sugary foods, such as cake or pastries, with those having less sugars, such as bread or crackers. In that way you can enjoy them within your calorie budget for the day.

● Go easy on foods with mostly sugars but few other nutrients. That includes foods from the tip of the Food Guide Pyramid such as candy, soft drinks, jelly, jam, and syrup. Enjoy them in moderation to add flavor and pleasure to eating.

● Use a light touch with the sugar spoon. Sweeten coffee or tea with just a bit of sugar. For a hint of "sweet" without the calories, try a touch of cinnamon. The same goes for sugar sprinkled on cereal or French toast. Use just a bit. Or sweeten with fresh fruit instead.

● Go "50-50"—and cut calories in half. Share a sugary dessert or snack with a friend. Or eat small portions. Perhaps eat a miniature-size candy, not a large candy bar. Then eat it slowly to get the most enjoyment.

● Try intense sweeteners to add flavor—yet few calories. *For tips on using these sweeteners, see "Cooking with Intense Sweeteners" later in this chapter.*

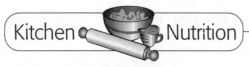

Kitchen Nutrition

Sweet Seasons

Bring out the flavors of foods with seasonings that offer the perception of sweetness: allspice, cardamom, cinnamon, ginger, mace, and nutmeg. If you add fruit, too, you'll get the benefits of their vitamins, minerals, fiber, and phytonutrients.

● Add ginger to a fruit glaze. Blend frozen raspberries with a pinch of ginger and a small amount of fruit juice concentrate or sweetener. Toss the glaze with fresh berries or sliced fruit.

● Add a "sweet" spice of your choice to dry coffee grounds before brewing.

● Add zest and sweet flavor to oatmeal and other cooked breakfast cereals with allspice, mace, or nutmeg. In place of water, cook it in fruit juice (or milk for more calcium and phosphorus)! Toss with dried fruits, such as cranberries or apricots. Or top with fresh fruit.

● For a hint of sweet flavor in rice, cook with cardamom, cinnamon, or ginger. You might substitute fruit juice for part of the cooking liquid. Perhaps toss in raisins, too!

● Add a touch of sweetness to cooked vegetables: for example, carrots with a hint of ginger, mashed sweet potatoes with cinnamon, and spinach with a sprinkle of nutmeg.

● Squeeze citrus juice—lemon, lime, grapefruit, or orange—over fresh fruit to enhance the flavor. Calorie-saving tip: You save about 45 calories with a "squeeze" of juice rather than one tablespoon of sugar.

● Create your own "syrup" for pancakes or waffles. In a blender, purée fresh, sliced peaches, berries, or apples with a little fruit juice, honey, and a pinch of cinnamon.

Pairing Sugars and Chocolate!

A love for chocolate can be traced through the centuries. Known as a food of the gods, chocolate was highly prized in the Americas in pre-Columbian times. Native Americans from what is now Mexico served chocolate to European explorers as early as the 1500s.

By itself, chocolate has a bitter taste. But sugar, transported from plantations in the American and Caribbean colonies, made chocolate tasty to the European palate. By the mid-1600s, the popularity of chocolate, sweetened with sugar, had spread throughout Europe. In 1847, milk chocolate was created, and quickly became popular around the world.

As an ingredient with a distinctive flavor, chocolate can fit within a healthful eating plan. It may add a flavor spark that makes nutritious foods, such as milk, more appealing. Chocolate, a plant-based ingredient, also contains a category of phytonutrients called polyphenols (specifically flavonoids), which may offer some health benefits. Research is exploring links to heart health; chocolate appears to have significant antioxidant potential.

The chocolate challenge? Sugary, chocolate-flavored foods become a problem when they crowd out more nutritious foods—for example, if a chocolate bar replaces fruit in your lunch bag—or when you can't control your chocolate urge. Much of the chocolate we consume is found in confectionery and baked products that are laden with fat, too.

White chocolate isn't chocolate. Even if it contains cocoa butter (the fat extracted from cocoa beans), it has no chocolate liquor (dark brown paste), made by processing cocoa beans. Usually white chocolate is sugar, cocoa butter, milk, solids, lecithin, and vanilla.

Melt Away Myths about Chocolate

Myth: Chocolate causes acne. That misconception has captured the attention of teens for years. However, hormonal changes during adolescence are the usual causes of acne, not chocolate.

Myth: Carob bars are more healthful than chocolate bars. Actually a carob bar has the same amount of calories and fat as a similar-size chocolate bar. Carob, a common substitute for chocolate, comes from the seeds of the carob tree, which are different from cocoa beans.

Myth: Chocolate has a lot of caffeine. While it's true that chocolate does supply caffeine, the amount is quite small. An 8-ounce carton of chocolate milk contains about 5 milligrams of caffeine, compared with 3 milligrams in 5 ounces of decaffeinated coffee. In contrast, 5 ounces of regular-brew coffee contain 115 milligrams of caffeine.

... if chocolate milk is okay for kids? Like unflavored milk, chocolate and other flavored milk supplies calcium, phosphorus, protein, riboflavin, and vitamin D that kids need. Flavored milk contains more calories from added sugars, but the sugars are no more cavity-promoting than any other carbohydrate.

... whether the FDA has guidelines for sugar substitutes? The FDA has set "acceptable daily intakes" (ADIs) for sugar substitutes used as food additives. The ADI for individual sugar substitutes, set at a very conservative level, is the amount that can be consumed daily over a lifetime without posing a risk.

... what fructo-oligosaccharides (FOS) are, and what they do? FOS, which are polymers of fructose, are found naturally in some foods. As prebiotics, they may help improve gastrointestinal health. Researchers are also exploring a possible link to reducing blood pressure and lowering blood cholesterol. See "Prebiotics and Probiotics: What Are They?" in chapter 4.

Myth: Some people are "chocoholics." Not true— although some people do have a stronger preference for chocolate than others, perhaps because of its taste, aroma, and texture. While popping chocolate candies may become a high-calorie habit with a pleasurable sensation, eating chocolate itself can't become truly addictive. Research is exploring any potential role of chocolate to brain neurotransmitters that regulate serotonin and dopamine, often referred to as "feel good" body substances.

Polyols: Sugar Replacers

Polyols, called "sugar alcohols" by scientists, are another category of nutritive sweeteners. Why nutritive? Like sugars, they provide energy, or calories, too. Usually they replace sugar on an equal basis. Why the term "sugar alcohol"? To clarify, "sugar" and "alcohol" refer only to their chemical structure. Polyols don't contain ethanol, as alcoholic beverages do. Polyols also may be referred to as "sugar replacers."

Polyols are naturally present in many foods you already enjoy, including berries, other fruits, and vegetables. In fact, polyols are carbohydrates. They're also a category of commercial ingredients derived from sucrose, glucose, and starch—for example, sorbitol, mannitol, and xylitol—and they offer several health benefits.

Sweet, Fewer Calories

Because polyols are carbohydrates, they supply energy, but fewer calories per gram than sugar does— for example, 2.6 calories per gram of sorbitol and 1.6 calories per gram of mannitol. As an energy source, however, polyols are absorbed slowly and incompletely, and require little or no insulin for metabolism. That's why foods made with polyols may offer alternatives for people with diabetes.

Their sweetness varies, from 25 percent to 100 percent as sweet as sugar. Sorbitol and mannitol, for example, may be half as sweet as table sugar; however, xylitol is just as sweet. Often polyols are combined with intense sweeteners, such as aspartame or saccharin, for a sweeter flavor.

Polyols are not cavity-promoting. Why? They aren't converted to acids by oral bacteria that produce cavities, so they offer a functional food benefit. In fact, the U.S. Food and Drug Administration has approved the health claim for gum, candies, beverages, and snack foods with sugar alcohols, noting that sugar alcohols in these foods do not promote tooth decay. For some people, sorbitol and mannitol may produce abdominal gas or discomfort or may have a laxative effect when they're consumed in excess. You might see this statement on food labels: "excess consumption may have a laxative effect." Eat foods with these sweeteners in moderation—perhaps with other foods, in case your tolerance is lower.

What about their safety? Sorbitol and xylitol are on the GRAS (generally recognized as safe) list of the U.S. Food and Drug Administration. Mannitol has been accepted, too, pending more health studies. And the GRAS petition for isomalt, lactitol, maltitol, hydrogenated starch hydrolysates (HSH), and erythritol has been accepted. Research is under way for their potential as a prebiotic, too. *See chapter 4 for a brief discussion of prebiotics in "Prebiotics and Probiotics: What Are They?"*

Polyols in Foods

Besides adding sweetness to some sugar-free foods, polyols add texture and bulk to a wide range of foods: baked goods, ice cream, fruit spreads, and candies. They also help foods stay moist, prevent browning when food is heated, and give a cooling effect to the taste of food. Baked foods made with polyols won't have a crisp brown surface unless it comes from another ingredient. Polyols also are used in chewing gum, toothpaste, and mouthwash.

How can you spot polyols on a food label? The ingredient list may give the specific name, perhaps sorbitol. If a nutrient content claim is made, perhaps "sugar-free," it must appear with the Nutrition Facts. Look for the grams of "sugar alcohols" or of the specific polyol. The label also may say that the food has fewer calories per gram than other nutritive sweeteners.

Anyone can enjoy foods made with polyols. However, a registered dietitian or other health professional can help people with diabetes fit them into a healthful eating plan. They're considered "free foods" on diabetic exchange lists—but only if one serving provides fewer than 10 grams of polyols.

Intense Sweeteners: Flavor without Calories

"Low in calories" and "sugar-free"! For many weight-conscious people and those with diabetes, these are sweet messages.

When it comes to sweetness, sugar is "top of mind." Yet intense sweeteners can deliver sweet taste with just a fraction of the calories, and they're many times sweeter than the same amount of sugar. With intense sweeteners, you need only a very small amount. *See "Sweet Comparisons" later in this chapter.*

Intense sweeteners also are known by other names: nonnutritive sweeteners, very-low-calorie sweeteners, or alternative sweeteners. They offer little if any energy, so the term "nonnutritive" is appropriate. In comparison, nutritive sweeteners, such as sugars and polyols, supply your body with energy in the form of calories.

Intense sweeteners can fit into healthful eating for just about anyone. Alone or blended with other sweeteners, they provide sweetness in foods such as yogurt and pudding without adding calories or compromising nutrients. The four intense sweeteners used today won't promote tooth decay, since they aren't carbohydrates.

Quintet of Sweet Options

Perhaps no ingredients have been scrutinized by researchers as much as intense sweeteners. Before being used in food—or as a tabletop sweetener—they're first tested extensively to meet the guidelines and safety standards of the U.S. Food and Drug Administration (FDA).

Currently in the United States, five intense sweeteners have been approved: aspartame, saccharin, acesulfame potassium, sucralose, and tagatose. But watch for news about others. Approval from the FDA is being sought for neotame, alitame, and cyclamate. If you travel abroad, you may hear of stevioside or thaumatin, too.

Aspartame

Aspartame is about two hundred times sweeter than table sugar, so a little goes a long way! Discovered in 1965 and approved by the FDA in 1981, aspartame was first marketed as NutraSweet and sold as the tabletop sweetener Equal. Aspartame is now available in a variety of tabletop sweeteners.

Aspartame isn't sugar. Instead, it's a combination of two amino acids—aspartic acid and the methyl ester of phenylalanine. While amino acids are the building blocks of protein, aspartic acid and phenylalanine are joined in a way that's perceived as sweet in your mouth. These same two amino acids also are found naturally in common foods such as meat, skim milk, fruit, and vegetables. When digested, your body treats them like any other amino acid in food.

Because aspartame contains phenylalanine, people with phenylketonuria (PKU) need to be cautious about consuming foods and beverages with it. On food labels look for "aspartame" in the ingredient list, as well as this statement: "Phenylketonurics: Contains Phenylalanine." PKU is a rare genetic disorder that doesn't allow the body to metabolize phenylalanine properly. It afflicts about one in every fifteen thousand people in the United States. In the United States, all infants are screened for PKU at birth. *For more about food sensitivities, see chapter 21, "Sensitive about Food."*

Because it's not heat-stable, aspartame is used mostly in foods that don't require cooking or baking. Most aspartame consumed in the United States is in soft drinks. Among other commercial uses are in puddings, gelatins, frozen desserts, yogurt, hot cocoa mix, powdered soft drinks, teas, breath mints, chewing gum, and tabletop sweeteners such as Equal and SweetMate.

Cooking tip: When aspartame is heated for a long time, it may lose its sweetness. When you prepare food with a tabletop sweetener containing aspartame, add it toward the end of the cooking process. Or sprinkle it on a cooked or baked product after removing it from the heat.

Saccharin

Discovered in 1879, saccharin has been used as a noncaloric sweetener for about a hundred years. It's produced from a naturally occurring substance in grapes. Today saccharin is used in soft drinks and in tabletop sweeteners such as Sweet'n Low and Sweet 10. The benefits? Calorie-free; not cavity-promoting, not metabolized by humans, and safe!

Being three hundred to five hundred times sweeter than table sugar, a small amount of saccharin adds a lot of flavor—without adding calories. Just 20 milligrams of saccharin give the same sweetness as one teaspoon (4,000 milligrams, or 4 grams) of table sugar. Because the body can't break it down, saccharin doesn't provide energy. Instead, it's eliminated in urine.

What about its bitter aftertaste? It's usually blended with other sweeteners to make the flavor pleasing.

After decades of research, saccharin was removed from the government's list of potential carcinogens. Scientific consensus in the U.S. government's year 2000 Report on Carcinogens deemed that cancer data on rats were not relevant to human physiology. In the past a few studies hinted that saccharin—in very large amounts (equivalent to 750 cans of soft drinks or 10,000 saccharin tablets daily)—may cause cancer in laboratory rats. No human studies have ever confirmed the findings. A warning label still appears on food with saccharin—until the FDA or Congress

removes it. As with any food or food substance, keep moderation in mind.

Cooking tip: Saccharin keeps its sweet flavor when heated, so it can be used in cooked and baked foods. Because it doesn't have the bulk that sugar has, it may not work in some recipes. *See "Cooking with Intense Sweeteners" later in this chapter.*

Acesulfame Potassium

Acesulfame potassium (or acesulfame K) entered the food world in 1967. Approved for use in the United States in 1988, acesulfame potassium is marketed under the brand name Sunette.

A white, odorless, crystalline sweetener, this intense sweetener provides no calories. Like saccharin, acesulfame potassium can't be broken down by the body, and it's eliminated in the urine unchanged. Again, no calories, and a potential benefit for people with diabetes.

Acesulfame potassium is two hundred times sweeter than table sugar, adding its sweet taste to candies, baked goods, desserts, soft drinks, and tabletop sweeteners such as Sweet One and Swiss Sweet. By itself in some foods, a high concentration of acesulfame potassium may leave a slight aftertaste, so it's often combined with other sweeteners, both traditional and intense.

Cooking tip: Because acesulfame potassium is heat-stable, you can use it in cooked and baked foods. Like saccharin, it doesn't give bulk, or volume, as sugar does, so it may not work in some recipes. *See "Cooking with Intense Sweeteners" later in this chapter.*

Sucralose

Of the low-calorie sweeteners, sucralose is the newest—and the only one that's made from sugar. It's actually six hundred times sweeter than sugar. Discovered in 1976 and approved in 1998 for U.S. use, sucralose is marketed as Splenda.

Unlike sugar, the body doesn't recognize sucralose as a carbohydrate. It's been modified to become a nonnutritive powder. As a result, it doesn't promote tooth decay and supplies no calories, either. Sucralose can't be digested, absorbed, or metabolized for energy, so it doesn't affect blood glucose levels or insulin production. Instead it passes through the body unchanged—a benefit for people with diabetes.

Cooking tip: Sucralose offers the sweet sugar flavor without the calories, and performs like sugar in cooking and baking. However, sucralose doesn't give bulk to baked goods. It's highly heat-stable, even for a prolonged time. And it keeps its flavor in foods, even when stored for a long time. Like sugar, it dissolves easily in water. Use sucralose as a tabletop sweetener in food preparation and beverages.

Tagatose

Approved by the U.S. FDA in 2001, tagatose is a low-calorie sweetener (1.5 calorie/gram) derived from lactose, which is found in some dairy foods. It may be used as a food and beverage ingredient; check the ingredient list to find out.

Intense Sweeteners: for Whom?

In the 1970s the baby boom generation became intent on slimness; in the 1980s, on fitness; then, in the 1990s and into this new century, diabetes and overweight became bigger issues, too. The growing use of intense sweeteners has paralleled these interests.

From a health perspective, almost anyone can consume foods and beverages flavored with intense sweeteners. It's a matter of personal choice.

Watching your weight? You can't lose weight just by using sugar substitutes! But, because they're usually lower in calories, foods sweetened with intense sweeteners can help you keep trim—if you control calories in your whole eating plan. Calorie control—from a variety of foods—is one part of the weight management formula; regular physical activity is the other.

For people with diabetes. Intense sweeteners can satisfy a taste for sweets without affecting insulin or blood sugar levels. They also can help with weight control.

During pregnancy and breast-feeding. Eating a variety of foods with enough calories and nutrients is the real issue. In moderation, foods with intense sweeteners can satisfy a desire for a sweet flavor without adding excess calories. That leaves room for nutritious foods.

Sweet Comparisons

Many ingredients have a sweet flavor—some much more than others. For intense sweeteners such as saccharin, a little bit goes a long way!

SWEETENER	COMPARING THE SWEETNESS TO SUCROSE (WHITE OR TABLE SUGAR)
Sorbitol	0.5–0.7
Mannitol	0.5–0.7
Tagatose	0.9
Sucrose	1.0
Xylitol	1.0
High-fructose corn syrup (HFCS)	1.5
Fructose (crystalline)	1.5
Cyclamate*	30
Aspartame	200
Acesulfame K	200
Saccharin	300–500
Sucralose	600
Alitame*	2,000
Neotame*	7,000–13,000

*Not yet approved for use in food or beverages in the United States

---

Children. Intense sweeteners are safe, but not intended, for infants and young children. Kids need ample calories for rapid growth and active play. Foods and beverages sweetened with intense sweeteners are okay occasionally—if children eat enough food variety from nutrient-dense foods.

Cooking with Intense Sweeteners

With their sugarlike flavor, intense sweeteners can be used in many recipes you already enjoy, perhaps to reduce calories. For example, sweetening an apple cobbler with saccharin rather than brown sugar might save 67 calories per serving (if a recipe to serve four calls for ½ cup of brown sugar).

If you use intense sweeteners, be prepared to adjust your recipe or food preparation technique. And remember, their unique cooking qualities differ from sugar. And they have limitations in baked goods.

● Check the food label on sweetener packages for usage. You'll see the sugar equivalents. Since some intense sweeteners have ingredients added to give them bulk, the substitution equivalents may vary.

● Know that recipes prepared with an intense sweetener may not turn out exactly like the same recipe made with sugar, especially if they don't have a bulking agent added. That's especially true of baked foods. Sugar has many functions other than sweetness. Check label directions for advice on using specific intense sweeteners.

● If intense sweeteners are new to you, experiment a little. Add just a little sweetener until you get the sweetness level you want. Adding too much can ruin the flavor.

● Use any intense sweetener in recipes that don't require heat, such as cold beverages, salads, chilled soups, frozen desserts, or fruit sauces. Be aware that intense sweeteners don't add bulk, or volume, as sugar does.

For cooked or baked foods, use saccharin, acesulfame potassium, and sucralose-based sweeteners according to package directions. They retain their sweetness when heated.

● Add aspartame-based sweeteners close to the end of the cooking or baking process. Prolonged and high heat breaks down aspartame, causing a loss of sweetness. But don't worry if it does get heated. Although you may lose flavor, aspartame still is safe to consume.

● Expect a lower volume when cooking and baking with intense sweeteners instead of sugar. Sugar adds bulk as well as sweetness. Intense sweeteners with a bulking agent help bring up the volume. Or go "50–50" by substituting saccharin- or acesulfame potassium-based sweeteners for half the sugar, according to package directions. However, the volume still won't be as high as with 100 percent sugar.

Need more guidance? Contact the manufacturers of intense sweeteners. Usually they'll provide tips and recipes for using their products to sweeten your palate.

Have You Ever Wondered

... why intense sweeteners don't cause tooth decay? As sweeteners, aspartame, acesulfame potassium, saccharin, or sucralose won't promote cavities because they aren't broken down by bacteria in plaque. Since they don't "feed" bacteria, no acids form. Sugarless gum, flavored with an intense sweetener, may actually promote dental health. First, it doesn't have any carbohydrates. Second, gum chewing increases saliva flow, which actually helps neutralize plaque acids.

... if aspartame is safe? Aspartame, approved as safe by the FDA, has been intensely studied for its safety to humans. Yet unreputable, unidentified scares appear on the Internet. No scientific evidence shows any link between aspartame and any health problems. That includes no link to seizures among children, or to difficulties with tasks among children with attention deficit disorder.

... what's stevia? It's a herb that's sweeter than sugar but calorie-free. It hasn't been approved by the FDA as a sweetener, but it's sold as a supplement. Like other supplements, talk to a health professional before using it.

Need more sweet strategies for healthful eating? Check here for "how-tos":

● Shop for less added sugars—see chapter 11.
● Sweeten food in your kitchen and cook for health, too—see chapter 13.
● Enjoy sweet flavors in restaurant foods—and eat smart, too—see chapter 14.
● Manage "carbs" if you're an athlete—see chapter 19.
● Handle carbohydrates in a diabetic eating plan—see chapter 22.

CHAPTER 6

Fiber

Your Body's Broom

Your ancestors probably consumed more fiber than you do!

Before the days of advanced milling technology, gristmills ground wheat, corn, and other grains into meal or flour. Using the power of a moving river, grain was milled between two coarse stones. Then it was sifted to remove the inedible chaff, or husk, leaving all the edible parts of the grain. The bran and the germ that contain fiber and many essential nutrients remained. Whole grains were the only grains people knew. In some parts of the world, that's still true today; in fact, some people still pound their grain by hand to make flour.

As technology improved, the bran and the germ were separated and removed, leaving refined white flour. With this new process came new status. White bread with its softer texture and high-class appeal became more desirable than coarser, darker bread. But it was more expensive and only available to those who could afford it. For the same reasons, white rice became more desirable than brown rice. Simply put, refined was "in"!

With this switch to refined grains, however, people became short-changed on many nutrients—including fiber—without knowing it. In the 1940s, recognizing the health consequences, manufacturers began enriching many grain products. Now, some nutrients lost during processing—thiamin, riboflavin, niacin, and iron—are added back. In some, fiber is added back, too. Since the late 1990s, enriched grain products have also been fortified with folic acid.

Only within the past thirty or so years have health experts realized that fiber offers more than bulk to food. It's loaded with health benefits; science continues to discover more. Today whole-grain products, along with other fiber-rich foods—vegetables, fruits, and legumes—are "in" again!

Just what is fiber—and how does it promote your health?

Fiber: An Important Nonnutrient

We talk about fiber as a single component of food, but it's not that simple. Actually, "fiber" is a general term, referring to complex carbohydrates that your body cannot digest or absorb into your bloodstream. Instead of being used for energy like other carbohydrates, fiber is eliminated.

Because fiber can't nourish your body, it's not a nutrient. But as a phytonutrient, it's still a component of food that promotes your good health in many other ways.

Fiber: Just What Is It?

Plants—and foods of plant origin—count on fiber for their shape. It's fiber that gives celery its rigid stalk and gives spinach the strong stems that hold up its leaves. That same structure "bulks up" the contents of your intestine.

Like starch, most fibers are made of many sugar units, so they're actually polysaccharides. But unlike

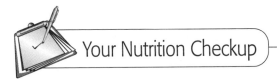

Your Nutrition Checkup

What's Your Fiber Factor— in Your Food Choices?

That's up to you—and what you choose to eat. If you had a choice, which would you pick for your meals or snacks?

1 medium unpeeled apple	or	½ cup applesauce
1 slice whole-wheat bread	or	1 slice white bread toast
3½-oz. cooked meat patty	or	½ cup baked beans
⅓ cup bran flakes	or	⅓ cup corn flakes
1 carrot stick	or	1 bread stick
½ cup white rice	or	½ cup brown rice
½ cup strawberries	or	½ cup grapes
½ cup spinach	or	½ cup peas
½ cup peanuts	or	1 oz. cheese
2 figs	or	2 dried plums (prunes)
2 tbsp. bean dip (hummus)	or	2 tbsp. sour cream
¾ cup orange juice	or	1 orange
1 baked potato with skin	or	½ cup mashed potatoes
1 tbsp. wheat germ	or	1 tbsp. wheat bran

Now check your answers . . .

For each pair, these foods contain more fiber: unpeeled apple, whole-wheat bread, baked beans, bran flakes, carrot stick, brown rice, strawberries, peas, peanuts, figs, bean dip (hummus), orange, baked potato with skin, and wheat bran.

To compare the specific amounts of fiber in these food pairs, see the chart "How Much Fiber?" later in this chapter. Give yourself 5 points each time you picked the higher-fiber choice; 70 points is the highest score you can get. The higher your score, the more fiber in your diet—if these foods truly would be your "picks" for the day!

starch, fiber's chains of sugars can't be digested in the human body into simple sugars. *For more about carbohydrates—their composition and digestion—see "Sugar: What Is It?" in chapter 5.*

In dairy cows, bacteria in digestive juices break down fiber in their grassy meals, providing energy they need to produce milk. However, human digestive enzymes cannot break fiber into units that are small enough for absorption. That's why fiber can't be converted into energy, or calories, in your body. That very quality gives fiber its own unique roles in keeping you healthy. (Technically, your body can digest very small amounts of some fibers. But the amount is much too small to count.)

Although not well studied, some nondigestible carbohydrates also come from animal-based foods. This type of fiber may have beneficial effects on human health, too.

Not All Fibers Are Alike!

Soluble and insoluble: two types of fiber with two different missions! What makes them unique? Soluble fiber dissolves in water, and insoluble fiber doesn't. These differing qualities allow them to keep you healthy in different ways. *"Foods for Fiber" later in this chapter lists foods that contain the two types of fiber.*

Insoluble Fiber: Aid to Digestion

Insoluble fiber: you know it as "roughage." This group of fibers—cellulose, hemicellulose, and lignin—gives structure to plant cell walls. Wheat bran, for example, is high in insoluble fiber.

Although they don't dissolve, insoluble fibers do hold on to water. And they move waste through the intestinal tract without being digested themselves, earning fiber its title as "nature's broom." By adding bulk and softness to stools, insoluble fibers promote regularity and help prevent constipation. By moving waste through the colon, insoluble fibers decrease transit time. That's the time that potentially harmful substances in food waste linger in the intestines and come in contact with the intestinal lining.

What Is a Whole Grain?

A whole grain is the entire edible part of any grain: wheat, corn, oats, and rice, among others. In the life cycle of plants, it's the seed from which other plants grow. Nutrients in these seeds supply the first nourishment for the plant . . . before the roots are formed. The whole grain, or seed, contains three parts: endosperm, bran, and germ.

The *bran* makes up the outer layers of the grain. It supplies large amounts of B vitamins, trace minerals, and dietary fiber.

The *endosperm,* which is the inner part of the grain, has most of the proteins and carbohydrates, and just small amounts of vitamins and minerals. White flour is ground from the endosperm.

The *germ* is small but very important. It sprouts, generating a new plant. It has B vitamins, trace minerals, and some proteins.

It's clear why whole-grain products have more fiber; the bran and the germ supply most of the fiber. When flour is milled to produce white flour, only the grain's endosperm remains. Both the fibrous bran and the germ are removed—along with important nutrients and phytonutrients, including fiber.

Soluble Fiber: Protective Benefits

Soft, liquid foods may have fiber, too. Surprised? Instead of giving a coarse texture to food, soluble fibers, such as those in oat bran, dissolve to become gummy or viscous. They're often used in low-fat and nonfat food to add texture and consistency. Fibers called gums, mucilages, and pectin are all soluble.

If you've ever made jam or jelly, you're probably familiar with pectin. Pectin gives them their thick, gel-like consistency. In your body, pectin plays a different role, binding to fatty substances and promoting their excretion as waste. This quality seems to help lower blood cholesterol levels. Soluble fibers also help regulate the body's use of sugars.

Fiber's "Benefit Package": A Closer Look

Unlike many nutrients, life doesn't depend on fiber— but your overall health may! Fiber's "benefit package" not only promotes health, it also may help reduce the risk for some chronic diseases. That's one reason why the Dietary Guidelines for Americans encourage con-

sumption of a variety of grains, especially whole grains, as well as fruits and vegetables, daily.

Fiber: Bundled with Nutrients and Phytonutrients

Fiber isn't a "lonely" component of food. And fiber's benefits in food can't be easily separated from the contributions of other nutrients and plant substances.

Most foods with significant amounts of fiber—such as legumes, whole-wheat bread, strawberries, and Brussels sprouts—are packed with carbohydrates (complex or simple) and other essential nutrients. For example, many fruits and vegetables contribute antioxidant vitamins (beta carotene and vitamin C), which may help protect against some types of cancer. Whole grains also contain antioxidant nutrients (such as vitamin E and selenium), iron, magnesium, zinc, and B vitamins. And legumes supply protein as well as B vitamins and iron. Foods with more fiber often have less fat, too.

Most fiber-rich foods are loaded with phytonutrients that offer a wide range of health-promoting benefits. Consider this: besides fiber, whole-grain foods supply lignan, which may block estrogen activity in cells and perhaps reduce the risk of breast, ovar-

Which Bread Is Whole Grain?

Being brown doesn't make bread whole wheat! Terms such as "7 grain" or "multigrain" are no assurance, either. It's true that whole-grain breads are browner than breads made with refined white flour. However, in some brown bread, the rich brown color comes instead from coloring, which is listed on the label, usually as "caramel coloring."

By law, any bread labeled "whole wheat" must be made from 100 percent whole-wheat flour. "Wheat bread," however, may contain some white refined flour and some whole-wheat flour; proportions vary from product to product. With a little label reading, you can get a general idea of the amounts of each type. The flour listed first in the ingredient list is present in the greater amount.

To find breads with more fiber, check the Nutrition Facts and the ingredient list on food labels. Look for those made with mainly whole-wheat flour or other whole-grain flour.

ian, colon, and prostate cancer. Whole grains also supply phytic acid, which, by binding to minerals, may prevent free radicals from forming and perhaps reduce cancer risk. *See the charts "Functional Nutrition: A Quick Look at Key Phytonutrients" in chapter 4, indicating those found in fruits, vegetables, and grain products, and "Functional Nutrition: A Quick Look at Fiber" below.*

Avoiding the Trio: Constipation, Hemorrhoids, Diverticulosis

You already read about the benefits of insoluble fiber—the kind in wheat bran. It holds on to water, helping to soften and add bulk to waste in the intestines. This action helps stools pass through the digestive system more quickly with normal frequency and ease. As a result, fiber helps prevent constipation and the discomfort that goes with it.

When soft stools easily pass out of the body, there's no need for strained bowel movements. As a result, hemorrhoids—a painful swelling of the vein near the anus—are less likely to form. Softer, bulkier stools put less pressure on the colon walls and so reduce the chance of hemorrhoids, too. With diverticulosis, tiny sacs form when the intestinal wall, especially in the colon, gets weak. These sacs may become infected and quite painful, a problem called diverticulitis.

For more about dealing with these health conditions, see "Gastrointestinal Conditions" in chapter 22.

Cancer Connection?

Eating plenty of fiber over the years may help prevent certain cancers, such as colorectal cancer. About thirty years ago scientists noted that these cancers were more common in Western countries where people ate less fiber. Today the majority of research studies show strong evidence linking fiber-rich foods (vegetables, fruits, and whole grains) to cancer prevention, although their protective role isn't yet clear.

Two recently published studies disputed the link between vegetables and colon cancer prevention. However, study participants consumed fewer than the recommended five vegetable and fruit servings daily. To reduce cancer risk, nutrition experts advise more: five or more vegetable and fruit servings daily. According to the American Institute of Cancer Research: "Evidence that diets rich in vegetables protect against cancers of the colon and rectum is convincing."

A high-fiber diet may help reduce cancer risk in several ways: (1) by speeding the time it takes for waste to pass through the digestive tract, (2) by forming a bulkier, heavier stool, and (3) by controlling the intestinal pH balance (the level of acidity or alkalinity). Slow movement of food waste through the digestive tract allows more time for potentially harmful substances to come in contact with intestinal walls. Bulkier stools help dilute the concentration of potential carcinogens. And insoluble fibers keep the pH at a level that reduces the ability of intestinal microbes to produce carcinogens.

Is it fiber that protects? Or is it something else? It's difficult to know. Many fiber-rich foods supply plenty of nutrients, including antioxidant nutrients and phytonutrients. The anticancer power of fiber-rich foods

---

FUNCTIONAL NUTRITION: A QUICK LOOK AT FIBER

DIFFERENT TYPES OF FIBER	WHAT THEY APPEAR TO DO	WHERE THEY'RE FOUND (SOME FOOD SOURCES)
Insoluble fiber	● May reduce risk of breast and/or colon cancer	● Wheat bran[†]
Beta glucan* (soluble fiber)	● Reduces risk of cardiovascular disease (CVD)	● Oats, oat bran[†]
Soluble fiber*	● Reduces risk of CVD	● Psyllium
Whole grains	● Reduces risk of CVD	● Cereal grains

*The U.S. Food and Drug Administration has approved a health claim for this food component.
[†]See "Foods for Fiber" later in this chapter for more food sources.

Source: International Food Information Council Foundation (2001). Reprinted with permission from the International Food Information Council Foundation.

Have You Ever Wondered

. . . which one to buy: wheat germ or wheat bran? They're two different parts of the grain, so their benefits differ. The germ is the nutrient-rich inner part, and the bran is the outer coating. From a nutritional standpoint, 1 ounce (⅓ cup) of wheat bran has a lot more fiber, about 13 grams, than 4.4 grams of fiber in 1 ounce (¼ cup) of wheat germ. Wheat germ has more protein, and more of some vitamins and minerals.

. . . what psyllium is? (When you pronounce it, the "p" is silent.) Psyllium—high in soluble fiber—is a seed husk used in some bulk-forming natural laxatives; it also has cholesterol-lowering qualities. Some supplements have it. Its source is plantago, a plant that grows in India and the Mediterranean. Although some people may be allergic to psyllium, in moderate amounts it's safe for most people.

may come from the interaction or the additive benefits of their many substances. In addition, a high-fat diet is associated with the risk for colon cancer. Since a high-fiber diet is usually lower in fat, it may be another reason why cancer risk seems to go down among people who eat more fiber.

"Waistline Watchers"

Fiber-rich foods may help your body keep trim! Often they're low in calories and fat. Because they take longer to chew, fiber-rich foods may help slow you down, so you eat less. With their added bulk, they help you feel full longer, making you less inclined to nibble too soon after eating. Fiber itself can't be fattening or provide calories—it isn't digested.

To make a fiber-rich diet work for your waistline, remember to keep your calorie intake low at the same time. (An active lifestyle is important, too.)

Help for People with Diabetes

For people with diabetes, soluble fibers—especially pectin and gums—may perform another important function. By helping to control the rise of blood sugar levels after a meal, soluble fibers may reduce the need for insulin, or medication, for some people. Incorporating at least one or two servings of beans, oats, or

other sources of soluble fiber as part of a total fiber intake of 20 to 35 grams per day may help to lower fasting blood sugar levels in some people with diabetes.

The reason why soluble fibers help lower blood sugar levels isn't fully understood. Perhaps it's because fiber makes the stomach contents more viscous (more sticky and gummy) and so prolongs its emptying time. Because carbohydrates break down more slowly, sugar is released and absorbed more slowly, too. That in turn slows the rise of blood glucose levels. *To learn more about blood sugar and its role in diabetes, see "What Is Diabetes?" in chapter 22.*

If you have diabetes and want to use more soluble fiber to help control blood sugars, talk to a registered dietitian.

Fiber—Heart Healthy, Too!

Another potential benefit: Soluble fibers (mostly beta glucan and pectin) may help lower the level of total blood cholesterol, mainly by lowering LDL cholesterol, or "bad" cholesterol. In the small intestine, soluble fiber acts like a sponge, binding cholesterol-rich bile acids. As a result, they can't be reabsorbed, but instead pass through the intestine as waste. As a result, the body absorbs less dietary cholesterol, and the liver pulls more cholesterol from the blood to replace the lost bile acids. That makes blood cholesterol levels drop.

Years of research with different groups of people show that soluble fibers in beans, psyllium, oats, flaxseed, and oat bran seem to help lower blood cholesterol levels in some people. In fact, there's enough sound research for the U.S. Food and Drug Administration to allow foods to carry health claims linking oats or psyllium with heart health. *See "Health Claims on the Label" in chapter 11 for more about health claims.* Those same high-fiber diets were lower in fat, too. What's more, these foods have other substances besides fiber that may affect the way the body uses lipids (fats). Yet another benefit: Fiber-rich foods may displace fattier foods in meals and snacks.

The benefits of fiber-rich foods for heart health are truly complex. Until more is known about lowering blood cholesterol levels, continue to consume fiber-rich foods of all kinds; decrease your intake of fat, especially saturated fat; maintain a healthy weight; and live an active lifestyle.

Tip: You need to consume a lot of soluble fiber for heart-healthy benefits. Research suggests that it takes 3 grams of beta glucan a day for a cholesterol-lowering effect. Here are some equivalents: 1½ cups of cooked oatmeal, *or* 1½ cups of some ready-to-eat oat bran cereals, *or* ¾ cup of uncooked oatmeal (added to meat loaf, salmon cakes, muffin batter, or as a topping for yogurt or fruit), or a combination.

For more about lowering blood cholesterol levels, see "Prevention: Cholesterol Countdown" on page 540.

Intestinal Gas: Part of Fiber's "Action"

Intestinal gas is a common complaint—and a normal side effect—of eating a high-fiber diet. If your eating plan has been typically low in fiber, minimize the discomfort that comes with "bulking up." Increase your fiber intake slowly over several months. Drink enough water, too, to help reduce the effects of intestinal gas and prevent impacted stools.

People especially complain—and sometimes joke—about beans and vegetables in the cabbage family: "They give me gas!" Gas forms in the intestines because humans lack the right enzymes to digest certain carbohydrates, leaving people feeling gassy and bloated. Other foods or ingredients reported to cause gas for some include milk, wheat germ, onions, carrots, celery, bananas, raisins, dried apricots, prune juice, and sorbitol. Sorbitol, which is slowly digested, is actually a sugar alcohol, not a sugar.

There are some techniques that may help to tame the gas caused by beans.

● When preparing dry beans, soak them overnight, then discard the soaking water. Some gas-producing carbohydrates get absorbed in the soaking water. For cooking the beans, use fresh water.

● Allow enough time to cook dried beans thoroughly. That makes them easier to digest.

● If bean dishes or other foods cause gas, take smaller helpings.

● "Degas" canned beans by draining off the liquid and rinsing the beans well. That also reduces the sodium.

If you need more relief from intestinal gas, several nonprescription products may help. Products containing charcoal, which are taken at the end of a meal, help absorb gas in the intestines. They can interfere with the absorption of medications, however, and are not recommended for children. Products with a food enzyme called alpha-galactosidase help convert gas-producing carbohydrates to more easily digestible sugars. They're sold in the form of tablets or drops taken before a meal. Products with simethicone help relieve gas symptoms but do not prevent them. This substance works by breaking large pockets of gas in the intestines into smaller bubbles.

Be aware that other gas-reducing or gas-preventing products are sold, some with questionable claims. You're wise to check with your doctor before using any gas-reduction products.

Fiber: How Much Is Enough?

If you're like most Americans, your day's meals and snacks come up short on fiber, supplying only about half the amount your body needs.

For their health benefits, many experts recommend eating more—20 to 35 grams of fiber daily. Unlike many vitamins and minerals, there's been no Recommended Dietary Allowance (RDA) for total fiber

---

Label Lingo

Fiber

Although the Nutrition Facts panel on a food label gives the specific amount of fiber in foods, "fiber lingo" on the label may offer a quick description. Look for these terms as you walk the supermarket aisles:

LABEL TERM ...	MEANS ...
High fiber	5 g or more per serving
Good source	2.5 to 4.9 g per serving
More or added fiber	At least 2.5 g more* per serving

*As compared with a standard serving size of the traditional food

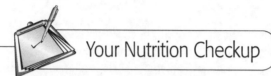

Your Nutrition Checkup

Do You Eat Enough Fiber in a Day?

Write in the Number of Daily Servings You Eat for Each Food Type*		*Multiply by* the Fiber (in grams)	*Total Your* Day's Fiber Intake (in grams)
Beans, lentils	_____ servings	× 6	_____
Fruits, vegetables, whole grain products, nuts	_____ servings	× 2.5	_____
Refined grain products (white bread, white rice, regular pasta)	_____ servings	× 1	_____
Other grain products (including breakfast cereal)	_____ servings	× _____ †	_____

*Check "The Food Guide Pyramid: Your Healthful Eating Guide" in chapter 10 for serving sizes

Total daily grams of dietary fiber _____

†Check the label for the number of fiber grams per serving

Adapted from: American Institute of Cancer Research, *The Facts About Fiber* (2001).

intake—or for amounts of soluble and insoluble fiber. For children (starting at age two) and teens, remember this fiber guideline: "Just add five." Add their age plus 5 to determine about how much fiber they need. For example, a seven-year-old needs about 12 grams of fiber (7 years + 5 = 12 fiber grams). New Dietary Reference Intakes, released in 2002, include fiber.

Although fiber comes from foods of plant origin, you don't need to eat huge amounts of whole-grain products, legumes, vegetables, and fruits to meet your fiber goal. By following the advice of the Food Guide Pyramid, your everyday food choices can supply all you need if you choose foods with more fiber. *Check the chart "How Much Fiber?" later in this chapter to quickly "guesstimate" your fiber intake.* You'll see that most of the grain products, fruits, and vegetables you eat have only 1 to 3 grams of fiber per serving.

However, when it comes to fiber, you can overdo a good thing! Too much fiber can move food through the digestive tract faster than some nutrients can be absorbed. By eating more than 50 to 60 grams of fiber a day, your body may lower the absorption of vitamins and minerals, among them zinc, iron, magnesium, and calcium. An excessive amount of fiber may cause gas, diarrhea, and bloating. By filling up with too many high-fiber foods or supplements, you may not have an appetite for other nutrient-rich foods.

How might you get too much fiber? By eating a lot of bran, very-high-fiber cereals, or perhaps using a fiber supplement in an eating plan that already has plenty of vegetables, fruits, and whole grains!

For Fiber—Variety!

As laboratory procedures have improved, consumers now know the "dietary fiber" content of food, which reflects both soluble and insoluble fiber content. Today you'll find dietary fiber listed on the Nutrition Facts panel on the labels of most packaged food products.

Foods for Fiber

Do you like to nibble on popcorn? It's a whole-grain snack that helps boost the fiber factor in your diet. Again, dietary fiber comes only from plant sources of food: fruits, vegetables, legumes, grains, nuts, and seeds. Plant-based foods actually contain a "mixed bag" of dietary fibers, having some of both types: soluble and insoluble. Good sources of soluble fiber may supply some insoluble fiber, too, and vice versa. For

. . . what grains are whole grain? Brown rice, bulgur, corn (hominy), oats, wheat berries, whole barley (not pearl barley), whole rye, and whole wheat. Cracked wheat is whole berry wheat, too—just broken into coarse, medium, and fine particles.

. . . what graham flour is? It's a whole-wheat flour that's a little coarser than regular whole-wheat flour. Try it in your cooking!

example, fruits and vegetables have both pectin (soluble) and cellulose (insoluble). However, fruit usually has more pectin; vegetables, more cellulose. Both oatmeal and beans have some of both: soluble and insoluble fiber. (Beta glucan is the soluble fiber in oats and barley.)

Here are some specific foods that provide significant amounts of insoluble and soluble fibers. Their texture is a clue to their presence.

- *Insoluble fibers:* whole-wheat products; wheat, oat, and corn bran; flaxseeds; and many vegetables (such as cauliflower, green beans, and potatoes), including the skins of fruits and root vegetables, and beans. In fact, their tough, chewy texture comes from insoluble fibers.

- *Soluble fibers:* dried beans and peas, oats, barley, flaxseeds, and many fruits and vegetables (such as apples, oranges, and carrots). When they're cooked, the soft, mushy texture comes from their soluble fibers. Psyllium seed husks also supply soluble fiber.

For the record: Any nondigestible carbohydrate in animal-based foods is not currently defined as "dietary fiber" on food labels. But stay tuned in the future for possible changes in fiber labeling on food.

From grain to grain, brans aren't all alike. The bran layers in different grains—wheat, rice, corn, oats, and others—have varying types and different amounts of fiber. Wheat bran, for example, has a higher concentration of fiber than most other bran, and its bran is mainly insoluble. To compare, oat bran contains mainly soluble fiber.

The fiber content of vegetables and fruits varies; some are better sources than others. A heaping bowl of fresh lettuce greens may seem loaded with fiber. However, one cup of lettuce contains just about 1 gram of fiber; instead, it's mostly water. In contrast, $\frac{1}{2}$ cup of a three-bean salad (mainly legumes) supplies more than 3 fiber grams.

Food preparation or processing may alter the fiber content of foods. Just as a sponge changes in its ability to hold water when it's chopped into very fine pieces, so properties of fiber may change a bit when the structure is altered by food processing or preparation. Fiber content drops, too, when the fiber-rich part of a food is removed. *See "Which Apple for Fiber?" later in this chapter to compare the fiber content in different forms of an apple.*

When it comes to making food choices, don't get hung up on which fiber is which—just consume enough overall. By adding a variety of fiber-rich foods to your meals and snacks, you usually get the health benefits of both soluble and insoluble fibers.

. . . if soybeans are a good fiber source, what about tofu? Half a cup of soybeans has more than 5 grams of fiber. That's great! But when soybeans are processed to make tofu, fibrous substances are strained out, and what's left is high in soy protein. Half a cup of tofu only has less than 1 gram of fiber.

. . . what's the difference between a lignin and a lignan? The terms often get confused. Classified as an insoluble fiber, lignin actually isn't a carbohydrate but a complex molecule that's a woody part of the stems and seeds of fruits and vegetables and the bran in cereals. Its properties may help prevent cancers. Lignans are phytonutrients found in whole grains and flaxseeds; research is examining their roles as phytoestrogens and anticancer agents.

. . . if oat bran has "magic" that defies heart disease? Since the early 1980s research has shown that soluble fiber in oat bran has a blood cholesterol-lowering effect. That's why it's been added to breakfast cereals, muffins, and other foods. Its soluble fiber may be just one of the heart-healthy benefits of foods made with oat bran. Regardless, no single food, not even oat bran, offers ultimate protection. Your overall eating plan, including oat bran and other high-fiber foods, along with less fat (especially saturated fat), offers the benefits!

Which Apple for Fiber?

Apple juice, applesauce, a whole apple—which has the most fiber? An apple of any variety with the peel on has more fiber than an apple without the peel. And as food changes form, its fiber content may change, too.

1 whole apple with peel	3.7 grams fiber
1 whole apple without peel	2.4 grams fiber
½ cup applesauce	1.5 grams fiber
¾ cup apple juice	0.2 gram fiber

Need a Fiber Boost?

Try to eat at least five servings of fruits and vegetables a day, and choose several servings of whole grains every day. Consume legumes often: different kinds and colors of fresh, frozen, dried, or canned beans. You can easily meet the 20- to 35-gram per day goal—and consume ample amounts of both soluble and insoluble dietary fibers, too.

If you boost your fiber intake, do so gradually! Give the bacteria in your stomach and intestines time to adjust. If you add more fiber to your diet too quickly—or consume too much on a regular basis—you may end up with gas, diarrhea, cramps, and bloating.

Drink plenty of water and other fluids, too, when you eat extra fiber. Remember that fiber acts like a large sponge in your colon. It holds water as it keeps waste moving along. That's how it helps prevent constipation and related intestinal problems. For fiber to do its job, you need to consume enough fluids. Set your goal for at least eight cups of liquids a day.

Caution: Before You Boost Fiber in Meals and Snacks . . .

For young children: Eating a lot of high-fiber foods may fill young children up too quickly. That may take away their appetite for other nutritious foods with nutrients their bodies need for proper growth. Excessive amounts of fiber also may interfere with their body's absorption of vitamins and minerals.

For elderly people and people who have had gastrointestinal surgery: If you're older than sixty-five or have had surgery on some part of your stomach, intestines, colon, or rectum, check with your doctor before adding fiber to your meals and snacks. You may feel the effects of added fiber more than others.

Supplement Watch: About Fiber Pills and Powders . . .

Should you take a fiber supplement—or not?

Depending on the supplement, adding a fiber pill or powder to the foods you already eat probably won't make much difference to your health, although it may help relieve constipation. So save the expense! Fiber-rich foods can supply more fiber than many fiber pills do. Also, supplements with more fiber may inhibit the absorption of some minerals—a problem for people whose diets are nutrient-deficient. If you decide to take fiber supplements for "regularity," your body might come to rely on them.

In contrast, fiber-rich foods—whole-grain foods, fruits, legumes, and vegetables—provide the added benefits associated with a high-fiber diet: little or no fat, especially saturated fat, and a good supply of other nutrients. Fiber pills and powders don't have any added benefits.

Most registered dietitians and doctors advise against taking fiber pills or powders as a primary source of dietary fiber.

Can fiber supplements help you lose weight and keep weight off? No scientific evidence supports this claim. You can't trick your appetite in the long run. Rather than fiber pills and powders, choose a low-fat, high-fiber diet with plenty of fruits, vegetables, whole-grain foods, and beans to get the fullness feeling. Research doesn't show a link between fiber supplements and reduced cancer risk, either.

Need more strategies for fitting fiber in? Check here for "how-tos":

● Shop for fiber—see chapter 11.
● Boost the fiber factor of your cooking—see chapter 13.

Ten Great Ways to "Fiber Up"!

Are you ready to eat more fiber—and hit the 20- to 35-gram daily target? The ten guidelines on page 140 can put your day's food choices within range.

How Much Fiber?

	Serving Size (1)*	Calories[†]	Fiber (g)[†]		
			Total	Soluble	Insoluble
Fruits					
Apple	1 medium	80	3.7	1.0	2.8
Applesauce	½ cup	95	1.5	0.5	1.1
Apple juice	¾ cup	85	0.2	0.1	0.1
Banana	1 medium	105	2.7	0.7	2.1
Blueberries	½ cup	40	2.0	0.2	1.7
Cantaloupe	½ medium	80	1.9	0.5	1.4
Cherries	10	50	1.6	0.5	1.1
Dates (dried)	5	115	3.1	0.5	2.6
Figs (dried)	3	145	5.2	2.2	3.0
Fruit cocktail	½ cup	55	1.3	0.7	0.6
Grapefruit	½ medium	40	1.4	1.2	0.3
Grapes	½ cup	55	0.8	0.3	0.5
Grape juice	¾ cup	115	0.2	0.2	0.0
Kiwi	1 medium	45	2.6	0.6	2.0
Orange	1 medium	60	3.1	1.8	1.3
Orange juice	¾ cup	85	0.4	0.2	0.2
Prunes (dried plums)	5	100	3.0	1.6	1.4
Peach	1 medium	35	1.7	0.7	1.0
Pineapple	½ cup	100	0.9	0.3	0.6
Pear	1 medium	100	4.0	2.2	1.8
Raisins	¼ cup	115	1.6	0.4	1.1
Raspberries	½ cup	30	4.2	0.4	3.8
Strawberries	½ cup	25	1.8	0.5	1.3
Watermelon	½ cup	25	0.4	0.2	0.2
Vegetables, cooked					
Asparagus	½ cup	25	1.8	0.7	1.1
Broccoli	½ cup	25	2.8	1.4	1.4
Brussels sprouts	½ cup	35	3.8	1.9	1.9
Corn	½ cup	65	2.0	0.3	1.7
Green beans	½ cup	20	2.0	0.9	1.2
Peas	½ cup	60	4.4	1.3	3.1
Potato (mashed)	½ cup	130	1.6	0.9	0.7
Potato (baked, plain, with skin)	1 medium	135	2.9	1.2	1.7
Spinach	½ cup	25	2.9	0.6	2.3
Sweet potato (baked, plain)	1 medium	115	3.4	1.3	2.2
Zucchini	½ cup	15	1.3	0.5	0.7
Vegetables, raw					
Carrot	1 medium	30	2.2	1.1	1.1
Celery	1 stalk	5	0.7	0.2	0.4
Cucumber (sliced)	½ cup	5	0.4	0.1	0.3
Lettuce (Romaine)	1 cup	5	0.7	0.2	0.5
Mushrooms (sliced)	½ cup	10	0.4	0.1	0.4
Spinach	1 cup	10	1.5	0.5	1.1
Tomato	1 medium	25	1.4	0.1	1.2
Legumes, cooked					
Baked beans (vegetarian)	½ cup	125	6.3	2.1	4.2
Garbanzo beans	½ cup	135	4.4	1.3	3.0
Kidney beans	½ cup	115	5.7	2.9	2.9
Lentils	½ cup	115	7.8	0.6	7.2
Navy beans	½ cup	130	6.5	2.2	4.3
Soybeans	½ cup	155	5.4	2.4	3.0

HOW MUCH FIBER? *(continued)*

	SERVING SIZE (1)*	CALORIES[†]	FIBER (G)[†]		
			TOTAL	SOLUBLE	INSOLUBLE
Breads, grains, pasta					
Bagel	½	80	0.6	0.3	0.3
Barley	½ cup	95	4.3	0.9	3.3
Bread, whole wheat	1 slice	70	2.0	0.3	1.6
Bread, pumpernickel	1 slice	65	1.6	0.8	0.8
Bread sticks	2 (4½-in.) sticks	40	1.1	0.2	0.9
Bread, French	1 slice	7	0.8	0.5	0.3
Bread, white	1 slice	65	0.6	0.3	0.3
Bun (hamburger or hot dog)	½	60	0.6	0.2	0.4
Pasta (cooked)	½ cup	100	0.9	0.4	0.6
Pita	½	60	0.6	0.3	0.3
Rice, brown (cooked)	½ cup	110	1.8	0.1	1.6
Rice, white (cooked)	½ cup	105	0.3	0.1	0.2
Breakfast cereals					
100% bran	1 oz.	70	9.7	0.8	9.0
Bran flakes	1 oz.	95	4.7	0.5	4.3
Corn flakes	1 oz.	110	1.0	0.1	1.0
Granola	1 oz.	135	2.4	1.4	1.1
Oatmeal (cooked)	½ cup	75	2.0	0.9	1.1
Puffed rice	1 oz.	115	0.5	0.1	0.4
Raisin bran	1 oz.	85	2.8	0.7	2.1
Whole grain oats cereal	1 oz.	105	2.9	1.3	1.5
Snacks					
Corn chips	1 oz.	155	1.4	0.0	1.4
Hummus dip	2 tbsp.	80	2.0	0.6	1.4
Peanuts (dry roasted)	¼ cup	210	3.4	0.7	2.7
Popcorn (air-popped, plain)	3 cups	90	3.6	0.1	3.5
Pretzels	1 oz.	110	0.9	0.3	0.7
Sunflower seeds	¼ cup	180	3.4	0.7	2.7
Walnuts	¼ cup	160	1.2	0.4	0.8
Added ingredients					
Flaxseeds	1 tbsp.	35	1.6	0.8	0.7
Gums	0.1 oz.	5	2.8	2.8	0.0
Oat bran	1 tbsp.	15	0.9	0.4	0.5
Psyllium	1 tbsp.	5	6.0	4.8	1.2
Rice bran	1 tbsp.	15	1.1	0.1	1.0
Seaweed	1 tbsp.	1	0.4	0.4	0.0
Wheat bran	1 tbsp.	10	1.6	0.1	1.5
Wheat germ	1 tbsp.	25	0.9	0.2	0.7

*The serving sizes correspond to the Food Guide Pyramid serving sizes from the USDA.

[†]Energy, carbohydrate, and fiber values determined from University of Minnesota Nutrition Data System Version 2.9/11/26.

The sum of the soluble and insoluble fiber values may not be equivalent to the total dietary fiber due to rounding.

Source: Marsha Hudnall, *Carbohydrates: What You Need to Know,* American Dietetic Association Nutrition Now Series (New York: John Wiley & Sons, 1998). This material is used by permission of John Wiley & Sons, Inc.

1. Eat a variety of foods. You'll benefit from a mix of fibers—both soluble and insoluble
2. Check the food label. Nutrition Facts on food labels can help you find foods with more fiber. Look for words such as "high in fiber" or "more fiber" on labels, too. *See "Label Lingo: Fiber" earlier in this chapter to see what these claims mean.* Spot fiber-rich ingredients on the ingredient list, too. For example, look for "bran," "whole grain," or "whole-wheat flour."

3. Remember breakfast—a good time for fiber-rich foods. Besides bran cereal or another fiber-rich breakfast cereal, enjoy oatmeal, whole-bran muffins, or whole-wheat waffles. Check food labels for a cereal with 5 or more grams of fiber per serving. Top with fruit for a little more fiber.

4. Switch to whole grains—in bread, cereals, buns, bagels, and pasta, to name a few—at least some of the time. Of your six to eleven Grains Group servings daily, make three whole grain! Besides the fiber, making sandwiches on a variety of whole-grain breads adds interest and taste. For breads, that includes cornbread from whole, ground cornmeal; cracked wheat bread; oatmeal bread; pumpernickel bread; rye bread; and the perennial favorite, whole-wheat bread. Eat breads made with bran, too, such as bran muffins.

5. Give brown rice a try sometimes, or mix half brown and half white rice

6. Plan to eat legumes two to three times a week. They're among the best fiber sources around. And they add flavor and texture to dishes.

7. Eat at least five servings of fruits and vegetables daily. Plan a cooked vegetable and a salad for dinner (that's two vegetable servings) and enjoy another for lunch. You have just two more to go!

8. Enjoy fruits and vegetables with the edible skin on. With the skin, a medium potato has 3.6 grams of fiber. Skinless, it has less—2.3 grams. Also enjoy the flavor and crunch of edible seeds—for example, in all kinds of berries, kiwi, and figs. They, too, supply fiber.

9. Choose whole fruit more often than juice. Fiber comes mainly from the peel and pulp; usually both are removed when juice is made (sometimes orange juice is processed with the pulp), so juice has almost no fiber.

10. "Fiberize" your cooking style. Substitute higher-fiber ingredients in recipes, such as using part whole-wheat flour in baked food. And fortify mixed dishes with high-fiber ingredients, perhaps bran or oatmeal added to meat loaf or ground flaxseeds added to baked goods.

Legumes: A Nutritious Fiber Source

All over the world, people eat and enjoy beans, peas, and other legumes! Legumes come from plants whose seed pods split on two sides when they're ripe.

Because they're a nutritious, flavorful, and inexpensive protein source and because they're easy to grow and store, legumes have been a staple food for thousands of years. Today we recognize another benefit. Besides their versatility, legumes are among the world's best fiber sources! No matter what the variety, legumes are loaded with nutrients: proteins, complex carbohydrates, and fiber, along with B vitamins (including folate), iron, other vitamins and minerals, and phytonutrients.

In the Food Guide Pyramid, legumes fit in the Meat and Beans Group. Like meat, they're good sources of protein. One-half cup of cooked legumes (beans or lentils) counts as 1 ounce of meat; 5 to 7 ounces of meat or meat alternate are recommended daily.

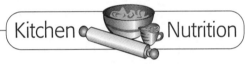

Cooking a Pot o' Beans

If you're short on time, go for canned, frozen, or fresh beans. If not, try the traditional way, by soaking them first. *Tip:* Dry legumes need soaking; lentils or split peas don't.

To soak the beans, do this:

● *Leisurely method.* Reduce cooking time by up to half by soaking beans for at least four hours or overnight in a pot filled with room-temperature water. Choose a pot that's big enough; beans expand!

● *Quick method.* Time short? Then bring water to a boil, and let beans soak in hot water for one to four hours, depending on the variety of beans.

To reduce the gas you might experience, rinse beans, discard the soaking water and any debris, and cook in fresh water. Not to worry—the beans, not the soaking water, retain most of the essential nutrients.

To cook, cover beans with fresh water: about 6 cups of fresh water for each pound of dry beans. Add seasonings to the cooking water. Salt toughens beans by taking out the moisture; and acid foods, such as tomatoes or vinegar, slow their softening. Wait until the end of the cooking time to add these ingredients.

Cover the pot partially. To keep legumes from foaming as they cook, add a little cooking oil (1/4 teaspoon) to the water. Simmer beans until they're cooked. *See the chart "Bean Bag" later in this chapter for simmering times.* Now add cooked beans or peas to your favorite dish.

BEAN BAG

Beans of all kinds are sold as dried, canned, frozen, and fresh. Each type has a distinctive appearance and flavor, varying cooking times, and somewhat different uses. Use of a variety bag that includes several types of beans is an easy way to taste the flavors of many types of different beans.

On average, 1 pound of dry beans equals about 2¼ cups of dry beans, or 5 to 6 cups of cooked beans. The yield for lentils is less; for 2¼ cups of dry lentils, figure about 3½ to 4 cups cooked. One can (15½ ounces) of drained, canned beans or lentils equals about 1⅔ cups cooked. As an aside, rinsing canned beans reduces the sodium content by about 40 percent.

BEANS AND PEAS	SIZE AND COLOR	FLAVOR	SIMMERING TIME (HOURS)*	COMMON USES†
Adzuki or azuki bean	Small, red, shiny	Slightly sweet	½ to 1	Salads, poultry stuffing, casseroles, soups
Black bean	Small, black, shiny, kidney-shaped	Slightly sweet	1½ to 2	Stew, soup, Brazilian *feijoada,* Cuban rice and beans
Black-eyed pea or cowpea	Small, cream-colored, ovals with black spots	Vegetablelike, full-flavored	1 to 1½	Southern dishes with ham or rice, bean cakes, curries, *Hoppin' John*
Cannellini or white kidney bean	Elongated, slender, creamy white	Mild	2	Soups, stews, salads, casseroles, Italian side dishes, *pasta e fagioli*
Chickpea, or garbanzo bean	Golden, hard, pea-shaped	Nutty	2¼ to 4	Casseroles, cooked with couscous, soups, stews, *hummus, caldo gallego*
Fava or broad bean	Broad, large, oval, light brown	Nutty	1½ to 2	Stews, side dishes
Flageolet or green haricot bean	Small to medium, pale green	Nutty	1½ to 2	Mixed bean salads, vegetable side dish
Great northern	Large, white	Mild	1 to 1½	Soups, casseroles, mixed bean dishes
Lentils‡	Yellow, green, or orange	Earthy	¾	Soup, *pease pudding, dhal,* curry dishes
Lima bean	Large or small, creamy white or pale green, kidney-shaped	Like chestnuts	1½	Casseroles, soups, salads, *succotash*
Mung bean	Small, olive green	Earthy	1	Soups, casseroles, purées, Asian and Indian dishes, "sprouted" for salads
Navy bean	Small, oval, white	Mild	1 to 1½	*Boston baked beans*
Pigeon pea	Small, round, slightly flat, beige, brown flecks	Mild	¾ to 1	Caribbean peas and rice
Pinto bean	Orange-pink, with rust-colored flecks, oval	Earthy, full-flavored	1 to 1½	*Mexican rice and beans, refried beans,* stew
Red kidney bean	Dark, red-brown, kidney-shaped	Full-flavored, "meaty"	1½ to 2	Stew, mixed bean salad, Cajun bean dishes, *chili con carne*
Soybean	Small, yellow or black	Full-flavored	3½ to 4	Side dish, soups, used to make tofu (bean curd), "sprouted" for salads

*Simmering time for dry beans.
†Traditional and ethnic dishes, italicized throughout the chart, commonly use the type of bean indicated.
‡Lentils don't require soaking, only shorter cooking times.

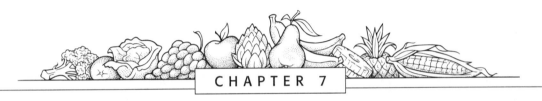

CHAPTER 7

Sodium

A Salty Subject

From your doctor, the media, and government experts, you've heard the messages: "Check food labels for sodium," "Cook with less salt," "Put away the salt shaker." These are today's headlines. Yet salt has made news for centuries!

Throughout recorded history, salt has played an important economic and political role—and has always been part of the world's food supply. Until the past two hundred years, salt was used heavily for preserving foods: meat, fish, vegetables, and even fruit. Cheese, too, was salted more than it is today. Especially in Mediterranean regions, cooks used herbs and spices to mask strong, salty flavors from preservation. Nations that controlled the salt trade also controlled distribution and preservation of food, especially in times of shortage.

The ancient Greeks valued salt so highly that they used it for currency. Salt was even traded for slaves, hence the phrase "He's not worth his salt." Originally Roman soldiers were given a handful of salt every day. Later they received money to buy their own salt, which was referred to as *salarium argentum;* that means "salt money." The word "salary" in English is derived from this Latin term.

Because of its value, salt historically has been used symbolically, too. To the ancient Romans, salt given to a newborn symbolized the giving of wisdom. In Europe, a pinch of salt tossed three times over the left shoulder helped fend off evil. Even today, we reflect our doubts with the comment "Take it with a grain of salt."

Until the late 1700s, salty flavors were common due to their use in food preservation. In the nineteenth century, tastes began to change, and people preferred less salty foods. Concurrently, other methods of food preservation got their start: canning, freezing, and refrigeration. By the twentieth century, commercially available canning, freezing, and refrigeration combined with the transportation system enabled people to have fresh foods at any time of year. Today most salt is used for industrial purposes rather than in the food supply.

In ancient times, salt's ability to preserve food helped provide a varied supply of nutrients to the population. Any other link to health or to ongoing health problems, such as high blood pressure, was unknown. As science has advanced, we've learned that the blood pressure of some people may be sensitive to salt, or to the sodium it's made from. We now recognize a link between sodium and high blood pressure among some people.

Did you know . . .

. . . 1 teaspoon of salt contains about 2,300 milligrams of sodium?

. . . most sodium that Americans consume comes from processed or prepared food, not from the salt shaker at the kitchen table?

. . . a preference for salty foods is acquired?

. . . you can cut back on salt in your food choices without giving up flavor?

Sodium and Your Health

Salt . . . or sodium? Although we often refer to them in the same breath, salt and sodium aren't the same thing. Table salt is actually the common name for "sodium chloride." It's 40 percent sodium and 60 percent chloride.

Sodium: You Need Some!

The link between sodium and high blood pressure is well publicized, yet few people know the flip side of the sodium story—why sodium is essential to health.

Sodium is a mineral that occurs naturally in food. Some of the most basic work your body does depends on sodium: maintaining proper fluid balance—controlling the movement of fluids in and out of your cells; regulating your blood pressure; transmitting nerve impulses; and helping your muscles, including your heart muscle, relax.

Sodium, along with other minerals such as chloride and potassium, are collectively described by another name: electrolytes. They get their name because they transmit electrical current in your body. You can compare them to electrically charged particles, or ions, in flashlight batteries.

If you lick your upper lip after sweating a lot, you know that body fluids have salt. You can taste it! Sodium, chloride, and potassium dissolve in body fluids, where they become separate ions. With their electrical charge, they transmit nerve impulses throughout your body. And they send messages from your brain to your muscles, causing them to relax or to contract.

Have you ever sprinkled salt on a sliced eggplant or potato, then watched the liquid come to its outer surface? Salt drew fluid out of the plant cells. That same reaction happens with electrolytes in your body. They control the balance of fluids in and out of cells. Sodium and chloride mostly work outside your body cells, and potassium works mainly inside. Together they regulate the balance of fluids.

Fluid balance—moving fluid in and out of cells—has important nutrition implications. Among them, electrolytes help move nutrients into cells and help take wastes away. Both nutrients and wastes are carried in body fluids.

For more about these minerals in health and in a variety of foods, see "Major Minerals: Electrolytes" in chapter 4.

Sodium: Keeping the Balance

Your kidneys regulate the sodium level in your body. If you're healthy, your body doesn't retain excess sodium—even when you consume more than you need. And excess amounts don't get stored.

Instead your body rids itself of the extra. Excess sodium passes out through urine and, to a much lesser extent, through perspiration. If, for example, you eat foods high in sodium, you may urinate more to get rid of the extra. Then you probably feel thirsty because you lost fluids, too.

Is extra sodium always removed? No. When kidneys don't work properly, perhaps due to kidney disease, extra sodium isn't excreted. This causes swelling, often in the face, legs, and feet. In medical terms, this swelling is called edema.

Can you have a deficiency of sodium? Yes, but this doesn't happen under normal circumstances. However, if a person vomits or has diarrhea for a prolonged period, or if he or she has some type of kidney problem, sodium levels might get too low. Unless sweating is profuse and extended over a long time, sodium levels will remain normal if you're healthy.

Link to High Blood Pressure

High blood pressure, or hypertension, is a major risk factor for heart disease, stroke, and kidney failure. It affects fifty million Americans—about one in four adults. Are you at risk? These are some factors linked to high blood pressure: family history of high blood pressure, overweight, excessive alcohol intake, advancing age, and smoking.

Why is attention given to sodium? Most people aren't affected by excess dietary sodium. Their bodies just get rid of the excess. However, up to 30 percent of America's population probably has blood pressure that's sodium-sensitive. For them, consuming too much sodium contributes to high blood pressure. Likewise, reducing their sodium intake may help to lower blood pressure if it's high.

Regarding blood pressure, there's another nutrition angle to consider. Three other minerals may be just as important in regulating blood pressure: potassium from fruits and vegetables; calcium from dairy foods and some vegetables; and magnesium from whole grains, legumes, nuts, and green vegetables.

In fact, the DASH (Dietary Approaches to Stop Hypertension) diet—an eating plan that's low in fat, with low-fat and fat-free dairy foods and plenty of vegetables and fruits—may help lower blood pressure, even among people within the "normal" range. The reason is unclear; it may be that the DASH approach to eating is high in potassium, calcium, and magnesium.

For some people, even 2,400 milligrams of sodium daily may be too much. In the DASH-Sodium study supported by the National Heart, Lung, and Blood Institute of the National Institutes of Health, people who followed the DASH diet and lowered their sodium intake to 1,500 milligrams daily had even better blood-pressure-lowering results—especially if they had hypertension. *To learn more, see "Blood Pressure: Under Control?" and specifically "DASH to Health" in chapter 22.*

Consider following the DASH diet whether or not you have high blood pressure. If you have it or some other health condition, your doctor might recommend less sodium than you consume now. Consult your doctor for the right sodium level for you, and a registered dietitian (RD) to help you fit this advice into your eating plan.

Have You Ever Wondered

. . . how you know if you're sodium-sensitive? There's no way yet to predict who may have blood pressure that's sodium-sensitive. Your best clue? Check your family history. If you have a blood relative who controls blood pressure with antihypertensive or diuretic drugs, or a low-salt diet, that's one hint. Often the condition is inherited. (Diuretics help the body get rid of excess fluids and so help control high blood pressure.) African Americans are at higher risk.

. . . if a high-salt diet is okay if you're not salt-sensitive? Moderation is always a better rule of thumb for anything you eat, so it's wise to be sensible. Choose and prepare foods with less salt, and hedge your bets with the DASH approach to eating: dairy foods, plenty of fruit and vegetables, and low-fat foods. The body excretes more calcium in urine when salt intake is high. To perhaps lower calcium loss, cut back on salt.

Potassium: Another Reason for "Five a Day"

Although the scientific reasons aren't fully understood, foods high in potassium may help protect against high blood pressure. Vegetables and fruits are among the best sources. Along with the other health benefits, their potassium content is another reason for consuming at least five servings of fruits and vegetables a day.

This partial list includes vegetables and fruits that are good potassium sources:

Apricot	Potato
Banana	Prunes (dried plums)
Broccoli	Raisins
Cantaloupe	Spinach
Carrot	Sweet potato
Dates	Swiss chard
Mushrooms	Watermelon
Orange	Winter squash
Parsnip	

Other sources: Dry beans, lentils, peas, almonds, and peanuts are good sources of potassium, too. Milk and yogurt are good potassium sources; they also supply calcium, another mineral, which may protect against high blood pressure.

Note: Potassium chloride, as a salt substitute, isn't recommended. Unless used under medical supervision, it can be harmful to health.

Research suggests another health benefit of cutting back on salt: possibly less calcium loss from bone, and as a result, reduced risk of osteoporosis and bone fractures.

How Much Is Enough?

To keep the body running normally, you need sodium. However, few Americans need to be concerned about getting enough. Instead, on average, most adults consume 4,000 to 6,000 milligrams of sodium daily, or about 4 to 6 grams (1,000 milligrams = 1 gram). That's significantly more than they likely need. There's no known advantage to consuming this much sodium. On the contrary, people with high blood pressure are better off with less.

You probably don't need extra salt even after strenuous physical activity. Although you lose sodium and some other minerals (electrolytes) through sweat, the amount is usually quite small. Meals and snacks eaten after exertion normally replenish these lost minerals. You probably don't need to salt your food, take a salt tablet, or drink a sports drink with electrolytes.

What's the recommendation, then? The National Institutes of Health and the American Heart Association recommend a limit on sodium intake: for the general population fewer than 2,400 milligrams of sodium daily. That's about the amount in 1 teaspoon of salt.

Moderation . . . Even for Healthy People

Moderation, along with variety and balance: these three qualities mark an overall healthful eating style that's good for your overall health and your heart, and that helps control your blood pressure.

As part of the moderation message, the Dietary Guidelines for Americans advise: *Choose and prepare foods with less salt.* It's the best way to cut back on sodium.

Why is that advice given to healthy people? For one, there's no way to tell if your blood pressure is sodium-sensitive. You may—or may not—develop high blood pressure from consuming too much sodium. Second, consuming less sodium or less salt certainly isn't harmful to healthy adults. Even if you don't have high blood pressure now, keeping your sodium intake within a moderate range may offer protection, just in case.

Note: Pregnant women shouldn't cut back on sodium to minimize water retention and swelling. During pregnancy women need more sodium than before. However, the amount of sodium in their prepregnancy eating plan probably provides enough extra.

Sodium in Your Food Choices

Salt and sodium—are they just in food for flavor? Or do they have other roles, too? It's easier to spot foods with salt or sodium if you know what they do.

Salt and Sodium: More than Flavor

Why are salt and other sodium-containing ingredients added in food preparation and processing? Flavor probably comes to mind first. Just a few grains of salt can bring out food's natural flavors—even in sweet

foods. However, sodium-containing ingredients play a broader role in the food supply.

● Before the days of refrigeration, people relied on salt to *preserve* many foods. Salt and sodium-containing ingredients preserve food by inhibiting the growth

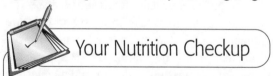

Your Nutrition Checkup

Sodium: A Healthful "Shake"

You know the guideline for healthful eating: *Choose and prepare foods with less salt.* How have you addressed this "salty issue"? Check off the tips that apply to your approach to eating. *Do you . . .*

☐ Shake a little salt on your food only *after* you taste it?

☐ Enjoy plenty of fresh and frozen fruits and vegetables?

☐ Keep the salt shaker in the cabinet, not on the table or kitchen counter where it's easier to use?

☐ Skip the salt in cooking water—for pasta, rice, and vegetables?

☐ Season food mostly with herbs, spices, or fruit juice?

☐ Read Nutrition Facts on food labels to check the amount of sodium in food?

☐ Consider the sodium content of restaurant food or fast food if you eat out regularly?

☐ Enjoy processed meats such as corned beef, ham, bacon, bologna, salami, hot dogs, and pastrami only occasionally?

☐ Buy brands of prepared foods and snack foods that have less sodium or salt?

☐ Go easy on condiments such as mustard, ketchup, soy sauce, and tartar sauce, or use brands with less sodium?

☐ Balance your food choices: if you enjoy some foods with more sodium, also eat others with less?

How many boxes did you check?

If you said yes to . . .

Nine to eleven items: you're likely consuming moderate amounts of sodium and salt. Read on for more ideas.

Six to eight items: you're controlling the sodium and salt in your food choices but may be able to "shake the sodium habit" even more. Read on.

Five or fewer items: it's time to read on and try the tips in this chapter to moderate the sodium and salt in your eating plan.

of bacteria, yeast, and molds—and so prevent food spoilage and foodborne illness.

Even today, many cured foods use salt or an ingredient made with sodium (such as sodium nitrate) as a preservative. For example, ham, sausage, corned beef, and Canadian bacon are cured meats. Another way to preserve vegetables is to soak them in brine, or a solution of water and salt. Eat pickles? Cucumbers and okra are pickled in brine.

● In many foods, salt *affects the texture*. For example, yeast breads with salt have a finer texture; salt-free yeast breads tend to be coarser.

● In some foods, such as cheese, bread dough, and sauerkraut, salt *controls the speed of fermentation*. Fermentation changes the chemistry of food, and as a result its appearance and flavor.

● In whipping egg whites or cream, a pinch of salt *increases and stabilizes the volume*.

● In processed meats, including sausage, salt and sodium-containing ingredients *also help hold the meat together*.

Where Does Sodium Come From?

Many people think their taste buds offer all the clues they need to the sodium content of food. However, you can't always judge the sodium content of food by its taste! Many foods with sodium don't have a salty flavor.

A shake here and a shake there—the amount of salt we sprinkle on food can add up quickly. The same is true for sodium-containing condiments such as soy sauce, mustard, and tartar sauce. However, only about

25 percent of the sodium in the food most people eat comes from the salt shaker or sodium-containing ingredients added to food.

Processed and prepared foods are the main sources of sodium in the average American diet: about 75 percent. Because salt and sodium-containing ingredients serve several functions in the food supply, it's not surprising that processed foods contain varying levels of sodium. For example, two cookies or crackers may have 25 to 270 milligrams of sodium. A frozen dinner might vary from 550 to 1,300 milligrams of sodium. And two slices of bacon may deliver 500 to 800 milligrams of sodium. Even "reduced-sodium" foods may be higher in sodium than you think!

For clues to the sodium in processed foods, check the label for sodium-containing ingredients. If an ingredient has *Na, salt, soda,* or *sodium* in its name, that's a clue for sodium. ("Na" is the scientific symbol for sodium.) Foods described as "broth," "cured," "corned," "pickled," or "smoked" usually contain sodium, too; cured ham often contains about 350 milligrams of sodium per ounce. Here are just a few sodium watchwords:

INGREDIENTS WITH SODIUM	WHAT THEY DO
Baking soda (sodium bicarbonate)	Leavening agent
Baking powder	Leavening agent
Brine (salt and water)	Preservative
Disodium phosphate	Emulsifier, stabilizer
Monosodium glutamate (MSG)	Flavor enhancer
NaCl (sodium chloride)	Flavor enhancer, preservative
Salt (sodium chloride)	Flavor enhancer, preservative
Sodium caseinate	Thickener, binder
Sodium citrate	Acid controller
Sodium nitrate	Preservative
Sodium propionate	Preservative, mold inhibitor
Sodium sulfite	Preservative for dried fruits
Soy sauce	Flavor enhancer
Teriyaki sauce	Flavor enhancer

Have You Ever Wondered

. . . *how much rinsing canned legumes reduces the sodium content?* If you rinse canned legumes in a strainer under cool running water, you can reduce their sodium content by about 30 to 40 percent. The rest remains in the beans. You also rinse away some nutrients, such as some B vitamins, that leach from the beans into the canning liquid.

. . . *if celery has a lot of sodium?* Many people think so. But a celery stalk has just 35 milligrams of sodium.

Salty Terms

When a recipe calls for salt, which one will you use? Most recipes call for table salt. How does table salt compare with other types of salt for nutrition and culinary uses?

- *Iodized salt:* table salt with iodine added. The human body needs just small amounts of iodine. By adding it to salt, people get enough iodine—even when they go easy on salt. An important nutrient, iodine helps prevent goiter, which is a thyroid gland condition.

- *Kosher salt:* coarse grain salt that adds a crunchy texture to some dishes and some drinks, such as margaritas. Kosher salt is also used to prepare meat by religious Jews. "Kosher salt" may have anticaking additives.

   Tip: ¼ teaspoon of kosher salt has somewhat less sodium than ¼ teaspoon of table salt. That's because kosher salt has a coarser grain, so less fits in the spoon. For the same saltiness in a cooked dish, you need the same amount by *weight*—and that has the same amount of sodium, kosher or not.

- *Lite salt:* salt that is "50–50": half sodium chloride (regular salt) and half potassium chloride. It has less sodium than table salt, but it's not sodium-free.

- *Pickling salt:* fine-grained salt used to make brines for sauerkraut or pickles. Unlike table salt, it has no iodine or anticaking additives. Additives would make the brine cloudy or would settle to the bottom.

- *Popcorn salt:* very finely granulated salt that sticks well to popcorn, fries, and chips

- *Rock salt:* large, chunky crystals of salt used in a crank-style ice cream maker or as a "bed" for serving foods such as clams or oysters. Not commonly used in recipes, rock salt contains some harmless impurities.

- *Salt substitute:* made of potassium chloride and contains no sodium. It may be recommended by a healthcare provider for people on a sodium-restricted diet.

- *Sea salt:* salt—either fine-grained or in larger crystals—produced by evaporation of seawater—for example, Black Sea, French, or Hawaiian sea salt. It has trace amounts of other minerals that may offer a somewhat different flavor. Still, it's sodium chloride. Even though sea salt is often promoted as a healthful alternative to ordinary table salt, the sodium content is comparable; the small amount of other minerals offers no known health advantages. As with other salts, use sea salt judiciously.

   Tip: With canning, trace minerals in sea salt may discolor food.

- *Seasoned salt:* salt with herbs and other flavoring ingredients added, such as celery salt, garlic salt, onion salt, or other seasoned salts. Seasoned salt has less sodium than table salt but more than herbs alone.

   Tip: For less sodium in cooking, use just herbs—for example, celery seed, garlic powder, or onion flakes. Check the ingredient list for salt.

- *Table salt:* fine, granulated salt commonly used in cooking and in salt shakers. An anticaking additive—calcium silicate—helps table salt flow freely and not get lumpy.

Because sodium occurs naturally, too, even unprocessed foods may contain sodium. But the amounts aren't high enough for concern.

How do you know if a food has a lot of sodium, or a little? Check the amount of sodium in one serving of a food, using the label's Nutrition Facts. If one serving contains 5 percent or less of the Daily Value (DV) for sodium, that's low. If it contains 20 percent or more DV, that's a lot. Remember, two servings double the sodium. *For tips on using food labels to compare sodium, see "Today's Food Labels" in chapter 11.*

Which food groups have the most sodium? The sodium content of foods varies—even in very similar foods. The difference comes from the way foods are prepared and processed. Foods in every group of the Food Guide Pyramid, including Fats, Oils, and Sweets, may contain sodium.

Flavor . . . with Less Salt and Sodium

Do you like the taste of salty snacks? Does food seem to taste better after a few shakes of the salt shaker?

Need more strategies to shake the salt habit? Check here for "how-tos":

● Shop for foods with less sodium—see chapter 11.

● Cut salt in your cooking—see chapter 13.

● Give food a flavor burst with herbs and spices, not salt—see chapter 13.

● Order restaurant foods with less sodium—see chapter 14.

● Follow the DASH diet—see chapter 22.

Most people eat what they like. According to consumer research, taste ranks first in making food choices. Good news: you can enjoy plenty of flavorful foods prepared with *less* salt and sodium.

"Salty"—an Acquired Taste

A preference for strong, salty tastes is acquired, probably starting in childhood. It's the saltiness that people like, not the sodium. In fact, chloride in salt may have more to do with flavor than sodium does.

Except for the sensory experience, the body adjusts easily to eating less salt. Interestingly, when people gradually cut back and learn to go with less salt in their food choices, the desire for salty tastes declines, too. Over time, the less salt they consume, the less they want.

For taste perception, no other foods truly substitute for the taste of salt. Even salt substitutes, suggested for some people, don't give the same taste sensation. They may taste somewhat bitter or sharp.

About Salt Substitutes

Is the use of salt substitutes a good way to moderate sodium in food choices? That depends. Salt substitutes aren't appropriate—and may not be healthful—for everyone.

Many salt substitutes contain potassium in place of all or some of the sodium. For some people, potassium consumed in excess can be harmful. For example, those with kidney problems may not be able to rid their bodies of excess levels of potassium. If you're under medical care—especially for a kidney problem—check with your doctor before using salt substitutes.

Rather than salt substitutes (potassium chloride), try herb-spice blends as a flavorful alternative to salt—or lemon or lime juice. Today's supermarkets carry a variety of salt-free seasoning blends. Remember to read the ingredient list and the Nutrition Facts on the

MSG—Another Flavor Enhancer

You probably know about monosodium glutamate, or more simply, MSG. Common in many types of ethnic cooking, MSG is a flavor enhancer. It blends well with salty or sour flavors . . . and brings out the taste of many prepared foods, such as "heat 'n' eat" meals, sauces, and canned soups.

Besides accenting the natural flavor of foods, MSG adds a unique taste of its own. Called "umami," its taste is described as "meaty" or "brothlike." Studies show "umami" actually elicits a fifth taste sensation, distinctive in cheese, meat, and tomatoes. Sweet, sour, salty, and bitter are the other four taste sensations. *For more about taste, see "'Flavor' the Difference" in chapter 13.*

As its name implies, monosodium glutamate contains sodium and glutamate or glutamic acid. Glutamic acid is an amino acid found naturally in our body and in high-protein foods. Meat, fish, dairy foods, and some vegetables contain glutamic acid.

Over the years, consumers have asked about the safety of MSG. The U.S. Food and Drug Administration considers MSG "generally recognized as safe" (GRAS) for consumption. Other GRAS substances include commonplace food "additives" such as sugar, salt, and baking soda. *See "Testing, Testing" in chapter 9 for more about the GRAS list. Also see "Have You Ever Wondered . . . if You Can Be Sensitive to MSG?" in chapter 21.*

MSG has nutrition-related benefits that may go unrecognized. Since a little goes a long way, MSG provides a bigger "bang" for the "shake." Because it contains only a third as much sodium as a comparable amount of salt, it may be an option for those controlling their sodium intake.

Adding MSG to foods such as soups and stews may make eating more enjoyable for older adults. As we grow older, our sense of smell may weaken and our taste buds decrease in number. As a result, foods lose some of their "taste appeal." The decline in smell and taste often causes seniors to lose interest in eating, putting them at nutritional risk. Adding MSG to certain foods can perk up the flavor! *See "Aging with 'Taste'" for more about taste and older adults in chapter 18.*

label. Some herb-spice blends are neither salt- nor sodium-free. As an alternative, make your own; *see "Kitchen Nutrition: Salt-Free Herb Blends" on page 151. For more about the sensations of taste and flavor, see "'Flavor' the Difference" in chapter 13.*

Taming Your Taste Buds

Enjoying what you eat is a top priority! Fortunately, healthful foods don't need to taste bland. And you don't need to give up your favorite high-sodium foods—just eat them in moderation. Here's how:

● Cut back on high-sodium foods gradually if you're accustomed to salty tastes. Because a preference for a salty taste is learned, it takes time to unlearn it, too—and to appreciate new flavor combinations.

● Taste food before salting it. Maybe it tastes great just as it is! Keep the salt shaker in the kitchen cabinet, not on the stove or the table. Use it as needed—not just as a habit.

● Enjoy plenty of fruits and vegetables. Most contain only small amounts of sodium (unless added in processing), and they're rich in potassium. Eat them as low-sodium snacks!

● Choose foods within a food group that have less sodium, such as fresh meats, poultry, fish, dry and fresh legumes, nuts, eggs, milk, and yogurt. Plain rice, pasta, and oatmeal don't have much sodium, either. Their sodium content only goes up only if high-sodium ingredients are added during their preparation.

● Season with herbs, spices, herbed vinegar, herb rubs, and fruit juices. *"A Pinch of Flavor: How to Cook with Herbs and Spices" in chapter 13 offers many ways to use herbs and spices. Or prepare the easy blends in "Kitchen Nutrition: Salt-Free Herb Blends" on page 151 to keep on hand.*

● Prepare food with less salt or fewer high-sodium ingredients. For example, skip the salt in cooking water for pasta, rice, cereals, and vegetables. Salt toughens many vegetables, especially beans, as they're cooked. Salt draws water out of the plant cells.

● Balance: if you eat high-sodium foods occasionally, balance them by eating foods with less sodium. How much salt and sodium you consume over several days is what counts.

● To buy processed and prepared foods with less sodium and salt, read Nutrition Facts on food labels. You'll find the sodium content in milligrams and the % Daily Value for sodium in a single serving. The Daily Value is based on 2,400 milligrams of sodium for the day.

Look at the Differences

To eat less salt and sodium, fresh foods are an ideal choice. You can enjoy processed and prepared foods, too.

Some processed foods have more sodium than others: cured and processed meats; many canned foods such as legumes, vegetables, and fish; cheese; condiments; boxed convenience foods such as pasta mixes or rice side dishes; and salted snack foods. For many, you can find lower-sodium versions. Read Nutrition Facts on food labels to compare similar products.

FOOD	SODIUM (MG)
2 oz. canned tuna	200
2 oz. low-sodium canned tuna	135
1 medium dill pickle	835
1 medium cucumber, marinated in vinegar	5
3 oz. ham	1,030
3 oz. reduced-sodium ham	700
3 oz. lean pork loin	75
3 cups regular microwave popcorn	190
3 cups air-popped popcorn	<5
3 cups salt-free microwave popcorn	0
1 oz. salted peanuts	100–160
1 oz. lightly salted peanuts	50
1 cup boxed convenience rice	1,600
1 cup plain brown or white rice seasoned with herbs	5
1 cup vegetable beef soup	840
1 cup reduced-sodium vegetable beef soup	50
½ cup canned green beans	170
½ cup canned no-salt-added green beans	<5
½ cup frozen green beans	5
½ cup fresh green beans	<5
1 cup chicken broth	1,005
1 cup low-sodium chicken broth	70

● Scan the nutrient content claims on the front of food labels as you walk the supermarket aisles. From soup, canned fish, vegetables, and vegetable juice to crackers, popcorn, and snack foods, you'll find a variety of food products described as "unsalted," "no salt added," "reduced sodium," "sodium-free," or "low in sodium." *To learn what these words mean, see "Label Lingo: Salt and Sodium" later in this chapter.*

● Buy foods with less sodium. Try reduced-sodium products, which may offer more flavor than low-sodium products. They're still lower in sodium than the traditional versions.

● Whether you eat in a four-star or a fast-food restaurant, be sodium-conscious if you eat out regularly. *See "Eating Out" on this page for simple ways to cut back.*

● Try lightly salted or unsalted nuts, popcorn, pretzels, and crackers if an urge for a salty flavor strikes.

Eating Out

Unlike foods you buy at the supermarket, you usually don't know the sodium content of items on a restaurant menu. Yet, if you eat out a lot, the sodium from restaurant meals and snacks could be significant. Try these simple ways to eat less salt from foods you order out:

● Move the salt shaker to another table, or taste before you shake. Ask for a lemon wedge, or bring your own herb blend to enhance the food's flavor if you feel the need.

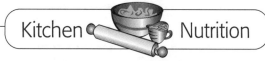

Salt-Free Herb Blends

Enhance the flavor of food with salt-free herb and spice combinations. To make ½ cup, combine the ingredients in a jar. Cover tightly and shake. Keep in a cool, dark, dry place. Then rub or sprinkle them on food for flavor. *(Tip:* They make great hospitality gifts!)

Chinese five-spice . . . for chicken, fish, or pork.

Blend ¼ cup of ground ginger, 2 tablespoons of ground cinnamon, 1 tablespoon each of ground allspice and anise seeds, and 2 teaspoons of ground cloves.

Mixed herb blend . . . for salads, pasta salads, steamed vegetables, vegetable soup, or fish.

Blend ¼ cup of dried parsley flakes, 2 tablespoons of dried tarragon, and 1 tablespoon each of dried oregano, dill weed, and celery flakes.

Curry blend . . . for rice, lentil, and vegetable dishes, and chicken.

Blend 2 tablespoons each of turmeric and ground coriander, 1 tablespoon of ground cumin, 2 teaspoons each of ground cardamom, ground ginger, and black pepper, and 1 teaspoon each of powdered cloves, cinnamon, and ground nutmeg.

Italian blend . . . for tomato-based soups and pasta dishes, chicken, pizza, focaccia, and herbed bread.

Blend 2 tablespoons each of dried basil and dried marjoram, 1 tablespoon each of garlic powder and dried oregano, and 2 teaspoons each of thyme, crushed dried rosemary, and crushed red pepper.

Mexican chili blend . . . for chili with beans, enchiladas, tacos, fajitas, chicken, pork, and beef.

Blend ¼ cup of chili powder, 1 tablespoon each of ground cumin and onion powder, 1 teaspoon each of dried oregano, garlic powder, and ground red pepper, and ½ teaspoon of cinnamon.

Greek blend . . . for seafood, poultry, and herbed bread.

Blend 3 tablespoons each of garlic powder and dried lemon peel, 2 tablespoons of dried oregano, and 1 teaspoon of black pepper.

Easy dip blend . . . for mixing with cottage cheese, yogurt cheese *(see "Kitchen Nutrition: Yogurt Cheese" in chapter 3),* or low-fat sour cream; also nice on chicken and fish.

Blend ¼ cup of dried dill weed and 1 tablespoon each of dried chives, garlic powder, dried lemon peel, and dried chervil.

● Recognize menu terms that may indicate a high sodium content: pickled, smoked, au jus, soy sauce, or in broth.

● Nibble on raw veggies rather than salty snacks.

● Go easy on condiments such as mustard, catsup, pickles, and tartar sauce for burgers, hot dogs, and sandwiches. Enjoy lettuce, onions, and tomatoes. Remember that bacon tends to be high in sodium.

● Ask the server to have your food prepared without added salt; or ask for sauces and salad dressings on the side, since they're often high in sodium. For a salad, use a twist of lemon, a splash of vinegar, or a light drizzle of dressing.

● Keep your order simple. Order broiled or grilled meat—without salty seasonings—rather than entrées cooked in sauces. Often special sauces and toppings add extra sodium to food. Order plain meat-type sandwiches with fresh vegetable toppings, too, rather than salads with dressing.

Have You Ever Wondered

. . . if drinking water has much sodium? The amount of sodium in drinking water varies from place to place. Unless you're on a sodium-restricted diet, you don't need to be too concerned. If you need or wish to know the sodium content, contact your local water department.

A water softener may add significant amounts of sodium to your water—7 to 220 milligrams per quart. Talk to the manufacturer of the water softener to find out how much sodium it adds to your water supply.

. . . if salting the cooking water will speed up the cooking? That's an urban legend. It's true that the boiling point of water may very slightly rise with added salt, but not enough to make a noticeable difference. Salt added to cooking water will, however, make food saltier.

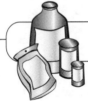

Label Lingo

Salt and Sodium

Does the term "sodium" or "salt" appear on the front of the food label? If so, here's what the descriptions mean. For the specific sodium content in a serving, check the Nutrition Facts.

LABEL TERM	MEANS	EXAMPLES OF FOODS
Sodium-free	Less than 5 milligrams of sodium per serving	Crackers
Very low sodium	35 milligrams or less of sodium per serving	Chips
Low sodium	140 milligrams or less of sodium per serving	Soup, cereal, crackers
Reduced or less sodium	At least 25% less sodium*	Soy sauce, soup, bacon, pretzels, crackers
Light in sodium	50% less sodium*; restricted to foods with more than 40 calories per serving or more than 3 grams of fat per serving	Crackers
Salt-free	Less than 5 milligrams of sodium per serving	Herb blends
Low-sodium meat	140 milligrams or less of sodium per 100 grams	Frozen dinner
Unsalted or butter, no added salt	No salt added during processing; does not necessarily mean sodium-free	Peanuts, butter, canned vegetables, microwave popcorn, crackers, breakfast cereal

*As compared with a standard serving size of the traditional food

CHAPTER 8

Fluids
Often Overlooked

ater? Unless your throat feels parched and sweat drips from your brow, you probably give little thought to water. Yet this clear, refreshing fluid is one of your body's most essential nutrients.

You've probably heard that water is vital to health—and to life itself. While you may survive for six weeks without food, you cannot live longer than a week or so without water. In fact, losing more than 10 percent of your body weight from dehydration, or water loss, causes extreme weakness and potential heat stroke. And a 20 percent loss is life-threatening. Water truly is the beverage of life!

A Fluid Asset

Water is the most abundant substance in the human body as well as the most common substance on earth. Like the oxygen you breathe, you can't live without it.

On average, body weight is 50 to 75 percent water—or about 10 to 12 gallons of water. The specific percentage varies from person to person, relating to body composition, age, and gender, among other factors.

Compared with body fat, lean tissue holds much more water, so the leaner you are, the higher proportion of water in your body. Males, with more muscle, carry a higher percentage of water in their bodies than females do. And younger individuals usually have more than older adults. Water accounts for about 75 percent of a newborn's weight, while the amount dwindles in the elderly to about 50 percent water weight.

Body tissues of all types contain water—some more than others. The fact that blood contains water is certainly no surprise; your blood is about 83 percent water. Lean muscle tissue is about 73 percent water; body fat, about 25 percent. Even though bones seem hard, they, too, contain water, about 22 percent by weight.

Water: An Essential Nutrient

What does water do in your body? Far more than satisfy your thirst! Thirst is actually more like a warning light that's flashing on the dashboard of your car. This physical sensation signals to you that your body needs more fluid to perform its many functions. To satisfy thirst, you drink fluids.

Water itself is a simple substance, containing just one part oxygen and two parts hydrogen. It supplies no calories. Yet every body cell, tissue, and organ, and almost every life-sustaining body process, needs water to function. In fact, water is the nutrient your body needs in the greatest amount.

Whether inside or surrounding your cells, nearly every function of the human body takes place in a watery medium. Water regulates your body temperature, keeping it constant at about 98.6° F. Many body processes produce heat, including any physical activity. Through perspiration, heat escapes from your body as water evaporates on your skin.

Water transports nutrients and oxygen to your body cells and carries waste products away. It moistens body tissues such as those in your mouth, eyes, and nose. Water is the main part of every body fluid, including blood, gastric (stomach) juice, saliva, amniotic fluid (for a developing fetus), and urine. By softening stools, water helps prevent constipation. And it helps cushion your joints and protects your body organs and tissues.

To keep your body functioning normally and to avoid dehydration, your body needs an ongoing water supply. During a strenuous workout, losing water weight is common, especially on a hot, humid day. Losing just one or two pounds of your body's water weight can trigger a feeling of thirst. With a little more fluid loss, the body loses strength and endurance; even mild dehydration can interfere with physical performance. With even more water loss and prolonged exposure to high temperatures, a person may suffer from heat exhaustion or risk heat stroke. With a 20 percent drop in the body's water weight, a person can barely survive.

Of all the nutrients in your diet, water is most abundant. Drinking water and other beverages are the main sources. But you "eat" quite a bit of water in solid foods, too—perhaps more than you think. Juicy fruits and vegetables such as celery, lettuce, tomatoes, and watermelons contain more than 90 percent water. Even dry foods, such as bread, supply some water. *The chart "Food: A Water Source" on page 155 shows the percentage of water in some common foods.*

Your body has still another water source. About 15 percent of your body's total water supply forms in your body cells when energy is produced from carbohydrates, proteins, and fats. Along with energy, water is an end product of your body's metabolism.

Fluids: How Much Is Enough?

The average adult loses about 2½ quarts (about 10 cups) of water daily through perspiration (even when sitting), urination, bowel movements, and even breathing. During hot, humid weather or strenuous physical activity, fluid loss may be much higher. Unlike some other nutrients, the human body doesn't store an extra supply of water for those times when you need more. To avoid dehydration and to keep your body working

---

Dehydration: Look for Body Signals!

The effects of dehydration, or loss of body water, are progressive: thirst, then fatigue, next weakness, followed by delirium, and finally death. Although you need to pay attention to the signals of water loss, all these steps won't happen in a single day.

PERCENT LOSS OF BODY WATER BY TOTAL BODY WEIGHT	PROGRESSIVE EFFECTS OF DEHYDRATION (PARTIAL LIST)
0 to 1	Thirst
2 to 5	Dry mouth, flushed skin, fatigue, headache, impaired physical performance
6	Increased body temperature, breathing rate, pulse rate
8	Dizziness, increased weakness, labored breathing with exercise
10	Muscle spasms, swollen tongue, delirium, wakefulness
11	Poor blood circulation, failing kidney function

---

normally, you must replace the fluids you lose through normal bodily functions.

How much water do you need each day? Your need for water depends on the amount of energy your body uses: for adults, 1 to 1½ milliliters of water per calorie of energy expended. That's 1 to 1½ liters for every 1,000 calories, or about 8 cups of water daily in a 2,000-calorie-a-day diet. (A liter is about as much as 1 quart.)

Most people need 8 to 12 cups of water daily—from drinking water, other beverages, and water in solid foods. Body weight is one factor affecting fluid need. Additional factors that may cause a need for more water include climate, level of physical activity, diet, and other physical differences. For example:

● When you're exposed to extreme temperatures—very hot or very cold—your body uses more water to maintain its normal temperature.

● With strenuous work or exercise, your body loses water through perspiration, or evaporation from your skin. To figure how much water you need daily, start with eight cups of water. Drink one to three more cups per hour as you increase the intensity and duration of your activity. *For signs that you need to drink more, see "Dehydration Alert!" in chapter 19.*

● When you're exposed to heated or recirculated air for a long time, water evaporates from your skin. For example, the dry, recirculated air on planes promotes dehydration.

● Pregnancy and breast-feeding increase the amount of fluid a woman's body needs.

● Being sick makes a difference, too. Fever, diarrhea, and vomiting all cause increased water loss. Follow the advice of your healthcare provider, and drink plenty of water and other fluids to prevent dehydration.

● If you eat a high-fiber diet, your body needs extra water to process the additional roughage and prevent constipation.

In healthy people, water intake and water loss balance out. If you consume more than you need, your kidneys simply eliminate the excess. You probably won't overdo on water. When you don't consume enough, your body may trigger a sensation of thirst.

Thirst signals the need for fluids, but it isn't a foolproof mechanism, especially for elderly people, children, and during illness, hot weather, or strenuous physical activity. Waiting until you feel thirsty to drink may be too long. By then, two or more cups of body fluids may be gone—even when you're healthy. *For more on fluids for older adults, see "Thirst-Quenchers: Drink Fluids" in chapter 18.*

To see if you're drinking enough fluid, check your urine. A small volume of dark-colored urine indicates that you aren't consuming enough fluid. Besides feeling thirsty, this is your signal to drink more. Urine that is pale or almost colorless means you're drinking enough.

As another option, weigh yourself before and after strenuous physical activity. For every pound of weight you lose, replace it with two cups of fluid.

Caution: If you always seem thirsty or urinate too much, talk to your healthcare provider. This may be a

---

Food: A Water Source

It's not easy to calculate just how much water you consume each day. While drinks—plain water and other beverages—supply a good portion of your water needs, solid food also provides a surprising amount.

FOOD	PERCENT WATER BY WEIGHT
Lettuce (½ cup)	95
Watermelon (½ cup)	92
Broccoli (½ cup)	91
Grapefruit (½)	91
Milk (1 cup)	89
Orange juice (¾ cup)	88
Carrot (½ cup)	87
Yogurt (1 cup)	85
Apple (1 medium)	84
Cottage cheese, low-fat (½ cup)	79
Tuna, canned, drained (3 oz.)	73
Potato, baked with skin (1 medium)	71
Rice, cooked (½ cup)	69
Kidney beans, boiled (½ cup)	67
Pasta, cooked (½ cup)	66
Chicken, roasted, no skin (3 oz.)	65
Beef, lean, roasted (3 oz.)	64
Whole wheat bread (1 slice)	38
Cheddar cheese (1 oz.)	37
Bagel (½)	32
Honey (1 tbsp.)	17
Butter or margarine (1 tbsp.)	16
Raisins (⅓ cup)	15
Pecans, dried (2 tbsp.)	5
Vegetable oil (1 tbsp.)	0

Source: Calculated from Jean A. T. Pennington, *Bowes & Church's Food Values of Portions Commonly Used,* 17th ed. (Philadelphia: J. B. Lippincott Company, 1998).

---

sign of diabetes. On the other hand, water retention, for reasons other than premenstrual syndrome, may suggest a kidney or a liver problem.

Water: In Balance

As an average adult, you probably lose about 2½ quarts (about 10 cups) of water daily. To maintain your body's fluid balance, you need to replace it each day. If you lose a little more, such as through perspiration, you'll need to drink more fluids to balance out.

Your body loses water daily through . . .

Urine	4 to 6 cups
Perspiration	2 to 4 cups
Breath (expired air)	1½ cups
Feces	⅔ cup

You replace water in your body daily through . . .

Water and other fluids	4 to 6½ cups*
Solid food	3 to 4⅓ cups
Water from metabolism	¾ to 1⅓ cups

*To be on the safe side, drink more fluids. Your body will excrete any extra.

Drinking for Health

To keep your body well hydrated, consume enough water—eight to twelve cups—throughout the day. Because milk, juice, and some other beverages are mostly water, they count toward your daily water intake. So does water from solid foods, although you can't really measure it.

Caffeinated beverages—coffee, tea, and some soft drinks—and alcoholic beverages aren't your body's best sources of water. Caffeine and alcohol act like diuretics, causing the body to lose water through increased urination. Decaffeinated beverages, however, don't have a diuretic effect.

If you need to increase your water intake . . .

● Take water breaks during the day instead of coffee breaks. If you're a subconscious "sipper," keep a cup of water on your desk.

● When you buy a vending machine or convenience store drink, reach for bottled water.

● "Water down" your meals and snacks. Complement food with water, milk, or juice. Occasionally, start your meals with soup.

● When you walk by a water fountain, take a drink!

● Refresh yourself at snack time with juice, milk, or sparkling water.

● Alternate sparkling water and alcoholic drinks at social gatherings.

● Before, during, and after any physical activity, drink water, especially in hot weather. Consume 4 to 8 ounces of water every fifteen to twenty minutes while you exercise. Don't wait until you feel thirsty! *For tips on fluids during exercise, see "Thirst for Success" in chapter 19.*

● Keep a bottle of water with you as you commute, while you work, as you run errands. Travel with a supply of bottled water, too, even for day outings. Airline travel promotes dehydration. *For tips on drinking fluids in flight, see "Dining at 35,000 Feet!" on page 358.*

Hydration for the Seasons

From the bone-chilling days of winter to the hot, sultry days of summer, your body needs water to maintain its normal temperature.

In hot, humid weather your body perspires, increasing water loss. Cool, refreshing drinks may help cool your overheated body. An interesting side note: Your body has a harder time cooling down in hot, humid weather than in hot, dry weather. That's because perspiration doesn't evaporate from your skin to cool you down. Instead your skin feels sticky and hot.

Dehydration may seem like just a summer issue. But keeping your body well hydrated during winter is just as important. When the weather turns chilly, most people head indoors. There heated air evaporates the moisture on your skin. Although you may not feel thirsty, you still need to replace water loss. Even in the cold outdoors, you may perspire . . . perhaps from the physical exertion of shoveling snow, skating or skiing, or from being bundled up with many layers of clothing.

What's to Drink?

Just plain water: it's the most available fluid around and often your best choice! Juice and milk make good beverage options, too, since they supply other nutrients besides water. For example, juice offers vitamins A or C, or both, and milk is calcium-rich. Other

The Fluoride Connection

Fluoride, a mineral, helps harden developing tooth enamel and so protects teeth from decay. Fluoride also may offer some protection from osteoporosis, or brittle bone disease. Many water systems contain a natural supply of fluoride. But in areas where fluoride levels are low, the water system may be fluoridated to levels recommended by the American Dental Association. The optimum fluoride level is 1 ppm—1 part fluoride per million parts water.

Fluoride is not only ingested through the water supply. In areas where water isn't fluoridated, or when bottled water without fluoride is consumed instead of tap water, dentists may prescribe fluoride supplements for children. If you're not sure about fluoride in your municipal water system, check with your local water department or public health department. If you have your own well, have it tested for fluoride. Some bottled water is fluoridated; check the label.

"Topical" fluoride—applied directly to teeth with toothpaste and mouth rinse, or in the dental office by gel treatments—also helps strengthen tooth enamel. According to oral health experts, topical fluoride is more effective when fluoride is also ingested. Check the labels on toothpaste and mouth rinse to see if they contain fluoride.

Be aware that consuming too much fluoride can cause the teeth to be mottled, or marked with brown spots, even though they're healthy in other ways. That most likely happens with excessive doses from a dietary supplement. The Tolerable Upper Intake Level for fluoride is 2.2 milligrams daily for children ages four through eight; from age nine through adulthood, it's 10 milligrams of fluoride daily.

For more about healthy teeth, see "Your Smile: Sugar and Oral Health" in chapter 5 and "Caring for Baby Teeth" in chapter 15.

beverage choices—coffee, tea, soft drinks, and alcoholic drinks—don't offer the nutrient benefits of milk, fortified soy milk, or juice.

Why drink water? For starters, water has no calories. If you're trying to avoid extra calories, that's a definite advantage. In other beverages, such as regular soft drinks and alcoholic beverages, calories really can add up. Water is also low in sodium and has no fat or cholesterol. Watching your caffeine intake? Unlike many coffees, teas, and some soft drinks, you won't find caffeine in water either.

Tap Water or Bottled Water?

Tap water or bottled water: Which should you drink? Both are regulated stringently by the government—tap water by the Environmental Protection Agency (EPA) and bottled water by the U.S. Food and Drug Administration (FDA). Especially when it comes from large municipal water systems, tap water is just as safe for drinking as bottled water.

Right from the Tap

Just turn on your faucet! Most drinking water in the United States comes right from the tap. Most of us take this for granted, but in many parts of the world, drinkable tap water is a luxury. If you live in an urban area, your tap water probably comes from a surface water source: river, lake, or reservoir, fed by a watershed, or land area. In a rural area, you likely drink groundwater that's pumped from an aquifer, an underground, natural reservoir. Either way, water must be treated with chemicals and filtered to ensure its quality and safety.

Treated: For Safety's Sake. No matter what the original source, water isn't naturally pure. Impurities dissolve or absorb in water as it flows through rivers and streams, filters through soil and rocks, and collects in lakes and reservoirs.

To make tap water safe from public health problems, the EPA has established standards for ninety contaminants that may occur in drinking water. Standards are set at a low enough level to protect most people, including children. Treatment protects you from microbes such as bacteria and viruses, inorganic contaminants such as chemicals, and lead, arsenic, and other minerals.

To find out about a public water supply, ask for the annual report, or Consumer Confidence Report, from your community water supplier. It indicates the water source, the presence or level of contaminants, and what you can do to protect your drinking water.

Water may be disinfected chemically, or by a physical process such as ultraviolet light. Chlorination is a tried-and-true method for effectively treating water and keeping you safe from most immediate microbial

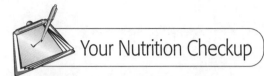

Your Nutrition Checkup

"Wet" Your Appetite?

Now that you've read about the value of water to your health, just how much fluid do you drink during a typical day?

If yesterday was typical for you, write down what you drank and about how much. Include beverages consumed with meals and snacks. Remember to include water you drank from a water fountain, tap, or dispenser on the refrigerator.

WATER	OTHER BEVERAGES	HOW MUCH?
Morning		
_____	_____	_____
_____	_____	_____
_____	_____	_____
_____	_____	_____
Afternoon		
_____	_____	_____
_____	_____	_____
_____	_____	_____
_____	_____	_____
Evening		
_____	_____	_____
_____	_____	_____
_____	_____	_____
_____	_____	_____

About how many cups of fluids did you drink? _____

For your good health, drink at least eight cups of fluid daily—more if you've been physically active or if it's a hot day. The rest of the water you consume comes from the food you eat. If you came up short, read on for ways you might drink a little more!

Tip: Caffeinated drinks and alcoholic beverages may not provide as complete a fluid-replacement benefit as noncaffeinated or nonalcoholic beverages because of their diuretic effect.

reactions such as diarrhea and vomiting, and from outbreaks of cholera, hepatitis, and other microbial diseases.

There's been some question about a by-product called trihalomethane (THM), created when chlorine reacts with organic matter in water. The very low amount of THM created in the process of making water safe to drink isn't enough to create a cancer risk. From a public health standpoint, protecting people from disease outbreaks far outweighs the insignificant effect of THM.

If you want to know the THM level of your water, check your municipal water quality report; home testing is unreliable. The THM standard from the EPA is an average (per quarter of the year) of 80 parts per billion (ppb) as of January 2002. Home water filters can reduce these compounds in your drinking water if you choose to use one.

Water quality is continually assessed for safety. For example, in a few spots in the nation, low levels of arsenic in drinking water (from natural and commercial sources), consumed over time, were identified as a potential cancer risk. For that reason, new standards for arsenic in drinking water were released in 2001. By January 2006, the arsenic level in water must be reduced from the maximum level of 50 parts per billion (ppb) to a maximum of 10 ppb. *For more information check http://www.epa.gov/safewater/arsenic.html—EPA's Web address.*

Hard or Soft? Surprisingly, water itself may not be the only nutrient in drinking water. Unless distilled, or demineralized, drinking water may contain minerals in varying amounts, such as fluoride, calcium, sodium, iron, and magnesium. The water source and how it's processed determine the actual composition of drinking water. Water from underground wells, springs, and aquifers may contain high mineral concentrations. As water from rain and snow seeps through rocks, gravel, and sand, it picks up minerals along the way. That's how some underground water becomes naturally fluoridated. *"The Fluoride Connection" earlier in this chapter describes the link between fluoridated water and oral health.*

Water may be described as "hard" or "soft" depending on its mineral content. Hard water contains more calcium and magnesium, while soft water has more sodium. With one exception there's essentially no difference in flavor between hard and soft water. Small amounts of iron give a metallic taste to hard water—but not enough to make it a significant source of dietary iron.

Where water is naturally hard, some consumers choose to use a water softener, which adds sodium and removes other minerals. The reason? The decision to soften water isn't a nutrition issue; instead, softening water can make soap work more efficiently, extend the life of a water heater, and avoid residue buildup in pipes. The amount of softening (salt added) depends on the hardness of the water. For well water that must be fully softened, the amount of sodium per cup of water is about 39 milligrams. Usually well water doesn't need to be fully softened; however, the average softened municipal water may contain about 22 milligrams of sodium per cup. Again, your own water supply may not be softened. For most people, the amount of sodium in softened water isn't significant enough for concern.

If you have your own water softener, you might soften only the hot water. Then, if you're sodium-sensitive, you won't have extra sodium in cold drinking water.

What about Bottled Water?

Do you carry a bottle of water? In recent years, consumption of bottled water has soared. The bottled-water industry began in the late 1950s, and by the

---

Water: In Case of Emergencies

Disaster can hit anyone, anywhere! To ensure a safe water supply for your family, disaster experts advise these precautions.

- Store a week's supply of bottled water for everyone in your family. Figure about 1 gallon of water per person per day.
- Store containers of water in a cool, dry place away from direct sunlight.
- Label bottles of water with the date. Replace them every six months to ensure freshness.

---

mid-1990s, Americans were consuming 2.9 billion gallons annually; that's projected to be about 6.8 billion gallons by 2004! With today's consumer demand, soft-drink companies have added bottled water to their line. The most common types include mineral water, purified water, sparkling water, spring water, and well water . . . plain or lightly flavored.

Since both tap and bottled water are safe, why drink bottled water? According to consumer research, some people prefer the taste. Bottled water usually doesn't contain chlorine, which can give water a slight flavor. It's convenient: portable for the office, a picnic, a drive, or a workout, and often easy to buy. For some, bottled water is a "chic," healthful beverage alternative. Many people drink bottled water for what it doesn't contain: calories, caffeine, or alcohol.

About Bottled Water. Bottled water that's sold state to state is regulated by the FDA to assure its quality, safety, and accurate labeling. Terms on labels for bottled water, such as "spring water" or "mineral water," are defined legally. If bottled water comes from a municipal water supply, the label must state that fact, unless it's been processed to be purified water. By regulation, bottled water can't contain sweeteners or additives—besides flavors, extracts, or essences from food or spices (less than 1 percent by weight). And it must be calorie- and sugar-free.

Instead of chlorine, bottled water usually is disinfected in other ways, including filtration; reverse osmosis; ultraviolet (UV) light; or ozone, a highly reactive form of oxygen. *See "Have You Ever Wondered?" later in this chapter for a brief background on*

Have You Ever Wondered

. . . where to get your water tested? Whether you're checking for lead, trihalomethanes, or other contaminants, or having a private well tested, skip home testing kits. They're imprecise and unreliable. Instead, contact the EPA or a state-certified laboratory.

. . . what you can do to help keep drinking water safe? Find out how to dispose of toxic trash such as household cleaners and batteries with lead or mercury. Your town may have a special collection site. Take used motor oil to a recycling center; don't discard it in your trash or storm sewer. Don't put any chemicals in places that seep into groundwater, such as septic systems, drainage wells, or dry wells.

water filtration systems. Depending on the method, bottled water may or may not be 100 percent pathogen-free. If you're at risk with suppressed immune function, talk to your healthcare provider to find bottled water that's pathogen-free.

Ever see "NSF-certified" or "IBWA Bottler Member" on bottled water labels? IBWA stands for International Bottled Water Association. These label statements indicate that a voluntary inspection, with standards set by the National Sanitation Foundation, has been conducted. The water source and finished product are checked against FDA regulations. Safe water may not have a label, since the inspection is voluntary. If you see "FDA-Approved" or "EPA-Certified," beware; neither agency conducts these inspections.

On bottled waters marketed for infants, you might see the term "sterile." That means the water meets the FDA's standards for commercial sterilization, making it safe from bacteria. If not, the label must state that the product isn't sterile and that it should be used to prepare infant formula only as directed by a doctor or according to infant formula preparation instructions. For safety, follow that guideline. Look for fluoridated bottled water if your child or infant consumes only bottled water.

Consumer Tips for Bottled Water. If you like it, buy it. But know that you may pay 240 to more than 10,000 times as much per gallon for bottled water that's no more healthful than most tap water.

Some people believe that bottled water is healthier than tap water. From a nutritional standpoint, there's no significant difference. In large municipal water systems, either bottled or tap water is safe and healthful. In fact, some bottled water *is* tap water, reprocessed to change its taste and composition.

Some bottled waters may be a good beverage choice for those at high risk; see *"Drinking Water: For Special Health Needs" later in this chapter.* In places where the lead or nitrate content of water is a concern, bottled water may be a good alternative, particularly for pregnant women or families with children. Bottled water doesn't contain lead.

Some cooks prefer bottled or filtered water for cooking. It usually doesn't contain chlorine, which may slightly alter the flavor of soups and stews. In

Label Lingo

Bottled Waters

Today's supermarket shelves offer bottled waters—some flavored, others plain. But what do the terms on the label mean? According to the FDA:

- *Artesian water* is a certain type of well water, collected without mechanical pumping. The well must tap a confined aquifer that has water standing much higher than the rock, gravel, or sand. An aquifer is an underground layer of rock or sand with water.

- *Well water* is collected from an underground aquifer, too, but with a mechanical pump.

- *Drinking water* is bottled water from an approved source. It must meet state and federal standards and go through minimal filtration and disinfection.

- *Mineral water* contains minerals at a standard level, no less than 250 parts per million (ppm) of total dissolved solids, or minerals. These minerals must be naturally present, not added. If the level is less than 500 ppm, it will be labeled "low mineral content"; if higher than 1,500 ppm, "high mineral content."

- *Purified water* has been processed to remove minerals and other solids. The process may be distillation, deionization, reverse osmosis, or another suitable process. *Tip:* "Purified" doesn't mean that purified water is any more "pure" or better for you than tap water.

- *Distilled water,* which is one type of purified water, has been evaporated to steam, then recondensed to remove minerals.

- *Sparkling water* is water with a "fizz." Either carbon dioxide is added, or water is naturally carbonated. If carbon dioxide is added, it can't have any more than its naturally carbonated level. It can be labeled as natural sparkling water only if there's no added carbonation. Seltzer, tonic water, and club soda are considered soft drinks, not sparkling water, and may contain sugar and calories.

- *Spring water* comes from an underground source and naturally flows to the surface. It must be collected at the spring or through a bored hole that taps an underground source of the spring. If it's collected by an external (not natural force), it must have the same composition and physical qualities (perhaps carbonated) as the naturally flowing spring water.

homes with lead pipes or lead solder, bottled water may be a good alternative in soups, stews, and other long-cooking dishes. During extended cooking times, any lead in tap water may become more concentrated.

Consider this: most bottled water isn't chlorinated. So if you sip from the bottle for several days, it's subject to bacterial contamination. Drink it right away; wash the bottle with soapy water if you plan to reuse it.

Safe Enough to Drink

For any nation, water safety is a top public health priority. In the United States, infectious disease spread by untreated water has been almost nonexistent, except during natural disasters such as floods, earthquakes, or accidental contamination of wells or municipal water. Any of these incidents can devastate a community's drinking water supply, so you're wise to know what to do in a water emergency.

When the safety of your water supply is in doubt, don't drink it! Instead, take steps to make it safe from bacteria that spread infectious disease.

● Report your concern to your water company or local public health department. They may test the water or refer you to a qualified private laboratory.

● If you rely on a private well or spring, have it tested annually by a certified water testing laboratory for coliform bacteria, nitrate, and perhaps other contaminants such as radon, pesticides, or industrial wastes. Do it more often if your sample exceeds the standard. People who draw their water from a private water source are responsible for the safety of their own water supply. *For tips on how to protect a private water supply, http://www.epa.gov/safewater/ is the EPA's Web site.*

● Purify contaminated drinking water by boiling tap water for at least one minute, then pouring the boiled water into a sterile container. At high altitudes, perhaps if you're camping, boil water longer. Why? At high altitudes water boils at a lower temperature, which may be less effective at killing bacteria.

● Use iodine or chlorine tablets to disinfect your water supply, strictly following directions on the package. These products are generally available in camp-ing stores. Campers, hikers, and others who rely on water supplied by lakes and streams in wilderness areas might use water filtration and purification devices as well as iodine or chlorine tablets.

● Contact the EPA's Safe Drinking Water Hotline or Web site; your state certification officer for referral to a certified water testing lab; or your local health department. *See "Resources You Can Use" at the back of this book.*

In some countries, contaminated water is an ongoing problem, spreading diarrhea and even life-threatening diseases such as cholera and hepatitis. For globe-trotters, water is a common source of travelers' diarrhea. *See "What's Safe to Drink?" in chapter 14 for guidance on safe drinking water for travelers.* For added safety in Third World areas, you might travel with a supply of iodine or chlorine tablets.

Drinking Water: For Special Health Needs

Some people are more vulnerable to microbial contaminants such as *Cryptosporidium* (or "crypto"), which isn't destroyed by chlorination. More often found in surface water than ground water, "crypto" may cause nausea, diarrhea, or stomach cramps when healthy people ingest it. For people who are more vulnerable, the symptoms may be more severe and perhaps life-threatening. That includes people with HIV/AIDS or other immune system disorders (such as lupus or Crohn's disease), organ transplants, the elderly, children, and those undergoing chemotherapy.

In 2001, new EPA standards put more controls on disinfecting procedures for microbial contaminants, including "crypto," for surface water. However, at-risk people should still talk to their healthcare provider and take careful precautions.

Boiling tap water and pasteurizing bottled water destroy "crypto." Filters with an "absolute 1-micron" rating are relatively effective; see *"Have You Ever Wondered? . . . if you need a water filter"* in this chapter. Bottled waters—processed by distillation or reverse osmosis, or commercially filtered with an NSF International Standard 53 filter before bottling—are safe. Not all bottled waters are handled in this way.

Get the Lead Out (and the Nitrates and Nitrites, Too)!

With the spread of infectious disease from drinking water under control, concern in the United States has shifted to certain compounds in water. Lead is a major issue.

Excessive lead in drinking and cooking water poses a serious health risk. Over time, too much lead consumed in food and beverages can build up in the body, potentially damaging the brain, nervous system, kidneys, and red blood cells. Infants, children, and unborn babies are more vulnerable to lead poisoning.

If the water supply is monitored, where does lead come from? Often, lead can come from plumbing inside the home or from service lines. In the past, many houses and multifamily dwellings were constructed with water pipes, fittings, or fixtures made of lead. Additionally, lead service lines in older communities may connect a house with the municipal water system. According to 1996 amendments to the U.S. Safe Drinking Water Act, all pipe, fittings, and fixtures introduced into commerce must be lead-free.

If you are concerned, check your pipes and water supply. Even copper pipes might use lead solder in the joints; brass faucets and fittings may contain lead, too. To have your water tested, contact your local public health department or water utility company. They may have a free testing kit, or may refer you to a government-certified laboratory that tests water safety.

If the lead problem in your water supply is severe, you might install a water filtering device or use bottled water for drinking and cooking. If less severe, follow these guidelines to help ensure the safety of your water:

● Avoid drinking water that has been in lead plumbing for six hours or more.

● For drinking and cooking water, let the cold water faucet run for sixty seconds or more to clear water that has been in the pipes and faucet. This will

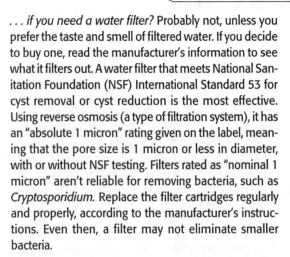

Have You Ever Wondered

. . . if you need a water filter? Probably not, unless you prefer the taste and smell of filtered water. If you decide to buy one, read the manufacturer's information to see what it filters out. A water filter that meets National Sanitation Foundation (NSF) International Standard 53 for cyst removal or cyst reduction is the most effective. Using reverse osmosis (a type of filtration system), it has an "absolute 1 micron" rating given on the label, meaning that the pore size is 1 micron or less in diameter, with or without NSF testing. Filters rated as "nominal 1 micron" aren't reliable for removing bacteria, such as *Cryptosporidium.* Replace the filter cartridges regularly and properly, according to the manufacturer's instructions. Even then, a filter may not eliminate smaller bacteria.

. . . if seltzer and club soda are the same as bottled water? No. Neither is required to meet the quality standards of bottled water. Some seltzer and club soda products contain sugar and sodium, whereas bottled water, by definition, cannot.

. . . what flavored waters really are? Flavored waters may have just a hint of flavor, derived from a natural fruit essence. Check the label carefully, though, because some clear beverages also contain sugar, other sweeteners, and artificial flavors. If they do, they're soft drinks or "water beverages," not bottled water. Remember, being clear doesn't mean that a beverage is simply water!

. . . if oxygen-enhanced drinks offer unique benefits such as a boost in athletic performance? No. It's just marketing hype.

First, consider "oxygen-enhanced" water. Under pressure, only a tiny amount (about the amount in one breath) of oxygen can be forced into water. It quickly bubbles out as soon as you open the bottle.

Even if some "extra oxygen" in water made it to your mouth, your digestive tract would get it, not your lungs. Your lungs, not your intestines, process oxygen that's captured by the heme (iron) portion of blood. Fortunately, there's enough oxygen in the environment to sustain life. To most efficiently use the oxygen you do breathe in, get regular aerobic activity.

help flush out water with the heaviest concentration of lead.

● For cooking and baby formula preparation, use cold water from your tap or bottled water. Hot water dissolves lead from the pipes more quickly than cold water does.

● To minimize lead in drinking and cooking water, install a water softening system only on your hot-water faucet. Hard water from your cold-water faucet won't pick up as much lead as soft water from your hot-water faucet.

● As another option, use bottled water for cooking and drinking.

As a precaution: The American Academy of Pediatrics and the Centers for Disease Control and Prevention advise initial lead screening for all infants and toddlers (nine to twelve months). After that, a follow-up schedule is generally recommended as needed. When children test above 10 micrograms per deciliter, sources of lead in the child's environment should be identified and corrected.

Another alert: If your water supplier alerts you to nitrate or nitrite levels that exceed EPA standards *and* if you have a child under six months of age, talk to your healthcare provider. Ingesting that water could cause "blue baby syndrome," which can be life-threatening without immediate medical attention. The symptoms are a blue appearance and shortness of breath.

Find a different and safe water source for preparing baby formula. Nitrates are inorganic and can't be destroyed like bacteria. As with lead, boiling water with nitrates just concentrates them and so increases the risk.

Juicy Story: Fruit Juice, Juice Drink, Fruit Drink . . . or Just Plain Water?

When you're thirsty, a refreshing, fruity beverage often hits the spot. Which will you reach for: fruit juice, juice drink, fruit drink, or water? All of these choices replace fluid. When you're choosing a "thirst quencher," go easy on juice or juice drinks, since their calories can add up; drink more water. A serving or two of juice per day (up to 12 ounces) is probably enough. For a flavorful refresher, dilute juice with water.

Depending on the fruits and perhaps the vegetables they're made from, juices and juice drinks supply varying amounts of vitamins A and C. When it comes to terminology: only 100 percent juice can be called "juice." If juice is diluted (<100 percent juice), the product label must identify it with a different name: "juice drink," "juice beverage," or "juice cocktail"; these terms can be used interchangeably. Or it may be called "diluted ____ juice"—for example, diluted apple juice. A "fruit drink" is simply flavored water (with no juice), perhaps fortified with vitamin C or other nutrients, phytonutrients, or herbs.

Does 100 percent juice make it better, with more vitamin C than a juice drink? Not necessarily. The percentage of juice is just part of the nutrition story. For example, some 100 percent fruit juices contain less than 100 percent of the Daily Value (DV) for vitamin C, while some juice drinks are fortified to supply at least 100 percent in a single serving:

Did You Stop to Think

. . . that with the incredible variety of bottled drinks on the market today, you really need to be a label reader? Serving sizes aren't always the same. A single bottle may have two or more servings, for at least twice the calories. And many water beverages, teas, and coffee drinks are high in added sugars.

. . . that a large, regular soda (32 ounces) from a convenience store or fast-food place adds up to about 400 calories? Drinking one drink that size three times a week adds up to 1,200 calories per week, or about 60,000 calories over a fifty-week work year. A pound of body fat is about 3,500 calories. Do the math! That adds up to several pounds of added body fat if you don't make other changes in your food or lifestyle habits!

. . . that "slow sipping" a regular soft drink, sweetened ice tea, or juice drink bathes your teeth in cavity-promoting sugars? And the effect continues for twenty to forty minutes after your last sip!

. . . that 8 ounces of milk at lunch provide a quarter to almost a third of your day's calcium recommendation? Great for bones! Drinking a 12-ounce can of diet soda instead provides "zero" calcium.

. . . that water is your best choice as a "staple beverage"? Great thirst quencher, calorie-free!

¾-Cup Serving	% Daily Value of Vitamin C
Orange juice	100
Fortified juice (such as cranberry)	100
Apple juice (unfortified)	2
Grape juice (unfortified)	50

To learn how to use Nutrition Facts on fruit juice and juice drink labels, see "Today's Food Labels" in chapter 11; you'll also find advice there on refrigerated juice safety.

All juice products contain water and sugar. Fruit juice contains naturally occurring fructose, or fruit sugar, whereas juice drinks have added sugars such as high-fructose corn syrup as well as some fructose. Scientific evidence shows that your body can't distinguish between naturally occurring and added sugars, so regardless of whether a juice or juice drink is naturally sweet or sweetened, its sugars are used by your body in the same way. *See chapter 5, "Sweet Talk: Sugar and Other Sweeteners."* Depending on the amount of sugars added, there may be a difference in the amount of calories per serving between fruit drinks and fruit juices.

On the label, 100 percent juices, such as orange juice, won't list sugar and water as separate ingredients. They're naturally present in juice. Sometimes tart juices, such as cranberry, are blended with other juices, water, and sweeteners to make them more pleasing. Some juice drinks are flavorful blends, such as cranberry-mango or tangerine-grapefruit. A nutritional difference between fruit juices and fruit drinks is that fruit juices often contain more of other important nutrients and phytonutrients, such as folate in orange juice or antioxidants in blueberry juice.

Does fruit come to mind first when you think of juice? Give vegetable juice, such as tomato juice or a vegetable juice mixture, a try, too.

For guidelines on fruit juice for infants and children from the American Academy of Pediatrics, see chapters 15 and 16.

Juicing Fruits and Vegetables

Some juice-machine promoters may lead you to believe that juicing makes fruits and vegetables healthier. Of course, their juices are healthful, offering most of the vitamins, minerals, and phytonutrients found in the whole fruit or vegetables. However, juices typically have less fiber; it gets left behind in the pulp. And in spite of the "cure-all" claims, simply changing the form of food by juicing can't deliver added benefits. Enjoy juice as one way to get the benefits of fruits and vegetables—but don't expect miracles!

Milk, Cocoa, and Flavored Milks: Calcium-Rich Choices

Like all beverages, milk supplies that essential nutrient water: about 89 percent by weight. And as one of the best calcium sources in the American diet, milk offers a lot more.

Along with water, milk supplies many essential nutrients; here's what just 1 cup (8 ounces) supplies. Do a little math to see what the recommended two to three Milk Group servings daily provide for you; for teens, the advice is three to four daily servings.

Nutrient	Daily Value (%)
Calcium (300 mg.)	30
Vitamin D (100 IU)	25
Vitamin A (500 IU)	10
Protein (8 g.)	16
Potassium (390 mg.)	11
Riboflavin (0.4 mg.)	23
Vitamin B_{12} (0.8 mcg.)	13
Phosphorus (200 mg.)	20
Niacin and niacin equivalents (2 NE)	10

Among the various types of milk—whole, 2 percent reduced-fat, 1 percent low-fat, and fat-free—the fat content varies, along with the calorie content. However, the contributions of other nutrients, including water, are about the same.

Flavored milk, perhaps fruit- or chocolate flavored, can be a healthful option. For chocolate milk, the only difference is an additional 60 calories per 8-ounce serving from the added sweetener, and chocolate or cocoa. Whether it's flavored or unflavored, milk supplies the same amounts of calcium, phosphorus,

. . . if sports drinks are good fluid replacers? The optimal drink for many sports activities is water! Sports drinks are meant to replace fluids, supply calories for energy, and replace sodium and potassium lost through perspiration. Most athletes don't need a sports drink unless they've exercised for an hour or more. Even then, the body mainly needs fluids. If you're more likely to drink a sports drink rather than water during physical activity, then by all means do. Just be aware that these drinks contain sugars, so they also supply calories. As a regular beverage choice, remember that their calories can add up: often 50 to 100 calories per cup in a sports drink. *For more information on fluids during athletic performance, see "Thirst for Success!" in chapter 19.*

protein, riboflavin, and vitamin D needed by people of all ages. *To compare the calories, calcium, fat, and cholesterol in various forms of milk, see "Milk: A Good Calcium Source" in chapter 10.*

The fact that many kids like flavored milk has prompted questions among some parents: Does the sugar and caffeine in chocolate milk cause hyperactivity? No scientific evidence suggests a link between sugar and hyperactivity, mood swings, or academic performance. The very small amount of caffeine in the chocolate or cocoa won't make a difference, either. Some soft drinks provide much more caffeine. *See the chart "Caffeine: What Sources, How Much?" later in this chapter.*

On cold winter days, hot cocoa can be another good beverage choice. Made with milk rather than water, hot cocoa supplies calcium along with the other nutrients in milk. For hot cocoa or cocoa made from a mix, use milk for the greatest nutritional benefit.

Drinks: With or without Caffeine?

Caffeine, a mild stimulant, has been part of the human diet for centuries. As far back as five thousand years ago, records suggest that the Chinese were brewing tea. About twenty-five hundred years ago, highly valued coffee beans were used in Africa as currency. And in the Americas, the Aztecs enjoyed chocolate drinks. Today, caffeine-containing foods and beverages are a growing part of our food pattern. Does coffee in the morning go with your "wakeup" routine?

A naturally occurring substance in plants, caffeine is found in leaves, seeds, and fruits of more than sixty plants, among them coffee and cocoa beans, tea leaves, and kola nuts. We consume these products as coffee, chocolate, tea, and cola drinks. Caffeine also is used as an ingredient in more than a thousand over-the-counter drugs as well as in prescription drugs, and as a subtle flavoring.

Coffee remains the chief source of caffeine in the United States. That includes drinks made with coffee, such as latte, mocha, and cappuccino. The amount of caffeine depends on the type of coffee, the amount, the brewing method, and whether it's caffeinated.

Soft drinks and teas are the main sources of caffeine for children and teens. Among soft drinks, cola isn't the only beverage with caffeine; some citrus-flavored beverages contain caffeine as well.

Caffeine acts as a mild stimulant to the central nervous system. Some people drink coffee just for that reason: to keep alert and prevent fatigue. Does caffeine improve physical performance? *See chapter 19 to find out.*

Caffeine: A Health Connection?

Over the years many studies have explored the connection between caffeine and health. No scientific evidence has been found to link caffeine intake to any health risks, including cancer (pancreatic, breast, or other types), fibrocystic breast disease (benign fibrous lumps), cardiovascular disease, blood cholesterol levels, ulcers, inflammatory bowel disease, infertility, birth defects, or osteoporosis.

Concerned about your blood pressure? Caffeine doesn't cause hypertension or a lasting increase in blood pressure. However, it may cause a temporary rise that lasts only a few hours and adds up to less than the rise from climbing stairs.

Caffeine may have a diuretic effect, increasing water loss through urination. However, the fluid in the beverage usually cancels out any diuretic effect. The diuretic effect depends on the amount of caffeine. Caffeinated drinks won't cause dehydration, either. If you have trouble with diarrhea, avoiding caffeine might be advised.

While caffeine can increase slightly the amount of calcium lost through urine and feces, it's the amount of calcium in about 1 teaspoon of milk that's lost for each cup of regular coffee. To help counter this effect and boost the calcium benefit, enjoy coffee drinks made with plenty of milk:

COFFEE DRINKS* (12 OZ.) (MADE WITH LOW-FAT/ FAT-FREE MILK)	CALCIUM (MG)	CALORIES	FAT (G)
Caffè latte	412	110	0
Caffè mocha	337	140	2
Cappuccino	262	60	0

Source: National Dairy Council (2001).

*Bottled coffee drinks may not have as much calcium and perhaps a lot of added sugar; read the Nutrition Facts on the label to find out.

By the way, you don't need to use whole milk to get a foam on cappuccino. Low-fat or fat-free milk and soy milk also will do the trick.

Moderate amounts of caffeine don't appear to raise the risk for osteoporosis. Although many people think a cup of coffee can help "sober up" someone who drinks too much alcohol, caffeine won't counteract the effects of drinking alcoholic beverages. Neither will a cold shower or a long walk. Only time can make someone sober.

In varying degrees, however, excessive caffeine intake may cause "coffee jitters," anxiety, or insomnia. Caffeine also may speed the heart rate temporarily. These physical effects of caffeine don't last long, since caffeine doesn't accumulate in the body. Within three to four hours, most is excreted in healthy people; for smokers, it's slightly faster. Some people are more sensitive to caffeine than others.

The definition of "excessive" caffeine intake is an individual matter. Your caffeine sensitivity depends on the amount and frequency of caffeine intake, body weight, physical condition, and overall anxiety level, among other factors. Tolerance to caffeine develops over time. A regular coffee drinker may not notice the effects as quickly as someone who drinks just an occasional cup. For most healthy adults, moderate amounts of caffeine—200 to 300 milligrams a day, or about two

Caffeine: What Sources, How Much?

The amount of caffeine in foods or beverages depends on several factors: the type of product, its preparation method, and the portion size. Caffeine occurs naturally in some products, such as coffee and chocolate, and is added as a flavoring agent in some others, such as soft drinks.

BEVERAGE	CAFFEINE (MG) TYPICAL	RANGE[†]
Coffee* (8-oz. serving)		
Brewed, drip method	85	60–120
Instant	75	60–85
Decaffeinated	3	2–4
Espresso coffee (1-oz. cup)	40	30–50
Tea (8-oz. serving)		
Brewed, major U.S. brands	40	20–90
Brewed, imported brands	60	25–110
Instant	28	24–31
Iced	25	9–50
Some soft drinks (8 oz.)	24	20–40
Cocoa beverage (8 oz.)	6	3–32
Chocolate milk beverage (8 oz.)	5	2–7
Milk chocolate (1 oz.)	6	1–15
Dark chocolate, semisweet (1 oz.)	20	5-35
Baker's chocolate (1 oz.)	26	26
Chocolate-flavored syrup (1 oz.)	4	4

*A coarse grind delivers about the same amount of caffeine as a fine grind.

[†]For coffee, these are average ranges. The plant variety of the bean, the roasting method, and the amount of ground coffee used in brewing are among the factors affecting the amount.

Source: International Food Information Council Foundation (1999). Reprinted with permission of the International Food Information Council Foundation.

to three cups of coffee—pose no physical problems.

Can you become addicted to caffeine? No, but caffeinated drinks may be habit-forming. If you drink them regularly, then suddenly stop, you may have some short-term symptoms—drowsiness, headache, perhaps less concentration—that disappear in a day or two.

According to the National Institutes of Health, caffeine affects children and adults in the same way. No studies show that caffeine causes attention deficit disorder or affects growth in children.

● *If you're pregnant or nursing* . . . it's wise to go easy on caffeine. Although most physicians agree on its safety, sensitivity to caffeine may increase during pregnancy. In breast milk, caffeine can pass to the baby, but the very small amount isn't enough to affect the infant.

● *If you have a medical problem* . . . ask your physician to guide you on caffeine consumption, particularly if you suffer from gastritis, ulcers, or high blood pressure, or if you're taking beta-blockers. People with stomach problems may be wise to steer clear of both caffeinated beverages and their decaffeinated counterparts. Substances in both stimulate the flow of stomach acids, potentially irritating the stomach lining.

● *If you're older* . . . your sensitivity to caffeine may increase with age.

● *At any age* . . . pay attention to the effects that caffeine may have on you, especially if coffee, tea, or soft drinks take the place of more nutritious foods or beverages.

For most people who choose caffeinated beverages, two to three cups of coffee (or that amount of caffeine) are likely reasonable. If you decide to reduce your caffeine intake, it's easy. Here's how:

● Cut back gradually—if you've been ingesting a lot of caffeine—to get your body accustomed to consuming less. For some people, abruptly cutting out caffeine can result temporarily in headaches or drowsiness for a few days. A gradual cutback helps avoid this problem.

● Try a mixture of half regular and half decaffeinated coffee.

● Drink decaffeinated coffee, which has almost no caffeine at all. Some bottled coffee drinks also are decaffeinated; check the label.

● Brew tea for a shorter time. A one-minute brew may contain just half the caffeine that a three-minute brew contains.

● Drink decaffeinated tea or caffeine-free herbal tea.

● Keep a cup of water handy to sip. If you drink coffee, tea, or soft drinks mindlessly, you may be drinking more caffeine than you realize.

● Read soft drink labels carefully. Approximately 75 percent of soft drinks consumed in the United States contain caffeine. If you drink soft drinks, look for decaffeinated drinks or those without caffeine. Color doesn't indicate the presence of caffeine; both clear and caramel-colored soft drinks may have caffeine. Caffeine is listed in the ingredient list if it is present in the product.

● Read medication labels carefully, or check with your pharmacist. One dose of an over-the-counter pain relief capsule can contain as much caffeine as one or two cups of coffee.

● For those with insomnia, avoid coffee or other caffeine sources in the evening.

Take Time for Tea

Tea: next to water, it's the most common beverage choice throughout the world. Whether it's black, green, or oolong tea, tea comes from the same plant, called *Camellia sinensis.* Differences in color and flavor depend on processing.

● For *black tea,* the most popular type in the United States, tea leaves are exposed to air. The natural biochemical process turns them a deep red-brown color and imparts a unique, rich flavor. Many flavored specialty teas start with black tea. As an aside, orange pekoe isn't made with orange flavor; instead "pekoe" or "orange pekoe" refers to the grade and size of the tea leaves.

● For *green tea,* typically served in Chinese and Japanese restaurants, the tea leaves are not processed as much. Instead, they're just heated or steamed quickly to keep their green color and delicate flavor.

● *Oolong tea* is an "in-between" tea: between black and green tea.

Teatime: Health Benefits?

Whether black or green or oolong, tea appears to have potential health benefits, perhaps derived from its flavonoids. Flavonoids and other polyphenols, which are phytonutrients, work as antioxidants that may help protect body cells from damage done by free radicals. Using the oxygen radical absorbency capacity (ORAC) score, which ranks the antioxidant potential of plant-based foods, tea ranks as high as or higher than many fruits and vegetables. *To learn more about antioxidants, the ORAC score, and phytonutrients, see chapter 4.*

Can tea drinking help keep you healthy? Maybe, but the research linking tea consumption and disease prevention is too new for certainty. And there's not enough evidence yet to offer specific advice about tea drinking. Some promising areas of study suggest that tea or tea's flavonoids may reduce risk of gastric, esophageal, and skin cancers and may offer protection from heart disease and stroke—if you consume enough (four to six cups a day). Some studies are investigating whether tea plays a role in relaxation or mental performance.

Tea may supply fluoride, which helps strengthen tooth enamel, if it's made with fluoridated water. Tea also may help fight cavities by reducing plaque formation and hindering cavity-forming bacteria. You still need to brush and floss!

For now, enjoy tea as a beverage choice; brew it for at least three minutes to bring out most of the flavonoids. Then stay tuned for science-based advice.

Creative Ways to Enjoy Tea

● Try bottled teas as a portable beverage choice. Many bottled or canned ice tea drinks have as much added sugars as a regular soda; read the label to check the calories. Look for those flavored with noncaloric sweeteners.

● Watching calories? Enjoy tea without added sugar or honey. For a touch of flavor in unsweetened tea, just add a slice of lemon or lime, fresh ginger, or fresh mint leaves.

● Add citrus juice for flavor and smart nutrition! Tea's flavonoids partly inhibit the absorption of nonheme iron (iron from legumes, grain products, and eggs). A squeeze of vitamin C-rich lemon, orange, or lime juice in your tea can counteract some of the action.

● For more calcium, enjoy "milk tea": hot or cold tea added to milk. With added milk, you may not get all the benefits of tea, however, because milk may inhibit the action of some phytonutrients.

● Experiment with culinary uses of dried tea leaves: as a flavor rub for a roast, for tea-marinated meat, or in homemade sorbet.

● Use tea—perhaps a flavored variety—in place of water as you bake breads, cookies, cakes, and brownies.

Pour a "Herbal"?

Have a sip of apple-cinnamon tea, mint tea, or ginger tea. Interest in herbal teas has been rising for those seeking an alternative to caffeinated beverages—and for those hoping for other health benefits.

To clear up a misconception: many branded herbal teas are really tea leaves with added herbs and perhaps fruit juice, honey, sweeteners, or flavor extracts; they have caffeine unless the label indicates "decaf." The ingredient list will include "tea." And some herbal teas on the market aren't tea at all. Instead, they're infusions made with herbs, flowers, roots, spices, or various other parts of many plants. The more correct term for them is "tisane," which means tealike substance.

When it comes to health benefits, herbal teas haven't been studied, so not much is known. Some research suggests that their polyphenols, one type of phytonutrient, may bind iron before it can be absorbed. Most major branded herbal teas are considered safe to drink. Still, you're wise to consume only common varieties sold by major manufacturers.

The basis of some medicines is herbs, so it's not surprising that some herbal teas interfere with over-the-counter or prescription medications. Talk to your doctor or pharmacist before drinking them when you're on medication.

Because of their potential harmful effects, be careful about using herbs to make "teas"—comfrey, lobelia, woodruff, tonka beans, melilot, sassafras root, and many others may be harmful in large amounts. For example, comfrey may cause liver damage. Woodruff, an anticoagulant, may cause bleeding. Lobelia may cause breathing problems. Even chamomile may cause an allergic reaction.

For more on herbal teas and remedies, see "For Herbal and Other Botanical Supplements . . ." in chapter 23.

Soft Drinks: Okay?

Flavored, carbonated drinks have been around for about two hundred years. And their popularity continues to grow—overtaking more nutritious beverages among some age groups.

The term "soft drink" originally was coined to distinguish these beverages from "hard" liquor. Yet a hundred years ago, consumers asked for "pop," named for the sound made by popping open the bottle cap. Today, "soft drink"—or "soda" in some parts of the United States—refers to a beverage made with carbonated water and usually flavoring ingredients.

What's in a soft drink? Whether they're regular or diet varieties, soft drinks contain water: about 90 percent for regular soft drinks and about 99 percent for diet soft drinks. Carbon dioxide, added just before sealing the bottle or can, gives the fizz. Regular soft drinks are sweetened with sugar, perhaps high-fructose corn syrup and/or sugar; diet drinks, with saccharin or aspartame. *See chapter 5 for more information on sugar and alternative sweeteners.* The additional flavor comes from artificial and natural flavors. Acids such as citric acid and phosphoric acid give a tart taste and act as preservatives. Coloring may be added; however, today clear soft drinks are popular, too. Some caffeine may be added to enhance the flavor, while other ingredients may add consistency.

As soft drink consumption goes up, the nutritional concerns are twofold:

● Too often soft drinks take the place of more nutritious beverages such as calcium-rich milk. Except for water and for carbohydrates in the form of sugars, soft drinks don't supply significant amounts of nutrients. A 12-ounce can of cola, for example, supplies water and about 150 calories (from almost 10 teaspoons of sugar), but little else. A diet soft drink is a source of water and has almost no calories.

● Too many regular soft drinks, especially with larger-than-ever drink portions, may lead to too many calories. That, in turn, may contribute to the growing problem of overweight and obesity.

● Soft drinks fortified with antioxidants have hit the market, too. Be wary. For the potential benefits, fruits, vegetables, and whole grain foods are much more effective sources. *See "Antioxidant Vitamins: A Closer Look" in chapter 4.*

As your best guideline, enjoy soft drinks in moderation—as long as you consume the nutrients you need from other sources and don't overdo on calories in your overall diet.

Functional Beverages

Improve your memory? Lift your mood? Relieve tension? Fight fat? Give you energy? A growing market of functional beverages—juice, tea, soft drinks, flavored water, isotonic drinks, enhanced with herbs, phytonutrients, and other functional ingredients—are marketed with promises to improve your health. But do they offer benefits?

Most functional beverages aren't likely to offer benefits to most healthy people Among the issues: Claims for most of these drinks aren't proven; *for what we know and don't know about the ingredients (gingko, kava, ginseng, and St. John's wort, among many others), see "Dietary Supplements: What Are They?" in chapter 23.* The amount of the added ingredient is neither standardized or identified on the label. And their safety—optimal doses, interactions, and long-term consequences—isn't known.

Will "energy drinks" really give you more energy? High caffeine and "carbs" are the so-called power behind their marketing hype. It's not the ideal drink for athletes, or for "grab-and-go energy." Extra caffeine may give a boost at first, but with too much caffeine, performance may suffer; *see "Which Fluids?" and "Sports Drinks" in chapter 19 for more about beverages for athletic performance.* The concentrated sugar content can slow the body's absorption of water, so energy drinks aren't the best fluid replacers. And as a mixer in alcoholic drinks, the stimulating effect of caffeine may mask the effects of too much alcohol—a potential danger. Energy drinks with the stimulant ephedrine can be harmful!

Remember that functional drinks won't counter dysfunctional eating or living. The best approach for health and for feeling energetic? Healthful eating, regular physical activity, enough rest—and learning to deal with stress!

Drink Smart—and Get Your Zzzzzzzs!

Do you wake up with a sleep deficit? Do you regularly have trouble sleeping? Adequate rest, along with good nutrition and regular physical activity, are part of any formula for fitness. Consider these tips for the "rest" of your life:

- If you're caffeine-sensitive, avoid caffeinated drinks six to eight hours before sleeptime. For meals and snacks later in the day, opt for milk, juice, water, or decaffeinated drinks.

- Don't expect a glass of wine or other alcoholic beverage to help you sleep well. A drink might help you feel drowsy at first, but even if you sip a drink two or three hours before bedtime, your sleep might be light instead of the deep, most restful kind of sleep pattern.

An added note: Promote rest through regular physical activity. Being active actually helps your body relax and sleep soundly. Just refrain from exercise too close to bedtime. Exercise speeds up your metabolism for a while, perhaps keeping you "pumped up" and unable to sleep right away.

Alcoholic Beverages: In Moderation

No one's sure who first invented beer, wine, or ale, but historians do know that societies have enjoyed these beverages throughout recorded history.

Today, moderate amounts still add pleasure to eating. For some, a single drink may be relaxing—perhaps in the company of another. For older adults and people with some chronic illnesses, a drink before a meal may enhance appetite. And evidence suggests that moderate drinking may lower the risk for heart disease among some people; healthful eating and active living are part of the equation, too.

The key to any potential benefits, however, is sensibility: moderation and an understanding of alcohol equivalency.

- *Moderation:* no more than one drink a day for women and no more than two drinks daily for men

- *Equivalency of one drink:* 12 ounces of regular beer (150 calories), *or* 5 ounces of wine (100 calories), *or* 1.5 ounces of 80-proof distilled spirits (100 calories). Each contains the same amount of alcohol—approximately 14 grams of pure ethanol. Distilled spirits include bourbon, brandy, gin, rum, vodka, whisky, and liqueurs.

The advice for most people who drink alcoholic beverages is: Enjoy them in moderation, with food. And never drink if it puts you or others at risk!

Alcoholic Beverages: The Health Effects

For most adults, one alcohol-containing drink or two during the day offers little risk for developing problems related to drinking. Are there any benefits? What are the risks?

Unlike nutrients, most alcohol isn't broken down through digestion. Its "pathway" to body cells moves much faster, including directly through the stomach lining and wall of the small intestine. With no food in the stomach to slow it down, absorption into the bloodstream is even faster (within about twenty minutes). From the bloodstream, it goes to every cell of the body, to some degree depressing cell activity.

Although some people drink to be the "life of the party," alcohol actually is a depressant, not a stimulant.

Have You Ever Wondered

. . . why you feel so thirsty after eating salty food? Salt is made of two minerals: sodium and chloride. When you eat a lot of salty foods, your body uses water to flush extra sodium away. With water loss, you feel thirsty, and you likely drink more. This explains why bars and cocktail lounges often serve salty snacks with drinks.

. . . if a few cold beers on a hot summer day are just as good as water to replace fluids? Not really. Alcohol is a diuretic, which increases urine output and so promotes dehydration—not the best fluid replacement when you're sweating already! If you enjoy a beer, drink water, too.

. . . what's rooibos tea? Pronounced ROY-boss, rooibos isn't a tea at all, but instead a herbal brew. First popularized in South Africa, this red brew in nutty, flowery, and fruity flavors is purported to have antioxidant benefits. Research doesn't back up the advertised claims. Like other herbals, be cautious.

The initial "lift" that may come with drinking is short-lived. By dulling various brain centers, alcohol may reduce concentration, coordination, and response time; cause drowsiness and interfere with normal sleep patterns; and result in slurred speech and blurred vision. Because alcohol has a diuretic effect, alcohol promotes water loss, too. That's why many people may feel thirsty after drinking a lot—perhaps the morning after.

The alcohol concentration in blood depends on the amount of alcohol consumed over a period of time as well as body composition, body size, metabolism, and medications. A healthy liver detoxifies much of the alcohol consumed—at a rate of about ½ ounce per hour. The higher the blood alcohol concentration level, the longer it takes. For two regular-size drinks consumed during a sixty-minute "happy hour," the body needs two to three hours to break it down.

A single alcoholic drink affects women more than men, due in part to differences in body size and metabolism. Alcohol is carried in the body's fluids, not in body fat. Because women have a smaller volume of water in their bodies than men do, the same amount of alcohol is more concentrated in the bloodstream and so potentially has a greater effect. The enzyme that helps metabolize alcohol in the body is also less active in women. As a result, women are at greater risk for problems related to alcoholism.

Caution: *The Risks.* The Dietary Guidelines for Americans notes risks related to alcoholic beverage consumption. Consuming more than one drink a day for women and two for men is linked to an increased risk for several health problems, including high blood pressure, stroke, and several forms of cancer, as well as motor vehicle crashes, other injuries, violence, and suicide. During pregnancy, drinking increases the chances for birth defects. For women, moderate drinking may slightly increase the risk for breast cancer.

Heavy drinkers may have social and psychological problems: for example, altered judgment and a potential dependency. Excessive drinking also can lead to brain and heart damage, cirrhosis of the liver, and an inflamed pancreas.

Potential Benefits? Moderate drinking may offer health benefits: lower risk for heart disease, mostly for men over age forty-five and women over age fifty-five. The benefits appear to come from any alcoholic beverage: wine, beer, or distilled spirits.

A little wine or beer before a meal may stimulate the appetite and make a meal more appealing. Talk to your healthcare provider if you have a health problem linked to appetite loss.

Watch the Calories, Mind Your Nutrients!

Alcohol is actually a fermentation product of carbohydrates: both sugars and starches. In beverages or food, it supplies energy, or calories. Alcohol provides 7 calories for every gram, compared with 4 calories per gram of carbohydrate and protein, and 9 calories per gram of fat. A 1-ounce jigger or "shot" of vodka, for example, may be 40 to 50 percent alcohol, or up

Red Wine: Heart-Healthy?

Does red wine protect against heart disease? There's no conclusive answer. Recent research suggests that a moderate amount of alcoholic beverages—red wine as well as white wine, beer, and distilled spirits—may help lower the risk for heart disease. Possibly a small amount may help increase HDL blood cholesterol, or "good" cholesterol, and it may prevent LDL, or "bad" cholesterol, from forming. However, factors other than ethanol (alcohol) also may play a role.

Phytonutrients such as resveratrol and tannins in wine may offer heart-healthy benefits, too. Resveratrol, a flavonoid found in the skins and seeds of grapes, has estrogenlike qualities that may help increase HDLs or increase the oxidation, or breakdown, of LDLs. (Grape skins are needed to make red wine.) Also speculated, resveratrol may boost the body's natural clot-dissolving enzyme; when blood platelets clot, they decrease blood flow, which can lead to a heart attack or a stroke. Tannins also may inhibit platelet clotting.

Scientists don't know enough to offer definitive advice, so if you don't drink, protecting your heart isn't a reason to start. If you do, a drink a day may offer a benefit. Remember, other lifestyle habits—such as healthful eating, regular exercise, not smoking, and keeping a healthy weight—offer the most protection against heart disease! *See "A Toast to Heart Health" in chapter 22.*

to ½ ounce of alcohol. That equals about 14 grams and contributes about 100 calories. The additional calories in beer, wine, or liqueurs come from carbohydrates.

The alcohol content of a single drink depends on the type of alcohol and the serving size. "Special" alcoholic drinks advertised on restaurant table tents usually contain more alcohol because they're bigger. The calorie content also is determined by the amount of alcohol and, for mixed drinks, the other ingredients in the drink. *See the chart "Alcohol and Calories: How Much?" later in this chapter for alcohol and calories in standard-size servings.*

Does drinking lead to weight gain? Probably not for moderate drinkers. In fact, a few scientific studies suggest that the body uses energy (calories) from alcohol differently than energy from other sources.

For some people, however, a "beer belly" is aptly named. Calories from alcoholic beverages can add up, contributing to excess body weight. For example, a six-pack of beer, consumed on a hot summer day, supplies 900 calories. To burn off those calories, a person would need to jog without a break for about two hours. A 5-ounce glass of dry wine before dinner supplies 100 calories, or 700 calories if consumed every day of the week. Within five weeks that adds up to a pound of body fat. (A pound of body fat equals 3,500 calories.) The mixers added to drinks make the calories add up even more, yet often add few nutrients; for example, the soft drink in a rum-and-cola drink; heavy cream in a grasshopper or brandy alexander; and sugar in a daiquiri or mint julep.

Although it supplies calories, or energy, alcohol isn't a nutrient. On the contrary, because alcohol may interfere with nutrient absorption, heavy drinkers may not benefit from all the vitamins and minerals they consume. Unless juice or milk beverages are used as mixers, alcoholic beverages themselves supply few if any nutrients.

Wine, beer, and distilled spirits don't count toward your fluid intake for the day. Beverage alcohol has a diuretic, or dehydrating, effect.

There's another nutrition issue. Poor nutrition is linked to drinking alcoholic beverages when they take the place of nutritious foods and beverages—for example, when a glass of wine with dinner takes the place of calcium-rich milk. By limiting beer, wine, and other alcoholic beverages, there's room in your eating plan for more nutritious foods and drinks. For the casual or moderate drinker, this may not be much of a problem; malnutrition is a significant concern for heavy drinkers.

Drinking: For Some Not Advised

The Dietary Guidelines for Americans advise: *If you drink alcoholic beverages, do so in moderation.* However, some people are wise to avoid alcoholic drinks entirely. Besides the risks mentioned earlier, avoid drinking . . .

. . . if you're a teenager or a child. Young people derive little if any potential health benefit from moderate drinking. Since the risk of alcohol abuse goes up when drinking starts at an early age, kids who drink can set themselves up for the same health-related risks that adults have. For inexperienced teenage drivers, alcohol and driving is a very risky combination. Besides, buying alcoholic beverages is illegal in the United States for anyone under age twenty-one.

. . . if you can't moderate your drinking. As part of a lifelong commitment, recovering alcoholics and prob-

---

Label Lingo

Alcoholic Beverages

You'll find this warning statement on the label of beverages containing alcohol. On wine and beer labels, you may also find information on sulfite content. *See "For the Sulfite-Sensitive . . ." in chapter 21. (Tip:* If you're sulfite-sensitive, sake, a type of rice wine, doesn't contain sulfites.)

GOVERNMENT WARNING:

(1) ACCORDING TO THE SURGEON GENERAL, WOMEN SHOULD NOT DRINK ALCOHOLIC BEVERAGES DURING PREGNANCY BECAUSE OF THE RISK OF BIRTH DEFECTS. (2) CONSUMPTION OF ALCOHOLIC BEVERAGES IMPAIRS YOUR ABILITY TO DRIVE A CAR OR OPERATE MACHINERY, AND MAY CAUSE HEALTH PROBLEMS.

CONTAINS SULFITES found in most wines to protect flavor and color.

lem drinkers should abstain from any alcoholic drink. Because of the genetic link to alcoholism, people with alcoholism in their family are wise to moderate their intake of alcoholic beverages, too—or avoid them altogether.

. . . if your project or work requires your attention, skill, or coordination. Alcohol affects productivity, which can affect your output on the job and your personal safety. Even with moderate drinking—a glass or two of wine or beer—alcohol stays in your blood for two to three hours.

. . . if you plan to drive or handle potentially dangerous equipment. Even low levels of blood alcohol from a single drink can make you more accident-prone for several hours. If you plan to drink, designate another driver from the start who won't be drinking!

. . . if you're pregnant or trying to get pregnant. In the United States, drinking during pregnancy is the leading cause of birth defects, or fetal alcohol syndrome. While there's not enough proof that an occasional drink is harmful, even moderate drinking may relate to low infant birthweight or a miscarriage. However, no safe level has been established for a woman any time during pregnancy, including the first few weeks. Too often, women drink before they even know they're pregnant, potentially compromising their baby for life. *See "Pregnancy and Alcoholic Beverages Don't Mix!" in chapter 17 for more on fetal alcohol syndrome.* Heavy drinking may not be wise for Dad, either. According to research, excessive alcohol may decrease sperm count and potency and so affect fertility.

. . . if you're on medication, even over-the-counter kinds. Alcohol may interact with medicine, making it either less effective or more potent. The medication itself may raise blood alcohol levels or increase its adverse affects on the brain. The result: a single drink will impair judgment, coordination, and skill faster. Check warnings printed on over-the-counter medications. And talk with your doctor, pharmacist, or healthcare provider about your own prescribed and over-the-counter medications. *See "Food and Medicine" in chapter 22.*

. . . if you suffer from allergies. Sulfites in wine may trigger histamine production and produce unwanted allergy symptoms.

Taking Control: Drinking Responsibly!

If you choose to drink alcoholic beverages, always do so responsibly. Here's how you can go easy . . .

● Start with a nonalcoholic beverage first. Satisfying your thirst first will help prevent you from gulping your drinks so you can enjoy your alcoholic beverage more slowly.

● Don't drink on an empty stomach. Eating a little food helps slow the absorption of alcohol.

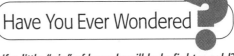

Have You Ever Wondered

. . . if a little "nip" of brandy will help fight a cold? On the contrary, if you have a cold or a chronic health problem that lowers your immunity, you're wise to abstain. Alcohol can impair the body's ability to fight infectious bacteria and may interfere with medication.

. . . if an alcoholic drink will warm you up in cold weather? No. Alcohol tends to increase the body's heat loss, making people more susceptible to cold. So if you're ice fishing, cross-country skiing, or watching outside winter sports, don't expect an alcoholic drink to keep you warm.

. . . what the term "80 Proof" means on a bottle of liquor? The term "Proof" is an indication of the amount of alcohol. The proof is twice the alcohol content. If a label on a bottle of liquor states "80 Proof," this means that the liquor contains 40 percent alcohol. The proof will vary depending on the type of liquor.

. . . if a nightcap will help you sleep? It may put you to sleep, but not help you stay asleep—with the deep, restful sleep you need. A drink with dinner probably won't affect your sleep habits.

. . . how much alcohol burns off or evaporates in cooking? That depends on the cooking time and the amount of distilled spirits, wine, or beer used. Added to uncooked foods, the alcohol content doesn't change. However, added to boiling liquid at the end of cooking, about 85 percent of the alcohol may be retained, compared to only about 5 percent if the dish was braised for 2½ hours. A flamed (flambé) dish may retain about 75 percent of its alcohol content.

. . . how cooking wine compares to regular table wine? Cooking wine is usually high in sodium. So cut back on salty ingredients if you use it. From a flavor standpoint, regular wine may be better.

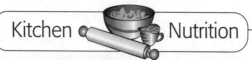

Substitutions for Alcoholic Ingredients

Baby back ribs, chicken, or seafood tenderized in a beer marinade, a touch of distilled spirits to enhance the flavor of cooking juices, light biscuits or bread made with beer, chicken braised in wine. Wine, beer, and distilled spirits can add to the flavor, tenderness, and texture of your culinary creations.

If you choose to avoid wine, beer, or distilled spirits, it's easy to make a quick, flavorful substitution. To equal the amount of liquid from the alcoholic ingredient, you may need to add water, broth, or apple or white grape juice.

IN A RECIPE THAT CALLS FOR . . .	USE THIS INSTEAD . . .
¼ cup or more white wine	Equal amount of: *In any dish:* white grape juice, apple juice, nonalcoholic wine* *In salad dressings:* lemon juice *In marinades:* vinegar *For savory dishes:* chicken, vegetable, or clam broth (Use ⅞ cup broth plus 2 tbsp. lemon juice or vinegar.) (*Add 1 tbsp. vinegar to balance sweetness.)
¼ cup or more red wine	Equal amount of: *In any dish:* red grape juice, cranberry juice, nonalcoholic wine* *In salad dressings:* lemon juice *In marinades:* vinegar *For savory dishes:* tomato juice, fruit-flavored vinegar, or beef, chicken, or vegetable broth (*Add 1 tbsp. vinegar to balance sweetness.)
¼ cup or more port wine, rum, brandy, sweet sherry	Equal amount of apple or apple juice plus 1 tsp. vanilla extract
¼ cup or more beer	*For soups, stews, and other cooked dishes:* Equal amount of nonalcoholic beer, apple cider, or broth
2 tbsp. almond-flavored liqueur, such as Amaretto	¼ to ½ tsp. almond extract
2 tbsp. bourbon	1 to 2 tsp. vanilla extract
2 tbsp. coffee liqueur, such as Kahlua	2 tbsp. double-strength espresso *or* 2 tbsp. instant coffee, made with 4 to 6 times the usual amount in a cup of coffee
2 tbsp. orange-flavored liqueur, such as Grand Marnier	2 tbsp. orange juice concentrate *or* 2 tbsp. orange juice plus a little orange rind
2 tbsp. chocolate/coffee-flavored liqueur	½ to 1 tsp. chocolate extract plus ½ to 1 tsp. instant coffee in 2 tbsp. water
1 tbsp. dry vermouth	1 tbsp. apple cider
2 tbsp. dry sherry or bourbon	2 tbsp. orange or pineapple juice *or* 1 to 2 tsp. vanilla extract
2 tbsp. rum or brandy	½ to 1 tsp. vanilla, rum, or brandy extract *or* 2 tbsp. orange or pineapple juice

● Decide ahead to limit drinks, preferably no more than one per day if you're a female or two per day if you're a male. If you choose to drink more, pace yourself. On average, the body can detoxify only one standard-size drink (about ½ ounce of alcohol) per hour. The rest continues to circulate until it's finally broken down.

● To slow your drinking pace, put your drink down. Socialize instead.

● If you have one alcoholic drink, make the next one nonalcoholic. When you do this, you consume less alcohol and give your body a chance to process the alcohol you've consumed already.

● Measure liquor for mixed drinks with a jigger. Use a 1-ounce jigger, not the 1½-ounce size. You'll likely use less with a jigger than if you pour from the bottle right into the glass.

● Make an alcoholic drink last longer; you'll less likely order another. Learn to sip, not gulp; perhaps use a straw for mixed drinks. Dilute drinks with water, ice, club soda, or juice to increase the volume. Tip: Frozen drinks often take longer to sip.

● If you feel thirsty, drink bottled water or a soft drink instead of another alcoholic beverage. Remember, alcohol actually has a diuretic effect.

● Prefer a wine cooler? Instead of commercial drinks, mix your own using less wine. For mixers, try sparkling water or fruit juice.

● Lighten up! Order low-alcohol beer or light wine instead. Both have less alcohol. Or try nonalcoholic beer.

● At the table, have a glass of water by your plate, too. You'll probably drink less wine or beer.

● Skip the last round before the bar closes! And, as a host, don't feel a need to refresh your guests' drinks.

● Order a "virgin" cocktail: nonalcoholic mixers without the liquor. Mix in juice, carbonated water, or a soft drink instead. Remember the garnish! *See "Kitchen Nutrition: Super Sippers" for more ideas.*

● Bring bottled water or soft drinks to a picnic or a sports event to be sure you have a nonalcoholic option.

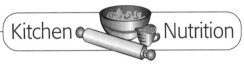

Kitchen Nutrition

Super Sippers

Hot-weather thirst quenchers:

● For a subtle citrus flavor in ice water, add slices of lemon, lime, or orange. Or add fruited or floral ice cubes: freeze fruit juice or edible flowers in your ice cube trays. *To learn about edible flowers, see "Please Don't Eat the Daffodils" in chapter 13.*

● Combine one 6-ounce can of grapefruit juice or cranberry-mango cocktail concentrate with two 12-ounce bottles of chilled club soda. Serve with a sprig of fresh mint. Serves four.

● Make a fruit smoothie. In a blender, purée berries, sliced kiwi, mango, or pineapple chunks, and frozen limeade concentrate. Perhaps add a little fresh mint. For convenience, try canned and frozen fruit for smoothies!

● Create your own shakes. In a blender, purée melon chunks or peach slices with buttermilk, crushed ice, and a touch of ginger or cinnamon until smooth.

● Use silken tofu as a great nondairy alternative in a creamy shake. Add a little juice and frozen fruit; purée until smooth.

Cold-weather belly warmers:

● Simmer cranberry-apple juice with cinnamon, cloves, allspice, and orange peel for about twenty minutes. Strain. Stir in fat-free dry milk powder and vanilla extract. Heat through.

● Add anise seeds, ground cinnamon, and ground cloves to ground coffee. Prepare hot coffee using the spiced ground coffee. Lighten with warm milk.

● Scoop praline or chocolate-swirl frozen yogurt into a mug. Pour hot cocoa or coffee over the top. Stir with a cinnamon stick.

Beer and Wine: What's in a Name?

Today these products appear on supermarket shelves. But just what do the descriptions mean, and how much alcohol do they contain?

Near beer: Malt beverage that has an alcohol content below 0.5 percent by volume. It also can be labeled a "malt beverage," a "cereal beverage," or when the label says "contains less than 0.5 percent alcohol by volume" as "nonalcoholic."

Alcohol and Calories: How Much?

Although their calorie content differs, these standard-size drinks each supply about the same amount of alcohol—about 14 grams of pure ethanol. (*Note:* alcoholic drinks are not 100 percent alcohol; that's why the volume differs.)

ALCOHOLIC DRINK	CALORIES
Beer, regular, 12 oz.	150
Beer, light, 12 oz.	100
Wine, dry, 5 oz.	100
Wine cooler, 12 oz.	180
Distilled spirits (80-proof), 1½ oz.*	100
Cordial or liqueur, 1½ oz.*	160

*An added mixer, such as a soft drink, adds more calories.

Low-alcohol or reduced-alcohol beer: Malt beverage with less than 2.5 percent alcohol by volume.

Alcohol-free malt beverage: Malt beverage that contains no alcohol.

Flavored malt beverage: Malt beverage (beer, lager, ale, porter, stout) flavored after fermentation, perhaps with juice, fruit, or juice concentrate—for example berry-, lemon-, or orange-flavored beer.

Aperitif wine: Wine with an alcohol content of 15 to 24 percent by volume, made from grape wine and added brandy, or alcohol flavored with herbs or other natural aromatic flavorings

Dessert wine: Wine that has brandy or distilled spirits added to it. Dessert wine has 14 to 24 percent alcohol by volume, more than table wine.

Table wine: Wine that has 7 to 14 percent alcohol by volume. Light wine, red wine, and sweet table wine are all types of table wine.

Low-alcohol wine: Wine, or fermented fruit beverage, that is less than 7 percent alcohol by volume. Low-alcohol wine isn't necessarily lower in calories; it may have more sugars than other wine.

Wine cooler: Diluted wine product (diluted with fruit juice, water, and/or added sugars) with an alcohol content of less than 7 percent by volume. Read the label's Nutrition Facts for calorie content per serving. Wine coolers may have more alcohol and calories than you think, since a serving is usually bigger: often 12 ounces, rather than a 5-fluid-ounce glass of table wine.

Sources: Bureau of Alcohol, Tobacco, and Firearms (2001); U.S. Food and Drug Administration (personal communication, 2001).

As an aside, most beers contain 5.0 to 5.5 percent alcohol by volume. In the United States and Europe, a pale beer (usually a lager), rather than a dark beer, may be referred to as a light beer. The alcohol content is about the same as in regular beer but the calories are somewhat less. An alcoholic beverage with more than 24 percent alcohol by volume is defined (and taxed) as a distilled spirit.

Need more strategies to boost your fluid intake? Check here for "how-tos":

- Buy the type of milk, including soy milk, that matches your needs—see chapter 11.
- Scout for nutrient-rich drinks when you eat out—see chapter 14.
- Get enough fluids when you're physically active—see chapter 19.
- Know how to fit milk in if you're lactose intolerant—see chapter 21.

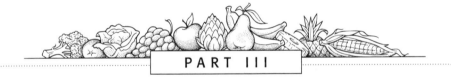

PART III

Smart Eating

The Consumer Marketplace

CHAPTER 9

What's on Today's Table?

From all the foods available for today's table, why do consumers—why do you—choose one food over another? Consumer research says taste is the top reason—followed by nutrition, food safety, price, and convenience!

In the past decade or two there's been a real "change of plate" on the family table. As a consumer, perhaps you've noticed a shift in available food products, or in your own shopping and cooking patterns, lifestyles, and attitudes about food and health. You may be more aware of eating to promote health. Like many others, you may be more adventuresome with food and want more flavor. Or in spite of ever better kitchens and cooking equipment, convenience and speed may be more important to you than before.

The diversity of foods in today's marketplace reflects the diversity of today's consumers. Rather than selling just to the mass market, food producers know the value of "different strokes for different folks." As a result, a variety of foods are produced and marketed to match unique needs: age, health, lifestyle, ethnic or religious background, and economic resources, among others.

Food: What's "in Store" for You?

Frozen skillet meals, bagged salad mixes, or marinated ready-to-cook beef roast for *convenience* . . . almond milk, ostrich tenderloin, blue potatoes, or doughnut-shaped peaches for *something new* . . .

hummus, guava juice, or vegetable curry for *ethnic adventure* . . . multigrain cereal with flaxseed, or juice with added antioxidants for their *health benefits*. You'll find these foods alongside your traditional favorites in today's supermarkets.

When it comes to food choices, consumers in the United States seem to have more variety of food to choose from every year—and more ways to eat healthy. A single supermarket stocks, on average, about fifty thousand different items, including nonfood items. In a typical year, about ten thousand new food products may be introduced in the marketplace. Yet only about 2 percent of all new food products make it past the consumer cut.

When you eat away from home, you may notice that fast-food menus are offering more variety—often more grain, fruit, and vegetable choices, and more broiled, steamed, and stir-fried, not just fried, foods. Many supermarkets sell fully prepared meals. Traditional restaurant menus and recipes for at-home cooking reflect an interest in healthful eating, ethnic cuisine, and a blending (or fusion) of ingredients and cooking styles.

More choices mean more decisions and more for you to know about your food supply.

Healthy Eating Sells!

Packaging promotes foods' health benefits: "lowers cholesterol," "promotes immunity," "builds bones." Nutrition Facts on labels display the calories, nutrient, cholesterol, and fiber content per serving. Signs in many produce departments remind you to eat at least five fruit and vegetable servings daily. You can hardly walk through a supermarket without being exposed to healthful eating messages!

Functional Foods: A New Wave

A new wave of foods is appearing on supermarket shelves: functional foods, perhaps the hottest food trend and the biggest ongoing nutrition news story today. Among the big sellers are green tea drinks and a soy version of almost everything! Traditional favorites such as tomatoes, oranges, oatmeal, yogurt, and tuna also have a new, functional message to share.

The term "functional foods" describes foods and beverages with special health benefits beyond (and in addition to) basic nutrition. A functional food or beverage may enhance your health, protect you from certain diseases, or do both. With functional nutrition, what you *do* eat, not what you *don't* eat, makes the difference!

Currently no legal definition for a functional food exists. Technically, many foods, in one way or another, are functional. That's why it's hard to estimate just how big the business of functional foods truly is. Using the definition here, functional foods account for more than a $20 billion business annually in the United States—a market that's rapidly growing!

Why the interest? Personal health is on the rise, and many people—perhaps even you—want control over their health, especially as healthcare costs go up. An aging population seeks avenues for health protection. Rapid advances in science provide a growing body of credible evidence for functional nutrition, and agricultural and food science technology can produce foods that offer potential functional benefits. In addition, changes in food regulation that began in the mid-1990s allow labels to include health claims and structure/function claims.

What makes foods functional? Food components that do more than nourish you! Consider a few examples:

- Many fruits, vegetables, and grain products have phytonutrients, or plant substances (carotenoids, flavonoids, isoflavones, or indoles, to name a few), that may reduce the risk for certain diseases

including prostate cancer, heart disease, and macular degeneration.

- Strong scientific evidence supports the belief that oats help lower cholesterol levels.

- Prebiotics/probiotics such as fructo-oligosaccharides in shallots and lactobacillus in some dairy foods may improve the balance of "good" intestinal bacteria.

- Fatty fish have fatty acids known as "omega-3s," which may lower your risk for heart disease and improve your mental performance.

- Dairy foods and some meat (beef, lamb) have another fatty acid, conjugated linoleic acid (CLA), which may help lower your risk for cancer.

- Calcium-rich foods such as dairy foods may protect you from high blood pressure and colon cancer.

- Soy protein in many soy-based foods may help lower your cholesterol levels.

In most foods, functional benefits probably come from several—perhaps many—food substances. The heart-healthy benefits of oats come not only from its soluble fiber (beta glucan) but also from its antioxidants, amino acids, and natural plant sterols. Cancer protection from legumes may come from fiber as well as isoflavones, saponins, and protease inhibitors.

Different types. "Tried and true" or "innovative and new," functional foods belong in several categories:

- *Unmodified whole foods* such as oats, carrots, tomatoes, grapes, salmon, and yogurt with active cultures.

- *Modified foods,* including those fortified or enriched with nutrients, or enhanced with phytonutrients or botanicals, such as high-fiber cereals, calcium-fortified orange juice, milk with added vitamins A and D, flour with added folic acid, and beverages with more vitamin E, even cereals with herbal additives.

- *New foods created for functional and other benefits* such as soyburgers, other foods with soy protein, and spreads with plant stanol or sterol esters that help lower blood cholesterol.

- *Foods produced through biotechnology* for functional benefits such as tomatoes with more lycopene, or rice with added beta carotene and iron.

See "Food Biotechnology: The Future Is Today!" later in this chapter.

Fitting functional foods in. Credible research shows that functional foods certainly play a role in wellness when combined with balanced food choices and plenty of physical activity. However, they're not "magic bullets" for health. And functional foods can't make up for a poor approach to eating or an unhealthy lifestyle.

Functional benefits of food—their bioactive components and their physiological action—are full of unknowns. To get their known benefits, as well as those that science may reveal in the future:

● Eat a *variety* of foods with potentially functional benefits, on a *regular basis,* and in *adequate amounts.* To be effective, you need enough over a period of time.

● Choose from all food groups of the Food Guide Pyramid. Foods in each group—plant- and animal-based foods—offer bioactive, potentially beneficial substances.

● For the functional benefits, enjoy food first, rather than supplements. Food has many more functional components that likely work best when eaten together, as nature provided.

● Choose wisely. Foods fortified for functional nutrition may not be the best choice, especially if they weren't naturally healthful to start with.

● Use claims on food labels to find foods that match your needs. *To understand what functional claims mean—and don't mean—see "Health Claims on the Label" and "Structure/Function Claims on the Label" in chapter 11.*

● Enjoy functional foods as part of your personal strategy for better health, not in place of appropriate medical care or medications. Tell your healthcare provider what you're doing.

● Be savvy with what you read about foods promoted with functional benefits. Junk science abounds! Nutrition research that's either misinterpreted or oversimplified often makes headlines. *To help you sort through the information maze see chapter 24, "Well Informed?"*

Functional Nutrition: What's in a Name?

With the advent of functional foods, new terms have entered our vocabulary. Although not legally defined, here's what they generally mean and how they differ.

● *Functional foods:* foods that provide health benefits beyond basic nutrition

● *Phytonutrients:* substances in plant-based foods with physiologically active components that have functional food benefits; also called phytochemicals

● *Prebiotics:* nondigestible food substance that may stimulate the growth and activity of health-promoting, or "good," bacteria in the intestine

● *Probiotics:* live bacteria that may promote health by improving the balance of "good" bacteria in the intestine

● *Synbiotics:* products with both prebiotic and probiotic substances that work together to keep the balance of "good" bacteria in the intestine

● *Zoonutrients:* a term sometimes used for substances, such as omega-3 fatty acids, with physiologically active components, in animal-based foods; also called zoochemicals

For more about phytonutrients, prebiotics and probiotics, and substances in animal-based foods that promote health, see chapter 4.

Nutrient-Modified Foods: "The Haves and the Have-Nots"

In today's supermarket, look for foods positioned for nutrition-conscious consumers. For example, you'll find plenty of "reduced-fat," "more fiber," and "calorie-free" foods. In many cases these newer foods are modified versions of traditional foods—often produced with less fat, saturated fat, cholesterol, sugar, or sodium, or with more fiber or certain vitamins or minerals. Fat-free taco chips and fat-free refried beans, high-fiber cereal, and reduced-sodium soup are some examples.

To create these foods, the food industry adjusts the "recipes." By modifying the nutrients, the qualities of food often change. For example, to cut back on fat, some foods may contain more carbohydrates, such as added sugar. That may change the flavor and the mouth feel of foods you're accustomed to. And formulating foods with less salt often makes them less flavorful, too—unless other flavor-intense ingredients, such as herbs or spices, are added.

How can you fit today's nutrient-modified foods into a healthful eating plan?

● Remember the big picture. Enjoy them as alternative choices in an overall way of eating that's varied, moderate, and balanced. For example, being "fat-free" doesn't mean calorie-free. And "calcium added" juice doesn't make it a substitute for all the nutrients in milk.

● Check the Nutrition Facts on food labels for foods with nutrient content claims. For example, cutting back on fat won't necessarily make a food low in calories. *See "Get All the Facts!" in chapter 11.*

● Count nutrient-modified foods in your eating plan just as you'd count their traditional counterparts. Either way, 1½ ounces of fat-free or of regular Cheddar cheese count as one serving from the Milk, Yogurt, and Cheese Group of the Food Guide Pyramid. *See "The Food Guide Pyramid: Your Healthful Eating Guide" in chapter 10.*

● Look for products with flavor-boosting spices, herbs, and other ingredients—for example, reduced-fat or low-fat sausages with herbs. Extra seasonings boost flavor in products with less fat or sodium.

The Multicultural Palate

With global communications, travel, and food imports, our "world of food" gets bigger, offering more ethnic and regional foods. But not that long ago, bagels, pita bread, pastas of every shape, and tortillas were considered trendy, ethnic foods—and salsa was a new flavor experience! Today these foods and many other ethnic foods are part of the supermarket mainstream.

What sparks interest in and availability of ethnic and regional foods? Perhaps a sense of curiosity and adventure as well as a desire to learn—and the search for nutritious, flavorful alternatives. Celebrity chefs entertain by preparing ethnic foods, even taking us via media to global markets and kitchens. Travel, cooking classes, Web sites, magazines, newspapers, cookbooks, and restaurants expose us to unique flavors: ingredients, seasonings, and dishes. Supermarkets stock their shelves with ethnic and regionally inspired foods, partly to meet the demand from recent immigrants, partly to match flavor trends.

As a result, consumers have more food variety, food combinations, and ways to eat for health and pleasure. Many ethnic and regional cuisines offer health benefits, especially those that focus on grains, vegetables, legumes, and fruits. *For many nutritious, good-tasting dishes in ethnic cuisines, see "Vegetarian Dishes in the Global Kitchen" in chapter 20.*

Our Edible Heritage

The idea of "ethnic food" isn't new. Throughout history, the foods of one culture have traveled to another, infusing cuisines with more variety and new flavors. Those foods also became new sources of nutrients and food energy.

The quest for flavor—exotic Eastern spices—launched the Age of Discovery and the exploration of the New World. Among the discoveries: a vast array of foods! Among other foods, the Americas contributed tomatoes to Italy, potatoes to Ireland, peanuts (or groundnuts) to West Africa, and hot chilies to Thailand. And foods unknown to the Americas five hundred years ago came from all parts of the Old World—for example, chickens, pigs, beef, wheat, oats, barley, okra, Asian rice, peaches, pears, watermelons, citrus fruits, bananas, and lettuce.

American cuisine has strong roots in its native foods: corn, legumes, pumpkins, peanuts, potatoes, tomatoes, peppers, pineapples, squash, wild rice, and turkey, among many others. Each wave of immigrants has contributed its own ethnic cuisine. In time, many ethnic foods were adapted and eventually became "typically American"—for example, pizza, tacos, and chop suey. That wave of "food immigration" continues as new waves of immigrants—mostly Latin Americans, Asians, Eastern Europeans, and Middle Easterners—influence American cuisine today.

Regional specialties develop as people adapt their cooking style to foods that are available. And many foods once eaten as regional specialties become nationally popular—for example, sweet potato pie, cooked collard greens, and black-eyed peas and rice from the South, created by African American cooks; crab cakes and clam chowder on the Atlantic coast; tamales, bean burritos, and cactus salad from the Southwest; and smoked salmon and berry cobblers from the Pacific Northwest.

A Fusion of Flavor

The blending of cuisines, sometimes called "fusion cuisine," is one of today's hot culinary phenomena. It combines the ingredients or cooking techniques of two or more cultures not geographically close together. The result: new cuisines, such as Thai-French, Southwest-Asian, Cuban-French, and unique dishes such as Moroccan couscous topped with Chinese stir-fried vegetables. Even fast-food menus reflect the trend, with Mexican pizza, chili in a pita pocket, or a Thai wrap tucked in a tortilla.

The fusion of ingredients and flavors isn't new. It's been going on for centuries as people gradually adapted their cuisines to the available food supply—sometimes by choice, often by necessity. Interestingly, about 50 percent of foods eaten in the world today originated in the Americas.

Today, fusion cooking brings an explosion of new dishes to the American table. In many cases, new "fused" dishes uniquely combine grain products, fruits, and vegetables. Their combinations may offer nutritional benefits for you. *For ways to "fuse" ingredients in your meals and snacks, see "Ethnic Table: For Variety, Health, and Eating Pleasure!" later in this chapter.*

Simply adding seasonings from an ethnic cuisine also creates fusion: perhaps a touch of curry powder from India blended in pumpkin soup . . . or basil and garlic, borrowed from Italian cooking, added to beef stew. *For more about seasoning combinations, see "Flavor Profile!" in chapter 13.*

What's New Is What's Old, Too

What's new on the table is also what's old. Grandma's meat loaf, mashed potatoes, soup, and biscuits are "dressed" with today's seasonings, such as sun-dried tomatoes, garlic, wasabi, lemon grass, and fresh herbs. Often sold in farmers' markets, heirloom vegetables and fruits—with their unique flavors, colors, shapes, and scents—add more variety to the table. "Heirlooms" are open-pollinated (grown from seed) cultivars grown for at least fifty years. Examples? Flavorful, pinkish-red Brandywine tomatoes (Amish); purple-striped Cherokee Trail of Tears pole beans (Native American); and sweet, lime-green Jenny Lind melons.

Culture on Your Plate

Moroccan or Lebanese, Nuevo Latino or Thai, Indian or Ethiopian, ethnic fare has captured consumer interest. Many people want to go beyond "ethnic" basics—Italian, Chinese, and Mexican—and explore regional ethnic foods: Tuscan, Liguria Roman, Calabrian, and Lazio (Italian); Sichuan, Peking, and Cantonese (Chinese); and Yucatán, Oaxacan, and Michoacan (Mexican). If you're among those who want to go beyond the basics . . .

● Try an ethnic or a regional restaurant; do "tastings" at community ethnic festivals. Order food that's new to you. *For restaurant tips, see "Eating Out Ethnic Style" in chapter 14.* Ethnic foods and other new food combinations often get introduced first in restaurants! If you're cautious, try an appetizer portion.

Take Your Taste Buds to the Mediterranean

There's no single cuisine for regions that border the Mediterranean Sea. The dishes of Greece, southern Italy, Spain, southern France, Tunisia, Lebanon, and Morocco, for example, are all distinctive. Yet they typically contain plenty of grain products, vegetables, legumes, nuts, and fruits; less meat and poultry; more fish; and moderate amounts of wine. Their fat is mostly monounsaturated (from olive oil). And yogurt and cheese offer other sources of animal protein.

Traditional Mediterranean eating may have several health benefits—especially for reducing risks of heart disease, and perhaps for some cancers. Studies show that the death rate from heart disease and the incidence of cancer are lower among many Mediterranean populations. And the incidence of these health problems has gone up among people who no longer eat in their traditional way. The reasons for this are not yet clear to scientists.

In general, the total fat intake of the Mediterranean diet isn't lower than the typical American diet. It's just shifted to more monounsaturated fat. Other dietary factors, not fully understood, may offer some protection.

Before you switch your eating style, be aware that the benefits of the Mediterranean lifestyle may go well beyond food. Traditionally, the people studied in the region were also more physically active. Body weight and genetics are factors, too. And the overall lifestyle was more relaxed.

● Shop from the ethnic food section of your supermarket. Or in an ethnic food store, shop and ask for advice on food preparation.

● Give yourself an ethnic cookbook; check one out from a library. Try a dish with more grains, vegetables, beans, or fruits—perhaps Mediterranean tabouli (bulgur salad) or cucumber-yogurt dip, Japanese

sukiyaki (stir-fried meat and vegetables) with udon noodles, Brazilian black bean soup, or vegetarian curries from India.

● Learn "hands on" about the ingredients, preparation, and flavors of ethnic dishes. Take a cooking class, or go on a culinary vacation.

Your Nutrition Checkup

Food Neophobia: Do You Have It?

Enjoying more variety of fruits, vegetables, and grain products puts more nutrients and phytonutrients on your plate! Measure your sense of food adventure.

1. How would you describe your willingness to try new foods?

I don't experiment.	1
I'll try if offered.	2
I'm a willing adventurer.	3

2. When was the last time you bought an unfamiliar vegetable or fruit at the store?

Last year or longer	1
Last month	2
Last week	3

3. When a new food product hits the market . . .

I'm rarely aware of it.	1
I give it a try after it's been on the market a while.	2
I try it right away—if it matches my needs.	3

4. I try to eat a wide variety of foods.

Never	1
Sometimes	2
Almost always	3

5. I look for new ways to prepare familiar foods . . . perhaps from cookbooks, magazines, newspapers, or from friends.

Never	1
Sometimes	2
All the time	3

6. The variety of foods becoming available due to today's agriculture . . .

Doesn't interest me	1
Mildly interests me	2
Intrigues me	3

7. When was the last time you ate at an ethnic restaurant (other than Italian, Chinese, or Mexican)?

Last year or longer	1
Within the past six months	2
Within the past month	3

8. If preparing an Italian meal, I would make . . .

Spaghetti noodles	1
Spaghetti noodles or some other type of pasta (e.g., whole wheat)	2
Any type of pasta, polenta, or risotto	3

How did you fare? Add up your points.

NOW SCORE YOURSELF

20 to 24: You're probably a "foodie" who enjoys food adventure and flavor. Being a food adventurer adds variety—along with more than forty different nutrients and phytonutrients—for your good health.

13 to 19: You're open to experiencing new foods . . . a healthy attitude toward eating! Be aware that the same food may taste different to different people, perhaps because they have a different number of taste buds. That may be why some people like spicy-hot flavors and others don't.

8 to 12: You're more comfortable with your "tried and true." But does your cautious approach mean missing out on a variety of nutritious foods? Don't be surprised if you don't like a food the first time you taste it. The more often you try a food, the more familiar it gets—and often, the more you like it!

Read on for new foods to add to your plate.

● Be adventuresome with food when you travel, rather than head for familiar fast-food fare.

● Learn from a friend: someone who prepares his or her own family's ethnic dishes.

What's "New"?

Supermarket shelves and restaurant menus feature a broad array of foods that weren't easily available a few short years ago—all offering more ways you can eat for health, flavor, convenience, and enjoyment! Trend watchers say today's table is filled with foods with:

● *More convenience.* You'll find more prepackaged foods—precooked meat and poultry, meal kits, speed scratch meals, and take-out—to help you serve a nutritious "home served" meal in record time.

● *More variety of fruits and vegetables.* With more health-consciousness, produce departments—even the canned and frozen aisles—stock a greater variety of fruits and vegetables year-round, including "exotics" and varietals. For example, an apple isn't just an apple anymore; it may be a Granny Smith, a Rome Beauty, or a Gala!

● *More variety of grains.* Interest in breads has shifted to more coarse-textured, denser, whole-grain breads. Breakfast cereals are made with more whole grains—and not just corn, oats, or wheat. And whole grains of all kinds are used in salads, soups, and mixed dishes. Eat at least three servings of whole grains a day—a choice made easier with so many new whole-grain products to select from.

● *More "fresh."* Even in mixes, you'll find more fresh foods—fresh salad mixes, stew and stir-fry mixes, vegetable snacks, and herbs. Mixes for breadmaking machines let you bake bread without effort. Fresh pasta is sold in refrigerated displays. And the fresh seafood department is more commonplace. Be aware that fresh foods aren't necessarily more nutritious. *See "Fresh vs. Processed: Either Way to Health" later in this chapter.*

● *More function. See "Functional Foods: A New Wave" earlier in this chapter.*

● *More vegetarian entrées.* With growing interest in vegetarian eating, you'll find more meatless, prepared entrées, such as bean burritos or vegetarian lasagna.

There's a greater variety of pasta, vegetables, and legumes (dry, canned, and fresh) for home-cooked vegetarian meals, too. Include legumes—perhaps in vegetarian entrées—in your overall eating plan several times a week.

● *More specialty foods.* With growing food sophistication, more gourmet and unique foods are available, too. But remember, being "gourmet" doesn't make food any better. Read the Nutrition Facts on the food label.

● *More flavor.* The influence of ethnic cuisine, herbs, and other flavor ingredients has put more flavor in canned and packaged foods, recipes, and restaurant foods. Consider the sales of hot sauces!

● *More indulgence.* There's a flip side to the growing array of foods marketed for health. There are now more indulgence foods: richer, higher-fat frozen desserts, bigger portions, and more high-calorie snack foods, among others. If you choose these foods, fit them into a smart strategy without overdoing on calories.

Keep your eyes open for new foods in the marketplace. Of the eighty thousand known edible plants, only about three hundred are cultivated for food! Only twelve are major food staples.

Garden of Eatin': Less Common Vegetables

Looking for new ways to eat "five a day" fruits and vegetables? Starting here, identify all the vegetables that you've never tried before. Then make a point of buying and trying one or two of them the next time you're in a supermarket or restaurant—and get their nutrient and phytonutrient benefits.

● *Arugula (ah-ROO-gu-lah)* is a green, leafy vegetable with a distinctive flavor. It's often used in mixed garden salads. It also may be cooked and tossed with pasta or risotto.

● *Bok choy (BAHK choy) (also called pak choi)* is one variety of Chinese cabbage. It doesn't form a head, but instead has several white, bunched stems with thick green leaves. It can be eaten raw or cooked, and is used often in stir-fry dishes.

● *Breadfruit* looks like a green, bumpy melon (brown when ripe) on the outside, and is creamy white on the inside. Like other starchy vegetables, it's peeled and prepared in many ways: baked, boiled, fried, grilled,

Ethnic Table: For Variety, Health, and Eating Pleasure!

Look for this multicultural array of foods in your supermarket aisles. Then enjoy these quick-to-fix dishes at home.

	Cuisine*	Serving/Preparation Ideas	Nutrient Contribution
Bread, Cereal, Rice, and Pasta			
Couscous (tiny, round pasta)	Moroccan	Serve hot with tomato sauce and Parmesan cheese, or serve cold as a salad with raisins, mandarin oranges, and spices.	Complex carbohydrates, B vitamins
Kasha (buckwheat kernels)	East European	Serve as a hot side dish with chicken or beef. Mix with pasta shapes.	Complex carbohydrates, B vitamins, fiber
Pozole (soup made with fermented corn kernels)	Mexican	Serve warm with diced onion, shredded cabbage, and a lime wedge.	Complex carbohydrates, vitamin C, fiber
Wonton wrappers (thin wheat dough used to wrap spring rolls)	Chinese, Vietnamese	Wrap thin strips of cooked lean barbecued pork or chicken, and shredded cabbage and carrots inside, then steam.	Complex carbohydrates, B vitamins
Vegetable			
Jicama	Mexican	Slice in thin strips and dip into salsa or reduced-fat or fat-free ranch dressing. Use to replace water chestnuts in stir-fry dishes.	Negligible
Collard greens	African American/Southern	Boil greens with chopped, smoked turkey, vinegar, and seasonings.	Beta carotene, fiber
Tomatillos	Mexican	Dice, and boil with jalapeño peppers for salsa. Dice, and combine with onions for an omelette.	Vitamin C, beta carotene, potassium, fiber
Shiitake mushrooms	Japanese	Add raw to salads and sandwiches, or toss in stir-fry dishes.	Negligible
Fruit			
Lychee	Chinese	Serve on top of frozen yogurt.	Vitamin C, potassium
Kumquat	Chinese	Pack a few for snacking, or slice for fruit salad.	Vitamin C, beta carotene, folate
Papaya	Mexican, Central American	Blend with pineapple for tropical juices, dice and add to salsas, or simmer in a chutney recipe.	Vitamin C, beta carotene, potassium
Plantain	Puerto Rican, Central American	Cube, and add to stews and soups.	Potassium, complex carbohydrates
Mango	Caribbean	Slice for fruit salads, or simmer in a chutney recipe.	Vitamin C, beta carotene, potassium

	Cuisine*	Serving/Preparation Ideas	Nutrient Contribution
Meat, Poultry, Fish, Dry Beans, Eggs, and Nuts			
Squid	Mediterranean, Asian	Slice in rings, and broil. Serve with marinara sauce. Or cook in stir-fry dishes.	Protein, iron, B vitamins
Veal, lamb	Mediterranean	Marinate in Italian vinaigrette, then grill.	Protein, iron, B vitamins
Hummus (mashed chick-peas)	Middle Eastern	Serve as a dip for raw vegetables or pita triangles.	Protein, B vitamins, fiber
Chorizo (sausage)	Mexican	Slice in bite-size pieces, add to omelettes or stews.	Protein, iron, B vitamins
Tofu	Japanese	Slice for stir-fry dishes, or dice for salads or soups.	Protein, calcium
Black beans	Latin American	Use in place of red beans in chili or soup, mash for homemade refried beans, or mix with rice.	Protein, B vitamins, fiber
Milk, Yogurt, and Cheese			
Plain yogurt	Middle Eastern	Top falafel sandwiches (chickpea- and vegetable-stuffed pita). Blend with mint as a dip or dressing for cucumbers.	Protein, calcium, riboflavin
Goat milk	Middle Eastern, African (some areas)	Drink goat milk plain. Make a thick drink by mixing with juice. Use it in place of cow milk in baking.	Protein, calcium, riboflavin
Ricotta cheese	Italian	Use in lasagna, or stuffed jumbo pasta shells.	Calcium, protein, riboflavin
Queso blanco (white cheese)	Mexican	Shred, and melt over enchiladas and quesadillas.	Calcium, protein, riboflavin

*Although these foods are identified with these cuisines, they may be used in the dishes of cuisines of other parts of the world as well.

Source: American Dietetic Association.

or cooked with stew and soup. Its flavor is somewhat sweet, yet mild. Some dishes from the Caribbean are made with breadfruit.

● *Cactus pads (nopales, or noh-PAH-lays),* which are cactus leaves, are used in a variety of Mexican and Southwest dishes. Their thorns are removed before cooking them. Then they're usually sliced, then simmered or cooked in a microwave oven. You also can buy canned nopales.

● *Cassava (kah-SAH-vah) (manioc, or MA-nee-ahk; yuca, or YOO-kah, root),* a starchy root vegetable, has a thick, brown peel, but inside it's white or yellow like a potato. It's often cooked in dishes similar to the way potatoes are used.

● *Celeriac (seh-LER-ee-ak),* a member of the celery family, is enjoyed for its root, not its stalks. It has a fibrous, brown, bumpy peel . . . and a sweet, celery flavor inside. Once peeled, it can be enjoyed raw, perhaps in salads, or cooked—boiled, steamed, or fried. Use it in soups or stews, too, perhaps in place of celery.

● *Chard,* actually a white-rooted beet, is grown for its leaves, and creamy-white or red stalks. With its mild yet distinctive flavor, it's used in food preparation much like spinach.

● *Chayote (cheye-OH-tay)* is a pale-green, pear-shaped vegetable with a mild flavor. Baked, boiled, braised, or stuffed, it complements the flavors of other ingredients and flavorings in mixed dishes. It can be used like squash.

● *Chicory (curly endive)* has a frizzy green leaf in a loose head of greens. Its bitter flavor adds a nice touch to salads—in small amounts.

● *Daikon (DEYE-kuhn)* is a Japanese radish that looks like a smooth, white parsnip. It has a stronger, more bitter flavor than a red radish. Often it's used to make sushi (fish rolled with rice in seaweed) and in vegetable carvings.

● *Dasheen (dah-SHEEN)* is a large, round root vegetable with a coarse, brown peel that's similar to taro. Usually prepared either boiled or baked, dasheen is starchy, somewhat like a potato.

● *Escarole (EHS-kah-role)* is a somewhat bitter-tasting salad green. Sometimes its green leaves have a reddish tinge. Unlike iceberg lettuce, it forms a loose head.

● *Fennel* looks somewhat like a squat bunch of celery with feathery leaves. Its flavor is distinctive, like a sweet, delicate anise. The bulb and stalks are often braised, steamed, sautéed, or used in soups. The feathery leaves may be used in salads, as a herb, or as an attractive garnish.

● *Jerusalem artichoke*—native to North America—has nothing in common with a globe artichoke, except for its name. Like a potato, it's a tuber, grown under the ground. But it is knobby and irregularly shaped, with a sweet flavor and a light brown or purplish-red peel. It's often cooked in its peel, but a little lemon juice in the cooking water keeps peeled Jerusalem artichokes from browning. Use them in dishes that call for potatoes, or eat them raw.

● *Jicama (HEE-kah-mah),* another root vegetable, is crisp and slightly sweet. It's often peeled, sliced, and eaten raw, perhaps in salads. Or it's cooked in stews and stir-fried dishes.

● *Kale* is a leafy vegetable that belongs to the cabbage family, but it doesn't form a head. It has a curly, purple-tinged, green leaf. Use it in salads and in ways that you would cook spinach.

● *Kelp* is brown seaweed, often used in Japanese cooking and wrapped around sushi.

● *Kohlrabi (KOLE-rah-bee),* a member of the cabbage family, looks and tastes somewhat like a turnip.

It's light green in color. It can be used in recipes that call for turnips, or sliced and used in stir-fry dishes, or peeled and eaten raw or in salads.

● *Leeks* are onions and look like a bigger, sturdier, flat-leaved version of green onions. Both the bulbs and the leaves are eaten. Bulbs usually are sliced and steamed in soups or baked in casseroles. The leaves are often used in salads. They need to be cleaned well to remove soil that gets between the leaves.

● *Lotus root,* which is the root of the water lily, often is peeled, sliced, then cooked—stir-fried, steamed, or braised, with mixed Chinese dishes. It has the texture of a potato and a flavor more similar to fresh coconut.

● *Plantain* actually belongs to the banana family, but it's longer and thicker, starchier, and less sweet. For that reason it's eaten as a vegetable—always cooked. It can be eaten at any of its three stages: green, yellow, or black, but it's sweetest when it's black. Plantains are cooked in or out of the peel. They may be baked, boiled, or fried, and often are mixed in stews.

● *Radicchio (rah-DEE-chee-oh)* is a small, purplish head of leaves with white ribs. It's somewhat bitter in flavor, and adds a nice touch to salads, or even to pasta and stir-fry dishes.

● *Rutabaga (ROO-tuh-bay-guh)* is another root vegetable, with a turniplike flavor and appearance. Use it in any recipe that calls for turnips—stews, soups, and casseroles, for example.

● *Seaphire* is a halophyte, or saltwater crop. With an asparagus-grass look, seaphire is crisp, crunchy, and salty. Since it's high in sodium, enjoy it in small amounts as a flavoring in salads, stir-fries, and vegetable dishes, especially if you're sodium-sensitive. Three ounces have 1,350 milligrams of sodium.

● *Seaweed,* used most often in Asian dishes and some Irish, Welsh, and Scottish dishes, includes a variety of types. Kelp may be the most commonly used in the United States. Another seaweed used in many Japanese dishes is nori (NOH-ree).

● *Taro (TAIR-oh)* is a rough, brown or purplish tuber vegetable that looks much like a yam, although some varieties look different. It has edible leaves, which are called callaloo in the Caribbean. Taro is peeled and usually boiled, baked, or fried, much like potatoes. Hawaiian poi is made from taro.

● *Tomatillo (tohm-ah-TEE-oh),* a member of the tomato family, has a paperlike husk. Under the husk it looks like a small green tomato. It's often used in food like a green tomato, although the flavor is more citruslike. It is often used in Southwest and Mexican dishes, including salsa and salads.

Fresh Ideas: Uncommon Fruit

Rather than reaching for fruit you know already, try something new! Many fruits aren't well known in the United States because they grow in tropical or subtropical areas. Fortunately, today's transportation systems are increasing the variety of fruits available from near and far—at all times of the year. Look for these or other unusual fruits in the produce department of your store, in the canned food aisle of your supermarket, or in Asian and Hispanic food stores.

Red bananas, amnazano bananas, apple bananas, plantains—not just yellow bananas! To help make "five a day" an adventure, try different varietals of common fruits, too—perhaps apples, bananas, oranges, plums, and pears—for their unique flavors, textures, and perhaps cooking qualities.

● *African horned melon,* also known as Kiwano, is unique in appearance: spiked, oblong shape, golden-orange color, with juicy green fruit inside that tastes like cucumber, banana, and lime.

● *Asian pear* looks like a yellow apple—and has a similar firm, crunchy texture. It's sweet and juicy and nice to eat as a whole fruit or mixed in salads.

● *Atemoya (a-teh-MOH-ee-yah)* is a cross between two fruits: cherimoya and sweetsop. With a green skin, it has a petal-like look. Inside, the cream-colored, custardlike pulp is studded with large black seeds and offers a mango-vanilla flavor.

● *Blood orange* is a tart, yet sweet orange with flesh that's either bright red or white with red streaks.

● *Cherimoya (chair-ih-MOY-ah) (custard apple)* has a custardlike consistency and flavor. On the outside it looks like a little green pineapple without the leaves. The inside has little black seeds. Its flavor can be compared to a mixture of other fruit flavors: strawberry, banana, pineapple, and mango. It's best to eat it as whole fruit; just cut it in half, remove the seeds, and scoop out the fruit.

● *Feijoa (fay-YOH-ah, or fay-JOH-ah)* looks like a kiwifruit without fuzz. Inside its cream-colored flesh is sweet, fragrant, and pearl-like. To eat it, remove the skin, which may be bitter, cut it in half, and scoop out the fruit. It's a great recipe substitute for apples or bananas.

● *Guava (GWAH-vah) (guayaba, or gwey-AH-bah)* is a sweet, fragrant fruit that's about the size of a lemon. Its peel varies in color from yellow to purple, and the fruit inside may be yellow, pink, or red. Eat guavas as whole fruit, or in sauces, salads, juices, frozen desserts, and jams.

● *Kumquat (KUHM-kwaht),* a member of the citrus family, looks like a small, olive-shaped orange. Because the peel is very thin, a kumquat is eaten with the peel on—either uncooked or cooked with meat, poultry, or fish. When sliced, it's nice as a garnish or in salads.

● *Longan (LONG-uhn)* is a small, round, cherry-sized fruit with a thick, nonedible brown shell. Inside, the white, juicy fruit, which surrounds a large black seed, is fragrant and sweet.

● *Loquat (LOH-kwaht),* a small, pear-shaped fruit, is light orange in color on the inside and the outside. Somewhat tart, it has a pit, which must be removed. Loquats are eaten whole, and often prepared in salads or in cooked poultry dishes.

● *Lychee (LEE-chee) (litchi),* a fruit that's just 1 or 2 inches in diameter and has a pink to red shell. Inside, the fruit is white and sweet with a consistency like a grape. Its seed isn't edible. Lychees make a nice snack or a dessert just as they are.

● *Mango,* a sweet-tart and juicy fruit, ranges in size and shape. It can be about 6 ounces to 5 pounds, and it may be round or long. Its inedible peel is orange when ripe, with orange fruit inside and a large seed. The best way to eat a mango is to either peel back the skin and eat it with a spoon . . . or remove both peel and seed and cut into pieces. Mangoes are eaten in fruit salads and may be prepared with cooked meat, poultry, rice, or grain dishes.

● *Mangosteen (MAN-goh-steen),* small in size, has leathery brown skin that cannot be eaten. Inside, the soft, white, juicy fruit divides into segments. This fruit is often hard to find.

● *Papaya (pah-PEYE-ah) (pawpaw)* may weigh from 1 to 20 pounds in an elongated, oval shape. Its inedible peel is yellow or orange, with an orange fruit inside and many black seeds. It has a tart, sweet flavor that is delicious as is or mixed in salads.

● *Passion fruit (granadilla, or gra-nah-DEE-yah)* is a small, spherical fruit with a leathery peel, which may appear shriveled. It has a perfumelike, sweet-tart flavor. The color varies from light yellow to reddish-purple. It may be eaten as a whole fruit or added to salads, sauces, desserts, or beverages.

● *Pepino (puh-PEE-noh),* ranging in size from a plum to a papaya, is a fragrant fruit with a smooth, golden skin that's streaked with purple. Inside, the yellow flesh is juicy sweet. Enjoy a peeled pepino whole, or cut for salads or garnishes.

● *Persimmon (puhr-SIHM-uhn)* looks somewhat like an orange-red tomato with a pointy end. If it's ripe, it's sweet. If not, a persimmon is mouth-puckering, bitter, and sour. It may be eaten as whole fruit or used in desserts and baked foods.

● *Pomegranate (PAH-meh-gran-uht)* is unlike any other fruit. It has a red, leatherlike peel; inside, membranes hold clusters of small, edible seeds with juicy red fruit around the seeds. The flavor is both tart and sweet. Pomegranate seeds are often used in salads and in many cooked dishes.

● *Pomelo (pom-EH-loh),* a huge citrus fruit, can be as big as a watermelon! But it's more commonly the size of a cantaloupe. In many ways it looks and tastes like a grapefruit, but the sections are not as juicy.

● *Prickly pear (cactus pear),* which is yellow-green to deep yellow, is the fruit of the cactus plant. It has a sweet, mild flavor. It should be peeled and seeded before eating. It may have small hairs or needles in the peel that can be uncomfortable if they get into your skin. The fruit itself is eaten fresh or used in salads, sauces, and other dishes.

● *Sapodilla (sah-poh-DEE-yah)* is a small, egg-shaped fruit that has a rough, brown peel. Only the creamy pulp inside is edible—when it's ripe. The flavor is mild, much like vanilla custard.

● *Starfruit (carambola, or kar-am-BOH-lah),* with its unique shape, forms stars when the fruit is sliced. The flavor varies from sweet to tart. It can be eaten as fresh fruit, in salads, or as a garnish.

● *Tamarillo (tam-uh-RIH-yoh),* with its tough but thin peel, is about the size and shape of a small egg. Because it's so tart, it is often sweetened with sugar. Often it is used in baked or cooked foods.

● *Ugli (UH-glee)* fruit is a cross between a tangerine and a grapefruit. It's sectioned on the inside but looks like a small grapefruit on the outside.

● *Zapote (zah-POH-tay) (white sapote)* is a sweet, yellowish fruit about the size of an orange.

Today's Grains

Looking for a creative, even exotic, way to eat more grains? Most of today's "new" grains are really as old as the hills. Although unfamiliar to many in the United States, some are staple foods that nourish millions of people around the world.

Today's grains are full of health benefits. Whole grains are good fiber sources that help to protect against cancer and heart disease, but also constipation, diabetes, and diverticular disease, along with other phytonutrients; they also supply B vitamins (including folate), vitamin E, and trace minerals such as copper and zinc. Refined grains are enriched with vitamins and minerals. What's more, all grains are rich in

Have You Ever Wondered ?

. . . if couscous is a grain? Actually, it's not. Instead, couscous is a form of pasta. Traditionally, couscous (made from ground millet) has been the pasta of northern Africa. In the United States it's made from ground semolina wheat and often used in salads, mixed with fruit, and used in other grain dishes. Because it's made from wheat, it's a good source of B vitamins. Look for whole-wheat couscous, too.

. . . what Quorn is? It's a mycoprotein, or a plant-based protein derived from the mushroom family. Sold in Europe for nearly two decades and now in the United States, this meat alternative is marketed as burgers, sausages, cold cuts, and other meat substitutes. Quorn supplies protein and fiber, with less fat and saturated fat than meat.

complex carbohydrates and low in fat. The fat they supply is mostly unsaturated—a heart health benefit. Seeds such as amaranth and wild rice are high in protein and often are used as grain substitutes.

Some grains and seeds are used mainly in distinctive ethnic dishes, and most also are used creatively in nutritious dishes that blend foods of two or more cultures.

● *Amaranth (AM-ah-ranth),* a seed rather than a true grain, is a protein-rich food. The seeds may be used as a cereal grain.

● *Arborio (ar-BOH-ree-oh)* rice, a plump medium- or long-grain rice, absorbs a lot of liquid. The result is a creamy-textured rice. Often it's used to make Italian risotto, a rice-based dish; the rice usually is cooked in broth.

● *Barley,* sold pearled (polished) and hulled, makes a hearty addition to stews, soups, salads, and casseroles. In its hulled form it offers more nutrients. Look for barley grits and barley flakes, too.

● *Basmati (bahz-MAH-tee)* rice, a long-grained aromatic rice, has a distinctive nutlike, fruity flavor. It's often used in Asian and Middle Eastern recipes—and in salads—because it's light and fluffy. Basmati rice may be polished or brown (whole-grain) rice.

● *Brown rice* is the whole grain of rice with only the inedible outer husk removed. Unlike refined white rice, brown rice still contains the bran, germ, and endosperm parts of the grain. *For more about whole grains and their nutrient content see "What Is a Whole Grain?" in chapter 6.* Any variety of rice—long-, medium-, or short-grain—can be brown rice.

● *Buckwheat,* which is a seed, not a grain, often is prepared like rice. The crushed, hulled kernels, called buckwheat groats, most commonly are used in dishes of Russian origin, such as kasha.

● *Bulgur,* whole wheat kernels that have been parboiled, dried, and crushed, has a variety of textures—from coarse to fine. It has a soft but chewy texture that's nice in many grain-based dishes such as pilaf and tabouli. Try adding it to bread dough, too. Bulgur isn't quite the same as cracked wheat.

● *Glutinous rice,* either black or white, is very sticky because it's high in starch, making it easier to pick up with chopsticks. The grain is either short- or medium-

grain. This is the type of rice typically served in Japanese and Chinese restaurants.

● *Hominy (HAH-mih-nee)* is the dried corn kernel with the hull removed. It's usually soaked in liquid to soften, then cooked, often in stews, casseroles, or other mixed dishes. *Note:* Although we eat corn as a vegetable, it's really a whole grain.

● *Jasmine (JAZ-mihn) rice,* another aromatic rice, is used in many Asian dishes. But it's equally nice whenever a subtle "sweet" side dish is called for, perhaps with pork or fruit-glazed poultry. A polished rice, it's often sold in specialty stores.

● *Kamut (kah-MOOT),* a high-protein wheat, has a nutty flavor. Its contribution of other nutrients is higher than traditional wheat as well.

● *Millet,* a small, round, yellow grain, is a staple grain in many parts of the world, including Europe, Asia, and northern Africa. It's less commonly used as food in the United States. Mild in flavor, millet cooks fast. It's used for mixed dishes such as pilaf or casseroles; for cooked cereal; and, when ground into flour, for bread such as roti from India.

● *Pearl barley* is an ancient, hardy grain used throughout the world. Pearl barley, with the bran removed, is the more polished and most common form of barley; the vitamins and minerals lost in processing are added back. Whole-grain barley is sold, too. Barley typically is served in soups.

● *Quinoa (KEEN-wah),* a grain native to South America, cooks much like rice but faster. Nutritionally it stands out because it's higher in protein than other grains, and it's a good source of iron and magnesium. The grain itself is small, ivory in color, and bead-shaped. With its bland flavor, quinoa can be used in soups, salads, and casseroles, and in any dishes that call for rice.

● *Texmati rice* (sometimes called popcorn rice), from Texas, is a cross between American long-grain rice and basmati rice. Less fragrant than basmati rice, it's a good all-purpose aromatic rice.

● *Triticale (trih-tih-KAY-lee)* is a modern grain, developed as a hybrid of both rye and wheat. The result: a nutty-flavored grain with more protein and less gluten than wheat alone. Cooked as a whole berry (not as flour), it is used in hearty grain-based salads, casseroles, and other grain dishes. Look for flaked and cracked varieties, too, which can be added to bread dough.

● *Waxy rice,* or sweet rice or sticky rice—either opaque white or deep, dark purple—is moist and very sticky when it's cooked. The purple variety has a subtle fruity flavor.

● *Wehani rice,* a basmati rice, is sold with the bran intact. When cooked it looks like wild rice.

● *Wheat berries* are whole grains that haven't been processed. They're often cooked and used in grain-based dishes. Cracked wheat isn't bulgur but instead is wheat berries that have been crushed. Also look for rye berries in specialty stores.

● *Wild rice* isn't a grain, but the seed of a water grass. With its nutlike flavor, it's often used in place of grains, or perhaps mixed with them. As a seed it's higher in protein and a good fiber source.

To learn how to prepare these grains, see "Cooking Grain by Grain" in chapter 13.

Need more strategies to enjoy the food variety from today's marketplace? Check here for "how-tos":

● Use label claims to get clued in to foods' functional and nutrient benefits—see chapter 11.

● Know how to fit all kinds of foods—including less common fruits, veggies, and grain products—into your eat-smart plan—see chapter 11.

● Add more food variety, perhaps functional ingredients, in your food "prep"—see chapter 13.

● Be more adventurous with food when you eat out—see chapter 14.

Ensuring Your Food Supply

The United States' food supply offers a safe, plentiful variety of food—anywhere, at any time of year. Compared with other nations, eating in the United States costs less: about 10 percent of our income, compared with 14 percent in Europe, 21 percent in Japan, and 48 percent in China! Even though food safety remains a consumer concern, strict regulations safeguard the U.S. food supply and minimize potential health risks.

Modern methods of agriculture, food processing, biotechnology, and transportation systems work together to put food on your table. In fact, the average U.S. farmer feeds you plus 127 other people here and in other nations; just 70 years ago, 1 farmer fed only 20 people. Despite that bounty, hunger still is a serious problem in the United States and certainly throughout the world.

Processing—Making Food Available

Throughout much of recorded history, people have processed foods to make them edible and to preserve them for times of scarcity. At opposite sides of the world ten thousand years ago, both Native Americans and ancient Egyptians ground grain into meal. In Europe and other parts of the world eight thousand years ago, foods were smoked and dried. In the Middle East, cheesemaking developed forty-five hundred years ago as a way to store milk. And about twenty-five hundred years ago, Europeans mastered skills needed to salt foods for preservation.

Modern processing methods began in the 1800s with canning, giving perishable food a longer shelf life. People finally could eat a variety of fruits and vegetables throughout the year. During the nineteenth century, pasteurization—a process of heating milk or other liquids to kill disease-causing bacteria—was developed. Today foods are still pasteurized, or perhaps ultrapasteurized at higher temperatures, to keep food safe and extend shelf life. Early-twentieth-century technology launched frozen foods. Later, lightweight, freeze-dried foods were developed for the space program; today backpackers and cyclists use them, too.

What are today's newer contributions to food processing? Many relate to health—for example, adding substances for their functional qualities . . . adding fat replacers and calorie-free sweeteners to cut back on fat and added sugars . . . and irradiating food for improved food safety.

Have You Ever Wondered

. . . why boxed fluid milk is sold on the grocery shelf, not the dairy case? Aseptic packaging, a relatively new food processing method in the United States, allows fluid milk to be stored on the shelf at room temperature for up to a year without preservatives. Sterilization is the key to preventing spoilage. Food is first heated quickly (three to fifteen seconds) to ultrahigh temperatures to kill bacteria. Then it's packaged in a sterilized container, such as a box, within a sterile surrounding. This process of flash heating minimizes loss of nutrients, texture, color, and flavor—and extends shelf life. Besides milk, look for many other grocery items sold in aseptic packaging—for example, soup, tofu, liquid eggs, tomatoes, soy drinks, juice and juice drinks, syrup, nondairy creamers, and wine. In the future, you'll find even more!

Fresh vs. Processed: Either Way to Health

The flavor of fresh produce is hard to beat: freshly picked, handled properly, and eaten right away! For convenience, their canned and frozen counterparts offer another option. Research shows that canned and frozen ingredients are as nutritious as fresh—sometimes even more so.

The moment you pick a fruit or a vegetable, or catch a fish, or milk a cow, food starts to change in texture, taste, perhaps color, and nutrient content. That's why food producers usually process food as fast as possible, while nutrient content and overall quality are at their peak. Immediate processing helps lock these qualities into food. For example, in canneries on board many fishing vessels, seafood is processed as it's brought in. Tomatoes are canned just yards away from the fields.

As long as processed foods are handled properly—from the food manufacturer to the supermarket to your home—there's little nutrient loss. Freezing, drying, and canning retain the nutritional quality of foods.

A processing method called fortification increases the nutritional value of food by adding nutrients, such as vitamins or minerals, not present naturally. Milk, for example, is fortified with vitamin D, which helps the body handle calcium for bone-building; grain

products are fortified with folic acid to reduce risk for birth detects. The nutritional quality of fresh fruit and vegetables depends on the care they receive after harvest. Handled improperly or stored too long, they may not be quite as nutritious as their canned or frozen counterparts.

Whether food is fresh or processed, it's up to you to minimize nutrient loss in your kitchen. Store, prepare, and handle all foods with care. *See "Food 'Prep': The Nutrition-Flavor Connection" in chapter 13.*

Irradiated Foods: Safe to Eat?

Like canning and freezing, irradiation is a food processing method that enhances an already safe food supply. It extends the freshness of food, helping to retain its quality and safety longer.

Since it uses no heat, yet destroys disease-causing bacteria, irradiation is called "cold pasteurization." Poultry and beef are irradiated to destroy pathogens that are especially harmful to children, the elderly, and people with weak immune systems. That includes *Escherichia coli 0157:H7, Salmonella,* and *Campylobacter.* Irradiation also slows ripening and retards sprouting—for example, in potatoes.

Irradiation destroys bacteria, mold, fungi, and insects by passing food through a field of radiant energy, much like sunlight passes through a window or like microwaves pass through food. It leaves no residue. A small number of new compounds are formed when food is irradiated, just as new compounds are formed when food is exposed to heat. These changes are the same as those caused by cooking, steaming, roasting, pasteurization, freezing, and other food preparation.

Irradiated foods generally retain their nutrient value. Like freezing, canning, drying, and pasteurization, irradiation results in minimal nutrient loss. The amount lost is often too insignificant to measure. Irradiation can't take the place of good food handling practices—nor improve the quality of food. As a consumer, you still need to store, prepare, and cook food in clean, safe ways to avoid foodborne illness.

Besides food safety, what are some other advantages of irradiation? Agricultural losses caused by insects, parasites, or spoilage can be cut dramatically. Foods that stay fresh longer can mean less food waste in your kitchen. Like other processing methods, irradiation is regulated and approved by the U.S. Food and Drug Administration (FDA). The level of radiant energy used in the United States is the most restrictive in the world—just enough to kill pathogens, yet pose no health risk.

By law, whole foods that have been irradiated must be labeled on the package. Look for the symbol and the phrase "Treated by Irradiation" or "Treated with Radiation." Irradiated ingredients in prepared, deli, or restaurant foods usually aren't labeled.

As a way to control foodborne illness, irradiation—studied for safety by the FDA for forty years—was approved in 1997 by the FDA for fresh and frozen meats, including beef, pork, lamb, and poultry. The process protects these foods from contamination by *Escherichia coli 0157:H7* and *Salmonella,* but doesn't compromise the nutritional quality of meat. *For more about foodborne illness, see chapter 12.* Irradiation also is used for vegetables, fruit, wheat flour, and spices. Research continues to evaluate irradiation as part of the overall system of ensuring food safety.

Additives: Safe at the Plate

Do you ever consider that most peanut butters don't separate? That products made from prepared baking mixes rise in the oven? That ice cream is smooth and creamy? And that breakfast cereal has been fortified with many vitamins you need for health? Probably not. Most likely you take many desirable qualities of food for granted. Even if you do, you may not attribute these qualities to food additives. Food additives are any substances added to food for specific purposes such as these.

Adding substances to food for preservation, flavor, or appearance is a centuries-old practice. Before refrigeration, salt preserved meat, fish, and poultry; vegetables were pickled in vinegar; and sugar was added to cut fruit to prevent spoilage. Ancient Egyptians used food colorings, and Romans used sulfites to help preserve wine. The spice trade among Asia, the Middle East, and Europe flourished because the pub-

Canned Food: Uncanny Safety and Nutrition Inside

Quick and convenient: more than fifteen hundred varieties of canned foods appear on today's supermarket shelves: traditional fare, along with a variety of nutritionally positioned products—for example, sodium-free, low-fat, no-added-sugar, and others. What are some benefits of canned foods?

- *Long shelf life.* Canned fruits and vegetables are preservative-free; the canning process (high temperatures and sterile containers) destroys organisms that would cause spoilage. Canned food remains safe as long as the container remains intact. Although most canned foods are coded with "use by" dates, you're wise to rotate them. Change your supply of canned products at least every other year.

- *Nutritious.* Canned foods—and dishes made with canned ingredients—are as nutritious as fresh, according to research, and perhaps more so, if fresh aren't handled properly. For lycopene (a carotenoid that protects against prostate cancer), canned tomatoes are better than fresh!

- *Tamper resistance.* Cans are very tamper-resistant. Any opening of the package is clearly evident. Rust spots on the outer surface or dents don't affect the contents of the can as long as the can doesn't bulge or leak.

- *Food safety.* Food is heated to destroy bacteria and then sealed in cans within hours of harvesting. Washing, peeling, and other steps in the canning process remove almost any pesticide residues left on unprocessed foods. For maximum flavor and nutritional value from canned foods, use the product immediately after opening it. Handle any leftover as a perishable food—stored in the refrigerator to retain taste and nutritional quality.

lic demanded the flavors that spices added to food.

Today about three thousand substances are used as food additives, *intentionally* added for certain functions. Many are common household ingredients: sugar, salt, and corn syrup. Very small amounts of other substances—called incidental additives—also may pass *unintentionally* into food during production, processing, distribution, or storage. One example is the small amount of packaging material that may come from the food container. Both intentional and incidental additives are subject to government safety regulations.

What do they do? Additives help foods retain their original qualities, which might otherwise change through temperature changes, storage, oxidation, and contact with microbes. The benefits include nutritional value, freshness and safety, food preparation and processing, and flavor appeal. Many additives offer qualities that you've probably come to expect. All additives are listed by name in the ingredient lists on food labels.

For Added Nutrition

Vitamins, minerals, or fiber are added to almost every category of processed foods to maintain or to improve their nutrition and health-promoting qualities. Until the past seventy-five years or so, nutritional deficiency diseases such as goiter, rickets, scurvy, and pellagra were relatively common. Adding nutrients to food has almost eliminated most nutrient deficiencies. Today nutrients are added to help protect against other health problems, too.

● *Enrichment:* replacing nutrients that are lost in processing. "Enriched" means that nutrients are added back to foods. Bread, flour, and rice, for example, are all enriched with B vitamins and iron.

● *Fortification:* adding nutrients and food substances not present before processing: for example, iodine in salt, vitamins A and D in milk and some soy milk, folic

acid in most grain products, calcium in some fruit juices, and fiber in breakfast cereal. Fortification adds nutrients often lacking in a typical eating pattern; for example, fortifying salt with iodine in the United States has eliminated goiter as a public health problem. Today fortification also enhances food's functional qualities.

What nutrients and food substances are added? Check the food label to find out. Any nutrient added to food shows up in two places on a food label: (1) the ingredient list, where the additive (nutrient) is listed, and (2) nutrition information on the Nutrition Facts panel, telling the total amount of that nutrient in a single serving of that food. *If it's a vitamin, mineral, or fiber, it's listed as % Daily Value. See "Get All the Facts!" in chapter 11.*

For Freshness and Safety . . .

Air, bacteria, fungi, mold, and yeast all promote food spoilage. Some additives, called preservatives, slow the process of spoilage and help maintain the appeal and wholesome qualities of food. You've likely heard of antioxidants. Some preservatives work as antioxidants, protecting food from chemical changes caused by contact with oxygen. Others are antimicrobials that inhibit the growth of mold, bacteria, and yeast. Some foods contain both.

● *Tocopherols (vitamin E), BHA, and BHT* help delay or prevent vegetable oils and salad dressing from becoming rancid. Working as antioxidants, they help protect nutrients that are naturally present in foods: essential fatty acids (linoleic and linolenic acids) and fat-soluble vitamins (A, D, E, and K). Studies have verified the safety of BHA and BHT listed as GRAS ("generally recognized as safe") substances.

● *Citric acid,* a natural component of citrus fruits, also works as an antioxidant, helping food keep its color. When you sprinkle sliced apples with lemon juice, you're doing the same thing—keeping fruit from turning brown. Ascorbic acid (vitamin C) does this, too.

● *Sulfites* help prevent color and flavor changes in dried fruits and vegetables. They're used to inhibit bacterial growth in wine and other fermented products. Some baked foods, snack foods, and condiments

Have You Ever Wondered

. . . if a breakfast cereal fortified with 100% Daily Value for nutrients is always your best choice? It's certainly one choice. But you may not need "100%" if you're already getting enough variety and balance in your day's food choices. Breakfast cereals fortified at a lower level may offer enough nutrition for you.

. . . if there's a difference between "natural" and "artificial" additives? Not when it comes to safety. Foods themselves are used to make some additives, such as soybeans and corn to make lecithin for product consistency, or beets to make food coloring. Others are man-made because they can be produced with greater purity, consistent quality, and perhaps more economically.

also may contain sulfites. Most people have no adverse reactions to sulfites. But packaged and processed foods containing sulfites are labeled for the small percentage of the population who are sulfite-sensitive. *For more on sulfites, see "For the Sulfite-Sensitive . . ." in chapter 21.*

● *Calcium propionate,* produced naturally in Swiss cheese, is a preservative that keeps bread and other baked foods from getting moldy too quickly.

● *Sodium nitrite,* used as a preservative in processed meats such as ham, hot dogs, and lunch meat, keeps the meat safe from botulism bacteria. It also adds to the flavor and pink color. *For more on botulism, see "Bacteria: Hard Hitters" in chapter 12.*

What foods have additives for freshness?

● *Antimicrobials* (to prevent spoilage from mold, bacteria, and yeast) . . . in baked foods, beverages, bread, cheese, cured meats, fruit juice, fruit products, margarine, pie filling, table syrup, and wine, among others.

● *Antioxidants* (to prevent rancidity or discoloration) . . . in baked goods, cereals, fats, oils, processed foods, salad dressings, and high-fat foods such as chips and doughnuts, among others.

For Food Preparation or Processing . . .

From helping bread rise . . . to keeping chocolate suspended in chocolate milk . . . to keeping seasoning blends from clumping, food additives fulfill a wide variety of tasks in food production. Without them, food manufacturers couldn't achieve many food qualities that consumers want.

● *Anticaking agents* keep seasonings, baking powder, confectioners' sugar, table salt, and other powdered or granular products flowing freely. Because they keep food from absorbing moisture, it won't lump together. Calcium silicate and silicon dioxide are two anticaking agents.

● *Emulsifiers* are mixers that keep ingredients and flavorings blended by holding fat on one end and water on the other end of their chemical structure. For example, they're used to keep the oil, vinegar, and seasonings in salad dressings from separating. In peanut butter, emulsifiers keep the peanuts and the oil from separating. Even in baked foods, they help keep the

dough uniform. Some emulsifiers come from food itself: for example, lecithin (from soybeans, milk, and egg yolks), alginates (salts from algae), and mono- and di-glycerides (from vegetables and beef tallow).

● *Humectants* such as glycerine or sorbitol, help foods keep their moisture and soft texture. Shredded coconut stays moist and marshmallows stay soft because a humectant is added.

● *Leavening agents* help create the light texture of waffles, bread, muffins, and other baked goods. Baking sodium (sodium bicarbonate) and baking powder (sodium bicarbonate and acid salts), as well as yeast, produce carbon dioxide that makes dough rise. Without them, the texture would be compact and heavy.

● *Maturing and bleaching agents* improve the baking qualities of foods made with wheat flour and improve the appearance of certain cheeses. When the yellow pigment of wheat flour is bleached, the dough becomes more elastic and the baking results, better. The white curd in some cheeses, such as gorgonzola and blue cheese, is the result of adding a bleaching agent to milk.

● *pH control agents* influence the texture, taste, and safety of foods by adjusting their acidity or alkalinity. Adding acids (acidulants) such as lactic acid or citric acid gives a tart taste to frozen desserts and beverages; they also inhibit the growth of bacteria in low-acid processed foods such as beets, and help prevent discoloration and rancidity. Alkalizers neutralize acids in foods such as chocolate so the flavor is milder.

● *Thickeners and stabilizers* give food a uniform texture. In ice cream they keep the texture smooth without forming ice crystals. In chocolate milk they allow the chocolate particles to stay in suspension. With stabilizers, oils that add flavor to food also stay in food. Carbohydrates in food—such as gelatin from animal bones, carrageenan from seaweed, and pectin from fruit—commonly are used as thickeners and stabilizers.

What foods have additives to aid food processing or preparation?

● *Anticaking agents* (to prevent lumping) . . . in baking powder, powdered foods, and salt, among others.

● *Emulsifiers* (to distribute particles evenly) . . . in

baked foods, bread, breakfast cereal, chocolate, chocolate milk, cocoa, frozen desserts, margarine, mayonnaise, nut butter, pie and pudding mixes, and salad dressings, among others.

● *Humectants* (to retain moisture) . . . in candy, shredded coconut, gum, and marshmallows, among others.

● *Leaveners* (to help food rise) . . . in baked goods such as bread, cake, freezer waffles, and muffins, among others.

● *Maturing and bleaching agents* (to improve baking quality) . . . in bread, cereal, some cheese, flour, and instant potatoes, among others.

● *pH control agents* (to control pH levels) . . . in baked goods, candy, chocolate, gelatin desserts, processed cheese, salad dressings, sauces, soft drinks, and vegetable oils, among others.

● *Stabilizers, thickeners, and texturizers* (for smooth, thick, uniform texture) . . . in baked goods, beverages, candy, cream cheese, frozen desserts, jam, jelly, pie filling, pudding, salad dressings, sauces, and soups, among others.

For Flavor and Appeal . . .

Some additives add adventure to eating. They may add color, provide flavor or enhance it, or sweeten food.

● *Colorings* won't affect the nutrients, safety, or taste of food, but they make a nutritional contribution when they make food look more appealing to eat. Cheese and margarine often get their yellow coloring from annatto, which comes from the tropical annatto tree. Ice cream and many baked foods also are among the many foods with added coloring.

Food colors may be added to food for many reasons: to restore the original color; to ensure a uniform color; to help protect flavor and light-sensitive vitamins, which may be destroyed during storage; to give an attractive appearance to foods; to help you identify it; and to help you visually recognize food quality.

Thirty-three colors are approved for use in food; only nine are synthetic. Synthetic colors are certified and named by color and number—for example, Yellow #5 and Red #2. More and more natural pigments from vegetables are being used to color food; they're exempt from certification but still meet regulations for safety and purity. For example, look for foods colored with annatto extract, beet juice, paprika, carrot oil, beta carotene, grape skin extract, or saffron. Only one food coloring is known to cause allergic reactions, in rare cases: Yellow #5. *See "Coloring . . . by Any Other Name!" in chapter 21 for more about it.*

● *Flavorings,* which may be natural or synthetic, make up about seventeen hundred of the additives

---

No Surprises

Additives in food are no secret to consumers. Just by reading the ingredient lists on food labels, you can identify specific additives in any food.

Emulsifier
to keep ingredients blended

Flavoring
to add sweetness

INGREDIENTS: **CRUST:** WHEAT FLOUR WITH MALTED BARLEY FLOUR, WATER, PARTIALLY HYDROGENATED VEGETABLE OIL (SOYBEAN AND/OR COTTONSEED OIL) WITH (SOY LECITHIN,) ARTIFICIAL FLAVOR AND ARTIFICIAL COLOR (BETA CAROTENE), SOYBEAN OIL, YEAST, (HIGH-FRUCTOSE CORN SYRUP,) SALT, (CALCIUM PROPIONATE) ADDED TO RETARD SPOILAGE OF CRUST, L-CYSTEINE MONOHYDROCHLORIDE; **SAUCE:** TOMATO PUREE (WATER, TOMATO PASTE), WATER GREEN PEPPERS, SALT, LACTOSE AND FLAVORING, SPICES, FOOD STARCH - MODIFIED, SUGAR, CORN OIL, (XANTHAN GUM,) GARLIC POWDER, **TOPPING:** LOW MOISTURE PART SKIM MOZZARELLA CHEESE (PASTEURIZED MILK, CHEESE CULTURES, SALT, ENZYMES.)

Preservative
to retard spoilage

Thickener
to give a uniform texture

approved for use in food. They include spices, herbs, essential oils and their extracts, fruit juices, caffeine, and other seasonings. To make artificial flavorings, food scientists carefully study the makeup of natural flavors, then approximate the complexity of the natural flavor. Natural flavors come from food itself after a minimum amount of processing. They're often taken from one food and added to another to enhance the flavor. The chemical structure of natural and artificial flavors is similar, although artificial flavors may not have all the complex elements that give a distinctive natural taste.

● *Flavor enhancers* don't add flavor of their own. Instead, they heighten natural flavors already present in food. The best-known flavor enhancer is monosodium glutamate (MSG). MSG comes from a common amino acid, which is a protein called glutamic acid. MSG comes mostly from vegetable proteins. *For more about MSG, see "MSG—Another Flavor Enhancer" in chapter 7.*

● *Sweeteners* are flavorings, but they're grouped separately from the others. Some, such as sucrose (table sugar), fructose, dextrose, and mannitol, are nutritive, which means they produce energy in your body. Besides adding a sweet flavor, these sugars add mouth feel and work as browning agents in food. And they may be used as a preservative. Intense, or nonnutritive, sweeteners such as saccharin and aspartame don't contribute calories, or food energy. *For more about sugars and other sweeteners see chapter 5, "Sweet Talk: Sugar and Other Sweeteners."*

What foods have additives to increase food appeal?

● *Colorings* . . . in baked goods, candy, cheese, gelatin mixes, ice cream, jam, jelly, margarine, pie, and pudding fillings, among others.

● *Flavorings* . . . in baked goods, candy, gelatin, pie filling, pudding, salad dressing mix, sauces, and soft drinks, among others.

● *Flavor enhancers* . . . in canned vegetables, gravy, processed meats, sauce mixes, and soups, among others.

● *Sweeteners* . . . in baked foods, canned and frozen fruit, frozen desserts, fruit yogurt, fruit juice drinks, gelatin mixes, jam, jelly, pudding mixes, and soft drinks, among others.

As a reference for specific additives, see "A Close-Up Look at Additives" in the Appendices.

Testing, Testing

Did you know that new additives must pass rigid safety tests before they can be used? During the past eighty years, the use of food additives has allowed a more varied and plentiful food supply. And beginning in 1938, government regulations have helped guide and ensure the safety of their use in food.

Today food additives are regulated more tightly than at any other time in history—with safety as the primary goal. In 1958 the federal government passed the Food Additives Amendment, which gave the U.S. Food and Drug Administration (FDA) responsibility for approving additives used in food. The FDA sets safety standards, determining whether a substance is safe for its intended use. If it's found to be safe, the FDA decides what types of foods the additive may be used in, in what amounts, and how it must be indicated on a food label.

Federal food laws distinguish among additives: those generally recognized as safe (GRAS), prior-approved additives, regulated additives, and color additives.

Have You Ever Wondered

. . . if food additives are okay for everyone? Except for a small number of reactions that occur in people with specific allergies, food additives are "safe at the plate." In fact, one of the primary uses of additives is protecting food quality and safety. For someone with a sensitivity to an additive, the reaction should be about the same whether the additive is natural or synthetic. The chemical makeup is quite similar. *For specifics about those rare cases of allergic responses, see "Sensitive to Additives? Maybe, Maybe Not" in chapter 21.*

. . . if people with gluten intolerance should avoid certain additives? Yes; they need to read food labels carefully. Some food additives contain gluten, a form of protein in wheat, rye, barley, and perhaps oats that people with gluten intolerance cannot handle. *See "Gluten Intolerance: Often a Lifelong Condition" in chapter 21.*

Generally recognized as safe (GRAS). In 1959 the FDA established a list of about seven hundred additives that were exempt from the regulatory process. This list—called the GRAS list—recognized that many additives had an extensive history or existing scientific evidence of their safe use in food. Additives that appear on the list include salt, sugar, spices, vitamins, and monosodium glutamate.

From time to time, GRAS ingredients are reevaluated by the FDA and the U.S. Department of Agriculture (USDA), and perhaps removed or reclassified. Sulfites are an example. In 1986 the FDA revoked their GRAS status for use on raw fruits or vegetables except potatoes. That occurred because research showed that some people are sensitive to sulfites. For more about sulfite sensitivity, see *"For the Sulfite-Sensitive"* in chapter 21.

Prior-approved substances. Before the 1958 Food Additives Amendment, some additives—such as nitrites used to preserve processed meat—had been approved by the FDA or the USDA. If used as originally approved, these substances didn't need to go through the approval process again; the government already had judged them safe.

As with the GRAS list, prior-approved substances are continually monitored. Current scientific evidence of their link to health is always reviewed, recognizing that the statutes of prior-approved substances can be changed.

Regulated additives. Any additive not considered as GRAS or prior-approved must be approved before it can be marketed and used in food. The burden of proof for additive safety falls on the manufacturer. These are the regulatory steps the food industry follows:

● First, the additive manufacturer must prove that the additive is effective—that the additive does what it is supposed to do, and that it can be detected and measured when put into a food.

● Second, the manufacturer must prove that large amounts of the food additive, when given to two kinds of test animals over an extended period of time, won't cause cancer, birth defects, or other problems. Results of human studies also may be submitted.

● The FDA reviews the results, then invites public response to the manufacturer's petition for the new additive.

● If approval is given, the FDA establishes regulations for the types of food in which the additive can be used, the maximum amount, and how the substance must be described on the label.

When the food industry proposes an additive for use in meat or poultry products, another approval also is required—this time from the U.S. Department of Agriculture's Food Safety and Inspection Service (FSIS), which applies different standards that consider the unique characteristics of meat and poultry. For example, the FSIS doesn't allow the use of sorbic acid, which is an approved additive, in meat salads because it could mask spoilage.

Color additives. In 1960 the federal government passed another law—the Color Additives Amendments, which required that dyes used in foods, drugs, cosmetics, and medical devices needed testing, similar to tests for regulated food additives. Before the law, nearly two hundred colors were used in foods. After the required testing, only thirty-three were approved for use today. Many have been withdrawn from the market.

Safety Check

Approval of additives, including those on the GRAS and prior-sanctioned lists, doesn't guarantee that they'll be used in food forever. The FDA continues to review all categories of food additives, and it judges them by the latest scientific standards. Based on new evidence, approval is either maintained or withdrawn.

As another safety check, the Food Additives Amendment also has a section called the Delaney Clause, which states that no additive known to cause cancer in animals or humans can be put in food in any amount. One artificial sweetener called cyclamate was removed from the GRAS list for that reason. Tests showed that large amounts were linked to cancer in test animals. The safety of cyclamate is currently being reevaluated; it is approved for use in some other countries.

To monitor and investigate complaints of adverse reactions to additives, the FDA also maintains the computerized Adverse Reaction Monitoring System (ARMS), which records updated safety data. Incidences of allergic reactions to food and color additives and to dietary supplements, reported by individuals or their doctors, are recorded, too. These reports help determine whether further investigation is warranted—and if action is required to maintain public health. *For more about adverse reactions to food additives, see "Sensitive to Additives? Maybe, Maybe Not" in chapter 21.*

Additives—Your Choice

With such a wide variety of foods available, consumers have considerable choice about food additives. If you have a history of food-related allergies, you may need to limit or avoid foods with ingredients, including additives, that you're sensitive to. Learn to read the ingredient lists on food labels. *See "A Word about Ingredients . . ." in chapter 11. If you have a food reaction and think it may be additive-related, talk to your doctor.*

Pesticides: Carefully Controlled

The vast array of safe, nutritious foods available in your supermarket throughout the year doesn't happen by chance. Successful growers carefully manage their croplands and orchards to control about eighty thousand plant diseases, thirty thousand weed species, a thousand species of nematodes, and more than ten thousand insect species! In the United States alone, about $20 billion of crops (10 percent of our production) are lost yearly with these problems. If you've ever struggled with mildew, insects, weeds, and rodents in your own garden, just multiply the problem! Pesticides help ensure an ongoing supply of high-quality fruits, vegetables, and grains for you and your family, the nation, and the world.

To produce high-quality produce with adequate yields, most farmers use some pesticides—either in the field or the grove, or just after harvest—to prevent mold or insect damage during transport or storage.

Without prudent use of pesticides, many farmers couldn't control crop damage from disease, insects, molds and fungi, weeds, and other pests. And their crop yields would be much lower. In spite of pesticide use, U.S. farmers annually lose a significant amount of crops because of damage from pests. That number would be far higher without careful use of pesticides.

About Pesticides . . .

Pesticides include a broad range of chemicals that protect crops. They're applied by dusting, fogging, spraying, or injecting them into the soil:

● *Herbicides* control weeds.

● *Fungicides* control mold, mildew, and fungi that cause plant disease, and inhibit molds that may be harmful to consumers.

● *Insecticides* control harmful insects, often those that damage crops or carry plant disease.

● *Rodenticides* control rodents in the field.

● *Disinfectants* act against bacteria and other disease-carrying microorganisms.

When people think of pesticides, synthetic chemicals often come to mind. However, naturally occurring chemicals in the environment, such as copper, nicotine, and sulfur, also are used to control pests. And many plants protect themselves by producing their own pesticides in low levels.

IPM—Best of Both Worlds

What does sex have to do with pest control? Interestingly, sex scents, called pheromones, can confuse pest mating patterns, allowing farmers to use less chemical pesticides. It's all part of a biological system of pest control.

IPM stands for integrated pest management—a contemporary farming approach that uses pesticides, biological control, and biotechnology to reduce crop damage. As farmers work in partnership with nature, they apply pesticides on crops selectively, ultimately using less.

IPM incorporates a variety of strategies—not just limited pesticide use—into pest management. For example:

● Crop rotation—for example, switching from soybeans to corn—helps limit pest buildup because insects lose their natural food source.

● Farmers may use living organisms to help control pest diseases, or use pest predators (when "good" bugs eat "bad" bugs).

• Growers may choose plant varieties that are more resistant to pests. Traditional plant breeding and genetic engineering can help crops develop their own natural resistance. *See "Food Biotechnology: The Future Is Today!" later in this chapter.*

• Computers can help growers forecast disease and weather conditions. The more they know, the more prudent they can be with pesticides.

Safety: Whose Job?

Safety starts with growers; most are prudent with pesticides for many reasons. One is cost. Pesticides are expensive, so farmers use them judiciously to remain profitable. Second, successful growers project toward the future. By using too much pesticide with one year's crop, they may cause crop damage in the future. Some pesticide residues remain in the soil. Third, today's farmers are more aware than ever of the environment (wildlife, groundwater, soil quality)—their livelihood depends on it. Most farmers are trained in the responsible, legal use of agricultural chemicals; some pesticides must be applied only by people certified or licensed to do so.

Pesticide manufacturers bear responsibility for the effects of pesticide use among consumers, farm workers, and the environment. If research indicates that pesticide use would not meet standards for toxicology, crop residues, or environmental impact, the Environmental Protection Agency (EPA) can stop or change its use. Several government agencies regulate and monitor pesticide safety in food:

• The *EPA* regulates the manufacture, labeling, and use of pesticides—and sets maximum levels, or tolerances, for pesticide residues. Before a pesticide can be used on crops, it must be thoroughly tested to assure that it's safe for the environment and for human health. If approved, the EPA may limit its use—amount, frequency, or crop—and require that these limitations be listed on the product label. Growers who misuse pesticides, even mistakenly, risk having their crop seized or destroyed. And the grower may be charged with a civil or a criminal lawsuit.

Regulations established in 1996 under the Food Quality Protection Act set even stricter safety standards. Among other measures, this law further protects children and infants from pesticide risk, requires testing and information about any estrogenlike effects of pesticide residues, and considers exposure of pesticides to drinking water.

• The *Food and Drug Administration (FDA)* monitors pesticide residues in most foods (not meat, poultry, and eggs)—both raw and processed—and enforces the tolerance levels set by the EPA. If residues exceed these levels, the food can be seized or destroyed, and a lawsuit may be filed. Any pesticide residues that remain on raw foods are usually removed during washing or peeling.

• Like the FDA, the USDA's *Food Safety and Inspection Service (FSIS)* monitors pesticide residues and enforces tolerance levels for meat, poultry, and eggs.

• Several states, including California, that grow many fruits and vegetables have their own regulations, too.

Tolerances, or maximum levels, for pesticide residues are set in parts per million, parts per billion, and parts per trillion. For example, 1 part per million would mean 1 gram of residue is the maximum allowed in 1 million grams of food. That equates to 1 cherry in about 20,000 1-pound cans.

Tolerances for pesticide residues are legal limits. In most foods, levels are well below that. Tolerances are a hundred to a thousand times lower than the amount that might pose a health risk, so there's a very wide margin of safety. FDA testing has shown that foods rarely exceed limits, and many samples are below the tolerance level or show no residues at all. To pass through U.S. customs, imported foods must meet the same stringent standards set for foods grown domestically.

Benefits vs. Risks

The presence of low levels of pesticide residues doesn't signal a risk. Tolerances are legal limits, not medical limits—set far below what is considered safe for the most sensitive part of the population, including infants and children.

In fact, the use of pesticides may reduce other risks related to food. For example, fungicides help control aflatoxin B2, a naturally occurring toxin in grains and peanuts. Most important, the prudent use of pesticides helps ensure a wide variety of fruits and vegetables, which supply important vitamins, minerals, dietary fiber, and other phytonutrients for human health.

There's no such thing as a risk-free world. The real issue is weighing the benefits against the risks—then deciding what's right for you.

What You Can Do . . .

Any pesticide residues in foods you buy are present at minimal levels. It's safe to say that they probably won't pose any risk to your health. You can add more to your safety net by the way you handle food in your kitchen . . . or by the way you grow fruits and vegetables in your own garden:

● Choose produce carefully. Avoid fruits and vegetables with cuts, insect holes, mold, or decay.

● Wash fresh fruits (including melons) and vegetables with water to remove residues on the surface and in the crevices. For foods such as carrots, squash,

apples, and pears, use a vegetable brush to clean them even more—if you eat the fiber-rich skin. Rinse well. Avoid soap, unless it's especially meant for produce, because it leaves its own residues. As an option, use a produce wash formulated to remove soil, wax, and pesticides. Rinse well after using a produce wash.

● Remove outer leaves of lettuce, cabbage, and other leafy vegetables.

● Although you could peel some fruits and vegetables, recognize what you'd be giving up—the nutrients and the fiber that the peel contains.

● Eat a variety of foods. Not only do you get the nutritional benefits of food variety, but you also minimize pesticide risks. Different crops require different pesticides, so variety limits exposure to any one type.

● If you're a home gardener, minimize your use of pesticides, and follow the directions for their safe use,

Have You Ever Wondered ?

. . . *what BST refers to?* BST, or bovine somatotropin (also called bovine growth hormone, or BGH), is a naturally occurring protein in all cow milk and meat. When given as a supplement in small, controlled doses it helps improve cows' efficiency in producing milk. Even without supplementation, BST naturally occurs in cow milk, in small quantities. It has no effect on humans. Like other proteins, it's broken down during digestion. With BST supplementation, a cow's milk production goes up, but the normal level of BST in milk itself doesn't change; the cow uses it up herself. In addition, there's no change in the flavor or nutritional qualities of milk produced from supplemented cows. As always, milk remains an excellent source of calcium, protein, vitamins, and other nutrients.

In 1990, the National Institutes of Health reinforced that BST is safe for humans. In 1993 the U.S. Food and Drug Administration approved BST supplementation based on its safety for humans, cows, and the environment. And regulatory agencies around the world have authorized milk and meat from cows receiving BST as safe for people of all ages.

. . . *if wax on fruits and vegetables is safe to eat?* Yes. There's no need to peel waxed produce. Just wash it

with water. You might use a brush to remove any dirt, bacteria, and pesticide residues. The thin, waxy coating on foods such as cucumbers and apples is applied after picking to replace natural wax and to help produce stay fresh and edible; a little fungicide often mixed with the wax helps control mold and rot. Wax helps by retaining moisture, protecting the food from bruising, and preventing spoilage. By long-standing federal law, waxed produce must be labeled.

. . . *if you should avoid any specific fruit or vegetable to reduce your exposure to pesticides?* No. For any crop, the use of pesticides varies with the time of year, the soil conditions, the climate, and the presence of pests. There's no way you can tell the difference. The best guideline is to wash produce thoroughly, and remove outer leaves on leafy greens—then enjoy the nutritional benefits that all fruits and vegetables provide.

. . . *if food grown in soil that's depleted of minerals or nitrogen is less nutritious?* No scientific evidence suggests that crops grown in depleted soil have fewer nutrients than those grown in fertilized soil. When soil lacks minerals or nitrogen, plants don't grow properly and may not produce their potential yield. If soil can grow crops, the food produced is nutritious.

storage, and disposal. Contact your county extension service if you need guidance. *See "Resources You Can Use" at the back of this book to help locate your local extension service.*

● Wash and sanitize your refrigerator produce drawer frequently.

● Remember, being "organic" doesn't guarantee safety. Clean organic produce well.

Organically Produced

If you've scanned the shopping aisles you know: organic foods, once available mostly from health food stores, now sell in mainstream supermarkets. Organic farming, mainly done by small-scale producers, is expanding fast—not only with fruits, vegetables, and grains, but also eggs, dairy foods, and to some extent meat and poultry. Just what are organic foods? And how do they compare with their conventionally produced counterparts?

The term "organic" is a misnomer. All foods come from living organisms—plant and animal. Because they all contain carbon, they're all technically organic. Foods referred to as "organic" are really "organically grown" or "organically produced"—with little or no synthetic fertilizers or pesticides and no antibiotics or hormones.

Perspective: Organically Produced Foods

Organic farming offers choice: an alternative to conventional agriculture and an alternative for you at point of purchase.

Pesticide-free? Maybe and maybe not. Organic farmers may use insects and crop rotation to control pests that damage crops. Certain insects, for example, are natural predators for other insects that cause crop damage. Or farmers may use chemicals found naturally in the environment, such as sulfur, nicotine, copper, or pyrethrins, as pesticides. When these methods don't work, organic farmers can use other substances (biological, botanical, or synthetic) from a list approved by the National Organic Program of the U.S. Department of Agriculture. To compare, pesticide levels with conventional farming are set low, so they're not harmful to health; *see "Pesticides: Carefully Controlled" earlier in this chapter.*

With organic farming, manure, compost, and other organic wastes fertilize crops; there are some allowed synthetic fertilizers. The soil is also managed with crop rotation, tillage, and cover crops. Although organic fertilizers are effective, plants can't distinguish them from synthetic fertilizers. Both types of fertilizer break down in the soil to nurture growing plants.

The criteria for organically raised livestock and poultry and for animals raised for milk and eggs are equally stringent. From the last third of gestation, or for poultry, the second day of life, animals are fed only 100 percent organic feed. Although vitamin and mineral supplements are allowed, hormones for growth and antibiotics are not. Any animal treated with medication can't be sold as organic.

Despite common perception, no scientific evidence shows that organically produced foods are healthier or safer for you. Both approaches—organic and conventional farming—supply nutritionally comparable foods. Climate and soil conditions, genetic differences, maturity at harvest, and the way food is handled—not the type of fertilizer—affect the nutrient content of raw foods.

How do taste and appearance compare? Studies show no significant flavor difference between organically grown and conventionally grown foods. Instead, taste differences appear to come from the food varietal, its growing conditions, and its maturity at harvest time. Unlike in the past, most of today's organic foods compare very favorably in appearance with conventionally grown foods.

Organically produced foods often cost more. That's usually due to higher production costs (more labor, transportation, processing, retailing), more crop losses, and smaller yields. In the future, costs may go down as organic farmers develop more cost-efficient techniques and farming systems and get larger yields.

On a large-scale basis, organic farming alone can't produce enough food for the world's exploding population. However, the marketplace does offer options if you prefer organically produced food.

Coming to Terms

The National Organic Program ensures that the production, processing, and certification of organic foods match a comprehensive standard. If you prefer organic foods, now you can be confident about what you buy.

... if antibiotics used in agriculture affect human health? Antibiotics have been used in animal agriculture for many years to prevent or cure diseases in animals. The FDA and the FSIS work together to provide consumers with a safe food product by ensuring the proper use of animal antibiotics in agriculture. The FDA regulates and monitors the use of animal antibiotics to ensure that any residues are minimal and at very safe levels. Currently, questions have been posed about the possibility of "antibiotic resistance" in humans if animal antibiotics are used in cattle production; definitive research is needed to determine any effect from the use of animal antibiotics on human health. (Penicillin, important to human health, is not used with cattle.) Meat and poultry may be labeled "no antibiotics added" or "raised without antibiotics" if there's enough substantiated proof to the FSIS that animals were raised without them.

... what are hydroponically grown foods? They're foods from plants raised in water, not soil; "hydro" means water. The hydroponic solution—which varies by crop and environmental conditions—supplies roots with elements found in soil and fertilizer. With hydroponic farming, high-quality food can be produced almost anywhere: a desert, outer space, and areas with poor soil. Nutritionally, hydroponically grown foods are comparable to those grown in soil; undamaged by weather, they may look better.

A few more terms in modern agriculture: aeroponics is a way of growing plants by spraying the roots with nutrient solution; aquaculture is raising fish in a controlled environment.

... if hormones used in beef production affect humans? The FDA and the FSIS work together to provide consumers with a safe food product by ensuring the proper use of hormones in cattle. In very small amounts, certain hormones have been approved by the FDA to improve the feed efficiency or weight gain of beef cattle and sheep. For naturally occurring hormones used in production, the amounts of hormone in meat must fit within the same range as for untreated animals. With the use of synthetic hormones, producers must show that any hormones in meat after treatment remain below a level that's too low to affect humans.

If you prefer meat from untreated animals, you have choices. Beef products may be labeled "no hormones administered"—if sufficient evidence is provided by the producer to the FSIS showing that hormones were not used to raise the animals. What about pork or chicken? Federal regulations prohibit the use of added hormones in raising hogs or poultry.

Under the Organic Foods Production Act, federal regulations require consistent and uniform standards. Organic farming or processing operations that take in more than $5,000 gross must be certified. Even smaller, uncertified organic operations must abide by the standards and may label their products. Certification allows organic labeling, with terms that have a consistent meaning: "100 percent organic," "organic," and "made with organic ingredients." The "USDA Organic" seal may appear on any foods that contain at least 70 percent organic ingredients. In organic food production, food irradiation, sewage sludge, and genetic engineering can't be used. A product with less than 70 percent organic ingredients can list only specific organically produced ingredients on the ingredient list. *For more about organic labeling, see chapter 11.*

Food Biotechnology: The Future Is Today!

In the twenty-first century your shopping cart will be filled with an array of new products: foods that taste fresher and more flavorful, more health-promoting varieties of foods, and a greater variety of produce all year long. Today's food biotechnology has already put some of these foods on your table: canola, corn, soybean, and cottonseed oil. Potatoes, squash, tomatoes, and others have been developed and could be available based on consumer demand.

What is food biotechnology? Today's modern biotechnology is simply applying plant science and genetics to improving food production—and food itself.

When did "traditional" biotechnology begin? Perhaps ten thousand years ago, as farmers raised animals and grew plants to produce food with desirable traits: higher yields, new food varieties, better taste, faster ripening, and more resistance to drought. Five thousand years ago in Peru, potatoes were grown selectively. In ancient Egypt—forty-five hundred years ago—domesticated geese were fed to make them bigger and tastier. About twenty-three hundred years ago, Greeks grafted trees, a technique that led to orchards and a more abundant fruit supply. In fact, products as commonplace as grapefruit and wine came from traditional biotechnology.

Over the years, farmers have replanted seeds or cross-pollinated from their best crops. And they've bred new livestock from their best animals. For example, within the past few decades, hogs have been bred to be leaner, in turn producing lean cuts of pork for today's consumers.

With traditional breeding, farmers changed the genetic makeup of plants and animals by selecting those with desirable traits. They then raised and selected again and again until a new, more desirable breed or food variety was established. Even in the "old days," all of this breeding resulted in genetic change.

Traditional cross-breeding takes time. Often it's unpredictable. Each time one plant pollinates another, or one animal inseminates another, thousands of genes cross together. Along the way, less desirable traits—and the genes that cause them—may pass with desirable ones. Several generations of breeding, perhaps ten to twelve years, may go by before desirable traits get established and less desirable qualities are bred away.

The "new" biotechnology offers a faster and more precise way to establish new traits in both plants and animals—and so provide improved foods that are safe, nutritious, healthful, abundant, and tasty.

Food Biotechnology Today: What's It All About?

In a nutshell, modern or "new" biotechnology refers to using living organisms—plants, animals, and bacteria—to develop new products,

not just for food, but also for medical treatment, waste management, and alternative fuels, among others.

Modern food biotechnology started about thirty years ago, as scientists learned more about DNA (deoxyribonucleic acid), genes, and the genetic code in living things, and applied this knowledge to plant and animal breeding practices. In fact, the latest advances in food biotechnology have spawned a new vocabulary. Popular media may use "genetically modified foods," or "GM foods," to refer to these foods. Other terms, such as "genetic engineering," "gene splicing," "cell culture," and "recombinant DNA," refer to some methods of biotechnology. Recombinant DNA is the process of inserting genes from one organism into the genetic code, or DNA, of another. That's how a trait is transferred.

To understand how today's food biotechnology works, think about writing a book on a computer. With a click of your keyboard, you can copy a single quote from one document to another, without merging the two, or you can highlight or delete a single phrase.

With food biotechnology, agricultural scientists can pinpoint specific genes that carry traits they want, such as disease resistance, better nutrient quality, or flavor. Then they can transfer a single gene from one plant or from an unrelated species, such as a bacterium, to another. Or they can extract a certain gene, leaving undesirable traits behind.

The latest advances in food biotechnology allow for a more efficient, more predictable, and less time-consuming method than traditional breeding—an approach that wasn't possible before we learned more about the biological world around us.

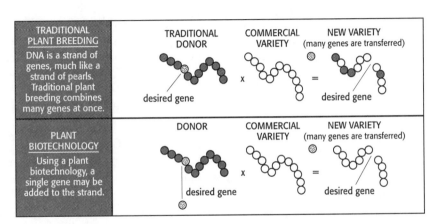

Source: American Dietetic Association.

Today's Meat

Through breeding, feeding, and management at the farm, hogs and beef cattle are leaner than ever. In addition, processing methods help create leaner meat. The reason? The need to provide products for consumers with high nutrient content, yet lower levels of total fat and saturated fat. For example, pork cuts sold in the supermarket today have an average of 43 percent less fat than they did in 1983, and compared with the 1970s, beef has 27 percent less trimmable fat.

One reason for leaner hogs is genetics. Some of the eight major hog breeds in the United States carry genes that produce leaner, meatier hogs. With selective breeding, hog producers have changed the fat and muscle composition of hogs, gradually producing leaner animals over the past few decades.

As with humans, a hog's food and "lifestyle" affect its body composition. With a scientifically balanced diet matched to its age, current weight, and nutrient needs, a hog is fed what it needs without excess.

The next step in producing lean meat is with the meat packers or processors. They usually trim the fat surrounding cuts of meat to ⅛ to ¹⁄₁₆ inch, rather than ½ to ¼ inch, as in the past. And, for example with beef, 40 percent of the cuts have no outside fat at all. There are often financial incentives offered by the packer to the farmer for producing lean animals. Even processed meat is being produced with less fat and cholesterol than ever before, yet it's still tender, moist, and flavorful. Look for low-fat ground beef and low-fat pork sausages: just 7 fat grams and 6 fat grams, respectively, per 3-ounce serving. That's about 50 percent less than for regular meat.

Finally, it's up to you to keep lean meat lean and flavorful . . . by using low-fat cooking methods and avoiding high-fat sauces, and by cooking to a safe internal temperature, without overcooking. *For more about preparing meat, see "Fat and Cholesterol Trimmers" in chapter 13. For tips on buying lean meat, see "Meat and Deli Case" in chapter 11.*

The Benefits Package

Food biotechnology also offers an approach for protecting the environment while producing a high-quality, abundant, more healthful, and inexpensive food supply. The benefits we already have are just the tip of the iceberg!

Healthier crops, higher yields. Crops produced using biotechnology are able to thrive with fewer pesticides. For the farmers, that means lower production costs, and for the environment, fewer residues.

For example, some varieties of corn have been enhanced through biotechnology to contain *Bacillus thuringiensis* (Bt), a common soil bacterium that allows the corn to protect itself from certain insects that eat and destroy plants. "Bt" itself isn't new, however. Organic farmers have sprayed it on their crops for forty years.

Enhanced farming is developing other crops to resist plant viruses and other diseases, or to require less herbicide or more environmentally friendly herbicides. Newly developed soybeans, as well as some corn, canola, cotton, and potatoes, flourish with less insecticides and herbicides.

Weather-resistant crops. Crops are being genetically improved to withstand severe weather, reducing crop loss for farmers and making more fresh fruits, vegetables, and grains available to consumers throughout the year.

Fresher foods, better flavor. By transferring desirable genetic traits, fruits and vegetables with different ripening qualities can be shipped longer and farther, without spoilage or damage: bananas and pineapples, for example, as well as strawberries that resist mold. This will mean fresher, better-tasting produce such as sweeter peppers, or potatoes with fewer dark spots, year-'round. And people living in remote places may have more fresh produce choices.

Healthier food. Food biotechnology can promote public health, providing fruits, vegetables, and grains with more nutritious benefits: more proteins, vitamins, and minerals, or less fat and saturated fat. In the near future, fruits and vegetables such as sweet potatoes with higher levels of antioxidants (vitamins C and E, and beta carotene) may help reduce heart disease and cancer risk. Already some vegetable oils have a better fatty acid profile—less saturated fat and more monounsaturated fat—for heart health.

Food biotechnology also has enhanced soybeans, so they can be grown with less saturated fat and more oleic acid, an unsaturated fatty acid that is a benefit to heart health.

In some regions of the world, nutrient-enhanced crops may help eliminate problems of malnutrition. For example, "golden rice" with beta carotene (vitamin A) and iron may address two health problems: blindness among children caused by a lack of vitamin A, and low iron intakes, harmful to many children and women.

Medical uses. Products of food biotechnology might treat health problems: bananas grown to include vaccines to deliver to developing nations. Other nonfood applications of biotechnology may result someday in new vaccines and medications to treat heart disease, cancer, and diabetes, among others, and the ability to produce human insulin to help treat diabetes.

Efficient food production. Foods can be grown in a better way to produce higher yields, reducing costs and efforts for farmers. One product under development is a sweeter, higher-yielding pea plant.

Food biotechnology also can use simple organisms to produce the same food components found in nature. One example is an additive called rennin. In fact, 70 percent of cheese produced in the United States is made with an enzyme available through biotechnology. Traditionally, rennet—an enzyme extracted from the lining of calves' stomachs—was used to form curds and whey from milk, a first step in making cheese. Through the use of food biotechnology, scientists have transferred the calf gene into "friendly" bacteria, where it produces the same enzyme. This enzyme is more active and more pure than rennet—and consistently available to food manufacturers.

New food varieties. Food biotechnology can extend advances in cross-breeding, allowing for new foods on your dinner plate: broccoflower, or green cauliflower, tangelos, and nectarines. In the future, look for small, single-serving melons without seeds. Through biotechnology, the thousands of edible plant species yet unexplored can more easily contribute to modern agriculture.

More food for the world. Food biotechnology can help farmers produce enough food to meet the world's rapidly growing population—expected to double in the next fifty years. Within just the next twenty years, the world will need 40 percent more rice, wheat, corn, and other grains!

Weather-resistant crops can turn regions with poor climate or soil conditions into productive agricultural land. Higher-yielding crops can feed more people, using less farmland, as more and more land is turned into housing and commercial space.

Protection for the environment. With enhanced farming, greater crop yields can reduce the need to clear forests for farmland. Opportunity for no-till or other forms of conservation tillage can lead to less erosion of valuable topsoil because the soil isn't turned over as much. Crops with traits that repel pests require fewer pesticides, and crops that take more nitrogen from the soil and air need less fertilizer. As a result, fewer residues pass into water supplies. And with "environmentally friendly" animal feed, less unwanted phosphorus passes into manure, then on to the water supply.

As another nonfood application, biotechnology also can provide options for renewable, nonpolluting sources of sources of fuel—for example, from corn. These fuel sources can reduce dependence on nonrenewable energy sources such as petroleum.

Now about Food Safety. . .

With any new technology, consumer safety is one of the first questions. The U.S. Food and Drug Administration subjects products of food biotechnology to the same stringent standards of labeling and safety as all foods sold in the United States.

Most foods enhanced through biotechnology don't differ in composition, nutritional quality, or safety from those that are conventionally produced—unless

Have You Ever Wondered ?

. . . if food developed through biotechnology can cause an allergic reaction? No more so than foods produced conventionally. To ensure safety, the FDA requires testing of foods enhanced through biotechnology for potential allergic reactions. Any food with an allergen introduced through biotechnology must carry a statement on the food label. Currently none of these foods are in production.

that's the trait specifically desired. And like other foods in the U.S. marketplace, any foods produced through biotechnology are rigorously tested and strictly regulated.

Who's responsible for safety? Several federal agencies and some state agencies regulate and ensure the safety of foods produced through biotechnology: the Food and Drug Administration (FDA), the Environmental Protection Agency (EPA), and the U.S. Department of Agriculture (USDA). The FDA's key role is assuring the safety of the product as a food for humans or as animal feed. The EPA regulates pesticides produced by the plant and their exposure to the environment. And the USDA takes responsibility for field trials.

Food manufacturers must conduct thorough research and demonstrate proof of testing for every crop brought to market—for example, showing proper nutrient levels, status of allergens or natural toxins, how the improved crop functions as food or animal feed, scientific procedures for product development, environmental effects, and the history of safe use. For substances that differ significantly from existing foods and ingredients, special testing is required. In fact, products are tested at many stages of development before they reach consumers.

With new technology come change and controversy. However, evaluation procedures used by manufacturers and regulators to ensure safety for consumers are endorsed internationally by the Food and Agriculture Organization (FAO) of the United Nations and the World Health Organization (WHO). In the United States, the National Research Council, the American Medical Association, and the American Dietetic Association support the safety of the foods produced by biotechnology.

Biotechnology Labeling: When You Need to Know

Most foods produced through biotechnology do not seem different from foods you enjoy already. They taste good, look fresh, and are available throughout the year. In addition, most of these foods do not need a special food label because they have been proven to be the same as other foods.

In fact, foods developed through biotechnology are subject to the same FDA labeling regulations and carry the same food labels as any other foods. Additional labeling is required on biotech foods, or foods with ingredients derived from biotechnology under some circumstances:

. . . *if a known allergen is introduced into the food.* Allergic reactions come from proteins in foods, and genes direct the production of proteins. So if a gene is taken from a food known to cause allergic reactions (such as peanuts), then transferred to another food (such as potatoes or corn), the new food must be labeled as potentially containing that particular allergen. No foods introduced to the food supply to date contain proteins that were introduced from known allergenic foods. (*Note:* Through biotechnology, research is under way to remove known allergens from food—for example, to develop allergen-free or allergen-reduced peanuts.)

. . . *if the nutritional content of the food changes.* Foods that are enhanced to change their nutritional content

Natural Toxins

Plants have their own built-in mechanism for pest control: fungi, insects, and animal predators. Unlike animals, plants can't flee when they sense danger, so they produce natural compounds—actually, low levels of pesticides—to protect against these invading organisms.

Of interest, the level of natural toxins in food may be many times higher than any level of synthetic pesticide residue, according to the National Academy of Sciences. And according to FDA estimates, Americans ingest ten thousand times (by weight) more natural pesticides than synthetic ones—with no apparent health risk.

Natural toxins are found in foods you eat every day—for example, oxalates in rhubarb, solanine in green potatoes, nitrates in broccoli, and cyanide in lima beans. At high levels, some might cause illness or may be carcinogenic (cancer-causing). However, in the amounts normally eaten in a varied diet, none has been shown to pose a cancer risk.

Through advances in biotechnology, scientists now can identify genes that produce natural toxins, then either remove them or suppress their action, to provide a health benefit.

must be labeled. Perhaps rice with more protein, an orange with more vitamin C, or cooking oil with less saturated fat.

. . . if the food changes composition substantially. Perhaps it would be labeled with a new varietal name; or maybe, like broccoflower, it would carry a new identity.

According to federal regulation, manufacturers may voluntarily label their foods as produced with or without the use of ingredients enhanced or produced through biotechnology. The phrases "derived through biotechnology" or "bioengineered" have been suggested by the FDA for labeling. A recent American Medical Association report indicates no scientific justification for labeling most foods.

Growing Possibilities . . .

Food biotechnology, which holds great promise for feeding the world, is developing in the global marketplace, not just in the United States. Gradually you might find these foods in your supermarket:

- Tomatoes with more lycopene, an antioxidant that protects against prostate cancer

- Low-fat potato chips or French fries, made from higher-starch potatoes that absorb less fat

- Vegetables and fruits with higher levels of antioxidants (vitamins C and E, and beta carotene) to help reduce risks for some health problems such as cancer and heart disease

- Rice with higher-quality protein (more amino acids) produced with genes from pea plants

- Vegetable oils—canola, corn, soybean, and others—with more stearate (a form of stearic acid, a saturated fat that doesn't appear to affect blood cholesterol levels) for use in margarine and spreads

- Garlic with more allicin, a phytonutrient that may help lower cholesterol levels

- Peanuts with less of the naturally occurring protein that causes allergic reactions

- Strawberries with more ellagic acid, a cancer-fighting phytonutrient

- Drought-resistant corn for growing in regions with extreme heat and drought

- Fruits that can deliver vaccines in regions of the world without adequate refrigeration to store vaccines.

CHAPTER 10

Planning to Eat Smart

Food, glorious food! We've explored how nutrients function in human health. But it's the wide array of food, not nutrients, that entices most people to eat. The aromas, flavors, textures, and appearance of all kinds of food stimulate the appetite, satisfy taste buds, and give the contented feeling that goes with a wonderful meal or a tasty snack.

Making healthful food choices has its own challenges: often lack of time, too much effort, and limited know-how. The goal is to satisfy your hunger, appetite, and desire for certain foods while ensuring that your meals and snacks have the food variety, balance, and moderation that help you maintain, and even enhance, your health. The solutions? Quick, simple, and convenient ways to eat smart and enjoy it, especially when you're short on time and energy!

The Food Guide Pyramid: Your Healthful Eating Guide

Looking for a simple, easy-to-remember strategy for smart eating? No matter what your eating style, the Food Guide Pyramid, which you've seen in many places, including on the packages of many food products, can be your personal guide for making healthful food choices. It's meant to make advice about food choices flexible, practical, and easy to use. It shows how you—and your family—can put the Dietary Guidelines for Americans into action.

The Pyramid is a guideline, not a rigid prescription. Based on sound science, it's meant for all healthy people, male or female, young or old—aged two years or more. It allows you plenty of flexibility to enjoy foods that match your lifestyle and your food preferences. Think of any food or beverage you've ever had. Whatever the food, it fits somewhere in the Food Guide Pyramid—either in one food group, or in more food groups if it's a mixed food, or in the Pyramid tip.

The Pyramid contains the building blocks of a healthful eating plan. Five food groups—in the three lower levels of the Pyramid—are filled with nutrient-rich foods, also with plenty of phytonutrients. Each group supplies some, but not all, of the nutrients your body needs. For example, milk provides calcium and vitamin B_{12}, but no vitamin C; oranges provide vitamin C, folate, and phytonutrients (flavones), but no calcium or vitamin B_{12}. Because their nutrients differ, foods in one food group can't replace those in another. In fact, no one food group is more important than another.

The Pyramid offers more advice: how to moderate the fats and added sugars in your day's food choices. Symbols on the Food Guide Pyramid show the categories of foods with naturally occurring and added fats (●) and added sugars (▼). Foods that are mainly fats, oils, and/or sugars are in the Pyramid tip. Foods within the five food groups may have varying amounts of fat or added sugars, too. When you're choosing foods, be aware: fats and added sugars are found in all food groups, not just those in the Pyramid tip.

Have You Ever Wondered

. . . if the Food Guide Pyramid applies to any cuisine? Asian, Mediterranean, Latin American, and soul food cuisines—in fact, any foods you enjoy—fit into the Food Guide Pyramid, which is used in the United States.

Other nations present their food guides differently, reflecting their own culture, their available foods, eating patterns, and food-related health concerns. For example:

● Food guide symbols "speak to" the culture. The United States, Panama, and Mexico use a pyramid shape; Canada, a rainbow. Guatemala uses a bean pot, since the pyramid shape symbolizes death. The United Kingdom and Costa Rica put their food guide on a plate; Germany, in a wheel. South Korea's food guide is shaped as a pagoda; the Philippines', a six-pointed star.

● Food guides reflect a culture's foods. The Chinese pagoda includes advice: more whole grains (since white rice is the main grain), and milk and bean products daily. Panama's food guide advises sufficient root vegetables. Zimbabwe's four-food-group square includes insects as one protein-rich food. Japan's six food groups recommend thirty different foods daily.

● Food guides address healthful eating for a range of individuals. That's why Canada's rainbow advises a wide range of servings—five to ten each day—for fruits and vegetables; fewer servings for young children and more for active teens and adults. Panama's food guide promotes breast-feeding for the first six months.

● Some food guides also focus on the pleasure of eating. Like many Asian food guides, the Philippine guide reminds people to savor their meals. The South Korean pagoda promotes harmony between diet and daily life. In the United Kingdom, the first guideline is "Enjoy your food."

Food Guide Pyramid
A Guide to Daily Food Choices

Fats, Oils, & Sweets
USE SPARINGLY

KEY
☐ Fat (naturally occurring and added)
▼ Sugars (added)

Milk, Yogurt, & Cheese Group
2–3 SERVINGS

Meat, Poultry, Fish, Dry Beans, Eggs, & Nuts Group
2–3 SERVINGS

Vegetable Group
3–5 SERVINGS

Fruit Group
2–4 SERVINGS

Bread, Cereal, Rice, & Pasta Group
6–11 SERVINGS

Source: U.S. Department of Agriculture/U.S. Department of Health and Human Services

Pyramid Power . . . For Variety, Balance, and Moderation

The Food Guide Pyramid conveys three main messages about healthful eating: variety, balance, and moderation.

● *For variety,* eat a variety of foods—fruits, vegetables, and grains—to get the nutrients you need. No one food supplies all the nutrients, fiber, and other substances your body needs. Variety also adds flavor, interest, and pleasure to meals!

● *For balance,* eat appropriate amounts—enough, but not too much—from each food group every day to get the nutrients and food energy your body needs. The range of servings for each group suggests how much based on age, gender, and activity level.

THE PYRAMID—FOR YOU

The Food Guide Pyramid is flexible and easily adapted to your individual food needs, regardless of age and culture.

- *Food Guide Pyramids with Popular Italian, Chinese, and Mexican Fare—see chapter 14.*
- *Food Guide Pyramid for Young Children—see chapter 16.*
- *Food Guide for Vegetarian Meal Planning—see chapter 20.*
- *Food Pyramid for Diabetes—see chapter 22.*

- *For moderation,* choose foods and beverages to meet your energy needs—without too much saturated fat, cholesterol, and added sugars. Moderation applies to alcoholic beverages, if you drink them. For example, to moderate fat, opt mostly for lower-fat choices. Eating in moderation helps you achieve or maintain a healthy weight and may help protect you from health problems such as diabetes, heart disease, and cancer later in life.

Although it's not in the Pyramid, remember taste, too! Healthful eating should add pleasure to your life!

Sizing Up Healthful Servings

How does your plate of pasta fit within the Pyramid? That large muffin you bought at the bakery? A deluxe fast-food burger? The refreshing 20-ounce fruit smoothie? An 8-ounce steak? A supersize soda? In this world of supersize portions from restaurants, delis, and convenience stores, many consumers are confused by serving sizes.

To follow Pyramid guidance and to eat enough calories to maintain a healthy weight, you need to know about servings: how many, what size, and how to use them. That's part of any strategy for smart eating.

Servings: Enough, but Not Too Much

The Food Guide Pyramid gives a range of servings, not a single amount. Being flexible, these guidelines help you choose enough servings to match your individual nutrient needs—without overdoing the calories and fat in your food choices.

Everyone age two or over needs at least the minimum servings daily from all five food groups. However, the specific number of servings for you depends on the amount of energy you need each day. The more energy (calories) your body uses, the more servings you need. If you're not very active, you probably need less. Your energy needs depend on your age, gender, health status, and level of physical activity.

Where do you fit within the serving ranges? The minimum servings from each food group can supply about 1,600 calories. That's about right for women who are less active and for some older adults. The midpoint in the serving ranges provides about 2,200 calories. That's an appropriate calorie target for children, teenage girls, active women, and less active men; women who are pregnant or breast-feeding may need somewhat more. Teenage boys, active men, and many athletes may eat from the top of the serving ranges, or about 2,800 calories. *For specific calorie recommendations for children and teenagers ages eleven to eighteen, see "The Pyramid for Teens" in chapter 16.*

Pyramid guidelines apply to young children (ages two and up). Like you, they need variety from all five food groups. But because their stomachs are small, younger children may not be able to eat the same size servings as older children and adults. While smaller servings are appropriate, to meet the energy needs of young children the total number of servings for the day should add up to the minimum Pyramid recommendations. For normal growth, their Milk Group servings should add up to two cups (16 ounces) of milk each day.

The chart "How Many Servings a Day for You?" in this chapter offers three plans—each at a different calorie level—for choosing a day's servings from the Pyramid. These plans are just guidelines. Your own choices probably will differ. Consume at least the minimum amount from each food group daily. If you don't need many calories, perhaps because you're not very active, aim for the minimum number of servings. *To estimate your energy needs, see "Your 'Weigh': Figuring Your Energy Needs" in chapter 2.*

Keep in mind that the Pyramid's recommendations do not change if you take a multivitamin supplement. Vitamin and mineral supplements are just what their name implies—supplements intended to supplement nutrients from the foods you eat. They don't replace

Need more specific strategies for healthful Pyramid eating? Check here for "how-tos":

- Shop the food groups in the supermarket—see chapter 11.
- Prepare food-group meals and snacks for the "health of it"—see chapter 13.
- Offer child-size servings to kids—see chapter 16.
- Adapt the Pyramid to vegetarian-style eating—see chapter 20.
- See how ethnic foods (Chinese, Italian, Mexican) fit into the Pyramid—see chapter 14.

food group servings. All healthy people need to follow food group guidelines first. Then, with the recommendation of a health professional, a supplement—not to exceed 100 percent of the Dietary Reference Intake for a nutrient—may be advised.

What Counts as One Serving?

What's one serving of fruit juice? Cooked pasta? Cheddar cheese? Raw salad greens? Ice cream? To make the Pyramid work, you need to know not only how many food-group servings you need daily, but also how much counts as a serving. In that way, your day's food choices will supply enough of the nutrients your body needs without overdoing it.

A food group isn't a helping, your portion, a plateful, or a small garnish. It's not the flavoring added to fruit-flavored yogurt or vegetable-flavored pasta (such as spinach pasta) either. And it's only sometimes the entire contents of one food package. Instead, food-group servings are specific, standardized amounts of food, meant to help you plan and judge your own portion size.

Serving sizes in the Pyramid differ among food groups, even among similar foods within food groups. The Pyramid's food group serving sizes are meant as general guides. It's okay to eat smaller or larger portions as long as you come close to the recommended totals on average over several days. If your portion is bigger than one food group serving, it counts as more than one serving; smaller amounts are partial food group servings. For example, one food group serving of cooked vegetables measures as $\frac{1}{2}$ cup. If you usually eat a $\frac{3}{4}$-cup portion of green beans, this counts as $1\frac{1}{2}$ food group servings of vegetables, and a $\frac{1}{4}$-cup portion counts as only $\frac{1}{2}$ serving.

HOW MANY SERVINGS A DAY FOR YOU?

FOOD GROUP	CHILDREN AGES 2 TO 6, MOST WOMEN, SOME OLDER ADULTS (ABOUT **1,600** CALORIES)*	OLDER CHILDREN, TEEN GIRLS, ACTIVE WOMEN, MOST MEN (ABOUT **2,200** CALORIES)*	TEEN BOYS, ACTIVE MEN (ABOUT **2,800** CALORIES)*
Grains Group, especially whole grains	6	9	11
Vegetable Group	3	4	5
Fruit Group	2	3	4
Milk Group—preferably fat-free or low-fat	2–3†	2–3†	2–3†
Meat and Beans Group—preferably lean or low-fat	2, for a total of 5 oz.	2, for a total of 6 oz.	3, for a total of 7 oz.

*These are the calorie levels if you choose low-fat, lean foods from the five major food groups and if you use foods from the fats, oils, and sweets group sparingly.
†Older children and teenagers (ages nine to eighteen) and adults over age fifty need three servings daily. During pregnancy and lactation, the recommended number of dairy group servings is the same as for nonpregnant women.
Source: Based on *Nutrition and Your Health: Dietary Guidelines for Americans* (2000).

Your Pyramid: Lopsided or Upside Down?

Does your Pyramid have a broad, firm base? Or is it distorted: lopsided, bulging in some spots, or turned upside down?

The base of the Pyramid is the foundation of healthful eating: plenty of grains, especially whole grains, fruits, and vegetables. Sugary and high-fat foods in the tiny Pyramid tip should be just a tiny portion of a healthful eating plan.

But many people don't eat that way! On average, Americans get 27 percent of their day's calories from fats, oils, and sweets at the tip of the Pyramid; 5 to 10 percent is probably enough! Choices from the Pyramid tip weigh you down with calories and fat, so the more you eat from the tip, the less room you may have for nutrient-rich, lower-calorie, and lower-fat foods from the five food groups.

The personal Pyramid for many Americans is distorted in another way! Vegetables, fruits, and calcium-rich dairy foods come up short. Besides their nutrients, the foods from these groups also supply fiber, antioxidants, and other substances that may protect you from heart disease, some cancers, osteoporosis, and other health problems.

The Nutrition Facts on a food label offers serving sizes, too. However, on food labels, the size may differ slightly from Pyramid servings. For example, on a Nutrition Facts label, a serving of cooked cereal, rice, or pasta is 1 cup; it's only ½ cup on the Pyramid. *"Get All the Facts!" in chapter 11 explains how serving sizes are used on food labels and how to use food labels to follow Pyramid advice.*

What's Inside the Pyramid?

Local foods, ethnic foods, your favorite foods, fast foods, snack foods, foods you grow yourself, supermarket foods—foods of every kind fit somewhere within the Food Guide Pyramid! Foods are grouped together because their nutrient content is similar. They promote health in comparable ways. In fact, each of the five food groups supplies your body with some, but not all, nutrients you need for energy, health, and for kids, growth.

Bread, Cereal, Rice, and Pasta Group (Grains Group)

The base of the Pyramid is filled with breads, cereals, rice, and pasta—all foods made from grains. Foods from plant sources, including foods from the Grains Group, are described as the foundation of the diet, perhaps because their complex carbohydrates are your body's best energy source. In fact, that's why six to eleven daily servings are recommended. *Read more*

Portion Distortion?

As restaurant portions and dinnerware get ever bigger, many people are clueless about sensible serving sizes. In fact, Americans tend to underestimate the amount they eat by 50 percent.

Today's megaportions promote: "eat until you feel stuffed, not just until you're satisfied." The problem? Adults and kids lose their ability to regulate how much they eat, as they listen less to hunger cues. Overeating leads to excess calories, fat, saturated fat, cholesterol, sodium, and added sugars. Besides leading to overweight, diet-related health risks go up with this approach to eating!

Not sure about the size of your helpings? Then take out the measuring cups and a kitchen scale. Serve typical helpings on a plate. Then measure or weigh them, and compare your portions to Pyramid servings. You might be surprised to find your helpings are bigger (maybe a lot bigger) or smaller than you think!

To overcome portion distortion and to downsize your helpings, try this:

● Get to know visual clues for servings. *See "Your Size Guide" on page 215.*

● Use smaller dishes, bowls, and cups, such as a lunch plate for your dinner, so less looks like more on your plate.

● Remember that meat, chicken, or fish don't need to take the biggest space on your plate. Let veggies, fruit, and grain products fill most of your plate.

● Eat from a plate, not a package, so you know how much you eat.

● Start with small helpings, and put the rest out of sight. Then eat slowly. Take a little more if you're still truly hungry.

For more ways to overcome supersizing, see the tips in chapters 11 and 14.

YOUR SIZE GUIDE

Do you know what 3 ounces of meat look like? How big is ½ cup of mashed potatoes or pasta . . . 1½ ounces of cheese . . . a serving of juice? To guesstimate the amount on your plate, get familiar with visual clues for Pyramid servings:

FOOD GROUP	ONE SERVING IS ABOUT THE SIZE OF . . .
Grains Group	1 slice bread, 1 pancake, or 1 waffle = stack of 3 computer diskettes
	1 cup dry cereal = baseball
	½ cup cooked pasta or rice = small computer mouse*
	1 bagel = hockey puck
	1 tortilla = 7-in. plate
	4 small cookies (vanilla wafers) = 4 casino chips
Vegetable Group	1 cup raw, leafy vegetables = baseball
	½ cup cooked vegetables = small computer mouse*
	10 French fries = deck of cards
	1 small potato = small computer mouse*
Fruit Group	½ cup sliced fruit = small computer mouse*
	1 medium fruit = baseball
	¾ cup juice = 6-oz. can
	¼ cup raisins = large egg
Milk Group	8 oz. glass of milk = small (8 oz.) milk carton
	8 oz. yogurt = baseball
	2 oz. cheese (mozzarella "sticks") = two Magic Markers
	1½ oz. hard cheese (Cheddar) = 2 9-volt batteries or a C battery
Meat and Beans Group	2 to 3 oz. meat, poultry, or fish = deck of cards *or* cassette tape
	2 tbsp. peanut butter = roll of film *or* Ping-Pong ball
	½ cup beans = small computer mouse*

*About the size of a deck of cards

about complex carbohydrates in "From Complex to Simple . . . " in chapter 5.

Grain products also supply B vitamins and iron (especially if they're enriched or whole grain), fiber, and other beneficial phytonutrients. Enriched means adding back nutrients that were lost in processing. Most grain products are enriched with B vitamins (thiamin, riboflavin, niacin) and iron and fortified with folic acid. The more whole grains or bran the foods contain, the higher the fiber content. Try to consume half your grain servings, or at least three servings daily, from whole-grain foods. Being plant sources of food, most grain products are low in fat and cholesterol. Exceptions are foods such as croissants, pastries, some crackers, and many muffins that are prepared with higher-fat and cholesterol-containing ingredients, as well as foods that are fried, such as doughnuts, hush puppies, fried rice, and regular tortilla chips. Remember, it's not bread, pasta, or rice that supplies fat, but instead what you serve with or put on them or how they're prepared!

Good news for health-conscious consumers: as long as you keep within your calorie level, consuming more complex carbohydrates, perhaps in place of a higher-fat food, helps to lower the percent of fat calories in your overall diet. *Consider the 2,200-calorie menu in "A Day's Menu for the Whole Family" in this chapter.* This menu gets 28 percent of its calories from fat. Just by choosing ¾ cup brown rice instead of ¾ cup French fries, the percentage of the calories from fat goes from 31 percent to 28 percent, even though the total calories consumed would be similar

The serving range—six to eleven servings from the Grains Group—may seem like a lot. But servings add up faster than many people realize. Starting with breakfast, one medium bagel counts as two Grains Group servings. (Depending on the size, a large bakery bagel can count for up to six Grains Group servings.) At lunchtime, a sandwich with two slices of whole-grain bread supplies two more servings. For dinner, ½ cup of rice pilaf and a dinner roll count as two servings. And for snacks, ½ cup of pretzels counts as one more serving. That's a total of seven Grains Group servings.

Pyramid Pointers

● Boost "carbs" by putting pasta, rice, or other Grains Group foods center stage at your meal or snack. Add flavor and interest with vegetables, small amounts of seafood, lean beef or skinless poultry, or fresh herbs.

● For fiber, choose foods made with whole grains (whole wheat, corn, multigrain) and bran each day: perhaps whole-grain bread, whole-grain cereal, bran flakes, oats, whole-grain corn, whole-wheat pasta, and brown rice. Recommendation: three whole-grain servings daily.

● Opt for breads made with less fat and added sugars, such as bagels, bread sticks, English muffins, Italian bread, hamburger buns, pita bread, or corn and flour tortillas. Go easy on those with more fat or sugars, such as croissants, doughnuts, and sweet rolls. Check the sodium content on the label, too.

● Try grain group foods that may be new to you, such as quinoa, buckwheat, millet, amaranth, or couscous. Enjoy grain-based salads, perhaps pasta salad, rice pilaf salad, or tabouli (made with bulgur). Or take your taste buds for northern Italian cuisine: enjoy risotto, made with arborio rice, or polenta, made with cornmeal. *See "Today's Grains" in chapter 9 for descriptions of various grains.*

● Look for crackers and crunchy snacks with less fat: air-popped popcorn, graham crackers, matzos, pretzels, rice cakes, saltines, breadsticks, zwieback, baked tortilla chips, and lower-fat crackers and cookies.

● Make ready-to-eat cereal or instant oatmeal a quick breakfast choice. Top with fresh fruit, yogurt, or milk for extra flavor and more nutrients.

Have You Ever Wondered ?

…where potato chips and corn chips fit in the Pyramid? Potato chips fit within the Vegetable Group, and corn chips fit within the Grains Group. Yet they're among those foods in the Pyramid groups that supply more fat and more calories per serving. Eating these foods occasionally is okay, but other foods in each food group supply more nutrients and less fat.

…if potatoes can substitute for bread since they're both high in complex carbohydrates? Potatoes are among the starchy vegetables that belong in the Vegetable Group. Breadfruit, cassava, corn, green peas, hominy, lima beans, rutabaga, taro, and yautia are some other starchy vegetables. Although high in complex carbohydrates, vegetables have a different nutrient and phytonutrient profile than foods in the Grains Group. Potatoes, for example, supply vitamin C, fiber, and a phytonutrient called quercetin, while many Grains Group foods supply some B vitamins, iron, fiber, and a phytonutrient called lignan.

● For sweet desserts from the Grains Group, choose angel food cake, gingersnaps, and low-fat cookies and cakes, which have less fat and sugar. Go easy on frosted cake, brownies, and pie.

● Snack on breadsticks, whole-wheat crackers, toasted pita bread points, or a bagel half. They're all good with vegetable dips or fruit spreads!

● Add cooked barley, other whole grains, rice, or pasta to soup, stir-fry dishes, or other mixed dishes.

● Check the ingredient list on food labels to find foods made with whole grains and to find grain products fortified with folic acid and other nutrients. *See "Which Bread Is Whole Grain?" in chapter 6 for ways to identify whole-grain foods.*

A Grains Group serving is . . .
● 1 slice enriched or whole-grain bread (1 ounce)
● ½ hamburger roll, bagel, pita bread, or English muffin
● 1 (6-inch) tortilla
● ½ cup cooked rice or pasta
● ½ cup cooked oatmeal, grits, farina, or Cream of Wheat cereal
● ½ cup cooked barley

- ½ cup cooked quinoa, bulgur, millet, or other whole grains
- 1 ounce (about 1 cup) ready-to-eat cereal
- 3–4 small crackers
- 1 (4-inch diameter) pancake or waffle
- 3 tablespoons wheat germ
- 2 medium cookies

Vegetable Group

How many Vegetable Group servings do you eat daily? And how many different vegetables do you eat regularly? The Food Guide Pyramid is filled with all kinds of varieties to choose from—*as you can see in the chart "Produce 'Package'" later in this chapter.*

Why eat a variety of vegetables? Different vegetables have different nutritional benefits. Dark-green leafy vegetables such as collard greens, broccoli, kale, and spinach are great sources of beta carotene, which your body converts to vitamin A, as well as vitamin C, folate, calcium, magnesium, and potassium. Deep yellow vegetables, such as sweet potatoes and carrots, supply beta carotene. Others, such as Brussels sprouts, bell peppers, and tomatoes, have more vitamin C. Many are rich in folate. Besides complex carbohydrates, starchy vegetables supply niacin, vitamin B_6, zinc, and potassium. Legumes provide protein as well as thiamin, folate, iron, magnesium, phosphorus, zinc, and potassium; and they also supply complex carbohydrates and fiber. *To learn about the phytonutrients in different vegetables, see "Phytonutrients—a 'Crop' for Good Health" in chapter 4 and "Paint Your Plate with Color" in chapter 13.*

Unless it's added during food preparation, vegetables have little or no fat, and they're cholesterol-free. In cases like the ever-popular French fries and fried onion rings, or salads with heavy dressing, the preparation methods or the toppings increase the fat content.

Vegetables are far more than a pretty garnish on a plate. For your good health, eat three to five servings from the Vegetable Group daily. If you're looking for nutritious, low-fat snacks, enjoy even more. This may be the place for a bigger portion!

Pyramid Pointers

- Eat a variety of types and colors of vegetables. Because vegetables supply varying amounts and types of nutrients, fiber, and other phytonutrients, variety makes good health sense.

- Eat a variety of dark green leafy and deep yellow vegetables (red, orange, and yellow), which supply carotenoids (such as beta carotene). Some carotenoids form vitamin A in your body. For example, make salads more interesting and more nutritious with a greater variety of darker greens: arugula, bibb lettuce, chicory, kale, leaf lettuce, romaine lettuce, spinach, and watercress. For fiber, keep the edible peels on vegetables such as potatoes, cucumbers, and summer squash.

- Enjoy the vegetables you've always eaten—just more of them! Broaden your personal vegetable menu beyond favorite standbys. Also try Brussels sprouts, Swiss chard, kale, parsnips, beets, bok choy, okra, and various squashes such as spaghetti, butternut, acorn, and dumpling squashes.

- Look for ways to add more vegetables to everyday meals. "Fortify" pasta dishes with steamed, sliced vegetables: zucchini, carrots, broccoli, and bell peppers. Add tomato or cucumber slices and sprouts to sandwiches. Tuck a can of tomato juice into your lunch or snack bag. Top a baked potato with vegetable salsa or stir-fried vegetables. Keep a bowl of cleaned, raw veggies in the refrigerator, ready for a quick nibble. *For more ways to "sneak" veggies in, see "Fruits and Vegetables: Food Prep for 'Five a Day'" in chapter 13.*

- If you want more legumes, enjoy some for Vegetable Group servings and others for Meat and Beans Group servings. Legumes have a "split personality." You can count them in either group, but the same bowl of beans can't count for two different food-group servings.

A Vegetable Group serving is . . .
- ½ cup chopped raw, nonleafy vegetables
- 1 cup leafy, raw vegetables (lettuce, spinach, watercress, or cabbage)
- ½ cup cooked vegetables
- ½ cup cooked legumes (beans, peas, or lentils)
- 1 small baked potato (3 ounces)
- ¾ cup vegetable juice

Fruit Group

What's in the fruit bowl? You'll find all of America's favorites: apples, oranges, and bananas. Some we

Have You Ever Wondered ?

. . . how much salsa counts as a serving? That depends on the ingredients. One-half cup of an all-vegetable salsa, perhaps made with beans, can count as one Vegetable Group serving. If the salsa is made with mango or another fruit, a ½-cup portion counts toward the Fruit and the Vegetable Groups. *Tip:* A squeeze of ketchup doesn't count as a vegetable serving.

. . . why "five a day" is advised for eating fruits and vegetables? Research shows that eating at least five servings of fruits and vegetables a day offers protection from 35 percent or more of all the causes of cancer. By eating more fruits and vegetables you may reduce your risk for heart disease and high blood pressure as well as other health problems.

How many Fruit Group servings do you need? The Pyramid recommends two to four servings daily. A versatile and "fast" food, whole fruits can be snacks, side dishes, or desserts. They may be sliced in a main-dish salad or in a meat, poultry, or seafood dish. Get your fruit servings from a variety of fruits and their juices.

Pyramid Pointers

● Every day, include vitamin C-rich fruit or fruit juice among your food choices: citrus fruits, berries, or melons.

● Keep frozen and canned fruit on hand, especially when many fruits are out of season.

● Go beyond the basics. Paint your plate with less common fruits: prickly pears, papayas, mangoes,

enjoy, yet eat less often: cherries, nectarines, pineapples, and honeydew melons. For more variety, the bowl has others you may rarely hear about, such as cherimoya, lychee, loquat, and mangosteen!

Like vegetables, Fruit Group foods supply varying amounts of carotenoids, including those that form vitamin A, as well as vitamin C, folate, potassium, fiber, and many other phytonutrients. *To learn about the phytonutrients in different fruits, see "Phytonutrients—a 'Crop' for Good Health" in chapter 4 and "Paint Your Plate with Color" in chapter 13.*

Citrus fruits (oranges, grapefruits, tangerines), melons, and berries are excellent sources of vitamin C. Many deep yellow fruits such as cantaloupes, apricots, mangoes, and peaches are rich in beta carotene (which forms vitamin A). Fruits, especially edible peels on apples, pears, peaches, other fruits, and dry fruits, provide fiber, too. Juices have little or no fiber. Many fruits also supply potassium and folate.

Fruit's sweet flavor comes from its natural sugar, a simple carbohydrate called fructose. Sometimes sugars are added to canned and frozen fruits and fruit juice as flavor enhancers or to help maintain quality. Since fruits are plant sources of food, most are low-fat and all are cholesterol-free. Not always thought of as fruits, avocados and olives contain fat—a monounsaturated fat. Avocados also supply beta carotene (which forms vitamin A).

What Are Cruciferous Vegetables . . . and What Do They Do?

A potential cancer-fighting benefit has focused attention on cruciferous vegetables. These members of the cabbage family derive their name from their four-petaled flowers, which look like a crucifer, or cross. They include a diverse selection of vegetables: arugula, bok choy, broccoli, Brussels sprouts, cabbage, cauliflower, collards, kale, kohlrabi, mustard greens, radishes, rutabaga, Swiss chard, turnip greens, turnips, and watercress.

Along with other vegetables and fruits, vegetables from the cabbage family may help protect against colorectal cancer. While the reasons are unclear, experts believe that cruciferous vegetables contain nutrients, compounds, and phytonutrients that seem to have a cancer-fighting component: beta carotene, fiber, and vitamin C, among others. Cruciferous vegetables also are fat-free. As an added bonus, cruciferous vegetables supply varying amounts of calcium, iron, and folate. For the potential benefits, try to consume cruciferous vegetables every day. The cabbage family of vegetables has something else in common: a strong cooking aroma. Proper food handling enhances the flavor of these vegetables without intensifying the aroma:

● Eat cruciferous vegetables soon after you buy them—raw or cooked.

● Cook them quickly, just until tender-crisp.

● Don't keep leftovers more than a day.

PRODUCE "PACKAGE"

Vegetables and fruits, each with a somewhat different combination of "good for you" components, are chock full of nutrients and phytonutrients. Here is a brief look at vegetables and fruits that are good* sources of several key nutrients and dietary fiber:

	CAROTENOIDS (VITAMIN A)	VITAMIN C	FOLATE	POTASSIUM	DIETARY FIBER
Vegetables					
Asparagus (½ cup)		X	X		
Beans, kidney (½ cup)			X	X	X
Beans, lima (½ cup)			X	X	X
Beets (½ cup)		X	X		
Black-eyed peas (½ cup)			X		X
Bok choy (½ cup)	X	X			
Broccoli (½ cup)	X	X	X		X
Brussels sprouts (½ cup)	X	X	X		X
Cabbage (½ cup)		X			
Carrots (½ cup)	X				X
Cauliflower (½ cup)		X			
Celery (½ cup)					
Chickpeas (garbanzos) (½ cup)			X		X
Collards (½ cup)	X	X			X
Corn (½ cup)					X
Cucumbers (½ cup)					
Eggplant (½ cup)					
Green beans (½ cup)		X			X
Green pepper (½ cup)		X			
Kale (½ cup)	X	X			
Lentils (½ cup)			X	X	X
Lettuce, iceberg (1 cup)					
Loose-leaf (l cup)	X	X			
Mushrooms, raw (½ cup)					
Okra (½ cup)		X	X		X
Onion (½ cup)					
Parsnips (½ cup)		X	X		X
Peas, green (½ cup)	X	X	X		X
Peas, split (½ cup)			X	X	X
Potato without peel (1 medium)		X		X	X
Potato, with peel (1 medium)		X		X	X
Spinach, cooked (½ cup)	X	X	X	X	X
Squash, winter (½ cup)	X	X		X	X
Sweet potato (1 medium)	X	X		X	X
Tomato (1 medium)	X	X			
Turnip greens (½ cup)	X	X	X		X
Turnips (½ cup)		X			
Zucchini (½ cup)		X			

PRODUCE "PACKAGE" (continued)

	CAROTENOIDS (VITAMIN A)	VITAMIN C	FOLATE	POTASSIUM	DIETARY FIBER
Fruits					
Apple, with skin (1)		X			X
Apricot, dried (3)	X	X			X
Avocado (1 medium)	X	X	X	X	X
Banana (1)		X		X	X
Blueberries (½ cup)		X	X		X
Cantaloupe (½ cup)	X	X			
Figs (2 medium)					X
Grapes (½ cup)					
Grapefruit (½)		X			
Grapefruit juice (¾ cup)		X			
Honeydew melon (½ cup)		X		X	
Kiwi (1 medium)		X			X
Mango (1 medium)	X	X			X
Orange (1)		X	X		X
Orange juice (¾ cup)		X	X	X	
Papaya (½ cup)		X	X	X	X
Peach (1 medium)		X			
Pear with skin (1)		X			X
Pineapple (½ cup)		X			
Plantain, cooked (½ cup)	X	X		X	
Plum (1 medium)		X			
Prune juice (¾ cup)		X		X	X
Prunes (dried plums) (4)	X				X
Strawberries (½ cup)		X			
Watermelon (1 cup)	X	X			

Note: A good source of a vitamin or mineral contributes at least 10 percent of its Daily Value (DV) in a selected serving size. A source of dietary fiber contributes at least 2 grams of dietary fiber in a selected serving size.

starfruit, figs, kiwis, or guavas. Try new-to-you varieties of apples, pears, plums, or melons.

● Keep dried fruits—raisins, dried plums (prunes), dried apricots, dried apple slices, dried cranberries—handy for healthful nibbling and pack-and-carry meals. Be aware: serving sizes of dried fruits are smaller than for fresh fruit because they don't have water; drying concentrates the calories and the nutrient content.

● Drink fruit juice as a snack beverage. Mix with sparkling water for a refreshing fizz.

● Enjoy a fruit smoothie from a fast-food restaurant, or make one at home. Just blenderize cut-up fruit (canned, fresh, or frozen), juice, and perhaps yogurt, frozen yogurt, or milk.

● Add fruits to all kinds of dishes. Toss orange slices, tangerine segments, grape halves, berries, and other fresh fruits with garden salads. Add crushed pineapple, raisins, or chopped apples to coleslaw. Sprinkle dried fruits of all kinds on breakfast cereal, pudding, or frozen yogurt. Blend them with stuffing and rice dishes. Or mix them in batters and doughs for homemade muffins and breads.

● Enjoy fruit as a sweet ending to your meals.

A Fruit Group serving is . . .

- 1 medium fruit (apple, orange, banana, or peach)
- ½ grapefruit, mango, or papaya
- ¾ cup fruit juice
- ½ cup berries or cut-up fruit
- ½ cup canned, frozen, or cooked fruit
- ¼ cup dried fruit

Milk, Yogurt, and Cheese Group (Milk Group)

Besides milk, foods made from milk—yogurt, cheese, cottage cheese, buttermilk, frozen yogurt, and ice cream—as well as pudding and milkshakes, all belong in the Milk Group.

Milk, yogurt, and cheese are our body's best sources of calcium and riboflavin. Without dairy foods, getting enough calcium for bone health can be difficult. Many dairy foods also are good sources of protein, phosphorus, potassium, vitamin A, and vitamin D.

The amount of fat and cholesterol in dairy foods varies. Fat-free (skim) milk contains 0.5 percent fat or less. Low-fat or light milk, or 1 percent milk, has 50 percent less fat than whole milk. Reduced-fat milk, or 2 percent milk, has 25 percent less fat than whole milk. And whole milk contains 3.25 percent fat. These percentages refer to the amount of fat by weight, not calories. *For the fat and cholesterol content of various types of milk, see "Milk: A Good Calcium Source" in this chapter.*

The many varieties of cheese vary slightly in fat content, although low-fat, reduced-fat, and fat-free varieties contain considerably less fat. Dairy foods with less fat usually have less cholesterol, too. Regardless of the fat content, the amounts of other nutrients—calcium, protein, phosphorus, and vitamin D—remain about the same.

Dairy foods may contain two types of sugars: naturally occurring sugar called lactose, and added sugars. Any added sugars in dairy foods come from flavorings such as those added to ice cream, flavored yogurt, and flavored milk.

A few dairy foods don't belong in this Pyramid group: butter, cream, cream cheese, and sour cream. These are made from the cream that naturally separates from unhomogenized milk. Unlike Milk Group foods, these foods contribute only small amounts of minerals, vitamins, and protein to the diet. Because they're high in fat, they belong with fats, oils, and sweets in the Pyramid tip.

Many people—teens and adult women especially—neglect the Milk Group. The Pyramid advises two to three Milk Group servings daily. However, nutrition experts suggest more to meet the calcium needs of older children, teens, and adults over age fifty.

Pyramid Pointers

- Look for ways to include calcium-rich Milk Group foods in meals and snacks: milk on breakfast cereal, cheese on a sandwich, yogurt dips with veggies, coffee au lait (with milk) or latte, shredded cheese on soups and salads, or cottage cheese as a side dish. Try flavored milk (chocolate, strawberry, or other flavors) if you prefer.

- Include calcium-rich dairy foods at snacktime. Yogurt, milk, and cheese cubes are three good choices. Dessert offers another chance; try frozen yogurt or pudding. Individual portions of pudding are easy to take along.

- Use evaporated fat-free (skim) milk instead of cream in coffee, on cereals, whipped as a topping, and in recipes calling for cream. Evaporated fat-free milk has a creamy texture and less fat, though it's light yellow in color.

Have You Ever Wondered

. . . where fortified foods fit on the Food Guide Pyramid? Fortified foods fit in the same food group as their unfortified counterparts. With their added nutrients, they simply provide a nutritional bonus. For example, calcium-fortified orange juice can't replace one Milk Group serving, since calcium is just one nutrient in milk. As with any juice, ¾ cup counts as one serving from the Fruit Group—with an added calcium bonus.

. . . if fruit drinks count as Fruit Group servings? No, even if fruit juice is one ingredient. Many fruit-flavored drinks fit in the Pyramid tip because they're actually water with fruit flavor and added sugars. Even a fortified drink made with a small percent of real juice won't supply all the nutrients, such as folate, that 100 percent juice contains.

● Add Milk Group servings by using plain, low-fat, or fat-free yogurt or cottage cheese (processed in a blender) in recipes as a substitute for sour cream.

● As a beverage alternative, drink thick and creamy buttermilk. Even with its "buttery" name, it's low in fat. Usually it's made from fat-free or low-fat milk.

● Start your day with dairy: yogurt or a yogurt-fruit smoothie with breakfast.

● Buy a carton of milk to go with food from a deli or fast-food restaurant.

● If you choose to avoid dairy foods, get your calcium from calcium-fortified beverages (juice and soy drinks) and other nondairy foods such as vegetables that are good calcium sources.

A Milk Group* serving is . . .

● 1 cup milk (flavored or unflavored) or buttermilk

● 1 cup yogurt

● ½ cup evaporated milk

● ⅓ cup dry milk

● 1 cup calcium-fortified soy beverage

● 1½ oz. natural cheese (Cheddar, mozzarella, Swiss, Monterey Jack)

● ½ cup ricotta cheese

● 2 oz. processed cheese (American)

Count ½ cup frozen yogurt or 1 cup cottage cheese as ½ serving. Count ½ cup ice cream as ⅓ serving.

*This includes lactose-free and lactose-reduced milk products. For any Milk Group food, choose fat-free or reduced-fat dairy products most often.

Meat, Poultry, Fish, Dry Beans, Eggs, and Nuts Group (Meat and Beans Group)

Even though we use its shortcut name, the Meat and Beans Group is much more than meat and beans! It's filled with a variety of foods, all excellent sources of protein: beef, veal, pork, chicken, turkey, finfish, shellfish, game, eggs, dry beans (legumes, lentils, and peas), soybean products (tofu, tempeh, soyburgers, and others), nuts, seeds, and peanut butter.

Besides protein, Meat and Beans Group foods supply varying amounts of iron, zinc, and B vitamins (thiamin, niacin, and vitamins B_6 and B_{12}). In fact, meat, poultry, and fish are some of the body's best sources of iron. The iron, called heme iron, in these foods is better absorbed than iron from plant sources of food. Looking at the symbols on the Food Guide Pyramid, you see that the Meat and Beans Group also is a source of dietary fat. Lean meat and skinless (not fried) poultry are lower-fat choices. But because they're animal products, meat and poultry also have varying amounts of cholesterol. Finfish—for example, flounder, cod, haddock, and catfish—have less fat, including less saturated fatty acids, and cholesterol than meat and poultry do, while shellfish tends to be very low in saturated fat and somewhat higher in cholesterol than finfish. Fatty varieties of fish (such as salmon, mackerel, swordfish, and herring) have another benefit—more omega-3 fatty acids. *See "Eat Your Omega-3s and -6s" in chapter 3.*

Milk: A Good Calcium Source*

Milk	Calories	Calcium (mg)	Fat (g)	Cholesterol (mg)
8 oz. . . .				
Buttermilk	100	285	2	10
Unflavored milk				
Fat-free	85	300	<1	5
1% low-fat	100	300	3	10
2% reduced-fat	120	295	5	20
Whole	150	290	8	35
Chocolate milk				
1% low-fat	160	285	2	5
2% reduced-fat	180	285	5	15
Whole	210	280	8	30
4 oz. . . .				
Eggnog	170	165	10	75
Evaporated milk				
Fat-free (skim)	100	370	<1	5
Whole	170	330	10	35
Sweetened				
condensed milk	490	430	13	50

*Figures are rounded.
Source: National Dairy Council.

Even though they're plant sources of food, dry beans—legumes and lentils—are part of the Meat and Beans Group. The reason? They're excellent sources of protein. Combined with grains, their protein is complete enough to substitute for protein from meat, poultry, or fish. Legumes also are a great source of complex carbohydrates, fibers, and other phytonutrients, and they're cholesterol-free and virtually fat-free! While nuts and nut butters supply protein and some vitamins, they're higher in fat (mostly unsaturated) and calories. Legumes actually lead a double life. One-half cup of dry beans can count toward the Vegetable Group or the Meat and Beans Group.

How much do you need from the Meat and Beans Group? Two to three servings per day (about 5 to 7 ounces) provide enough protein for most people. This may surprise people who sometimes eat much more.

Pyramid Pointers

● Include a variety of Meat and Beans Group foods—lean meat, skinless poultry, fish, and legumes.

● Enjoy fish two or three times a week. Include some fatty fish.

● Consider the size of meat and poultry portions. Usually, a portion that fills about one-quarter of your plate is enough. Remember, you need only 5 to 7 ounces a day. While it's okay to occasionally eat large portions of meat or poultry, an 8- or a 12-ounce steak probably is more than you need at one sitting.

● Make legumes—dry beans, peas, lentils—or tofu the "center of your plate" several times a week. Try vegetarian chili or lasagna, vegetable tofu stir-fry, or a bowl of bean soup—or mix canned legumes with a vegetable salad.

● Enjoy eggs as a meat alternate. To control cholesterol, eat egg yolks and whole eggs in moderation—up to one a day if you keep your total cholesterol intake under 300 milligrams daily. That includes eggs used in prepared and baked foods. Since egg whites and egg substitutes have no cholesterol and little or no fat, you may use them freely. You can use egg substitutes or egg whites in recipes that ask for whole eggs.

● Eat nuts and nut butters in moderate amounts. Just a small handful adds variety to meals and snacks. For example, tossed chopped nuts into a vegetarian stir-

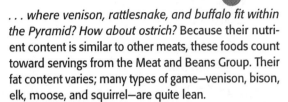

Have You Ever Wondered

. . . where venison, rattlesnake, and buffalo fit within the Pyramid? How about ostrich? Because their nutrient content is similar to other meats, these foods count toward servings from the Meat and Beans Group. Their fat content varies; many types of game—venison, bison, elk, moose, and squirrel—are quite lean.

Ostrich tastes like red meat, even though it's poultry. From a nutritional standpoint, it's quite lean—fewer than 3 grams of fat in 3 ounces, which is less than chicken with skin and beef round. It's also a good source of protein and iron.

. . . if nuts are okay on a low-fat diet? You bet! Although higher in fat than many other Meat and Beans Group foods, nuts contain mostly unsaturated fat. Although high in calories, nuts are cholesterol-free and provide good sources of protein, phosphorus, zinc, and magnesium, as well as vitamin E and selenium (two antioxidant nutrients). They have phytonutrients such as omega-3 fatty acids, which may have other health benefits. As long as portions are small, they're a healthful choice within the Meat and Beans Group—especially for people on strict vegetarian eating plans.

fry, casserole, salad, or pasta dish. Or sprinkle some on your morning cereal or lunchtime yogurt.

A Meat and Beans Group serving is . . .

● 2 to 3 ounces cooked lean meat, poultry, or fish (4 ounces raw meat, poultry, or fish equal 3 ounces when cooked)

● 2 to 3 ounces lean sliced deli meat (turkey, ham, beef, or bologna)

● 2 to 3 ounces canned tuna or salmon, packed in water

. . . for a total of 5 to 7 ounces each day.

Count as 1 ounce meat:

● ½ cup cooked lentils, peas, or dry beans

● 1 egg

● ¼ cup egg substitute

● 2 tablespoons peanut butter

● 1/3 cup nuts

● ½ cup tofu

● 2½-ounce soyburger

Count as 2 ounces meat:

- ½ cup tuna or ground beef
- 1 small chicken leg or thigh
- 2 slices sandwich-size meat

Count as 3 ounces meat:

- 1 medium pork chop
- ¼-pound hamburger patty
- ½ chicken breast
- 1 unbreaded 3-ounce fish filet
- Cooked meat, about the size of a deck of cards

Fats, Oils, and Sweets

What's in the tip of the Pyramid? Salad dressings, oils, cream, butter, gravy, margarine, cream cheese, sugars, soft drinks (soda or pop), fruit drinks, jams and jellies, candies, sherbet, gelatin desserts, and bacon and pork rinds. In small amounts, they add flavor and pleasure to your meals and snacks.

As the symbols on the Pyramid show, foods in the Pyramid tip have high proportions of naturally occurring or added fats, or added sugars, or both. Because they supply mostly calories and few nutrients, the guideline is: use fats, oils, and sweets sparingly. For this reason, no serving ranges or serving sizes are given.

Pyramid Pointers

- Limit dressing on salads to 1 or 2 tablespoons, or switch to low-fat or fat-free varieties.
- Go easy on fatty or sugary spreads, toppings, gravies, and sauces that add fat or sugars to foods from all five food groups.
- Go easy on cream cheese, sour cream, and margarine—or try low-fat varieties. Cream cheese and sour cream are also sold in fat-free versions.
- Enjoy soft drinks, fruit drinks, and candies occasionally, if you like.
- Skip the sugar and the cream in coffee or tea, or use less sugar and cream. Use a sugar substitute, fat-free half-and-half, or milk instead.

Build Your Personal Pyramid

Eating smart isn't just for today! To keep fit, you need to make wise food choices for a lifetime. *To see how your food choices stack up, take the nutrition checkup "How Did You Build Your Pyramid?" on page 225.* If you need to make changes, here's how to start eating smarter:

1. *Modify your food choices gradually.* That may be easier than overhauling your whole eating plan at one time. Perhaps start with one meal or snack . . . or try working with just one food group for a few months. Then move on gradually from there.

2. *Choose foods each day from the five major food groups.* Build your Pyramid from the bottom up—with plenty of grains, fruits, and vegetables. And fit in some low-fat dairy foods and lean or low-fat foods from the Meat and Beans Group each day.

How might your dinner plate look? Divide your plate into four sections. Fill three sections with vegetables, fruits, and grains, and the fourth with a serving from the Meat and Beans Group. Then add a glass of low-fat milk.

Do you avoid all foods from any of the five food groups (perhaps as a strict vegetarian)? *If so, see chapter 20, "The Vegetarian Way," for tips on filling your plate for health and flavor!* Or seek advice from a registered dietitian.

Pizza: What Food Group?

Pizza, fajitas, lasagna, and cioppino (fish stew) . . . many foods don't fit neatly into a single food group. Prepared with ingredients from several food groups, mixed foods count as partial servings from two or more food groups. Use your best guesstimate to determine how many servings they represent.

Pizza, topped with ground beef, cheese, tomato sauce, and green peppers, offers a good example. The crust counts toward the Grains Group, and the toppings add partial servings to the Meat and Beans Group, the Milk Group, and the Vegetable Group. If you change the toppings—perhaps to a Hawaiian pizza with ham (Meat and Beans Group) and pineapple (Fruit Group)—food group servings change.

For fajitas, chicken or beef (Meat and Beans Group) is stir-fried with peppers and onions (Vegetable Group) and served inside a soft tortilla (Grains Group). The cioppino, with its seafood and vegetables, counts toward the Meat and Beans Group and the Vegetable Group.

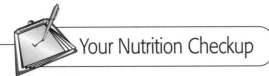
How Did You Build Your Pyramid?

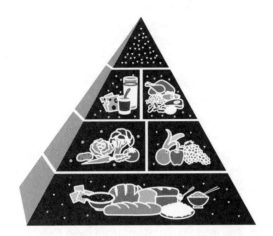

Step One. Jot down all the foods and beverages you consumed yesterday for meals and snacks. Include the portion size and where it fits on the Pyramid.

	FOODS AND BEVERAGES	PORTION SIZE	FOOD GROUP(S) OR PYRAMID TIP
Breakfast			
Lunch			
Dinner			
Snacks			

Step Two. Approximate your calorie level using the chart "How Many Servings a Day for You?" earlier in this chapter.

I need about _____ calories a day.

Step Three. Total the number of servings you consumed from each food group. Then compare the number of servings you consumed with the serving amounts on page 211. Remember, if your portion is bigger than one Pyramid serving, it counts as more than one serving; smaller servings count as partial servings. *Pyramid serving sizes are listed earlier in this chapter.*

HOW MANY SERVINGS ARE RIGHT FOR YOU?	HOW MANY SERVINGS DID YOU CONSUME?
(circle one)	
Grains Group	
6 7 8 9 10 11	_____
Vegetable Group	
3 4 5	_____
Fruit Group	
2 3 4	_____
Milk Group	
2 3	_____
Meat and Beans Group (oz.)	
5 6 7	_____

Step Four. Take a few moments to look at your food record. Write down some changes you could make for a healthier eating style. You might start with small changes, such as adding an extra serving of vegetables or using less dressing on your salad, then make more changes gradually until healthful eating becomes your habit. Or if you do best by making major changes, it's okay to do them all at once . . . as long as you succeed over time.

Source: Adapted from "The Food Guide Pyramid," *Home and Garden* bulletin 252 (Washington, D.C.: U.S. Department of Agriculture/

3. *Make moderation, not elimination, your goal.* Eat foods lower in fat and calories more often than those that have more. Make trade-offs to keep your meals and snacks in balance. It's okay to enjoy fats and sweets occasionally, as long as you go easy.

4. *Go for variety within the food groups.* Take your taste buds on an adventure by trying new foods. Besides the nutritional benefits, food variety makes meals and snacks more interesting and tasty.

5. *Consider your lifestyle . . .* and how much food energy you need daily. Then, from each food group, eat enough servings—at least the minimum daily—to maintain a healthy weight.

The beauty of the Food Guide Pyramid is its flexibility. As you get older or as your lifestyle, health condition, or activity level change, simply adjust how many servings you eat. Or pick different food-group foods.

Source: Adapted from *The Food Guide Pyramid: Your Personal Guide to Healthful Eating* (International Food Information Council Foundation, U.S. Department of Agriculture/Center for Nutrition Policy and Promotion, and Food Marketing Institute, 2000).

Health-Wise Eating Strategies

Do you prefer a hearty breakfast or a light morning bite? A big meal at lunchtime or at dinner? Snacks or no snacks? Three meals a day or several mini-meals? There's no one pattern for smart eating. However, following are some strategies to help you and your family follow Pyramid guidelines.

Quick, Easy Trade-offs

Are some of your favorite foods higher in fat, sugars, calories, or salt? You don't need to give up your favorite foods—just trade them off!

What is a trade-off? It's simply considering your food choices over the course of the day. In other words, if you choose foods higher in fats, sugar, or salt sometimes, then choose foods with less fats, sugar, or salt at other times. At the same time, keep within nutrient and Pyramid guidelines for your good health. Just watch how much and how often you consume different types of foods, especially those high in fats, sugars, or salt. Remember, your goal isn't to eliminate foods, but to moderate and balance your day's meal and snack choices.

Trading off . . .

Consider these easy trade-offs, then apply the strategies. Remember, when you trade off for fat, you trade off for calories, too.

. . . for fat

● Enjoy a baked potato (without a high-fat topping) for supper rather than French fries to save on fat. Spend some of the savings on a small dish of ice cream for dessert.

● Top homemade pizza with reduced-fat, rather than regular, mozzarella. Then spend some of the savings on cookies and milk later in the day.

. . . for sugars

● Top French toast with sliced fresh peaches rather than syrup. Fruit contains natural sugars along with carotenoids (vitamin A) and vitamin C; the syrup likely has sugars only.

● Enjoy fruit canned in natural juices as a snack, rather than fruit packed in syrup, to save on calories. Then use those calories on jam or honey on your dinner biscuit.

To make trading off easier, read the Nutrition Facts on food labels.

Meal Skipping: Poor Option!

People give all kinds of excuses for skipping meals: "no time," "nothing to eat," "tied up in meetings," "had to work out instead," "didn't bring any cash," "woke up too late," "eating alone is no fun," "on a diet," and "not hungry," among others.

As a regular habit, skipping or skimping on meals usually catches up with you. For one thing, meal skipping usually affects productivity: less concentration, more difficulty with problem solving, and increased fatigue—serious problems for children and adolescents. Often, meal skipping leads to missed food-group servings and nutrients during the day, too. If you have to skip a meal, try to make up for what you missed during other meals or with snacks. Moreover, skipped meals often lead to overeating at snacktime or the next meal. The bottom line is this: skipping meals doesn't make good nutrition sense!

Quick-to-Fix Meal Tips

Like most of today's consumers, you may spend forty-five minutes or less preparing a family meal (compared with 2½ hours forty years ago). In fact, marketing research shows that 60 percent of American women want to spend less than fifteen minutes preparing a meal! Like others, you may not decide on the menu until the end of the workday. Sound familiar? When time is short, don't give up on healthful eating. Just take shortcuts to save time and energy!

● When you have time to cook, make a double or a triple batch. For example, simmer enough pasta for two days. Serve it hot on one night with meat sauce, then chilled for a salad with tuna, parsley, and low-fat salad dressing the next.

● Buy prepared foods for "speed scratch" cooking: for example, grated cheese; precut stir-fry vegetables; shredded cabbage; skinless chicken strips; mixed salad greens; prewashed spinach; and chopped onion. Even thin-sliced, lean deli meat is quick for stir-fried recipes.

Often more costly, "meal solutions" sold in many of today's supermarkets simply need to be cooked, heated, or assembled on your plate. Just make a simple side dish, perhaps a tossed salad—and you're ready to eat!

● Plan ahead: prepare ingredients ahead of time yourself. For example, wash and trim broccoli florets. Skewer kebobs with vegetable and meat pieces the night before. Cook lean ground meat ahead for soft tacos.

● Stock your kitchen with quick-to-fix foods: pasta, rice, frozen and canned vegetables, canned fruits, bread, lean deli meats, salad ingredients, salsa, canned beans, milk, yogurt, and cheese, among others.

● Cook on weekends; save food "prep" time on weekdays. Freeze leftovers in individual meal containers for quick thawing midweek.

● Use quick cooking methods. Stir-frying, broiling, grilling, and microwaving usually are faster than baking or roasting. Slice meat and poultry in thinner slices for faster cooking.

● Use cooking equipment to cut food preparation time. Rinse and dry vegetables in a salad spinner. Slice hard-cooked eggs and mash avocados with a pastry blender. Shred small amounts of cheese with a vegetable peeler. Crush crackers (in a plastic bag) with a rolling pin. Thaw foods quickly in a microwave oven.

● Prepare meals that pack variety in just one dish. Try chicken fajitas in a soft taco. Stuff tuna and vegetable salad into a pita pocket. Prepare a ham and spinach quiche. Make a chef's salad requiring no cooking at all. Or prepare risotto with seafood, Swiss chard, and shredded cheese, or stir fry with noodles, tofu, and vegetables.

● Keep a variety of prepared foods on hand. Check the Nutrition Facts on the food label to choose those that match your family's nutrition needs. Prepare them along with fresh foods—for example, prepared pasta sauce heated with cooked ground meat, then served over pasta or a microwave-baked potato. Or try a heat-and-eat pot roast sold in the meat case of the supermarket; just serve with a microwaved potato and green beans.

● Serve assemble-your-own menus: perhaps deli sandwiches, minipizzas on English muffins, or burgers with veggies and cheese toppings that your family can assemble in your kitchen.

Breakfast: Off to a Healthy Start!

You've heard it many times before: breakfast is the healthful way to start the day. Forty years of breakfast-related studies show that jump-starting the day with breakfast benefits everyone—children, teens, and adults.

However, despite its benefits, breakfast may be the meal most often neglected and skipped. Some people

---

Does Your Dinner Pass the Tests?

● *The "Color Crunch" Test.* Try to choose foods with a variety of colors and textures at each meal.
● *The Pie Test.* Think of your plate as a pie: 75 percent of the pie is made of fruits, vegetables, and grains; 25 percent of other foods, such as dairy products or other protein foods.
● *The Five-a-Day Test.* Five servings of vegetables and fruits each day are important for your good health. Count them as you go along.

Source: American Dietetic Association.

A Day's Menu for the Whole Family

Food Choices	1,600 Calories (Child 4-6 Yrs.)	2,200 Calories (Active Mom)	2,800 Calories (Active Dad)
Breakfast			
Bran flakes	1 oz.	1 oz.	1 oz.
topped with low-fat fruit yogurt or 1% milk	½ cup	½ cup	½ cup
Whole-wheat toast	½ slice	1 slice	2 slices
with jam	2 tsp.	1 tbsp.	1 tbsp.
Orange juice	¾ cup	¾ cup	¾ cup
Coffee	0	6 oz.	6 oz.
Lunch			
Sandwich with			
Rye bread	1 slice	2 slices	2 slices
Lean beef	1 oz.	2 oz.	2½ oz.
Colby cheese	0	1 oz.	1 oz.
Lettuce	¼ cup	¼ cup	¼ cup
Tomato	1 slice	1 slice	1 slice
Mustard	1 tsp.	1 tsp.	1 tsp.
Broccoli florets	½ cup	½ cup	1 cup
Banana	½	1	1
Milk, 1%	1 cup	1 cup	1 cup
Snack			
Grapes	½ cup	½ cup	1 cup
Peanuts	⅓ cup	⅓ cup	⅓ cup
Dinner			
Broiled chicken (skin removed)	3 oz.	3 oz.	4 oz.
Herbed brown rice	½ cup	1 cup	1 cup
Carrot coins	½ cup	¾ cup	¾ cup
Tossed green salad	1 cup	1 cup	1 cup
with low-fat dressing	1 tbsp.	1 tbsp.	1 tbsp.
Whole-wheat roll with	1	1	2
margarine or butter	1 tsp.	1 tsp.	2 tsp.
Angel food cake	1 slice	1 slice	1 slice
Milk, 1%	1 cup	1 cup	1 cup
Snack			
Oatmeal cookies	2	2	2
Food Group Servings			
Grains	6	9	11
Vegetable	3½	4	5
Fruit	2½	3	4
Milk	2½	3	3
Meat and Beans	5 oz.	6 oz.	7 oz.
Fat grams	47 g	74 g	93 g

blame their body clock for not feeling hungry when they wake up. With today's hectic lifestyles, others come up short on time and energy first thing in the morning. And some falsely believe that skipping breakfast offers an effective strategy for weight control.

Why Breakfast?

Breakfast is your body's early-morning refueling stop. After eight to twelve hours without a meal or a snack, your body needs to replenish its glucose, also called blood sugar. A new supply of food produces more glucose. The brain needs a fresh supply of glucose, its main energy source, because it has no stored reserves. Sustained mental work—in school or in the workplace—requires a large turnover of glucose in the brain. Your muscles also need a replenished blood glucose supply for physical activity throughout the day.

Actually, you may not feel hungry by midmorning if you skip breakfast. Conversely, you may feel hunger pangs even if you do eat early in the day. That's because your body reverts back to its normal metabolic response. Hunger pangs are a healthy signal. You need to respond to, not deny, them. Denying often leads to bingeing later.

Are you a breakfast skipper, skimper, or eater? According to research, breakfast skippers often feel tired, irritable, or restless in the morning. On the flip side, breakfast eating is associated with better attitudes toward work or school and higher productivity in the late morning, as well as better ability to handle tasks that require memory. Breakfast eaters tend to have more strength and endurance, and better concentration and problem-solving ability. What about breakfast skimpers? Eating even small amounts of food helps restore glucose stores.

The Nutrient Connection. Breakfast contributes Pyramid servings and nutritional benefits. The good news: total nutrient intake for the day is usually higher for those who eat a morning meal, especially for children and women. A whole-grain cereal, milk, and citrus juice can provide 100 percent of the vitamin C; 33 percent of the calcium, thiamin, and riboflavin; and 10 percent or more of your needs for fiber, iron, folate, and other nutrients for a day. Break-

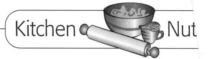

"Jazz Up" Cooked Cereal

For a "great grain" breakfast, add flavor and nutrition to cooked cereals (instant or not) such as oatmeal, Cream of Wheat, grits, rice, or couscous:

● Use fruit juice—apple, orange, or any other juice— or milk for some or all of the cooking liquid.

● To cooked cereal, blend in grated cheese, chopped fruit (apples, peaches, bananas, kiwis), dried fruit (chopped apricots, papaya, dates, raisins), or nuts.

● Fortify cooked cereal with dry milk for more calcium.

● Liven it up with spices: cinnamon, nutmeg, allspice, or cloves.

● Top it with fresh fruit of any kind!

fast skippers may never make up the nutrients they miss without a morning meal.

Breakfast and Learning. Breakfast prepares children and teens to meet the challenges of learning. Those who regularly eat a morning meal tend to perform better in school, often scoring higher on tests. While adults may condition themselves to overcome symptoms caused by breakfast skipping, children cannot. They experience the very real effects of transient, or short-term, hunger.

Nutrition experts note that morning hunger significantly affects learning since it reduces concentration, problem-solving ability, and muscle coordination. That's especially hard on young children because basic skills—reading, writing, and arithmetic—are often taught first thing in the morning. Consider the long-term effects of transient hunger on learning. When children can't reach their learning potential day after day, they can get farther and farther behind.

Kids who eat breakfast are more likely to be in the classroom. Stomach aches or hunger pangs caused by breakfast skipping or skimping are the main reason for morning visits to the school nurse. And breakfast skippers tend be tardy or absent from school more often. Breakfast eaters often behave better in school.

If your child doesn't eat breakfast at home, encourage school breakfast, if it's available to you. Many schools throughout the nation provide breakfast in the morning. *For more about school breakfast, see "For Kids Only—Today's School Meals" in chapter 16.*

Breakfast for Better Health. Among breakfast benefits: a jump start on your "five-a-day fruits and vegetables" and perhaps fiber-rich whole grains. Orange juice for breakfast offers more than vitamin C; it's also a good source of potassium, shown to lower the risk of high blood pressure and stroke. Whole-grain and other fiber-rich cereals and breads can boost soluble fiber and folate intake, also linked to heart health. Consuming enough folate, important for women of childbearing age, also reduces the risk of birth defects.

Studies suggest two other reasons for being a breakfast convert: weight control and reduced risk for heart disease. Breakfast eaters are less likely to be ravenously hungry for midmorning snacks or lunch; overall they tend to eat less fat during the day, too. Compared to breakfast eaters, studies show that those who skip breakfast tend to have higher blood cholesterol levels, which is a risk factor for heart disease. Further research is needed to explore this link. For those who choose ready-to-eat breakfast cereals in the morning, their eating pattern typically has more vitamins and minerals, less total fat, saturated fat, and cholesterol, and fewer calories.

An Energizing Start

Even if you've committed to eating breakfast, consider this: what you choose for breakfast can make a difference in your energy level for the morning. When a breakfast consists mostly of sugary foods such as fruit, fruit juice, candy, or soft drinks, a quick rise in your blood sugar occurs, causing a surge in energy. After about an hour, blood sugar and energy decline, bringing on symptoms of hunger. This scenario is depicted on the left side of the figure below.

When a varied breakfast, consisting of foods containing carbohydrates, proteins, and fats, is consumed, a sustained release of energy occurs. This delays symptoms of hunger for several hours and maintains blood sugar levels. This scenario is depicted in the figure below at the right.

For more choices, see "Breakfast on the Road" in chapter 14.

Beating Breakfast Barriers

Every excuse or apparent barrier to breakfast actually has an easy solution! If you have kids, breaking breakfast barriers takes on another importance. You're their best role model for smart breakfast habits. Kids who see their parents eat breakfast are more likely to eat breakfast, too.

Not hungry in the early morning? Start with a light bite, perhaps juice or toast. Later, when you are hungry, have a nutritious midmorning snack: a hard-cooked egg, milk, yogurt, cheese, or a bagel. You can pack a breakfast that goes with you.

Short on time? Keep quick-to-fix foods on hand: breakfast cereal, instant breakfast mix, bagels, toaster

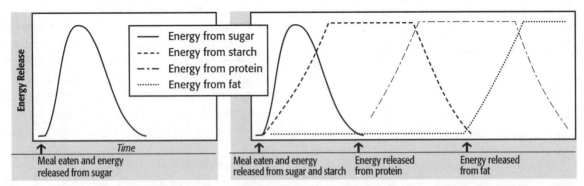

Sugary foods, such as fruit, fruit juice, candy, or soda pop, eaten in place of a meal cause a quick rise in blood sugar and energy. About an hour later, blood sugar and energy decline rapidly, bringing on symptoms of hunger.

A balanced breakfast containing sugar, starch, protein, and fat (like a typical school breakfast containing fruit or juice, toast or cereal, and 2 percent or whole milk) gives a sustained release of energy in children, delaying symptoms of hunger for several hours.

waffles, bread for toast, yogurt, canned and fresh fruit, juice, milk, cheese, and cottage cheese. Get breakfast foods ready the night before, such as mixing a pitcher of juice. Or plan on a breakfast that goes with you: a carton of yogurt; a bagel spread with peanut butter; or grapes, crackers, and cheese. If all else fails, set your alarm clock a few minutes earlier.

Think you'll gain weight? There's no evidence to support this belief. To be on the lean side, choose grain products, fruits, juice, lean meat, and lower-fat dairy foods. Go easy on higher-fat breakfast foods such as bacon, breakfast sausage, hash browns, and biscuits with gravy.

Don't like traditional breakfast foods? That's okay. Breakfast can be any food you like, even a slice of pizza, chicken sandwich, or soup. Leftover macaroni and cheese, heated in a microwave oven, makes a fine breakfast. Or try something new to make breakfast more interesting—perhaps a new yogurt flavor, or an exotic fruit on cereal. Just make your meal count

toward food-group servings. *For mo[...] "Easy Breakfasts for Kids to Make" i[...]*

That Snack Attack!

At the office, in the car, by the television set, at a sports event, in a movie theater—snacking is part of the American lifestyle. We often chide ourselves for between-meals nibbling, sometimes with good reason. Too often, people snack mainly on high-calorie, high-fat foods, then skimp on meals. Then they come up short on overall nutrition for the day—and perhaps overdo on calories.

Calcium is a case in point. Compared with moderate snackers, research suggests that people who frequently consume a lot of soft drinks and sugary snacks take in less calcium. They're likely substituting these foods for servings from the Milk Group, the best sources of calcium.

Carefully chosen, snacks promote good health and add pleasure to life. They can supply needed nutrients

---

SIMPLE "ONE MINUTE" BREAKFASTS

Each easy breakfast is packed with nutrients from three or more food groups.

G = Grains, **V** = Vegetable, **F** = Fruit, **M** = Milk, **MB** = Meat and Beans

Ready-to-eat cereal topped with sliced banana and yogurt	G	F	M
Bran muffin and yogurt topped with berries	G	M	F
Peanut butter or hummus on whole-wheat toast or soft tortilla, and milk	MB	G	M
Cheese pizza slice *and* orange juice	M	G	F
Instant oatmeal topped with dried cranberries and grated cheese	G	F	M
Breakfast smoothie (milk, fruit, and a teaspoon of bran, whirled in a blender)	M	F	G
Toasted whole-wheat waffle topped with fruit and yogurt	G	F	M
Toasted whole-wheat waffle topped with ricotta cheese, granola, canned peaches, and cinnamon	G	M	F
Bagel topped with fruit chutney, baby carrots, *and* milk	G	V	M
Lean ham on a toasted English muffin, vegetable juice	MB	G	V
Low-fat yogurt with granola or wheat germ, and cut-up fruit mixed in	M	G	F
Heated leftover rice mixed with beans, peppers, and cilantro, *and* vegetable juice	G	MB	V
Heated leftover rice with chopped apples, nuts, and cinnamon, *and* fruit juice	G	F	MB
Breakfast wrap with cut-up fresh or canned fruit and low-fat cream cheese rolled in a whole-wheat tortilla, *and* chocolate milk	F	G	M

TWO-FOOD-GROUP SNACKS

Each easy snack is packed with nutrients from two food groups.

G = Grains, **V** = Vegetable, **F** = Fruit, **M** = Milk, **MB** = Meat and Beans

● Whole-grain cereal and milk	G	M
● Fruit smoothie (fruit or juice blended with milk or yogurt)	F	M
● Yogurt and fresh fruit	M	F
● Peanut butter on whole-wheat crackers	MB	G
● Pita bread and hummus (chickpea dip)	G	MB
● Apple or pear slices topped with cheese	F	M
● Bagel chips (oven-baked) and salsa	G	V
● Dried cranberry and peanut mix	F	MB
● Pita bread stuffed with lettuce, tomato, cucumber, and low-fat salad dressing	G	V
● Raw veggies with a cottage cheese or yogurt dip	V	M
● Light microwave popcorn and fruit juice	G	F
● Quesadilla (soft tortilla and cheese, folded and heated)	G	M
● Flaked tuna and chopped celery tossed with low-fat mayonnaise	M	V
● Microwave-baked potato topped with salsa and cheese shreds	V	M

---

such as vitamins A and C, and calcium, as well as fiber and other phytonutrients, without adding too much fat or too many calories. If you haven't eaten for three or more hours, a snack may even help bring up your blood sugar.

For children and teens especially, snacks supplement meals. Because their stomachs are small, kids may need to eat more often than adults do, perhaps every three to four hours. Teenagers, who are active and growing rapidly, need the calories that snacks supply. *For more about snacking for kids and teens, see "Healthful, No-Cook Snacks for Kids" and "Great Snacking!" in chapter 16.* Adults may enjoy a snack as a break in the day and as a way to satisfy midday hunger. Older adults with small appetites or limited energy may find several small meals easier to handle. And almost everyone enjoys the social value of snacking with others.

Myths about Snacking

Despite what they know about nutrition, many people feel guilty about snacking. To them, snacks seem like a questionable extra, rather than a part of healthful eating. Good nutrition sense, however, challenges the popular myths about snacking.

Myth: Snacking makes you fat!

Fact: There's no direct link between snacking and body weight. The issue is total calories, not how often you eat. (Watch for megasize snack containers.) Your calorie, or energy, balance at the end of the day—based on the number of calories you ate and the number you burned—determines whether you gain, lose, or maintain weight.

Snacking, in fact, may have weight-control advantages. Eaten well before mealtime, snacks help take the edge off hunger, helping you avoid overeating at meals. Smart snackers choose foods carefully to match their calorie target—without going over.

Myth: Snacking causes cavities.

Fact: Frequent snacking can promote cavities. The longer teeth come in contact with food, particularly carbohydrate foods, the more time bacteria in plaque have to produce acids that damage tooth enamel.

However, you can control a plaque attack. Consume the whole snack at one time rather than nibble constantly. Then brush and/or floss when you finish snacking to remove food that sticks to and between teeth—or rinse your mouth with water to help remove food particles. Enjoy snacks such as Cheddar cheese with properties that protect teeth from cavity formation. *For more about oral health, see "Your Smile: Sugar and Oral Health" in chapter 5.*

Myth: Snacking gets in the way of good nutrition.

Fact: Snacks can contribute to a healthful eating style. Snack foods include any variety of foods and beverages from all five food groups. Food-group snacks help fill in the nutrition gaps from meals, helping to balance food choices for the day.

Myth: Snacking isn't a good habit for kids to learn.

Fact: With their high-energy needs and small stomachs, most children need snacks. And so do teens. Three daily meals often aren't enough to provide all the nutrients and food energy they need. The advice for parents: keep food group snacks that kids enjoy on hand, and encourage kids to snack to satisfy hunger without overeating.

Myth: Healthful snacking means giving up some fun foods.

Fact: Any food can be eaten as a snack. You can eat foods such as chips and soft drinks occasionally and still eat for health. Balance higher-fat or higher-calorie snack foods with lower-fat and lower-calorie choices at meals. For example, if you snack on two chocolate chip cookies, enjoy chicken-vegetable stir-fry for dinner, rather than fried chicken and creamy slaw.

Remember: one snack, one meal, or one day of high-fat or high-calorie eating won't make or break your health. It's your food choices over the long term that count!

Snacking Smart

Chosen wisely, snacks can work for you. As with other food choices, snack with variety, balance, and moderation in mind. These ten smart-snack tips can make between-meal eating a valuable part of your eating style!

1. *Make snacks part of your personal Pyramid for the whole day.* Rather than thinking of them as "extras," choose snacks as minimeals that con-

> ### Did You Know
>
> . . . munching on a handful of baby carrots will meet your vitamin A needs for the entire day?
>
> . . . preschoolers get nearly a third of their energy from snacks?
>
> . . . a planned snack can help prevent overeating?
>
> . . . watching television tends to increase snacking—particularly of high-fat, high-calorie "goodies"?
>
> . . . larger snack containers add up to more calories? People eat more when the package is bigger!
>
> *Source:* American Dietetic Association.

tribute food-group servings to your personal Pyramid. Fruits and vegetables boost your vitamin, mineral, and fiber profile. Caffè latte, "milk tea," or fat-free yogurt add calcium.

2. *Choose snacks for variety.* Add to the enjoyment and nutritional quality of your diet; consume a variety of snack foods within each food group. Even try snacks with an international flavor: spring rolls, bean burritos, or foccacia bread.

3. *Snack only when you're hungry.* Skip the urge to nibble when you're bored, frustrated, or stressed. "Feed" that urge to munch by walking the dog, checking your e-mail, or talking to your family.

4. *Make snacking a conscious activity.* Without realizing it, you can overeat easily when you absent-mindedly snack while doing something else, such as watching television or surfing the Internet.

5. *Eat small snacks well ahead of mealtime.* A light bite eaten two to three hours before meals probably won't interfere with your appetite. Instead, it may divert the temptation to overeat at dinner.

   If you want to stave off hunger longer, pick snacks with protein and fat such as peanut butter on celery, or cheese and crackers. Proteins take longer to digest, and fats help slow the release of food from your stomach to your intestines. For short-term satisfaction pick carbohydrate-rich snacks such as fruit, vegetables, and grain products, which digest quicker.

6. *Eat snack-size portions.* Snacks aren't meal replacers. Smaller portions usually are enough to

take away between-meals hunger pangs without interfering with your mealtime appetite. Control your portions to avoid overeating: snack from a single-serve container; put a small helping in a bowl, rather than eat directly from the package; and skip megasize or supersize drinks and snacks.

7. *Match snack calories to your activity level.* A physically active person or growing teenager can consume more substantial snacks—with more calories—than an armchair sports fan can. Whether from snacks or meals, calories can add up unless you watch what you eat and maintain physical activity.

8. *Consider snacks in your fat budget.* Balance snacks with mealtime foods to keep the total amount of fat you consume to no more than 30 percent of your day's energy intake. To check the fat content of snacks, read the Nutrition Facts on the food label, and check the serving size, too!

9. *Go easy on snacks from the Pyramid tip.* Enjoy candy, juice drinks, and soft drinks in small amounts, but snack mostly on nutrient-dense foods from the five food groups. *To compare juice and juice drinks see "Juicy Story: Fruit Juice, Juice Drink, Fruit Drink . . . or Just Plain Water?" in chapter 8.*

10. *Plan ahead for smart snacking.* Keep a variety of tasty, nutritious, ready-to-eat snacks on hand at home, at work, or wherever you need a light bite to take the edge off hunger. In that way you won't be limited to snacks from vending machines, fast-food restaurants, convenience stores, or your own randomly stocked kitchen.

Check Your Snack Options

Satisfy your "snack tooth" anytime, anywhere with these easy, convenient, and healthful choices.

● Stock your fridge and freezer: yogurt, cottage cheese, cheese, lean deli meats, whole fruits, cut-up raw veggies, fruit and vegetable juices, milk, frozen juice bars, frozen yogurt.

● Stash snacks at work—in case of late or busy workdays: instant vegetable or bean soup, pretzels, soy nuts, snack-size cereal boxes, minicans of water-packed tuna, boxes of raisins, instant oatmeal or couscous,

dried fruit or single-serve fruit cups, whole-wheat crackers, nuts.

● Find vending machines with food-group snacks: peanuts, raisins, trail mix, granola bars, whole fruit, fruit juice, milk (flavored or unflavored).

● Stock up for microwave snacks: single-serving soups; pocket bread or English muffins with tomato sauce, Italian herbs, and mozzarella cheese for instant pizza; bean dip or salsa, with tortillas; Cheddar cheese for a microwave-baked potato; plain sweet potato (great for microwaving).

● Pack a snack sack: canned or boxed juice, crackers and cheese, pretzels, soy nuts, air-popped popcorn, nuts, whole fruit, dried fruit, oatmeal-raisin cookies, fig bars, graham crackers, or raisin-nut mixes.

● Choose smart at convenience stores or malls: soft pretzels, bagels (go light with cream cheese), frozen yogurt, fruit smoothies (small size), fruit juice.

● Quench your thirst: water, milk, fruit juice, vegetable juice, juice spritzers (juice and mineral water), fruit smoothies (fruit or juice, blended with milk or yogurt), hot chocolate. (Be aware that fruit-flavored waters may be high in added sugars.)

"Grazing" for Good Health

Many Americans have moved away from "three square meals" a day. Instead, they eat several minimeals, sometimes called "grazing," which matches their active, on-the-go lifestyle. As with traditional meal patterns, the goals for grazing remain the same: variety, balance, and moderation throughout the day.

Have You Ever Wondered **?**

. . . if canned liquid supplements or meal replacements are good snacks for you? Despite advertising messages, you don't need pricey liquid nutrition to supplement your meals if you're healthy. Your kids don't, either. Foods—fruit, smoothies, whole-grain crackers, yogurt—taste better, and they provide nutrients and other beneficial substances that canned liquid "meals" lack. If you think you need a supplement, stick with a multivitamin/mineral supplement tablet. For a fraction of the price, you get the same nutrient benefits.

Little meals aren't snacks eaten between larger meals; instead they're several small portions eaten throughout the day. As long as food choices add up to Pyramid recommendations without overeating, eating five or six minimeals can be as healthful as three meals a day.

Little meals are nothing new. Instead, they're part of the traditional eating style in many places outside the United States. A variety of small portions of traditional Spanish dishes are served as *tapas.* In Greece, Turkey, and Egypt they're called *mezze.* A little meal, or *spuntino,* in Italy might be a minipizza, grilled bread with tomatoes and cheese, or small skewers of meat and vegetables. And *dim sum,* which means "to do (or touch) the heart" in Chinese, is a savory snack of spring rolls, pot stickers, and steamed dumplings, to name a few types of *dim sum.*

Eating a series of minimeals may have several benefits. Like traditional eating styles, minimeals contribute full or partial food-group servings. For some people, especially those with small appetites, little meals match their personal needs and lifestyles. Eating fewer calories more frequently may burn a few extra calories; the reason may be that eating and digesting food has a thermogenic, or calorie-burning, effect for a short time. Some researchers also say that spreading the same number of calories in four to six meals throughout the day, rather than at three meals, may relate to somewhat lower blood cholesterol levels, too. But these findings aren't conclusive.

For Healthful "Grazing" . . .

● **Total it up.** To avoid overeating, yet still satisfy your appetite, pay attention to your small helpings and to the amount you eat in all your minimeals.

● Choose appetizer-size portions in restaurants and at home. That's about right for minimeals.

FUNCTIONAL FOODS: FAST AND EASY

Foods from every food group have functional health benefits that go beyond basic nutrition. Try these quick, easy, and convenient ways to fit functional foods in. *For more about the benefits of functional foods (in italics in this chart), see "Phytonutrients—a 'Crop' for Good Health" in chapter 4 and "Functional Foods: A New Wave" in chapter 9.*

BREAKFAST

● Top *oatmeal* with *blueberries.*
● Mix *yogurt* with *whole-grain dry cereal.*
● Spread *soy nut butter* on *whole-grain toast.*
● Drink sparkling *purple grape juice* with breakfast.
● Blend *soy milk* with fresh *pineapple.*

HEALTHFUL MEAL IDEAS

● Mix *tuna* salad with grated *carrots, red peppers, onions,* and *garlic.*
● Serve *whole-grain pasta* with *tomato sauce* and fresh *herbs.*
● Cook *leeks* and *onions* with *tomatoes* as a side dish.
● Grill *salmon* and serve with fresh *greens* and *yogurt* salad dressing.
● Try low-fat cream of *carrot, spinach,* and *broccoli* soups.
● Enjoy *green tea* with a marinated *tofu* sandwich.
● Stir-fry fresh *vegetables* with extra *garlic.*

SNACK ON THE GO

● Grab a piece of fresh *fruit.*
● Mix *soy nuts* and *dried fruit* together and hit the trail.
● Grab a glass or a box of *tomato, cranberry,* or *orange juice.*
● Try fresh *broccoli, cauliflower,* and *carrots* with a *tofu dip.*
● Mix *bananas* with fresh *raspberries.*

Source: University of Illinois Functional Foods for Health Program.

● Use the power of the Food Guide Pyramid. The real challenge with this eating style is keeping within Pyramid guidelines—eating enough servings, yet not too much. If you're not careful, overgrazing can be your source of excess fat, salt, and calories.

Eat Healthy, Work Smart

Today's world of work demands increasing productivity. To reduce stress yet increase your own productivity, eat for success!

● Start your workday with breakfast. You'll replenish your body's blood sugar stores, needed for sustained mental work and physical activity throughout the day. You'll also stave off midmorning hunger, which may reduce your concentration.

● Take short stress breakers. Take a brisk, ten-minute walk. Stretch your muscles, and hold for thirty seconds. Relieve tension in your shoulders and neck by tilting your head from side to side and from front to back. Or switch tasks for a while. Avoid the urge to nibble for stress relief.

● Take time for a lunch break—even when you're under pressure. Lunch may help you avoid a dip in your afternoon energy level.

Feel sleepy in the afternoon anyway? Your overall sleep habits, age, and body cycle may cause your drowsiness. New research also suggests that a midafternoon slump may be normal and induced by hormones. For some people, high-carbohydrate meals may increase serotonin, contributing to drowsiness. To stay alert all day, regularly rest well at night. If you feel sleepy in the afternoon, try a ten- to twenty-minute nap to renew your energy (if your workplace allows).

● When you go out for lunch, order a nonalcoholic beverage. For a business lunch, sparkling water with a lemon twist is a great "cocktail." Alcoholic drinks can make you feel drowsy—a problem when you need to feel alert at work. The effects of just one beer or glass of wine can last about an hour. Blood-alcohol levels from two drinks may stay with you the better part of the afternoon. When you handle potentially dangerous equipment or drive as part of your job, the combination of drinking and working is risky.

● Need a snack break? Stash nutritious foods in your desk drawer or in the workplace fridge. But control any urge for mindless nibbling at the computer.

● If you're caffeine-sensitive, limit coffee, tea, and soft drinks with caffeine. Enjoy a cup if that helps wake you up in the morning. But switch to "decaf," milk, water, or juice if caffeine bothers you.

● What about office celebrations? Enjoy just a small piece of cake. When it's your turn to bring doughnuts, bring bagels and fruit.

● Get your coworkers moving with you. Walk or take a strength-training class over the lunch hour. Or team up for an after-work volleyball, baseball, golf, or bowling league.

Healthy Eating from Your Home Office

Work from an office at home? More and more of us do. If you've accustomed to a company cafeteria or a nearby deli, you may need to redesign your approach to eating. Start here:

● Keep routine in your life. Instead of rolling out of bed and into your home office at the computer, start with breakfast. And try to set a regular lunchtime.

● Need a work break? Opt to walk outside rather than automatically checking out the refrigerator

● Make time to move. When you work at home, your chance for routine physical activity may go down, and, for example, there's no need to walk from the parking lot, bus, or train. Instead, you're blessed with other ways to take an action break—for example, walk the dog, dig in the garden, swim in the neighborhood pool. Look for opportunities!

● Keep food on hand for quick workday meals and snacks. With a kitchen handy, you have almost any food options you plan for.

● Occasionally give yourself a treat. Make a workday lunch day with others who work at home, or with those who work in traditional settings. The social contact that goes with eating out is "good for your head."

● Take advantage of working at home for other food preparation. As a work break, start making after-work meals. Perhaps simmer bean soup, or put a turkey breast in the oven.

CHAPTER 11

Supermarket Smarts

With about fifty thousand items available in today's supermarkets, it's no wonder you have so many decisions to make! From food labels, to brochures and posters, to "in-store" consumer affairs professionals and computer kiosks, you have more food facts at your fingertips than ever before. That's good for informed shoppers. With facts and plenty of choices available, you can shop for taste, nutrition, safety, price, and convenience, all at the same time. Food labels with Nutrition Facts appear on virtually all food products, and claims about nutrients and health, as well as food safety tips, appear on many.

Supermarkets comprise most of the retail food business, but that's not the only place where you can buy food to prepare and eat at home. Today, specialty stores, warehouse and bulk food stores, wholesale clubs, health food stores, restaurants, convenience stores, department stores, drugstores, farm stands, farmers' markets, mail order, and even on-line shopping services sell food to eat at home.

No matter where you shop, look for qualities of excellence in a food store:

● The store should be clean—that means the display cases, the grocery shelves, and the floor. And it should have a pleasing smell.

● Produce, meat, poultry, fish, and dairy foods should show qualities of freshness. Read on for ways to spot the signs of freshness in a variety of foods.

● Refrigerated cases should be cold. Freezer compartments should keep food solidly frozen.

● Bulk bins, salad bars, and other self-serve areas should be clean and properly covered.

● Workers handling raw and unpackaged food should wear disposable gloves, and change them after handling nonfood items and again after handling raw food.

Beyond these minimum standards, today's supermarkets may offer other useful services: home delivery, electric carts, cooking classes, consumer newsletters, video rental, banking and postal facilities, pharmacies, photo finishing, florists, in-store restaurants, and recycling programs, to name just a few.

Today's Food Labels

At the store, food labels are your best sources of consumer information. Food labels tell the basics. They identify the food, the amount inside the package, and the manufacturer.

If you need to eat less fat, more calcium, or more fiber, Nutrition Facts labels can help you. Nutrition information on labels helps you choose foods to meet recommendations of the Dietary Guidelines for Americans and the Food Guide Pyramid. The ingredient list, safety guidelines, preparation tips, and freshness dating—food labels tell still more about food inside the package.

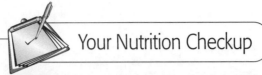

What's in Your Shopping Cart?

According to annual supermarket surveys done by the Food Marketing Institute, consumers rank taste, nutrition, safety, storability, and convenience as important reasons for making decisions in the store. If that's true for you, just how do your supermarket smarts stack up? Check here before you read this chapter.

Do You . . .	**ALWAYS** (3 PTS.)	**USUALLY** (2 PTS.)	**SOMETIMES** (1 PT.)	**NEVER** (0 PT.)
For nutrition . . .				
Read the Nutrition Facts on a food label?	____	____	____	____
Use nutrient content claims and health claims to quickly spot foods you want?	____	____	____	____
Check the % Daily Values to get specific information after you read a nutrient content claim?	____	____	____	____
Use food labels to compare the nutrients and ingredients in similar foods?	____	____	____	____
Look for nutrition information displayed near fresh foods: produce, meat, poultry, and fish?	____	____	____	____
Know how to use the "5–20 guide" to quickly check Nutrition Facts?	____	____	____	____
Use Nutrition Facts including serving sizes on food labels to plan healthful meals and snacks?	____	____	____	____
Subtotal for nutrition	____	____	____	____
For safety . . .				
Look for dates printed on packages to buy foods at their peak?	____	____	____	____
Check packaging and cans to be sure they're clean and not damaged?	____	____	____	____
Take perishable foods home within thirty minutes of shopping, and immediately refrigerate or freeze them?	____	____	____	____
Check to be sure that frozen foods are solid and that refrigerated foods are cold?	____	____	____	____
Know how to spot qualities of freshness in produce and raw meat, poultry, and fish?	____	____	____	____
Put fresh meat, poultry, and fish in separate bags when you can so they don't drip on other foods in your cart?	____	____	____	____
Put foods that need to be refrigerated in separate bags to help maintain a cooler temperature when they're bagged?	____	____	____	____
Subtotal for safety	____	____	____	____
For cost savings . . .				
Use unit price codes on shelves to compare the cost of similar products?	____	____	____	____
Take advantage of cents-off coupons and in-store specials?	____	____	____	____
Buy only the amount you'll use to avoid waste?	____	____	____	____
Shop for seasonal produce?	____	____	____	____
Pay attention to the price as the cashier scans each item?	____	____	____	____
Consider carefully before buying a new food after you sample it or see an attractive display?	____	____	____	____
Subtotal for cost savings	____	____	____	____
For convenience . . .				
Keep a shopping list to use as you shop?	____	____	____	____
Shop during off-hours to save time and avoid crowds?	____	____	____	____

Do You ...	**ALWAYS** (3 PTS.)	**USUALLY** (2 PTS.)	**SOMETIMES** (1 PT.)	**NEVER** (0 PT.)
Buy foods that are partly or fully prepared?	____	____	____	____
Buy single-portion or small-sized packages when you're feeding one or two?	____	____	____	____
Keep shopping trips to a minimum—no more than once or twice a week?	____	____	____	____
Subtotal for convenience	____	____	____	____

Count up your "supermarket smarts" category by category, then add up the total. *Total score* _____.

For nutrition and safety, a perfect score is 21 for each. For cost savings, it's 18; for convenience, 15. That adds up to 75 points.

If you come close to a perfect score in any category, count yourself as "supermarket smart" in that area. And make it your goal to be a well-rounded shopper—with top scores in every category! *Read on for more ways to shop smart and boost your score.*

What's on the Label?

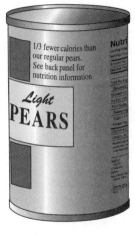

Wrapped around almost every packaged food in the supermarket you'll find nutrition information. Today's food labels may carry up to five different types of nutrition and health information, to help you make choices and fit foods you like into your meals and snacks. Read on for more about . . .

● A *nutrient content claim* such as "low fat" or "high fiber" helps you easily find foods that meet your specific nutrition goals. *See "Label Lingo" in this chapter to find out what specific nutrient content claims mean.*

● The *Nutrition Facts* give specifics about the calories and nutrients, such as fat, cholesterol, sodium, fiber, and certain vitamins and minerals, in a single serving of the food. This information must appear on virtually all food labels.

● The *ingredient list* on packaged food gives an overview of the "recipe," with the ingredients listed from most to least.

● A *health claim* describes the potential health benefits of a food, nutrient, or food substance, such as reducing the risk for a health problem.

● A *structure/function claim* describes the way a nutrient or a food substance maintains or supports a normal body function, such as "helps maintain bone health" or "supports a healthy immune system."

Nutrition Facts and the ingredient list appear on almost every packaged food in the supermarket. Today many fresh fruits and vegetables, as well as meat, poultry, and seafood, may be labeled voluntarily with nutrition information, too, either on the package or on a poster or a pamphlet displayed nearby. If you don't find this information in your supermarket, ask the store manager to start providing it.

Food labels let you make nutrition-related decisions as you shop—and at home:

● Use labels to compare the nutrient content of similar foods and to choose foods that fit in an overall healthful way of eating.

● Use Nutrition Facts to make trade-offs so you can fit any food into a healthful way of eating.

The Language of Labels

Imagine rolling your shopping cart through the supermarket. Your eyes dart from one food product to another. Some canned peaches say "no added sugar." Certain breakfast cereals are "high in fiber"; others are "fortified." On packages of luncheon meat you see the term "lean." The words "high in calcium" on a milk carton catch your eye. You can choose "lite" salad dressing. And a box of cookies says "fewer calories." What does all this label language mean?

Known as nutrient content claims, these terms describe the amount of nutrients, cholesterol, fiber, or calories in food. But they don't give exact amounts.

Usually they appear on the front of food labels, where you can use them for quick comparisons.

For example, suppose you're comparing fat in Italian salad dressing. Terms such as "reduced fat" and "fat-free" offer a general idea of the fat content. To find the exact amount in one serving, check the Nutrition Facts, usually found on the package's side or back.

Nutrient content claims mean the same thing for all foods, no matter what food or manufacturer. That's because they're defined strictly by regulation. Like Nutrition Facts, nutrient content claims are defined for a single serving. That's a standard serving size set by the government—not necessarily what *you* consider one helping.

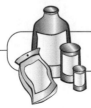

Label Lingo

What Do These Nutrient Content Claims Mean?

LABEL TERM ...	MEANS ...
Free	It's an amount so small that it probably won't have an effect on your body—for example, "calorie-free," "fat-free," or "sodium-free." Other terms: "no," "zero," "without," "trivial source of," "negligible source of," "dietarily insignificant source of," "non" (nonfat only).
Low	It's an amount specifically defined for each term, such as "low-calorie," "low-fat," or "low-cholesterol." *Other terms:* "few," "contains a small amount of," "low source of," "low in," "little," "a little."
Reduced	It's an amount used to describe a food with at least 25 percent less calories, fat, saturated fat, cholesterol, or sodium than a comparable food. Look for information about the food it's being compared to. *Other terms:* "reduced in," "___% reduced," "fewer," "lower," "lower in," "less."
High	It's an amount that's 20 percent or more of the Daily Value* for a nutrient—for example, "high in vitamin C" or "high-calcium." *Other terms:* "excellent source of," "rich in."
Good source	It's an amount that's 10 to 19 percent of the Daily Value* for a nutrient—for example, "good source of fiber." *Other terms:* "contains," "provides."
More	It's an amount that's 10 percent or more of the Daily Value*—for example, "more fiber" or "more iron." You won't find it on meat or poultry products. *Other terms:* "enriched," "fortified," "added."
Light	It's a food with a third fewer calories or 50 percent less fat than the traditional version. A "low-calorie" or "low-fat" food with 50 percent less sodium might also be called "light." *Other term:* "lite."
Healthy	It's a food that's low in fat and saturated fat, 60 milligrams or less cholesterol per serving, 480 milligrams or less sodium per serving, and at least 10 percent of the Daily Value per serving of vitamin A, vitamin C, calcium, iron, protein, and fiber. Raw, frozen, and canned fruits and vegetables are exceptions; they can be labeled "healthy" without having 10 percent of the DV or more of these nutrients per serving.

On seafood, meat, or poultry, look for:

Lean	It's a food with less than 10 grams total fat, 4 grams saturated fat, and 95 milligrams cholesterol per 3-ounce serving.
Extra lean	It's a food with less than 5 grams total fat, 2 grams saturated fat, and 95 milligrams cholesterol per 3-ounce serving.

*When compared with a standard serving size of the traditional food.

Nutrient content claims are optional, however. Many foods that meet the criteria don't carry these terms on the label. Their use is up to the food manufacturer. So if you need—or want—to know about the food, read the Nutrition Facts! *For definitions of nutrient content claims, see "Label Lingo" on page 240. You'll find more specific definitions of label lingo in other chapters.*

Get All the Facts!

Let's get specific. Nutrition Facts differ from nutrient content claims. Nutrition Facts specifically state the amount of nutrients and calories in one serving of a food, while terms such as "low in fat" or "more fiber" are quick-to-read descriptions.

For making quick, informed food choices, read the Nutrition Facts on food labels:

● To know the nutritional content of one serving of that food.

● To compare calories (food energy) and nutrients in similar foods.

● To see how calorie and nutrient amounts change when your portions are smaller or larger than the serving size listed.

● To find foods that help you manage your weight; promote your health; reduce your risk for chronic diseases; or manage diabetes, cardiovascular disease, or hypertension.

● To help you make food trade-offs. (If you want one high-fat snack today, Nutrition Facts can help you to trade off—find other foods with less fat.)

Nutrition Facts on food labels offer information in two parts: (1) specific information (serving size, calories, and nutrition content) for the food, and (2) general nutrition information in the footnote on the bottom.

Start with servings. The label gives both the serving size and number of servings in the package. Given in both familiar kitchen measures (e.g., teaspoon, tablespoon, cup) and metric amounts, the serving size depends on how much most people actually eat, not necessarily the recommended amount or the portion you usually eat.

Remember, the Nutrition Facts apply to the serving size (amount for one serving) on the label, not necessarily to all the food in the container.

To know the calorie and nutrient amounts in your portion, compare your portion to a serving size on the label. If a label serving is one cup and you ate two cups, you consumed twice the amount of calories and other nutrients listed. Also bear in mind that serving sizes on food labels may differ from Pyramid servings.

Check the calories. Calories are a measure of food energy. Look for the number of calories in a single serving—and how many of those calories come from fat. Remember that if you eat two servings, you get twice as many calories from fat, too.

Tip: Avoid confusing the number of "calories from fat" in one serving with the dietary advice "Eat no more than 30 percent of total calories from fat." The dietary advice applies only to your overall food choices, not to a single food or meal. Percent of calories from fat does not appear on the food label.

Note the nutrients. Of all the nutrients in food, only a few are listed on the label—those that relate to today's most important health issues. You'll find some you probably need to limit and others you may need in greater amounts.

Fat, saturated fat, cholesterol, and sodium are nutrients people often consume in excess. The concern? Eating too much of these nutrients may increase your chances for developing some chronic diseases, including heart disease, some cancers, and high blood pressure.

Fiber, vitamins A and C, calcium, and iron are listed because they often come up short. So make food choices that help you eat enough of these nutrients. It's a way to help improve your health, stay healthy, and perhaps reduce your risk of some health problems such as osteoporosis or anemia.

Unless their amounts are insignificant, some nutrients must appear on the label: fat, saturated fat, cholesterol, total carbohydrate, sugars, protein, vitamins A and C, calcium, and iron. Other nutrients may be listed voluntarily.

If you see a nutrient content claim, perhaps "fortified with vitamin D" or "high in folate," you'll find that nutrient on the Nutrition Facts panel. Nutrients added to a food such as fortified breakfast cereal must be listed.

Refer to the % Daily Values (DV). That's where you'll see if a single serving has a little or a lot of different nutrients. These percentages give you a general idea of how one serving contributes nutritionally to a 2,000-calorie-a-day diet. Remember that % DV refers to a whole day, not to a single meal or a snack.

Depending on your age, gender, and activity level, you may need more or less than 2,000 calories a day, so for some nutrients, you may need more or less than 100% DV. *To estimate how much food energy, or calories, you need daily, see chapter 2.* Even if you don't know how many calories you need a day, the % DV offers a reference point. *For Daily Values used in food labeling, see the Appendices.* In your whole day's food choices, use the Nutrition Facts to help limit some nutrients and get enough of others:

● *For fat, saturated fat, cholesterol, and sodium,* try to limit how much you consume to 100% DV or less for the day. Total fat includes all types of fat: saturated fat as well as polyunsaturated and monounsaturated fat.

● *For fiber, vitamins A and C, calcium, and iron,* try to consume a variety of foods that add up to 100% DV per day for each one. Be aware that 100% DV may or

> *Use the "5–20 guide" as a quick guide to label reading. For any nutrient:*
>
> ● *5% or less is low:* For nutrients you need to limit, eat plenty of foods with 5% or less Daily Value.
>
> ● *20% or more is high:* For nutrients you need more of, eat plenty of foods with 20% or more Daily Value.

may not be the optimal amount recommended for you. For example, on food labels, the DV for calcium is 1,000 milligrams and the specific Dietary Reference Intake (DRI) recommended for adults to age fifty is also 1,000 milligrams daily. However, teens through age eighteen are urged to consume 1,300 milligrams of calcium daily, and for adults over age fifty, the advice is 1,200 milligrams of calcium daily

Daily Values footnote. This reference chart shows some Daily Values. For two calorie levels (2,000 calories and 2,500 calories), it shows the maximum amounts recommended for total fat, saturated fat, cholesterol, and sodium—and the target amounts for total carbohydrate and fiber. Depending on your calorie needs, you may need less or more. This footnote is the same on every food label because it's general nutrition advice.

> *Metric conversion key:*
>
> ● 28 grams (g) = 1 ounce
> ● 1,000 milligrams (mg) =1 gram

Calories-per-gram conversion. You may see the number of calories in 1 gram of fat, carbohydrate, and protein. Notice that fat supplies more than twice the calories per gram (9 calories) than carbohydrate and protein (4 calories each).

A Word about Ingredients . . .

Imagine that you're reaching for a can of beef stew. The ingredient list, like a recipe, tells what's in the stew.

How to Use the Nutrition Facts Label

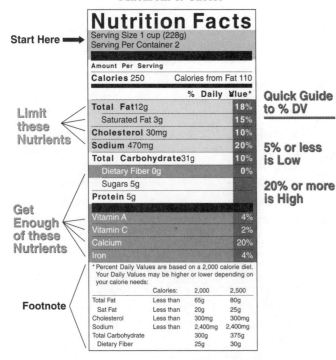

Macaroni & Cheese

Start Here ➡

Nutrition Facts
Serving Size 1 cup (228g)
Serving Per Container 2

Amount Per Serving

Calories 250   Calories from Fat 110

% Daily Value*

Total Fat 12g	18%
Saturated Fat 3g	15%
Cholesterol 30mg	10%
Sodium 470mg	20%
Total Carbohydrate 31g	10%
Dietary Fiber 0g	0%
Sugars 5g	
Protein 5g	
Vitamin A	4%
Vitamin C	2%
Calcium	20%
Iron	4%

Limit these Nutrients

Get Enough of these Nutrients

Footnote

Quick Guide to % DV

5% or less is Low

20% or more is High

* Percent Daily Values are based on a 2,000 calorie diet. Your Daily Values may be higher or lower depending on your calorie needs:

	Calories:	2,000	2,500
Total Fat	Less than	65g	80g
Sat Fat	Less than	20g	25g
Cholesterol	Less than	300mg	300mg
Sodium	Less than	2,400mg	2,400mg
Total Carbohydrate		300g	375g
Dietary Fiber		25g	30g

... why you don't see % Daily Values for protein? Getting enough protein isn't a health concern for people age four and over, so it usually isn't listed with a % DV. If the food is touted with a nutrient content claim—perhaps "high in protein"—then protein must be shown. Foods meant for infants and children under age four show % DV for protein on the Nutrition Facts panel.

... why a food label that says "no sugar added" shows some grams of sugars on the Nutrition Facts? Many foods—fruits, vegetables, milk, cereals, grains, and legumes—have naturally occurring sugars. "Sugars" in the Nutrition Facts include both added and naturally occurring sugars. There's no DV for sugars because there's no daily recommendation. To find out about the added sugars, check the ingredient list.

... if foods sold in health food stores or a supermarket's natural-food department are any more nutritious? The nutritional quality of foods sold as "health foods" isn't necessarily superior. In fact, the unregulated term "health food" is technically a misnomer. Check the Nutrition Facts and ingredient list to compare foods.

What's the difference? Perhaps price. Specialty stores or departments may charge more for similar foods. In most health food stores, the overall variety of foods is limited, too. But health food stores or natural-foods departments also may carry foods you won't easily find elsewhere: perhaps amaranth, quinoa, millet, or a wider variety of legumes.

Some health food stores set their own guidelines for food products they choose to sell—for example, foods with few or no preservatives, more organically produced foods, or foods from local growers, among others. The decision of what foods to stock in a health store isn't regulated.

By regulation, any food made with more than one ingredient must carry an ingredient list on the label. Food manufacturers must list all ingredients in descending order by weight. Those in the largest amounts are given first. For example, canned tomato soup that lists tomatoes first contains more tomatoes by weight than anything else. Next time you reach for canned stew, check what ingredients are listed first, second, and third.

The ingredient list is also useful for people with special food needs; for example:

● People with a food sensitivity (allergy or intolerance), perhaps to peanuts, eggs, lactose (milk sugar), wheat, or sulfites. If you're sensitive to artificial color, know that the colors are named individually, not just listed as "coloring." If the ingredient list isn't clear to you, write or call the food manufacturer. *See chapter 21, "Sensitive about Food," for more information on food sensitivities.*

● People who avoid pork, shellfish, or other meat for religious or other reasons

● People who prefer vegetarian eating, including vegans who choose to avoid any food made with ingredients from animal sources

In some cases the ingredient list gives the source of the ingredients. For example, on the label for Mark's Cheese Pizza (*see below*), you'll see that "partially hydrogenated vegetable oil" is followed by "soybean and/or cottonseed oil" and that "tomato puree" is water and tomato paste. What is part-skim mozzarella cheese made from? The ingredient list says pasteurized milk, cheese cultures, salt, and enzymes.

For more about food additives, see "Additives: Safe at the Plate" in chapter 9 and the list of additives and their functions in the Appendices.

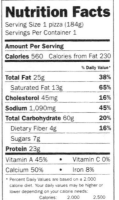

Nutrition Facts

Serving Size 1 pizza (184g)
Servings Per Container 1

Amount Per Serving

Calories 560   Calories from Fat 230

	% Daily Value*
Total Fat 25g	**38%**
Saturated Fat 13g	**65%**
Cholesterol 45mg	**16%**
Sodium 1,090mg	**45%**
Total Carbohydrate 60g	**20%**
Dietary Fiber 4g	**16%**
Sugars 7g	
Protein 23g	

Vitamin A 45%	•	Vitamin C 0%
Calcium 50%	•	Iron 8%

* Percent Daily Values are based on a 2,000 calorie diet. Your daily values may be higher or lower depending on your calorie needs:

	Calories:	2,000	2,500
Total Fat	Less than	65g	80g
Sat Fat	Less than	20g	25g
Cholesterol	Less than	300mg	300mg
Sodium	Less than	2,400mg	2,400mg
Total Carbohydrate		300g	375g
Dietary Fiber		25g	30g

Calories per gram:
Fat 9 • Carbohydrate 4 • Protein 4

MARK'S Cheese Pizza

MICROWAVE OVEN DIRECTIONS

1. **Open pizza carton carefully.** Remove frozen pizza and microwave disk; unwrap pizza. For best results, do not add additional toppings.
2. **Reclose carton by inserting tab into slot.** Place carton in center of microwave oven. Place disk silver side up on carton.
3. **Center frozen pizza on top of disk. Microwave at HIGH 3 to 4½ minutes,** or until most of cheese is melted, rotating carton ½ turn after 2 minutes.
4. **Remove pizza from oven by holding** sides of carton. Loosen pizza from disk with spatula.
CAUTION: Disk and pizza will be very hot.
NOTE: Microwave directions were developed using 600 to 700 watt ovens.

INGREDIENTS: CRUST: WHEAT FLOUR WITH MALTED BARLEY FLOUR, WATER, PARTIALLY HYDROGENATED VEGETABLE OIL (SOYBEAN AND/OR COTTONSEED OIL) WITH SOY LECITHIN, ARTIFICIAL FLAVOR AND ARTIFICIAL COLOR (BETA CAROTENE), SOYBEAN OIL, YEAST, HIGH FRUCTOSE CORN SYRUP, SALT, CALCIUM PROPIONATE ADDED TO RETARD SPOILAGE OF CRUST, L-CYSTEINE MONOHYDROCHLORIDE; **SAUCE:** TOMATO PUREE (WATER, TOMATO PASTE), WATER, GREEN PEPPERS, SALT, LACTOSE AND FLAVORING, SPICES, FOOD STARCH - MODIFIED, SUGAR, CORN OIL, XANTHAN GUM, GARLIC POWDER. **TOPPING:** LOW MOISTURE PART SKIM MOZZARELLA CHEESE (PASTEURIZED MILK, CHEESE CULTURES, SALT, ENZYMES.)

Manufactured by Mark's Pizza, Silver Spring, MD 20000

Health Claims on the Label

Another bit of nutrition information might appear on food labels: a health claim. Health claims link food—or food components—in your overall eating plan with a lowered risk for some chronic diseases. Since this information is optional, many foods that meet the criteria don't carry any health claim on their label.

Strictly regulated by the U.S. Food and Drug Administration (FDA), only health claims supported by scientific evidence are allowed on food labels. So far these health claims have been approved on food, linking food, food substances, or nutrients to these health conditions:

- *Calcium* and osteoporosis
- *Sodium* and hypertension
- *Dietary fat* and cancer
- *Saturated fat and cholesterol* and the risk of coronary heart disease
- *Fiber-containing grain products, fruits, and vegetables* and cancer
- *Fruits, vegetables, and grain products that contain fiber, particularly soluble fiber,* and their risk of coronary heart disease
- *Fruits and vegetables* and cancer
- *Folate* and neural tube defects
- *Sugar alcohol* and dental caries (cavities)
- *Soluble fiber from certain foods* and the risk of coronary heart disease
- *Soy protein* and the risk of coronary heart disease
- *Plant sterol/stanol esters* and the risk of coronary heart disease
- *Whole-grain foods* and the risk of heart disease and certain cancers
- *Potassium* and the risk of high blood pressure and stroke

Each health claim has specific regulations for the food (or nutrients in the food) and for the wording of the claim. *(A few other health claims are approved for supplement labels; see chapter 23.) See the Appendices for specifics about each approved health claim.*

When you read health claims, remember: your food choices are just one factor that can reduce your risk for certain health problems. Heredity, physical activity, and smoking are among other factors that affect your health and risk for disease.

Structure/Function Claims on the Label

Structure/function claims such as "helps promote urinary tract health" describe how a nutrient or a food substance may affect your health; these claims *cannot* suggest any link to lowered risk for disease. Unlike health claims, structure/function claims don't need to be approved or reviewed by the U.S. Food and Drug Administration, and they have no specific standards that regulate the wording. However, they still must be truthful and not misleading. Labels with structure/function claims must carry a disclaimer: "This statement has not been evaluated by the FDA. This product is not intended to diagnose, treat, cure or prevent any disease."

Food Labels: Food Safety and Handling Tips

For your good health, some food labels offer guidance on food safety and handling. To reduce the risk of foodborne illness, raw and partially cooked meat and poultry products must be labeled with guidelines for safe handling. *See the following "Safe Handling Instructions" label.* Each of the simple graphics—a

---

Safe Handling Instructions

This product was prepared from inspected and passed meat and/or poultry. Some food products may contain bacteria that could cause illness if the product is mishandled or cooked improperly. For your protection, follow these safe handling instructions.

 Keep refrigerated or frozen.
Thaw in refrigerator or microwave.

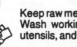 Keep raw meat and poultry separate from other foods. Wash working surfaces (including cutting boards), utensils, and hands after touching raw meat or poultry.

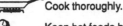 Cook thoroughly.

Keep hot foods hot. Refrigerate leftovers immediately or discard.

refrigerator, hand washing, fry pan, and meat thermometer— represents a safe handling tip.

Cartons of shell eggs also have safe-handling instructions to help control *Salmonella* contamination. The statement reminds you:

> SAFE HANDLING INSTRUCTIONS: To prevent illness from bacteria: keep eggs refrigerated, cook eggs until yolks are firm, and cook foods containing eggs thoroughly

Besides food safety, following these guidelines helps food retain its appealing flavor, texture, and appearance. *For in-depth information on food safety and handling, see chapter 12, "The Safe Kitchen."*

More Reading on the Food Label

If you take a few more moments with food labels, you'll learn even more about the food inside the package.

Type of food. The product name lets you know exactly what's in the container. Besides naming the specific food, it tells the form it's in, perhaps smooth or chunky, sliced or whole, or miniature size—important to know when you're following a recipe.

Quantity. Food labels tell you the total amount in the container, either in volume, count, or net weight. Net weight refers to the amount of food inside the container, including any liquid, but it doesn't include the weight of the container.

For juice products, total percent juice content. This tells you how much juice and how much water the beverage contains. Keep reading for the Nutrition Facts. Compare nutrients, such as vitamin C, along with sugars and calories, before making your selection.

A "100 percent" juice may—or may not—supply 100 percent of the Daily Value for vitamin C. For example, a 6-ounce serving of orange or grapefruit juice provides more than 100 percent of the Daily Value for vitamin C, while the same amount of 100 percent grape juice supplies about 50 percent; unfortified apple juice, much less. Juice may be fortified with vitamin C.

Juice "drinks," "beverages," or "cocktails" (with some juice, but not 100 percent juice) may be fortified

to provide 100 percent of the Daily Value for vitamin C, too. Typically these beverages have added sugars, but probably not all the other nutrient and phytonutrient benefits of 100 percent juice. To the body, the sugar in fruit, called fructose, and added sugars in juice drinks can't be distinguished. They're used in the body in the same way. *For more on the differences between juice and juice drinks, see "Juicy Story: Fruit Juice, Juice Drink, Fruit Drink . . . or Just Plain Water?" in chapter 8.*

Name and address of the manufacturer, packer, or distributor. With this information you can contact a food company with your consumer questions and concerns. Look for a consumer service phone number or Web site address, too. If the food is imported, the country of origin must be shown; this import regulation comes from the U.S. Department of the Treasury.

Food product dating. You can't see inside the food package; how do you know if it's fresh? Many foods, such as dairy products, have a date on the package, often given as numbers, such as "12-15" or "1215" or as "Dec. 15" to mean December 15. Food manufacturers and retailers use three types of dates you can read:

● *"Sell by" or pull date:* That's the last day a food should be sold if the food is to remain fresh for home storage.

● *Pack date:* That's when the food was manufactured, processed, or packaged.

● *"Best if used by" date:* For optimal quality, use the food by this date, but it's not a safety date. For example, the label may indicate, "Best if used by 12-31-03." Depending on the food and if it has been stored properly, it will likely be safe beyond this date.

For guidelines on home storage, see "The Cold Truth: How Cold, How Long?" in chapter 12.

Organic labeling. The Organic Foods Production Act and the National Organic Program ensure that the production, processing, and certification of organic foods are standardized. The term "organic" now has a legal label definition so you know what you're buying if you prefer organic foods. Foods may also bear the "USDA Organic" seal. Here's what the term "organic" means on food labels:

● *"100 percent organic"*: The product must contain only organically produced ingredients (except for water and salt).

● *"organic"*: The product must contain at least 95 percent organically produced ingredients (except for water and salt). The other 5 percent are ingredients that aren't available in organic form or that appear on an approved list.

● *"made with organic ingredients"*: Processed foods may bear this label if they contain at least 70 percent organic ingredients—for example, "soup made with organic peas, potatoes, and carrots." The regulation also identifies certain production methods that can't be used, either.

If it's labeled organic, you can find other label information. In the ingredient list look for the organically produced ingredient. The name and address of the organization that certifies the product as organic will appear, too.

Organic labeling regulations don't change food labeling regulations, administered by the U.S. Food and Drug Administration or the U.S.D.A.'s Food Safety and Inspection Service.

Organic foods aren't necessarily more healthful or more nutritious than other foods. Using them is really a consumer preference. *For more about organically grown foods, see chapter 9.*

Grading and inspection symbols on some products. These symbols indicate that foods have met certain standards set by the government:

● *Inspection stamps* on meat, poultry, and packaged meats mean the food is wholesome and was slaughtered, packed, or processed under sanitary conditions.

● *Food grades*—for example, on some types of meat, poultry, eggs, dairy foods, and produce—suggest standards of appearance, texture, uniformity, and perhaps taste. With the exception of marbling fat in meat, food grading does not suggest nutrient value. *Keep reading for specific information on grading for meat, poultry, and eggs.*

Preparation instructions. Some products suggest oven or microwave times and temperatures, or perhaps other preparation or serving tips. Some offer recipes.

Universal Product Code (UPC). This series of black bars, which identifies the manufacturer and the food, is used by the food industry for inventory control and price scanning.

Kosher symbols. The term "kosher" means "proper" or "fit" in Hebrew. Kosher symbols indicate that the food has met the standards of a Jewish food inspector, done in addition to government safety inspection. The kosher code, which may appear on foods throughout the store, doesn't imply any nutritional qualities.

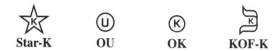

Often the word "Pareve" is written next to these symbols, meaning the food has neither meat nor dairy ingredients. During March and April a large "P" next to the symbols means it's kosher for Passover.

Halal and Zabiah Halal symbols. Products prepared by federally inspected meat packing plants, and handled according to Islamic dietary law and under Islamic authority, may bear Halal and Zabiah Halal references.

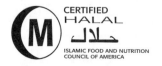

Health warnings for special conditions. A few foods carry health warnings for people with special needs. For example:

● Foods and beverages made with aspartame (a non-nutritive sweetener) offer a warning for people with phenylketonuria (PKU). Aspartame contains the amino acid phenylalanine, which people with PKU cannot metabolize.

● You'll find "Contains Sulfites" on beer and wine labels for those who are sulfite-sensitive.

● Alcohol-containing beverages also carry warnings for pregnant women.

See chapter 21 for more information on PKU and other food sensitivities.

Note: Any food with an allergen introduced through biotechnology must carry a statement on the food label. Currently none of these foods is in production.

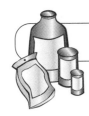

Label Lingo

Besides nutrition and health claims, some labels carry other label terms.

LABEL TERM . . .	REFERS TO . . .
Fresh	Food in its raw state. The term can't be used on food that has been frozen or heated, or on food that contains preservatives.
Fresh frozen	Food that is quickly frozen while very fresh shortly after harvest
Homogenized	Process of breaking up and separating milk fat. This makes the texture of milk smooth and uniform.
Natural	Product with no artificial ingredient or added color and that is minimally processed. The label must explain the use of the term "natural" (e.g., "no added colorings or artificial ingredients"; "minimally processed")
Pasteurized	Process of heating foods such as raw milk, raw eggs, and fresh juice to a temperature high enough to destroy bacteria and inactivate most enzymes that cause spoilage
Ultrapasteurized	Process of heating food such as cream to a temperature higher than pasteurization. This extends the time it can be stored in the refrigerator or on the shelf.
UHT (Ultra-High Temperature)	Process similar to ultra-pasteurization. With high heat and sterilized containers, food can be stored unopened without refrigeration for up to three months. Once opened, it needs refrigeration.

Diet exchanges. Some foods provide diet exchanges for help in managing diabetes or weight. The label probably will note that these exchanges are calculated from the system of exchange lists developed by the American Diabetes Association and the American Dietetic Association.

Labels—and You

What nutrition information do you use to make food selections—food labels or the Food Guide Pyramid? Use both!

● *The Food Guide Pyramid* helps you choose a variety of foods—and helps you know about how much (serving sizes and number of servings) you need.

● *Nutrition Facts* on food labels offer nutrition information to help you choose foods within each food group and the Pyramid tip.

Suppose you're shopping for dinner. You want a vitamin A-rich vegetable or fruit. Using food labels, you see that frozen broccoli fits the bill, and it can supply one serving from the Vegetable Group of the Food Guide Pyramid. But which package of frozen broccoli? Again read the label. Broccoli with sauce has more calories and fat than plain broccoli. You pick the one you prefer and that fits within your day's energy needs and fat budget.

Or suppose you're buying spaghetti sauce. Made with tomatoes, it counts toward the Vegetable Group. If you need to control your sodium intake, check the

Have You Ever Wondered

. . . what the code on the lid or the bottom of canned foods means? A series of letters or numbers identifies the plant location, exact date, and perhaps work shift or time of processing. Codes differ from one processor to another. If you can't read the code but wish to, contact the food company, using the toll-free number, Web site address, or address on the label.

. . . what the term "wholesome" on food labels really means? Nothing legally. It may capture your attention, but it has no legal definition on a food package.

Nutrition Facts panel for the exact sodium content per serving. The label also may offer other information, such as "reduced sodium" or "low sodium." And if you're curious, the ingredient list shows what ingredients contribute sodium.

Nutrition Facts help you make trade-offs. For example, a switch from regular to lean hot dogs likely saves both fat grams and calories without giving up protein. The label tells how much. Feeling indulgent? "Spend" some of the savings on ice cream for dessert. *See "Quick, Easy Trade-offs" in chapter 10.*

Supermarket Psychology

Understanding food labels can help you shop for wellness and nutrition, but that's just part of your smart shopping strategy. Following a few more practical tips can save you time, money, and hassle on grocery store trips.

Nutrition $ense

How can you get the most nutrition for those food dollars? Be an educated consumer and plan ahead. Know exactly what you need. And be aware of marketing ploys that may encourage you to buy beyond your shopping list.

● Keep a shopping list—and stick to it! A list jogs your memory and saves time as you walk the supermarket aisles. With a list, you're less likely to spend money on items you really don't need.

For time management, keep a running list in your kitchen of items you need to replace. Organize by category to match the store layout—for example, produce department, dairy case, meat counter, deli, bakery, frozen, and grocery shelves.

● Avoid extra shopping trips. If possible, shop just once or twice a week. You'll spend less on impulse items—and save time, too.

● Check supermarket specials printed in newspaper inserts. Then plan menus around them. If the store runs out of an item on special, ask for a rain check. Be aware that "limit" signs ("limit three per customer") and messages such as "two for $5.00" (not

"$2.50 each") are marketing ploys to get consumers to buy more. Research shows they work!

● Clip coupons for items you really need. Be aware that items with coupons aren't always the best buy. Another brand or a similar food might be cheaper, even without a coupon.

● Try not to shop when you're hungry. You'll less likely succumb to impulse items, including more expensive and less nutritious snack and dessert foods.

● Take advantage of seasonal produce. In season, the price for fresh fruit and vegetables may be lower, and the produce, more flavorful. Depending on where you live, you might even go directly to the farm where they grow.

● Use food labels as you shop. Remember that label information can help you find foods that match your needs, provide Nutrition Facts for comparison shopping, and help you get the most nutrition for your food dollar.

● Decide what quality food you need. For example, if you're making a casserole, chunky tuna may be fine. But more expensive solid-pack tuna has more eye appeal in a tuna-vegetable salad.

● Buy the economy size or family packs only if you can use that much. There's no savings if food spoils and must be discarded. For foods that freeze, take time to repackage food into smaller amounts in freezer bags, then freeze for later use.

● Compare prices using unit pricing on supermarket shelves. To make comparisons easier, especially for similar foods in different-size containers, prices are given as cost per unit rather than price per package or container. The unit might be an ounce, a quart, or some other measurement. If the foods themselves and the units being compared are the same, the best value is the lowest price per unit.

● Compare the prices of national brands, store brands, and generic brands. Store brands and generic products may cost less than national brands, since they don't have the same promotional costs. But the quality may not be as consistent, so watch for store specials when the prices may be comparable. Convenient, innovative packaging such as squirt bottles and ready-to-serve pouches often add to the cost; decide if the benefits are worth any extra cost.

● If available, and if you qualify, take advantage of senior citizen discount days.

● Stock up on canned and other nonperishable foods when they're on sale. At home, rotate your food supply so that the "first in" is the "first out."

● Buy perishable foods in amounts that will be consumed during their peak quality. An extra bunch of broccoli that spoils in the refrigerator is no savings.

● Consider foods sold in bulk bins. Without the expense of packaging or branding, bulk foods often cost less, and they're usually the same foods you find on supermarket shelves. Perhaps the best advantage: you can buy just the amount you need. Foods such as dry fruits, rice, pasta, other grains, snack mixes, and spices are among those sold in bulk.

● Consider the cost for convenience. Prepared, presliced, and precooked foods usually cost more. Depending on your schedule, labor-saving and step-saving ingredients may be worth the price.

● Remain flexible as you shop. If you see a better bargain or a new food (perhaps a vegetable or a fruit), adjust your menu.

● Shop during off-hours. If time is at a premium, shop when stores aren't crowded—often early in the morning, late in the evening, or midweek rather than on weekends. It may be a less stressful time to shop, too.

● Pay attention at checkout. See that prices ring up as advertised or as indicated on the shelf label, especially for sale items.

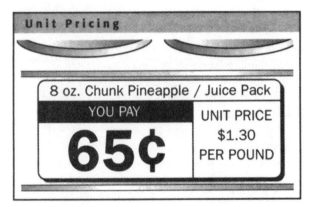

"Small-Scale" Shopping

How do small households maximize their food dollars? Besides general cost-saving tips, you might save in other ways if you're a household of one or two:

● Buy frozen vegetables and fruit in bags, not boxes. As long as they aren't thawed, you can pour out as much as you need, then reseal and return the package to the freezer.

● Look for foods sold in single servings: juice, yogurt, frozen meals, soup, and pudding, among others. In that way you can have a greater variety of food on hand. Because small households are a big segment of the consumer market, more and more products now are available in single-size servings.

● To take advantage of the savings of economy-size packages, share your food purchases with a friend.

● Shop from bulk bins. In that way you can buy small amounts.

● Repackage meat, poultry, and fish into single portions in freezer wrap or plastic freezer bags. Freeze these portions to use later.

● Ask the butcher or the produce manager for a smaller amount of prepackaged fresh meat, poultry, or produce. Usually they can repackage food.

● Buy produce that keeps longer in the refrigerator: broccoli, Brussels sprouts, cabbage, carrots, parsnips, potatoes, sweet potatoes, apples, grapefruit, melons, oranges, pears, and tangerines.

● Shop for convenience. Often mixed salad greens (perhaps from the salad bar) or raw vegetables, already cut and mixed for stir-fry dishes or salads, cost less than buying individual foods in quantity.

● Buy small loaves of bread, or wrap and freeze what you won't use right away.

Your Shopping Guide

Filling your shopping cart? Choose plenty of foods from the five food groups and then add a few extras. Overall, the foods you buy should allow you to make meals and snacks with variety, moderation, and balance.

Shopping for Freshness!

For Fruit . . .

Apples: firm with smooth, clean skin and good color. Avoid fruit with bruises or decay spots.

Apricots: plump with as much golden-orange color as possible. Blemishes, unless they break the skin, will not affect flavor. Avoid fruit that is pale yellow, greenish-yellow, very firm, shriveled, or bruised.

Bananas: plump with uniform shape at desired ripeness level. Avoid produce with blemished or bruised skins.

Blueberries: plump, firm berries with a light-grayish bloom. The bloom is the thin coating on the surface.

Cantaloupes: slightly oval fruit, 5 inches or more in diameter, with yellow or golden (not green) background color. Signs of sweetness include pronounced netting on the rind and a few tiny cracks near the stem end. Smell the melon; it should be noticeably strong and sweet. At home, check for ripeness before you eat it; the stem area will be slightly soft when ripe.

Cherries: plump, bright-colored sweet or sour cherries. Sweet cherries with reddish-brown skin promise flavor. Avoid overly soft or shriveled cherries or those with dark stems.

Grapefruits: firm, thin-skinned fruit, full-colored, and heavy for their size. The best grapefruits are smooth, thin-skinned, and flat at both ends. Avoid fruit with a pointed end or thick, deeply pored skin.

Grapes: plump grapes firmly attached to pliable green stems. Color is the best indication of ripeness and flavor. Avoid soft or wrinkled fruits and those with bleached-looking areas at the stem end.

Honeydew melons: melons weighing at least 5 pounds, with waxy white rind barely tinged with green. Fully ripe fruit has a cream-colored rind. When ripe, the blossom end should give to gentle pressure.

Kiwifruit: softness similar to a ripe peach. Choose evenly firm fruit.

Lemons: firm, heavy fruit. Generally, rough-textured lemons have thicker skins and less juice than fine-skinned varieties.

Mangoes: usually quite firm when sold and need to be ripened further at home before eating. Avoid those with shriveled or bruised skin. Once ripened, they will give to gentle pressure.

Nectarines: orange-yellow (not green) background color between areas of red. Ripe nectarines feel slightly soft with gentle handling, but not as soft as ripe peaches.

Oranges: thin-skinned, firm, bright-colored fruit. Avoid oranges with any hint of softness or whitish mold at the ends.

Papayas: fruit with the softness of peaches and more yellow than green in the skin. Most papayas need to be ripened further after purchase in a loosely closed paper bag at room temperature. Avoid bruised or shriveled fruit showing any signs of mold or deterioration.

Peaches: creamy or yellow background color. Ripe peaches feel slightly soft with gentle handling. Avoid green, extra-hard, or bruised fruit.

Pears: fruit with firm skin. Pears gradually ripen after picking.

Pineapples: large, plump, fresh-looking fruit with green leaves and a sweet smell. Avoid fruit with soft spots, areas of decay, or fermented odor.

Plums: fruit that is full-colored. Ripe plums are slightly soft at the tip end and feel somewhat soft when handled gently. Avoid fruit with broken or shriveled skin.

Raspberries: firm, plump, well-shaped berries. If soft or discolored, they are overripe. Avoid baskets that look stained from overripe berries.

Strawberries: firm, plump berries that are full-colored.

Watermelons: fruit heavy for its size, well shaped, with rind and flesh colors characteristic of the variety. Ripe melons are fragrant and slightly soft at the blossom end. A melon that sloshes when shaken is probably overripe. The stem should be dry and brown, not green. When thumped, you should hear a low-pitched sound, indicating a full, juicy interior.

For Vegetables . . .

Artichokes: tight, compact heads that feel heavy for their size. Surface brown spots don't affect quality.

Asparagus: firm, brittle spears that are bright green almost their entire length, with tightly closed tips.

Beans (green or waxed): slender, crisp beans that are bright and blemish-free. Avoid mature beans with large seeds and swollen pods.

Beets: firm, smooth-skinned, small to medium beets. Leaves should be deep green and fresh-looking.

Bok choy: heads with bright white stalks and glossy dark leaves. Avoid heads with slippery brown spots on the leaves.

Broccoli: compact clusters of tightly closed, dark green florets. Avoid heads with yellow florets or thick, woody stems.

Brussels sprouts: firm, compact, fresh-looking sprouts that are bright green. They should be heavy for their size.

Cabbage: firm heads that feel heavy for their size. Outer leaves should have good color and be free of blemishes.

Carrots: firm, clean, well-shaped carrots with bright, orange-gold color. Carrots with their tops still attached are likely to be freshest.

Cauliflower: firm, compact, creamy-white heads (without brown spots), with florets pressed tightly together. A yellow tinge and spreading florets indicate overmaturity. Leaves should be crisp and bright green.

Celery: crisp, rigid, green stalks with fresh-looking leaves. Avoid celery with limp stalks.

Corn: fresh-looking ears with green husks, moist stems, and silk ends free of decay or worm injury. When pierced with a thumbnail, kernels should give a squirt of juice. Tough skins indicate overmaturity.

Cucumbers: firm, dark green cucumbers that are slender but well shaped. Soft or yellow cukes are overmature.

Eggplants: firm, heavy for their size, with taut, glassy, deeply colored skin. Stems should be bright green.

Greens: fresh, tender leaves that are free of blemishes. Avoid bunches with thick, coarse-veined leaves.

Jicama: firm, well-formed tubers free of blemishes. Size does not affect flavor, but larger roots do tend to have a coarse texture.

Kohlrabi: young, tender bulbs with fresh green leaves. Avoid those with scars and blemishes. The smaller the bulb, the more delicate the flavor and texture.

Leeks: clean, white bottoms and crisp, fresh-looking green tops.

Mushrooms: blemish-free mushrooms without slimy spots or signs of decay.

Okra: small to medium pods that are deep green and free of blemishes. Pods should snap or puncture easily with slight pressure.

Onions: green onions with crisp, bright green tops and clean white bottoms. Choose firm, dry onions with brittle outer skin, avoiding those with sprouting green shoots or dark spots.

Parsnips: small to medium, smooth, firm, and well shaped. Avoid large roots because they may have a woody core.

Peas: small, plump, bright green pods that are firm, crisp, and well filled.

Peppers: bright, glossy, firm, and well shaped. Avoid those with soft spots or gashes.

Potatoes: firm, smooth, with no wrinkles, sprouts, cracks, bruises, decay, or bitter green areas (caused by exposure to light).

Rutabagas: small to medium, smooth, firm, and heavy for their size.

Salad greens: crisp, deeply colored leaves free of brown spots, yellowed leaves, and decay.

Sprouts: crisp buds still attached.

Summer squash: yellow squash and zucchini of medium size with firm, smooth, glossy, tender skin. Squash should be heavy for their size.

Sweet potatoes and yams: firm, well shaped, with bright, uniformly colored skin.

Tomatoes: smooth, well formed, firm, not hard.

Turnips: firm, smooth, small to medium size, that are heavy for their size.

Winter squash: hard, thick-shelled.

Source: Adapted from M. J. Smith, *The Miracle Foods Cookbook* (Minneapolis: Chronimed Publishing, 1995). This material is used by permission of John Wiley & Sons, Inc.

Now let's tour the supermarket, department by department, focusing on shopping tips for high-quality, nutritious, and safe foods—that match your needs.

Produce Department

Today's supermarkets offer a great variety of fresh fruits and vegetables—about three hundred different types of produce in the average store. *See chapter 9 for new fruits and vegetables you might try.* Because fruit and vegetables are most nutritious and best-tasting at their peak quality, shop with savvy.

● Check the produce department. Besides being clean, organized, and appealing, fresh fruits and vegetables should be held at a proper temperature. Most are kept chilled; a fine mist helps keep lettuce and other greens crisp.

● For fresh fruits, consider ripeness. If you're buying fruits to eat today, buy ripe. For tomorrow or the next day, look for fruits that need just a little ripening. If you don't plan to eat them until later in the week, buy fruits that aren't yet ripe. *Tip:* To hasten the ripening of some fruits such as pears and peaches, put them in a loosely closed paper bag at room temperature.

● Buy the amount you need. Even when properly stored, produce is perishable. The freshest produce contains the most nutrients.

● Look for nutrition information. If packaged, the label on produce may carry Nutrition Facts. If not, check for a poster or a pamphlet with this information nearby. Ask the store manager to provide this information if it's not available. *For fruits and vegetables that are good sources of beta carotene (which forms vitamin A), vitamin C, potassium, folate, and fiber see "Produce 'Package'" in chapter 10.*

● Go for variety! That includes fruits and vegetables rich in beta carotene or vitamin C or both. Rather than just the old standbys, add a new fruit or vegetable to your shopping cart each week or two; try some that are locally grown. The store may have preparation and handling tips for unfamiliar produce.

Explore different varieties of a familiar food. For example, try different apples: perhaps Cortland, Granny Smith, Newtown Pippin, and Rome Beauty. Or choose one of each variety of plums: perhaps Laroda, Queen Ann, Santa Rosa, and Wickson.

● Look for signs of quality. Bruised or wilted produce suggests that it hasn't been handled properly or that it's past its peak. Some nutrients may be lost as a result. *Refer to the chart "Shopping for Freshness!" earlier in this chapter for signs of quality in commonly eaten fruits and vegetables.*

● For flavor, buy small. Small fruit is often sweeter than larger pieces of the same fruit.

● Handle fresh fruits and vegetables gently. Damage and bruising hasten spoilage. Place produce in the shopping cart where it won't get bruised. At the checkout, make sure produce is packed on top or in separate bags.

● Consider choosing your own produce rather than buying it prepackaged. In that way you can examine and pick out items at their peak of quality.

● Look for other items in the produce department, such as fresh herbs, herbs in jars, and sun-dried tomatoes, among others. Fresh herbs are often prepackaged; choose those that look fresh, not wilted. Dried fruits are a nonperishable option, often sold in the produce department; they supply the same nutrients as fresh fruit. If you're sensitive to sulfites, check the label; sulfites are used to prevent browning in many dried fruits.

● Shopping at a farm stand? Be aware that the produce sold may not be fresh from the field. Ask to find out. Sometimes produce is brought in from the same commercial markets used by supermarkets, then sold as "farm fresh."

Meat and Deli Case

Through advanced breeding and feeding practices, today's animals are leaner than ever. Leaner cuts are available also because of closer trimming of beef, veal, pork, and lamb cuts. The average thickness of fat

Have You Ever Wondered

. . . how safe are the refrigerated juices purchased from the store? Most packaged juices and juice drinks—refrigerated, frozen, and shelf-stable—have been heat-treated (pasteurized) or processed in other ways to destroy harmful bacteria and naturally occurring enzymes that hasten spoilage.

If sold in interstate commerce, fresh juice and juice products that have *not been pasteurized* or appropriately treated must show this warning on the package label.

> WARNING: this product has not been pasteurized and, therefore, may contain harmful bacteria that can cause serious illness in children, the elderly, and persons with weakened immune systems.

Juices made locally, such as apple cider from a nearby orchard, aren't required to provide this warning unless there is a state ruling. Juice bars and restaurants that sell freshly squeezed juice in glasses to drink right away don't need to provide this warning, either.

around the edge of steaks and roasts has trimmed down from ½ inch to ¾ inch twenty-five or more years ago to less than ⅛ inch trim today. *See "Today's Meat" in chapter 9.*

For the "lean advantage"—and the other nutrients that meat supplies (especially protein, B vitamins, iron, and zinc)—consider these shopping tips:

● *Shop for meat's "skinny" cuts.* Certain cuts of meat are leaner than others. Use this rule of thumb in selecting lower-fat cuts of fresh meats: Look for the words "round" or "loin" in the name when shopping for beef, and the words "loin" or "leg" when buying pork or lamb. Here are some examples of lean cuts.

  ● *Beef:* eye of round, top round steak, top round roast, sirloin steak, top loin steak, tenderloin steak, and chuck arm pot roast

  ● *Veal:* cutlet, blade or arm steak, rib roast, and rib or loin chop

  ● *Pork:* tenderloin, top loin roast, top loin chop, center loin chop, sirloin roast, loin rib chop, and shoulder blade steak

  ● *Lamb:* leg, loin chop, arm chop, and foreshanks

If you're not sure of the cut, check the meat label. It identifies the kind and cut, along with the net weight, unit price, and cost per package.

● Choose leaner grades of meat. "Select" grades of beef have the least marbled fat (or thin streaks of fat between the muscle) followed by "choice" cuts, then "prime" beef cuts. Veal and lamb 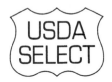 use the same grading system; however, the term "good" is used instead of "select." Grading, which is determined by the U.S. Department of Agriculture, is based on fat content, appearance, texture, and the age of the animal. Pork is not graded.

The more costly "prime" grade of beef—more often on restaurant menus than sold in supermarkets—has more marbled fat, which helps make the meat juicy and flavorful. However, with moist methods of cooking and proper carving, the leaner "select" and "choice" meats can be tender, juicy, and flavorful, too.

Nutritionally speaking, nutrients in meat—protein, thiamin, niacin, iron, and zinc, among others—are the same, regardless of grade.

● Buy well-trimmed meat: ⅛-inch fat trim or less. "Trim" refers to the fat layer surrounding a steak or other cut of meat. *Note:* Marbled fat cannot be trimmed away. Only cooking methods can remove some, but not all, marbled fat.

● Check the "numbers" for ground meat—look for packages that have the greatest percent lean to percent fat ratio. Ground beef labeled as 95 percent lean also may include the nutrition description "Lean" because it meets the definition of a lean product. *Note:* "Percent lean" refers to the weight of the lean meat in relation to the weight of the fat.

On ground meats you also may see other names. Ground round is the leanest, followed by ground sirloin, ground chuck, then regular ground meat. If you don't see ground round, the butcher can grind meat for you from a round cut of meat, or you can grind it yourself in a food processor.

● Buy enough meat without overdoing on portion size. For moderate-size portions (3 ounces cooked), figure 4 ounces of uncooked, boneless meat per person. *Refer to the chart "Meat Buying Guide" later in this chapter to help you decide how much meat to buy.*

● Use nutrition labeling to find lean packaged meats. By regulation, packaged deli meats must carry nutrition labeling. That helps you find today's leaner hot dogs, luncheon meats, and sausage patties.

Also check out the lean options from the deli case. When buying ready-to-slice luncheon meats from a deli, ask for nutrition information if you're unsure of a product's leanness. Some lean products will be identified with a nutrient content claim such as "low-fat," "___% fat-free," or "lean."

● Look for nutrition information for fresh meat, poultry, and seafood. Single-ingredient raw meat, poultry, and seafood may be labeled with Nutri-Facts. Look for this information on materials (poster or pamphlet) near the meat or seafood counter for forty-five commonly consumed meat and poultry cuts and twenty seafood items. You'll see nutrition information for meat with and without trimmable fat. The Nutri-Facts program is voluntary, so it may not appear in all supermarkets.

● When shopping for bacon, try Canadian bacon or turkey bacon. Canadian bacon is lean, much like ham, and fits in the Meat and Beans Group of the Food Guide Pyramid. In contrast, traditional bacon is mainly fat and fits in the Pyramid tip, not in the Meat and Beans Group. If you're watching your sodium intake, check the label.

● Occasionally choose organ meats, also called variety meats. Brain, chitterlings (pig intestines), heart, kidney, liver, sweetbreads (thymus gland), tongue, and tripe (stomach lining of cattle) are all organ meats. Organ meats are good sources of many nutrients; liver, in particular, is high in iron. However, most are higher in cholesterol than lean meat. And some, such as chitterlings, sweetbreads, and tongue, have more fat than others.

● For convenience, look for meat that's already seasoned, prepared, and ready to cook, such as meat and vegetable kebobs or marinated pork loin. You may also find precooked, packaged heat-and-eat meats in the refrigerated case. Be aware that these meats may be higher in sodium.

Reading Meat Labels

1. The kind of meat—Listed on every label

2. The primal (wholesale) cut—Tells where the meat came from on the animal

3. The retail cut—Tells from what part of the primal cut the meat comes

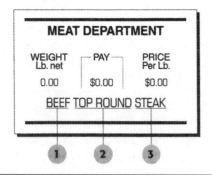

● Recognize the qualities of fresh meat. The color of meat indicates its freshness. Beef is typically a bright red color. Both young veal and pork are grayish-pink. Older veal is a darker pink. And lamb can be light to darker pink, depending on how it was fed.

● Check food product dating on meat. Only buy fresh and processed meats that still will be fresh when

you're ready to eat them. Or plan to freeze immediately for later use.

● Notice the safe food handling label. *A sample label is shown in this chapter. For more about the safe handling of meat, see chapter 12, "The Safe Kitchen."*

Poultry Counter

Besides being economical, chicken and turkey offer high-quality protein, and they're usually very lean. Consider these tips as you choose poultry for your shopping cart:

● Choose mostly lean varieties of poultry—turkey and chicken. Domesticated duck and goose are higher in fat. A 3½-ounce cooked portion of roasted, skinless chicken (light and dark meat) has about 7 fat grams compared with 11 fat grams in the same portion of roasted, skinless duck. Pheasant and quail, especially without the skin, are lean, too.

● To trim fat, shop for skinless poultry—chicken and turkey. You'll cut the grams of total fat and saturated fat in half. Or buy poultry with the skin on if it costs less, then take the skin off at home.

Meat Buying Guide

How much raw meat should you buy? If you figure about 3 ounces of cooked, lean meat per person, that's about 4 ounces of raw meat per person. For some meats you'll need to take the amount of bone and fat into account.

TYPE OF MEAT	SERVINGS PER POUND*
Boneless or ground meat	4
Meat with a minimum amount of bone (steaks, roasts, chops, etc.)	2 to 3
Meat with a large amount of bone (shoulder cuts, short ribs, neck, etc.)	1 to 2

*Three ounces of cooked trimmed meat equal one serving.

Source: Adapted from Nutrition, Health, and Food Management Division, American Association of Family and Consumer Sciences, *Food: A Handbook of Terminology, Purchasing, and Preparation* (Alexandria, Va.: American Association of Family and Consumer Sciences, 2001), pp. 139-143. Copyright 2001 by the American Association of Family and Consumer Sciences. Reprinted with permission.

Poultry Buying Guide

How much poultry? Here's how many servings come from 1 pound of uncooked chicken, duck, goose, game hens, or turkey.

POULTRY	SERVINGS PER POUND*
Whole chicken (broiler-fryer or roaster)	2
Boneless chicken breast	4
Duck, whole	1
Goose, whole	1½ to 2
Rock Cornish game hen, whole	1
Whole turkey, bone in	2
Boneless turkey roast	3
Ground turkey	4

*Amounts are based on 3 ounces of cooked poultry without bone per serving.

Source: Adapted from Nutrition, Health, and Food Management Division, American Association of Family and Consumer Sciences, *Food: A Handbook of Terminology, Purchasing, and Preparation* (Alexandria, Va.: American Association of Family and Consumer Sciences, 2001), pp. 139-143. Copyright 2001 by the American Association of Family and Consumer Sciences. Reprinted with permission.

For less fat, choose light meat such as the turkey or chicken breast. Compare the difference: 3½ ounces of roasted, skinless, dark-meat chicken have about 10 fat grams and 3 grams of saturated fat; the same amount of roasted, skinless, light-meat chicken has about 3 fat grams and 1 gram of saturated fat. The cholesterol content is about the same.

● When you buy whole turkey, know that self-basting varieties are higher in fat. Self-basting turkeys are moist because they're injected with fat—which may be high in saturated fatty acids. Instead, you can baste turkey regularly with broth, juice, or juices from the poultry. *Hint:* Roasting any whole bird with the breast side up makes it moister.

● Is ground meat on your shopping list? Look for lean ground turkey breast, too. Ground turkey breast can be as lean as 99 percent fat-free. The fat content is higher if it's ground with dark meat and skin.

● Recognize the qualities of fresh poultry. Look for meaty birds with skin that's creamy-white to yellow and that are free of bruises, tiny feathers, and torn or dry skin. Check for food product dating on food labels, too.

● Read the Nutrition Facts before you buy turkey dogs, turkey ham, or turkey bologna. They may—or may not—be low in fat. Compare the sodium content with that of traditional processed meats; processing typically adds sodium. For fresh cuts of poultry, look for Nutri-Facts, which may be posted in the retail case.

● For cost savings, buy a whole bird. You'll usually save money if you carve a chicken in parts yourself.

Have You Ever Wondered

. . . if free-range chickens have less fat? It's a common misperception that free-range chickens—those that "roam the barnyard and forage for food"—are always leaner than chickens raised in coops. Whether they're raised in a coop or a barnyard, their exercise level often is about the same. Genetic stock, age, and growth rate have greater influence on fat levels. Older, larger chickens and those that grow faster tend to have more fat. That's true of all chickens, no matter how they're raised.

According to the USDA's Food Safety and Inspection Service, which regulates poultry labeling, the terms "free-range" and "free-roaming" may be used on poultry labels if the producers can demonstrate that the poultry has been allowed access to the outside for a significant portion of their life. Some people are willing to spend more for free-range chickens because they perceive a taste difference; blind taste tests don't show differences in flavor perception.

. . . if the tiny red spots on finfish are safe to eat? These spots are bruise marks, not contamination. They occur when fish is not handled gently, either when it's caught or in the supermarket. It's safe to eat. But be aware that bruised areas often deteriorate faster.

. . . how the fat and cholesterol in surimi compare with crabmeat? Surimi is imitation crabmeat, made from pollock or another mild-flavored fish. The fish is processed by rolling "sheets" of fish and adding color so it looks like crab legs. The nutrient content reflects the fish it's made from. Surimi is comparable in fat content but lower in cholesterol than crabmeat.

● Buy enough poultry for moderate portions. *The chart "Poultry Buying Guide" earlier in this chapter shows how much to buy per person for 3-ounce cooked portions.*

Fish Counter

There's increased attention to seafood these days, often for its nutritional benefits. Besides being a good protein source, most seafood is low in fat, especially saturated fat. Fatty fish offers potential health benefits from omega-3 fatty acids; that's why health experts recommend eating seafood several times a week. *See "Eat Your Omega-3s and -6s" in chapter 3.*

The many varieties of fish on the market today can offer great taste and versatility in menu planning. So learn to shop for seafood confidently; choose high-quality, safe seafood that also matches your personal needs and preferences.

A few definitions before you start shopping: seafood includes both finfish and shellfish. Catfish, cod, haddock, flounder, mahimahi, snapper, tuna, and trout are among the many types of finfish. Shellfish are both crustaceans (crab, crayfish, lobster, and shrimp) and mollusks (clam, mussel, oyster, scallop, octopus, squid, abalone, conch, and snail).

● Check the fish counter before you buy. Always buy seafood from a reputable source, probably not a pickup truck. Seafood should be displayed with food safety in mind: properly iced, well refrigerated, and in clean display cases. To reduce the chance of spoilage, fish should be displayed "belly down" to drain away melting ice. Be sure that the seafood is wrapped separately, in a leakproof package.

Check for general cleanliness and quality: clean look and smell; free of insects; employees wearing disposable gloves (changed after handling nonfood and again after handling raw fish); and knowledgeable workers who can answer your questions about the freshness of the seafood. Ask when and how often fresh and flash-frozen fish come in. Try to be flexible with your menu; buy the freshest fish if you don't need a specific type.

● Recognize the different fat contents of various fish. In general, most fish has less fat than other protein-rich foods, including meat and poultry with skin. And most fat in seafood is polyunsaturated.

Fish that's white or light in color, such as orange roughy, perch, snapper, and sole, has less fat than fish that is firm and darker in color, such as mackerel, salmon, and bluefin tuna. Fattier fish have more omega-3 fatty acids than lean fish or shellfish; omega-3s may offer heart-healthy benefits. Try to eat fatty fish twice a week.

● Choose fish that's best for the recipe. Lean fish is great for baking, microwaving, and poaching. Fish with more fat tends to be better for grilling and roasting because it doesn't dry out as quickly and because it holds its shape better. For example, salmon and tuna are better for kebobs. Mild-flavored fish tends to be the lowest in fat, while fish with more fat usually has a fuller flavor.

● Learn to recognize the qualities of fresh seafood.
  ● *Finfish*. At peak quality, whole finfish have a fresh ocean-breeze scent, not a fish or ammonialike smell. They're naturally firm to the touch, with stiff fins and scales that cling tightly to the skin. The skin

Seafood Buying Guide

TYPE OF SEAFOOD	APPROXIMATE AMOUNT OF RAW SEAFOOD NEEDED PER ADULT SERVING*
Whole fish	¾ pound
Dressed or pan-dressed fish	½ pound
Fish fillets	¼ to ⅓ pound
Fish steaks with bone	½ pound
Fish steaks without bone	⅓ pound
Live clams and oysters	6 to 8
Shucked clams and oysters	⅓ to ½ pint
Live lobsters and crabs	1 to 1½ pounds
Cooked lobster or crabmeat	¼ to ⅓ pound
Scallops	¼ to ⅓ pound
Shrimp, headless and unpeeled	⅓ to ½ pound
Shrimp, peeled and deveined	¼ to ⅓ pound

*The smaller amounts in the ranges shown provide a cooked portion that is approximately 3 ounces when prepared by most common cooking methods.

Source: Ken Gall, *Seafood Savvy.* Information Bulletin 1041B226 (Ithaca, N.Y.: Cornell Cooperative Extension, Cornell University, 1992).

is shiny and "metallic," not dull. The gills are pink or bright red and free from mucus or slime. If undamaged, their eyes are clear, bright, and protruding. Walleyes are among the few fish with naturally cloudy eyes. Fish fillets or steaks also have a mild scent, firm and moist flesh, a translucent appearance, and no browning around the edges. If wrapped, the packaging should be tight and undamaged.

● *Shellfish*. Crustaceans and some mollusks are sold live. In fact, unless frozen, canned, or cooked, crabs, crayfish, and lobsters should be alive when sold. They'll move slightly if they're alive, and live lobsters curl their tails a bit when handled. For food safety, buy shellfish from a reputable source.

If their shells are still on, clams, mussels, and oysters must be sold alive, too, for food safety sake; shells shouldn't be damaged. When these mollusks are alive, their shells are slightly open, but they close tightly when tapped. As another easy test, hold the shell between your thumb and forefinger and press so that one part of the shell slides across the other. If the shells move, it isn't fresh.

Freshly shucked mollusks (shells removed) have a mild, fresh scent. A somewhat clear liquid—not too milky or cloudy—should cover the shucked "meat."

Scallops are removed from their shells at sea. They vary in size and color, from creamy white to light orange, tan, or somewhat pinkish. When fresh, they're not dry or darkened around the edges.

Regardless of size and color, fresh, raw shrimp will have a mild odor. For all fish—finfish and shellfish—use your nose. A strong "fishy" odor is a sign that fish is no longer fresh.

● Know the qualities of frozen fish, too. Frozen seafood should be solidly frozen, mild in odor, and free of ice crystals and freezer burn. Freezer burn is indicated by drying and discoloration. The package shouldn't be damaged or water-stained, and it should be stored below the frost line in the store's display freezer. These qualities apply to both frozen fish and frozen prepared items such as crab cakes and breaded shrimp.

● Check the food product dating on the label of fresh, frozen fish. Choose packaged seafood that doesn't show signs of thawing, then refreezing. Check the "sell by" date, if it has one, for a quality product. *See information about food product dating earlier in this chapter.*

● Choose cooked shrimp, lobsters, crabs, and crayfish that are moist with a mild odor and a characteristic color. The shells of cooked shrimp should be pink to reddish. For other crustaceans, the shells should be bright red.

● For safety, don't buy cooked seafood that's displayed alongside raw seafood. Bacteria from raw fish can contaminate cooked fish, creating a potential for foodborne illness. *To learn more about cross-contamination and food safety, see "Checklist for a Clean Kitchen" in chapter 12.*

● Choose smoked fish, such as smoked salmon or smoked trout, that is bright, glossy, and free of mold. Since it may not be cooked before serving, smoked fish should be wrapped and kept away from raw fish to avoid cross-contamination.

● Substitute one fish for another. When the store doesn't have the seafood you want or if it costs more than you anticipate, don't despair; just make a switch. For example, when a recipe calls for flounder, almost any mild finfish (probably one that's low in fat, such as haddock, halibut, or perch) can take its place.

Be aware of differences in nutritional content when you make substitutions. Squid, shrimp, and lobsters, for example, have more cholesterol than clams, crabs, mussels, and scallops do. Three ounces of boiled shrimp supply about 165 milligrams of cholesterol, while the same amount of scallops have about 55 milligrams of cholesterol.

● Whether it's sold at the seafood counter or from the freezer section, go easy on breaded items such as shrimp and fish sticks, which typically contain more fat and calories.

● For nutrition information check the Nutrition Facts on packaged seafood products. For fresh seafood you'll find this information displayed nearby.

● Buy the amount of seafood you need. Because of waste, you need more when preparing whole or dressed fish. A dressed fish has the head, tail, and fins removed. Usually fish steaks, fillets, and shellfish, which have less waste, cost more per pound. *The chart "Seafood Buying Guide" earlier in this chapter helps you estimate how much you need for a cooked 3-ounce portion.*

Refrigerated Case

Although you'll find tortillas, refrigerator rolls, and yeast among the many products in the refrigerated case, dairy foods and eggs take the most prominent spots. For both food categories, you have many choices.

Dairy Foods

Milk

● Choose milk that matches your needs. No matter what type, milk is an excellent source of calcium, with one cup supplying 30 percent of the Daily Value. Milk also provides protein, riboflavin, vitamins A and D, phosphorus, and other vitamins and minerals. How do the various forms of milk differ? Fat content is the main difference. *The chart "Milk: A Good Calcium Source" in chapter 10 makes some nutrition comparisons. See "Which Milk for You?" in this chapter for the definitions of types of milk.*

● If you're sensitive to lactose, or milk sugar, look for lactose-reduced or lactose-free milk. By adding the enzyme lactase, manufacturers can produce dairy foods with much less lactose. *See chapter 21 for more information on lactose intolerance.*

Yogurt

Like milk, yogurt comes in whole, low-fat, and non-fat varieties. The fat and calorie content reflect the milk it's made from. Yogurt also may be flavored with fruit, fruit preserves, or extracts such as vanilla or coffee. If you're watching calories, reach for yogurt flavored with a low-calorie sweetener, such as aspartame.

Yogurt is made with "friendly" bacteria, which give a distinctive taste and consistency. As an added benefit, active, live cultures may offer health benefits, perhaps in boosting immunity or in helping the body digest milk's sugar. However, the research on the health benefits of active, live cultures in yogurt isn't conclusive.

Yogurt with labels that state "made with active cul-tures" may not contain live cultures if it's been heat-treated. Frozen yogurt may contain live active cultures; if they're present, freezing slows their action.

● If you want the potential benefit of active live cultures, look for the *"Live and Active Cultures"* seal, administered by the National Yogurt Association, on regular and frozen yogurt containers. The ingredient list shows the presence of the probiotic, or live cultures; those most commonly used are *Lactobacillus acidophilus, L. casei, L. reuteri,* and *Bifidobacterium bifidum (Bifidus).*

● Look for different types of yogurt—fruit-flavored or plain, and whole, low-fat, or nonfat. Yogurt is another high-calcium, high-protein dairy food. In fact, 8 ounces of either yogurt or milk supply about 300 milligrams of calcium. If you don't drink much milk, you might buy more yogurt to get the calcium you need.

● Enjoy flavored yogurt-juice beverages—another source of calcium. Or look for the yogurt drink called kefir, often sold in health food stores. Ingesting thick and frothy kefir is somewhat like drinking yogurt. It's a cultured dairy beverage usually made from cow or goat milk and the active, "friendly" kefir bacteria.

Cheese

● Check out the wide variety of the more than four hundred varieties of cheese sold today. Cheese is milk in concentrated form; about 10 pounds (5 quarts) of milk are used to make every pound of Cheddar cheese. That's why cheese is a great source of milk's nutrients: protein; calcium, phosphorus, zinc, vitamin A, riboflavin, and vitamin B_{12}.

● To cut back on fat and still get plenty of nutrients, you might look for lower-fat cheeses such as low-fat ricotta, part-skim mozzarella, string cheese, or varieties of reduced-fat cheese. Many cheeses have considerably more fat per serving than a serving of milk does. As a rule of thumb, any cheese made with fat-free milk will likely have less fat.

● *Low-fat cheese* has 3 grams or less fat per serving; that's 1 ounce for most cheese and 4 ounces for cottage cheese.

● *Reduced-fat cheese* has 25 percent less fat than the same full-fat cheese.

● *Fat-free cheese* has less than 0.5 gram of fat per serving.

Cheese with less fat usually has less cholesterol, too, but you need to check the label to be sure.

● Consider buying shredded cheese and sharp-flavored cheese. For cheese shreds you may pay a little more per ounce for the convenience of "preprep." When it's grated you may use a little less cheese in recipes than if you had used sliced or chunk cheese. That's another way to savor the flavor yet control fat. *Tip:* Using stronger-flavored cheese such as Parmesan, feta, or sharp Cheddar delivers more flavor with less cheese than mild cheese does.

● Look for reduced-sodium cheeses if you're watching your sodium intake. Traditional cheese has sodium because it's a key ingredient in cheesemaking.

Cream, Sour Cream, Spreads

● Buy them—just go easy on how much you use. Both are high in fat and deliver very little calcium.

● For less fat and fewer calories, try lower-fat and nonfat varieties. Try half-and-half rather than cream; another option is fat-free half-and-half (mostly made of fat-free milk). Choose sour half-and-half or fat-free sour cream. Read the labels, since the fat content among products varies.

● Look for spreads—butter, margarine, and cream cheese—in the dairy case. From a fat and calorie standpoint, butter and margarine are the same, with about 35 calories and 4 grams of fat per teaspoon. Both are primarily fat; only the source differs. Butter

Have You Ever Wondered

. . . how cow milk and soy milk compare? The nutrient content of soy milk isn't the same as in cow milk. Unless fortified, soy milk, made by pressing ground, cooked soybeans, is significantly lower in calcium. As a substitute for cow milk, choose soy milk that's calcium-fortified. Soy drinks range from 80 to 500 milligrams of calcium per cup; read the Nutrition Facts on the label. Research indicates that the form of calcium in fortified soy beverages isn't as bioavailable, or absorbed as well in the body; to equal the calcium benefits of 1 cup of cow milk (300 milligrams calcium) you may need to consume 500 milligrams of calcium from fortified soy milk.

Compared with cow milk, soy milk is lower in protein and riboflavin, and has little vitamin A or D naturally; some soy milk is fortified with vitamins A and D and riboflavin. As a phytonutrient, soy protein may offer unique benefits from phytoestrogens; *see "A Quick Look at Key Phytonutrients" in chapter 4.* Soy milk is cholesterol-free. The fat content of soy milk is similar to 2 percent cow milk; also look for low-fat versions of soy milk.

. . . why cottage cheese has less calcium than other cheese? During processing, the whey is drained away, along with 50 to 75 percent of the calcium. Check food labels for cottage cheese processed with extra calcium. Good news: it still provides plenty of protein and riboflavin, without much fat.

contains more saturated fats than most margarines. Because margarine is made from vegetable oil, it has no cholesterol.

● For a spread with less saturated fat, buy soft tub margarine, rather than stick margarine with more trans fatty acids. Whipped versions of butter or margarine have less fat per tablespoon, too; air adds to the volume. However, they can't be substituted for regular butter or margarine in recipes that require baking or frying. Reduced-fat butter and margarine are sold, too, but they aren't suitable for some recipes because they have more moisture. Use them as spreads. Other less-saturated-fat options: squeezable, liquid margarine and spray margarine.

● Enjoy small amounts of cream cheese, but don't confuse its nutrient content with other forms of

Cream: How Much Fat? How Many Calories?

CREAM	% MILK FAT CONTENT	FAT GRAMS PER TABLESPOON	CALORIES PER TABLESPOON
Half-and-half	10.5 to 18	2	20
Light or coffee cream	18 to 29	3	30
Light whipping cream	30 to 36	5	44
Heavy cream	36 or more	6	52

Which Milk for You?

From a nutritional standpoint, the differences among whole, 2 percent reduced-fat, 1 percent low-fat, and fat-free milk are the fat and the calorie contents. Because milk solids make up at least 8.25 percent of each of these types of milks, their nutrient content is about the same. (Milk solids are the part of milk that's neither milk fat nor water.) Keep in mind that the percentages of milk fat used to distinguish different types of milk refer to the percent milk fat by weight and not by calories. *See chapter 10 to compare the calorie, fat, and calcium differences.*

In the refrigerator case . . .

- *Whole milk* contains not less than 3.25 percent milk fat and may be fortified with vitamin D.

- *2 percent reduced-fat milk* has 2 percent milk fat. It's also fortified with vitamins A and perhaps D.

- *1 percent low-fat milk,* also called light milk, has just 1 percent milk fat. It must be fortified with vitamins A and D.

- *Fat-free, also referred to as nonfat or skim, milk,* has less than 0.5 percent milk fat. Like low-fat milk, fat-free milk must be fortified with vitamins A and D. Most labels now list fat-free or nonfat terms first and may or may not include the word "skim."

- *Chocolate milk* can be whole, 2 percent reduced-fat, 1 percent low-fat, or fat-free milk with added chocolate or cocoa, and sweetener. Fruit-flavored milk is available, too. Look for strawberry, orange, banana, and other flavors. These milks may not be vitamin-D fortified.

- *Cultured buttermilk* is made by adding "friendly" bacteria cultures to milk, usually fat-free or low-fat milk. The bacteria cultures produces its unique flavor, aroma, acidity, and thick texture. Salt is often added for more flavor. Despite its name, butter isn't added.

- *Eggnog,* sold around certain holidays, is a blend of milk, pasteurized eggs, sugar, cream, and flavors. Because eggnog is higher in calories and fat, some people prefer eggnog-flavored milk, made with fat-free or 2 percent reduced-fat milk.

- *Acidophilus milk,* a fermented dairy food that's usually made from 1 percent low-fat or fat-free milk, is processed with "friendly" bacteria, which gives it a distinctive flavor. Although research isn't conclusive, "friendly" bacteria in fermented dairy foods may help improve lactose digestion and promote healthy bacteria in the gastrointestinal tract.

- *Lactose-free and lactose-reduced milks* (whole, 2 percent reduced-fat, 1 percent low-fat, and fat-free) are treated with the lactase enzyme. Because lactose, the sugar in milk, converts to glucose and galactose, people with lactose intolerance can drink it. To be considered "lactose-reduced," the lactose level must be reduced by 70 percent. Lactose-free milk is 100 percent lactose-reduced.

- *Protein-fortified milk* is milk that has nonfat milk solids added so the milk solids level reaches 10 percent. These solids are often added to fat-free or 1 percent low-fat milk for a fuller flavor and to improve the nutrient content. Often both protein and calcium are added.

- *Low-sodium milk* has most of the sodium removed. Per 8-ounce serving, it has 25 milligrams of sodium, which is 80 percent less than in nonflavored milk. This is an option for those on a sodium-restricted diet.

On the grocery shelf . . .

- *Nonfat dry milk* is milk with the fat and the water removed. It has the same nutrients as fat-free milk.

- *Shelf-stable milk* has been processed quickly by very high heat to destroy bacteria. That allows it to be aseptically packaged and stored on a shelf until it's opened. Once opened, it needs refrigeration.

- *Sweetened condensed milk* is concentrated whole milk, with 8 percent or less milk fat, and added sweetener. You also can buy sweetened condensed fat-free milk.

- *Evaporated milk* has been concentrated with about 60 percent of the water removed. It's sold as both skim and whole evaporated milk and has no less than 20 percent milk solids. Evaporated milk is fortified with vitamins A and D. Once it's opened, it needs refrigeration.

Source: Milk Product Sheet, National Dairy Council (2000).

cheese. Cream cheese is mainly milk fat, with very little milk solids. If you want the creamy texture with less fat, look for reduced-fat or fat-free cream cheese. Or buy regular cream cheese, then spread a little less on your morning bagel. Whipped cream cheese is often easier to spread, so you may be able to use less.

● As another alternative, look for cholesterol-lowering spreads that contain plant stanol and sterol esters. *See chapter 3 for more about them.*

For fluid milk and other dairy foods, products that are properly refrigerated in the store won't spoil as quickly. Check the "sell by" date on the carton.

Eggs

If you're looking for an economical, convenient, and easy-to-prepare source of high-quality protein, try eggs. A single egg supplies about 10 percent of the protein you need in a day, along with good amounts of vitamins A, D, and B_{12} choline, as well as phytonutrients (lutein and xeaxanthin). Although eggs are high in cholesterol, 213 milligrams per large egg, they have 5 grams of fat—no more than an ounce of cheese. Shell color—brown or white—doesn't affect the nutritional quality of eggs; the color varies with the breed of hen. The color of the yolk depends on the feed and doesn't affect the quality, flavor, nutritive value, or cooking characteristics.

From jumbo to small eggs: What size should you buy? The bigger the egg, the more it has of everything: nutrients, cholesterol, and calories. *As a shopping and food preparation tip:* Four jumbo eggs equal five large eggs or six small eggs. Usually recipes are written for large eggs.

The size is different from the grade printed on the label. Eggs are graded AA, A, and B. Grading refers to the interior and exterior quality of eggs when they're packed. Most eggs sold in supermarkets are Grade A; they're almost the same as Grade AA eggs, which are considered slightly higher in quality.

● To check the freshness of shell eggs, look for the date on the carton. If the egg carton comes from a USDA-inspected plant, it displays a number (called a Julian date) for the packing date. A Julian date will be between 1 (January 1) and 365 (December 31). You can refrigerate fresh shell eggs for four to five weeks beyond the Julian date, in their carton, without losing

quality. The carton also may carry an expiration date; after that it can't be sold. When you use eggs, the yolks of fresher eggs hold their shape when they're cracked open. As eggs age, the white thins and the yolk flattens.

● Open egg cartons before you buy. Are the eggs clean and whole? Avoid cartons with cracked eggs. They may be contaminated with *Salmonella.*

● Buy eggs that are refrigerated, not kept at room temperature in the aisle. Even though eggs are stored in their own natural package, they spoil quickly when they're not refrigerated.

● Need to limit egg yolks because of their cholesterol content? Try cholesterol-free or reduced-cholesterol egg substitutes. The yolk, which contains the cholesterol, is left out. Other ingredients, such as nonfat milk, tofu, and vegetable oils, take its place; for coloring, it may contain some beta carotene. You'll find egg substitutes in either the freezer or the refrigerated section of the store.

Since cholesterol is in the yolk and not the white, you also can buy eggs and use just the whites to replace some or all of the whole eggs. *For more about cholesterol, see "Cholesterol: Different from Fat" in chapter 3.*

Have You Ever Wondered

. . . if fertile eggs, organic eggs, or free-range eggs have nutritional advantages? No. Fertile eggs, which can become chicks, won't keep as long, and they cost more. Organic eggs, produced by hens on organic rations, cost more, too, but the nutrient content is the same regardless. And free-range eggs, raised outdoors or with daily access to the outside, also are more costly without extra nutritional benefits.

. . . if modified-fat eggs or lower-cholesterol eggs are worth the extra cost? That depends on your overall food choices. Hens on feed that's high in flaxseed can produce eggs with more omega-3 fatty acids; flaxseed is a great source of omega-3 fatty acids, which may offer health benefits. *See "Eat Your Omega-3s and -6s" in chapter 3 for more about omega-3 fatty acids.* Shell eggs produced with less cholesterol are available as well; however, you may save money by buying whole eggs and tossing out some yolk.

● Want convenience? Consider frozen and refrigerated whole egg products. They're pasteurized; use them immediately after you open the container.

Freezer Case

Bagels and bread dough, waffles and cookies, fruit and fruit juice, pizza and burritos, vegetables and full dinners, fish and poultry, ice cream and frozen yogurt—the freezer case is stocked with every kind of convenience food. Many of these foods are preportioned, or partly or fully cooked, so you can serve these foods with little or no work.

Frozen Vegetables and Fruits

● To control fat and calories, choose frozen plain vegetables or those made with low-fat sauces. Some sauces mixed with frozen vegetables add fat, saturated fat, and calories; check the Nutrition Facts on the label.

● Look for frozen fruits as an option when berries and other fruits are out of season; they're sold in both sweetened and unsweetened varieties. To help frozen fruit keep its shape, serve while it's still somewhat frozen. Frozen fruit bars make a nutritious snack, too; read the label to know if they're made with juice or just flavored water.

● Buy fruit and vegetables in loose-pack plastic bags. You'll only need to pour out what you need; then immediately return what you don't use to the freezer.

● Choosing frozen juice concentrate? *The tips in "More Reading on the Food Label" in this chapter apply.* Read the label to compare products. Bear in mind that juice concentrates often cost a bit less that juice sold in cartons—and you can store them longer.

Frozen Meals and Entrées

● Use nutrition labeling to compare frozen prepared meals and entrées. Along with traditional foods, you'll find many products with fewer calories and with less fat, cholesterol, and sodium—even pizza, lasagna, enchiladas, and burritos! When you're comparing the nutrients in one frozen dinner with another, check the serving size. For example, some may be 7-ounce dinners; others, 11 ounces.

● Whether vegetables, fish, or poultry, go easy on breaded and fried frozen foods. They supply more fat and calories. When you buy them, check the package directions for oven heating rather than deep-fat frying, to control calories and fat.

Frozen Desserts

● For frozen desserts, compare frozen yogurt, various ice creams, and sherbet. The fat and calories in frozen yogurt (hard-frozen or soft) depend on its main ingredient: whole, 1 percent low-fat, or fat-free milk. Although frozen yogurt is made with lactic acid cultures, it may or may not have active, live cultures; to find out, look for the seal indicating active, live cultures; the seal is administered by the National Yogurt Association.

Most frozen yogurt has less fat than ice cream—although you'll also find lower-fat brands of ice cream in today's freezer section, too. In a half-cup serving:

● *Reduced-fat (2 percent) ice cream* has at least 25 percent less fat than regular ice cream.

● *Low-fat (1 percent) ice cream* has 3 grams or less of fat.

● *Light ice cream* has at least 50 percent less fat.

● *Fat-free ice cream* has less than 0.5 fat grams per serving.

To get the whole story, check the Nutrition Facts for the calories and fat grams in one serving.

You may prefer the creamy texture and rich flavor of premium ice cream, which contains more fat and thus more calories. If so, cut back on fat somewhere else so you can enjoy premium ice cream, or eat a smaller helping than you normally would.

Sold alongside ice cream and frozen yogurt, sherbet is sweetened fruit juice and water, 1 to 2 percent milk fat, and 2 to 5 percent milk solids, and stabilizers such as egg white and gelatin. While it has less fat,

Have You Ever Wondered

. . . how frozen custard differs from ice cream? It's about the same. The only difference is that more egg yolks are used in custard.

it contains more sugar than ice cream and belongs in the Pyramid tip. Fruit sorbet—whipped and frozen fruit juice—is sold commercially, or you can make it at home; it may be counted as a Fruit Group serving.

● Buying a whipped topping? Frozen whipped toppings are convenient to keep in the freezer. Many have the same calories and contents as real whipped cream. If they're made with palm and coconut oils, frozen whipped toppings are high in saturated fat. If you enjoy the taste of the real thing, buy it—then use just a dollop, not a heaping spoonful. Or look for light or low-calorie versions of frozen whipped toppings.

Grocery Aisles

By going up and down the inside aisles of the supermarket, you'll find an immense variety—convenience foods, ethnic foods, baking ingredients, snack foods, seasonings, and beverages.

Canned Fruits and Vegetables

● For a nonperishable supply of fruit and vegetables, buy canned varieties. They're great to have on hand for boosting vegetables and fruits in mixed dishes and for convenience—especially when their fresh counterparts aren't in season. (*Tip:* In many mixed dishes such as in soups, stews, other cooked dishes, and smoothies, the flavor and appeal from canned and fresh ingredients are comparable, according to consumer research.) Canned beans are faster to prepare than soaking dry beans overnight. Look for flavorful, newer products, too, such as raspberry-flavored peaches, cinnamon-flavored pears, and corn with chopped peppers. Stock up on some "gourmet" items—perhaps canned or jarred artichokes, olives, and roasted peppers.

● For canned fruit, examine the label. You'll find descriptions such as "packed in its own juices," "packed in fruit juice," "unsweetened," "in light syrup," or "in heavy syrup." Fruits packed in juices have less sugar than fruits packed in syrup and so fewer calories. If you prefer the flavor of fruit packed in syrup, just be sure the extra calories match your own calorie target.

● Canned juice, juice cocktail, or juice drinks— which should you buy? *For tips, see "More Reading*

on the Food Label" in this chapter. Tip: Juices may cost less per serving than soft drinks—and juice is more nutritious.

● Canned vegetables: if you're cutting back on sodium, which should you buy? Read the Nutrition Facts for sodium content, or look for descriptions such as "no salt added."

● For less fat, look for vegetarian or fat-free baked beans and refried beans. Compared with traditional products, you may cut the fat by 50 percent or more. Some canned beans are reduced in sodium, too. *Note:* Refried beans may be made with lard, which contains saturated fat and cholesterol.

Canned Fish

● Be aware that tuna, salmon, sardines, crabs, clams, mackerel, and other fish are canned in water or oil (typically vegetable or olive oil). Even when the oil is drained away, fish packed in oil have significantly more fat than water-packed varieties. However, with oil-packed canned fish, some omega-3 fatty acids transfer to the oil, which may be discarded. Besides the fat and calorie difference, fish packed in spring water has a milder flavor, but it has a drier texture.

● Compare the fat and calories in 3 ounces of water-packed and oil-packed tuna. *For more about omega-3 fatty acids, see "Eat your Omega-3s and -6s" in chapter 3.*

3-OUNCE SERVING	CALORIES	FAT GRAMS
Water-packed tuna, drained	110	2
Oil-packed tuna, drained	160	7

● For more calcium, buy canned fish (salmon and sardines) with edible bones. Three ounces of salmon eaten with the bones have about 200 milligrams of calcium, almost as much as 6 ounces of milk. (Not all canned salmon has edible bones—check the ingredient list.) The canning process softens bones, making them edible. Canned tuna and crabmeat don't have edible bones.

● Although tuna outsells other canned fish, give your-self a change in flavor with canned salmon or sardines. Besides adding variety to your eating pattern, salmon is higher in omega-3 fatty acids. Use it in salads, stir-fries, soups, and pizza toppings.

Soups, Stews, and Convenience Foods

● As a main dish, choose stews and hearty soups; because they're made with nutrient-rich foods, they usually provide plenty of nutrients. Use the Nutrition Facts and the ingredient list to find out. Clear soups and stews are usually lower in fat and calories than creamy varieties or stew with gravy. Another option for creamy soups: low-fat and fat-free versions of cream of celery soup and cream of mushroom soup, among others.

● If you're heating a quick meal at the office, look for ready-to-eat soup or dehydrated soup. Unlike con-densed soup, ready-to-eat soup doesn't need added liquid—open the can, heat, then serve. For dehydrated soup, just add hot water.

● For quick meals, buy canned and shelf-stable microwaveable entrées: perhaps pasta with meat or cheese, or chili con carne. If you eat them regularly, look for varieties with less fat and, depending on your needs, less sodium.

● If you're watching how much sodium you eat, read the Nutrition Facts for sodium content. Many canned and instant soups, as well as canned stews, are high in sodium. Check grocery shelves, though; you'll see many that are prepared with less sodium.

For instant noodles (Oriental noodles) and entrée mixes (macaroni and cheese), consider using half of the seasoning packet to cut back on sodium. Depend-ing on your overall food choices for the day, you might toss in some chopped vegetables for more vitamins and fiber, too. Or if you need to reduce fat, use less but-ter or margarine than the directions call for.

● To cut back on fat, look for defatted broth. Or put a canned soup or stew in the refrigerator prior to use. The fat will congeal so you can skim it off.

Pasta, Rice, and Other Grains

● For meal appeal, buy a variety of pasta shapes. For thick sauces, use thicker pastas: fettuccine, lasagna,

How Much Pasta? How Much Rice?

Because dry pasta and rice cook to a larger volume, use these general guidelines when deciding how much to buy.

Pasta or Rice	Uncooked	Equal Cooked
Egg noodles	8 oz. (2 cups)	4 cups
Spaghetti, fettuccine, other long shapes	8 oz. (1½-in. diameter bunch)	4 cups
Macaroni, shells, bow ties, penne, other small to medium shapes	8 oz. (2 cups)	4 cups
Brown rice	½ lb. (1¼ cups)	4⅓ cups
Polished, long-grain white rice	½ lb. (1¼ cups)	3¾ cups
Converted white rice	7 oz. (1 cup)	3½ cups
Instant white rice	8 oz. (2 cups)	4 cups

and tagliatelle. Chunky sauces are best with sturdy pasta shapes: fusilli (twists), farfalle (bow ties), mac-aroni, rigatoni, and ziti. With smooth, thin sauces, use thinner strands of pasta: cappellini (angel hair), ver-micelli, and spaghetti. The refrigerated section of the store also sells fresh pasta; use it right away or freeze it.

● Look for whole-grain pasta: spaghetti, lasagna, macaroni, and fettuccine. Like traditional pasta, whole-wheat pasta is high in complex carbohydrates. And the fiber content is almost three times higher; half a cup of whole-wheat pasta has about 3 grams of fiber, compared with about 1 gram of fiber in traditional pasta.

For more variety, savor the appeal of vegetable and herbed pasta. The addition of tomatoes, beets, carrots, spinach, and other vegetables adds a variety of colors and flavors to pasta dishes. And herbs add a delicate flavor. What about the nutrients? Tomato pasta and spinach pasta don't count toward servings from the Vegetable Group. The nutritional contribution of vegetable purees used to make commercially flavored pasta usually is quite small. It's the vegetables or tomato sauce tossed with pasta that carry extra nutrients.

● Experiment with Asian-style noodles. They're made with many ingredients besides wheat flour, including potato flour, soybean starch, rice flour, and buckwheat flour. Japanese soba noodles are made with buckwheat and wheat flour; Japanese wheat noodles are udon (thick noodles) and somen (thin noodles). Look for rice noodles, mung bean noodles, wonton wrappers (sheets of wheat dough), and rice paper (a thin dough used somewhat like a tortilla). Ramen noodles, which are Japanese instant-style deep-fried noodles, are often packaged with dehydrated vegetables and broth mix; the broth mix is typically high in sodium.

● Wonder about the fat content of egg noodles? While pasta is made from flour and water, noodles also contain eggs, egg yolks, or egg whites. Nonegg pasta contains no cholesterol and very little fat. Egg noodles may have small amounts of cholesterol and a little more fat but still are considered low in fat and cholesterol.

● Try different forms of rice. Use the label to compare their nutrients. Brown rice contains slightly more nutrients, followed by polished white rice, then instant white rice. Because it's a whole grain, brown rice—with 1.5 grams of fiber per half cup—has about three times the fiber of white rice. When you read the label, check for uncooked and cooked rice; it may give the nutritional content for prepared rice with added butter or salt.

Change the flavor and the texture with specialty rices. Jasmine and basmati rice have a fragrant flavor and aroma, especially nice with Thai and Indian food. Arborio rice, a short-grain rice, gives Italian risotto its creamy texture.

Despite its name, wild rice is actually a long-grain marsh grass. From a nutritional standpoint, wild rice has a little more protein, riboflavin, and zinc, and a little less carbohydrate than brown rice. The fiber content is about 0.5 gram per half cup. For its nutty flavor, serve wild rice in salads, stir-fries, soups, stuffing, and side dishes. Or mix it 50–50 with regular or brown rice.

What about rice mixes? If you need to watch sodium, consider using just half the dry seasoning mix.

● Browse the grocery shelves for other grain products: barley, bulgur, couscous, kasha, and quinoa, to name a few. *See "Today's Grains" in chapter 9. In "Cooking Grain by Grain" in chapter 13 you'll find guidelines for cooking with other grains.*

● How much should you buy? Base the amount of dry pasta and rice on their cooked volume. And remember, you may eat more than one serving, so figure the nutritional contribution based on the amount you really eat.

Breakfast Cereals

● Stocking up for quick breakfasts? Choose from the huge variety of ready-to-eat breakfast cereals. Besides being fortified with vitamins and minerals, you'll also find many high-fiber cereals. Because cereals use different parts of the grain—bran, germ, and endosperm—in differing amounts, their nutritional content varies. Use the Nutrition Facts to compare.

Adding milk or yogurt makes cereal a great vehicle for delivering calcium and other nutrients in milk. For this reason, cereal labels often give the Nutrition Facts for cereal only and for cereal with added milk.

When buying sweetened cereals, use the same criteria for choosing any cereal—sweetened or unsweetened. Read the Nutrition Facts for the nutrient and fiber content in one serving, then make your choice. Sweetened cereals are no more cavity-causing than unsweetened cereals; both complex carbohydrates in all kinds of cereal and sugars can linger on tooth surfaces and promote cavities. Choose the cereal that matches your family's preferences and needs, and encourage good oral hygiene.

● Look for clues to breakfast cereals with more fiber. They may carry label terms such as "high fiber," "whole grain," or "bran." If the label gives a nutrient content claim, check the Nutrition Facts for specific nutrient information. Cereals that are good fiber sources supply at least 2.5 grams of fiber per serving; whole-grain cereals typically have more. The ingredient list reveals the whole grains and bran in the cereal's "recipe."

● Check the nutrients in fortified cereals. Most supply about 25 percent of the Daily Value for vitamins and minerals. And some have much more—100 percent—making these cereals comparable to a nutrient supplement. Remember, a variety of other foods supply these nutrients, too. Like any food, consider fortified cereal as part of your whole day's eating plan.

Like many other breakfast cereals, bran cereals usually are fortified. Although high in fiber, bran lacks the vitamins and minerals supplied by the germ portion of grain.

Tip: Because many vitamins and minerals may be sprayed onto cereals, they can be lost if all the milk in the bottom of a cereal bowl isn't eaten along with the cereal.

● Check the variety of cooked cereals, too: Cream of Rice, grits, rolled oats, and toasted wheat. Many are low in fat and sodium.

Think cooked cereals take too long to prepare? With today's packaging, you'll find microwave instructions for quick preparation. And many to-be-cooked cereals—oatmeal, grits, Cream of Wheat—are sold in instant varieties. The nutritional content is comparable to their traditional counterpart, although sodium may be higher in instant cereals. Read the label to compare.

● Check the Nutrition Facts on cereal labels. The nutritional content varies from product to product, brand to brand. "Natural" cereals or granola may have more fat, sugars, or sodium than you'd think; many contain more saturated fats from palm and coconut oils. For something different, try muesli, made with grains, nuts, and dried fruit.

Beans, Nuts, and Peanut Butter

● Add a variety of legumes (beans and lentils) to your shopping list: adzuki, cannellini, garbanzos, navy beans, soybeans, and pinto beans, to name a few. With the demand for low-fat, high-fiber recipes and the interest in ethnic cooking, today's supermarkets stock a greater variety of beans and lentils—both dry and canned. You may even find fresh legumes in the produce department and frozen beans in the freezer case.

If the store doesn't carry the type you're looking for, you usually can substitute another. For example,

pinto, adzuki, and black beans can substitute for kidney beans, giving a dish a slightly different look. Cannellini, lima beans, and navy beans are the same color, just a different size. Nutritionally, most legumes are about the same, even though their appearance, texture, and flavor may differ somewhat. *To explore the varieties of legumes, see "Bean Bag" in chapter 6.*

● For freshness, look for these qualities in dry beans: no pinhole marks or discoloration, beans with a bright color, and bags that aren't torn.

● When food preparation time is short, opt for canned, rather than dry, beans. Unlike canned varieties, dry beans require cooking and perhaps soaking time. If your blood pressure is sodium-sensitive, be aware that salt is added to canned beans; check the Nutrition Facts and the ingredient list to compare similar products. *Tip:* Rinse canned beans under cold running water to reduce sodium.

● Read labels on peanut butter. Peanut butter is simply peanuts that are roasted and ground into a paste. The style—smooth, chunky, or crunchy—doesn't affect the nutritional content. All are good sources of protein, but the added ingredients may make a difference. To the ground peanuts, salt or small amounts of sugar may be added for flavor; unsalted and sugar-free varieties also are sold. You'll also see reduced-fat varieties, which may not be lower in calories; sugar and other ingredients may be added to enhance flavor and texture. The small amount of naturally occurring oils in peanut butter may be hydrogenated for spreadability, making them somewhat more saturated. *For more about hydrogenated (trans) fats, see "About Trans Fats" in chapter 3.*

Have You Ever Wondered

. . . if dry-roasted nuts or peanuts are lower in fat than oil-roasted nuts or peanuts? An ounce of dry- or oil-roasted nuts has about the same amount of fat and calories—almost 14 fat grams per ounce. Nuts and peanuts don't absorb much oil when they're roasted. The fat comes from the nuts and peanuts themselves. They also are a good protein source and provide fiber and other phytonutrients.

To keep oil and solids from separating, stabilizers usually are added to peanut butter. However, in "natural" peanut butter, the oil separates out. At home, avoid the urge to make peanut butter lower in fat by pouring that fat away. Your peanut butter will become too stiff to spread. Instead mix it well, or turn the jar upside down to let the oil run through.

● Be aware that nuts often are sold in salted and unsalted varieties. Unsalted nuts typically are found in the baking aisle; salted nuts, with snack foods. Try ground or chopped nuts; you can use less—but still get the nutty flavor. Remember, different nuts offer different phytonutrient benefits!

Beverages

● Enjoy flavored waters. Peach, lemon, mango, and other fruit-flavored waters are refreshing. For the "fizz," some are made of sparkling water and juice. Others are flavored with sweeteners but contain little juice. Unlike plain water, they may not be calorie-free. *See "What about Bottled Water?" in chapter 8.*

● For a no-calorie beverage, look for club soda, mineral water, and plain seltzer. Don't confuse these beverages with tonic or quinine water, which has 125 calories per 12 ounces.

● For carried meals, camping, and emergencies, stock up on boxed, or UHT, milk. Because boxed milk is ultrapasteurized, or heated to an ultrahigh temperature (UHT), then sealed in a sterile container, it can be stored unopened at room temperature for about three months without spoiling or nutrient loss. For added appeal, simply chill it before drinking. Once opened, UHT milk is as perishable as milk sold in the refrigerated dairy case.

● For more convenience, try nonfat dry milk or evaporated, canned milk. They're both shelf-stable. Nonfat dry milk powder has the same amount of nutrients as fat-free fluid milk—without the water. When reconstituted and chilled, it's a nutritious beverage. *Tip:* For 1 cup of fluid milk, combine ¾ cup of water with ⅓ cup of dry milk powder. Dry milk powder also can be used to fortify casseroles and other mixed dishes with calcium and other nutrients from milk. It costs less than fat-free fluid milk, too.

Evaporated milk has about 60 percent of the water removed, so its nutrients are more concentrated than regular fluid milk. If reconstituted, the nutrients are equivalent to the same-size serving. Evaporated milk may be whole or fat-free (skim). Sweetened condensed milk—whole or fat-free—is concentrated, too, but because sugars are added, it's higher in calories. *See the chart "Milk: A Good Calcium Source" in chapter 10 to compare the calories, fat, cholesterol, and calcium in evaporated milks.*

Tip: Once evaporated milk is opened and dry milk is reconstituted, both should be refrigerated for safety.

● *Be aware:* Nondairy creamers, either dry or liquid, may not be low in saturated fat. Although nondairy creamers are made with vegetable oil, the fats—often coconut or palm oil—are highly saturated. To lighten your coffee or tea, nonfat dry milk or evaporated fat-free (skim) milk are both good substitutes from the grocery aisle—or use fluid milk or fat-free half-and-half instead.

● Sensitive to caffeine? Then look for decaffeinated coffee and tea, and caffeine-free soft drinks. Also, seltzer, sparkling water, and most fruit-flavored soft drinks have no caffeine. *See "Drinks: With or without Caffeine?" in chapter 8.*

● *Note:* Flavored coffee mixes may contain sugars and coconut oil, which is high in saturated fatty acids.

● For soft drinks, know the calorie differences as you shop. A regular soda has 150 to 200 calories per 12-ounce can—with carbohydrates and water as the only significant nutrients. Diet sodas may quench thirst, too, and they're essentially calorie-free. *For more about including soft drinks in your overall eating plan, see "Soft Drinks: Okay?" in chapter 8.*

Have You Ever Wondered

. . . if a beverage is made with corn syrup or high-fructose sweetener, does it have fewer calories? Not necessarily. Used in the same amount, these sweeteners are equal in calories to table sugar, or sucrose. They are slightly sweeter than sucrose, however, so a little less might be used.

Soft drinks and other beverages with nonnutritive, or intense, sweeteners, carry nutrition labeling. If you're sensitive to their nonnutritive sweetener, avoid these products. In moderation, nonnutritive sweeteners are fine. *See "Aspartame" in chapter 5.*

● Buy single-serving containers of juice and boxed milk. They're handy for packing along to lunch, meetings, or a spectator sport. Rather than rely on a vending machine, you'll have a nutritious option on hand to go with you. Be aware that single soft drinks are getting bigger; 20-ounce plastic bottles are becoming as common as smaller cans. Ask yourself if you need that much.

● If you enjoy the taste of alcohol-containing drinks but choose to cut back, look for low-alcohol versions of beer and wine. The taste compares favorably. Regarding calories, you'll need to check the label. *For more about alcoholic beverages, see "Alcoholic Beverages: In Moderation" in chapter 8.*

Crackers and Snack Foods

● For meals or snacks, consider the growing array of crackers, including those with "less fat" or "less sodium." A few popular crackers are typically low in fat, or even fat-free: packaged breadsticks, graham crackers, melba toast, rice crackers, matzos, rusk, saltines, and zwieback. For more fiber, look for whole-wheat crackers, too!

● Many snack foods are made with oil—but what kind of oil? Check the ingredient list and the Nutrition Facts. Those made with partially hydrogenated vegetable oils may have more saturated fats.

● For a low-fat, crunchy snack food, buy pretzels or plain popcorn. They have less fat than potato chips, corn chips, bagel chips, or buttered popcorn. If your blood pressure is sodium-sensitive, look for unsalted snack foods such as unsalted pretzels. For a lower-fat option look for oven-baked tortilla and potato chips; 1 ounce of baked tortilla chips has about 1 fat gram compared with about 7 fat grams in the same amount of regular tortilla chips. And check the label on microwave popcorn. Some contain high-fat flavorings.

● When it comes to cookies, explore the growing variety of reduced-fat and fat-free varieties. If calo-ries are your challenge, read the label for calorie content, too, to see if the calories really are less. Even fairly small calorie and fat savings can be significant if you eat these cookies frequently. On the other hand, bigger helpings may "spend" any calorie or fat savings! Some types of commercial cookies are typically lower in fat: animal crackers, fig bars, gingersnaps, and vanilla wafers.

● If you buy candy, look for small, portion-controlled packages. In that way, it's not as easy to overindulge. To check the calories, read the Nutrition Facts. Some sugar-free candies have calories. And remember, candy bars may have fat, too.

Dressings, Sauces, Oils, and Condiments

● Mayonnaise or salad dressing? For less fat, choose "light," "reduced-fat," "low-calorie," or "fat-free" varieties. Fat-free dressings typically have 5 to 20 calories per tablespoon, compared with 75 calories and 6 to 8 fat grams in 1 tablespoon of regular salad dressing. Typically vinegar and water are the first two ingredients in fat-free dressing.

● Buy dry blends for mixing your own salad dressing. Then you can control the amount of oil and vinegar you add. Often you can use less oil and more vinegar, water, or other flavorful liquid than the package directions call for.

● Shopping for a prepared pasta sauce? Alfredo, clam, meat, marinara, and primavera—you'll find sauces of all kinds. The type of sauce doesn't indicate nutrient content (although creamy sauces such as alfredo and clam usually have more fat). Read the Nutrition Facts. *See "Gourmet's Guide to Sauces" in chapter 14.*

● If you're trying to cut back on sodium, look for soy sauce, teriyaki sauce, chile sauce, and marinades that are "reduced-sodium." Their traditional counterparts may be quite high in sodium.

● Look for nonstick cooking sprays. With these sprays you can use less oil in a fry pan or casserole dish, or on a baking pan.

● Remember that all vegetable oils contain the same amount of calories: about 120 calories per tablespoon.

And while the amounts of saturated, monounsaturated, and polyunsaturated fatty acids differ, all vegetable oils are cholesterol-free. "Light" oil refers to the color or mild flavor, not the fat content.

● Oils high in polyunsaturated fatty acids include corn, safflower, and sunflower oils. And those high in monounsaturates include olive, flaxseed, and canola oils. *See "Fats and Oils: How Do They Compare?" in chapter 3 for a comparison of various vegetable oils.*

● Experiment with stronger-flavored oils: for example, sesame, walnut, herb-infused, or chile-flavored oils. Just a splash adds a distinct flavor to salads, stir-fries, pasta, rice, and other dishes.

● Stock your kitchen with a variety of vinegars to pair with oils in saladmaking: red wine vinegar, herb vinegars, apple cider vinegar, and fruit-flavored vinegars. The strong flavor of sweet balsamic vinegar complements salad greens. Vinegars are fat-free.

● Buy ketchup, mustard, and pickle relish as tasty spreads, with just 2 fat grams or less per tablespoon. Check the label for sodium content if you're watching your sodium intake. Unless prepared with less salt or sodium, most of these condiments provide 150 to 200 milligrams of sodium per tablespoon. For more flavor with fewer calories, buy prepared horseradish. And look for chutney—a condiment made with fruit or vegetables, vinegar, spices, and sugar—that's low in sodium and fat.

Have You Ever Wondered

. . . if virgin olive oil has fewer calories than pure olive oil? No matter what the type, olive oil is high in monounsaturated fatty acids, and the calories are the same. Terms that may confuse consumers, such as "virgin" and "extra virgin" olive oil, refer to the acid content—not the nutrient content. Extra virgin olive oil has less acid and a fruitier flavor than "pure" or "virgin" olive oil. Because it has more aroma and flavor, you can use less.

What about light olive oil? The term "light" refers to the color and fragrance, not to the calories, fat content, or if it has an olive-oil flavor.

● Remember salsas. They're low in calories and bursting with flavor. Experiment with the different levels of spiciness—usually labeled as mild, medium, or hot—to see which you like best.

● Fruit jams and jellies—from a nutritional standpoint they're much the same. Check the label. You'll see that both have relatively small amounts of nutrients. *Hint:* Fruit jams and jellies belong in the Pyramid tip, not the Fruit Group. Fruit spreads—sweetened with juice—can have the same number of calories as jam or jelly, or they may have less sugar. And they provide some nutrients. Check the label's Nutrition Facts.

Baking Aisle

Flour

● Recognize different types and qualities of wheat flour before you buy. Whole-grain flour contains more fiber than refined wheat flour because the bran layer of the grain is still intact; that's where most of the fiber comes from. Unlike refined flour, whole-grain flour also contains the germ layer, which provides many vitamins and minerals. *For more on the different parts of a whole grain, see "What Is a Whole Grain?" in chapter 6.*

Refined flour, used in about 80 percent of baked goods, including white bread, is made only from the endosperm of the grain. While the flour has a snowy-white appearance, almost all of the fiber and many of the vitamins and minerals are lost. Refined flour may be bleached or unbleached. Bleaching simply whitens the somewhat yellowish unbleached flour. From a nutritional standpoint, bleached and unbleached flours are almost the same.

When flour is enriched, four nutrients that were lost in processing—thiamin, riboflavin, niacin, and iron—are added back. Flour also is fortified with folic acid. The amounts of these nutrients compare to those of whole-grain flour.

The label also may describe the flour as "all-purpose," "bread," "cake," or "self-rising."
● *All-purpose flour* is a mixture of high-gluten hard wheat and low-gluten soft wheat.
● *Bread flour* is mainly high-gluten hard wheat, suitable for yeast bread.

Have You Ever Wondered

... if all brown bread is whole wheat? Whole-wheat bread is always brown, but brown bread may not be whole wheat. Instead, the color may come from molasses or caramel coloring, and the flour may be mostly white flour. To be labeled "whole wheat," bread must be made from 100 percent whole-wheat flour. You'll know because "whole wheat flour" will appear first in the ingredient list.

● *Cake, or pastry, flour* made from low-gluten soft wheat has a finer texture that makes pastry and cakes more tender.

● *Self-rising flour* is all-purpose flour with baking powder and salt already added for making quick breads.

Although bread can be made with only 100 percent whole-wheat flour, the result will be a dense, heavy loaf. For a lighter texture, use a combination of whole-wheat and white flour.

● Look for other types of whole-grain flour in the supermarket and specialty stores: barley, buckwheat, corn, oats, brown rice, rye, and triticale. Triticale flour, with less gluten than all-purpose flour, makes a denser bread; triticale is a blend of wheat and rye flour. To lighten the texture of baked goods, go "50–50" with triticale and bread flour. Corn flour, made from the whole kernel, is finely ground cornmeal; masa harina is a specialty corn flour used to make tortillas. Yellow corn flour—and other yellow cornmeal—have more vitamin A than white corn flour.

● Try other types of flour, such as corn and rice flours, especially useful for people who have a wheat allergy or are sensitive to gluten. *See "Gluten Intolerance: Often a Lifelong Condition" in chapter 21.*

Sugar

● Know the difference in various types of sugar. Most cooking and baking are done with granulated, refined sugar. Superfine sugars, more finely granulated, may be used in meringues or in recipes that call for granulated sugar. Powdered or confectioners' sugar is granulated sugar that's been crushed into a fine powder. *See chapter 5 for information on honey, brown sugar, and raw sugar.*

Baking Mixes

● Choose baking mixes—cakes, breads, waffles, muffins, etc.—that allow you to add ingredients. When you add the fat, eggs, and liquid, you can control the type you use. If you need to watch cholesterol carefully, you might add an egg substitute rather than an egg. Or to cut back on saturated fats, you could use soft margarine rather than butter. Check the label; some manufacturers provide tips for preparing mixes with less fat and less cholesterol.

Breads and Bakery Items

Breads help to form the foundation of the Food Guide Pyramid. They provide carbohydrates, fiber, and other nutrients, and many are low in fat.

● Look for "whole grain" and "whole wheat" bakery products. Other label terms may suggest whole grain—for example, oatmeal and multigrain—but check the label to be sure. Whole-wheat flour must be first on the ingredient list.

Just because it's called "wheat bread" doesn't mean it's whole grain. Instead it may be made mostly from refined wheat flour. Terms such as "stone ground," "cracked wheat," or "100 percent wheat" don't mean whole wheat, either. And most store-bought rye and pumpernickel breads are made mostly from white flour, too. For more fiber, check the Nutrition Facts and the ingredient list for those made with mainly whole-wheat flour.

On the Nutrition Facts you'll see that a 1-ounce slice of whole-wheat bread has about 1.6 fiber grams compared to 0.5 to 1 gram of fiber in the same-size slice of enriched white bread. Bakery products that supply 2.5 or more grams of fiber per serving are a good fiber source.

● For white bread and rolls, look for "enriched" products. Like whole-grain breads, white bread made from enriched flour is another good source of complex carbohydrates, B vitamins (including folic acid), and iron. Whole-wheat products still have a nutrition advantage. When flour for white bread is enriched, B vitamins and iron are added back—but not fiber or other vitamins and minerals. Most grain products also are fortified with folic acid.

● Choose mostly bread and other bakery products with less fat. Most Italian bread, French bread, bagels, pita bread, kaiser rolls, English muffins, rye bread, corn tortillas, and pumpernickel bread have 2 grams of fat or less per serving. Check the Nutrition Facts for serving size and nutrient content.

● Go easy on bakery products with more fat: croissants, many muffins, doughnuts, sweet rolls, and many cookies and cakes. Although croissants make a tasty sandwich bread, half of a croissant has 5 fat grams compared with 1 fat gram in half of an Italian roll. And a doughnut has about 10 fat grams compared to 2 fat grams in a cinnamon raisin bagel.

● Check the product date on the label for freshness. Packaged bakery products, with preservatives added, may have a longer shelf life than those baked in the in-store bakery. *See "Additives: Safe at the Plate" in chapter 9.*

Seasonings: Dry or Fresh

Herbs and spices enhance the flavor of food without adding sodium. Dry or fresh, add them to your list.

● Buy herbs and spices in the amounts you need. Fresh herbs last in the refrigerator for only a short time. Dry herbs can be stored for up to a year to retain their peak flavors. *Tip:* Ethnic food stores often sell herbs and spices in bulk at lower prices.

● Know that seasoned salts are high in sodium. This includes garlic salt and onion salt. As an alternate choice, look for garlic powder and onion powder. To check the sodium content, read the ingredient list.

● Look for salt-free herb blends. Different combinations of herbs, such as Italian herb blend, or herbs de Provence (typical in French cooking), take the guessing out of seasoning.

● Be adventuresome—buy seasonings that may be new to you: perhaps sage for chicken soup, tarragon with peas, fresh ginger for sweet potatoes, or cumin in chili.

● Try liquid smoke. It adds the smoky flavor of cured meat without the salt that's added during the curing process.

For tips on using herbs and spices in food preparation, see "A Pinch of Flavor: How to Cook with Herbs and Spices" in chapter 13; check "Salty Terms" in chapter 7 for more about different types of salt.

Take-out Foods

Consumers increasingly shop at supermarkets for the most convenient home-served meals of all, foods that are ready to eat: salad bars, rotisserie chicken, steamed shrimp, sushi bar, and deli sandwiches, as well as a variety of heat-only main dishes, appetizers, and side dishes. The food industry puts these foods in a broad new category called "meal solutions."

If you're time-pressed, buy your main dish—or a whole meal—already prepared. Then just heat and serve as your own healthful eating solution on a hectic day! Guidelines for supermarket take-out foods are similar to buying and handling foods from a carry-out restaurant. *See "Safe Take-out" in chapter 14.*

Food Safety: Start at the Store

While the safety of the food supply has been monitored and regulated all along the food chain, it's your responsibility to select foods carefully at the store, then keep them safe until they're eaten.

● Only buy food from reputable food businesses that follow government regulations for food safety.

● Check the package. The packaging shouldn't have holes, tears, or open corners. If you suspect food tampering, report it to a public health authority. Frozen foods should be solid, and refrigerated foods should feel cold. Frozen foods shouldn't show signs of thawing.

● Check safety seals and buttons. Safety seals often appear on milk, yogurt, and cottage cheese. Jars of foods often are vacuum-sealed for safety. Check their safety seals with your finger. If the indented safety button on the cap pulls down, it's still in place; if it's up, don't buy or use the food. Report the incident to the manager of the local store.

● Reject cans that are swollen, damaged, rusted, or dented. These are warning signs for the bacteria that cause botulism. *See "Bacteria: Hard Hitters" in chapter 12 for information on botulism.*

● When possible, put raw poultry, meat, and fish in separate plastic bags before placing them in your cart. Occasionally their packaging may leak and drip onto unprotected foods.

● Pay attention to "sell by" and "use by" dates on perishable foods. If the "sell by" date has passed, don't buy the product. The "use by" date applies to its use at home. Purchase only those that will be fresh when you're ready to eat them. *See "More Reading on the Food Label" earlier in this chapter for more about food product dating.*

● Select perishable foods such as meat, poultry, and seafood last before checkout.

● In the checkout line, pack cold foods together, preferably in paper bags, which keep foods cold longer than plastic bags do. They'll stay chilled longer for the trip home.

● Take groceries home immediately, and store them right away. If you must run a few quick errands, bring a cooler with chill packs for perishable foods if you'll be longer than thirty minutes. That's especially important in warm weather. The temperature of refrigerated food can go up 8 to 10 degrees Fahrenheit on a typical trip home from the supermarket. That goes higher as the time gets longer. *For guidelines on keeping food safe once you get home, see chapter 12, "The Safe Kitchen."*

What's "Soy" Good?

Soybeans! Made into many food products, they're very versatile and nutritious. Compared with many other legumes, soybeans have more protein, fat, and calcium, and they're lower in complex carbohydrates. Whole soybeans also contain polyunsaturated fatty acids, which often are extracted as soybean oil. Read the Nutrition Facts and the ingredient list to find out about and compare these products.

In the past, soybean products (except for soy oil) mostly attracted vegetarian consumers. Today we know that they're good sources of nutrients as well as phytonutrients (including isoflavones) for any eating style. These are among the many products made with soy:

● *Egg replacers.* Made from potato starch and lecithin, a soy-based product.

● *Miso* (MEE soh). Fermented soybean paste, most commonly used as a flavoring in Japanese cooking. With a consistency like peanut butter, miso can be used as a condiment, but it's also prepared in dips, marinades, sauces, and soups. Depending on the amount used, miso adds protein, calcium, and some B vitamins to dishes. Unless it's a low-salt variety, miso tends to be high in sodium.

● *Meat analogs.* Products made from soybeans that resemble meat products—for example, soyburgers, soy bacon, soy sausages, and hot dogs.

● *Soy cheese, yogurt, and sour cream.* Dairylike products made from soybeans. Soy yogurt is made by adding live bacteria cultures to soy milk. Soy cheese (tofu cheese) is lower in fat and is cholesterol-free, but it doesn't have the same characteristics as cheese made from cow milk.

● *Soy flour.* Flour that's much higher in proteins but lower in carbohydrates than wheat flour. In baking, soy flour is usually mixed with other types of flour because it has less gluten.

● *Soy grits.* Usually sold near whole-grain flours and hot breakfast cereals.

● *Soy mayonnaise.* Typically made with tofu. Read the ingredient list to find out if it's made with eggs.

● *Soy milk.* Nondairy beverage made from crushed, cooked soybeans. Soy milk is a good source of protein, but unless it's calcium-fortified, it provides much less calcium than cow milk does. Like cow milk, soy milk may be fortified with vitamins A and D. Check the Nutrition Facts panel on the carton to find out the calcium and vitamin content per serving.

● *Soynuts.* Crunchy, roasted snack somewhat like peanuts.

● *Soynut butter.* Like peanut butter, but made from soybeans.

- *Soy oil and margarine.* Unsaturated fat extracted from whole soybeans. The most commonly available vegetable oil is made from soy.

- *Soybeans (removed from the pod).* Purchased canned, frozen, dry, or fresh. They can be cooked for soups, stews, and casseroles. For a snack, fresh soybeans can be roasted

- *Soybeans (in the pod).* Picked immature and sold frozen or fresh. Edamame (ed-ah-MAH-may) are soybeans cooked in the pod and eaten as a snack.

- *Soy sauce.* A condiment used in many Asian dishes, it also comes from fermented soybeans. Although it adds flavor, it's not a significant protein source. Tamari is a wheat-free variety; shoyu is not.

- *Tempeh* (TEHM peh). Soybeans mixed with rice, millet, or other grain, then fermented into a rich soybean cake. Tempeh has a smoky or nutty taste that adds flavor to soups, casseroles, chili, or spaghetti. It can be grilled or marinated. Like tofu, tempeh is a good protein source but has somewhat less calcium.

- *Textured soy protein, or TSP.* Soy flour that's high in protein and often sold as granules, flakes, or chunks. You can use TSP to replace or extend meat or poultry. Vegetableburgers and sausages often are made with TSP, too.

- *Tofu* (TOH foo), *or soybean curd.* A cheeselike curd made from curdled soybean milk and pressed into soft cakes. Tofu easily takes up the flavor of other ingredients in a dish, including stir-fries, chili, tacos, salads, noodle dishes, and pizza. You also can buy flavored tofu such as smoked, teriyaki, Mexican, and Italian tofu.

  Tofu is sold in several forms: *soft or silken* for dressings, smoothies, soups, dips, shakes, and sauces; *medium-soft* for puddings, cheesecakes, pie fillings, and salads; *firm or extra-firm* for grilling, marinating, slicing, or stir-frying and in casseroles, soups, and sandwiches; and *baked* for stir-frying and grilling. Tofu sold in bulk (not packaged) or in water needs to be refrigerated and used within a week because it's very perishable. It should be kept in water that's changed daily. Bought in an aseptic package, tofu doesn't need refrigeration until it's opened. You also can freeze tofu for up to three months for a chewier texture.

  Tofu is a good source of protein. Its calcium content is highest when it's calcium-fortified. Look for calcium sulfate on the ingredient list and on the label.

- On today's supermarket shelves, look for soy protein combined in many other foods: pasta, yogurt, cheese, meat sausages, to name just a few.

CHAPTER 12

The Safe Kitchen

America's food supply is one of the safest in the world. All those along the food chain—farmers, food manufacturers, supermarkets, and restaurants—are required by law to follow strict food safety regulations, which are carefully monitored. Once food leaves the grocery store, the responsibility for food safety is up to you. Because of the risks posed by foodborne illness, the Dietary Guidelines for Americans remind us: *Keep food safe to eat.*

We've all heard the most important rules for handling food safely: Keep all food clean, keep hot foods hot, and keep cold foods cold. But just what is the temperature connection? How can you keep foods clean and safe . . . for "goodness sake"? And most important, how does food safety affect your health?

Foodborne Illness: More Common than You Think!

Imagine . . . an upset stomach, diarrhea, and fever. Do you have the flu? Disguised as flu, your illness actually may be foodborne illness, not flu (a respiratory viral infection).

Foodborne illness, sometimes called food poisoning, comes from eating contaminated food. But the symptoms can easily be mistaken for other health problems. In fact, symptoms vary from fatigue, chills, a mild fever, dizziness, headaches, an upset stomach, and diarrhea, to dehydration, severe cramps, vision problems, and even death. Although actual incidence is unknown, foodborne illness may lead to a small percentage of some long-term health problems, too, including arthritis and Guillain-Barré syndrome.

Since 1996 food safety and health experts at the Centers for Disease Control and Prevention (CDC) have estimated that seventy-six million people get sick, more than three hundred thousand are hospitalized, and five thousand Americans die each year as a result of foodborne illness. Foodborne illnesses that result in more severe symptoms and death usually are diagnosed. However, the less severe "nuisance" symptoms more likely go unreported. While many reported cases are caused by food prepared outside the home, small outbreaks in home settings are considered to be far more common.

The ways people react to foodborne bacteria and contaminated food differ. One person may show no symptoms; another may get very ill. The reaction depends on the type of bacteria or toxin, how extensively the food was contaminated, how much food was eaten, and the person's susceptibility to the bacteria.

Anyone can be a victim of foodborne illness, but some people are at increased risk. They may include friends and families you entertain, perhaps at holiday parties or casual gatherings. You may not be aware that someone you offer food to is at high risk; always make food safety a high priority! *See "Who Is at High Risk for Foodborne Illness?" in this chapter.*

Bacteria cause most cases of foodborne illnesses, usually due to improper food handling. But foods also can be contaminated by viruses, parasites, and toxic chemicals such as cleaning supplies stored near food. With proper hand washing when preparing and handling food, nearly half of all cases of foodborne illness can be prevented. (With government, industry, and consumer food safety efforts, CDC reported in 2002 that the incidences of foodborne illness may be declining.)

Bacteria Basics

Life begins at 40! Between 40° F and 140° F, a single bacterium can multiply to become trillions in just twenty-four hours! Why the exponential leap? Under

the right conditions, bacteria double in number every twenty to thirty minutes.

Even with so many, you can't see bacteria without a microscope. Unlike microorganisms that cause food to spoil, you can't taste or smell most bacteria. Yet they live everywhere—in many foods, on your skin, under your fingernails, on other surfaces, and on pets and other live animals. Foods of animal origin—raw meat, poultry, fish, eggs, raw (unpasteurized) milk—are the most common food sources of bacteria. Although less common, harmful bacteria also can be transferred to fresh produce, perhaps through contaminated water or soil residue.

Because they're everywhere, you can't avoid harmful bacteria completely. Fortunately, from a food safety standpoint, most adults don't need to worry about harmful bacteria—at least not in small numbers. Your body can handle small amounts with no threat to your health. However, you are at risk for foodborne illness when bacteria multiply to very large numbers—which can happen when you mishandle food. **Caution:** Young children, the very old, and people whose immune systems don't function normally are at greater risk, even for small amounts of harmful bacteria.

To survive and multiply, bacteria need time and the right conditions: food, moisture, and warm temperature. Many need oxygen, too. Bacteria thrive on protein. Foods with protein—meat, poultry, fish, eggs, milk—offer the medium for bacteria to grow. The ideal temperatures for bacterial growth are between 40° F and 140° F. Above 160° F, heat destroys bacteria. Refrigerating foods below 40° F slows their growth. Freezing stops but doesn't kill bacteria. *Check "The Danger Zone" on page 276.*

Mishandling food—improper preparation, cooking, or storage—is the culprit action that allows bacteria to grow and multiply in your kitchen. With its rich supply of nutrients and often moist quality, food offers the perfect medium for bacteria to grow in.

Most bacteria won't harm you. Some, such as the ones used to make yogurt, some cheeses, and vinegar, are actually helpful.

Yet harmful bacteria are the main sources of foodborne illness in the United States. That's why keeping bacteria under control is so vital to your health.

If you suspect that food is contaminated, don't even

Have You Ever Wondered **?**

. . . how much you need to worry about mayonnaise in picnic foods and brown-bag lunches? Mayonnaise is a perishable spread, so it must stay chilled. Homemade mayonnaise, made with uncooked eggs, is potentially more hazardous than its commercial counterpart and isn't considered appropriate for people at high risk. Commercial mayonnaise and salad dressings, made with pasteurized ingredients, also contain salt and more acid, which slow bacteria growth. In unrefrigerated mayonnaise-based salads such as chicken, tuna, or egg salad, it's usually not the mayonnaise that poses the risk but rather the chicken, tuna, or eggs.

. . . if fish you catch are safe to eat? About 20 percent of fish eaten in the United States are caught by people for personal use. There's no safety problem if fish is caught in safe waters. However, seafood toxins, which occur naturally in some waters, and fish contaminated by chemicals in the water pose health risks. Check with authorities from your local and state health department, state fishery agency, or Sea Grant office for a current safety status. Follow the advisories.

. . . how food irradiation affects food safety? Food irradiation breaks down the DNA molecules in harmful organisms such as *Salmonella, E. coli,* and other foodborne bacteria. In that way it can dramatically reduce or eliminate disease-causing bacteria and other harmful bacteria, and so reduce or prevent outbreaks of foodborne illness. With that in mind, you still need to handle food properly to keep it safe to eat. *See "Irradiated Foods: Safe to Eat? in chapter 9.*

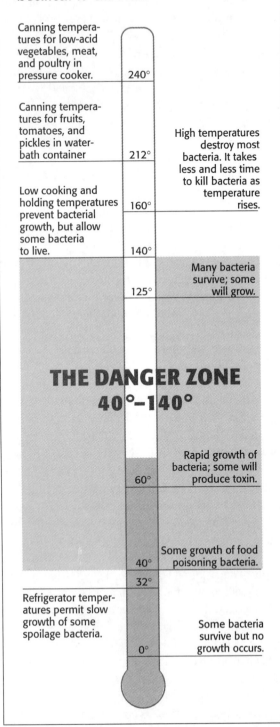

The Danger Zone

Effects of temperature (°F) on growth of bacteria in food. The most dangerous zone of temperature is between 40° and 140°F.

Canning temperatures for low-acid vegetables, meat, and poultry in pressure cooker. — 240°

Canning temperatures for fruits, tomatoes, and pickles in water-bath container — 212°

High temperatures destroy most bacteria. It takes less and less time to kill bacteria as temperature rises.

Low cooking and holding temperatures prevent bacterial growth, but allow some bacteria to live. — 160°

140°

Many bacteria survive; some will grow. — 125°

THE DANGER ZONE
40°–140°

Rapid growth of bacteria; some will produce toxin. — 60°

Some growth of food poisoning bacteria. — 40°

32°

Refrigerator temperatures permit slow growth of some spoilage bacteria.

Some bacteria survive but no growth occurs. — 0°

taste it! You can't see, smell, or taste bacteria that cause foodborne illness. Securely wrap the suspected food, and discard it where neither humans nor animals can get at it.

Bacteria: Hard Hitters

Although as many as a hundred bacteria cause foodborne illness, these are among the worst trouble-makers: *Salmonella, Staphylococcus aureus, Campylobacter jejuni, Clostridium perfringens, Clostridium botulinum, Escherichia coli 0157:H7, and Listeria monocytogenes.* You also may hear about *Shigella, Vibrio vulnificus,* and *Yersinia enterocolitica,* three other bacteria that cause foodborne illness.

Salmonella, the second most common cause of foodborne illness, is found mostly in raw or under-cooked poultry, meat, eggs, fish, and unpasteurized milk. Control is simple enough—proper cooking kills *Salmonella.* Combat this bacterium by cooking foods thoroughly, especially eggs, poultry, and meat; by keeping foods clean; and by consuming only pasteurized milk.

Raw milk, even if it's certified, may not be a wise choice because it isn't pasteurized. Pasteurized milk is quickly heated to a temperature high enough to kill harmful bacteria such as *Salmonella.* Raw milk isn't widely available to consumers.

Staphylococcus aureus (staph) spreads from someone handling food. It's carried on the skin, nose, and throat and in skin infections; then it spreads to food. Toxins, or poisons, produced by staph aren't killed by ordinary cooking. That's why personal hygiene and cleanliness in the kitchen are so important!

Campylobacter jejuni is estimated to be the major bacterial cause of diarrhea in the United States. Like *Salmonella, Campylobacter jejuni* can be transferred to raw and undercooked poultry and meat, unpasteurized milk, and untreated water.

The good news is that *Campylobacter jejuni* can be destroyed easily through safe food handling and water treatment systems. To protect yourself, always cook food thoroughly and avoid cross-contamination by washing utensils, cutting boards, and hands after handling raw poultry or meat. Avoid raw, unpasteurized milk. And if you're camping, always treat water from streams or lakes.

Clostridium perfringens is present everywhere, growing where there's little or no oxygen. Sometimes called the "buffet germ," it grows fastest in large portions—such as casseroles, stews, and gravies—held at low or room temperatures in "the danger zone." Chafing dishes that aren't hot enough and large portions that don't cool quickly in the refrigerator are breeding grounds. To slow the growth of this bacterium, replace buffet table servings often, rather than putting out large portions for an extended time, and refrigerate leftovers quickly.

Clostridium botulinum is rare. Yet, left untreated, botulism is often fatal! It requires immediate medical attention. Botulism-causing bacteria can come from home-canned or commercially canned foods. Usually these are low-acid canned foods such as meats and vegetables that haven't been processed or stored properly. Foods improperly canned at home, as well as improperly handled home-prepared herbal oils, pose a higher risk.

To combat this bacterium, look for warning signs: swollen or dented cans or lids, cracked jars, loose lids, and clear liquids turned milky. Beware of cans or jars that spurt when they're opened. Never eat—or even taste—these foods. For home canning, always use approved methods. Heat home-canned meats and vegetables thoroughly, about fifteen to twenty minutes, before serving. And serve or refrigerate baked potatoes and grilled vegetables right away. Cooked root vegetables held at room, instead of refrigerated, temperature can be a problem. That's especially true when they're wrapped in foil; botulinum spores thrive without the air!

Escherichia coli (E. coli), a common bacterium, exists in your intestinal tract. For the most part, it's harmless. However, some strains are associated with travelers' diarrhea caused by contaminated drinking water, as well as with diarrhea among infants.

One strain—*E. coli 0157:H7*—has received much attention because its effects can be so severe. This strain, associated with eating raw or undercooked ground beef, or drinking unpasteurized milk or unpasteurized cider, can result in life-threatening health problems: hemorrhagic colitis with severe abdominal cramps, bloody diarrhea, nausea, and vomiting and perhaps hemolytic uremic syndrome (HUS), which may cause kidney failure, brain damage, strokes,

Who Is at High Risk for Foodborne Illness?

- Pregnant women
- Young children
- Older persons
- People with weakened immune systems or certain chronic illnesses

If you're at high risk, follow general advice for food safety and take *extra* precautions:

- Do not eat or drink unpasteurized juice, raw sprouts, raw (unpasteurized) milk, and products made with unpasteurized milk.
- Do not eat raw or undercooked meat, poultry, eggs, fish, and shellfish (clams, oysters, scallops, and mussels).
- Avoid soft cheeses such as feta, Brie, Camembert, blue-veined, and Mexican-style cheeses.

New information on food safety is constantly emerging. Recommendations and precautions for people at high risk are updated as scientists learn more about preventing foodborne illness. *If you are among those at high risk,* be aware of and follow the most current information on food safety. For the latest information and precautions, talk to your healthcare provider, check the government's food safety Web site *(http://www.foodsafety.gov),* or *call the government information numbers listed in the Appendices.*

Source: *Dietary Guidelines for Americans* (2000).

If you or someone you know is at high risk and needs help with meals, find out about services such as home-delivered meals in your community. Check to be sure that the service follows food safety regulations. *To find services in your community, see "To Find Food and Nutrition Services" in chapter 24.*

seizures, and death, especially in young children and the elderly.

To combat all strains of *E. coli,* cook and reheat meat thoroughly. Be especially careful of ground meat—for example, hamburgers—because bacteria on the surface of the meat get mixed into the center of the meat, which takes longer to cook. Keep cutting surfaces clean. Avoid cross-contamination of raw food, or transferring bacteria from one food to another with dirty utensils, cutting boards, plates, and hands. Raw milk and produce also may be sources.

Listeria monocytogenes can cause a less common but potentially fatal foodborne illness called listeriosis. Pregnant women, infants, the elderly, and those with weakened immune systems are more susceptible. *Listeria* are part of your everyday surroundings, including places where food is processed. It can grow even under proper refrigeration.

Because *Listeria* is commonly found in milk and in cheese made from unpasteurized milk, it's wise to avoid unpasteurized milk products. *Listeria* also can be found in raw and undercooked meat, poultry, seafood, and eggs, and in produce. As with any packaged food product, follow the "keep refrigerated" advice on the label, the "use by" date on the package, and the reheating instructions. To avoid *Listeria*, high-risk individuals are advised by the U.S. Food and Drug Administration to avoid soft cheeses (such as Brie, Camembert, feta, and Mexican-style cheeses); hot dogs or luncheon meats unless they're reheated until they're steaming; refrigerated pâtés and meat spreads; and smoked seafood (such as lox, jerky, or nova-style) that requires refrigeration.

Shigella, one source of bacterial diarrhea, is transmitted from improper handling of either food or water. It originates in the feces of infected humans and easily passes from one person to another through improper hand washing. Proper cooking eliminates it; uncooked food such as potato, tuna, or chicken salad is more likely the source.

Vibrio vulnificus, a bacterium in shellfish, especially in mollusks, can be fatal within two days of developing the condition. Symptoms include sudden chills, fever, nausea, vomiting, and stomach pain. Although this bacterium is destroyed in the intestinal tract or in the immune system of most healthy people, this form of foodborne illness can be very serious, even fatal for high-risk individuals. These bacteria multiply even during refrigeration. Thoroughly cooking shellfish destroys them.

Yersinia enterocolitica, a bacterium found in contaminated food, is most often found in contaminated raw or undercooked pork products (including chitterlings, or pork intestines). The most common symptoms: for young children, fever, abdominal pain, and diarrhea, often bloody, and for older children and adults, fever and abdominal pain that feels like appendicitis. Unpasteurized milk or untreated water also may transmit this bacterium. In most cases the body can handle a yersiniosis infection without antibiotics. As prevention, avoid eating raw or undercooked pork and unpasteurized dairy foods, practice good hand washing, avoid cross-contamination, and dispose of animal feces in a sanitary way. If you're making chitterlings, have someone else care for your children. *For cooking pork, see "Safe Internal Temperatures" later in this chapter.*

From Parasites and Viruses, Too

Bacteria are responsible for most cases of foodborne illness. However, parasites and viruses—other tiny organisms that contaminate food—are culprits, too. Parasites such as *Trichinella spiralis, Toxoplasma gondii, Cryptosporidium parvum, Entamoeba histolytica,* and *Giardia lamblia* survive by drawing on the nutrients of a living host. Viruses such as hepatitis A act like parasites. Through the food chain, both parasites and viruses can infect humans.

Trichinosis is contracted by consuming undercooked pork or game that has been infested with trichina larvae. With careful controls in the food industry, trichinosis is much less common today than in the past. However, still cook pork, game, and other meat to the recommended internal temperature to destroy any live trichina larvae. *See "Safe Internal Temperatures" in this chapter.*

Toxoplasmosis is caused by a parasite indirectly linked to undercooked meat or poultry. It's also directly transferred to humans from cat feces. Pregnant women are at special risk because they can pass the parasite to their unborn baby. The disease can severely affect the central nervous system, causing mental impairment and visual disorders. To combat this parasite, cook meat, especially pork, lamb, and poultry, thoroughly. For pregnant women, limit exposure to cats and cat litter boxes; if you do handle cats, wash your hands well with soap and water.

Cryptosporidium, traditionally linked to travelers' diarrhea in developing nations, has become a more common parasitic illness in the United States. It enters the environment through the feces of warm-blooded animals, including humans. Contaminated water or ice usually is the source. Municipal water filtration controls this parasite; chlorine doesn't destroy it.

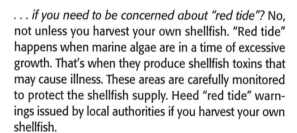

Have You Ever Wondered

. . . if you need to be concerned about "red tide"? No, not unless you harvest your own shellfish. "Red tide" happens when marine algae are in a time of excessive growth. That's when they produce shellfish toxins that may cause illness. These areas are carefully monitored to protect the shellfish supply. Heed "red tide" warnings issued by local authorities if you harvest your own shellfish.

. . . if mercury in seafood is risky? Mercury is naturally present in all living things as well as in soil, air, and water. Pollution also releases into the air mercury that falls into water or on land, then washes into lakes, rivers, and oceans. Bacteria in water change mercury to methyl mercury, which is toxic. Over time methyl mercury can build up in long-lived larger fish. Because methyl mercury is a potential risk to the developing nervous system of the fetus or the child, the U.S. Food and Drug Administration has offered this advice: Women who are pregnant or who might become pregnant, nursing mothers, and young children should avoid eating shark, swordfish, king mackerel, and tilefish. Eating about 12 ounces of other cooked fish—shellfish, canned fish, smaller ocean fish, and farm-raised fish—is safe.

. . . if your food is safe from "mad cow disease" and "foot and mouth" disease? These are two different diseases, but neither has been found in livestock in North America, so the U.S. food supply is safe from these diseases.

Although foot-and-mouth disease (FMD) is highly contagious among livestock and is economically disastrous, it poses no human risk. Because travelers who visit agricultural areas can bring it back, the government prohibits import of agricultural products by people entering the United States who've been on a farm abroad or in contact with livestock abroad, and inspects their baggage. Before returning to the United States from FMD-infected areas, the U.S. Department of Agriculture (USDA) advises: Avoid agricultural areas five days before returning to the United States; clean and disinfect footwear with detergent and bleach; wash or dry-clean clothing; and avoid contact with livestock or wildlife for five days after returning to the United States. As other safety measures, the USDA regularly monitors U.S. cattle herds and has banned animals and animal products from infected areas.

"Mad cow disease," or bovine spongiform encephalopathy (BSE), can infect humans, affecting the nervous system; it may be linked to a brain-wasting illness in humans known as Creutzfeldt-Jakob disease. To protect the U.S. supply, government regulations have created a triple "firewall" system: (1) import bans to make sure no live cattle or products from these animals are imported from areas where BSE is known to exist, (2) a ban on most mammalian protein in cattle feed, and (3) a USDA surveillance program. If you travel to Europe, where BSE is known to exist, your risk for getting this disease is very small, according to the National Institutes of Health. If you're concerned, however, avoid beef or beef products, or eat only solid pieces of meat rather than ground-beef products such as burgers or sausage.

Proper hand washing and food handling are extra controls you can take at home. People with compromised immune systems and children are among those at higher risk. *See "Drinking Water: For Special Health Needs" in chapter 8.*

Giardiasis, most often caused by drinking untreated water, also may be transmitted by uncooked food contaminated with *Giardia* or by passing the parasite from hand to hand on surfaces. In recent years, giardiasis has become one of the most common causes of waterborne disease among humans in the United States. Another source of gastrointestinal symptoms, it more likely strikes campers and hikers, travelers, diaper-age children who go to day-care centers, and others who drink untreated water from contaminated sources. Symptoms typically appear one to two weeks after infection and may last several weeks. Boiling destroys *Giardia* in water; chlorine may not if the

Need more strategies for food safety? Check here for "how-tos":

- Find out how to eat out safely—see chapter 14.
- Take food safety precautions when you travel—see chapter 14.
- Purify unsafe water—see chapter 8.

chlorine concentration isn't high enough. Good hand washing habits are essential to its control. If you travel or camp in areas where the water may not be safe, only drink from a safe water supply, and wash and peel produce before eating it.

What if there's a giardiasis outbreak in your child's day-care center? If it continues despite control efforts, children with or without symptoms might be screened and perhaps treated. If your child has symptoms (diarrhea, abdominal cramps, nausea), contact your health-care provider. The American Academy of Pediatrics doesn't advise treatment for children diagnosed with giardiasis who don't have diarrhea—unless poor appetite, weight loss, or fatigue are observed

Amebiasis (*Entamoeba histolytica*) also comes from polluted water and vegetables grown in soil polluted with human feces. It's a problem mostly for

Should You Call Your Doctor?

Suppose you suspect foodborne illness. You or a family member has an upset stomach, diarrhea, vomiting, fatigue, abdominal discomfort, or a fever. Symptoms of foodborne illness can appear from thirty minutes to three weeks after eating contaminated food. Most often, though, symptoms appear within four to forty-eight hours after eating. Symptoms usually pass within twenty-four to forty-eight hours; rest and plenty of fluids are the best ways to treat most incidences of foodborne illness. Some foodborne illnesses can affect your health for weeks, months, even years. Talk to your healthcare provider if you think that food has made you sick. In some circumstances it's especially important that you receive care from a doctor:

● When diarrhea is bloody. This may be a symptom of *E. coli O157:H7.*

● When diarrhea or vomiting is excessive. This may lead to dehydration if fluids aren't replaced.

● When these three symptoms all appear: stiff neck, severe headache, and fever. The victim may have *Listeria,* which can be life-threatening.

● When you suspect foodborne illness from *Clostridium botulinum* or *Vibrio vulnificus,* which can be fatal.

● When the victim is at high risk—perhaps a young child, an elderly person, or someone whose immune system is compromised due to illness.

● When symptoms persist longer than three days.

What Do You Do if You Suspect Foodborne Illness?

● Call or see a medical professional. Physicians and laboratories are responsible for contacting the appropriate health department to report diagnosis of foodborne illness. However, most cases of foodborne illness aren't diagnosed; the symptoms simply are treated to relieve discomfort.

● Report the incident to your local health department as soon as possible if the suspected food came from a public place or large gathering—a restaurant, sidewalk vendor, employee cafeteria, company picnic, or grocery store, among others.

● If you are reporting the incident, try to preserve the suspected food. Ask authorities for instructions for packaging and storing the food until it can be collected by them. If you can, keep the packaging, too, because it identifies where the product was produced. Mark it with a warning label so no one else consumes it.

If you suspect that a food has been contaminated by a household chemical:

● Check the label for an antidote or a remedy. Likely you'll find an "800 or other toll-free" number for first-aid advice, too. Follow the advice.

● Call the national hotline to reach a poison control center: 1-800-222-1222. This number will automatically link you to the closest poison control center. Another option: Contact your local health department or use a local poison control center number. As a safety precaution, post their phone numbers by your telephone. You'll have them handy if household chemicals do contaminate food or are misused in any way.

travelers in less-developed areas. Symptoms include intestinal cramps and diarrhea.

Hepatitis A virus comes from food that's been contaminated by feces. The conditions caused by hepatitis, such as jaundice and liver problems, can be severe. Sometimes hepatitis A comes through the food chain from shellfish that's been harvested from contaminated waters—perhaps where raw sewage is dumped. More commonly, an infected person who handles food without properly washing his or her hands can transmit the disease—often from a restaurant or other food-service operation. Cooking may not kill the

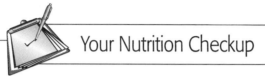

Kitchen Safety

How's your food safety savvy? Are you clean and careful enough to keep foodborne illness out of your kitchen? Take this kitchen safety checkup to find out.

Do You . . .	ALWAYS	USUALLY	SOMETIMES	NEVER
Wash your hands with warm, soapy water before and after handling food?	____	____	____	____
Change your dishtowels and dishcloths every few days?	____	____	____	____
Clean up splatters in your microwave oven immediately with hot, soapy water?	____	____	____	____
Sanitize cutting boards after each use with a chlorine bleach-water solution?	____	____	____	____
Clean your refrigerator each week, discarding foods that are too old?	____	____	____	____
Put dates on frozen foods?	____	____	____	____
Thaw foods in the refrigerator, not on the counter?	____	____	____	____
Rotate foods in your freezer and cupboards, with the oldest foods in front?	____	____	____	____
Check foods in cans and jars for bulging or leaking before opening?	____	____	____	____
Marinate meat, poultry, and seafood in the refrigerator?	____	____	____	____
Grill food so it cooks evenly inside and outside?	____	____	____	____
Use a clean plate and fork to take cooked food from the grill to the table?	____	____	____	____
Clean your picnic cooler with hot, soapy water before you use it?	____	____	____	____
Use leftovers within three or four days?	____	____	____	____
Remove stuffing from chicken and turkey before refrigerating leftovers?	____	____	____	____
Avoid the urge to use the stirring spoon for a quick taste?	____	____	____	____
Use a clean knife and cutting board for vegetables after cutting meat, poultry, or seafood?	____	____	____	____
Use a meat thermometer to cook meat and poultry to a safe internal temperature?	____	____	____	____
Use pasteurized eggs in recipes calling for eggs that won't be cooked?	____	____	____	____
Put leftovers in the refrigerator within two hours of cooking?	____	____	____	____
Cook hamburger patties until they're 160° F and no longer pink inside?	____	____	____	____
Heat leftovers until they're steaming hot?	____	____	____	____
Clean the outdoor grill after every use?	____	____	____	____
Remove perishable foods from a buffet after two hours?	____	____	____	____
Store poultry, meat, and fish on the bottom of your refrigerator in containers that won't leak?	____	____	____	____
Subtotal	____	____	____	____

Now score yourself:

"Always": 4 points
"Usually": 3 points
"Sometimes": 2 points
"Never": 1 point

Your total score _____

When it comes to food safety, you need a perfect score—100 points! Anything less and you're putting yourself—and anyone who eats with you—at risk for foodborne illness. It's safe to assume that the higher your score, the lower the risk.

For any item on which you scored "3" or less, exert a conscious effort to make a change to "always." Keep reading!

Take Control of Home Food Safety

1. Wash hands often.
2. Keep raw meats and ready-to-eat foods separate.
3. Cook to proper temperatures.
4. Refrigerate promptly below 40° F.

Source: *Home Food Safety . . . It's in Your Hands* (American Dietetic Association and ConAgra, Inc., 2000).

virus. As a precaution, always choose a restaurant that appears clean. And eat only well-cooked seafood.

Checklist for a Clean Kitchen

From top to bottom, a clean kitchen offers a main line of defense against the spread of colds, flu, and food-borne illness. Before you work with food, eliminate the breeding grounds for harmful bacteria:

Hands. Wash your hands—front and back, between your fingers, under your fingernails—in warm, soapy water for at least twenty seconds before and after every step in preparing foods. That includes your kitchen helpers, including children. Teach kids to sing "The Alphabet Song" while they wash their hands; that takes about twenty seconds. Use disposable paper towels or a clean cloth to dry your hands.

Why is hand washing so important? Bacteria live and multiply on warm, moist hands. Hands pick up germs, spreading them from surface to surface, food to food, and person to person. One of the best ways to control the spread of illness is thorough proper hand washing.

Work surfaces. Clean them often to remove food particles and spills. Use hot, soapy water. Keep nonfood items—mail, newspapers, purses—off the counters and away from food and utensils. Wash the counter carefully before food preparation.

Utensils. Wash dishes and cookware carefully in the dishwasher or in hot (at least 140° F), soapy water. Rinse well. Be aware that chipped crockery and china can collect bacteria.

Towels and dishcloths. Change them often, and wash them often in the hot cycle of your washing machine.

And allow them to dry out between each use. Being damp, they're the perfect breeding ground for bacteria. Throw out dirty sponges, or wash them in a bleach-water solution.

Appliances. On any appliance, clean up spills right away. Wash appliance surfaces with hot, soapy water. Pay special attention to the refrigerator and the freezer—shelves, sides, and door—where foods are stored. (Pack perishables in coolers while you clean or defrost your refrigerator and freezer.) Splatters inside your microwave oven can harbor bacteria, too. Keep it clean!

Safe from Cross-Contamination

Cross-contamination happens when bacteria in one food spread to another, often from a cutting board, knife, plate, spoon, or your hands. For example, drippings from raw meat, poultry, and seafood left on a cutting board can transfer bacteria to vegetables, which are being sliced next.

Wash Your Hands More Often

Before you:
- Handle or prepare food
- Eat meals
- Feed children

After you:
- Prepare food
- Touch raw food, especially meats
- Switch food preparation tasks
- Touch eggs and egg-rich foods
- Use the rest room
- Change a diaper
- Cough or sneeze
- Handle garbage or dirty dishes
- Smoke a cigarette
- Pet animals
- Use the phone
- Touch face, hair, body, other people
- Touch a cut or a sore
- Clean or touch dirty laundry

Source: *Home Food Safety . . . It's in Your Hands* (American Dietetic Association and ConAgra, Inc., 2000).

Cutting boards. Whether you choose plastic, acrylic, glass, marble, or wood, keep cutting boards clean. After each use, wash them in hot, soapy water, rinse, and dry well, perhaps in the dishwasher. Rinsing or wiping them isn't enough!

Clean a cutting board after using it to cut raw meat, poultry, or seafood. If you prefer wooden cutting boards, keep one just for raw meat, poultry, and seafood. Mark it to avoid confusion. Discard wooden boards with deep grooves and knife scars that can't be cleaned easily.

To sanitize cutting boards, use a chlorine bleach-water solution after each use. To make the solution, mix 2 teaspoons of bleach in a quart of water. Let the cutting boards air-dry. Brush to reach grooves and other hard-to-reach places.

Utensils. Unless it's cleaned well in between, avoid using the same knife to slice meat and chop vegetables.

Although hard to resist, remind everyone who ventures in the kitchen—never taste with the stirring spoon! If children reach for a finger-licking taste, be sure they wash their hands before continuing to help in the kitchen. There's another reason to resist tasting: if food (perhaps meat sauce) isn't cooked through yet, it may still harbor harmful bacteria!

Other reminders. Store produce in clean bags or containers after you wash it, not in the store bag. If you have an open cut or sore, wear latex gloves to handle food. Open food bags with a clean knife or scissors.

Safekeeping

Store food in the right container, in the right place, at the right temperature, for the right length of time.

Have You Ever Wondered

... if you should switch to antibacterial soap or detergent? An antibacterial product may be a good choice if you or someone in your family is at risk for infection, perhaps recovering from an illness or surgery. In normal circumstances, regular soap or detergent products are fine. Overused, antibacterial products lose their effectiveness as bacteria become resistant to them.

Common Food Safety Mistakes

- Countertop thawing
- Leftovers left out of the refrigerator
- Unclean cutting board
- Room-temperature marinating
- Store-to-refrigerator lag time
- BBQ blunder: same platter for raw and grilled meats
- Restaurant "doggie bag" delay
- Stirring-and-tasting spoon
- Shared knife for trimming raw meat and chopping vegetables
- Hide-and-eat Easter eggs
- Undercooked high-risk foods such as eggs, meat, poultry, and fish

Adapted from: Plating It Safe: A Market-to-Mealtime Checklist to Help Keep Food Safe (© Cattlemen's Beef Board and National Cattlemen's Beef Association, 1994).

Foods maintain their quality, safety, and nutrients when they're stored properly and used within a certain time. Besides, you stretch your food dollar when you don't need to discard spoiled food. *To determine the freshness of a packaged food product, see "More Reading on the Food Label" in chapter 11.*

In the Cupboard

How long do nonrefrigerated foods keep their quality? That depends on how carefully you store them. For safe, dry storage, store food for keeps!

● Keep your cupboards and pantries clean, dry, dark, and cool—preferably away from heat-producing appliances. Ideally 50° F to 70° F is the best storage temperature range. High temperatures (over 100° F) lower the quality of canned foods.

● Organize your cupboards with older cans up front for first use. The good news is: canned foods do have a long shelf life. Stored properly, most unopened canned foods stay edible and keep their nutritional quality well beyond two years. Although the food is still safe to eat for a long time, the color and texture of the food may change after a while.

● Be alert for signs of food spoilage. Never use food from cans that are cracked, bulging, or leaking or that spurt liquid when opened. The food may be contaminated with the deadly botulism organism. Toss—don't taste!

● Store opened packages of food in dry, airtight containers. That keeps out insects and rodents. Well-sealed containers also keep one food from absorbing the odors of others.

● Store foods away from kitchen chemicals and refuse. As important, keep chemicals and refuse away from places where food is prepared and eaten.

In the Fridge

Do "science experiments" ever grow in your refrigerator? Is yesterday's meat loaf hiding behind tomorrow's juice carton? Has that special cheese become as dry as old leather? With the hustle and bustle of today's living, these things happen, even in the best kitchens. To keep perishable food safe and out of the "danger zone," wrap it and store it right. Follow safe handling instructions on food packages and labels. *For an example of a safe food handling label found on fresh meat and poultry items, see "Safe Handling Instructions" on page 244.*

● Keep your refrigerator cold—between 34° F and 40° F. In this temperature range, bacteria that spoil food grow slowly. Below 32° F, which is freezing, bacteria survive but won't grow. Temperatures fluctuate, especially from season to season. Use a refrigerator thermometer to check; buy one at the supermarket. Remind your family to make their refrigerator raids quick so the door doesn't stay open too long.

● Store all foods wrapped or in covered containers. Seal storage containers well to prevent moisture loss and absorption of off-odors. Unless the package is torn, leave food in its store wrapping. The less you handle food, the better. Store washed produce in a clean container, not the store bag.

● Transfer opened canned food to a clean container. It's safe to refrigerate food in covered cans after opening, but off-flavors may develop.

● Keep packages of raw meat, poultry, and fish in separate plastic bags, in a bowl or a pan, on the lowest

Have You Ever Wondered

. . . if molds on cheese are dangerous? Not usually. Few molds on cheese produce toxins, or poisons. But just to be on the safe side, discard one inch of the cheese on all sides where mold is visible. Re-cover the food with fresh, clean wrap. Soft cheeses such as cream cheese, Brie, and cottage cheese, and other foods with mold on them, should be discarded. The exceptions are mold-ripened cheeses such as blue, Gorgonzola, Roquefort, and Stilton. Check the color and the pattern of the mold. If it's different from the usual blue or green veins and you see furry spots or white, pink, blue, green, gray, or black flecks, discard the cheese. Mold spores may have spread throughout the cheese.

refrigerator shelf. That keeps the juices from dripping onto other foods. The lowest refrigerator shelf usually is the coldest.

● Store food quickly. Avoid keeping perishable foods at room temperature for long: supermarket foods as well as leftovers. Cool leftovers and food cooked for later use in the refrigerator or freezer, not on the counter. Leftovers shouldn't be left at room temperature for longer than two hours.

● For faster cooling, store cooked food in small portions and in shallow containers. Large portions can take a long time to drop below 40° F.

● Keep leftovers where you'll see them. Then use them up within three or four days at the most. Toss them out if you can't remember when you stored them.

● Avoid overloading your refrigerator. Cold air needs room to circulate.

● Use special compartments in your refrigerator. The meat keeper keeps meat extra cold so it stays fresher longer. And crisper bins help produce retain its moisture. Keep eggs, however, in their carton, not in the egg tray or door shelf, to keep them fresher longer. And use them within four to five weeks of the Julian date on the carton. *See "Eggs" in chapter 11 for how to read the date on an egg carton.*

● Eat perishable foods while they remain at peak quality. Discard foods, rather than risk foodborne illness, after they've passed their prime. Use beefsteaks, roasts, deli meats, and poultry within three to four days. Use ground meat, ground poultry, and fish within one to two days. You may notice that the interior of ground beef often is purplish-red in color. The color doesn't mean the meat is spoiled. Instead, it hasn't been in direct contact with oxygen. As it's exposed to air, meat will turn the familiar bright red. *Check the chart "The Cold Truth: How Cold, How Long?" in this chapter.*

● If you're not sure about a food's safety, toss it out! Never trust the odor or the appearance. Food may look, taste, and smell okay—even when it's no longer safe to eat. When in doubt, throw it out!

● Discard moldy food "under wraps." Put food in a bag or a wrapper so mold spores don't spread. Then clean the container and the refrigerator well.

● Refrigerate or freeze whole grains, since they tend to get rancid faster.

In the Freezer

In freezer storage, the colder, the better. Freezing extends the shelf life of all kinds of foods.

● Keep your freezer "iceberg" cold! For long-term storage, maintain a freezer temperature of 0° F or less. A free-standing freezer can stay that cold. However, the freezer compartment of most refrigerators usually won't; plan to use foods stored there more quickly. To check the temperature, install a freezer thermometer, available at many kitchen stores or supermarkets.

● Store foods purchased frozen in their original packaging. Commercial packaging usually is airtight.

● Freezing home-prepared foods? Take time to properly package them. Use freezer containers, foils, and moistureproof paper, plastic bags, or other wraps. Traditional plastic wraps aren't suitable. Use freezer tape to help keep the package airtight and free of freezer burn. For storage that's longer than a few days, fresh meat retains its quality best when it's rewrapped or overwrapped.

● Before freezing, label each package with the food, date, and the number of servings. When you open your freezer, you'll be able to identify the foods on hand and their freshness.

Caution—Decorative Dishes

For years lead has been an ingredient in the glaze, or coating, on ceramic bowls, dishes, and pitchers. With proper firing, or heating in a kiln, glazes with lead are safe. However, when dishes are fired incorrectly or when copper is added to the glaze, hazardous amounts of lead can leach from dishes into food. Lead is harmful to health, collecting in bones and some soft tissues. Among other problems, lead poisoning can cause learning disabilities, organ damage, and even death. Children and pregnant women are particularly sensitive to the toxic effects of lead.

To be sure your dishes are safe enough for food, follow these guidelines:

● Inspect the surface of ceramic dishes. The surface that contacts food should be smooth and shiny, not rough or painted on top of the glaze.

● Check both sides of dishes, bowls, and pitchers. If it says "Not for Food Use" or "For Decorative Purposes Only," don't use it for food!

● Don't store food in ceramic dishes or leaded crystal. Lead can leach out when acidic foods and beverages such as coffee, tomato juice, fruit, or wine come in contact with glaze or leaded crystal over time.

● Beware of ceramicware made by untrained potters. For the most part, today's hobbyists are well aware of the problems of lead glazes.

● Beware of ceramicware brought back from foreign travel and of older dishes, imported before government monitoring.

● To check your own dishes, purchase a lead-test kit. Hardware or hobby stores are the best places to find one.

● Organize your freezer. Rotate foods, keeping the oldest foods in front so they're used first. Stack similar foods together—they'll be easier to find.

● Remember that some foods don't freeze well: bananas, fresh tomatoes, lettuce, celery, gelatin salads, custard, mayonnaise, hard-cooked eggs, sour cream, cream (unless it's whipped), raw potatoes, unblanched vegetables, and foods made with these ingredients. Freezing affects their quality, not the safety.

● Blanch vegetables to lengthen their freezer life. Blanching is immersing foods in boiling water for one to three minutes, then plunging them in cold water to stop the cooking. Freeze in airtight plastic bags after draining well.

To Thaw Safely

● Thaw foods in the refrigerator, not on the counter. Bacteria thrive at room temperature. Put thawing food in a plastic bag or on a plate to collect any juices. If you need a fast thaw, remove the store wrap first; put meat, poultry, or fish in a microwave-safe container; and defrost on "low" or "defrost" settings in your microwave oven. Or thaw frozen meat, poultry, or fish in cold water that's changed every thirty minutes. Cold water chills the surface. Then cook the food right away!

● Plan ahead to defrost frozen meat in the refrigerator. Here's how long it takes:
  ● Large roast—four to seven hours per pound
  ● Small roast—three to five hours per pound
  ● 1-inch-thick package of ground beef—twenty-four hours
  ● 1-inch-thick steak—twelve to fourteen hours

● To thaw, especially small amounts of food, in a microwave oven, use the "defrost" setting. Once thawed, cook food right away. The time for microwave thawing depends on the amount of food you need to thaw.

When Your Power Goes Out

Suppose a storm, an accident, or another event shuts off power to your home—along with your refrigerator and freezer. You may not need to toss out food if you take a few precautions.

Keep the refrigerator and freezer doors closed so heat stays out and cold stays in. Unopened, most refrigerators stay chilled for at least four to six hours, depending on the warmth of your kitchen. If the power is out longer, you might buy a block of ice to keep the refrigerator cool.

Frozen foods can hold for about two days in a full, freestanding freezer if it stays closed. Half full, a freezer remains cold for about one day. Freezers are well insulated; each frozen food package is an ice block, protecting foods around it.

Have You Ever Wondered

. . . if freezer burn on food is harmful? Freezer burn, which is the white, dried-out patches on improperly wrapped frozen food, won't make you sick, but it will make food tough and tasteless. To prevent freezer burn, wrap food that hasn't been previously frozen in proper freezer wrap (aluminum foil, heavy freezer paper, or plastic freezer bags), push the air out, then seal with freezer tape. Well-sealed freezer containers work, too; before putting on the lid, cover food with plastic wrap to avoid freezer burn from air inside the container.

. . . if partially thawed food can be refrozen? Yes, with caution—if it still has ice crystals and has been kept in the refrigerator for one day or less. Be aware that quality may be lost with refreezing. Try cooking the food first, then refreezing it.

Once the Power's Back On

Avoid using appearance or odor as your guide to food safety. Instead, follow these guidelines:

● If foods in the freezer still have ice crystals, refreeze them right away. Then use them as soon as you can.

● Discard perishable foods held at room temperature for more than two hours: meat, poultry, and fish; milk, soft cheese, and yogurt; soups; leftover prepared foods; cooked pasta; mayonnaise; and many refrigerated desserts. In that time, bacteria can multiply enough to cause illness. Dispose of these foods safely—where animals can't eat them.

● If the power's been out for only a few hours, keep less perishable foods. Fresh fruits and vegetables, peanut butter, nuts, hard and process cheeses, condiments, butter, and margarine often keep for several days at room temperature. Toss food out, however, if it turns moldy or smells bad.

Plan for Unexpected Emergencies

No matter where you live, experts advise a three-day supply of food and water for you, your family—and your pets.

● Stock up on nonperishable foods: ready-to-eat canned meat, fruits, juices, milk, soups, and

THE COLD TRUTH: HOW COLD, HOW LONG?

How long can refrigerated food keep safely and remain at top quality? Freezer and refrigerator times vary. As long as the food is properly packaged, these are basic guidelines:

FOOD	REFRIGERATOR (40° F)	FREEZER (0° F)
Eggs		
Fresh eggs, in shell	4 to 5 weeks	Don't freeze
Hard-cooked eggs	1 week	Don't freeze; they don't freeze well
Liquid pasteurized eggs or egg substitutes,		
Opened	3 days	Don't freeze
Unopened	10 days	1 year
Dairy products		
Milk	1 week	3 months
Cottage cheese	1 week	Doesn't freeze well
Yogurt	1 to 2 weeks	1 to 2 months
Commercial mayonnaise (refrigerate after opening)	2 months	Don't freeze
Vegetables, blanched/cooked		
Beans	3 to 4 days	8 months
Carrots	2 weeks	10 to 12 months
Celery	1 to 2 weeks	10 to 12 months
Lettuce, iceberg	1 to 2 weeks	Don't freeze
Lettuce, leaf	3 to 7 days	Don't freeze
Spinach	1 to 2 days	10 to 12 months
Squash, summer	4 to 5 days	10 to 12 months
Squash, winter	2 weeks	10 to 12 months
Tomatoes	2 to 3 days	2 months
Frozen Dinners and Casseroles		
Keep frozen until ready to serve		3 to 4 months
Deli and Self-Serve Foods		
Store-prepared (or homemade) egg, ham, chicken, tuna, macaroni salads	3 to 5 days	Don't freeze
Entrées, cold or hot	3 to 4 days	2 to 3 months
Hot Dogs*		
Opened package	1 week	In freezer wrap, 1 to 2 months
Unopened package	2 weeks	In freezer wrap, 1 to 2 months
Lunch Meats		
Opened	3 to 5 days	1 to 2 months
Unopened	2 weeks	1 to 2 months
Fresh Meat		
Beef—steaks, roasts	3 to 5 days	6 to 12 months
Pork—chops, roasts	3 to 5 days	4 to 6 months
Lamb—chops, roasts	3 to 5 days	6 to 9 months
Veal—roast	3 to 5 days	4 to 6 months

THE COLD TRUTH: HOW COLD, HOW LONG? *(continued)*

FOOD	REFRIGERATOR (40° F)	FREEZER (0° F)
Fresh Poultry		
Chicken or turkey, whole	1 to 2 days	1 year
Pieces	1 to 2 days	9 months
Giblets	1 to 2 days	3 to 4 months
Fresh Fish		
Lean fish (cod, flounder, etc.)	1 to 2 days	6 months
Fatty fish (salmon, etc.)	1 to 2 days	2 to 3 months
Ham and Corned Beef		
Canned ham (label says keep refrigerated)	6 to 9 months	Don't freeze
Ham, fully cooked, and corned beef (half and slices)	3 to 5 days	1 to 2 months
Corned beef, in pouch with pickling juices	5 to 7 days	Drained, wrapped, 1 month
Hamburger, Ground and Stew Meats		
Hamburger and stew meats	1 to 2 days	3 to 4 months
Ground turkey, veal, pork, lamb, and mixtures	1 to 2 days	3 to 4 months
Bacon and Sausage		
Bacon	1 week	1 month
Sausage, raw (pork, beef, turkey)	1 to 2 days	1 to 2 months
Precooked, smoked breakfast links, patties	1 weeks	1 to 2 months
Hard sausage (pepperoni, jerky sticks)	2 to 3 weeks	1 to 2 months
Variety Meats		
Tongue, brain, kidneys, liver, heart, chitterlings	1 to 2 days	3 to 4 months
Vacuum-Packed Products		
Commercial-brand, vacuum-packed dinners with USDA seal	2 weeks, unopened	These products don't freeze well.
Leftovers		
Cooked meat, meat dishes, egg dishes, soups, stew, vegetables	3 to 4 days	2 to 3 months
Gravy and meat broth	1 to 2 days	2 to 3 months
Cooked poultry and fish	3 to 4 days	4 to 6 months

Fresh Produce

● Raw fruits are safe at room temperature, but after ripening they will mold and rot quickly. For best quality, store ripe fruit in the refrigerator, or prepare and freeze. After cooking, fruits must be refrigerated or frozen within two hours.

● Some dense, raw vegetables such as potatoes and onions can be stored at cool room temperatures. Refrigerate other raw vegetables for optimum quality and to prevent rotting. After cooking, vegetables must be refrigerated or frozen within two hours.

*Some may have package dates that may not be consistent with these guidelines.

Adapted from: To Your Health: Food Safety for Seniors (Washington, D.C.: U.S. Food and Drug Administration and U.S. Department of Agriculture, 2000).

vegetables. Canned foods are better than foods in glass bottles or jars because they won't break in a disaster. Choose single-serving portions, too; you may have no way to keep leftovers cold. Keep some high-energy foods on hand, too, such as peanut butter, nuts, and trail mix.

● Rotate your emergency food and water supply every year or so. In that way it's fresh when you need it.

● Buy either commercially bottled, well-sealed water, or store your own water in sanitized, food-grade containers (not milk cartons or jugs). Plan for 1 gallon of water per person per day. *See "Safe Enough to Drink" in chapter 8 for advice on making contaminated water safe to drink.*

● Keep manual can openers on your emergency shelf. A well-stocked emergency shelf with no way to open food cans doubles any disaster!

For more advice about handling food in disasters (fires, floods, hurricanes), contact experts: the U.S. Food and Drug Administration Food Safety Hotline (1-888-SAFE-FOOD), the U.S. Department of Agriculture's Meat and Poultry Hotline (1-800-535-4555), your local American Red Cross chapter, Cooperative Extension Service, Civil Defense, or emergency management office.

Safe Preparation and Service

Preparing, cooking, and serving can't make your food safe—if it hasn't been handled properly from the very start. But, assuming food's been cared for safely all along, you can ensure its quality as you prepare and serve it.

"Prep" It Safe

● Wash fresh fruits and vegetables to remove any pathogens from dirt or handling—even if you discard rinds or peels—with clean, running water, but not soap. Porous surfaces of produce can absorb ingredients in soap products. If appropriate, use a brush. Cutting through unwashed produce can carry bacteria from its surface in the inside flesh. Remove bruised or damaged spots because they may harbor bacteria or mold. "Rust" spots on lettuce aren't harmful; they occur as cells in the leaf break down naturally after harvest.

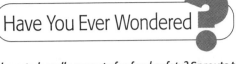

Have You Ever Wondered

... how to handle sprouts for food safety? Sprouts tend to harbor *E. coli* and *Salmonella;* the moist conditions that sprouts need to grow are perfect for breeding bacteria. The Centers for Disease Control and Prevention advise that sprouts (alfalfa, clover, radish, other sprouts) be thoroughly cooked before eating them to destroy bacteria and that high-risk individuals avoid sprouts altogether; the U.S. Food and Drug Administration also recommends cooking sprouts. Even carefully washed sprouts can harbor bacteria. Especially if you're at high risk, be aware that sandwiches and salads in restaurants may be made with raw sprouts.

To reduce your risk for foodborne illness if you choose to eat them raw, handle sprouts with care: refrigeration to slow bacterial growth; and washing under cold, running water. Buy them fresh, with the buds still on.

... about the safety of wild mushrooms? Stick with exotic mushrooms from the store if you're a mushroom-lover. Telling the difference between edible and poisonous (some deadly) mushrooms takes a lot of expertise. Unless they're gathered by a trusted mushroom expert, the best advice is to avoid them.

... if blood spots on eggs are okay? Yes, they happen naturally while the egg is forming, sometimes when a blood vessel on the yolk ruptures. Remove them if you prefer.

● Check canned and jar foods before opening them. Make sure that safety buttons on jar lids are depressed and that canned goods are still safe, not bulging or leaking. Wash the tops of canned goods before opening them so particles don't fall into food. Vacuum-packed canned foods may hiss softly when they're opened. That's probably the normal release of air pressure. A loud hiss or spurting may indicate food spoilage. Wash can openers after each use.

● Rinse poultry and seafood in cold water; check for off-odors, too. Deveining shrimp is up to you. Cooking destroys any bacteria in shrimp, including in the intestinal vein. However, for cosmetic purposes you may want to remove it. In large shrimp the vein may contain a lot of grit.

Disaster Planning: Emergency Supply Checklist

Stocking up now on emergency supplies—and rotating them regularly—can add to your safety and comfort during and after a disaster. Store enough supplies for at least seventy-two hours.

FOOD AND WATER*

- Water: 1 gallon per person per day
- Ready-to-eat canned meats (tuna, chicken, beef, chili), beans, soups, spaghetti
- Canned fruits, vegetables, juice; dried fruit, raisins
- Evaporated, powdered or ultrapasteurized milk
- Crackers, ready-to-cereals, pretzels, instant oatmeal, pasta, rice
- Peanut butter, jelly, granola bars, trail mix, nuts
- Instant coffee, teabag, hot chocolate, pudding, cookies, candy
- Staples: sugar, salt, pepper, mustard, catsup, mayonnaise, creamer

COOKING

- Barbecue grill, camp stove, pots/pans
- Fuel for cooking (charcoal, propane, etc.)
- Plastic knives, forks, spoons
- Paper plates and cups
- Paper towels
- Heavy-duty aluminum foil
- Matches (waterproof)
- Can opener (manual)

SANITATION SUPPLIES

- Large plastic trash bags for trash, waste, water protection
- Large trash cans
- Bar soap and liquid detergent
- Hand sanitizer, wet wipes
- Shampoo
- Toothpaste and toothbrushes
- Feminine and infant supplies
- Toilet paper
- Household bleach
- Newspaper (to wrap garbage and waste)

SAFETY AND COMFORT

- Sturdy shoes, socks
- Heavy gloves for clearing debris
- Candles and matches
- Change of clothing, sweatshirts
- Knife or razor blades
- Garden hose—siphoning and fire fighting

OTHER SUPPLIES

- First-aid kit—freshly stocked
- First-aid book
- Suntan lotion, hats
- Blankets or sleeping bags
- Portable radio, flashlight, and spare batteries
- Essential medication and spare glasses
- Fire extinguisher: A-B-C type
- Ax, shovel, broom
- Crescent wrench for turning off gas
- Screwdriver, pliers, hammer
- Coil of ½-inch rope
- Plastic tape
- Tent
- Money
- Food, water, and essential medication for pets
- Toys for children

*In case distribution is disrupted after an emergency, store a two-week supply if you have special food or medical needs.

Source: Adapted from American Red Cross WIC Program, San Diego, CA. "Emergency Supply Checklist." Governor's Office on Emergency Services, Sacramento CA.

● Keep juices from raw meat, poultry, or fish from coming in contact with other foods—cooked or raw. Use separate cutting boards, plates, trays, and utensils for cooked and uncooked meat, poultry, and fish.

● Marinate meat, poultry, and seafood in covered, nonmetallic containers—in the refrigerator! Many marinades have acid-containing ingredients—wine, vinegar, and citrus juice—that react with metals. These metals can leach into food.

● If marinades have been in contact with raw meat, poultry, or seafood, boil the marinades for at least a minute. Then they're safe to use as a sauce for cooked food. Better yet, make a double batch of marinade. Use half to marinate, then discard it after marinating. Reserve the rest for a sauce at serving time.

● Avoid mixing dark-colored sauces into ground meat or poultry. Dark-colored sauces such as teriyaki sauce, soy sauce, barbecue sauce, and Worcestershire sauce make it hard to judge the doneness of ground meat. Instead, brush sauces on cooked patties when they're almost cooked. When ground beef is cooked to the proper and safe inside temperature, the juices run clear; use a meat thermometer to check.

● Avoid eating raw seafood, meat, poultry, and eggs, or foods containing these foods. Foods with raw eggs include some recipes for homemade mayonnaise, homemade eggnog, homemade ice cream, Hollandaise sauce, and Caesar salad dressing. For people with a compromised immune system, even lightly cooked egg dishes such as soft custards and French toast can be risky. *See "Is Raw Seafood Safe to Eat?" on this page if you choose to enjoy raw seafood occasionally.*

● If you stuff poultry, do so just before roasting, and stuff loosely. Be sure that the internal temperature of the meat reaches 180° F and the center of the stuffing reaches 165° F before removing from the oven. As an option, cook stuffing separately from chicken or turkey. Never cook stuffed poultry in a microwave oven. Always refrigerate leftover poultry and stuffing separately.

● If you infuse oil with herbs or garlic, use it right away rather than store it. Botulism has been linked to consuming some home-prepared herb and garlic oils.

Commercially prepared herb and garlic oils are required to contain protective additives to prevent possible foodborne illness. As an added precaution, always store commercial herb and garlic oil products in the refrigerator.

Is Raw Seafood Safe to Eat?

With sushi bars and with seviche (a popular Mexican and Caribbean appetizer), many people have come to enjoy raw and uncooked marinated seafood. With careful control, they can be safe; read on to learn how.

Shellfish, especially mollusks (oysters, clams, mussels, and scallops), may carry the bacterium *Vibrio vulnificus,* which multiplies even during refrigeration. Other viruses in uncooked or partly cooked mollusks also can cause severe diarrhea. *See the early part of this chapter for more about the risks related to* Vibrio vulnificus.

A few precautions reduce the risk of eating raw seafood:

● High-risk individuals—those with HIV, impaired immune systems, liver and gastrointestinal disorders, kidney disease, inflammatory bowel disease, cancer, diabetes, or steroid dependency—should avoid eating any raw or partly cooked fish. Pregnant women, the elderly, infants, and those with alcohol problems also are considered to be at high risk.

● If you prepare raw fish at home, start with high-quality seafood—very, very fresh, and use it within two days. Buy from a licensed, reputable dealer. For mollusks (clams, mussels, oysters), you can ask to see the certified shipper's tag. If you harvest your own, make sure the waters of origin are certified for safety. Follow the rules for safe food handling described in this chapter. Even at that, eating raw fish at home isn't advised. You're wiser to cook fish to an internal temperature of 145° F to destroy parasites.

● If fish is sushi-grade or high-quality, sushi, sashimi, seviche, and oyster bars are generally safe. Reputable restaurants have highly trained chefs who not only know how to buy fish that meets safety and sanitation standards but also know how to handle fish safely. *See chapter 14 for tips on Japanese cuisine.*

See chapter 11 for more guidelines on buying fresh seafood.

● Direct your coughs and sneezes away from food. Coughs and sneezes spread germs. Cover your mouth and nose with a tissue when you sneeze or cough. Then wash your hands with warm, soapy water.

Cook It Safe

● Keep hot food hot. Cook and hold cooked foods at temperatures higher than 140° F. High temperatures (160° F to 212° F) kill most bacteria. Temperatures between 140° F and 159° F prevent their growth but may let bacteria survive.

● Get the right tools for the job: a meat or "instant-read" thermometer to see when foods are thoroughly cooked; an oven thermometer to check your oven heat; and a timer to time the cooking accurately.

● Check the internal temperature of food, especially roasts, thick steaks (more than 2 inches thick), large cuts of meat, whole chickens or turkeys, and large casseroles. Put the thermometer or oven temperature probe into the center of the thickest part of the food, but not near the bone or fat. After each use, wash the thermometer stem well in hot, soapy water. *See the chart "Safe Internal Temperatures" for recommended internal temperatures, and "Using a Meat Thermometer"—both in this chapter—for guidelines on inserting and reading a meat thermometer.*

● Cook ground meat and poultry thoroughly—until no longer pink inside, juices run clear, and the internal temperature reaches 160° F. Thorough cooking is especially important with ground meat; bacteria on the outside get mixed inside as meat and poultry are ground and mixed.

Have You Ever Wondered

...how you store live mollusks? For the very short time you may keep them (within two days), refrigerate them in a container with a damp cloth over the top. Be sure other foods don't drip on them. Do not store them in an airtight container or in water. Remember, they're saltwater fish that need air to stay alive. Scrub them with a stiff brush just prior to shucking or cooking them.

Safe Internal Temperatures

For food safety—and the best flavor—cook meat and poultry to the right internal temperature. To check, use a meat or "instant-read" thermometer.

FOOD ITEM	INTERNAL, COOKED TEMPERATURE (° F)
Beef, Veal, and Lamb	
Ground products such as hamburger (as patties, meat loaf, meatballs, etc.)	160
Nonground products such as roasts and steaks	
Medium rare	145
Medium	160
Well done	170
Fresh Pork	
All cuts, including ground products	
Medium	160
Well done	170
Ham	
Fresh, raw ham	160
Fully cooked ham, to reheat	140
Fish	145
Poultry	
Ground chicken, turkey	165
Whole chicken, turkey	180
Boneless turkey roasts	170
Poultry breasts and roasts (white meat)	170
Poultry thighs, wings and drumsticks (dark meat)	180
Duck, goose	180
Stuffing (cooked alone or in bird)	165
Eggs	Yolks and whites are firm.
Egg dishes, casseroles, and cheesecakes	160
Leftovers, reheated	165

Source: Adapted from and consistent with guidelines from the U.S. Department of Agriculture and the U.S. Food and Drug Administration.

● Instead of "rare," cook beef until "medium rare" (to an internal temperature of 145° F) for safety. Steaks, roasts, and other cuts of beef cooked to a "rare" doneness increase your risk for foodborne illness.

● When in doubt, cook ham. If the label says "cooked ham," it's okay to eat without cooking or heating. If not, don't take chances; cook it before eating it. Words such as "smoked," "aged," or "dried" are no guarantee of safety without cooking. The smoked flavor may come from added flavoring, not curing.

● Follow the "ten-minute" rule for cooking finfish— whole fish, steaks, and fillets. For every inch of thickness, cook fish for ten minutes at 425° F to 450° F. If the fish is cooking in a sauce or foil wrap, cook for five minutes longer. The internal temperature should reach 145° F. If one end is thinner than another, fold it underneath so the thickness is uniform. This rule applies to broiling, grilling, steaming, baking, and poaching. Cooking times for frying and microwaving are generally faster ways to cook. If fish is cooked from a frozen state, double the cooking time. Cooked fish is opaque and flakes easily with a fork.

● Cook shellfish properly. Scallops and shrimp take three to five minutes, depending on their size. Scallops turn white and firm; shrimp turn pink. Boiling lobsters takes five to six minutes per pound after the water comes back to a boil; when fully cooked, they'll turn bright red.

● Be sure that mollusks are still alive before you cook them. If the shells don't close tightly when you tap them, toss them! Cook them in a pot that's big enough to cook all the shellfish thoroughly—even the shells in the middle. Discard any that don't open during cooking. For live clams, mussels, and oysters: boil water for three to five minutes after the shells open, or steam them for four to nine minutes. *If they're shucked:*

  ● Bake them for about ten minutes at 450º F
  ● Boil for at least three minutes or until the edges curl
  ● Fry for at least ten minutes at 375º F
  ● Broil them for at least three minutes

● Know the visual signs of doneness: egg yolks and whites that are firm; fish that is opaque and flakes easily; juices from meat and poultry that aren't pink; and poultry joints that move easily.

● If you've been basting, or brushing sauces on food, as you cook, switch to a clean brush and fresh sauce for cooked foods. In that way you won't transfer bacteria from raw to cooked foods. Discard the marinade used for raw meat, poultry, or fish, or boil it for at least one minute before using on cooked food.

● Avoid very low oven temperatures (below 325° F) for roasting meat, or long or overnight cooking for meat. With oven cooking, these low temperatures encourage bacterial growth before the meat is cooked.

● If using a slow cooker, know how to use it safely. Even though the food is cooked at a lower temperature, food prepared in a slow cooker is safe because the moist heat used to cook foods in this way is more lethal to bacteria than dry heat, such as oven cooking. Set the cooker on high until the food begins to bubble, then turn to a simmer or "low" setting to continue cooking. Use the lid, and check the internal temperature, which should be at least 160° F. Always choose a recipe that contains a liquid. When adding meat, use small pieces of thawed meat. Avoid filling the cooker to more than two-thirds of its capacity. A slow cooker is not for reheating.

● Cook food through at one time. Don't cook it partially, then finish later. Partially cooked food may not get hot enough inside to destroy bacteria; these conditions may encourage bacteria to grow.

● Heat leftovers to 165° F or until steaming hot. Reheat sauces and gravies to a rolling boil for at least one minute.

Play It Microwave-Safe

Today, a microwave oven is as common as a television set in our homes, workplaces, schools, and even recreational vehicles! For most people, the main reason is cooking speed. However, microwaving also has nutri-

> **For the Mile-High Cook**
>
> If you live at an altitude of 1,000 feet or more, you may need to cook food longer to kill bacteria. At higher altitudes, water boils at a lower temperature, which makes it less effective for killing bacteria. Most cooking and canning temperatures are based on food preparation at sea level.

tion benefits. Faster cooking helps retain nutrients and allows food to be cooked without added fat.

General cooking guidelines apply to microwave cooking. Since foods cook differently in a microwave oven, follow these special precautions:

● Use only microwave-safe containers. To see if your glass bowls, dishes, or cups are safe, place each one empty in the microwave oven with a separate cup of tap water. Microwave it on high for one minute. If the empty container stays cool, it's microwave-safe; slightly warm, use it for reheating only. Any bowls, dishes, or cups that get hot shouldn't be used in a microwave oven. Unless it says "microwave safe," avoid microwaving food in the container it came in. That includes margarine or butter tubs, other plastic tubs, polystyrene boxes or trays, plastic bags, brown paper bags, paper towels, paper plates, and paper napkins. Chemicals from these products may transfer to food. Containers from store-bought microwave meals are meant for one-time use; toss them.

● Cut food so the pieces are the same size. This helps ensure even cooking.

● Keep food well covered while cooking. Use waxed paper, microwave-safe plastic wrap, or a lid that fits. This keeps food from drying out and helps ensure even cooking. For safety, allow a little space for some steam to escape.

● Rotate food for even cooking. Halfway through cooking, do one of the following: turn the dish; stir or reposition the food on the plate or bowl; turn large foods over; or reposition the dish on the turntable. Check for cold spots

● Allow for standing time. Food keeps cooking after the microwave oven turns off, spreading the heat more evenly. In fact, the internal temperature can go up several degrees as food stands.

● Check for doneness—after the standing time. Then, as with food cooked in the oven, check the internal temperature and the visual signs of doneness. Check in several places, but not near the bone.

● Be aware of differences in the power, or wattage, of microwave ovens. Cooking times may differ. Use a thermometer to check for doneness.

● Follow microwave instructions on food packag-

ing. By law, package directions are approved by the U.S. Food and Drug Administration; however, recipes on packages may not be approved.

● Avoid using your microwave oven for canning. The pressure that builds up inside the jar may cause it to explode.

For more on microwave oven safety, see "Play It Safe: Warming Baby's Bottle and Food" in chapter 15 and "Microwave Oven Safety for Kids" in chapter 16.

Grill It Safe

Before you put another burger on the grill, take some precautions:

● Adjust the grill so the food cooks evenly—inside and outside. When meat or poultry are too close to the heat, the outside surfaces cook quickly and may appear to be done, but the inside may not be cooked well enough to destroy bacteria.

● Transfer food to a clean plate once it's cooked—with a clean utensil! Don't use your fingers. To avoid cross-contamination, carry cooked meat to the table on a clean dish—not the unwashed dish you used to bring raw meat to the grill.

● Clean the grill between each use. Removing charred food debris from the grill reduces exposure to bacteria and possible cancer-causing substances.

● If you're grilling at a picnic site, do all the cooking there—from start to finish. Partially cooked meats transported there may contain bacteria.

● Grill on both sides. Turn meat, poultry, and fish over at least once for even cooking. If fish is less than ½ inch thick, you don't need to turn it.

Have You Ever Wondered

. . . if liquid smoke is safe to eat? Bottled liquid smoke is sold alongside herbs and sauces in many supermarkets. It gives a smoky flavor without grilling. The flavoring is created by burning wood, then trapping the smoke; most potential carcinogens are removed. About 60 percent of processed meats sold in supermarkets are "smoked" with liquid smoke.

● Grill meat, poultry, and fish until they're cooked through but not charred. The charring—for example, on a well-done steak—is a possible cancer-causing compound called heterocyclic amines, or HCAs. While the research on health effects is inconclusive, you're smart to avoid the "black stuff." Instead, cook meat to medium, rather than well done. Marinating meat first may help reduce HCAs; precooking meat, then quickly grilling for flavor, may, too. Grill poultry and fish until the internal temperature reaches its target but the surface isn't blackened. Scrape off any charred areas before you eat.

● Control hot coals to avoid flame flare-ups. The smoke caused by fat dripping on hot coals contains another possible cancer-causing compound, called polycyclic aromatic hydrocarbons. Again, the research as a health risk isn't conclusive. These compounds may not pose a cancer risk, but you're still wise to trim visible fat from meat before cooking, drain any high-fat marinades, and have a spray bottle with water for flare-ups.

Where to Place the Meat Thermometer?

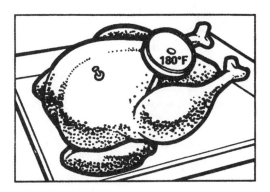

Poultry (Whole Bird)

Insert the meat thermometer into the inner thigh area of the breast but not touching bone.

If stuffed, stuffing temperature must reach 165° F. Do this near and at the end of the stand time.

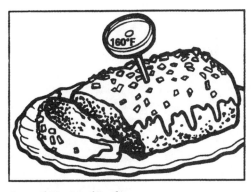

Ground Meat and Poultry

The thermometer should also be placed in the thickest area of ground meat or poultry dishes such as meat loaf. The thermometer may be inserted sideways in thin items such as patties, reaching the very center with the stem.

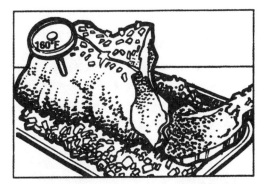

Beef, Pork, Lamb, Veal, Ham (Roasts, Steaks, or Chops), and Poultry Pieces

The thermometer should be inserted into the center of the thickest part, away from bone, fat, and gristle.

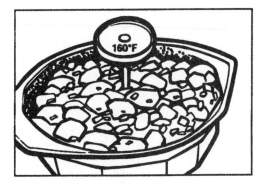

Casseroles and Egg Dishes

The thermometer should be inserted into the center or thickest part.

Using a Meat Thermometer

Using a meat thermometer takes the guesswork out of cooking. Besides helping to prevent foodborne illness, a meat thermometer helps to prevent overcooking and can help to hold foods at a safe temperature. Use a meat thermometer every time you prepare poultry, roasts, ham, casseroles, meat loaves, and egg dishes.

Types of Meat Thermometers

● *Regular, ovenproof:* Inserted into food at the beginning of cooking and remains there throughout cooking. Easy to read; placement is important.

● *Instant-read and digital:* Not intended to stay in food while cooking; gives a quick reading when the stem is inserted into food about 2 inches. For very thick foods, these thermometers cannot measure temperature accurately because they cannot reach the cold center.

● *Pop-up:* Often found already inserted into poultry; also may be purchased for other types of meat. Verify that meat is done by checking the temperature with a conventional thermometer as well.

● *Microwave-safe:* Designed for use in microwave ovens only.

● *Disposable thermometer:* Use once and toss. Meant for grilling at picnics and tailgate parties, they're inexpensive. Find these thermometers for burgers or chicken in the meat case of your supermarket.

Note: When buying a meat thermometer, read the package label carefully to be sure you are buying the type designed for use with meat, and not other food items such as candy. Look for a thermometer made of stainless steel, with an easy-to-read dial and a shatterproof clear lens.

"Egg-Stra" Cooking Tips for Food Safety

If they're not handled properly, eggs and egg-rich foods are a perfect medium for *Salmonella* to grow. To enjoy all the benefits that eggs provide, take these precautions:

● Toss any cracked or dirty eggs.

● Cook eggs until they're done—slowly over gentle heat. *See "How Do You Know When Cooked Eggs Are Done?" on this page for visual signs of doneness.*

● Prepare soft meringues and mousse made with slightly cooked eggs to destroy any *Salmonella*. To

prepare, put the egg whites in a double boiler or a heavy pan. Add 2 tablespoons of sugar for each egg white. Cook over low heat, beating on low speed as you cook until the whites reach 160° F, then turn the speed to high and beat until soft peaks appear. Then proceed with the recipe as directed.

● Avoid foods with raw eggs, such as Caesar salad or homemade ice cream, mayonnaise, or eggnog—unless they're made with an unopened carton of pasteurized eggs. However, once pasteurized eggs are open, they must be treated like any other eggs because they can be contaminated by bacteria. How about

How Do You Know When Cooked Eggs Are Done?

Cooking eggs? Look for these signs of doneness to ensure that *Salmonella* are destroyed.

COOKING METHOD	SIGNS OF DONENESS
Scrambled, omelettes, frittata	No visible liquid egg remains
Poached, fried over easy, sunny side up	White completely set; yolk starting to thicken but not hard (*Hint:* For sunny-side-up eggs, cover with lid to ensure adequate cooking.)
Soft-cooked	White completely set; yolk starting to thicken but not hard (Bring to a boil; turn off heat. Let eggs stand in water for four to five minutes.)
Hard-cooked	White and yolk completely set (Bring to a boil; turn off heat. Let eggs stand in water for fifteen minutes.)
Stirred custard, including ice cream and eggnog	Mixture coats the spoon; temperature reaches 160° F
Baked custard, including quiche	Knife placed off-center comes out clean (*Note:* cheese in a properly cooked quiche will leave particles on the knife, too.)

FOR SAFETY'S SAKE: HOW LONG CAN YOU REFRIGERATE LEFTOVERS?

PERISHABLE FOOD	KEEPS REFRIGERATED UP TO
Cooked fresh vegetables	3 to 4 days
Cooked pasta	3 to 5 days
Cooked rice	1 week
Deli counter meats	5 days
Greens	1 to 2 days
Meat	
● Ham, cooked and sliced	3 to 4 days
● Hot dogs, opened	1 week
● Lunch meats, prepackaged, opened	3 to 5 days
● Cooked beef, pork, poultry, fish and meat casseroles	3 to 4 days
● Cooked patties and nuggets, gravy, and broth	1 to 2 days
Seafood, cooked	2 days
Soups and stews	3 to 4 days
Stuffing	1 to 2 days

When in doubt, throw it out!

Source: Home Food Safety . . . It's in Your Hands (American Dietetic Association and ConAgra, Inc., 2000).

homemade cookie dough? If it contains raw eggs, there can be risk. Commercially prepared dressing, mayonnaise, cookie dough, and cookie dough ice cream all use pasteurized eggs.

● As another option, use cooked yolks in recipes that call for raw eggs. Cook the yolks in a double boiler or a heavy skillet with liquid from the recipe: 2 tablespoons of liquid for each yolk. Beat it while it cooks until the yolk coats a spoon, or bubbles form around the edges, or the temperature reaches 160° F.

● Keep eggs and egg-rich foods at 40° F to 140° F for no longer than two hours, including serving time. Otherwise, keep them refrigerated. Use leftovers made with eggs within two or three days.

● Store Easter eggs in the refrigerator. Handle eggs carefully while decorating; cracked eggs invite bacteria. Hide them so they stay clean from pets, dirt, and other sources of bacteria. Toss any that get cracked or dirty or go unfound (unrefrigerated) for more than two hours. Hard-cooked eggs don't keep as well as raw shell eggs; use hard-cooked eggs within a week. Like other high-protein foods, hard-cooked eggs shouldn't sit out at temperatures of 40° F or higher for longer than two hours. If they do, toss them.

Plate It Safe

● Use clean dishes and utensils for serving—use nothing that touched raw meat, fish, or poultry unless it was cleaned in hot, soapy water first.

● Avoid keeping perishable foods on a serving table or at room temperature for longer than two hours (one hour in hot weather 90° F or above). That includes cooked meat, poultry, fish, eggs, and dishes made with these ingredients.

● For buffet-type service keep cold foods cold and hot foods hot. Serve cold foods on ice, at a temperature of 40° F or below. Use heated servers such as a chafing dish to keep hot foods hot. After two hours even these foods should be discarded.

● When replenishing serving dishes don't mix fresh food with food that's been sitting out already. *For more about* Clostridium perfringens *contamination on buffets, see "Bacteria: Hard Hitters" earlier in this chapter.*

● Refrigerate leftovers as soon as you're done eating.

Carry It Safe

Picnic Foods

It's summertime. The season's "ripe" for picnics—and foodborne illness. Keep food fit to eat in your fresh-air kitchen with the three basic food-safe rules: Keep food clean, keep hot food hot, and keep cold food cold.

● For perishables, use clean, insulated coolers chilled with ice or chemical cold packs. As a rule of thumb, pack your cooler with 75 percent food and 25 percent ice or frozen cold packs. Freeze cold packs at least twenty-four hours ahead so they stay cold as long as possible. Chill the cooler ahead, too. Secure the lid. Then keep the cooler closed—no peeking!

● Store nonperishable foods in a clean picnic or laundry basket—with the heaviest foods on the bottom.

If You or Someone Else is Choking

Perform the Heimlich Maneuver. If a victim can't talk, can't breathe, is turning blue in the face, or is clutching at his or her throat, get behind the person and wrap your arms around his or her waist. Making a fist, put the thumb side of the fist against the victim's upper abdomen, below the ribs and above the navel. Grasp your fist with your other hand and press into the victim's upper abdomen with a quick upward thrust. Repeat until the object is expelled. (Don't slap the victim's back. This can make matters worse.)

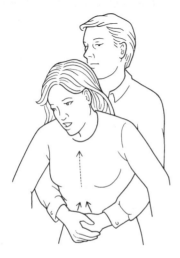

When you choke and no one is there to help, use the same technique as described above. You can also lean over a fixed horizontal object (a chair, a table edge, a railing), pressing your upper abdomen against the edge until the object is expelled.

Source: Courtesy of The Heimlich Institute, Cincinnati, Ohio.

● Seal all foods tightly in bags, jars, or plastic containers. That keeps out moisture and bugs.

● Pack foods that are cold or frozen already. Don't assume your cooler can cool foods adequately if they're packed at room temperature. Pack perishable foods between ice or cold packs; they'll stay cold longer.

● Pack uncooked meat, poultry, or fish carefully—in well-sealed containers—for grilling at the picnic spot. Put them in the bottom of the cooler so any juices won't leak onto other foods. Bring a meat thermometer.

● Keep your cooler in a cool place—not in the hot trunk or in the sun. Instead, place it under a tree or a picnic table.

● Return perishable foods to the cooler immediately when you're done serving, and serve only the amount of food you'll eat right away. Keep the rest in the cooler until it's needed.

● For picnics nearby that will be eaten right away, consider a hot dish—covered and wrapped well. Wrap the dish in several layers of newspaper, then in an insulated container. Baked beans are a popular choice.

● Bring premoistened towelettes to wash up after handling meat, poultry, or chicken—or any food, for that matter. Or bring soap and a bottle filled with clean water to wash your hands and cooking surfaces. *Another option:* a hand sanitizer, usually formulated with alcohol, which kills bacteria on your hands; you don't need soap and water.

● Be prepared to clean the grill at the picnic site—unless you bring your own clean grill. Pack a brush, soap, and perhaps water.

● After the picnic, toss perishable leftovers. Or repack them in a cold cooler if they have been out for less than two hours (one hour at 90° F or warmer) and are clean (no flies, dirt, or improper handling).

Carried Meals and Snacks

Whether you pack it at home or buy ready-to-eat take-out foods, any time perishable foods are left at room temperature for two hours or more, there's risk for foodborne illness. That's especially true when it's stuffed in a school locker with a dirty gym bag or left on a warm windowsill at the office!

● Order take-out food just before lunch or dinner, then eat it right away. Or keep it in the refrigerator at work or wherever else you may be.

● Use a clean insulated bag or a lunch box. Tuck in a small refreezable ice pack to keep food cold. Or freeze a juice box or small plastic container of water to keep the lunch box and the food cold. Pack a hand sanitizer, too, if there's no chance for hand washing.

● For cold beverages, refrigerate an insulated vacuum bottle ahead. Then fill it with milk or juice to carry with you. If your meal goes to work, keep a carton of juice or milk in the fridge at work.

● For hot soups, stews, and chilies, heat an insulated container ahead. Fill it with boiling water, then let it sit for several minutes before pouring it out. Be sure the food is very hot when it's put into the container. Then keep the container closed until you eat the food.

● Assemble your meal the night before, and chill the meal well. You'll "buy" a little more time in the morning!

● Keep carried, perishable food in a clean, cool place—away from sunlit windowsills, radiators, or warm vehicles. If a refrigerator is available, use it.

● Pack nonperishable foods: unopened canned soup or stew to heat up in the microwave oven at work, dried raisins or apple slices, crackers and peanut butter, boxed juice or milk, beef jerky, to name a few. For canned foods, remember to tuck in a can opener! Fresh fruit doesn't require refrigeration.

● Discard any perishable, carried food that isn't eaten.

● Launder your lunch bag or wash your lunch box with soapy water after every use.

Ship It Safe

Food safety is an issue if you buy food on-line or mail order, call for home-delivered groceries, or ship perishable food as a gift.

● *To place an order,* ask how and when perishable foods will be sent. Ask that the food be packed with dry ice or cold packs, and order for overnight delivery. Record the order number for tracking—just in case!

● *If you're packing a perishable food gift,* freeze it solid or refrigerate until cold before packing it. Pack food in an insulated cooler or a heavy corrugated box with cold packs or dry ice. (Check the phone book for a place to buy dry ice; talk to your shipper or the post office about proper forms and warning labels for shipping packages with dry ice.) Mark the properly addressed package as "Perishable—Keep Refrigerated." Use overnight delivery. And let the recipient know it's coming so the package won't sit on the doorstep.

● *If you receive a food gift,* open it right away. Some mail-order foods, such as dry-cured ham and hard salami, don't require refrigeration. Other meats (including most hams), poultry, fish, and other per-ishable foods should arrive just as cold as they would be in your refrigerator. If it's cold enough, put the food in the freezer or the refrigerator. If it's not, toss it out, and contact the mail-order company for a replacement or a refund.

Quick Tips for Injury Prevention

Kitchen safety is more than preventing foodborne illness. Keep your kitchen safe from hazards that cause injury:

● Wipe up spills immediately. Someone who enters the kitchen may not notice water or grease on the floor before he or she slips.

● Avoid teetering on a chair or a bar stool to reach a high cabinet. Invest in a stable stool.

● Keep cabinets, drawers, and doors closed so you don't bump into them. Put safety catches on drawers so they won't fall out when they're opened too far.

● Keep pot holders handy—and use them. Be careful if they get wet; water conducts heat.

● Turn the handles on pots and pans inward and away from the edge of the stove where they may be knocked . . . or where children can grab them.

● Avoid overfilling pots and pans. Too much hot soup, stew, or pasta can quickly burn if it spills on you.

● Be careful with the hot-water tap, especially if you have small children.

● Allow enough time for the pressure to release if you use a pressure cooker.

● Avoid dropping water into hot oil. The splatters may burn you. Remember, water and oil don't mix!

● Douse grease fires with baking soda—not water! Or "put a lid on it" to control the flame.

● Avoid electrical fires. Keep electrical cords away from burners on your stove.

● Use a safety latch on cabinets with household chemicals, alcoholic beverages, matches, plastic bags, and sharp utensils (knives, toothpicks) so they're out of reach of children.

● Handle knives for safety. Store them carefully, perhaps in a knife holder. Avoid leaving them in the dishpan where you can't see them. Use sharp knives; dull knives are harder to use and promote injury. Always cut away from you, using a cutting board.

● Watch out for broken glass. Remove it immediately. If glass breaks in the sink, empty the water so you find all the pieces before you cut yourself.

● Watch your fingers near your garbage disposal! Teach children to use it safely.

The "Eco Kitchen"

Along with food safety, you and your family are wise to follow practices for kitchen ecology—conserving energy and water—and minimizing and properly disposing of waste.

Water in the "Eco Kitchen"

● Choose the proper size pots and pans for cooking. Utensils that are too big use more cooking water.

● Cook in a microwave oven or a pressure cooker to conserve water—and time.

● Cut down on evaporation of liquid—and nutrient loss—by covering pots with tight-fitting lids during cooking. To heat water for cooking or beverages, use a teakettle or a covered pot.

● Prepare vegetables in a small amount of water to save water and nutrients!

● Time foods that need to boil or simmer so you don't lose too much water through evaporation.

● Washing dishes? Turn the faucet on and off as you rinse, rather than allowing the water to run continually.

● Wait until your dishwasher is full before running a full cycle.

● Repair your faucet if it leaks.

Energy Savers

● Preheat your oven right before you use it.

● To make your freezer more energy-efficient, defrost it regularly.

● Turn off lights when you leave the kitchen.

● Avoid the habit of leaving the heat under the coffeepot all day. Turn it off when it's no longer needed.

● Buy energy-efficient appliances. Dishwashers that use less hot water save energy, too.

● Keep the oven and the refrigerator doors shut. Each time you peek inside, your appliance needs to use power to regain its set temperature. For the refrigerator, decide what you want before you open the door. When using the oven, use a timer. *Tip:* An open oven isn't efficient or safe for heating your kitchen!

● Keep appliances in good condition: tight gaskets around the oven and refrigerator doors. For efficiency, a gas stove should burn with a blue, not a yellowish, flame in the pilot light.

● Use equipment to speed cooking time, such as a microwave or convection oven or a pressure cooker. Consider new speed cooking microwave ovens that also use radiant or halogen heat.

● Trim the flame. Use a burner that matches the cooking pot.

● Arrange baking pans in the oven so air circulates. You'll get more even baking, and your food will cook faster and more efficiently.

● Use the self-cleaning feature on your oven judiciously—when it really needs cleaning. For a head start, start it while the oven is still hot from baking.

Resource Conservation

● Resist the urge to buy food you don't need. To avoid excessive food waste, buy only the amount of food your family will eat.

● Look for products in packaging that can be recycled, such as aluminum cans, steel cans, glass containers, recycled plastic, and paperboard cartons that are gray on the inside. On plastic containers, look for the recycling symbol with a number in the center. Lower numbers are recycled more easily.

● Recycle. Keep a recycling bin for food containers. Dispose of recyclables according to the regulations and services of your municipality.

● Reuse glass or plastic food packages. Clean them well with hot, soapy water if they're used for food storage.

● If you grow your own vegetables, make a compost heap. Add kitchen waste—for example, corn husks and melon rinds—to your compost heap.

● Keep your refrigerator in check. Use perishable foods before they spoil and need to be discarded.

CHAPTER 13

Kitchen Nutrition

Kitchen nutrition—cooking for health—isn't new. About 150 years ago, *The Book of Household Management* described the kitchen as "the great laboratory of the household . . . much of the 'weal and woe' as far as regards bodily health, depends on the nature of the preparations concocted within its walls."

Now, in this new century, we still identify the kitchen as the place where foods are transformed into nourishment for the body. Yet foods, food preparation methods, and recipes have changed dramatically, and so have lifestyles.

"Resetting" Your Table . . . for Taste and Health

What are your favorite foods? And why do you like them so much? Taste is likely a major reason!

Taste actually is a bigger nutrition issue than many of us realize. According to consumer research, taste tops nutrition as the number one reason why consumers buy one food over another. There's a lot wrapped up in why you prefer certain foods, including a multitude of social, psychological (emotional), and physical reasons. In any case, the foods you enjoy are likely the ones you eat most. The more often you eat them, the more important their nutritional impact on your overall health.

For most Americans, enjoyment is an important reason for eating; it may even be *the* reason. If you're also nutrition-savvy, it's okay to make food appeal a major kitchen priority. When it comes to nutrition, think about taste . . . and when it comes to taste, think about nutrition!

"Flavor" the Difference

Relax for a moment, and imagine . . . the aroma of homemade, whole-wheat bread baking in your oven . . . the sweet, juicy taste of a ripe peach or strawberry—just picked . . . the cool sensation of an ice-cold glass of milk . . . the crispy crunch of a raw carrot; the smooth, creamy texture of chocolate ice cream; or the fiery feeling of a hot chile pepper!

There's no question: foods that appeal to your senses are probably those you enjoy most! Just what is flavor? And how does it contribute to nutrition?

Flavor is actually several sensations closely linked together: taste plus smell, as well as touch (temperature and mouth feel). With one sensation diminished, your flavor experience is entirely different. As an experiment, hold your nose so you can't smell, then bite an onion. It may taste somewhat sweet, more like an apple. Or think about the taste of food when your nose is stuffed up—not much flavor and not much pleasure either. Eighty percent of food's flavor is really its aroma.

As an average adult, you have about ten thousand taste buds, which respond to different tastes: sweet, sour, salty, bitter, and also umami (the brothy, meaty, and savory flavor of glutamate). You can sense *all* these tastes on *every* part of your tongue. However, some parts of the tongue may be especially sensitive to certain tastes—for example, bitter will taste stronger at the back of the tongue. Even the lining of your mouth, the back of your throat, your tonsils (if you still have them), and your epiglottis (a flap of tissue that covers your larynx, preventing food and liquids from entering the airway) have some taste buds, especially in childhood.

Aromas that waft through the room get picked up by smell receptors high up in your nasal passages. Temperature, mouth feel, even the "irritation" from a jalapeño pepper or the "numbing" effect from a persimmon also affect your perceptions of food and its flavor—and what you may describe as its "taste."

Not surprisingly, we're born with an ability to perceive, and a preference for, sweet tastes. To some degree, we can perceive all tastes at birth—sweet, sour, bitter, salty, and umami. Flavor preferences are learned—starting from the early years.

Are You a Supertaster?

Why do you like the foods you like? The reasons are partly genes and age. Even in the same family, people experience tastes differently. The intensity of taste depends partly on how many fungiform papillae (tiny, smooth red bumps) a person has on his or her tongue.

Supertasters, who have a lot of papillae, tend to strongly like or dislike certain foods. They pick up bitter flavors, perhaps in pungent vegetables, tea, coffee, and grapefruit juice, more intensely, too. Those with few papillae tend to be indifferent to one flavor over another, and those in the middle are likely to enjoy all kinds of food if prepared well.

Children have more papillae than adults, perhaps one of many reasons why a child may be a picky eater. Taste sensitivity seems to decline with age, which is explained by the decrease in the number of papillae.

Have you ever burned your tongue on steamy hot soup, or the roof of your mouth on cheese topping a hot pizza? Hot foods may burn your mouth and damage papillae. Fortunately, your body repairs its papillae fairly quickly.

Are you a supertaster? Find out. First punch a hole (with a hole punch) in a small piece of wax paper. Put the hole on the tip of your tongue; wipe it with blue food coloring. With a mirror, magnifying glass, and flashlight, count the papillae. Nontasters only have five or six, but supertasters have dozens of them! (More women are supertasters than men are.)

Have you ever wondered why the same food may be too spicy for some but not for others? People may sense the same foods very differently. Among the factors that make a difference: saliva (affected by diet, heredity, and other factors), the number of taste buds, medications, some illnesses, and smoking. The senses of taste and smell diminish with age. That's why older people may say that foods just don't taste the way they remember. *For more about flavor in foods for older adults, see "Less Sense-Able" in chapter 18.*

Today, taste and smell are getting more attention in the scientific world—in part because flavor is a priority for food choices. Since people eat for taste, there's good reason to think of nutrition and taste together. That's why research is being done—for example, to make food more flavorful for older adults; to find ways to magnify salty tastes while lowering levels of sodium in food; and to use biotechnology to develop more flavorful fruits and vegetables.

To get the most flavor from foods:

- Eat foods when they're at their peak of freshness.
- Include a variety of foods with different flavors at a single meal to stimulate taste buds.
- Prepare food to retain and enhance its flavor.
- Take time to savor the flavor of food. Enjoy its aroma. Chew it well to release taste and aroma.
- Serve food at the temperature that most enhances its flavor.

Variety: A Meal with Appeal

Like a well-decorated room or a beautifully landscaped garden, an appealing meal follows basic principles of design. Different foods add a variety of color, flavor, texture, shape, and temperature to meals or snacks. At the same time, a variety of foods supplies different nutrients to your eating style.

Vary the color. Contrast the visual differences: meat loaf, mashed potatoes with gravy, corn, and applesauce . . . compared with meat loaf, baked sweet potato with chopped chives, asparagus, and spinach salad with orange slices. Which one has more interest? The meal with an artist's palette of color!

Vary the flavor. Within a meal, offer foods with different flavors: sour, sweet, bitter, and salty. All of these flavors come naturally in food, including sweet and salty tastes. Instead of serving orange-glazed chicken with candied sweet potatoes and fruit compote, complement chicken with wild rice pilaf and a fresh garden salad for more flavor, variety, and interest.

Vary the texture. Crunchy foods offer a nice contrast when served with soft foods—for example, chopped nuts in brown rice, or raw veggies with herbed cottage cheese dip. Think about the two meat loaf dinners described earlier. Variety of texture adds appeal as much as variety of color!

Vary the shape. Round meatballs, round peas, round new potatoes, and round grapes may look somewhat boring if they're all plated together. Perhaps add variety to the plate with finger carrots instead of peas, pasta spirals instead of potatoes, or sliced apple wedges instead of grapes.

Vary the temperature. Meals don't require foods with different temperatures. For example, a cold summer supper or a picnic from the cooler can be refreshing. However, a warm whole-wheat roll offers a nice contrast to a cool chef's salad. And frozen yogurt makes a nice ending to a hot dinner.

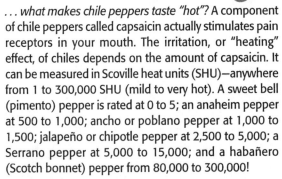

... *what makes chile peppers taste "hot"?* A component of chile peppers called capsaicin actually stimulates pain receptors in your mouth. The irritation, or "heating" effect, of chiles depends on the amount of capsaicin. It can be measured in Scoville heat units (SHU)—anywhere from 1 to 300,000 SHU (mild to very hot). A sweet bell (pimento) pepper is rated at 0 to 5; an anaheim pepper at 500 to 1,000; ancho or poblano pepper at 1,000 to 1,500; jalapeño or chipotle pepper at 2,500 to 5,000; a Serrano pepper at 5,000 to 15,000; and a habañero (Scotch bonnet) pepper from 80,000 to 300,000!

... *how to reduce the "fire" caused by eating hot chile peppers?* Try dairy foods! Caesin, the main protein in milk, washes away the substance in hot chiles that makes your mouth and throat "burn." Hot chile peppers do "fire up" the flavors of Thai dishes, Mexican salsas, and Cajun foods, among others. To tone down the heat, remove the seeds and inner membranes of hot chiles. To avoid a burning sensation on sensitive skin as you handle hot chiles, use rubber gloves. Never touch or rub your eyes—or any other sensitive areas—when you're handling them.

Paint Your Plate with Color!

Toss blueberries in your yogurt. Garnish your salad with sliced beets. Tuck spinach leaves in your sandwich. Color offers much more than eye appeal to a wonderful meal! A rainbow of fruits and vegetables creates a palette of nutrients and phytonutrients, or plant chemicals, on your plate, each with a different bundle of potential benefits: from oxidizing free radicals that may damage healthy cells, to having anti-inflammatory qualities, to lowering LDL cholesterol. *See "Phytonutrients—a 'Crop' for Good Health" in chapter 4.*

Research has just begun to uncover the benefits of the pigment-related phytonutrients—and the colorful fruits and vegetables that supply them.

● *Orange and deep yellow:* sweet potatoes, carrots, apricots, winter squash, cantaloupes, and mangoes. These fruits and vegetables get their color from beta carotene, a carotenoid that may offer protection from heart disease, some cancers, and macular degeneration, among other potential benefits. The deeper the color, the more carotenoids they contain. Beta carotene converts to vitamin A in your body, offering its benefits as an antioxidant.

● *Red:* tomatoes, pink grapefruit, and watermelons. Lycopene, another powerful carotenoid, may offer protection from some cancers, including prostate cancer. When cooked or canned, lycopene in tomatoes is more available.

● *Dark green:* spinach, collard or turnip greens, romaine lettuce, and other dark green leafy vegetables. They supply lutein and zeaxanthin (two carotenoids that may lower the risk of macular degeneration) as well as vitamin C, folate, vitamin K, and other nutrients.

● *Purple, dark red, and blue:* eggplant, blueberries, raspberries, other berries, beets, red and purple grapes, cherries, beets, and red-skinned potatoes. Anthocyanin, one of many flavonoids, is the pigment that provides their color. Flavonoids may promote heart health by lowering LDL blood cholesterol, among others.

● *What else?* Aside from their pigments, citrus fruits (oranges, grapefruits, and tangerines), vegetables in the allium family (leeks, garlic, and onions) and cruciferous vegetables (cabbage, Brussels sprouts, broccoli, and cauliflower) also add visual appeal as well as nutrients, fiber, and phytonutrient benefits.

Food "Prep": The Nutrition-Flavor Connection

Nutrition and flavor go hand in hand. You don't need to sacrifice one for the other. Proper food storage and handling enhance the natural flavors of food and keep nutrient loss to a minimum.

● Start with high-quality ingredients. These don't need to be the most expensive foods in the store. But they do need to be handled properly all along the food chain—right to your kitchen.

● Store foods properly until they're prepared. Cooking can't improve poor-quality food, but it can enhance the flavors of already high-quality foods. *Chapter 12, "The Safe Kitchen," offers many tips for keeping food fresh and safe in your kitchen.*

For a Taste Lift

● Grill or roast your veggies in a very hot oven or grill. They take on a sweet, smoky flavor. Brush or spray them lightly with oil so they don't dry out. Sprinkle with herbs, too.

● Caramelize sliced onions to bring out their natural sugar flavor. Just cook them slowly over low heat in a small amount of oil. Use them to make a rich, dark sauce for meat or poultry.

● Spark up sauces, soups, and salads with a splash of flavored, balsamic, or rice vinegar. *See "Herbed Vinegars" in this chapter for ways to make your own herb and fruit vinegars.* Balsamic vinegar gets its sweet, pungent flavor when grape juice is aged in special wooden barrels. Rice vinegar, often used in Asian dishes, comes from fermented rice.

● Add a tangy taste with citrus juice or grated citrus peel: lemon, lime, or orange.

● Pep it up with peppers! Use red, green, and yellow peppers of all varieties—sweet, hot, and dried. Or add a dash of hot pepper sauce.

● Give a flavor burst with good-quality condiments such as horseradish, flavored mustard, chutney, and salsas of all kinds!

● Concentrate the flavors of meat, poultry, and fish stocks. Reduce the juices by heating them—don't boil! Then use them as a glaze. It's a flavorful substitute for gravy.

More Taste Lifters

● For grains that absorb fluid (rice, buckwheat, and barley), cook them in defatted, perhaps reduced-sodium, chicken or beef broth. Risotto, an Italian rice specialty, typically is prepared by cooking arborio or white short-grain rice in broth, along with herbs and other ingredients.

● Blend herbs, spices, sun-dried tomatoes, and shredded cheese into bread dough before baking it.

● Experiment with herbs and spices. Add flavor with basil, chives, cilantro, rosemary, savory, garlic, ginger, caraway, and cumin.

● Sharpen up the flavor with cheese. Even a little Parmesan, sharp Cheddar, Romano, feta, Asiago, or blue cheese—sprinkled on vegetables, rice, or pasta—goes a long way in adding a distinctive flavor.

● Add intense flavors with dried ingredients: sun-dried tomatoes, dried mushrooms, dried cranberries, dried apricots, dried plums (prunes), and red pepper flakes. Plump up sun-dried tomatoes and dried mushrooms in broth or cooking wine, and dried cranberries or dried plums (prunes) in apple juice.

● Cook to retain nutrients, flavor, color, texture, and overall taste appeal. *For quick flavor enhancers, see "For a Taste Lift" and "More Taste Lifters" on this page.*

High temperatures and long cooking times can destroy heat-sensitive nutrients such as B vitamins, vitamin C, and folate. Some minerals and water-soluble vitamins dissolve in cooking water; they're lost when cooking water is discarded. And light destroys riboflavin (vitamin B_2) and vitamin A. Proper cooking techniques keep nutrient loss to a minimum and food quality at its peak. *For ways to minimize vitamin loss, see "Simple Ways to Keep Vitamins in Food" later in this chapter.*

Beyond Parsley . . . Quick, Easy Garnishes

Garnishes do more than add eye appeal to food; they also offer flavor, color, and texture contrasts and, if eaten, some nutritional value. Garnish food with edibles that complement the ingredients in the food.

For example, a sprig of basil goes with many Italian dishes; a slice of lemon or lime complements many seafood dishes. Arrange the garnish artistically around, under, or on top of the food.

Parsley, which may be the most common garnish, dresses up a plate and serves as a natural breath freshener. While having less flavor than flat-leafed varieties, curly parsley adds texture to the plate, too, and both varieties have some beta carotene (which forms vitamin A) and vitamin C! To garnish, go beyond parsley and "paint your plate" with other foods, too:

On salads . . . capers; fennel slices; pomegranate seeds; red onion slices; red, green, and yellow pepper strips; toasted, chopped walnuts or pecans; chopped apple (tossed with lemon juice to prevent browning); watercress; mandarin orange sections; blueberries or raspberries; grated cheese; snow peas; shredded jicama; or marigold petals. *For edible flowers as garnishes see "Please Don't Eat the Daffodils" in this chapter.*

On soups . . . an avocado slice dipped in lemon; shredded carrot; minced chives; sprigs of fresh herbs; minced fresh herbs; snow peas; a dollop of plain yogurt; orange peel strips; a thin slice of lemon; croutons; pesto sauce; edible flowers; shredded green, yellow, and red peppers; grated cheese; or plain, air-popped popcorn.

Give It a Little Salsa

Salsa is simply the Spanish word for "sauce." With today's cuisine, salsa has become a lot more sexy! By combining a variety of chopped vegetables, fruits, herbs, and even hot sauce, there's a salsa for every flavor mood.

Tomato salsa: Combine chopped plum tomatoes, onions, canned green chiles, cilantro, and lime juice. Add red pepper flakes or hot sauce for more zip. Chill. *Tip:* Plum tomatoes, especially when they're in season, often have more flavor than salad tomatoes.

Pineapple salsa: Combine chopped, fresh pineapple with chopped cilantro, fresh lime juice, and a touch of sugar and minced garlic. Chill.

Black bean salsa: Combine canned, drained black beans with chopped tomato, chopped onion, chopped cilantro, and a little jalapeño and red wine vinegar. Chill.

On cooked vegetables . . . toasted, sliced almonds; toasted pine nuts; grated Parmesan cheese; stir-fried onion slices; stir-fried mushroom slices; chopped lean ham; chopped olives or pimiento; or chopped fresh herbs.

In beverages . . . a mint sprig; scented geranium leaves; orange, lime, or lemon slices; fresh, whole berries; sliced starfruit (carambola), apple, or kiwi; or a cinnamon stick.

With meat, poultry, or fish . . . tomato slices; a small bunch of grapes; lemon and lime wedges; crab apple slices; a grilled peach or pear half; baby corn; baby beets, squash, and carrots; or chutney or salsa in endive, a lettuce cup, or a lemon slice.

Recipes: Judge for Yourself!

Each year, seemingly hundreds of new cookbooks appear on bookstore shelves. Many focus on healthful eating. Besides cookbooks, you find recipes of all kinds in magazines and newspapers, on supermarket racks, package labels, and computer software, and at on-line Web sites. To find a cookbook or a food magazine that matches your needs, read its introduction for starters. How can you sort through their recipes and endless combinations of ingredients?

Look at the main ingredients and the portions. You'll get an idea of how just one recipe portion fits within your personal Pyramid for the day and whether it's high in fat, sugar, or salt.

Check the nutrient analysis of the recipe—if it's provided. Unlike food labels, nutrition information and serving sizes for recipes aren't standardized. Recipes may list some, but not all, the nutrients you find on a label. Usually the nutrient analysis in a recipe is provided for a single portion, but not always. A portion, perhaps of lasagna, in one recipe might be bigger or smaller than a serving of the same food in another recipe. And neither one might equal one labelsize serving of a frozen version. Computerized cookbooks offer the advantage of technology. With some, you can plan meals for the whole day—with recipes from the cookbook—then total up the calories and nutrients. Changing the menu for your nutrient and calorie needs is as easy as a few computer keystrokes!

Please Don't Eat the Daffodils

Edible flowers add a distinctive flavor (*sweet* lilac, *spicy* nasturtium, *minty* bee balm) and a unique splash of color to all kinds of foods. But you can't eat just any flower!

Some are poisonous; even edible flowers may be contaminated by chemicals if they weren't grown for eating. Don't eat flowers you buy from a florist or a greenhouse—or that you pick along the road. Don't use them as a garnish, either. There's a long list of flowers that aren't edible: buttercup, delphinium, lily of the valley, foxglove, goldenseal, periwinkle, oleander, sweet pea—and daffodils, to name just a few!

For edible flowers, either grow your own or buy them in the produce section of your supermarket. They should be labeled as "edible flowers." Only eat flowers if you're *absolutely* sure of their safety! *Tip:* If you have hay fever, allergies, or asthma, be cautious about eating flowers.

Try growing these edible flowers in the kitchen garden outside your back door: bee balm, calendula (pot marigold), borage, chrysanthemum, day lilies, dianthus, marigolds, nasturtiums (enjoy leaves and blossoms), pansies, roses, scented geraniums, squash blossoms, sunflowers, tulips, and violets. Enjoy the blossoms from any herb plant, too; try basil, chive, lavender, oregano, sage, savory, and thyme blossoms.

Fertilize your flowers as you would a vegetable garden. Then, when harvesting, wash them well, and gently pat them dry.

To keep edible flowers for a few days, refrigerate them. Just keep the stems in water, or put short-stemmed blossoms in a plastic bag or between damp paper towels. For most flowers, remove the stamens, pistils, and sepals, and enjoy the petals. *Bon appétit!*

Choose recipes to complement the whole meal—in fact, meals and snacks for the whole day! Consider variety of color, flavor, texture, taste—and nutrition. Nutrients and calories in any one recipe aren't the whole picture. If the recipe you choose has more fat or sodium, then plan your menu with other foods that have less.

Most important, choose recipes that appeal to you. No matter how nutritious a recipe sounds, the end result should be something you enjoy—or a food you're willing to experience, perhaps for the first time.

Recipe Makeovers

Ready to limit calories, fat, or sodium . . . or boost calcium, fiber, or complex carbohydrates? You can transform almost any recipe, even Mom's specialties. A few subtle modifications may improve their nutrition content without much flavor change. Or experiment more dramatically by adding more fruits, vegetables, or whole grains to your recipes!

Chefs and test-kitchen food experts change recipes all the time. There's nothing sacred about most recipes (except perhaps Mom's). Recipes get altered when new ingredients come on the market, when cooking equipment changes, when consumers want recipe shortcuts, when ingredients are in or out of season or become more or less costly, and when consumers shift their food preferences. Nutrition and food safety are reasons for recipe changes, too.

In your own "test kitchen," you can modify recipes in several ways: change the ingredients, modify the way the recipes are prepared, cut portion sizes, or do all three. Even one or two small recipe changes can net a significant difference in the nutrition content. This chapter has plenty of ideas to get you started!

Whatever your approach to recipe makeovers, keep flavor, texture, and appeal as priorities. Remember that moderation in your overall food choices counts, not what's in one dish. A single dish that's high in fat, sugar, or salt may not need a makeover—*if* you don't eat it often; *if* the rest of your day's choices have less fat, sugar, or salt; or *if* you eat just a small amount.

1. *Change the ingredients.* You might use less of one or more ingredients . . . or substitute one ingredient for another . . . or take an ingredient out entirely . . . or add something new.

● *Start by reviewing the recipe and the ingredient list.* Does it really need to be adjusted? Decide what ingredients might be changed to achieve your goals, perhaps to cut back on fat, boost calcium, use leftovers, add flavor, take advantage of a supermarket sale, or match a family food preference.

● *Consider the ingredients' functions before you switch.* To get an appealing result, make suitable substitutions. For example, in meat, poultry, fish, and vegetable dishes, salt enhances taste; herbs make flavorful substitutes. Regular ground beef is a key ingredient in hot chili, but lean ground turkey

An Easy Makeover: Tuna-Noodle Bake

Compare these two recipes for Tuna-Noodle Bake. How has the traditional recipe been changed to make it lower in fat, cholesterol, and sodium, yet higher in vitamins A and C and fiber?

ORIGINAL RECIPE

8 oz. egg noodles
2 tbsp. butter
2 cans (7 oz. each) tuna, packed in oil, drained

1 cup sour cream

¾ cup whole milk
1 can (3 oz.) sliced mushrooms

1 tsp. onion salt
½ tsp. salt
¼ tsp. pepper
¼ cup plain, unseasoned bread crumbs
⅓ cup grated Parmesan cheese
2 tbsp. butter, melted

Preheat oven to 350° F. Cook noodles in salted water as directed on package. When cooked, drain and rinse. Return noodles to pot; add butter or margarine. Stir in tuna, sour cream, milk, mushrooms, onion salt, salt, and pepper. Pour into a greased 2-quart casserole. Combine bread crumbs, Parmesan cheese, and melted butter. Sprinkle over casserole. Bake uncovered for thirty-five minutes. Makes six servings.

Nutrition information per serving:
480 Calories (235 Calories from Fat)

	% Daily Value
Total fat: 26 g	39%
Saturated fat: 13 g	64%
Cholesterol: 102 mg	34%
Sodium: 1,100 mg	46%
Total carbohydrate: 34 g	11%
Dietary fiber: 0 g	1%
Sugars: 3 g	
Protein: 28 g	
Vitamin A	21%
Vitamin C	1%
Calcium	19%
Iron	15%

MAKEOVER RECIPE

8 oz. whole-wheat noodles

2 cans (7 oz. each) tuna,* packed in spring water, drained
½ can (10½-oz.) cream of mushroom soup
½ cup pureed low-fat (1%) cottage cheese
¾ cup fat-free milk
½ cup chopped celery
½ cup shredded carrot
¼ cup chopped green pepper
1 tsp. onion flakes
¼ tsp. each paprika and tarragon
¼ tsp. pepper

⅓ cup grated Parmesan cheese

Preheat oven to 350° F. Cook noodles in unsalted water as directed on package. When cooked, drain. Return noodles to pot; add tuna, soup, cottage cheese, milk, celery, carrot, green pepper, onion flakes, paprika, tarragon, and pepper. Pour into a nonstick 2-quart casserole. Sprinkle with Parmesan cheese. Bake uncovered for thirty-five minutes. Makes six servings.

Nutrition information per serving:
295 Calories (45 Calories from Fat)

	% Daily Value
Total fat: 5 g	8%
Saturated fat: 2 g	10%
Cholesterol: 25 mg	8%
Sodium: 640 mg	27%
Total carbohydrate: 35 g	12%
Dietary fiber: 2 g	8%
Sugars: 3 g	
Protein: 29 g	
Vitamin A	32%
Vitamin C	19%
Calcium*	17%
Iron	16%

*Use canned salmon in place of canned tuna to increase calcium to 32% Daily Value.

Daily Values are used with food labeling. To help you compare these two recipes, Daily Values are used with this nutritional analysis. *To learn about Daily Values on the Nutrition Facts of food labels, see chapter 11.*

works just as well. And low-fat yogurt can take the place of sour cream in dips, potato toppers, and some creamy sauce.

Here's where you can learn more about the functions of:

1. *Fat: "Why Foods Contain Fat," in chapter 3*
2. *Sugar: "Sugar: More than Sweeteners," in chapter 5*
3. *Salt: "Salt and Sodium: More than Flavor," in chapter 7*

● *Pick ingredients you might reduce or eliminate.* In many baked foods, you may cut back on sugar by a third and still enjoy good results. With sautéed foods or with foods cooked in a small amount of oil, try using less cooking oil. Optional ingredients are easy to take out; removing others may alter the appearance or the flavor. Season with extra herbs or spices if you cut back on salt.

● *To boost nutrients, decide what ingredients to add.* For example, fortifying casseroles with wheat germ or dry milk powder may go unnoticed. Adding shredded carrots to mashed potatoes, or dried cranberries to muesli, gives extra flavor and color, along with more nutrients and phytonutrients.

● *As easy substitutions, buy modified ingredients.* For example, use cholesterol-free egg products, reduced-fat cheese, or sodium-reduced chicken broth in some recipes. Follow package directions if the product needs to be prepared differently.

● *Experiment a little at a time, perhaps with just one ingredient.* That's especially important when the ingredient has functional purposes, such as eggs or sugar in baked foods. When the recipe makeover works, jot it down—right in the cookbook or in your recipe file.

2. *Modify the way food is prepared.* Simple changes in cooking techniques may require little or no extra investment in your time—just know-how. For example, skim fat that collects on stews, scrub rather than peel fiber-rich potato skins, skip salt in cooking water, or oven-bake frozen French fries rather than fry them.

3. *Reduce portion sizes.* If a recipe is high in fats or sugars, try serving less. For example, instead of ¼ cup of cheese sauce on a baked potato, use just two

Culinary Lingo

Braise: to simmer over low heat in liquid—water, broth, or even fruit juice—in a covered pot for a lengthy time

Broil: to cook with direct heat, usually under a heating element in the oven

Grill: to cook with direct heat directly over hot coals or another heat source

Panbroil: to cook uncovered in a preheated, nonstick skillet without added fat or water

Poach: to cook gently in liquid, just below boiling

Roast: to cook uncovered with dry heat in the oven

Sauté: to cook quickly in a small amount of fat, stirring so the food browns evenly

Simmer: to cook slowly in liquid, just below the boiling point

Steam: to cook with steam heat over (not in) boiling water, or wrapped in foil or leaves (such as lettuce or banana leaves) packets, over boiling water or on a grill

Stew: to cook in liquid, such as water, juice, wine, broth, or stock, in a tightly covered pot over low heat

Stir-fry: to cook small pieces of meat, poultry, fish, seafood, and/or vegetables in a very small amount of oil, perhaps with added broth, over very high heat, stirring as you cook

tablespoons—and add some steamed, chopped vegetables and/or herbs for flavor.

Simply Nutritious, Simply Delicious

Modifying recipes without compromising taste doesn't require extra time—just quick, easy kitchen know-how. Tips here offer many ways to prepare foods with less fat (including saturated fat), cholesterol, sugars, and sodium. You'll also find ways to add fruits, vegetables, fiber, and calcium to your food preparation—and keep vitamins in. Now cook for the health (and taste) of it!

Fruits and Vegetables: Food Prep for "Five a Day"

As a child, you probably enjoyed fruits and vegetables for their vibrant colors, crunch, and wonderful flavors. You probably also learned that fruits and vegetables were good for you. Today, science has a better understanding of the reasons why they should be part of a varied, balanced, and moderate diet. Although their nutrient content varies, fruits and vegetables:

● Supply many essential nutrients: (which becomes vitamin A inside yo min C, folate, vitamin B_6, potassium, nesium, and selenium, as well as naturally occurring sugars, complex carbohydrates, and fiber.

Stocking the Kitchen . . . with Easy Nutrition

Keep a variety of foods on hand—and make nutritious meals and snacks quick and easy to prepare. Buy fresh ingredients as you need them! Many of these foods are sold with reduced amounts of fat or sodium—or they're fat- or sodium-free. Decide which form to buy to fit your overall goals for your meal and snack choices.

To Store in Your Kitchen Cabinet . . .
Whole-grain breakfast cereal
Rice (white and brown)
Brown and wild rice pilaf mix
Pasta (spaghetti, macaroni, others)
Couscous
Bulgur or barley
Gingersnaps or vanilla wafers
Whole-wheat or mixed grain bread and rolls
Beans (dry and canned)
Peanut butter
Tuna or salmon (canned, packed in spring water)
Refried beans (canned, fat-free, reduced-fat, vegetarian)
Fruit (canned in own juice or light syrup)
Vegetables (canned)
Fruit (dried)
Vegetable soup (canned and dry mix)
Nonfat dry milk powder
Evaporated fat-free (skim) milk
Salsa or picante sauce
Pasta sauce
Chicken or beef broth (canned, reduced sodium and fat)
Fruit spread
Mustard
Ketchup
Vinegar
Vegetable oil (olive and others)
Salad dressing (perhaps reduced fat)
Vegetable oil cooking spray
Herbs and spices
Flour (whole-wheat, bleached white)
Sugar (granulated, powder)

Brown sugar
Cornstarch
Baking powder
Baking soda

To Keep in a Cool, Dry Place . . .
Baking potatoes
Onions

To Store in Your Refrigerator . . .
Apples
Oranges
Tortillas
Milk (fat-free, low-fat, perhaps whole milk)
Yogurt
Parmesan cheese
Cheese (regular, perhaps reduced-fat cheese)
Sliced smoked turkey breast or chicken, deli meat
Eggs (or in your freezer, egg substitute)
Bottled lemon juice
Bottled garlic (minced)

To Keep in Your Freezer . . .
Fruit juice concentrate (or fresh juice in your refrigerator, or juice boxes on the shelf)
Frozen vegetables
Frozen green pepper (chopped)
Frozen onion (chopped)
Frozen waffles or whole-wheat bagels
Frozen fish fillets
Lean ground beef
Pork loin chops
Chicken breast (perhaps skinless)
Frozen yogurt or fruit sorbet

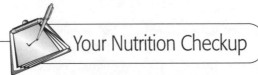

Your Nutrition Checkup

Kitchen Nutrition IQ

Do you cook with nutrition, as well as flavor, in mind? Test your kitchen nutrition IQ to see if what you know shows up in how you cook!

Do You . . .	Always	Usually	Sometimes	Never
Trim visible fat from meat and poultry?	_____	_____	_____	_____
Keep edible peels on fruits and vegetables—just wash, not peel them?	_____	_____	_____	_____
Remove the skin from poultry before eating it?	_____	_____	_____	_____
Use garnishes to make food look more appealing?	_____	_____	_____	_____
Cook vegetables until they're just tender-crisp?	_____	_____	_____	_____
Skip the salt in cooking water for pasta, rice, other grains, and vegetables?	_____	_____	_____	_____
Cook with whole grains?	_____	_____	_____	_____
Try to include foods with different colors and tastes in a meal?	_____	_____	_____	_____
Add canned or cooked legumes to salads, soups, or other foods?	_____	_____	_____	_____
Sprinkle cheese on salads, soups, and vegetables for more calcium?	_____	_____	_____	_____
Cook vegetables with the lid on the pot—in just a small amount of liquid, or steam or microwave them?	_____	_____	_____	_____
Sweeten foods with fruit, fruit juice, or fruit purees?	_____	_____	_____	_____
Use ingredients with less fat, such as low-fat yogurt, lean ground meat, and defatted broth?	_____	_____	_____	_____
Boost calcium in soups, cooked cereals, and casseroles with dry milk powder?	_____	_____	_____	_____
Drain fat off meat after it's cooked?	_____	_____	_____	_____
Use herbs, spices, or lemon juice, rather than salt, to flavor food?	_____	_____	_____	_____
Prepare foods with vegetables that have more calcium, such as broccoli and greens (such as kale or collards)?	_____	_____	_____	_____
Use lower-fat cooking methods: broil, grill, roast, stir-fry, steam, microwave, or braise?	_____	_____	_____	_____
Taste before adding salt to foods?	_____	_____	_____	_____
Use cooking water from vegetables for soups, stews, or sauces?	_____	_____	_____	_____
Subtotal	_____	_____	_____	_____

Now score yourself:

"Always": 3 points

"Usually": 2 points

"Sometimes": 1 points

"Never": 0 point

Your total score _____

With 50 to 60 points, you're "kitchen nutrition-savvy."

With 40 to 49 points, improving your food preparation skills would make a nutrition difference! Read on.

With 21 to 39 points, you've got the hang of it. Now turn those "sometimes" answers to "usually" and "always." Read the rest of the chapter for "food prep" tips.

With 20 points or less, read the chapter. There's lots to learn!

● Are naturally low in fat, especially saturated fat, and sodium. They're also cholesterol-free.

● Provide an array of phytonutrients, or plant chemicals.

As a daily guideline, the Food Guide Pyramid advises three to five servings of vegetables and two to four servings of fruit a day. That adds up to at least "five a day" servings for health! Here's how you might use them in food preparation:

● *Try some "grate" ways.* Add grated, shredded, or chopped vegetables such as zucchini, spinach, and carrots to lasagna, meat loaf, mashed potatoes, and mixed meat, poultry, pasta, rice, and other grain dishes.

● *Be saucy with fruit.* Puree berries, apples, peaches, or pears for a thick, sweet sauce on grilled or broiled seafood or poultry, or on pancakes, French toast, or waffles.

● *Get creative with pizza.* Order or make it "deluxe" with vegetable toppings: broccoli florets, carrot shreds, thinly sliced zucchini, chopped spinach, red and green bell pepper strips, chopped tomatoes, or other firm veggies!

● *Bake with fruits and vegetables.* Use pureed fruit such as applesauce, dried plums (prunes), bananas, or peaches in place of about half the fat in recipes for homemade breads, muffins, pancakes, cookies, and other baked goods. For flavor, texture, and nutrients, blend in shredded zucchini, carrots, or dried fruits.

● *"Sandwich" in fruit and vegetables.* Add pizzazz to sandwiches by layering on sliced pineapple, apple, raisins, peppers, cucumbers, sprouts, or tomatoes.

● *Combine it with veggies.* Make a quick stir-fry or combine pasta or rice with just about any vegetables, or add them to soup—great ways to use fresh vegetables before they spoil. *Hint:* Add canned, frozen, or cooked legumes.

● *Experiment.* Substitute a new-to-you fruit or vegetable in a favorite recipe. Try broccoli rabe (broccoli variety with smaller heads, also called rapini) in stir-fries or yautia (a starchy vegetable) in stew. Or try a new recipe with fruit or vegetables.

● *Take a fruit to lunch!* Make a habit of tucking an apple, a tangerine, two plums or kiwis, grapes, cherries, dried fruits, or other fruit into your briefcase, tote bag, or lunch bag. Fruit is a great traveler for snacks, too.

● *Stuff an omelette with veggies.* For a hearty meal, fill it with crisp, tasty vegetables like broccoli, squash, carrots, peppers, tomatoes, or onions.

● *Toss up a vegetable salad.* Add extra cut-up vegetables, legumes, and fruits (such as berries, kiwis, or mandarin oranges) to salads. Even if you prefer iceberg lettuce, which delivers less nutrients than other greens, pair it with other veggies in your garden salad for a nutritional boost!

● *Count your beans.* If you consume enough protein-rich foods from the Meat and Beans Group of the Food Guide Pyramid, legumes can count as a serving from the Vegetable Group. Try adding cooked, canned, or frozen beans, peas, or lentils to salads, casseroles, and pasta dishes. Or puree cooked beans as a low-fat base for spreads, sauces, and soups.

● *Make dips and spreads with vegetables and fruit.* Spicy salsas can be made with tomato, bell peppers, onions, and cilantro. For a tangy twist, also look for salsas with pineapples, mangoes, papayas, or peaches. Try hummus, made with mashed chickpeas; or caponata, made with eggplant and tomato; or baba ghanouj, made with eggplant.

● *Toss in raisins and other dried fruits:* dried cranberries, apples, dried plums (prunes), bananas, papayas, mangoes, apricots, pears, or pineapples. They're great in stuffing, rice dishes, tossed salads, main dish salads, homemade breads, and casseroles; even desserts!

● *Focus on veggies.* Enjoy 3-ounce portions of cooked meat, poultry, and fish; fill the rest of the plate with vegetables, fruits, and grain products. A vegetable-meat kebob is one way to do it. It's great for grilling!

● *Feature vegetables with grains in casseroles.* Let meat, poultry, or fish enhance the dish but not take center stage.

● *Stock up.* Fill your fridge with raw vegetables and fruits—"nature's fast food"—cleaned, fresh, and ready to eat. Try baby carrots! And keep canned and frozen vegetables and fruit on hand for convenience's sake.

For more ideas, see "Garden of Eatin': Uncommon Vegetables" and "Fresh Ideas: Less Common Fruit" in chapter 9, and "Pyramid Pointers" in chapter 10.

Simple Ways to Keep Vitamins in Food

- Clean thick-skinned vegetables and fruits well with a soft brush and water. Avoid soaking them as you wash. Some vitamins dissolve in water.

- Leave edible skins on vegetables and fruits—for example, on carrots, potatoes, or pears. And trim away as little as possible. Most vitamins and minerals are found in the outer leaves, skin, and area just below the skin—not in the center. Peels also are natural barriers that help protect nutrient loss.

- Cook vegetables or fruits in a small amount of water—or better yet, steam them in a vegetable steamer or a microwave oven. Steaming retains most of the nutrients because vegetables usually don't come in contact with cooking liquids.

- Cut vegetables that need to be cooked longer, but in larger pieces. With fewer surfaces exposed, less vitamins are lost.

- Eat vegetables and fruits raw. Or cook many vegetables, such as asparagus, green beans, broccoli, and snow peas, as quickly as possible—just until tender-crisp. Some vitamins, such as B vitamins and vitamin C, are destroyed easily by heat. The shorter the cooking time, the more nutrients are retained.

   Short cooking times help vegetables keep their bright color and flavor, too. The flavors of strong-flavored vegetables, such as Brussels sprouts and turnips, can get even stronger when they're overcooked.

- Cook vegetables and fruits in a covered pot. In that way steam doesn't escape, and cooking time is faster.

- Just reheat canned vegetables on the stovetop or in the microwave oven. If they've just been opened, canned vegetables don't need to be cooked again. They would lose flavor and nutrients!

- Save liquid from cooking vegetables for soups, stews, and sauces; perhaps freeze it for later use. That's one way to "recycle" water-soluble vitamins and minerals that otherwise would be tossed with the cooking water.

- For beets and red cabbage, add a little lemon juice or vinegar to the cooking water. This helps retain their bright-red color. Don't add baking soda! Although the alkali in baking soda keeps vegetables looking greener, it also destroys some vitamins.

- Microwave! Why? First, because microwaving is so fast, heat-sensitive nutrients aren't subjected to heat for long. Second, microwaving doesn't require added fat. There's a flavor advantage, too: unless overcooked, vegetables retain the color and tender-crisp qualities that make them appealing.

- Keep milk in opaque containers—and in the refrigerator. Leaving it in a clear, glass pitcher on the table allows some riboflavin to be destroyed by sunlight.

- Skip the urge to rinse grains, such as rice, before cooking. That may wash nutrients down the drain.

Have You Ever Wondered

. . . if cooking ever makes vegetables or fruits more nutritious? Cooking itself won't add nutrients (unless ingredients are added) to a food, but can make food safer and perhaps more edible and appealing. For example, you probably prefer eating a potato that's cooked, not raw.

   For some foods, cooking may enhance the nourishment. For example, lycopene, a phytonutrient, in tomatoes, is absorbed in the body better from cooked or processed tomatoes; lycopene may offer protection from some cancers. Carotenoids (which form vitamin A) are more available for absorption when cooked.

Fat and Cholesterol Trimmers

Hardly a day goes by without a new magazine or newspaper article giving tips for trimming fat, saturated fat, and cholesterol in foods prepared at home. And with good reason—many people consume more fat, especially saturated fat, than their bodies need for health.

   We know that many health conditions—heart disease, cancer, and obesity, among others—are linked to high-fat diets. Instead, learn to prepare food with less fat, so your overall food choices provide no more than 30 percent of total calories for the day—and with less saturated and trans fats, too.

   Fats have many roles in traditional recipes. For one,

they carry, blend, and stabilize flavor. With less fat, flavors may be more volatile, and not hold up as long as you might like. In baked foods, fat also tenderizes, adds moisture, holds air in so they're light, and affects the shape—for example, in cookies. In sauces, fats keep foods from curdling and form part of an emulsion, so that water and fats don't separate. Fat in recipes also conducts heat—for example, when sautéeing and stir-frying; fat lubricates so food doesn't stick to the pan, and fat seals in moisture when foods are basted. Fat in food also carries some nutrients from food into your body.

Although it doesn't make cooking sense or health sense to cut all the fat, preparing food with less fat does. With simple changes you can cook "leaner"—and still prepare great-tasting food.

Meat, Poultry, and Fish: Lean Cuts and Low-Fat Cooking Methods

	Dry Heat					Moist Heat			
	Roast	**Broil**	**Grill**	**Panbroil**	**Stir-fry**	**Braise**	**Stew**	**Steam**	**Poach**
Beef									
Eye round*		X					X	X	
Top round*	X	X	X	X	X				
Round tip*	X	X	X	X	X	X	X		
Bottom round*	X					X	X		
Sirloin	X	X	X	X	X				
Top loin	X	X	X	X	X				
Tenderloin	X	X	X	X	X				
Flank*		X	X		X				
Ground round	X	X	X	X	X				
Pork									
Tenderloin	X	X	X	X	X				
Boneless top loin roast	X	X	X						
Loin chop		X	X	X					
Loin strips					X				
Boneless sirloin chop		X	X	X					
Boneless rib roast	X		X			X	X		
Rib chop		X	X	X					
Boneless ham	X	X	X	X	X				
Poultry†									
Whole chicken	X		X			X	X		
Whole turkey	X		X			X			
Cornish game hen	X		X			X	X		
Breast	X	X	X	X	X				X
Drumstick	X	X	X						
Fish									
Cod	X	X	X	X	X		X	X	X
Flounder	X	X	X	X				X	X
Halibut	X	X	X	X	X		X	X	X
Orange roughy		X	X	X	X			X	X
Shrimp		X	X	X	X		X	X	X

*May be cooked by dry heat methods if they are tenderized first by marinating or pounding.
†White meat has less fat than dark meat. Skin should be removed before eating.
Source: ©National Cattlemen's Beef Association Culinary Center, 2002.

Lean Tips . . . for a Variety of Foods

● Use cooking methods that require little or no added fat; try to broil, grill, roast, braise, stew, steam, poach, stir-fry, or microwave foods, rather than fry them, most of the time. *For a definition of these cooking techniques, see "Culinary Lingo" in this chapter. You'll also find in this chapter the techniques explained in detail: "Meat Cookery: Dry Heat Methods" and "Meat Cookery: Moist-Heat Methods."*

● Stretch higher-fat ingredients. For example, grate cheese so less looks like more. Spread 1 tablespoon of peanut butter on toast rather than 2 tablespoons.

● Use tempeh, tofu, or legumes as a low-fat but high-protein ingredient in stews, soups, pasta dishes, and other mixed foods. *For more about tempeh and tofu, see "What's 'Soy' Good?" in chapter 11.*

● Substitute reduced-fat and fat-free products in many recipes. *See chapter 11, "Supermarket Smarts," for suggestions throughout the supermarket.*

● Coat cooking pans with a thin layer of oil, then wipe with a paper towel. Two tablespoons of oil add up to 240 calories and 28 fat grams; a thin coating of vegetable oil spray has just 10 calories and 1 fat gram. Using nonstick pans makes it easier to use less fat.

● Prepare yogurt cheese as a substitute for higher-fat spreads. *To learn how to make it, see chapter 3.*

● Drain pan-fried foods on a paper towel to absorb extra grease. Go easy on the oil.

● When adding ingredients to packaged mixes (such as macaroni and cheese, scalloped potatoes, or brownies), try low-fat options. Use half the margarine or butter in packaged macaroni and cheese or scalloped potatoes, extra-lean ground beef in casserole mixes, or fat-free milk in brownies or instant pudding.

Lean Tips . . . for Meat, Poultry, and Fish

● Cook with lean meats (round, sirloin, and loin cuts), skinless poultry, and fish. *See chapter 11, "Meat and Deli Case," "Poultry Counter," and "Fish Counter" for buying tips. To decide how to cook them, see "Meat, Poultry, and Fish: Lean Cuts and Low-Fat Cooking Methods" in this chapter.*

● Use smaller amounts of processed meats that tend to have more fat: bacon, hot dogs, and luncheon meats. Or use leaner versions, such as 95 percent fat-free.

● When recipes call for bacon, use lean ham, Canadian bacon, or smoked turkey. You'll still get the smoky flavor.

● Trim away any visible fat on meat and poultry. Even on lean meat, you'll find some fat. Trimming the fat removes some, but not all the cholesterol; cholesterol is in both the lean tissue and the fat in meat, poultry, and fish. On whole birds you'll find the most fat near the opening of the cavity.

How Much Fat and "Sat-Fat" in the Skinniest Beef Cuts?

The Skinniest Seven Beef Cuts

Cut	saturated fat	total fat
Chicken breast	0.9	3.0
Eye round	1.5	4.2
Top round	1.4	4.2
Round tip	2.1	5.9
Top sirloin	2.4	6.1
Bottom round	2.1	6.3
Top loin	3.1	8.0
Tenderloin	3.2	8.5
Chicken thigh	2.6	9.2

grams of:
saturated fat
total fat

Source: USDA, ARS. Nutrient Database for Standard Reference, Release 13. Nutrient Data Laboratory homepage (www.nal.usda.gov/fnic/foodcomp), 1999.

All cuts are based on 3-ounce cooked servings, all grades, 1/4 inch trim, separable lean only. All chicken cuts are based on 3-ounce cooked servings, skinless.

Source: ©Cattlemen's Beef Board and National Cattlemen's Beef Association (2000).

● Go "skinless" on poultry. Under the skin there's a layer of fat. Remove the skin before or after cooking it to cut the fat content about in half; there's not much difference, as long as you remove the skin before you eat it! *Tip:* Cooking poultry with the skin on helps keep it tender and moist. The same is true for beef and pork; trim remaining fat after cooking.

● Drain off fat from ground-meat crumbles as they're cooked. To reduce fat further, transfer cooked ground-meat crumbles to a large plate lined with 3 layers of white, recycled paper towels. Blot top of meat and let sit one minute. Place meat in a strainer or a colander. Pour about 1 quart of hot tap water over the meat. Drain five minutes. You can rinse away 2 to 5 grams of fat per 3-ounce serving.

Meat Cookery: Dry Heat Methods in Three Easy Steps

Roasting

1. Heat oven to recommended temperature (varies based on cut of meat).

2. Place roast (straight from refrigerator) fat side up, on rack in shallow roasting pan. Season before cooking as desired. Insert ovenproof meat thermometer so tip is centered in thickest part of roast, not resting in fat or touching bone. Do not add water; do not cover.

3. For beef, pork, veal, and lamb, roast to 5 to 10° F below desired doneness.* Transfer to carving board; tent loosely with aluminum foil. Let stand fifteen to twenty minutes. (Temperature will continue to rise 5 to 10° F to reach desired doneness.) For whole poultry, cook until desired temperature is reached.*

Broiling

1. Preheat broiler for ten minutes.

2. Place meat, poultry, or fish on rack in broiler pan. Season with herbs or spices as desired. Position thinner pieces (3/4 to 1 inch) so that surface of meat is 2 to 3 inches from the heat; thicker pieces, 3 to 6 inches from the heat.

3. Broil to desired doneness, turning once.* After cooking, season with salt if desired.

Grilling

1. For gas grilling, set heat to medium. For charcoal grilling, coals should be ash-covered and medium temperature; allow about thirty minutes. (To test cooking temperature for charcoal grill: Spread coals out in single layer. Carefully hold palm of hand above the coals at cooking height. Count the number of seconds you can hold your hand in that position before the heat forces you to pull it away—approximately four seconds for medium heat.)

2. Season meat, poultry, or fish with herbs or spices as desired. For smaller pieces of meat, poultry, or fish (chops, steaks, burgers, breasts, fillets, or kebobs), place on cooking grid directly over coals. For roasts, thick steaks, or chops, whole chicken or turkey, the meat is placed on the grid, with coals or heat source on each side.

3. Grill to desired doneness, turning occasionally.* After cooking, season with salt if desired.

Panbroiling

1. Heat heavy nonstick skillet over medium heat (meats 3/4 inch or thicker) or medium high heat (meats 1/2 inch or thinner) until hot, about five minutes.

2. Season meat, poultry, or fish with herbs or spices as desired. Place in preheated skillet. Do not crowd. Do not add oil or water. Do not cover.

3. Cook to desired doneness, turning once.* For thicker pieces, turn occasionally. Remove excess drippings as they accumulate. After cooking, season with salt if desired.

Stir-Frying

1. Partially freeze meat, poultry, or fish (about 30 minutes) for easier slicing. Cut into thin, uniform strips or pieces. Marinate to add flavor or tenderize while preparing other ingredients if desired.

2. Heat small amount of oil in wok or large heavy nonstick skillet over medium high heat until hot.

3. Stir-fry in 1/2-pound batches (do not overcrowd), continuously turning with a scooping motion, until cooked to desired doneness. Add additional oil for each batch if necessary. (Cook meat and vegetables separately, then combine and heat through.)

*See "Safe Internal Temperatures" in chapter 12.

Source: ©National Cattlemen's Beef Association Culinary Center (2002).

● Blot cooked ground-meat burgers, meatballs, and meat loaf with several layers of clean paper towels.

● Brown meat, poultry, and seafood in a nonstick skillet with little or no added fat, except for vegetable oil spray. Compare the difference: 2 tablespoons of oil, used to brown meat, carry an extra 240 calories from fat (28 fat grams), compared with less than 10 calories (1 fat gram) from vegetable oil spray.

● Grill, broil, or roast meat and poultry on a rack so fat drips through. In that way, fat drippings aren't reabsorbed.

● Marinate meat, poultry, and fish in marinades with little or no fat: orange, lime, or lemon juice; defatted

Have You Ever Wondered

. . . how the fat content of deep-fried turkey compares to roasted turkey? If the cooking oil stays high enough—350°F for the entire frying process—it makes little difference. A 3½-ounce portion of deep-fried turkey with the skin on has about 12 grams of fat, compared with 10 grams in a 3½-ounce portion of roasted turkey (white and dark meat) with the skin on. However, if the cooking oil remains at 340°F or less, more oil seeps into the turkey meat, adding to the fat content. For the record, without the skin, the same amount of roasted turkey (white and dark meat) has 5 fat grams.

Meat Cookery: Moist-Heat Methods in Three Easy Steps

Braising

1. Slowly brown meat or poultry on all sides in small amount of oil in heavy pan. Pour off drippings. Season as desired.
2. Add small amount (½ cup to 2 cups) of liquid such as broth, water, juice, beer, or wine.
3. Cover tightly and simmer gently over low heat on top of the range or in a preheated 325° F oven until meat or poultry is fork-tender. (The cooking liquid may be reduced or thickened for a sauce after removing fat as desired.)

Stewing

1. Lightly coat meat, poultry, or fish with seasoned flour if desired. Slowly brown on all sides, in small amount of oil, if necessary, in heavy pan. Pour off drippings. Season as desired.
2. Add liquid such as defatted broth, water, juice, beer, and/or wine to pan. (Use ½ cup to 2 cups liquid for chili type/shredded beef dishes; enough liquid to cover for stews and soups.) Bring to a boil; reduce heat.
3. Cover tightly and simmer gently over low heat on top of the range, or in a preheated 325° F oven until meat, poultry, or fish is fork-tender. (Cooking soups in the oven is not practical.) Thicken or reduce defatted liquid as desired.

Poaching

1. Season meat, poultry, or fish as desired. For roasts, tie with heavy string at 2-inch intervals if needed. Brown on all sides in nonstick pan. Pour off excess drippings.
2. Cover meat, poultry, or fish with liquid such as defatted broth, juice, water, beer, or wine. Season with additional ingredients if desired.
3. Bring to a boil. Reduce heat, cover, and simmer until fork-tender.

Steaming

1. Place fish on a steamer pan or a perforated tray. Vegetables, such as onions, leeks, celery, and bok choy, can be added.
2. Set steamer into pan above simmering liquid.
3. Cover pan and continue simmering over low heat until fish flakes.

Microwave

1. Place fish in a microwave-safe dish in spoke fashion for even cooking.
2. Add a small amount of liquid or seasoned vegetables if desired. (Some vegetables may take longer to cook; choose vegetables with similar cooking times, or cook vegetables separately.)
3. Cover with microwave-safe plastic wrap, venting or lifting one corner.
4. Following manufacturer's directions, microwave on high until fish flakes and any added vegetables are tender.

Source: National Cattlemen's Beef Association Culinary Center (2002).

Degreasing Pan Juices, Soups, and Gravies

Remember your science lessons? Fat rises to the top because it's lighter than water. The same thing happens in cooking. Fat in pan juices, soups, gravies, and canned broth collects on top, making it easy to skim off. Every tablespoon of fat you discard removes about 120 calories and 13 fat grams from the dish you're preparing.

- Remove fat from meat and poultry juices with a wide-mouthed spoon or a fat-separating pitcher.
- Refrigerate soups and stews before they're served. Do the same with homemade and canned broth, soups, and chili. Fat, which hardens when chilled, is easy to remove with a spoon.
- When time is short, add a few ice cubes to the broth. Fat will rise and congeal around the ice, but the ice may dilute the broth slightly.

broth; wine; tomato juice; salsas; fat-free or reduced-fat salad dressings; plain, low-fat yogurt; or buttermilk. Add fresh herbs to the marinade.

- To keep fish or chicken moist, steam fillets in heavy aluminum foil with fruit, herbs, onions, vegetables, and other flavorings. Secure the "package" and then bake it in the oven or on the grill. For the oven, you can also wrap and cook meat, fish, or poultry in parchment paper (chefs call this *en papillote,* or paper package) or leaf packets (such as banana leaves).

- Oven-fry fish or chicken. Dip it first in egg whites, then coat with seasoned bread crumbs. Bake on a nonstick baking pan coated with vegetable oil spray.

- As a quick, low-fat main dish, bake fish with a splash of white wine, chopped tomatoes, and fresh basil or oregano.

Lean Tips . . . for Egg Dishes

Eggs, which supply protein and iron to the diet, contribute toward your Pyramid servings from the Meat and Beans Group. While nutritious, health experts advise healthy Americans to eat whole eggs and yolks in moderation to control dietary cholesterol (to keep cholesterol intake less than 300 milligrams daily).

Egg yolks, not whites, contain fat and cholesterol.

That's why you can use egg whites liberally in place of egg yolks in many foods. Here's how to enjoy eggs in moderation:

- Use two egg whites in place of one whole egg in breads, pancakes, casseroles, French toast, cookies, cheesecake, pudding, and other recipes that call for whole eggs. Although one egg white can substitute for one yolk, recipes that require egg yolks, such as puff pastry, are best made with whole eggs.

- As another option, use a cholesterol-free liquid egg product in place of whole eggs. Usually ¼ cup egg product equals one whole egg; check the package label to be sure.

- In recipes that call for two or more eggs, substitute just some of the whole eggs with egg whites. For example, for two whole eggs, instead use two egg whites and one whole egg. That way you'll get the color and the flavor of the yolk, but less cholesterol and less fat. This ideas works well for scrambled eggs, quiche, and omelettes.

Lean Tips . . . for Vegetables

- For vegetables, "sauté" with a little liquid, not oil. Cook them in a little defatted broth, juice, wine, or water in a covered, nonstick pan. It's great for onions and mushrooms, which are sautéed for many recipes!

- Cook vegetables by steaming, stir-frying (in a nonstick wok or skillet), simmering, or microwaving. If you really enjoy the crispiness of French fries and fried onion rings, oven-bake them instead of frying them.

- Puree or mash potatoes, sweet potatoes, and other vegetables with milk, reduced-sodium chicken broth, or liquid left from cooking them. Go easy on butter or margarine. Boost the flavor and the nutrients by blending in some shredded carrots or zucchini!

- For the flavor of butter on vegetables, add a smaller amount—but just before serving. (Add herbs and garlic, too.) Cooking dilutes the flavor. You need less if you add it last. As another just-before-serving option, try a butter-flavored spray or powder.

- Sprinkle some Parmesan or Romano cheese on vegetables. It adds a lot of flavor but not much fat.

● Roast or grill vegetables (sliced eggplant, bell pepper chunks, sliced zucchini) as a low-fat way to bring out the flavor. Coat them lightly with vegetable oil spray. Then roast in the oven at 400° F or grill for about 15 minutes until tender-crisp.

Lean Tips . . . for Salads

● Flavor salads with lower-fat commercial dressings, or make your own with less oil and more vinegar.

● On taco salads, use lots of salsa—bottled or homemade with tomatoes, chiles, onions, herbs, and lime juice. Use a lighter touch with sour cream by going "50–50": 50 percent sour cream and 50 percent plain, low-fat yogurt. Or use reduced-fat or fat-free sour cream.

● Instead of creamy coleslaw made with regular mayonnaise, moisten cabbage and other shredded vegetables with low-fat or fat-free yogurt or mayonnaise with seasonings. Or use vinaigrette dressing.

● Adjust the proportions in homemade vinaigrette. Make it with three parts vinegar to one part oil (e.g., ¾ cup vinegar to ¼ cup oil) instead of the other way

---

EASY SUBSTITUTIONS TO CUT FAT AND/OR CHOLESTEROL

WHEN COOKING CALLS FOR . . .	USE . . .
Sour cream	Plain low-fat yogurt, or ½ cup cottage cheese blended with 1½ tsp. lemon juice, or light or fat-free sour cream
Whipped cream	Chilled, whipped evaporated fat-free (skim) milk, or a nondairy whipped topping
Cream	Evaporated fat-free (skim) milk, fat-free half-and-half
Whole milk	Fat-free (skim), 1 percent, or 2 percent milk as a beverage or in recipes
Full-fat cheese	Low-fat, part skim-milk cheese, cheese with less than 5 grams of fat per ounce, or fat-free cheese (be aware that cooking qualities differ)
Ricotta cheese	Low-fat or fat-free cottage cheese or nonfat or low-fat ricotta cheese
Ice cream	Low-fat or fat-free ice cream, or frozen low-fat or fat-free yogurt, frozen fruit juice products such as sorbet
Ground beef	Extra-lean ground beef, or lean ground turkey or chicken
Bacon	Canadian bacon or lean ham
Sausage	Lean ground turkey, or 95% fat-free sausage
Whole egg	Two egg whites, or ¼ cup cholesterol-free liquid egg product, or 1 egg white plus 2 tsp. oil
One egg yolk	One egg white
One egg (as thickener)	1 tbsp. flour
Mayonnaise	Low-fat, reduced-fat, or fat-free mayonnaise or whipped salad dressing, or plain low-fat yogurt combined with pureed low-fat cottage cheese
Salad dressings	Low-fat or fat-free commercial dressings, or homemade dressing made with less saturated oil (peanut, soy, olive, others), water, and vinegar or lemon juice
Cream soups	Defatted broths, or broth-based or fat-free milk-based soups
Nuts	Dried fruit such as raisins, chopped dried apricots, or dried cranberries
1 ounce unsweetened baking chocolate	3 tbsp. cocoa powder and 1 tbsp. oil
Butter, lard	Soft, tub margarine, squeeze margarine

around. Experiment with different types of flavored oils and vinegars or make your own herbed vinegars. *See "Herbed Vinegars" earlier in this chapter.*

Lean Tips . . . for Grain Dishes and Breads

● Skip the oil when cooking pasta, but use plenty of water. Don't rinse, just drain cooked pasta; toss with sauce immediately so pasta won't stick together; use a lower-fat sauce such as tomato-based or other vegetable sauces. For more flavor, add herbs instead of oil, or used flavored pastas, such as basil or garlic.

● Cook couscous, rice, and other grains with herbs, defatted broth, or juice instead of adding fat. And don't rinse rice; you'll wash away some vitamins, especially B vitamins, which are added to enriched and fortified grain products.

● Serve breads, rolls, muffins, bagels, and biscuits with low-fat spreads—fruit butter, chutney, jam, mustard, reduced-fat margarine spread, nonfat mayonnaise, reduced-fat or nonfat cream cheese, or pureed beans such as garbanzos. *For a list of condiments with less than 1 gram of fat per tablespoon, see "Lighter Condiments" in this chapter.*

Lean Tips . . . for Soups, Stews, and Sauces

● Skip gravy and rich sauces; enhance the flavors with fat-free ingredients: garlic, ginger, lemon juice, onions, tomatoes, herbs, and spices, among others. Before cooking, use a herb rub on meat, poultry, or fish; for a spicy taste, rub a mixture of cumin, chili powder, coriander, red and black peppers, and cinnamon on a pork roast. Or coat meat, poultry, or fish with salsas or chutneys. *See "Rub Combos" in this chapter for herb rubs and salsa ideas.*

● Cut back on or eliminate oil in homemade marinades. Or marinate with reduced-fat or fat-free salad dressing.

● "Sauce" up the flavor of vegetables, poultry, fish, and pasta with pureed vegetables rather than cream-based sauces. To create a creamy texture, add milk, plain or low-fat yogurt, or low-fat cottage cheese to vegetables as you process them in the blender or food processor. To warm, reheat gently.

● Try these "creamy" sauces. Blend fresh dill into fat-free, plain yogurt as a sauce for seafood or chicken. Blend horseradish with plain yogurt to serve with lean beef. For an easy sauce, braise poultry, fish, and meat in low-fat canned soups. Then heat to reduce the liquid to sauce consistency.

● Skim fat from pan juices, soups, and stews. *For quick techniques see "Degreasing Pan Juices, Soups, and Gravies" in this chapter.*

● Thicken soups with pureed beans, potatoes, or other vegetables and nonfat dry milk powder; or puree part of the soup and add it back as a thickener. Added vegetables can boost the vitamin and phytonutrient content; adding dry milk powder "ups" the calcium. Neither adds fat. For another "creamy" ingredient, try buttermilk or evaporated fat-free (skim) milk.

● If the recipe calls for a rich sauce, go easy. You want to add flavor, not overwhelm the food, with sauce. Serve sauce on the side.

Lean Tips . . . for Baked Goods

● Follow good baking techniques. In that way you'll test your recipe adjustment, not your baking skills. Have your oven checked for proper calibration. Bake according to the temperature and the time in the recipe. Check for doneness signs.

● Experiment a little. Take out some fat—but not all. In baked breads, cakes, muffins, and brownies, try substituting an equal amount of applesauce, mashed bananas or dried plums (prunes), other pureed fruit, or cottage cheese for at least half the oil, margarine, or butter in recipes. For bar and drop cookies, this substitution works well.

Try buttermilk or nonfat or low-fat yogurt in place of sour cream, butter, and margarine in biscuits, muffins, and other breads. Remember that some recipes work well with less fat; others don't. For example, with less fat, baked goods may not brown as well. Shortbread, butter cakes, butter cookies, and many pound cakes need fat for the flavor and texture you expect.

● Enjoy a nutty flavor? Use less nuts than called for, but toast or chop them for the most flavor. For even more flavor (or to extend it), yet no more fat, mix in chopped dried fruits, too: dried apricots, dried apples, raisins, dried cranberries, or dried plums (prunes).

● Coat baking pans very lightly with nonstick spray rather than margarine, butter, or oil.

● Instead of whipped cream toppings, whip chilled evaporated fat-free (skim) milk—with just a touch of sugar—for a creamy topping. Serve it right away since it's less stable and may get runny! Evaporated fat-free milk can be substituted in many recipes that call for heavy cream.

● Skip the frosting on a cake, or frost it lightly. Why not dust it with powdered sugar, or top with fresh fruit or fruit puree?

● Instead of flaky pastry shells with their high-fat content, make desserts with graham cracker crumb crusts. Prepare crumb crusts with half the margarine or butter called for in the recipe. If the crumbs seem dry, add just a little liquid to moisten.

● As another pastry option, prepare single-crust pies. Either make an open-face pie, or arrange the fruit in the pie pan first, then put the crust on top. *Another tip:* Top with uncooked oatmeal mixed with a few finely chopped nuts.

● As an easy substitution, use low-fat and fat-free dairy products.

● To cut down on saturated fat, experiment with cooking oil instead of margarine, butter, or lard. Be aware, however, that the texture of baked goods will differ, being coarser, mealier, and perhaps more oily. In fact, this substitution isn't suggested for quick breads, pastry, or sweet baked goods that are higher in fat to start.

Oil has more shortening power than solid fat, without the small amount of water that most solid fats contain. The recipe probably needs less oil than the amount of solid fat called for. Use this substitution:

FOR SOLID FAT ...	TRY LIQUID OIL ...
1 tbsp.	¾ tbsp.
⅓ cup	4 tbsp. (¼ cup)
½ cup	6 tbsp.
¾ cup	9 tbsp.
1 cup	12 tbsp. (¾ cup)

● Replace some (not all) whole eggs with whites. Baked goods can be rubbery with only whites.

Try This: Give It a Shake!

How much salt do you typically add to food? Take the "shaker test" to find out. Cover a plate or a bowl with foil or plastic wrap. Now pretend your dinner is on the plate—or that the bowl is filled with popcorn. Salt your "food" just as you would if the bowl or plate was full of food. Now measure how much salt you added. If you shook as much as ¼ teaspoon of salt, you added almost 600 milligrams of sodium to your meal or popcorn.

Salt "Shakers"

Cooking with salt may seem so natural that it goes unnoticed. If you're an average American, about 25 percent of your sodium comes from food preparation or salt you add at the table. A preference for salt, and the habit of cooking with salt, are learned. You can unlearn them, too.

You don't need to eliminate sodium from your cooking. In fact, you probably can't—and you shouldn't! Sodium occurs naturally in many foods, and it's a nutrient your body needs in limited amounts. *For a quick review of sodium see chapter 7, "Sodium: A Salty Subject."*

Especially if your blood pressure is sodium-sensitive, learn to cut back and use salt in moderation. Do so gradually . . . especially if you're a salt lover. After a while, your taste for salt probably will change. You might even be surprised when some foods seem too salty! Except for recipes with yeast, you can cut back on salt, in most recipes, perhaps by 50 percent—or even eliminate it altogether. Baked goods made with yeast need salt to control the rising of the dough.

● Taste before you reach for the salt shaker. Food may taste great just as it is!

● Shake the habit! Remove the salt shaker from the kitchen counter and the table. A ⅛-teaspoon "salt shake" adds more than 200 milligrams of sodium to your dish. Many health experts advise a limit on sodium intake for the general population: less than 2,400 milligrams a day.

● Instead of added salt, spark up the flavor with herbs and spices, garlic, onions, and citrus juice. *For food preparation tips, see "A Pinch of Flavor: How to Cook with Herbs and Spices" in this chapter.*

● Make a little salt go a longer way. Salt your food lightly just before serving. When it's on the surface of food, the salty taste seems more intense. Instead of salt, add a touch of flavor with foods that contain some salt and a little fat, such as olives, Parmesan or Romano cheese, and salted nuts. The fat helps keep the salty taste in your mouth longer.

● Drain liquid from some salty canned foods such as canned beans or vegetables. Rinse and cook in tap water or defatted broth.

● Reduce or skip the salt in cooking water . . . even if a package label says to add salt. Salt won't make water boil any faster. Instead, season pasta, rice, vegetables, and cereals with spices and herbs after they're cooked.

● Substitute prepared ingredients with those that have less sodium—perhaps low-sodium broth, no-salt-added canned vegetables, light soy sauce, and salt-free seasoning mixes. Read the label. If foods have ingredients with salt or sodium already, you don't need to add more.

Fiber Boosters

Does your plate lack fiber? You're not alone. With so many refined ingredients in breads, pasta, and other grain products and too few fruits and vegetables, many people come up short. Yet a few easy changes in your cooking style can boost your fiber factor—and add interest and flavor, too!

Why boost the fiber in your eating plan? Although it's not a nutrient, fiber promotes your health in many ways—by aiding digestion and by reducing the risks for intestinal problems, some types of cancer, and heart disease. In food, fiber is often bundled with essential nutrients, too. *To brush up on fiber and high-fiber foods, see chapter 6, "Fiber: Your Body's Broom."*

● Keep peels on fruits and vegetables. A medium baked potato with the skin on has about twice the fiber of a "naked" potato: 5 fiber grams compared to 2.5 fiber grams!

● Add legumes and lentils to all kinds of dishes. For convenience, use canned or frozen. *Check "A Word about Legumes . . . " in this chapter for ideas!*

● Substitute whole-grain pasta—lasagna noodles, macaroni, spaghetti, and other whole-grain pastas—in

all kinds of dishes. Use brown or wild rice (2 grams and 1.5 grams of fiber, respectively, per ½ cup cooked) in place of white rice (<0.5 fiber grams per ½ cup cooked), too—or use a combination.

● Experiment with unfamiliar whole grains: barley, buckwheat, bulgur, millet, quinoa, rye berries, and wheat berries. *To learn about these grains, see "Today's Grains" in chapter 9. The chart "Cooking Grain by Grain" in this chapter shows how to prepare them.*

● Add bran or wheat germ to casseroles, meat loaf, and dry or cooked cereal. Or blend some with yogurt for a little crunch. Each tablespoon of bran adds a little more than 1 gram of fiber.

● In dough and batter, substitute whole-wheat flour for half of the white flour. Don't go 100 percent, though; the texture will be too dense.

● Try oat flour in baking, too. Whirl dry oatmeal in a blender to make oat flour. Use it to replace up to ⅓ of white flour in a recipe.

● Add extra vegetables to casseroles, soups, salads, pizza, sandwiches, and pasta and rice dishes. For example, adding ½ cup of broccoli to a pasta dish adds 2 grams of fiber. A quarter cup of cooked spinach, mixed in soup or risotto, adds 2 grams of fiber. And half a medium-size carrot, shredded as a salad topping, adds 1 gram of fiber.

● Get whole-grain goodness on sandwiches. Use whole-grain breads, whole-grain bagels, and whole-grain pita pockets.

● Enjoy the fiber factor of fruits. Use all kinds of fruit in salads, cooked cereals, and as toppings on frozen desserts and angel food cake. For example, try sliced berries, pears, or peaches. Half a cup of strawberries and half of a pear (skin on) each add 2 grams of fiber!

Have You Ever Wondered

. . . how to cook with flaxseed? To get the benefit of flaxseed, you need to grind it in a blender, food processor, or coffee grinder. Then add it to dough and batter, or use it as a topping on puddings, cereal, and other food. Flaxseed is high in fiber and omega-3 and -6 fatty acids, yet has little saturated fat.

COOKING GRAIN BY GRAIN

Wonder how to cook whole grains? You can use the same simple steps for all these whole grains. Bring the cooking water to a boil; stir in the grain. Cover, reduce heat, and simmer. Let stand, covered, if indicated below. Then use these wonderful cooked grains in salads; as side dishes flavored with sauces or seasonings; or in soups.

1 CUP UNCOOKED GRAIN	COOKING WATER (CUPS)	COOKING TIME (MINUTES)	STANDING TIME (MINUTES)	YIELD (CUPS)	COMMON USES
Amaranth	3	25	–	3½	Cereal, side dish
Buckwheat (kasha)	2	20	10	3	Side dish (buckwheat groats flour also used in baked foods)
Bulgur	1½	*	30	2½	Side dish, stew, salad (tabbouleh)
Hominy (corn) (soak 8 hours)	4	30	5	3½	Side dish, stew, soup, cereal
Millet	2¾	30	15	3	Side dish, bread
Pearl barley	3	40	5	3½	Side dish, cereal, soup
Quinoa (rinsed)	2	15	–	3	Side dish, stuffing, soup, salad, stew
Rice, brown	2½	45	5	3	Wherever rice is used
Rice, wild[†]	3	55	–	3½	Side dish, stuffing, soup, salad
Rye berries	2	60	–	2¾	Side dish, bread
Triticale (wheat and rye) (soak overnight)	2½	40	–	4	Side dish, soup, cereal, bread
Wheat berries (soak overnight)	2	45	–	2½	Side dish, bread

*Bulgur isn't cooked. Put bulgur in a bowl, pour boiling water over it, and let it stand until the water is absorbed.
[†]Wild rice is actually a seed, not rice.

Sources: Compiled from *L. C. Peterson, "The ABC's of Whole Grains," Food Management* (March 1993):108; J. E. Brody, *Jane Brody's Good Food Book* (New York: Bantam Books, 1987).

● Add oatmeal, nuts, and seeds (sesame seeds, poppy seeds) to mixed dishes: pudding and fruit toppings, meat loaf, stuffing, salmon patties, crab cakes, burgers.

● Mix dry fruit—raisins, dried cranberries, apricots, and dried plums (prunes)—into breads, cookies, salads, and other dishes. One-quarter cup of raisins adds 2 grams of fiber; three dried plums have almost as much!

● Choose whole grain breakfast cereals. Look for the words "whole-grain" on the package. Other label clues are a "good source of fiber" or "rich in fiber." Oats in cereal are whole grain, too. *See chapter 11 for more on label reading.*

A Word about Legumes . . .

Legumes—dried beans, peas, and lentils—are packed with fiber! A half-cup serving of cooked legumes supplies 4 to 10 grams of fiber. (As a healthy adult, you need 20 to 35 grams of fiber a day.) Legumes also are packed with proteins, other nutrients, and phytonutrients, yet little fat and no cholesterol, so adding them to meals and snacks several times each week is well worth it. If you use canned products, they don't need to take any effort.

Have you heard this complaint in your family? "I don't like beans!" When boiled and served plain, they don't have much flavor. But when combined with other foods, they're versatile, taking on many flavor dimensions.

● Make minestrone soup with drained, canned kidney or garbanzo beans and vegetables. Add beef or chicken broth or canned tomatoes and their juice for flavor.

● Fill tacos or burritos with drained, cooked or canned pinto beans. Accent the flavor with a little grated cheese and lots of salsa, tomatoes, onions, and/or chopped lettuce or cabbage.

● Top green salads with drained, canned or cooked beans. Or mix up a three-, four-, or five-bean salad!

● For an easy lunch, open a can of split pea, navy bean, or lentil soup. Some shredded carrot or apple tastes great on top!

● As an easy side dish, baked potato topping, or pasta sauce, simply heat canned beans, combined with a tasty sauce of tomatoes, molasses, or jalapeño peppers.

● Use legumes as a meat substitute in many mixed dishes: kidney beans in chili, lentils in meat loaf, pinto beans in enchiladas, black beans in chunky soups, mashed kidney or pinto beans in meatballs, lentils in curry, soybeans in casseroles, and white beans in stews.

● Create a high-fiber pasta sauce that's low in fat, too! In a blender or a food processor, puree drained, canned beans with beef or chicken stock. White cannellini beans make a creamy white sauce, but any variety of beans will do. Add a blend of fresh herbs: basil, chives, garlic, marjoram, and oregano, among others. Fresh tomatoes or tomato sauce add a nice flavor and color, too. Heat and toss with your favorite pasta!

See "Kitchen Nutrition: Cooking a Pot o' Beans" in chapter 6 and "Vegetarian Way: Legumes and Other Meat Alternates" in chapter 20 for more tips on cooking with beans.

Calcium Boosters

If you're like many Americans, the calcium in your diet needs a boost! People of all ages need calcium for healthy bones and teeth, and for other body functions. Yet too many of us just don't consume enough servings from the Milk Group of the Food Guide Pyramid.

Like that for younger children, the Dietary Reference Intakes (DRI) for adults ages nineteen to fifty is

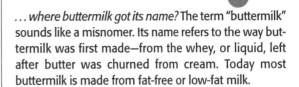

Have You Ever Wondered

... where buttermilk got its name? The term "buttermilk" sounds like a misnomer. Its name refers to the way buttermilk was first made—from the whey, or liquid, left after butter was churned from cream. Today most buttermilk is made from fat-free or low-fat milk.

1,000 milligrams of calcium daily; over age fifty, it's 1,200 milligrams of calcium. For young children and teens ages nine to eighteen, it's 1,300 milligrams of calcium daily. Dairy foods are the best source of calcium—in fact, they supply about 75 percent of the calcium in the U.S. food supply. But small amounts come from other food groups too. *See "Calcium: A Closer Look" in chapter 4 for more information.*

To boost the calcium in your diet, consume two to three Milk Group servings daily. Fat-free and lower-fat varieties are good choices for fat-conscious individuals. Use these food preparation tips to add a little more calcium here and there. You'll help ensure that your bones—in fact, your whole body—get the calcium needed.

● Fortify mashed potatoes, casseroles, vegetable purees, and thick soups with nonfat dry milk powder, evaporated fat-free milk, or plain yogurt. Dry milk added to meat loaf won't even be noticed! One-quarter cup of nonfat dry milk powder adds 375 milligrams of calcium to a whole recipe for meat loaf.

● Sprinkle shredded cheese on salads, soups, stews, baked potatoes, and vegetables. One ounce of Cheddar cheese (¼ cup) has 200 milligrams of calcium.

● Make cooked cereal and hot cocoa with milk instead of water. One-half cup of milk adds 150 milligrams of calcium to your day's food choices. You

How Much Cheese?

1 cup shredded cheese = 4 ounces*
1 cup grated cheese (Parmesan, Romano) = 3 ounces

*A Pyramid serving is ½ cup (2 ounces) of shredded processed cheese, or about ⅓ cup (1½ ounces) of natural cheese such as Cheddar or mozzarella.

might fortify them with extra nonfat dry milk powder, too. Calcium-fortified soy milk also adds calcium.

● Puree cottage cheese in a food processor or a blender. Add herbs, then use it as a dip or a bagel spread.

● Instead of black coffee (regular or decaffeinated) in the morning, buy caffè latte (made with milk, perhaps fat-free) at the coffee shop. It's made with steamed milk. One-half cup (4 ounces) of milk added to coffee adds 150 milligrams of calcium.

● Use plain yogurt for some of the mayonnaise in salad dressings, sandwich spreads, and dips.

● For something different, try goat cheese. It has a strong and unique flavor. A half-ounce portion of semisoft goat cheese has about 42 milligrams of calcium. Serve it on crackers, on salads, or as a vegetable garnish. A half ounce of hard goat cheese has 127 milligrams of calcium. *Hint:* You might find herb-flavored goat cheese in your supermarket.

● Add vegetables that have more calcium to many dishes: soups, salads, and stews, for example. One serving of broccoli, collard greens, kale, mustard greens, okra, and turnip greens all provide calcium, although not as much as a serving of milk.

● For main dish salads and sandwich spreads use canned salmon with bones as an occasional change from tuna. Fish with edible bones—salmon, sardines, perch—all supply calcium to the diet.

● If you boost calcium with reduced-fat or fat-free cheese, recognize that it doesn't blend or melt as well as whole-milk cheese. For best results shred lower-fat cheeses finely or use them in a mixture with whole-milk cheese. Blend them with other ingredients rather than just sprinkling them on top.

● Boost calcium, not fat, with yogurt cheese. Made by draining the whey from the solids in plain yogurt, it makes a great substitute for cream cheese or sour cream. *See "Kitchen Nutrition: Yogurt Cheese" in chapter 3.*

● Make stir-fried dishes with tofu (soybean curd), preferably with a tofu variety that's made with calcium sulfate. One-quarter cup of tofu with calcium sulfate has about 130 milligrams of calcium. The same amount of tofu without calcium sulfate has 65 milligrams of calcium.

Sugar Savers

"Just a spoonful of sugar," as Mary Poppins knew, adds flavor! Besides the taste, sugar adds to the aroma, texture, color, and body of a variety of foods. Sugar is the "food" for yeast that helps bread rise. In baked foods it contributes to the light brown color and crisp texture. In canned jams and jellies, sugar helps inhibit the growth of molds and yeasts. In many baked foods and other products, sugar contributes to a food's bulk and texture.

Like other ingredients in food, eating added sugars in moderation is part of a healthful eating plan. Sugars are one source of food energy. For some people, moderation means controlling sugar they add to foods, perhaps to cut back on calories. *For a quick review of sugars, see Chapter 5, "Sweet Talk: Sugar and Other Sweeteners."*

Before you change the sugar in a food you're preparing, think about its function and whether reducing or eliminating sugars will give the baking or cooking result you want. Then if you need to cut calories, use sugars in moderation in your cooking:

● In cakes, cookies, breads, and other baked goods, try using less sugar. Often you can reduce sugar by a fourth to a third, yet hardly notice the difference. *Be aware, however, that many recipes have already done this for you. Check the chart "Baking with Sugar" below as your guide.*

● "Sweeten" recipes with extracts such as vanilla or peppermint, or so-called sweet spices such as cinnamon or allspice. This enhances the sweetness of food. Warm these spicy foods; they'll taste sweeter! Other

---

Baking with Sugar

To ensure good results when reducing sugar in baked foods, use this guideline.

Baked Foods	For Each Cup of Flour Use
Cakes and cakelike cookies (cookies made with juice, milk, water)	½ cup sugar
Muffins and quick breads	1 tbsp. sugar
Yeast breads	1 tsp. sugar

spices that give the perception of sweetness include cardamom, coriander, ginger, mace, and nutmeg. *For more tips see "Kitchen Nutrition: Sweet Seasons" in chapter 5.*

● Briefly broil or microwave peach, pear, or grapefruit halves. Sprinkle with a small amount of sweetener or sweet spice . . . or just enjoy the natural flavor. The warm temperature enhances their sweet flavors!

● Sweeten with fruit pureed in a blender or a food processor. Too thick? Add a little fruit juice. Fruit purees are great on pancakes, waffles, French toast, fruit salads, angel food cake, and frozen desserts. They're also a tasty glaze for chicken and poultry! You can use applesauce or pureed baby-food fruits, too.

● Instead of fruit-flavored yogurt, add your own fruit flavoring to plain yogurt with fresh, canned, or frozen fruit. Blend in chopped fruit, berries, or fruit puree.

● As a way to get your "five a day" (fruits and vegetables), enjoy a baked apple or a pear for dessert. Poach it in fruit juice and any "sweet" spice.

● Buy processed foods with less added sugars—canned fruits in natural juices and unsweetened cereals.

● In some foods you can use intense sweeteners such as aspartame or saccharin. They're almost calorie-free! However, because they don't function in food like sugars do, their use is limited. *See "Intense Sweeteners: Flavor without Calories" in chapter 5 for more about cooking with these sweeteners.*

● Making a gelatin salad or a dessert? Rather than using flavored gelatin, dissolve unflavored gelatin in fruit juice. Then sweeten with an intense sweetener.

Well Equipped–for Healthful Cooking!

To cook the "lean" and healthful way, equip your kitchen with a few simple utensils and appliances!

Cheese grater. With a grater, a little cheese goes a longer way. When cheese is grated, a smaller cheese portion still adds plenty of flavor. It's also a "grate" idea for shredding vegetables such as carrots and summer squash, or for grating lemon, lime, and orange rinds for flavor.

Coffee grinder. It's great for grinding small amounts of nuts, seeds, and grains as well as dry herbs and spices.

Egg separator. An egg separator helps yo͜ arate the yolks from the whites. That's imp͏ you're cutting back on dietary cholestero͝. egg separator has a food safety benefit, too. ͜ to the technique of transferring the yolk back and forth between the two shell halves, using an egg separator reduces the chance of transferring bacteria from the outside of the shell to the uncooked egg.

Fat-separating pitcher. With the position of the spout, a fat-separating pitcher lets you pour out the liquid from the bottom, leaving the fat behind.

Food processor or blender. With this countertop appliance you can puree low-fat cottage cheese to the consistency of thick cream; chop, grate, or puree vegetables for use in soups, sauces, salads, and side dishes; or puree fruit, yogurt, and milk for a thick yet low-fat milk shake.

Hot-air popcorn popper. This type of popcorn popper requires no oil or butter, so popcorn can be a quick, low-fat, low-calorie snack.

Indoor grill. Indoor grills either fit over the burners on your stove or they may be free-standing appliances. Either way, you can easily discard the excess fat, which drips through the grates into a drip pan.

Instant-read thermometer. An instant-read thermometer helps you cook food to a safe internal temperature. *See chapter 12 for tips on using a meat thermometer.*

Kitchen scale. A scale that measures in ounces helps you figure portion sizes. If you have a hard time determining the size of your meat, poultry, fish, or cheese servings, a kitchen scale is helpful.

Kitchen scissors. Along with knives, kitchen scissors come in handy for trimming visible fat from meat and poultry.

Microwave oven. A microwave oven cooks food fast, without the need for added fat. The fast cooking time also helps food retain vitamins and minerals. Why so speedy? Microwaves, which cause food molecules to vibrate and create friction, travel fast; the friction heats and cooks food.

Nonstick pots and pans. Some cookware is specially coated, allowing you to cook with little or no added fat. Although today's nonstick finishes last a long time, you need to care for them properly. Use nonmetal utensils to prevent scratching, and avoid abrasive cleaners that strip away coatings. Many nonstick finishes are dishwasher-safe.

Pastry brush. A small pastry brush lets you just lightly coat meat, poultry, fish, and baked goods with fats or oils.

Pressure cooker. Among other time-saving benefits, you can cook dry beans in it quickly. (Cooked dry beans have less salt than canned beans.) It cooks food quickly without much water, helping with vitamin retention.

Pump spray bottle. A refillable oil pump can be filled with the type of oil you like, for use as a vegetable oil spray. By spraying olive oil on bread you may use less.

Ribbed frypan. The ribs on the bottom surface let meat or poultry cook above the fat drippings so less fat gets absorbed.

Rice cooker. With this countertop appliance, rice cooking is easy! Just add rice, the liquid of your choice (perhaps juice or broth), and herbs and flip a switch. It turns off automatically when the rice is cooked.

Roasting pan with a grate. With a grate, roasted and broiled meat or poultry can't absorb fat drippings. They collect in the pan below.

Slotted spoon. A slotted spoon allows you to lift food out of the pan, leaving any fat drippings behind.

Slow cooker. This countertop appliance cooks food with low, steady, moist heat. It can be used to make tougher cuts of meat more tender and appealing. Casserole-type dishes and soups work well in a slow cooker.

Steamer. Rather than fry foods, steam them. Actually there are several kinds of steamers to choose from: an electric steamer for vegetables, rice, fish, or chicken; a stackable bamboo steamer set that fits in a wok or a stockpot; or a small aluminum vegetable steamer that fits in a saucepan.

Strainer. With a microwave-safe plastic strainer you can cook ground meat in a microwave oven, collecting fat drippings in a container underneath.

Wok. A wok's sloped sides allow food to cook fast without much oil. Unless it has a nonstick surface, "season" a new stainless-steel wok to keep food from sticking. Here's how: First coat the cooking surface with vegetable oil, then heat the pan in a 350° F oven for about an hour. The oil will work its way into the porous surface of the wok.

Yogurt cheese strainer. A fine mesh strainer allows you to drain away the liquid in yogurt and use the thickened yogurt as a substitute for sour cream. *See chapter 3 for tips on making yogurt cheese.*

Add Life to Your Spices— and Herbs, Too!

With today's cuisine, we've discovered a new world of taste. Innovative uses of herbs and spices offer a flavor advantage as we trim fat and sodium from cooking. And the result is a new fusion of flavors!

Herbs and spices have a long culinary tradition. If you're a history buff, you know that spices have been traded throughout the Mediterranean and the Middle East for more than two thousand years. In the first century, Apicus, who was a Roman epicure, described herb combinations to enhance the flavor of food. Spices were the motive for Christopher Columbus' forays across the ocean. Now, with our nutrition interest and a world that's smaller than ever, we use more herbs and spices—in new combinations—than ever before.

Many people confuse the terms "spice" and "herb." There is a difference. Spices, which grow in tropical areas, come from the bark, buds, fruit, roots,

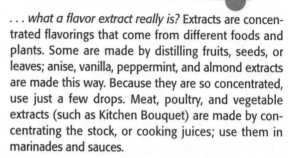

Have You Ever Wondered

. . . what a flavor extract really is? Extracts are concentrated flavorings that come from different foods and plants. Some are made by distilling fruits, seeds, or leaves; anise, vanilla, peppermint, and almond extracts are made this way. Because they are so concentrated, use just a few drops. Meat, poultry, and vegetable extracts (such as Kitchen Bouquet) are made by concentrating the stock, or cooking juices; use them in marinades and sauces.

. . . about cooking with wine, beer, or distilled spirits? They all can enhance the flavor, tenderness, and texture to food preparation. *See "Have You Ever Wondered . . ." in chapter 8.*

seeds, or stems of plants and trees. Usually they're dried; garlic and gingerroot are two common exceptions. Herbs, which grow in temperate climates, are the fragrant leaves of plants. The same plant may supply both. For example, the seeds of coriander are used in curry powder, while the leaves of the same plant are called cilantro, a favorite seasoning in Mexican dishes.

Locking in Flavor: How to Store Herbs and Spices

Your herbs and spices won't keep indefinitely—even dried! To lock in the aromatic flavors of fresh and dry herbs, you need to store them carefully.

● Store dry herbs and spices in tightly covered containers—in a cool, dry, dark place (not the refrigerator). Avoid placing your spice rack near a window or above the stove. Heat, bright light, and air destroy flavor. Moisture can cause herbs and spices to mold.

● Date dry herbs and spices when you buy them. Then use them preferably within a year. After a while, even properly stored seasonings lose their full "bouquet."

● To check the freshness, rub seasonings between your fingers, and smell the aroma. If there's not much, get a new supply. Buy just enough dry herbs for a few months for the most freshness.

● One way to keep fresh herbs longer: treat them like a bouquet of flowers! Snip the stem ends, then stand them in a glass of water. Cover them with a plastic bag, and store in the refrigerator. Change the water every couple of days.

● Growing your own herbs? Preserve them for those long, cold weather months. Either freeze, dry, or add fresh herbs to oils and vinegars. Be aware that some herbs are better dried—for example, bay leaves, marjoram, oregano, and summer savory.

　● *To freeze herbs*... Wash and dry them well; then seal them in plastic freezer bags. Or snip herbs, then freeze them with water in ice cube trays. Adding a "herb ice cube" to soups and stews is easy! Basil, chives, dill, fennel, parsley, rosemary, and tarragon are among the herbs that freeze well.

　● *To dry herbs in the oven*... Wash the herbs first, blot them dry, and remove the leaves from the stems. Place the herbs on baking trays in a single layer. Heat them in the oven at 100° F for several hours with the door slightly open. Remove the leaves before they get browned. Cool, then store in tightly covered containers.

　● *To dry herbs in the microwave oven*... Wash the leaves first, then place them between paper towels. Then dry the herbs on the lowest setting for two or three minutes.

A Pinch of Flavor: How to Cook with Herbs and Spices

Add a pinch of this and a pinch of that. Used carefully, herbs and spices make many foods distinctive and "simply flavorful"!

Dry or fresh—which herbs should you use? Nothing beats the delicate flavor of fresh herbs. But they're not always available. And unless you have your own herb garden in your backyard or on your windowsill, fresh herbs can be expensive. Whether you use fresh or dry seasonings, use them carefully to gain their best flavor advantage:

● Before using fresh herbs, wash them! Then pat them dry with paper towels.

● If fresh herbs have woody stems, strip off the leaves before using them. Discard damaged leaves. If the stems are soft and pliable, use them, too. Stems often carry a lot of flavor and aroma.

● To harvest herbs, pick them at their peak of flavor. That's just before they bloom. Remember, the flowers on many herb plants are very flavorful, too.

● To release more flavor and aroma, crumble dry, leaf herbs—basil, oregano, savory, and tarragon, among others—between your fingers. Or use a mortar and pestle or coffee grinder. Finely chop fresh herbs.

● In dishes that require a long cooking time, such as soups, stews, and braised dishes, add herbs toward the end of cooking. In that way their flavor won't cook out.

● For chilled foods such as salads and dips, add seasonings several hours ahead. That allows time for their flavors to blend.

Flavor Profile!

Would you combine tomato with basil, or with cinnamon, or with chile powder? The subtle blend of the two ingredients often defines the distinctive flavor of an ethnic cuisine . . . in this case, Italian, or Middle Eastern, or Mexican.

Many ethnic cuisines are defined partly by their mix of seasonings.

Italy	Tomato, olive oil, garlic, and basil
Mexico	Tomato and chile
West Africa	Tomato, peanut, and chile
Middle East	Lemon and parsley
Greece	Olive oil, lemon, and oregano
India	Curry, cumin, ginger, and garlic
Hungary	Onion and paprika
China	Soy sauce, rice wine, and ginger
Morocco	Cinnamon, cumin, coriander, ginger, and fruit
France	Thyme, rosemary, sage, marjoram, and tomato

● When substituting fresh for dry herbs, use this equivalent: 1 tablespoon of fresh herb equals 1 teaspoon of dried herb. Dry herbs are stronger than fresh; powdered herbs are stronger than crumbled herbs.

● Add dry herbs and spices to liquid ingredients. They need moisture to bring out their flavors.

● Chop fresh herbs very fine. Kitchen shears are great for mincing and snipping. With more cut surfaces, more flavor and aroma are released.

● Use seasonings with care—especially if you're not familiar with their flavor. They should enhance, not disguise, the aroma and taste of food. Start with ¼ teaspoon of dry herbs for 1 pound of meat or 1 pint of sauce. You can always add more herbs and spices, but you can't take them away!

● Avoid overwhelming a dish with seasonings. A few simple herbs and spices bring out the flavor of food without confusing your taste buds.

● If you're doubling a recipe, you may not need to double the herbs. Use just 50 percent more. If you triple the recipe, start by doubling the seasonings.

● Vary herbs and spices in your meal. Variety is the spice of a pleasing meal!

● Use seasoning blends, including curry, fine herbes, and bouquet garni. Each one is really a blend of herbs—and maybe spices, too. *Curry powder* is a pulverized mixture of as many as twenty different spices, herbs, and seeds. The spice turmeric is the ingredient that makes curried dishes so yellow. *For a recipe to make your own curry, see "Kitchen Nutrition: Salt-Free Herb Blends" in chapter 7. Fine herbes* usually refers to a mixture of chopped herbs, such as chervil,

Herbed Vinegars

Although today's supermarket shelves are stocked with herbed vinegars, why not make your own? They're less costly—and very satisfying to make. They also make great gifts from your kitchen!

● To sterilize, simmer the bottle for ten minutes, and let it cool. Wash the cap or obtain a clean cork.

● Insert a combination of fresh herbs (stems and leaves) and spices into the bottle. Three or four herb sprigs per pint are usually enough.

● Fill the bottle with vinegar. You can use any vinegar as a base: white, red wine, or cider vinegar. Herbs and spices may go better with some vinegars than others. For example, try tarragon and garlic cloves in red or white wine vinegar, and delicate herbs in distilled white vinegar.

Is wine or rice wine vinegar okay to use? Be aware that a protein they contain may promote bacteria growth if the herbed vinegar isn't stored properly.

● Put on the cap, or insert the cork. Store the bottle in a cool, dark place. Allow the flavor to develop for two to three weeks.

● Try these flavorful combinations: fresh tarragon in cider vinegar; garlic cloves, fresh rosemary or sage, and lemon peel in white wine vinegar; and fresh mint and orange peel in cider vinegar. For fun, make herbed vinegar with edible flowers—for example, nasturtiums with peppercorns, garlic cloves, whole cloves, and cider vinegar.

Have You Ever Wondered **?**

. . . if homemade herbed oils and garlic oils can pose a food safety risk? Yes, for *Clostridium botulinum* bacteria! (See chapter 12.) If you make them at home, use immediately! The U.S. Food and Drug Administration advises that home-prepared mixtures of garlic in oil be made fresh for any meal or snack and not be left at room temperatures. Refrigerate and use leftovers within ten days; after that, discard.

chives, parsley, and tarragon. *Bouquet garni* is a bundle of fresh and/or dried herbs, often parsley, bay leaf, and thyme, that's added to soups, stews, and braised meat or poultry. Usually they're tied up in cheesecloth or placed in a metal teaball. In that way bouquet garni is easy to remove later.

● If you grow a herb garden, experiment with less common varieties: pineapple sage, orange mint, burnet, lemon basil, and coriander, among others.

● Grow scented geraniums, too: apple-, lemon-, peppermint-, and rose-scented geraniums, to name a few. Their aromatic leaves and flowers offer a nice garnish and flavor to sauces, salads, vinegars, and baked foods. Besides, they'll give your garden a wonderful scent!

Rub Combos

Experiment with your own favorite blend of herbs and spices for all sorts of great rubs. You don't need a recipe; just combine flavors that taste good together. Use rubs on tender cuts of meat, poultry, and fish. To apply the rub, gently press the mixture onto the surface of the meat prior to cooking. Flavors usually become more pronounced the longer the seasoning mixture is on the meat. Try these for starters:

Citrus rub. Combine grated lemon, orange, or lime peel (or a combination) with minced garlic and cracked black pepper.

Pepper-garlic rub. Combine garlic powder, cracked black pepper, and cayenne pepper.

Italian rub. Combine fresh or dried oregano, basil, and rosemary with minced Italian parsley and garlic.

Herb rub. Combine fresh or dried marjoram, thyme, and basil.

The chart "Quick Reference: Herbs and Spices" in this chapter suggests the herbs and spices that complement a variety of foods. See the chart "Flavor Profile!" on page 328 for the unique seasonings that define various ethnic cuisines. Also see "Kitchen Nutrition: Salt-Free Herb Blends," in chapter 7.

Foods for All "Seasons"!

For a few easy ideas to use herbs and spices in food preparation, start with these tips:

● For baked chicken, fill the cavity with herbs and citrus peel—perhaps rosemary and sliced lemon—then roast it in the oven. Lemon grass or lemon scented geranium leaves are nice, too.

● Cook strong-flavored vegetables, such as cabbage, with savory to cut down on the strong aroma yet enhance the flavor.

● Add flavor with herb and spice rubs. *See "Rub Combos" on this page.* For a simple rub, just combine garlic and lemon pepper. Use herbed yogurt as a flavorful dip or vegetable topping. To get started, blend dill, parsley, chives, and garlic into low-fat yogurt.

● Make no-fat marinades with an acid ingredient— vinegar or fruit juice—and herbs or spices. For example, orange juice and nutmeg make a nice combination. A splash of herbed vinegar adds a flavor spark to salads and soups.

● Flavor mineral water, iced tea, lemonade, and spritzers with the leaves of scented geraniums, sprigs of fresh herbs, or edible flowers. Allow enough time for the infusion of their flavors and aromas. *For more about edible flowers, see "Please Don't Eat the Daffodils" in this chapter.*

Looking for more food preparation tips for healthy eating? Check here for "how-tos:"

● Boost the phytonutrient benefits when you prepare fruits, veggies, and grains—see chapter 4.

● Find more creative food "prep" ideas—see "Kitchen Nutrition" in many chapters.

Quick Reference: Herbs and Spices

Not sure what herbs and spices to use? Use this quick reference to enhance the flavor of foods in every part of your meal. This is just a partial list—add your flavor creativity to this list, too.

IN THESE FOODS . . .	TRY THESE HERBS AND SPICES!
Bread	
Sweet breads, rolls	Allspice, cinnamon, cloves, ginger, lavender, nutmeg
Other breads, rolls	Any herb, spice, or seed
Eggs	Basil, black pepper, chervil, chives, cilantro, garlic marjoram, oregano, tarragon, thyme
Fish and Seafood	
Finfish	Basil, bay leaf, chile powder, dill, fennel, ginger, oregano, paprika, sage, tarragon, thyme
Shellfish	Basil, black pepper, curry powder, dill, garlic, ginger, tarragon
Fruit	Cinnamon, cloves, ginger, lavender, mint, nutmeg, rosemary
Meat	
Beef	Bay leaf, basil, black pepper, celery seeds, curry powder, fennel (in sausage dishes), marjoram, oregano, onion, savory, thyme
Ham	Cloves, ginger, mustard seeds, tarragon
Lamb	Garlic, marjoram, mint, oregano, rosemary
Liver	Basil, onion
Pork	Cayenne pepper, chile powder, cinnamon, cloves, fennel (in sausage dishes), sage, thyme
Veal	Basil, curry powder, lemon grass, oregano, rosemary, sage, thyme
Poultry	
Chicken, turkey	Curry powder, ginger, marjoram, sage, tarragon
Stuffing	Basil, marjoram, onion, parsley, sage, savory
Pasta, Rice	
Pasta (including couscous)	Basil, chives, marjoram, oregano, saffron
Rice (white)	Cumin, fennel, onion, parsley, saffron, turmeric
Rice (brown and wild)	Ginger, onion, parsley
Salads	
Chicken or turkey	Chives, celery seeds, oregano, tarragon
Egg	Marjoram, onion, parsley, tarragon
Fish or seafood	Chives, curry, powder, ginger, marjoram, oregano, tarragon
Fruit	Cinnamon, ginger, lavender, mint
Greens	Basil, black pepper, chervil, chives, cilantro, garlic, marjoram, mint, onion, parsley, tarragon, thyme
Vegetables or legumes	Basil, oregano, onion, parsley, tarragon

In These Foods . . .	Try These Herbs and Spices!
Sauces	
Cheese	Chervil, chile powder, chives, paprika, parsley
Cream (milk-based)	Basil, curry powder, marjoram, tarragon, thyme
Tomato	Basil, bay leaf, cayenne pepper, cilantro, fennel seed, oregano, paprika, parsley, sage, thyme
Soups	
Chicken or poultry	Bay leaf, lemon grass, mace, marjoram, paprika, parsley, sage, savory, thyme
Clear broth	Basil, lemon grass, paprika, parsley
Cream (or milk based)	Chervil, chives, rosemary, sage, tarragon, white pepper
Fish or seafood	Bay leaf, celery seeds, chives, curry powder, ginger, saffron, tarragon, thyme
Legume	Bay leaf, celery seeds, saffron, tarragon, thyme
Meat	Basil, clove, coriander (cilantro), oregano, rosemary, savory, thyme
Mushroom	Basil, bay leaf, garlic, marjoram, onion, oregano, parsley, tarragon, thyme
Potato	Chives, curry powder, dill
Vegetable	Allspice, basil, bay leaf, black pepper, cloves, garlic, marjoram, sage
Vegetables	
Asparagus	Chervil, savory
Baked beans	Allspice, chile powder, cinnamon, cloves, mace, parsley, red pepper
Broccoli	Oregano
Brussels sprouts and cabbage	Caraway, celery seeds, dill, marjoram, mint, sage, savory, tarragon
Carrots	Basil, bay leaf, ginger, marjoram, mint, oregano, parsley, thyme
Cauliflower	Marjoram, nutmeg, parsley
Corn	Chile powder, chives
Green beans	Basil, cloves, marjoram, parsley, sage, savory
Lima beans	Marjoram, sage, savory
Mushrooms	Marjoram, oregano, parsley, tarragon, thyme
Onions	Basil, oregano, sage, thyme
Peas	Basil, chervil, marjoram, mint, oregano, parsley, sage, tarragon, thyme
Potatoes	Basil, caraway, chives, dill, garlic, parsley
Spinach	Marjoram, ginger, nutmeg, parsley, savory
Tomatoes	Basil, bay leaf, cilantro, cloves, marjoram, nutmeg, oregano, sage
Winter squash and sweet potatoes	Allspice, cinnamon, cloves, ginger, nutmeg, savory, thyme

Lighter Condiments

Consider adding chutneys and sauces, made with little or no fat, to the kitchen cupboard to spice up the looks and flavor of light menus. The following all have less than 1 gram of fat per tablespoon. Some are high in sodium.

Barbeque sauce	Pickle relish	Chili sauce	Seafood cocktail sauce
Cranberry-orange chutney	Soy sauce	Horseradish	Teriyaki sauce
Ketchup	Worcestershire sauce	Dijon mustard	

CHAPTER 14

Your Food Away from Home

Whether it's a rushed, fast-food meal, lunch in the company cafeteria, an order of pizza, a casual dinner at a family restaurant, or an elegant evening of fine dining in a relaxing atmosphere, eating out is no longer just for special occasions. It's become part of our everyday lifestyle!

According to the National Restaurant Association, Americans (age eight and over) eat out more than four times a week on average—or about 225 meals a year: mostly lunch and dinner, but breakfast continues to gain more of our food-service dollars. Overall, food service currently gets about 46 percent of every dollar that U.S. consumers spend on food, with projections expected at 53 percent by 2010. In fact, in 2002, about $408 billion are expected in restaurant industry sales, up about 4 percent from 2001. *The data are clear: there's good reason to give eating out your careful attention!*

Food service includes any food that's not prepared in the home kitchen. So who's cooking for us?

In growing numbers, consumers want fast, easy, and flavorful food to fit their busy lifestyles. Take-out, delivered food, and fast-food restaurants do the job so you have time for other things. In the late 1970s, fast-food sales amounted to about $9 billion annually in the United States. In 2002 that figure was projected at about $115 billion.

Despite our reliance on quick food, consumers also flock to full-service restaurants, which are projected to take in $147 billion in 2002. Why? Chances to socialize with family, friends, and coworkers; to enjoy their leisure time; and to experience flavors that aren't prepared at home.

Hungry or not, food bombards our senses almost everywhere we go today. The broad array of restaurants offers an explosion of dining-out options to choose from: traditional family cuisine; regional, ethnic, and fusion cuisine; vegetarian cuisine; coffee cafés; bagel and doughnut shops; and sushi bars, to name a few.

Supermarkets cook, letting us "take out" to "eat in." We also eat from convenience stores, bookstores, drugstores, recreational centers, institutions (schools, hospitals, businesses, and others), sports and cultural events, hotels and cruise ships, airlines, and vending machines, among others.

Where do you typically eat out—and how often? Whatever your answer, the more you eat away from home, the greater the impact food-service meals and snacks make on your overall food choices, health, and well-being.

Dining Out for Health and Pleasure

Eating out? You've got choices—plenty of them! It's up to you decide what foods to enjoy, where, and how much. With a little forethought and menu savvy, the meals and the snacks you eat away from home can be great-tasting, enjoyable, even adventuresome—and healthful, too.

What are your eating-out challenges: "too big" portions, the urge to splurge, no time to eat smart away from home? If you're a frequent restaurant diner, take stock of the big picture of eating with health in mind.

Restaurant Eater's Tip List

No matter where you choose to eat, the same smart-eating strategies can guide your eating: plan ahead, consider the menu, and choose foods carefully to match your needs. Remember, though, that an occasional meal with elegant, creamy sauces or a rich dessert pastry needn't upset your overall plans for low-fat eating.

Plan Ahead

How can your restaurant choices fit into your whole day's eating plan—without overdoing on calories and fat? And how can you enjoy the variety of food available in today's restaurant scene?

● Map out your restaurant plan of action. Perhaps plan for a light dinner out if you just ate a big lunch, or decide ahead of time to split a dessert, even before you see the menu. If you know ahead that your restaurant meal will have more calories or fat, just trade off: cut back during other meals that day or the next. If a menu item tempts you, this chapter offers ways to enjoy it and still stay on track.

● Avoid skipping breakfast or lunch to "save up" for a fancy restaurant dinner. This strategy often backfires. It's easy to overindulge at the restaurant when you're over-hungry. Eating small meals earlier in the day is a better approach.

● Looking for convenience, saving time, a flavor adventure, or a "leaner" meal? Patronize a restaurant that can meet your needs. Some offer more food variety, ethnic cuisine, unique dishes, smaller portions, and leaner cuisine than others. A restaurant that prepares food to order allows more control for any special requests; call ahead to find out. A handful of today's restaurants even let you call or fax any special requests ahead so the kitchen is ready for you.

● Go with a "smart eating" mind-set, which may help you sort through the menu faster and avoid straying from your plan.

Learn Menu Language

Primavera, béarnaise, al dente. What do all these menu terms mean? Knowing menu terms and cooking basics makes ordering easier, especially if you need to control calories, fat, and other nutrients, or handle any food sensitivity. *For the meanings of menu terms check the chart "Menu Language" in this chapter. For menu items typically prepared with less fat, see "May I Take Your Order?" and check "On the 'Leaner' Side" in this chapter.*

● Generally, look for foods with simple preparation, such as steamed vegetables or broiled chicken, if you need to lower fat and calories. For instance, the term "al dente" is used to describe how pasta and vegetables are cooked—only until firm when bitten, not soft or overdone. Literally translated, it means "to the tooth." Vegetables cooked "al dente" retain more nutrients than those that are cooked longer.

● Check menus for nutrient content claims. With new government regulations, terms such as "lean" and "light" on restaurant menus are defined consistently. Menu terms have roughly the same meaning as the same terms on food labels. *For more on label terms see "Label Lingo" in chapter 11.*

Have It Your Way!

Do you have unique food and nutrition needs or preferences? Many restaurants honor requests. It's up to you to be assertive, ask menu questions, make special requests in advance—and be realistic, too. Service-oriented restaurants are eager to please. They want you back!

Ask how the food is prepared or served, especially if the description isn't clear or the food is unfamiliar. Today's servers are accustomed to the questions of more sophisticated diners. Find out about ingredients and any substitutions. You might ask:

● How are the vegetables seasoned? Are they salted? Is butter or margarine added?

● Is the fish grilled, broiled, breaded, or fried? Is it cooked with butter, margarine, or some other fat?

● How is the sauce prepared?

● Can I have the sauce (or salad dressing or whipped topping) on the side?

● Is the soup clear (broth) or cream-based?

● Can I substitute a baked potato, rice, pasta, or a salad for the fries?

● What is mole sauce (in a Mexican dish)? Galangal (in a Thai dish)? Or cassava (in a Caribbean dish)?

Have You Ever Wondered

. . . what's "slow food"? It's the idea of enjoying food traditions and high-quality food, and taking time in your busy life to enjoy it. Consider how time at the table may add pleasure, great flavors, and social time to your lifestyle!

. . . if Caesar salad on the menu is safe to eat? Probably so, but ask how it's prepared. In the past, a Caesar salad, made with a raw egg, was often prepared right at your table. Today most Caesar salads are made in the kitchen with a pasteurized egg product or cooked salad dressing, following safe food-handling techniques. Some Caesar salads are eggless.

On the "Leaner" Side

Not sure what to order? For leaner cuisine, try this:

Appetizers	Fresh fruit cup, broth, bouillon, or consommé, fruit or vegetable juice, marinated vegetables, crudités, or raw vegetables, with a yogurt or salsa dip, seafood cocktail
Breads	Hard rolls or whole-wheat buns, French or Italian bread, breadsticks, melba toast, or saltine crackers
Salads	Salads with dressing on the side
Vegetables	Steamed vegetables, plain or with a lemon wedge, grilled or roasted vegetables
Entrées	Lean meat, fish, and poultry that are broiled, grilled, or roasted, with any sauces served on the side (remove visible fat and poultry skin); vegetarian dishes that go easy on cheese or cheese sauces
Desserts	Fruit ice or sorbet, fresh fruit, angel food cake with fruit, low-fat frozen yogurt, cappuccino

---

Ingredients in sauces confuse many restaurant-goers. What, for example, is the difference between a béarnaise sauce and a bolognese sauce? Which one is apt to be lower in fat? What's a reduction sauce? *For a quick description of common sauces see "Gourmet's Guide to Sauces" on page 337.*

● Find out about portion sizes. Big portions tend to be today's hallmark of restaurant service. For example, a 5- to 6-ounce portion of meat, poultry, or fish probably is enough for the whole day, especially if you eat other Meat and Beans Group servings during the day. If the menu offers a choice—a 12-ounce steak or a 6-ounce filet mignon—go for the smaller portion. You'll save on calories, fat, and money. *See "Restaurant Portions: You're in Control" in this chapter for ways to handle restaurant portions.*

● Don't see anything that's right for you? Ask to order "off the menu." For less fat and calories, you might request broiled fish or chicken breast seasoned with herbs and lemon juice, or fresh fruit for dessert, or low-fat milk if it's not on the menu. *See "On the*

'Leaner' Side" in this chapter for common menu items with less fat.

● Choose a meal with food variety when you eat out, just as you would at home. That's easy to do with an à la carte menu. (Remember the Food Guide Pyramid as you choose.) À la carte means that each item is separately ordered and priced. Be specific about a special menu request—for example, rather than ask for a "low-fat plate," ask if the chef can "broil fish without butter," "bring dry toast," or "serve dressing on the side."

● If you don't plan to eat a side dish or sauce, ask to have it left off your plate—perhaps skip tartar sauce served with fish, or chips served with a sandwich.

● If you choose a higher-fat entrée, balance it with a lower-fat side dish and dessert. Perhaps balance fettuccine alfredo, which is high in fat, with fresh fruit to end the meal. Remember that no food is off-limits. Just make trade-offs: if you eat foods with more fat or sodium when you dine out, cut back at home.

● If the food isn't prepared as you ordered, send it back. Ask for something else if necessary.

Help Yourself

Practice the art of enjoying food variety, balance, and moderation when you eat out.

● Can't resist the urge to overindulge on tortilla chips or the basket of bread served when you're seated? Do you nibble mindlessly on snacks such as pretzels and chips, brought to the table with a beverage order? Take a few and then move them, or ask to have them removed from the table.

● Go easy on dipping oils—even though they're usually olive oils (often herb-infused). A slice of bread may soak up 3 or 4 teaspoons of oil, or 14 to 19 fat grams, compared 4 to 8 fat grams in 1 to 2 teaspoons of butter or margarine spread on a bread slice.

● If you need help in curbing a big appetite, order a salad or appetizer crudités (raw vegetables) right away. And go easy on dressings and dips.

MAY I TAKE YOUR ORDER?

Variety on the menu? The choices on the left have fewer fat and calories than their counterparts on the right.

ENJOY MORE OFTEN	ENJOY SOMETIMES
Consommé, gazpacho	Cream soups, soups topped with cheese, bisques
Vegetable plate with salsa, steamed vegetables	Pâté, quiche lorraine, stuffed appetizers
Garden, tossed, or spinach salad with dressing on the side, crisp and crunchy vegetables	Salads with large amounts of dressing, bacon, avocado, cheese, croutons, and mayonnaise-laden salads such as potato, macaroni, and tuna
Grilled meats, broiled or flame-cooked	Breaded or batter-dipped meat or extra gravy
Broiled, steamed, poached, roasted, baked, Cajun, or blackened	Breaded, fried, sautéed, au gratin, escalloped, en croûte, creamed, en casserole, or Kiev entrées
4- to 8-oz. steak	More than 8-oz. steak
Au jus, Provençal or fruit sauces	Gravy, alfredo, béarnaise, béchamel, beurre blanc, carbonara, hollandaise, pesto, and velouté sauces
Baked potatoes (plain or with a small amount of margarine or sour cream), red skin potatoes	Home-fried and deep-fried potatoes, twice-baked potatoes, croquettes, butter noodles
Sandwiches on whole-wheat, pita, or rye with mustard or low-fat mayonnaise	Sandwiches on croissants or biscuits
Plain whole-wheat or multigrain rolls or breadsticks	Garlic bread, cheese spreads, flavored butters
Fruit, fruit sorbet	Cheesecake, French pastries, pie, ice cream

● Eat slowly, and stop eating before you feel too full. That gives you time to get in touch with your satiety cues. Ask the server to remove your plate when you're done, even if a little food is left.

● If you drink, enjoy alcoholic beverages, including wine and beer, in moderation. Healthful eating guidelines advise no more than one (if you're a woman) or

MENU LANGUAGE

Looking for foods with less fat or sodium? Check the menu. Although they offer no guarantee, descriptive terms often give clues to more or less fat or to more sodium. See "Eating Out" in chapter 7.

Menu Clues: Less Fat

Baked	Lightly sautéed
Braised	Poached
Broiled	Roasted
Cooked in its own juices	Steamed
Dry broiled (in wine or lemon juice)	Stir-fried
Grilled	

Menu Clues: More Fat

Au gratin or in cheese sauce	French-fried
Batter-fried	Hollandaise
Béarnaise	Marinated (in oil)
Breaded	Pan fried
Beurre blanc	Pastry
Buttered	Prime
Creamed	Rich
Crispy	Sautéed
Deep-fried	Scalloped (escalloped)
Double crust	With gravy
En croûte	With mayonnaise
Escalloped	With cream sauce

Menu Clues: More Sodium

Barbecued	Smoked
Cured	Teriyaki
In broth	With cocktail sauce
Marinated	With creole sauce
Pickled	With soy sauce

Restaurant Portions: You're in Control!

If restaurant portions seem too big for you, remember this: you have choices. You control portions by what you order and how you handle what comes on your plate.

● Order first, before your meal companions do, if possible. Then you won't be influenced by their order.

● Choose the portion size you want. Many restaurants offer appetizer portions, half portions, and full portions. Or try tapas, "little plates," or dim sum, and just order one or two dishes to share at a time.

● Split a dish with someone else. Ask for two plates.

● Order à la carte. You won't be tempted by more food than you need.

● Turn today's dinner into tomorrow's lunch. Most restaurants have take-away containers. That gives you a time-saving strategy for your next meal. *Tip:* Store perishable foods in the refrigerator within two hours, or within one hour if the temperature is over 90° F.

● For double benefits, look for restaurants with "early bird" specials. They may offer smaller portions for a lower price. Or eat out midday for a lunch-size portion.

● Leave some food on the plate; it's okay to do this. Why pay twice: your pocketbook *and* your waistline?

● Plan ahead if you're going for a trendy, multicourse tasting menu. Enjoying many small portions can add up to a lot of food!

● Pass on all-you-can-eat specials, buffets, and unlimited salad bars if you tend to eat too much. Unless you pay attention to your hunger and satiety cues, food bars easily add up to too many calories.

● If buffet-style eating is your choice, try this. Fill up on salad (easy on dressing) and vegetables first to take the edge off your appetite. Take no more than two trips to the buffet: one for veggies, fruit, and salads, one for anything else. Use the small plate, which holds less food.

two (if you're a man) alcoholic drinks per day. Besides their calories, a drink or two may increase your appetite and lessen your personal discipline at the table. As an option, try mineral water or club soda with a twist of lemon or lime.

Gourmet's Guide to Sauces

What's in the sauce? Use this list as a quick reference to make you a savvy restaurant patron.

Alfredo. Creamy Italian sauce, typically prepared with butter, heavy cream, and Parmesan cheese.

Béarnaise. Thick French sauce made with white wine, tarragon, vinegar, shallots (onions), egg yolks, and butter.

Béchamel. Basic white sauce made with flour, milk, and butter, and flavored with onion.

Bolognese. Italian meat sauce made with ground beef and sometimes pork and ham and sautéed in a small amount of butter and/or olive oil with tomatoes, other vegetables, herbs, and sometimes wine. Also referred to as a ragú bolognese sauce.

*Bourguignonne.** French sauce made with red wine, carrots, onions, flour, and a little bacon.

Buerre blanc. Thick, smooth sauce whisked with wine, vinegar, shallot reduction, and cold butter.

Carbonara. Italian sauce made of cream, eggs, Parmesan cheese, and bits of bacon.

*Demi-glace.** Reduction sauce that gets its intense flavor by slowly cooking beef stock and Madeira or sherry to a thick glaze.

Hollandaise. Thick sauce made with white wine, vinegar, or water; egg yolks; melted butter; and lemon juice.

*Marinara.** Italian tomato sauce made with tomato and basil and perhaps other seasonings such as onions, garlic, and oregano.

Pesto. Uncooked sauce made of fresh basil, garlic, pine nuts, Parmesan or Pecorino cheese, and olive oil. It's a favorite with Italian pasta.

*Reduction sauce.** Sauce of usually broth or pan juices boiled down to concentrate the flavor and thicken the consistency. Unlike in many other sauces, flour or other starches aren't used as thickeners.

*Sweet-and-sour.** Sugar and vinegar added to a variety of sauces; typically added to Chinese and German dishes.

Velouté. Light, stock-based white sauce. Stock is the broth left from cooking meat, poultry, fish, or vegetables. It's thickened with flour and butter; sometimes egg yolks and cream are added.

*Vinaigrette.** Oil-and-vinegar combination.

*These sauces tend to be lower in fat. But the ingredients vary, and so does the fat content.

● Trying to control calories? If you choose to resist rich desserts, don't even peek at the dessert tray when the server brings it by. If you're tempted, share it with someone else.

Enjoy, Enjoy, Enjoy!

Eating is an occasion that can "nourish" the soul as well as the body. In fact, eating out can be one of life's pleasures.

● Take your palate on a taste adventure. Order something you've never tried before—or that you usually don't eat at home. Feeling cautious about something new? Try an appetizer portion. Restaurants are a great place to try new foods!

● Savor each bite and enjoy food—and the layers of flavor—at a leisurely pace, especially if you've had a tiring or stressful day.

● If you're eating with others, enjoy the social time. Make it a relaxing chance to keep in close touch with your family and friends. *Check "Eating Out with Kids" in chapter 16 for ways to make eating out pleasant with young children.*

● Whether you eat with others or dine alone, appreciate the ambience (decor, aroma, and sounds) of the restaurant, and all the other pleasures that go with a meal "on the town."

Sizing Up Salad Bars

A salad bar can serve up a healthful meal all by itself—or as a great side dish. The rainbow of vegetables and fruits often is loaded with vitamins A and C, folate, fiber, and an array of phytonutrients.

Did you know: A do-it-yourself salad, chosen from the salad bar, often has more calories than a deluxe burger, fries, and a shake, or a steak-and-potato dinner? An average salad bar plate can top out at more than 1,000 calories, depending on your choices and portions. Not so surprisingly, then, salads have been reported to be a main source of dietary fat for many women.

Where do excessive amounts of calories, fat, even sodium come from? Not from the lettuce, tomatoes, cucumbers, and other fresh vegetables. Depending on the amount, regular salad dressings, along with many higher-fat toppings such as cheese, croutons, bacon bits, nuts, chow mein noodles, and olives, can heap

BUILD A HEALTHFUL SALAD

Imagine a salad bar with bowls and bowls of ingredients. Your plate is empty. How would you build your salad? Choose the ingredients from the list below—and decide how much you'd take of each one. When your salad plate is full, add up the calories and the fat. You may be surprised.

Food	Amount	Calories*	Fat (g)	Food	Amount	Calories*	Fat (g)
Greens				*Meat, Poultry, Fish, and Eggs*			
Bean sprouts	¼ cup	8	trace[†]	Eggs, chopped	2 tbsp.	25	2
Lettuce	1 cup	10	trace	Lean ham, chopped	1 oz.	35	1
Spinach	1 cup	10	trace	Popcorn shrimp	1 oz.	30	<1
Other Veggies				Surimi	1 oz.	30	<1
Artichoke hearts	¼ cup	20	trace	Tuna in spring water	1 oz.	35	<1
Beets	¼ cup	15	0	Turkey in strips	1 oz.	35	<1
Bell peppers	2 tbsp.	3	trace	*Cheese*			
Broccoli	¼ cup	6	trace	Cheddar cheese, grated	2 tbsp.	55	5
Carrots, shredded	¼ cup	15	trace	Cottage cheese, creamed	¼ cup	60	3
Cauliflowers	¼ cup	6	trace	Cottage cheese, 1% low-fat	¼ cup	40	<1
Cucumbers	¼ cup	4	trace	Parmesan cheese	2 tbsp.	45	3
Green peas	2 tbsp.	30	trace	*Others*			
Mushrooms	¼ cup	5	trace	Bacon bits	1 tbsp.	25	2
Onions	1 tbsp.	8	0	Chow mein noodles	1 tbsp.	50	2
Radishes	2 tbsp.	2	trace	Croutons, seasoned	2 tbsp.	25	1
Tomatoes	¼ cup	15	trace	*Mixed Salads*			
Fruits				Potato salad, made with mayonnaise	¼ cup	110	9
Avocados	¼ cup	75	8	Three-bean salad in vinaigrette	¼ cup	60	0
Canned peaches, in juices	¼ cup	25	0	Tuna salad, made with mayonnaise	¼ cup	190	10
Fresh melons	¼ cup	15	trace	*Dressings*			
Fresh strawberries	¼ cup	10	trace	Blue cheese, regular	2 tbsp.	155	15
Mandarin oranges, segments in juice	¼ cup	25	0	French, regular	2 tbsp.	135	15
Olives, ripe	2 tbsp.	30	4	Italian, low-calorie	2 tbsp.	15	0
Raisins	2 tbsp.	60	0	Italian, regular	2 tbsp.	160	15
Beans, Nuts, and Seeds				Lemon juice	2 tbsp.	8	0
Chickpeas	¼ cup	40	<1	Oil and vinegar	2 tbsp.	100	8
Kidney beans	¼ cup	55	trace	Thousand Island, regular	2 tbsp.	120	10
Sunflower seeds	1 tbsp.	80	7	Vinegar	2 tbsp.	4	0
Tofu (raw, firm)	¼ cup (about. 3 oz.)	90	6				

*Nutrient values have been rounded.

[†]"Trace" on all the vegetables and fruits is about .05 to 0.2 gram of fat.

calories on a bed of raw vegetables. "Dressed" side dishes (potato salad, pasta salad, ambrosia, and macaroni salad), creamy soups, cheese and crackers, even desserts—all with more calories—line up on the salad bar, too.

To control calories and fat in your salad concoctions and to fill your plate with nourishment:

● Pace yourself. Check out the salad bar from end to end before you even begin filling your plate.

● Use a small salad plate, not a dinner plate, if you're tempted to overdo.

● Start with greens. Dark-green leafy vegetables such as spinach and romaine supply more nutrients than iceberg lettuce does.

● Spoon on plenty of brightly colored vegetables (broccoli, peppers, beets, carrots, to name a few), legumes (such as kidney and garbanzo beans), and fruits for their nutrient, fiber, and phytonutrient benefits. They're low in fat, too.

● Make it a hearty salad with protein-rich ingredients: legumes, lean meat, turkey, crabmeat or surimi, tuna, eggs, and cheese. Cottage cheese, other cheese, and yogurt on the salad bar also add calcium to your salad.

● Lighten up on higher-fat toppings and mayonnaise-based side salads.

● Dress your salad for success! A 2-tablespoon ladle of French, Italian, blue cheese, or Thousand Island dressing adds about 150 calories to an otherwise low-calorie salad. Too often, people spoon on double or triple that amount and overpower the delicate flavor of the salad ingredients. Go easy, try a low-fat or fat-free dressing—or sprinkle on just a splash of flavored vinegar or lemon juice.

Eating Out Safely!

Almost nothing can ruin a trip or a pleasant meal out more than foodborne illness. Although restaurants in the United States, Canada, and many other developed nations must pass strict public health regulations, you're still wise to double-check for cleanliness. Any restaurant can have an occasional lapse in sanitation procedure, and in some parts of the world, these regulations may not exist. Hotel staff often can recommend restaurants with high standards.

These tips can help ensure that the meal you eat away from home won't come back to "bite you":

● Check for cleanliness. Although you probably can't see into the kitchen, you can learn a lot about a restaurant by looking at the public areas. Look for:
  ● Tables that are wiped clean—using clean cloths
  ● Well-groomed servers
  ● Clean silverware, tablecloths, glasses, and dishes
  ● Adequate screening over windows and doors to keep out insects
  ● No flies or roaches, which can spread disease
  ● Clean rest rooms with soap, hot water, and towels or air dryers
  ● A clean exterior with no uncovered garbage outside

● Before you eat from a food bar, check the temperature. A hot buffet should be piping hot. And a cold salad bar should be well chilled or placed on ice.

● Order food from food bars and displays only if the food is properly covered with a sneeze guard or a hood. This includes desserts and appetizers.

● Avoid eating raw meat; it may carry bacteria and parasites. These menu items are served raw: steak tartare (raw ground beef and raw eggs), carpaccio (thin-sliced raw beef), and sashimi (raw fish). Sushi, often made with raw fish, is popular among many restaurantgoers. *See "Is Raw Seafood Safe to Eat?" in chapter 12 for specific guidance on sashimi.*

● Check your burger. It should be cooked until the center is no longer pink and the juices run clear, usually "medium" or "medium-well." If it's not cooked thoroughly, send it back!

Safe Take-out

Take-out foods are becoming essential to today's busy lifestyles. Because many buy-and-go foods are perishable, you need to handle them with care to avoid foodborne illness. Keep hot foods above 140° F and cold foods at 40° F or below. Discard any perishable foods kept at room temperature for more than two hours. If the temperature inside or outdoors tops 90° F, toss it after one hour.

For hot foods . . .

● Make sure the food is hot when you get it. Then eat it within two hours.

● If the food won't be eaten for more than two hours, refrigerate it in shallow, covered containers. Then reheat it to a temperature of 165° F, or until it's hot and steaming. Check the temperature with a meat thermometer. *See "Using a Meat Thermometer" in chapter 12.* Or reheat it, covered and rotated for even heating, in a microwave oven. Then let the food stand for two minutes for more thorough heating.

● Keep hot take-out food in the oven or in a slow cooker at 140° F or above—but not if you'll hold it much longer than two hours. Food loses its appeal if it's held longer. Cover it with foil to keep it moist. And check the temperature with a meat thermometer.

For cold foods . . .

● If you don't eat cold take-out foods right away, refrigerate them, or store them in chilled, insulated coolers

● For deli platters that stay on the buffet, keep the platters on bowls of ice.

For more information on foodborne illness—and how to prevent it—see chapter 12, "The Safe Kitchen."

Fast Food, Healthful Food

Dependence on fast foods goes back thousands of years. In the Roman Forum more than two thousand years ago, urban consumers ate sausages and honey cakes. The Chinese ate stuffed buns in the twelfth century. And five hundred years ago, Spaniards encountered tacos in the marketplaces of today's Mexico.

Fast food has been part of the American food culture for many more years than most people realize. If your great-grandparents traveled by train in the early 1900s, they likely devoured "fast food," or quick meals, from the dining car. When the automobile took over, the dining-car concept was transformed and reinvented as fast-food restaurants, dotting the roadside. Eating in the car isn't new, either; the popular "drive-in" restaurant of the 1950s evolved into the "drive-through" window today.

As we know it today, the so-called fast-food chain, or quick-service restaurant, is a phenomenon that's

Have You Ever Wondered

. . . how to feel comfortable when you dine alone? Any discomfort from eating alone shouldn't make you skip a meal. In reality, you're likely the only one who notices that you're a solo diner. If you feel conspicuous, ask for a table off to the side. Take an avid interest in your surroundings. Talk with the server; study the menu and the decor. While you wait, be productive: read, write a letter, jot down your "to do" list, do a little office work, or simply reflect on your day. Once your meal is served, put down your book or office work; eat slowly and savor the flavors. When you're traveling and truly need to let down and be alone, choose a hotel with room service!

. . . what spa cuisine is? Although the term isn't regulated, spa cuisine often refers to health-positioned food preparation, perhaps promoted in resorts or health club cafés. On a menu that offers "spa cuisine" you may find foods with less fat or calories, more fruits, vegetables, and fiber-rich grains, or perhaps smaller portions. Like any cuisine, you need to ask questions about the menu and order with consumer savvy.

only about fifty years old, launched for a post-World War II, fast-oriented, mobile society. At that same time, eating out became more than an occasional treat. At the start, fast food was limited to mainly fried chicken, hamburgers, French fries, ice cream, shakes, and soft drinks.

Today's fast-food menus offer far more options than traditional fare. From grilled chicken sandwiches, wraps, and broiled fish, to salads, to low-fat milk and fruit smoothies, you have plenty to choose from, including lower-calorie, lower-fat, and fresh menu items. You might even find pizza, seafood, pasta, Tex-Mex food, stuffed baked potatoes, noodles, and deli items along with quick ethnic cuisine. Breakfast also has become a big fast-food business. Even convenience stores where you gas up your car sell fast food—truly the "dining car" of the highway!

Are fast-food meals healthful? Overall, yes—if you choose wisely. Because menus are so varied, no overall comment can describe their nutritional value. Traditional meals—a burger, fries, a fried fruit turnover, and a soft drink, or fried chicken, biscuit, creamy slaw, and mashed potatoes with gravy—remain *high* in calories and fat, including saturated fat, and sodium, but *low* in vitamins A and C, calcium, and fiber, and *short* on fruits and vegetables. In response to consumer demand, many of today's fast-food restaurants also offer more varied menus—and lower-fat options.

Fast-Food Pointers

If you're a regular at the fast-food counter, keep these pointers in mind. As general advice for healthful

eating, order more fruits and vegetables, more foods with bone-building calcium, less fat and added sugars, and reasonably sized portions.

To watch your portions . . .

● Be aware of portions that may be larger than you need: "deluxe," "super," and "mega" may be different sizes of "big." Whether it's a sandwich, fries, a milk shake, or another menu option, bigger portions mean

 Your Nutrition Checkup

How Do Your Fast-Food Meals Measure Up?

Reflect back on your last fast-food meal or snack. What did you order? Did you consider how your menu choices fit within your overall diet? Take a moment to rate your food choices.

● On the following chart, write in the last fast-food meal or snack you ordered and the portion size for each menu item.

● *Using the chart "FFF—Fast Food Facts" in this chapter,* find out how your food choices measured up. Write in the amount of calories, fat, saturated fat, cholesterol, and sodium for each menu item you ordered. Then total the amounts at the bottom of

the chart. Check the restaurant's Web site for the nutritional breakdown of their current menu.

● Go a little farther. Using information from the Food Guide Pyramid in chapter 10, write the food group and the serving(s) from each menu item.

● Surprised by the results? What did you learn about your fast-food choices? What might you change if you order this meal or snack again?

There's no right or wrong answer to fast-food eating. The best meal or snack for you depends on you—your needs, your health, and the overall food choices you make every day!

WRITE IT DOWN

MENU ITEM	SERVING SIZE	CALORIES	FAT (G)	SATURATED FAT (G)	CHOLESTEROL (MG)	SODIUM (MG)	FOOD GROUP/SERVING
TOTALS:							

Fast Food: Beyond Burgers

If you're in a fast-food rut, look around for some quick and different approaches to fast-food eating:

- Sushi bar
- Submarine sandwich spot
- Wrap restaurant
- Bakery-shop deli
- Noodle shop

more calories and likely more fat, cholesterol, and sodium. For most people, the small or regular size is enough.

- Think before you buy. Order takers often promote with marketing questions—for example, "Would you like fries with that?" or "Do you want the value size?" It's okay to say "No."

- Go easy on snacks. A large order of fries and a large soft drink can add a hefty 650 or more calories to your day's intake!

- Split your order. Halve the calories and double the pleasure by sharing your fries or snack sandwich with a friend!

- Decide *before* you order whether the "value meal" is a good deal. If you don't need the extra food, there's really no extra value; smaller may cost less. Sharing may be a good deal.

For more food variety . . .

- For flavor and nutrition, consider the other foods you have eaten—or will eat—during the day. Order fruits, vegetables, calcium-rich foods, and even whole grains if you can.

- Select a side order of salad, raw vegetables, or coleslaw for added vitamins A and C, and fiber. Boost your calcium intake with a carton of reduced-fat, low-fat, or fat-free milk.

- Try different types of fast foods, not the same foods every day.

- Enjoy fast-food outlets that serve ethnic foods: perhaps Chinese stir-fry dishes, a Mexican burrito, Japanese domburi, or a vegetable-stuffed pita with cucumber-yogurt dressing. Often food courts in shopping malls allow you to travel the world of flavor without leaving home.

Trim the fat and calories . . .

- Learn to spot high-fat foods—then go easy.

- On sandwiches and salads, go easy on condiments, special sauces, and dressings. Just one packet of mayonnaise (about 1 tablespoon) adds about 60 calories and 5 fat grams. The same size packet of tartar sauce has about 70 calories and 8 fat grams. And a 1½-ounce packet of French dressing contains about 185 calories and 17 fat grams. Ask for mustard, catsup, salsa, or low-fat or fat-free condiments, spreads, and dressings (mayonnaise, sour cream, or cream cheese).

- For fried foods, pay attention to the oil used for frying. Most fast-food chains use 100 percent vegetable oil, which may be identified on the menu. Vegetable oil is cholesterol-free and high in polyunsaturated fatty acids; the oil used for frying in the fast-food industry is often high in trans fatty acids. *See "About Trans Fats" in chapter 3.* And when French fries and other foods are fried in fat that's partly beef tallow, these foods contain more cholesterol and saturated fats.

- Better yet, choose fried foods only as "sometimes" foods. Rely mostly on grilled, broiled, steamed, or microwaved fast foods instead.

Eating and Driving: A Safety Issue?

With Americans' hectic lifestyles, more people eat in the car—and more than 70 percent use the drive-through window, according to the National Restaurant Association. However, eating and driving can pose a personal safety risk!

When time is short, many people assume that the fastest food comes from the drive-up window. Not so. Many times the drive-through line is longer than that for counter service. Beyond that, eating or drinking while driving not only can be messy, it's also dangerous when one hand is on the wheel and the other hand is holding a burger or a steaming hot beverage. If the cell phone rings at the same time, you may really be in trouble!

If you do eat in the car, pull over in a parking lot, city park, or by the curb. Then enjoy those few minutes of eating without thinking about driving, too. Better yet, relax with your food in a mall or on a park bench. Then take a brisk walk.

• Read on for more fast-food tips. *Check "FFF—Fast Food Facts" in this chapter,* or look for nutrition information on posters or printed in brochures.

Lighten up on salt . . .

Many fast foods are high in sodium—a challenge if you're sodium-sensitive. For less salt and sodium, ask for unsalted fries. Skip the special sauces, pickles, olives, and relish as well as the bacon, sausage, ham, and deli meat.

Break-FAST

Breakfast out—with the more hectic pace today, it's not surprising that more and more consumers, particularly those heading to work, buy breakfast on the run. It may be a quick breakfast sandwich from the drive-up window, a sit-down meal of eggs and hash browns, or pancakes from the fast-food counter, or coffee and a deli muffin or a bagel to eat at the desk. However, when these quick breakfasts become a regular eating pattern, it's time to take stock of their nutritional impact!

Fast-food menus usually offer fewer options for breakfast than for lunch and dinner. Many of the choices are high in calories, fat, cholesterol, and sodium. Here's some breakfast menu savvy:

• Order the fastest breakfast of all: dry cereal and milk. Cereal offers a serving from the Grains Group, along with complex carbohydrates and B vitamins and almost no fat. If you choose a whole-grain or bran cereal, you get more fiber, too. A carton of milk, which equals one Milk Group serving, supplies about 300 milligrams of calcium; that's about 25 to 30 percent of the calcium you need daily. Pour some on your cereal, perhaps some in your coffee—and drink the rest!

• Start your day with a stack of pancakes. For less fat, use syrup and skip the margarine or the butter. Enjoy half the bacon, or ask for Canadian bacon, which is leaner.

Breakfast: Cut Down on Fat and Sodium

• Go easy on breakfast sandwiches. A typical bacon, egg, and cheese biscuit sandwich has about 475 calories, 30 fat grams, and 1,260 milligrams of sodium. Go for a breakfast (bean and cheese) burrito with 375 calories, 12 fat grams, yet 1,170 milligrams of sodium.

• Ask to skip the bacon or the sausage on your breakfast sandwich. Or substitute ham or Canadian bacon for less fat.

• Order your sandwich on an English muffin, bagel, or even a hamburger bun. To compare, a typical fast-food breakfast biscuit can have about 18 fat grams, and a croissant, about 10 fat grams, compared to 1 fat gram in an English muffin.

• Instead of a doughnut, order an English muffin, bagel, toast, or even a plain soft baked pretzel. To save on fat grams, order cream cheese, margarine, or butter on the side, and spread it on lightly. Or use jam or jelly.

• Be sizewise about muffins and bagels, as well as about croissants and biscuits. Even muffins can be higher in fat than you'd think when they are big. A typical muffin has about 5 fat grams—10 to 15 fat grams or more if it's jumbo-size! And a large bakery bagel can count toward as many as 6 Grains Group servings.

• If you're a fast-food regular, go easy on egg entrées. The reason? A large egg has 213 milligrams of dietary cholesterol. Health experts advise that healthy people consume 300 milligrams of cholesterol or less per day, and eat yolks and whole eggs in moderation. A two-egg breakfast has at least 425 milligrams of cholesterol!

• Order juice as your breakfast beverage. With just one cup or 8-ounce carton of orange juice, you'll get more than 100 percent of the vitamin C your body needs in a day.

• At a deli? Ask for yogurt to go with your bagel and juice. An 8-ounce carton of low-fat fruit yogurt supplies about 315 milligrams of calcium, 225 calories, and just 2 to 3 fat grams.

Burgers, Chicken, or Fish?

Hamburgers may be America's all-time favorite fast food. But chicken and fish have gained a significant market share, in part because consumers perceive them as lower in fat. It's true that chicken and fish sometimes have a lean advantage. However, fast-food preparation—breading, battering, and frying—bump up the calorie and fat content significantly. As a result, a fried fish or fried chicken sandwich may supply more calories and fat than a hamburger.

To keep the lean advantage of hot sandwiches and to boost the contribution of other nutrients, consider this advice:

● Boost the nutrients in all kinds of hot sandwiches—burgers, chicken, or fish—by adding tomato slices and other vegetables. If you're coming up short on calcium, add cheese. For a fiber boost, ask for a whole-wheat bun.

● Cut calories by ordering sandwiches without higher-fat condiments and special sauces, such as mayonnaise-based spreads and tartar sauce. Instead use mustard, relish, or ketchup. As a rule of thumb: calories go up with the number of "extras."

● Skip the super-size sandwich; go for the regular, junior, or single size instead. The bigger size can about double everything, including the calorie, fat, and sodium content. A large hamburger, for example, supplies about 510 calories and 28 fat grams compared with 275 calories and 12 fat grams in a regular hamburger. A regular burger has about 2 ounces of cooked meat, compared with 3 to 4 ounces in a larger sandwich. Double patties are bigger still.

● To lower the calories and the fat, remove the crispy crust from fried chicken and the skin from rotisserie chicken. Get grilled, skinless chicken. If you prefer fried chicken, order the regular variety rather than "extra-crispy," which soaks up more oil when cooked. The batter or the breading may have a high-sodium seasoning, too, so you can lower the sodium by removing the crust. And eat just one piece, rather than a two- or three-piece order. Chicken nuggets are usually fried and may contain skin and meat (white and dark). Poultry skin is high in fat.

● Choose broiled or baked fish if you have a choice. But be aware that the fillets on most fish sandwiches are battered and fried. Go easy on tartar sauce; ask for tomato-based cocktail sauce instead.

On the Side

Food variety adds nutrients, so round out your fast-food meal with veggies, fruit, and calcium-rich foods—perhaps a salad, baked potato, carrot sticks, fruit, juice, milk, or frozen yogurt. In most fast-food restaurants your options are limited. Get the most nutrition mileage from the choices you have.

Spuds

● Order a baked potato as a side dish or an entrée. Served plain, a baked potato is fat-free and cholesterol-free, with almost no sodium. It also supplies complex carbohydrate, fiber, vitamin C, and other vitamins and minerals.

● Go easy on higher-fat toppings: bacon, sour cream, and butter. For more nutrients and usually less calories and fat, top with broccoli, salsa, chili, or cottage cheese. Along with a salad and milk, a broccoli-cheese spud or a chili spud make a nutritious meal!

● Go easy on fries to limit calories and fat in an already higher-fat meal. Or ask for the small order, then share. French fries offer some vitamin C.

● If you have the option, ask for a plain baked potato or mashed potatoes to control fat. Ask for gravy on the side to control how much you add. Find out how mashed potatoes with gravy are prepared; check the nutrition information if it's posted.

● As alternative to fries, fried onion rings, fried okra, and hush puppies, order corn on the cob, green beans, or baked beans if you can.

Salads

● Order a garden salad with dressing on the side. Use a reduced-fat or fat-free dressing. *For tips on eating from the salad bar, see "Sizing Up Salad Bars" earlier in this chapter.*

● Go easy on prepared salads made with a lot of mayonnaise or salad dressing, such as creamy coleslaw, potato salad, or macaroni salad. They have more fat than salads prepared with a vinaigrette dressing, such as coleslaw or three-bean salad in an oil-and-vinegar dressing.

● Order a container of raw veggies or fruit chunks, or whole fruit if you can.

Beverages

● Make beverages count! For both flavor and nutrients, round out your meal with milk or juice. Many fast food chains offer reduced-fat and fat-free milk. For a flavor switch, try chocolate or other flavored milk.

   ● An 8-ounce carton of milk supplies about 300

milligrams of calcium as well as protein, riboflavin, vitamin D, and other nutrients.

● An 8-ounce carton of orange juice supplies 75 milligrams of vitamin C, which more than meets your daily need.

● Go easy on soft drinks. Reasonable amounts are okay sometimes for their fluids, food energy, and enjoyment. They don't, however, contribute other nutrients supplied by milk, or fruit or vegetable juice. Large-size drinks can add up to a lot of calories: 150 for every 12 ounces of regular soft drinks, or 800 calories for a 64-ounce cup! Diet drinks supply essentially no calories—and no nutrients (except water).

● If the added calories match your eating plan, enjoy a milk shake as part of your fast-food meal or snack. A shake of any flavor is a good calcium source—if it's made from milk. A 10-ounce strawberry shake contains about 320 calories. It can serve double duty—as both your beverage and dessert. Super-size shakes, with their 18 ounces, may supply a hefty 575 calories. Some places sell low-fat shakes.

● Try a smoothie bar for a thick blend of juice, fruit, and perhaps yogurt. Consider size. A smoothie that's 20 ounces or more may supply more than you need—including calories. Beware that some smoothies are made with fruit syrup that adds sugar, but not all the nutrients that fruit contains; ask about the ingredients before you order.

● Order a latte, cappuccino, or coffee or hot tea with milk. Milk, rather than cream, is the calcium booster. Creamers are typically high in saturated fats, too. Remember, sweetened ice tea and many flavored coffee drinks have added sugars, too.

● For an ideal thirst quencher, choose water. For added flavor, add a lemon wedge if you can. Unless bottled, it's usually offered free as a customer service—if you ask!

Have You Ever Wondered

... about herbal mix-ins in smoothies? Bee pollen, ginseng, and other herbal mix-ins may cost extra in smoothies, yet not offer the benefits you think. *See "Herbals and Botanicals: Help or Harm?" in chapter 23.*

Desserts

● Go easy on fried fruit fritters or turnovers—eat them only if they fit within your daily calorie and fat budget. They're usually more sugar and fat than fruit.

● Check to see if fresh fruit is available. As another option, bring fresh fruit from home, perhaps an apple, banana, pear, or grapes.

● For a refreshing dessert, enjoy frozen yogurt—or a scoop of ice cream. You may find low-fat versions on the menu. Either way, the small or kids' size offers a taste without indulging. For fewer calories, go easy on fudge sauce, candy pieces, or syrup toppings. A little of these toppings goes a long way. Ask for cut-up or dried fruit, nuts, or granola instead.

Pizza—as You Like It!

Pizza is nutritious fast food with the nutritional benefits of three or more food groups in one or two slices. The crust supplies complex carbohydrates and B vitamins, the cheese is a good source of calcium

PIZZA TOPPINGS

ENJOY MORE OFTEN	ENJOY SOMETIMES
Artichoke hearts	Anchovies
Bell peppers	Bacon
Broccoli florets	Extra cheese
Canadian bacon or lean ham	Pepperoni
Crabmeat	Prosciutto
Eggplant slices	Sausage
Green onions, chopped	
Jalapeño peppers	
Lean ground meat	
Mushroom slices	
Onion slices	
Pineapple chunks	
Shrimp	
Spinach	
Tomato slices	
Tuna	
Zucchini slices	

and protein, and the tomato sauce and vegetable toppings add vitamins A, C, and phytonutrients. Meat or seafood toppers add protein, iron, and some vitamins, too.

The actual nutrient content depends on what you put on top—and the type of crust you order. The good news is: You can be the architect of your pizza, controlling the toppings along with the nutrient and calorie content and the flavor.

● Consider the crust. For more fiber, build your pizza on a whole-wheat crust. To trim the calories, order a thin-crust pizza rather than a thick-crust or deep-dish pizza. A stuffed-crust pizza can have considerably more calories and fat than a thinner-crust pizza; for example, 1 slice of a large stuffed-crust pizza may have 20 fat grams or more, and 450 calories or more.

● Load up on vegetable and fruit toppings for less fat, more fiber, and more vitamins. *Check out "Pizza Toppings" in this chapter for low-fat choices.*

● Go easy on higher-fat toppings: bacon, pepperoni, prosciutto, sausage, olives, anchovies, and extra cheese. If you like higher-fat toppings, try to stick with just one. If your blood pressure is sodium-sensitive, know that these foods add sodium, too. Many combination or deluxe pizzas have several high-fat toppings.

● Choose lean toppings from the Meat and Beans Group, such as lean ham, Canadian bacon, or shrimp.

● Enjoy the variety of toppings and new combinations available in some pizza parlors. Many new toppings are vegetables—artichoke hearts, broccoli florets, eggplant, red bell peppers, and asparagus spears, as well as salmon, tuna, chicken, and shrimp! Want more flavor? Sprinkle on hot pepper flakes for no calories but lots of flavor.

● Order a salad to complement your pizza. Salad not only adds nutrients and fiber, it also helps you fill up. You may be less likely to eat another pizza slice.

● Order a reasonable-size pizza. Limit yourself to two or three slices—or one slice if you're really watching calories. Calories from any pizza, even a veggie pizza, add up when you eat just one more slice. A typical slice—an eighth of a 12-inch thin-crust meat and cheese pizza—supplies about 185 calories.

● If a bigger size is the better deal, wrap up the extra

for the fridge before you start eating. You'll enjoy pizza again—and save time with lunch—the next day!

● Go halfzies. Order half the pizza your way if someone else prefers toppings with more fat. In that way you both get what you want.

● For a different flavor, enjoy wood oven-baked pizza, or pizza with a regional twist: perhaps a Southwest pizza; a Cajun-style pizza; or a Hawaiian pizza with pineapple and lean ham.

Deli Sandwiches and Wraps

Sandwiches, subs, and wraps, as well as yogurt, fruit, salads, soups, bagels and muffins, milk, flavored waters, coffee, and tea—the deli bar sells an array of foods and beverages. Of the many foods, the sandwich takes center stage. The great thing is that you often can order a deli sandwich just as you want it!

● Just start with bread. Choose a whole-grain bread, roll, or pita pocket for more fiber. Or try a bagel or herbed foccacia.

● Next, the filling—2 to 3 ounces of lean meat or poultry contribute protein, iron, and other nutrients. Add a slice of cheese to boost the calcium content. For fillings with less fat, order lean roast beef, ham, chicken breast, or turkey. Some delis use meats that are 90 percent or more fat-free—just ask. Request tuna, ham, or egg salad made with less mayonnaise or with reduced-fat or fat-free dressing if available.

● Have your sandwich made to order with a spread that adds flavor, such as mustard or fat-free dressing. To control fat and calories, ask the server to go easy on higher-fat spreads.

● Layer on vegetables: perhaps red or green peppers, jalapeños, tomatoes, sprouts, cucumbers, carrot shreds, onions, or grilled veggies. They're low in fat, and they supply vitamins A and C, fiber, and other nutrients.

● Choose sandwich accompaniments to fit your healthful eating style. To cut down on fat, ask for carrot or green pepper sticks rather than chips or creamy slaw. For less sodium, enjoy a cucumber spear instead of a pickle.

● Look for a sandwich "wrap" in a soft tortilla. Often the fillings are low in fat, perhaps rice blended with

FFF—Fast Food Facts

Menu Item	Portion Size	Calories	Fat (g)	Saturated Fat (g)	Cholesterol (mg)	Sodium (mg)
Breakfast Items						
Egg and sausage biscuit	1 (180 g)	580	39	15	300	1,140
Egg and cheese croissant	1 (127 g)	370	25	14	215	550
Danish, cheese	1 (91 g)	355	25	5	20	320
Danish, fruit	1 (94 g)	335	16	3	20	330
English muffin with butter	1 (63 g)	190	6	2	15	390
English muffin with egg, cheese, and Canadian bacon	1 (146 g)	385	20	9	235	790
French toast sticks	5 (141 g)	515	29	5	75	500
Hash brown potatoes	½ cup	150	9	4	10	290
Pancakes with butter and syrup	3 (232 g)	520	14	6	60	1,100
Chicken						
Chicken nuggets	6 pieces (102 g)	290	18	6	60	540
Fried chicken, dark meat	drumstick and thigh	430	27	7	165	760
Fried chicken, white meat	side breast and wing	495	30	8	150	980
Chicken fillet sandwich	1 (182 g)	515	30	9	60	960
Rotisserie chicken white meat, quarter with skin	5 oz.	330	18	5	150	530
Rotisserie chicken dark meat quarter with skin	5 oz.	330	22	7	150	450
Grilled chicken breast sandwich	1	310	9	1	60	890
Fish						
Fish fillet, fried	3 oz. (91 g)	210	11	3	30	480
Fish sandwich with tartar sauce	1 (158 g)	430	23	5	55	620
Sandwiches						
Bacon cheeseburger, large	1 (195 g)	610	37	16	110	1,040
Cheeseburger, regular	1 (102 g)	320	15	6	50	500
Hamburger, regular	1 (90 g)	230	8	3	35	475
Hamburger, large, with lettuce and tomato	1 (218 g)	510	27	10	85	830
Hamburger, double meat patty	1 (226 g)	540	27	10	120	790
Submarine sandwich	1 (228 g)	455	19	7	35	1,650
Roast beef sandwich	1 (139 g)	345	14	4	50	790
Hot dog	1 (98 g)	240	15	5	45	670
Chili dog	1 (114 g)	295	13	5	50	480
Mexican						
Taco, small	1 (171 g)	370	21	11	55	800
Taco salad, large with shell	21 oz.	905	61	19	80	910
Burrito, bean and cheese	2 (186 g)	375	12	7	30	1,170
Burrito, beans and meat	2 (230 g)	510	18	8	50	1,340
Enchilada, beef and cheese	1 (192 g)	325	18	9	40	1,320
Frijoles (refried beans) with cheese	1 cup (167 g)	225	8	4	35	880
Nachos with cheese	6–8 nachos (113 g)	345	19	8	20	820
Nachos with cheese, beans, beef, and peppers	6–8 nachos (255 g)	570	31	13	20	1,800

FFF—Fast Food Facts (continued)

Menu Item	Portion Size	Calories	Fat (g)	Saturated Fat (g)	Cholesterol (mg)	Sodium (mg)
Other						
Pizza, cheese	⅛ of 12-in. pie (63 g)	140	3	2	10	340
Pizza, meat and vegetables	⅛ of 12-in. pie (79 g)	185	5	2	20	380
Pizza, pepperoni	⅛ of 12-in. pie (71 g)	180	7	2	15	270
Chili con carne	1 cup (253 g)	255	8	3	135	1,010
Sides						
Coleslaw	¾ cup (99 g)	145	11	2	5	270
French fries, fried in vegetable oil	30–40 fries (115 g)	355	19	6	0	190
	20–25 fries (76 g)	235	12	4	0	120
Onion rings	8–9 rings (83 g)	275	16	7	15	430
Potatoes, mashed, with gravy	½ cup (136 g)	120	6	1	0	440
Potato, large, baked, plain	1 (8.8 oz.)	270	<1	Trace	0	20
Potato, large, baked, with cheese and broccoli	1 (339 g)	400	21	9	20	480
Potato, large, baked, with cheese and chili	1 (335 g)	480	22	13	30	700
New potatoes	1 cup (4.6 oz.)	130	4	<1	0	20
Salad, vegetables without dressing*	1½ cups (207 g)	30	<1	0	0	50
Salad with egg and cheese, without dressing*	1½ cups (217 g)	100	6	3	100	120
Salad with chicken without dressing*	1½ cups (217 g)	105	2	<1	70	210
Vegetables, steamed	1 cup (3.7 oz.)	30	<1	Trace	0	10
BBQ baked beans	¾ cup (156 g)	130	3	1	5	760
Pasta salad, tortellini	1 cup	430	25	5	55	660
Desserts						
Cookies, animal crackers	1 box	300	9	4	10	270
Cookies, chocolate chip	1 box	235	12	5	10	190
Sundae, hot fudge	1 (158 g)	285	9	5	20	180
Ice milk, soft serve	1 cone (103 g)	165	6	4	30	90
Fruit pie, fried	1 pie (85 g)	265	14	6	15	330
Beverages						
Milk, whole	8 oz.	150	8	5	35	120
Milk, 2% reduced-fat	8 oz.	120	5	3	20	120
Milk, fat-free	8 oz.	85	<1	<1	5	130
Milk, chocolate, 2% reduced-fat	8 oz.	180	5	3	15	150
Soft drink, cola, regular	12 oz.	150	0	0	0	10
Soft drink, cola, calorie-free	12 oz.	1	0	0	0	10
Iced tea, sweetened	12 oz.	135	0	0	0	10
Iced tea, unsweetened	12 oz.	5	0	0	0	<10
Orange juice	8 oz.	105	<1	0	0	6
Shake, chocolate	10 oz.	360	11	7	35	270
Shake, low-fat, chocolate	10 oz.	320	2	<1	10	240
Coffee, black	6 oz.	5	0	0	0	<10
Coffee with 1 tbsp. half-and-half cream	6 oz.	25	2	1	5	10

See "Build a Healthful Salad" in this chapter for nutrition information about salad dressings.

seafood, shredded chicken, or vegetables, or grilled vegetables and chicken breast.

● When sandwiches, subs, and wraps get big, buy one to split. Then share or keep some in the fridge for the next day.

Eating Out Ethnic Style

As a nation of immigrants, the United States has always been home to ethnic cuisine. The real interest in "foreign theme" restaurants grew in the 1960s with pizza parlors and Japanese tabletop cooking. From there, our exposure to ethnic foods became more sophisticated. We added Mexican and more Asian flavors to our restaurant repertoire. Today, ethnic restaurants of one kind or another appear in almost every city and town.

What ethnic cuisines are most popular? Italian, Mexican, and Chinese (Cantonese), say trendtrackers. In fact, they're so mainstream today that they're no longer considered ethnic. French and fine Italian cuisines have been upscale restaurant cuisine for years. According to the National Restaurant Association, our appreciation for ethnic flavors is growing, with more restaurants featuring Japanese (sushi), Thai, Caribbean, and Middle Eastern cuisines. From every corner of the globe, urban areas offer even more ethnic flavors to try!

For fun, find the restaurant pages of your phone book. Now count—how many different ethnic cuisines could you enjoy? To expand the variety in your eating style, try a new cuisine the next time you eat out!

Italian . . . Not Just Pizza and Pasta!

Italian cuisine is the most popular restaurant food in the United States. Two-thirds of all restaurants feature Italian dishes—and not just pizza and pasta. With foods from every region, Italian foods are simple, flavorful, and nourishing.

Italian food is one of several Mediterranean cuisines receiving attention from both food and nutrition experts. Featuring pasta, risotto (rice dish), and polenta (cornmeal dish), Italian food is high in complex carbohydrates. The cuisine relies on smaller meat portions, and cheese is used to flavor many dishes.

Have You Ever Wondered

. . . what "primavera" and "fresco" on menus mean? Translated from Italian, "primavera" means "spring style." In cooking terms it refers to dishes prepared with raw or lightly cooked fresh vegetables. "Fresco" means fresh.

Particularly with the foods of southern Italy, olive oil is the primary cooking fat, in contrast to butter, used in many northern Italian dishes. High in monounsaturated fatty acids, olive oil has some nutritional benefits. Regardless, go easy; any oil is still fat, with the same number of calories per ounce as margarine and butter. *For more about this cuisine, see "Take Your Taste Buds to the Mediterranean" in chapter 9.* Consider these tips the next time you order Italian foods in any restaurant:

● Enjoy crusty Italian bread—a slice or two, but not the whole basket! For less fat, go easy on butter or on olive oil for dipping, or enjoy the flavor of fresh bread as it is, without a spread. *Hint:* Garlic bread usually is lathered in high-fat spreads, Parmesan cheese, and garlic before it arrives at your table. Plain bread is a lower-calorie, lower-fat choice.

● Go easy on antipasto. "Antipasto" means "before the pasta," and it usually refers to a variety of hot or cold appetizers. In the Mediterranean tradition, they include cheese, olives, smoked meats, and marinated vegetables and fish. While they're nutritious, some may be high in fat and sodium. Nibbling appetizers, followed by a heavy meal, may add up to more calories than you expect.

● Order a fresh garden salad, or "insalata," to round out your meal, with salad dressing, perhaps herbed vinegar and olive oil, served on the side. Salads in Italian restaurants often are tossed with a variety of raw vegetables and mixed greens, including arugula, radicchio, bell peppers, tomatoes, and onions. As an entrée, salad with bread makes a nice, light meal.

● Look for traditional bean and vegetable dishes on many Italian menus. Minestrone is a hearty, tomato-based soup with beans, vegetables, and pasta. White beans, called "fagioli," are featured in soups and risotto (rice dishes). "Florentine" dishes are prepared with spinach.

● Know menu lingo. For example, dishes described as "fritto" (fried) or "crema" (creamed) are higher in fat. "Primavera" refers to dishes prepared with fresh vegetables and herbs. Sometimes primavera dishes are served with a creamy sauce; ask your server.

● For enjoyment, order different types of pasta dishes—in shapes and sizes you may not find on supermarket shelves. Made of flour and water, pasta is a carbohydrate-rich food. Fat comes from the sauces and other ingredients tossed with pasta. Did you know that a tomato-based sauce usually has fewer calories than a creamy white pasta sauce or a pesto sauce? Look for marinara and other tomato-based sauces that usually have more vegetables and less fat, too, than creamy white sauces such as alfredo and carbonara. *See "Gourmet's Guide to Sauces" earlier in this chapter.*

● As a change of pace, order polenta, gnocchi, or risotto instead of pasta. Ask how these are made before ordering.

● *Polenta,* similar to a cornmeal mush, typically is served with sauce, vegetables, and meat; some ingredients may have more fat.

● *Gnocchi,* usually made from potatoes or flour, means dumplings; sometimes eggs, cheese, or chopped vegetables are mixed into the dough. After they're cooked in boiling water they may be baked or fried, then served with a flavorful sauce.

● *Risotto,* typically made from arborio rice, usually is cooked in broth and perhaps butter, often with meat, seafood, cheese, and vegetables. If your blood pressure is sodium-sensitive, be aware that the broth may be salty.

● As another option, order ravioli, which are square "pillows" of pasta filled with meat, seafood, cheese, or vegetables. Usually they're served with a sauce. Ask about preparation before you order; as appetizers, they may be fried.

● Watch portion size. If you know the restaurant offers generous servings, order an appetizer portion, or share with someone else.

● If you need to watch fat carefully, go easy on veal scaloppini, and chicken or veal parmigiana, which are sautéed or pan-fried. Parmigiana entrées—made with Parmesan cheese—also are breaded, so they absorb more fat. As an alternative and a lower-fat option, order chicken or veal cacciatore, marsala, or piccata.

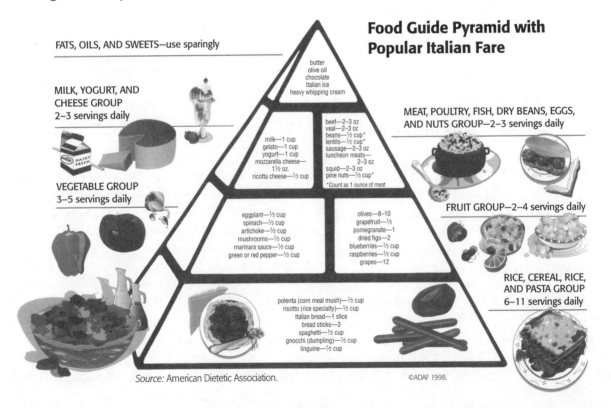

Food Guide Pyramid with Popular Italian Fare

FATS, OILS, AND SWEETS—use sparingly

butter
olive oil
chocolate
Italian ice
heavy whipping cream

MILK, YOGURT, AND CHEESE GROUP
2–3 servings daily

milk—1 cup
gelato—1 cup
yogurt—1 cup
mozzarella cheese—1½ oz.
ricotta cheese—½ cup

MEAT, POULTRY, FISH, DRY BEANS, EGGS, AND NUTS GROUP—2–3 servings daily

beef—2–3 oz
veal—2–3 oz
beans—½ cup*
lentils—½ cup*
sausage—2–3 oz
luncheon meats—2–3 oz
squid—2–3 oz
pine nuts—⅓ cup*
*Count as 1 ounce of meat

VEGETABLE GROUP
3–5 servings daily

eggplant—½ cup
spinach—½ cup
artichoke—½ cup
mushrooms—½ cup
marinara sauce—½ cup
green or red pepper—½ cup

olives—8–10
grapefruit—½
pomegranate—1
dried figs—2
blueberries—½ cup
raspberries—½ cup
grapes—12

FRUIT GROUP—2–4 servings daily

RICE, CEREAL, RICE, AND PASTA GROUP
6–11 servings daily

polenta (corn meal mush)—½ cup
risotto (rice specialty)—½ cup
Italian bread—1 slice
bread sticks—3
spaghetti—½ cup
gnocchi (dumpling)—½ cup
linguine—½ cup

Source: American Dietetic Association.   ©ADAF 1998.

Cacciatore is a tomato-based sauce; marsala is broth-based and cooked with wine; and piccata is pan drippings, lemon juice, and chopped parsley.

From the Italian Menu

Enjoy more often:

- Minestrone soup
- Garden salad
- Breadsticks
- Vinegar and oil dressing
- Pasta with red sauce, such as marinara
- Chicken cacciatore
- Cappuccino (Ask your server to have it made with fat-free or low-fat milk.)
- Italian fruit ice or fruit

Enjoy sometimes:

- Antipasto plates
- Buttered garlic bread
- Creamy Italian dressing
- Pasta with white sauce such as alfredo or carbonara
- Italian sausage and prosciutto
- Fried dishes such as eggplant Parmesan
- Cannoli (Cannoli, cannelloni, and cannellini often get mixed up. Cannoli are deep-fried pastry shells filled with ricotta cheese or whipped cream and perhaps chocolate bits, nuts, and candied fruit. Cannelloni are pasta tubes filled with meat and cheese and topped with sauce. Cannellini are white kidney beans.)

It's Greek Food to Me!

Another Mediterranean cuisine is popular: Greek food. For many consumers, experience with Greek restaurants comes from fast-food courts in shopping malls. The popular gyro sandwich, souvlaki, Greek salad, rice pilaf, moussaka, and baklava are best known. But like other cuisines, full-service restaurants offer far more variety. To order smarter, consider these menu tips:

- For a creamy dressing on salads, or a sauce on pita sandwiches, enjoy tzatziki. It's made with yogurt, garlic, and cucumbers. Sometimes tzatziki is listed on the menu as a salad. Try tzatziki as an appetizer dip with pita bread, too.

- Enjoy smaller amounts of baba ghanouj, a higher-fat dip made with eggplant and olive oil, and of hummus, made with mashed chickpeas and sesame seed paste.

- Flavorful olive oil for dipping is often served with a basket of pita bread. Again, go easy. Although low in saturated fat and cholesterol-free, olive oil contains just as much fat as butter or margarine. Bread often can soak up a lot of oil!

- Ordering saganaki as an appetizer? Saganaki is thick kasseri cheese that's fried and sometimes flamed in brandy. To trim the fat, share with someone else.

- For nutritious fast food order pita bread stuffed with Greek salad, lean meat, tabouli, or other ingredients. Tabouli is bulgur wheat mixed with chopped tomatoes, parsley, mint, olive oil, and lemon juice. For more fiber ask for whole-wheat pita. Another popular use of the pita is the gyro, which is minced lamb molded and roasted vertically. When cooked, the lamb is sliced and tucked into pita bread with grilled onions, bell peppers, and tzatziki sauce.

- As a main dish, look for broiled and grilled meat, poultry, and seafood. The menu might have shish kebob, which is skewered and broiled meat and vegetables; souvlaki, which is lamb marinated in lemon juice, olive oil, and herbs, then skewered and grilled; or plaki, which is fish broiled with tomato sauce and garlic.

- As another menu option, try dolmas, or stuffed vegetables. Grape leaves are most commonly stuffed with ground meat; other vegetables, such as bell peppers, cabbage leaves, eggplant, and squash, are stuffed with mixtures of ground meat, rice, dried fruit, and pine nuts. Because they're steamed or baked, fat usually isn't added with cooking.

- To boost fiber, order dishes made with legumes. In a full-service restaurant you'll likely find mixed dishes and soups made with fava beans and other legumes.

- Order a Greek salad to go with meals. Ask for dressing on the side. And go easy on the higher-fat, higher-sodium ingredients: anchovies, kalamata olives, and feta cheese.

● Go easy also on rich Greek desserts such as baklava. Made with phyllo and plenty of butter, honey or sugar, and nuts, this sweet, compact pastry is very high in calories. It's wonderful-tasting, but a small serving is enough to satisfy a sweet tooth!

From the Greek Menu

Enjoy more often:
- Broiled, grilled, simmered, or stewed dishes
- Greek salad
- Tabouli
- Dolmas
- Tzatziki
- Fresh fruit
- Pita bread

Enjoy sometimes:
- Pan-fried dishes
- Vegetable pies such as spanakopita and tyropita
- Baba ghanouj (a Middle Eastern dish that appears on some Greek menus)
- Baklava
- Deep-fried falafel

Mexican Food: Tacos, Tamales, and More

From fast-food establishments to full-service restaurants, Mexican food and its Tex-Mex offspring are among America's favorite ethnic foods. One-fourth of all restaurants today feature foods with a Mexican flavor. The staples—tortillas, beans, and rice—are great sources of complex carbohydrates, and pinto or black beans supply fiber as well. Moderate portions of meat and poultry contribute adequate, but not lavish, amounts of protein. And beans and rice, or beans and tortillas when eaten together, also supply high-quality protein.

Depending on the choices, Mexican or Tex-Mex cuisine can be high in fat—and sodium, too. In most restaurants, vegetable oil (no longer lard) is the fat used in cooking (except perhaps in refried beans). With vegetable oil, the saturated fat may be lower, but not the calories or the total fat. As with foods of every culture, enjoy variety, but go easy on foods with more fat, cholesterol, and sodium.

Mexican Menu Language

Learn to speak Mexican menu talk. Look for descriptions that offer clues to the fat content.

Menu clues—less fat:
- Asada (grilled)
- Mole sauce (chile-chocolate sauce)
- Served with salsa verde (green chile sauce)
- Simmered
- Tomato sauce, picante
- Topped with lettuce and tomato
- Veracruz-style (tomato sauce)
- With chiles
- Wrapped in a soft tortilla

Menu clues—more fat:
- Crispy
- Fried
- Layered with refried beans
- Mixed with chorizo (Mexican sausage)
- Served in a crisp tortilla basket
- Smothered in cheese sauce
- Topped with guacamole and sour cream
- Chile con queso

● Order guacamole and sour cream on the side so you can control the amount. Or ask for low-fat or fat-free sour cream. For more vitamins A and C, use a heavy hand with tomato-based salsa. Because it's made with tomatoes, onions, chiles, and herbs, it's virtually fat-free, yet bursting with flavor. So are the cilantro, hot sauce, and crushed peppers!

● Ask for soft tacos. Crispy tacos and tostadas are deep-fried.

● Ordering a taco salad? Enjoy, but go easy on the big, crisp tortilla shell it's served in—or the taco chips on top—to trim fat and calories. Enjoy warmed, soft tortillas on the side. And dress it with salsa!

● Go easy on nachos and cheese, or chile con queso, especially if it's just the appetizer before the meal. To cut in half the fat and the calories from cheese, ask for half a ladle of cheese sauce, or half as much cheese shreds. For the starter of chips and salsa, enjoy one basket or less, then have it taken away if you can't resist the urge to nibble.

● Order a low-fat appetizer: gazpacho (chilled tomato soup), jicama and salsa, tortilla soup, or black bean soup.

● Since portions in Mexican meals tend to be large, choose the regular plate, not the "deluxe combo" plate. For most people, the regular plate is plenty! Ask for more shredded lettuce and tomato instead.

● Choose mostly baked or stir-fried entrées such as enchiladas or fajitas served on a soft tortilla. Go easy on fried entrées such as chiles relleños, chimichangas, or flautas.

Although tacos, tamales, enchiladas, and burritos are among the most popular items, especially in Tex-Mex restaurants, Mexican and Southwest restaurants offer a far broader menu. Next time, check the menu further. You may find salads with nopales, or cactus pads; chayote and jicama, which are starchy vegetables; and tomatillos, or green tomatoes. For prepared foods look for Veracruz-style seafood dishes, which are cooked in a herbed tomato sauce; or chile verde, which is pork simmered with vegetables and green chiles.

From the Mexican Menu

Enjoy more often:

● Jicama with fresh lime juice

● Salsa

● Soft tacos

● Burritos, enchiladas, tamales, fajitas

● Red beans and rice*

● Spanish rice*

● Refried beans (no lard)

● Steamed vegetables

● Black bean soup, menudo (spicy soup made with tripe and hominy), gazpacho

● Arroz con pollo (chicken with rice)

● Fruit for dessert such as guava, papaya, or mango

● Flan or pudding

* The fat content varies depending on the ingredients and the preparation method.

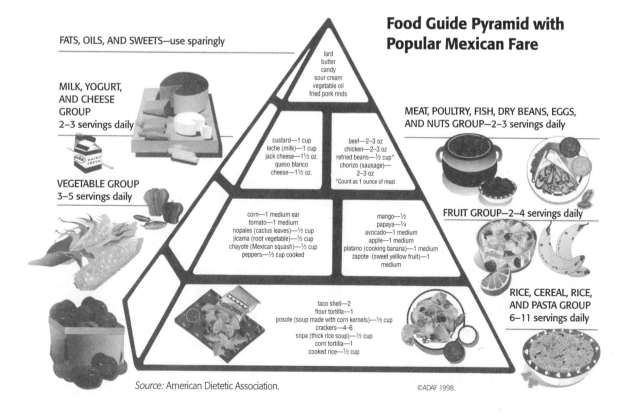

Food Guide Pyramid with Popular Mexican Fare

FATS, OILS, AND SWEETS—use sparingly

lard
butter
candy
sour cream
vegetable oil
fried pork rinds

MILK, YOGURT, AND CHEESE GROUP
2–3 servings daily

custard—1 cup
leche (milk)—1 cup
jack cheese—1½ oz.
queso blanco
cheese—1½ oz.

beef—2–3 oz
chicken—2–3 oz
refried beans—½ cup*
chorizo (sausage)—
2–3 oz
*Count as 1 ounce of meat

MEAT, POULTRY, FISH, DRY BEANS, EGGS, AND NUTS GROUP—2–3 servings daily

VEGETABLE GROUP
3–5 servings daily

corn—1 medium ear
tomato—1 medium
nopales (cactus leaves)—½ cup
jicama (root vegetable)—½ cup
chayote (Mexican squash)—½ cup
peppers—½ cup cooked

mango—½
papaya—¼
avocado—1 medium
apple—1 medium
platano (cooking banana)—1 medium
zapote ·(sweet yelllow fruit)—1
medium

FRUIT GROUP—2–4 servings daily

taco shell—2
flour tortilla—1
posole (soup made with corn kernels)—½ cup
crackers—4–6
sopa (thick rice soup)—½ cup
corn tortilla—1
cooked rice—½ cup

RICE, CEREAL, RICE, AND PASTA GROUP
6–11 servings daily

Source: American Dietetic Association.

©ADAF 1998.

Enjoy less often:

- Guacamole dip with taco chips
- Sour cream and extra cheese
- Crispy, fried tortillas
- Crispy tacos, taco salad
- Tostadas, chile relleños, quesadillas, chimichangas
- Refried beans (cooked in lard)
- Honey-sweetened pastry and sopapillas
- Fried ice cream

Chinese Fare

Most of us have said, "I know a great Chinese restaurant!" Chinese restaurants—full-service or take-out—are among the three most popular for ethnic dining. From a culinary standpoint, Chinese cuisine is complex and highly developed, offering significant contributions to the world's food experiences. With its focus on vegetables, rice, and noodles, Asian-style cooking also has earned its place as a nutritious option in a healthful eating pattern.

Chinese cuisine reflects the different cooking styles, ingredients, and flavorings of China's many regions. Restaurants may specialize in foods from Canton, Hunan, Peking (Beijing), Shanghai, or Szechuan, for example. Cantonese-style cooking is the most popular in the United States, largely due to the number of Cantonese immigrants in the mid-1800s who brought their cooking styles with them. Cantonese cuisine of southeastern China features roasted and grilled meat, steamed dishes, stir-fried dishes, and mild flavors. Szechuan and Hunan foods tend to be hot and spicy, and perhaps higher in fat. Peking cuisine of northeastern China is noted for skillful, subtle uses of seasonings. Shanghai-style has more seafood. The term "Mandarin" on menus usually refers to aristocratic cuisine, featuring the finest aspects of all regional cuisines.

Unlike other cuisines in the United States, Chinese meals emphasize rice or noodles, and vegetables, with their contribution of complex carbohydrates. Vegetables are good sources of fiber, beta carotene (which forms vitamin A) and vitamin C, and phytonutrients, too. Meat, poultry, and seafood are served in small portions, often sliced and cooked with vegetables.

Tofu, or soybean curd, is a common, high-protein, low-fat, cholesterol-free ingredient, too. Many Chinese dishes are roasted, simmered, steamed, or stir-fried, so they're likely to be low in fat.

From a nutritional standpoint, the areas of caution in Chinese dining are the fat and the sodium content. Deep-fat frying is a common cooking technique for many menu items. Sometimes foods are stir-fried in large amounts of oil. For those who are sodium-sensitive, know that two ingredients with more sodium—monosodium glutamate (MSG) and soy sauce—often are used to flavor foods. Even MSG, however, has a third the sodium of table salt. *For more information, see "MSG—Another Flavor Enhancer" in chapter 7.*

Calcium-rich foods are limited on Chinese menus since milk, cheese, and yogurt aren't part of the traditional cuisine. Most calcium comes from fish with edible bones and from vegetables such as broccoli and greens, although the amount of calcium per serving is much lower than a serving of milk.

Whether you eat in or carry out, keep these ordering tips in mind at a Chinese restaurant:

- Enjoy the flavorful soups as a starter or a main dish. Many are made with clear broth with small amounts of meat and vegetables. Made by cooking eggs in the broth, egg drop soup and hot-and-sour soup are higher in cholesterol; the amount, however, is small, since there's not much egg in a single serving.

- Go easy on fried appetizers at the start of your meal. Fried wontons, crab rangoon, and many egg rolls are deep-fat fried. As an option, order steamed spring rolls or egg rolls.

- Enjoy the variety of vegetables in Chinese dishes! Besides the familiar bell peppers, broccoli, cabbage, carrots, chile peppers, green onions, mushrooms, and bean sprouts, Chinese dishes are prepared with bamboo shoots, bok choy, lily pods, napa, snow peas, and other vegetables. For more choices flip to the vegetarian section of the menu, where you'll find dishes featuring tofu and legumes.

- For less fat look for dishes that are braised, roasted, simmered, steamed, and stir-fried (with little or no oil). Ask that stir-fried dishes be cooked in just a small amount of oil.

● Order plain rice and noodles rather than fried versions. Plain rice and noodles usually are lower in sodium, too, than fried versions, which are flavored with soy sauce. Crispy skin on poultry dishes such as Peking duck is high in fat.

● Be aware that the meat, poultry, or fish in sweet-and-sour dishes is typically breaded and deep-fat fried. Instead, ask for roasted or grilled meat with sweet-and-sour sauce to cut down on fat.

● If you're watching your sodium intake, go easy on foods prepared with MSG, soy sauce, or high-sodium sauces such as black bean, hoisin, and oyster sauce. Ask the server to have your dish prepared to order without high-sodium seasonings or sauces. You might ask for light or reduced-sodium soy sauce that you can add yourself. Or instead, choose dishes prepared with hot-mustard, sweet-and-sour, plum, or "duck" sauce, which have less sodium.

● For a small bite, enjoy dim sum. Translated as "little heart," these small portions include steamed dumplings and steamed spring rolls. Go easy on fried dim sum dishes. To order dim sum, you choose your dishes from a server, who passes your table with one dish after another. As a result, you can easily overeat!

● Enjoy your fortune cookie—and the fortune inside! A single cookie has just 15 calories and 0 fat gram. Typically, Chinese meals don't give much attention to sweet desserts. Usually you'll have ice cream, fresh fruit, or almond cookies.

● Control the urge to overeat. In Chinese restaurants portions are often quite ample. For a sit-down meal order the amount you need, not necessarily a meal special with several courses. Ask for half a portion if you can. Plan to share a dish; perhaps order two or three dishes to serve four people. Or take leftovers home with you. Skip popular Chinese buffets, or go easy.

From the Chinese Menu

Enjoy more often:

● Wonton soup
● Hot-and-sour soup
● Steamed spring rolls
● Chicken, scallops, or shrimp with vegetables
● Whole steamed fish
● Steamed rice
● Steamed dumplings and other dim sum
● Soft noodles

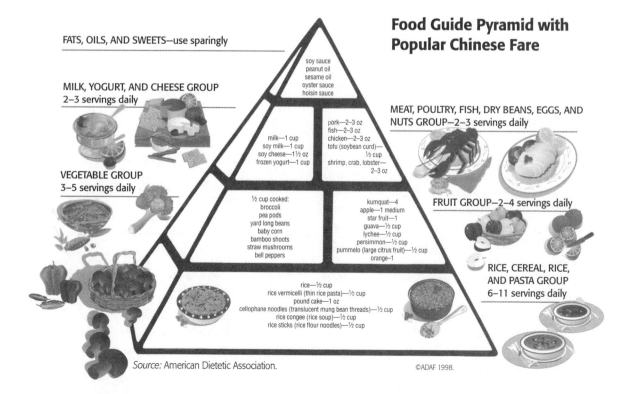

Food Guide Pyramid with Popular Chinese Fare

FATS, OILS, AND SWEETS—use sparingly

soy sauce
peanut oil
sesame oil
oyster sauce
hoisin sauce

MILK, YOGURT, AND CHEESE GROUP
2–3 servings daily

milk—1 cup
soy milk—1 cup
soy cheese—1½ oz
frozen yogurt—1 cup

MEAT, POULTRY, FISH, DRY BEANS, EGGS, AND NUTS GROUP—2–3 servings daily

pork—2–3 oz
fish—2–3 oz
chicken—2–3 oz
tofu (soybean curd)—½ cup
shrimp, crab, lobster—2–3 oz

VEGETABLE GROUP
3–5 servings daily

½ cup cooked:
broccoli
pea pods
yard long beans
baby corn
bamboo shoots
straw mushrooms
bell peppers

kumquat—4
apple—1 medium
star fruit—1
guava—½ cup
lychee—½ cup
persimmon—½ cup
pummelo (large citrus fruit)—½ cup
orange—1

FRUIT GROUP—2–4 servings daily

RICE, CEREAL, RICE, AND PASTA GROUP
6–11 servings daily

rice—½ cup
rice vermicelli (thin rice pasta)—½ cup
pound cake—1 oz
cellophane noodles (translucent mung bean threads)—½ cup
rice congee (rice soup)—½ cup
rice sticks (rice flour noodles)—½ cup

Source: American Dietetic Association.

©ADAF 1998.

- Stir-fried dishes*
- Steamed and simmered dishes
- Tofu
- Fortune cookies

Enjoy less often:

- Fried wontons
- Fried egg rolls or spring rolls
- Peking duck
- Fried fish with lobster sauce
- Fried rice
- Fried dim sum
- Fried noodles
- Fried "crispy" dishes, sweet-and sour dishes with breaded, deep-fried ingredients

* If cooked in just small amounts of oil, they can be quite low in fat. Stir-fry dishes, however, can be quite oily (e.g., lo mein).

Thai and Vietnamese Cuisine

For restaurant patrons who enjoy an Asian kitchen, "spicy hot" defines many Thai dishes. Similar to Thai dishes in many ways, Vietnamese dishes are not known for their spiciness. Both cuisines also are noted for plenty of fruits, vegetables, rice, and noodles. The fresh, unique flavor of these cuisines comes from the contrasting seasonings, unique herbs and spices, and fresh ingredients.

Rice is a staple that's simply cooked or enjoyed as an ingredient in rice noodles, rice flour, and rice "paper." Enjoy it plain: long-grained jasmine rice with its perfumelike flavor; or sticky, plump rice. Try a dish in moistened rice "paper," used to wrap chopped, cooked vegetables; meat, seafood, and poultry; and fresh herbs. Or order translucent rice noodles, tossed in salads and stir-fried dishes. You'll find wheat flour noodles on the menu, too.

Vegetables and fruits add flavor, nutrients, and interest to Thai salads, soups, and mixed dishes. Look for dishes made with less familiar fruits and vegetables such as bamboo shoots, banana blossoms, bananas, bitter melons, green mangoes, pomelos, or straw mushrooms, as well as the familiar: cucumbers, bean sprouts, eggplant, green peppers, or snow peas. Thai restaurants are unique for Asian cuisine because you can order a salad!

In this mixed style of cooking, the portions of meat, poultry, and seafood are reasonable. Look for all kinds of seafood, including shrimp, mussels, and scallops, as well as beef, pork, chicken, and duck.

If you choose to go meatless, look for dishes made with tofu or egg, or combinations of noodles or rice, and vegetables. The popular pad Thai (with noodles, sprouts, tofu, eggs, scallions, and peanuts) may be a good choice; just leave off the eggs and some shrimp on top to cut the cholesterol.

What's the special flavor in Thai cooking? In menu descriptions you'll find a unique variety of herbs native to Thailand that add flavor but no sodium: coriander, ginger, galangal, kaffir lime leaves (citrus leaf), lemongrass, and Thai basil. Look for spices in curry dishes. Peanuts and cashews, common to Thai cooking, may add texture and flavor as well as protein to your dish.

The small, green or red bird's eye chiles (prik kii noo suan) are viciously hot and distinctively Thai. But they aren't the only chiles used in Thai cooking. Check the menu for clues to the "heat." If you can't take the heat, ask for "toned-down Thai." Many dishes can be prepared to suit your taste.

Consider the nutritional bounty in Thai cuisine—especially because it has less fat and sodium—and great flavor! Keep these points in mind:

- If you enjoy Thai food often, go easy on soups, curries, desserts, and other dishes made with a Thai staple: coconut milk or cream. The fat in coconut milk is highly saturated and high in calories. The popular satay (grilled chicken or meat skewers) usually are marinated in curried coconut milk and served with a sauce made of peanuts and coconut milk. To control the amount, ask for the peanut sauce to be served on the side.

- Find out what type of oil the kitchen uses. If it's lard or coconut oil, ask to have vegetable oil substituted.

- Look for stir-fried, sautéed, braised, grilled, and steamed dishes. In Thai cooking you'll also find deep-fried foods and ingredients. Go easy.

- Ask for a light touch with nam bla (Thai fish sauce), a high-sodium sauce, and with soy sauce. Or see if they can use light soy sauce in place of either one. The distinctive flavors of Thai curries come from a blend of nam bla with chiles, garlic, and other unique seasonings: coriander, cumin, and turmeric in Indian-type curries, and gingerroot, lemongrass, and shrimp paste in South Asian-style dishes. Go easy on dishes made with salty condiments such as salty eggs, dried shrimp, and fish paste, too.

If you pick a Vietnamese restaurant, the cuisine is similar, also based on rice, noodles, similar vegetables, seafood, and meat, so order with the same mind-set. Vietnamese cuisine also is flavored with fish sauce but contains more fresh coriander root and leaf (cilantro) and less garlic and chile pepper.

From the Thai and Vietnamese Menu

Enjoy more often:

- Broth-based soups such as tom yum koong
- Spring rolls in moistened rice paper
- Stir-fried noodle dishes such as pad Thai
- Stir-fried or sautéed vegetables with meat, poultry, fish, or tofu
- Broiled or steamed dishes
- Steamed rice
- Tropical fruits and juices
- Grilled or charbroiled meat, chicken, or seafood

Enjoy less often:

- Soups made with coconut milk such as tom ka gai
- Fried spring rolls
- Peanut-coconut milk sauce
- Dishes (including curries) made with coconut milk
- Deep-fried tofu or eggplant
- Dishes with deep-fried fish, duck, or meat
- Fried rice and fried noodles
- Fried banana
- Desserts made with coconut milk

Japanese Cuisine

Although Chinese restaurants have a long history in the United States, interest in Japanese-style restaurants is much newer. It all started with the Japanese steak house. There, Americans experienced the flair of tabletop, stir-fry cooking, seated around the grill. In either full-service or fast-food restaurants, today's Japanese menu offers far more variety.

With its use of rice, noodles, tofu, vegetables, seafood, and small meat portions as staples, and limited use of oils, Japanese cooking is noted for being low in fat. Glazes and sauces are typically made with ingredients that are low in fat: broth, soy sauce, rice vinegar, and sake (rice wine). While some foods are fried, the more common cooking methods are low in fat and include braising, broiling, grilling, simmering, and steaming. Rice, noodles, and vegetables contribute complex carbohydrates, and vegetables supply fiber, beta carotene, and vitamin C. Meat, poultry, seafood, and tofu are high-protein ingredients, usually served in moderate-size portions. Calcium-rich foods are limited. For those whose blood pressure is sodium-sensitive, the use of high-sodium flavoring is a nutrition concern.

To the Japanese cook, artistry ranks as important as nourishment. Edible garnishes of ginger or vegetables, or seaweed carefully wrapped around raw fish and rice, or an artful food arrangement on a plate are among the aesthetic touches that make Japanese food beautiful. Enjoyment of food has always been an important dietary guideline for the Japanese diet!

The language of a Japanese menu might be new to you. Use these guidelines to sharpen your menu savvy:

- Know that tempura is a popular battered, fried dish. Agemono and katsu dishes are also breaded and fried. To control fat and calories, go easy on fried dishes, but don't avoid them altogether or you'll miss some outstanding taste treats! Just balance these foods with other, lower-fat choices.

- Look for menu terms that suggest less fat, such as *nimono* (simmered), *yaki* (broiled), and *yaki-mono* (grilled). Two examples of this for meat, poultry, or fish: yakitori, which is skewered, then grilled or broiled; and teriyaki, which is marinated in soy sauce and mirin (rice wine), then grilled.

- Looking for another low-fat choice? Try sashimi (raw fish) or sushi (vinegared rice, prepared with seaweed, raw fish, and/or vegetables). If sodium is a concern, go easy on the soy sauce for dipping. *See "Is Raw Seafood Safe to Eat?" in chapter 12 for tips on choosing a sushi restaurant.*

- As another meal in a bowl, try domburi, or rice

covered with vegetables, meat, or poultry, and perhaps egg. To cut back on cholesterol, ask that this dish be prepared without the egg.

● If you're watching your sodium intake, go easy on high-sodium sauces such as soy sauce, miso sauce, or teriyaki sauce, as well as broth and pickled vegetables. Many dishes, such as soup, noodle dishes, and stir-fried dishes, also are flavored with soy sauce. As an alternative, ask for dishes prepared without soy sauce, such as shabu shabu, foods that are not marinated, or steamed seafood; then dip them in a low-sodium soy sauce. For flavor without sodium, use a bit of the shredded or mashed green wasabi, which is a very strong and hot horseradish. Beware—a very little wasabi goes a long way!

● For more vegetables, order a salad as a side dish. Try edamame (fresh, steamed soybeans in the pod). For less sodium, ask for a lemon slice to squeeze on your salad, rather than miso dressing. Miso, a common flavoring in Japanese cooking, is derived from fermented soybean paste and is high in sodium.

● As a switch from rice, enjoy Japanese noodles—udon (wheat noodles) or soba (buckwheat noodles). Noodles are often served under cooked dishes such as sukiyaki or in soups.

● Enjoy fresh fruit for dessert. You won't find rich pastries on Japanese menus.

● Take time to enjoy the aesthetics of a Japanese meal in a full-service restaurant. Learn to use chopsticks. They may slow down your eating, and that can be a good part of the dining experience!

From the Japanese Menu

Enjoy more often:
- Stir-fried dishes such as sukiyaki
- Simmered dishes such as shabu shabu
- Grilled dishes such as yakitori
- Stir-fried tofu
- Clear soups such as miso and suimono
- Steamed rice
- Sashimi and sushi

Enjoy less often:
- Deep-fried dishes such as tempura
- Breaded and fried dishes such as tonkatsu
- Fried tofu

Eating for Travelers

Does eating on the road challenge your waistline and good nutrition sense? Overdoing is all too easy—especially when portions are big; the desserts are rich; and the menus, tantalizing. Dehydration and food safety are other issues that demand consideration and action for travelers.

Dining at 35,000 Feet!

What's to eat at 35,000 feet? Food service depends on the carrier, where you sit on the plane, and the length and time of your flight. Usually the meal is lighter in coach than in business or first class. As airlines cut back to control costs, portions have gotten smaller on many carriers, and meal service may be just a light snack, or a pack of pretzels or peanuts, and a beverage.

Whether you're a frequent flier or an occasional passenger, plan ahead so the plane "fare" fits into your eating style—and promotes your health.

● Don't count on an airline meal. Instead, check with your travel agent or the airline before the flight to verify the type of food service.

● If there's no meal served, take your own food on board. In any case, that may be your best bet, especially if you travel with small children. Dried fruit such as apricots; an apple or a banana; raw vegetables; packaged crackers and sliced cheese; muffins; bagels; pretzels; and peanuts are among portable foods that travel well. For safety's sake, don't keep a sandwich with meat or other perishable food for too long at cabin temperature—no more than two hours.

● Want a special meal? If you or your travel agent call at least twenty-four hours before your flight, you can arrange for special meals on major carriers: vegetarian, kosher, low-calorie, low-fat, low-sodium, diabetic, and fruit plate, among others—for no extra cost if the flight has meal service. Often special meals are available for infants and children. On some carriers you can order a Hindu, Muslim, or Asian meal.

● For frequent fliers, your travel agent can keep your meal request in your client profile, along with your

PASSPORT TO FLAVOR: SIX MORE ETHNIC CUISINES

Add variety and adventure to eating out. Try these cuisines, too! Enjoy menu items with fewer calories and less fat more often. Go ahead and enjoy a higher-fat food if you prefer; share or have a smaller portion. This are just a few menu items to whet your appetite:

ENJOY MORE OFTEN	ENJOY LESS OFTEN
Caribbean	
● Beans and rice dishes	● Fried fish
● Chicken and rice	● Fritters (conch fritters)
● Grilled meat and chicken (jerk chicken or goat)	● Fried plantain
● Vegetable stews (callaloo)	
Middle Eastern	
● Bean and bulgur salad	● Baba ghanouj
● Cold yogurt soup	● Fried chickpea cakes (falafel)
● Couscous	● Fried meat-bulgur patties (kibbeh)
● Fatoosh (bread salad)	● Rich pastries, often with honey (baklava)
● Lamb and vegetable stew	
● Rice and lentil/bean dishes	
German	
● Cooked cabbage	● Breaded and fried meat and poultry (schnitzel)
● Dumplings	● Creamy soup
● Potato salad with a sweet-sour dressing	● Noodle and cheese dishes
● Roast pork (lean) with gravy on the side	● Sausages
	● Thicky, creamy gravy
French	
● Broth-based fish soup (bouillabaisse)	● Cheese
● Demiglace sauces	● Cream soups
● Poached fruit	● Creamy sauces
● Roasted or braised meat, poultry, or fish	● Croissants
● Salad greens with vinaigrette	● Goose or duck liver (foie gras)
● Steamed vegetables	● French fries (pommes frites)
● Vegetable casserole (ratatouille)	● Rich desserts (mousse, Napoleon)
	● Soups with gratinée (cheese)
Russian	
● Boiled or baked dumplings (pelmeni)	● Blini
● Broiled meat skewers (shaslyk)	● Dishes made with sour cream gravy (stroganoff)
● Kasha	● Fried dumplings
● Meat-stuffed cabbage	● Salads with mayonnaise or sour cream
● Whole-grain breads	● Soups made with cream or sour cream (borscht)
Indian	
● Baked roti (bread, such as naan)	● Dishes, such as curry dishes, made with coconut milk
● Dishes prepared with yogurt	● Fried bread (poori, paratha)
● Lentil dishes	● Fried dishes (samosa, shami)
● Roasted chicken or fish dishes with vegetable sauces	● Ghee (clarified butter)
● Tandoori cooked chicken	

seating preference. In that way your request is automatic. In fact, the most efficient time to place your request is when you make your reservation.

● Remember: it's okay to say "no." You don't need to eat an airline meal or snack just because it's offered. If you just ate lunch or plan a nice meal when you get on the ground again, let the serving cart roll by.

● To avoid dehydration, drink plenty of fluids (even if you're not thirsty)—8 ounces of fluids for every hour of your flight. Juice and water are great choices. For the same reason, go easy on alcoholic drinks. With the low humidity and recirculating air within the pressurized cabin, airline travel can be dehydrating; you lose body fluids through evaporation on your skin. Rushing to catch a plane may work up a sweat that already puts you in a "fluid deficit." Dehydration only

Your Anti-Jet Lag Plan

The best advice: Organize yourself so you're well rested and relaxed before you travel. Avoid skipping meals as you rush to prepare for your trip; stick to a healthful meal pattern.

When flying, being dehydrated actually promotes jet lag. To minimize the effects, drink a glass of water or juice before your airline flight, then each hour in flight. Alcoholic beverages also can promote dehydration and may increase jet lag. Go easy if you drink them. During long flights, get up, stretch, and walk around the cabin.

Once you're on the ground, keep on drinking fluids. After a long flight, drink extra fluids for several days. Immediately adjust your meals and sleep to the new time if you've traveled over several time zones. If your body clock skips from late afternoon to early morning and you lose the night (as you often do with overseas flights), take a short nap when you arrive if you need to, then continue with a normal day—lunch, dinner, and an early evening. If, instead, you leave in the morning and arrive at night, have dinner and go to bed—even if your body clock says it's just midday.

Be aware that no evidence shows anti-jet lag formulas or diets are effective. You may have heard anti-jet lag claims about a dietary supplement called melatonin. While this claim may be partially true, the amount of melatonin that promotes sleep is far less than the amount in over-the-counter products. *For more information on melatonin and other supplements, see chapter 23.*

aggravates the symptoms of jet lag and causes fatigue. Pack some bottled water in your carry-on luggage as an extra supply. Especially on a long trip, drink plenty of liquids before, during, and after flying.

● Want to relax or sleep on the flight? If you're sensitive to caffeine, avoid caffeinated beverages: coffee, tea, and colas. For some people, too much caffeine can promote sleeplessness, anxiety, and overstimulation . . . especially for those anxious about flying anyway!

● If you drink alcoholic beverages, go easy—even if you have free drink coupons or you're in first class, where they're free. It's wise to stop after one or two drinks. On a long flight, wine or cocktails may not help you sleep—and may not relax you, either. Instead, larger amounts may have the opposite effect, making you more restless.

● When the beverage cart rolls by, make your choice count as one serving from the Food Guide Pyramid—especially if you may come up short during the day. Ask for fruit juice, tomato juice, or milk.

● Especially on a long flight, get out of your seat and move around. Even a little exercise, such as walking the aisles, will help you feel better than just sinking into the seat with your headset on or with a good book.

Travel Fare—on the Ground

For the businessperson, eating on the road can be an "occupational hazard." For the leisure traveler, calories add up, too, especially when food is the main event. Eating just 500 extra calories a day can add up to 3,500 extra calories a week. Unless you compensate with more physical activity, those 3,500 extra calories can turn into a pound of body fat!

● Whether traveling on business or leisure, be a wise restaurant consumer. *As with any meal out, the "Restaurant Eater's Tip List" and "Fast Food, Healthful Food" in this chapter apply to eating when you travel.*

● On an expense account? Avoid the urge to overeat just because you aren't paying the bill. Promising to "cut down when I get back home" may not be enough to keep trim, especially if you're a frequent traveler.

● Schedule your wake-up call to allow time for breakfast. An early morning meal is, after all, a smart way to start any day. If you're in a hotel with room service, order breakfast the night before. *For some quick and nutritious breakfast menus, check "Breakfast on the Road" below.*

● When you work during a meal or a cocktail hour, be as attuned to your food and drink as you are to business issues. Overordering is easy when you're not paying attention to your body's hunger and satiety signals. A second round of drinks or another basket of chips can appear without much notice.

Drinking is often part of the social side of business travel, or viewed by the traveler as a way to relax. However, calories in a cocktail or two, and perhaps wine with dinner, add up fast. Depending on the size, a single drink can supply 10 percent of your day's calorie needs—so go easy. Moreover, be careful that cocktails and salty snacks don't replace a nutritious meal.

Too often people complain that travel upsets their physical activity routine. As a leisure or business traveler, make time to move: explore museums, historic spots, parks, and shops on foot. Take time to use athletic facilities at the hotel or local park. *For tips on fitting physical activity into our travel schedule, see "When You're on the Road" in chapter 19.*

Breakfast on the Road

A 2-egg omelet, 3 strips of bacon, ½ cup hash browns, 1 slice of toast with 2 teaspoons of butter or margarine, ¾ cup of fruit juice, and coffee: this hearty restaurant breakfast can total up to 685 calories and 40 fat grams. For a quick, nutritious start on your day, order one of the following breakfasts instead for 400 calories or less:

● Fresh fruit, bagel with jam, low-fat milk

● Cereal (hot or cold) with low-fat milk, fresh berries or banana, coffee or tea

● Low-fat yogurt, whole-wheat English muffin with spread served on the side, fruit juice or fresh fruit, coffee or tea

● Whole-wheat pancakes topped with fruit; hot cocoa made with milk

● One poached egg, whole-wheat toast with jam, ½ grapefruit, fat-free milk

Ordering just a Continental breakfast (bread, juice, and coffee)? For breads with less fat, ask for a bagel, toast (perhaps whole-wheat or rye), or an English muf-

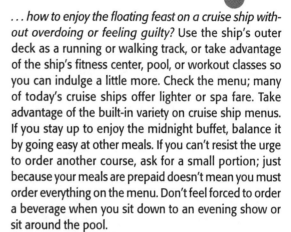

Have You Ever Wondered

… how to enjoy the floating feast on a cruise ship without overdoing or feeling guilty? Use the ship's outer deck as a running or walking track, or take advantage of the ship's fitness center, pool, or workout classes so you can indulge a little more. Check the menu; many of today's cruise ships offer lighter or spa fare. Take advantage of the built-in variety on cruise ship menus. If you stay up to enjoy the midnight buffet, balance it by going easy at other meals. If you can't resist the urge to order another course, ask for a small portion; just because your meals are prepaid doesn't mean you must order everything on the menu. Don't feel forced to order a beverage when you sit down to an evening show or sit around the pool.

Have a problem with seasickness? Skipping food entirely isn't the answer. Instead, ask the passenger services desk for motion sickness medication, and eat something light, perhaps crackers, to keep something in your stomach.

fin with jam or with butter or margarine served on the side. Skip doughnuts, sweet rolls, croissants, and other pastries to cut down on fat.

Have Food, Will Travel

If your job, vacation, or weekend outings take you on the road, brown-bag it—or fill a cooler—to eat as you go. By taking a "survival kit," you don't need to rely on vending machines, convenience stores, fast-food chains, or snack bars.

● Fill sealable plastic bags with vegetable finger foods: raw vegetables (broccoli and cauliflower florets, jicama and carrot sticks, zucchini and bell pepper circles, or snow peas, among others). Take all kinds of seasonal fresh fruit. Besides taking the edge off hunger, fruit can be a thirst quencher.

● Tuck in single-portion beverages: canned or boxed fruit juice, canned tomato juice, boxed milk, and bottled water. Take other portable, nonperishable foods—for example, crackers, peanut butter, raisins, small boxes of ready-to-eat cereal, other dried fruit, pretzels, or plain popcorn. Tuck in packages of instant oatmeal for a quick, easy, hot breakfast in your hotel.

● Stock an insulated cooler with perishable foods: deli sandwiches, yogurt, and cheese, among others. Keep fresh fruit and raw vegetables in the cooler, too, to keep them crisp. *For more tips, see "Carry It Safe" in chapter 12.*

● When you're hungry, stop to eat. Get out of the car. Stretch. Take a short walk. You'll enjoy your meal more—and feel more relaxed as you continue driving. To help prevent constipation—a frequent complaint on long-distance car trips—stop every hour or two for a brisk walk and drink of water.

Food in Faraway Places

From cozy cafés, small food stores, and open-air markets . . . to rice paddies, hillsides with tropical fruit trees, and fishermen hauling in their nets . . . food offers a unique cultural experience for the curious traveler. Americans' growing enjoyment of ethnic foods comes in part from their travel experiences. Savvy travelers take the opportunity to try the adventure of new foods and flavors.

As the world continues to grow smaller, more business and pleasure travelers venture to places where sanitation standards are not as high as in the United States. In certain environments, bacteria, parasites, and viruses can transfer to food from poor sanitation or agricultural practices. To help control the spread of disease, immigration forms for entering the United States ask if you've visited a farm; travelers and their baggage also may go through an agricultural inspection.

No matter what you call it—Montezuma's Revenge, *turista,* or something else—travelers' diarrhea most often is caused by contaminated food and/or water. Typically, it lasts no more than three to four days, but that's enough to upset or even ruin an otherwise wonderful vacation—and certainly puts a business trip into a tailspin. The first bout won't "immunize" you from the next. But the good news is that you can reduce your risk by being cautious and careful. Pay attention to everything you eat and drink.

Food Safety: Ounces of Precaution

Like other types of foodborne illness, travelers' diarrhea is most commonly caused by bacteria—probably 80 percent of the cases. For travelers, improperly handled, contaminated food and drink also can cause *E. coli* infections, hepatitis, giardiasis, shigellosis, and other contagious diseases. *To avoid foodborne illness, the guidelines in "Eating Out Safely!" in this chapter apply no matter where you eat away from home.* In less developed areas, you need to take added precautions: "boil it, cook it, peel it, or forget it." *For more about foodborne illness, see chapter 12.*

● Start several weeks before you go. Especially if you're traveling to developing or rural areas, ask your physician and county health department about immu-

---

TRAVELING ABROAD? EATING FOR SAFETY'S SAKE

BE CAUTIOUS—SKIP THESE FOODS . . .	EAT THESE FOODS INSTEAD . . .
Salads, fruit with peels, raw vegetables (in uncertain areas)	Fruit peeled by you, cooked vegetables
Raw, rare, or partly cooked meat, poultry, or fish	Well-cooked meat, poultry, or fish
Softly scrambled or sunny-side up eggs (unless the egg is well cooked)	Well-cooked scrambled eggs or hard-cooked eggs
Unpasteurized milk	Canned or ultrapasteurized (UHT) boxed milk, or pasteurized milk from a large commercial dairy (ask to be sure)
Cheese made from unpasteurized milk	Cheese made from pasteurized milk
Food and drinks sold by street vendors	Only commercially bottled drinks and commercially packaged foods from vendors

nizations and preventive medication suggested for your travel destination. The Centers for Disease Control and Prevention (*http://www.cdc.gov/travel*) provides food, water, and immunization alerts and advice for travelers in many regions of the world. If you're traveling with an infant, child, or someone at high risk *(see chapter 12),* immunizations are a must.

● Avoid buffets for travelers if food is just rewarmed after sitting for a while, or if it's been kept at ambient, or room, temperature for longer than 1 to 2 hours.

● Be aware: A few fish and shellfish contain toxins even when they're cooked; avoid barracuda and puffer fish. Especially in tropical waters of the West Indies, Pacific, and Indian Oceans, a few other fish are occasionally toxic, such as: tropical reef fish, red snapper, amber jack, grouper, and sea bass. Especially if you're at high risk, be careful.

● Like at home, always wash your hands before eating! Remember, your hands can transfer diarrhea-causing bacteria to your mouth. Carry an antibacterial hand wash, wet wipes, and maybe a small bar of soap.

● When you aren't sure what you may encounter, carry packable foods. Single-serve foods, sold for lunch boxes, are great for travelers.

● Check travel guides and talk to staff in the better hotels, or to your tour guide, to find restaurants with high sanitation standards. Restaurants in better hotels usually have high standards.

● If you travel with a baby, breast milk guarantees food safety. If your infant takes formula, prepare it from commercial powder, and boiled or commercially bottled water. *For more about handling infant formula, see "Another Healthful Option: Bottle-Feeding" in chapter 15.*

What's Safe to Drink?

You're always smart to play it safe. In developed countries, tap water should be fine.

Better hotels in lesser-developed areas also may filter and chlorinate their tap water to make it safe. Before you use water from the faucet, find out if the hotel has a water purification system. When you're not sure, don't drink or brush your teeth with tap water.

Instead, use commercially bottled or canned water with the seal or cap intact. Keep a bottle or can of water in your carry-on bag.

Soft drinks, canned or bottled juices, beer, and wine are safe to drink. Coffee, tea, and other hot beverages are usually safe because the long heating time destroys most and perhaps all of the bacteria, viruses, and parasites that might be present in the water. You also can boil or chemically treat water you drink. *For guidelines on treating water to make it safe for drinking, see "Safe Enough to Drink" in chapter 8.*

In less-developed areas, avoid beverages made with water or ice cubes—unless you know that commercially bottled water was used. Also avoid bottled water served to you without an intact seal or cap; it may have been refilled with local tap water. Be cautious of locally bottled water because the standards may not be high for bottling. Even crystal-clear water in wilderness areas anywhere, including the United States and Canada, should be treated before drinking it.

If You Do Get Sick . . .

● For most cases of travelers' diarrhea, dehydration is the biggest concern. If it strikes you, increase your fluid intake—with plenty of safe water, canned juice, and soup. Canned soft drinks (preferably without caffeine) are okay, too.

● If the problem persists (more than three or four days) or if your symptoms are severe, seek qualified medical care. Your hotel or tour guide should be able to suggest a physician.

● Be prepared before you travel; talk with your physician at home, and take along any medication he or she recommends. *For more about dealing with diarrhea, see "Gastrointestinal Conditions" in chapter 22.*

Need more tips on eating out? Check here for "how-tos":

● Eat out with kids and deal with their "fussy" restaurant eating—see chapter 16.

● Eat out vegetarian-style—see chapter 20.

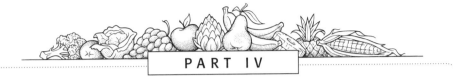

PART IV

Food for Health

Every Age, Every Stage of Life

CHAPTER 15

Off to a Healthy Start

"Should our baby be breast-fed or bottle-fed?" "Can solid foods be given too soon?" "How do I know if my baby has eaten enough?" "Do I give my baby juice from a cup or a bottle?" "Should solid foods be warmed?"

New and experienced parents ask so many questions! Wouldn't it be great for parents and other caregivers if newborns were delivered into their parents' arms with a "how-to" manual filled with feeding instructions? Still, it's amazing how fast infant feeding becomes routine. However, as soon as babies and parents master one feeding stage, they're both ready to move on and learn the next.

As you feed your baby, keep two main goals in mind: provide enough food energy (or calories) and nutrients to support your baby's optimal growth and development . . . and nourish the emotional bonds between you and your baby.

Learning baby feeding basics takes the guesswork out of infant feeding. Practical guidance from your pediatrician, pediatric nurse, registered dietitian, and other parents is a blessing. Your own patience, time—and creativity—build warm, memorable feeding experiences for your baby, your family, and you.

Breast-Feeding Your Baby

Nature provides ideal nourishment for babies: breast milk. Medical and nutrition experts highly recommend breast-feeding for an infant's first year of life, especially during the first few weeks after birth. Breast milk alone can provide enough nourishment to support your baby's optimal growth and development during the first four to six months of life. Then when solid foods are introduced, breast milk can continue to be an important part of your baby's diet until his or her first birthday—and even longer.

The decision to breast-feed is a personal one. It takes into account the mother's lifestyle, economic situation, and cultural beliefs, along with her own physical ability to do so.

For Good Reasons . . .

Breast-feeding offers a host of physical, emotional, and practical benefits for both baby and mother. The benefits of breast-feeding are greatest when mother's

Breast-Feed or Bottle-Feed?

If you're a new parent, either approach—*breast- or bottle-feeding*—can provide adequate nourishment and the strong emotional bond that your growing baby needs. Whenever possible, though, breast milk is best for baby during the first year of life. If you're not sure which approach to use, start with breast-feeding. If it isn't right for you, switch to bottle-feeding. Starting with a bottle, then trying later to breast-feed is difficult. *If you choose to breast-feed, you'll find guidance in "Breast-Feeding Your Baby" on this page. For bottle-feeding, see "Another Healthful Option: Bottle Feeding," also in this chapter.*

milk is your baby's exclusive source of nourishment for at least the first four months; and continues when solids are introduced. However, your baby benefits even when breast-feeding lasts for only a short time, perhaps only during your six- to eight-week mater-nity leave. Let's start with the advantages of breast milk for baby.

Breast milk is a specialized liquid food designed to meet the growth, development, and energy needs of infants. And as a baby matures and grows, the

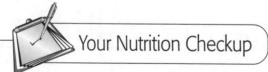

Your Nutrition Checkup

Do You Baby Your Baby?

There's a lot to know about feeding an infant and a toddler—and about ensuring a positive eating experience from day one.

Check yourself out on these baby-feeding basics. Which infant-feeding practices do you follow (or have you followed) when feeding your baby—or perhaps when helping a new parent?

YES	No	
☐	☐	1. Count the number of wet diapers (six or more every twenty-four hours) to make sure your breast- or formula-fed baby is getting enough to eat.
☐	☐	2. Offer breast milk or formula, not cow milk, to your baby up to twelve months of age.
☐	☐	3. If your baby is bottle-fed, choose an iron-fortified formula—unless your baby's doctor advises otherwise.
☐	☐	4. Discard unused expressed breast milk or infant formula after a bottle feeding.
☐	☐	5. Wait until at least four months of age before starting solid foods.
☐	☐	6. Always wash your hands before feeding your baby.
☐	☐	7. Clean all baby-feeding equipment with hot, soapy water, and rinse well.
☐	☐	8. Avoid putting your baby to bed with a bottle.
☐	☐	9. Offer infant cereal that's iron-fortified.
☐	☐	10. Start with single foods—one new food at a time.
☐	☐	11. Monitor your baby's reaction to a new food, in case of a reaction.
☐	☐	12. Offer your baby enough to eat, rather than trying to restrict calories or fat.
☐	☐	13. Check the temperature of food or bottles that are heated to be sure they're evenly warmed, not hot!
☐	☐	14. Try new foods several times, rather than giving up after one or two tries.
☐	☐	15. Let your baby—not you—set the feeding pace.
☐	☐	16. Remain patient as your baby learns to feed himself or herself.
☐	☐	17. Offer smooth foods until your baby is ready for mashed or finely chopped foods.
☐	☐	18. Always stay with your baby while he or she is eating.
☐	☐	19. Discard unused food after a feeding.
☐	☐	20. Make infant feeding a special time to nurture and enjoy your baby—these days don't last!

Now Score Yourself:
Give yourself—and your baby—a big hug if you said "yes" to all twenty items. If you said "no" to any item, read on. Then practice what you learn. Your baby's health depends on it!

composition and amount of breast milk from a healthy mother naturally changes.

For most nutrients, what a mother eats has little if any effect on the nutritional content of breast milk. Selenium and some vitamins are exceptions. But if the mother's nutrient intake is low, her body's own stored nutrients may be used for breast milk, putting her at potential nutritional risk. That's especially true for calcium and the B vitamin folate. For overall health, a nutritious diet during breast-feeding is important, as it was during pregnancy. *For more information, see "For Those Who Breast-Feed" in chapter 17.*

Breast-fed babies get protection from both allergies and common illnesses. Unlike formula, breast milk is rich in antibodies and other substances that help protect an infant from illnesses such as middle ear infections, pneumonia, allergies, intestinal infections, and perhaps sudden infant death syndrome (SIDS). In fact, human milk contains at least a hundred ingredients that infant formula doesn't have!

Colostrum, which is the clear or yellow fluid secreted for two to four days after delivery, is rich in protein and vitamin A, and has higher levels of antibodies than the mature milk that follows. It helps protect a newborn's intestines from infection during the first few months. Think of colostrum as a newborn's first immunization. Colostrum also helps a baby pass his or her first stool.

Breast milk changes with baby's changing needs. From about the third to the tenth day after delivery, the body produces transition milk—a mix of colostrum and mature milk. And then mature milk, bluish in color and thinner in consistency, comes in.

Breast milk is easy for babies to digest. It's clean and safe. Babies may react to something their mothers eat, but they're rarely allergic to their mother's milk. Breast-feeding requires more sucking than bottle-feeding. This helps strengthen and develop the baby's jaw.

An older child who was breast-fed may be less likely to develop certain chronic diseases, including diabetes, some types of cancer, and certain stomach and intestinal diseases. Research in this area is not conclusive, but it is promising.

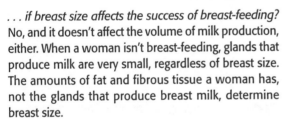

Have You Ever Wondered

. . . if breast size affects the success of breast-feeding? No, and it doesn't affect the volume of milk production, either. When a woman isn't breast-feeding, glands that produce milk are very small, regardless of breast size. The amounts of fat and fibrous tissue a woman has, not the glands that produce breast milk, determine breast size.

. . . if premature babies can breast-feed successfully? Many premature babies can. But if your baby is born prematurely, get help from a lactation counselor, pediatric nurse, or your doctor. You may need to express milk at first; you'll still feed your milk to your baby, perhaps mixed with a nutrient supplement for preterm infants. For premature babies, breast milk offers benefits that help them grow and stay free from illness. There's another reason to start right away: you need to establish your milk supply if you plan to nurse.

. . . if the foods you eat during pregnancy or breast-feeding increase your baby's risk for food allergies? Plenty of research indicates that breast-feeding reduces the risk for food allergies, particularly if there's a family history of allergies. In fact, food allergies are less common in breast-fed babies than in formula-fed babies.

No conclusive evidence shows that all pregnant or nursing mothers should avoid certain foods to protect against allergies. However, as a precaution against potential allergens in breast milk, the American Academy of Pediatrics suggests that nursing mothers of susceptible infants (with a family history of allergies) are wise to skip peanuts and peanut-containing foods.

. . . what to do if your baby reacts to something you eat? Be watchful. If your baby seems to react poorly after you eat certain foods, including those with known allergens, stop eating them for a while. Any allergic reaction usually comes from a protein in a food that a mother consumes, not from breast milk itself. If your pediatrician identifies an allergy, eliminate that food or ingredient in your diet until your baby is weaned. *See "Food Allergies: Commonly Uncommon" in chapter 21.*

How about Mom?

Besides knowing that your baby is well fed, you as a nursing mom get many benefits from breast-feeding, too. The longer a woman breast-feeds, the greater the benefits to both baby and mother.

Breast-feeding nurtures a close bond between mother and baby. That's often a gratifying, emotionally fulfilling extension of pregnancy.

Always ready to feed, breast milk doesn't need measuring, mixing, or warming. So it's easy, especially in the wee hours of the night. With no bottles to prepare or wash and no infant formula to shop for, nursing moms have more time to relax with the baby, or to catch a nap as baby sleeps.

Breast-feeding also may help a new mother regain her prepregnancy figure. Because nursing stimulates the release of oxytocin, a hormone that helps the uterus to contract and shrink, a mother's abdomen trims down more quickly. Her body also uses the fat pad that was deposited on her hips and thighs during pregnancy as some fuel for milk production. Gradual weight loss during breast-feeding doesn't affect milk production.

Breast-feeding is economical, too—even when you account for the extra food a mother eats. The average cost of infant formula is about $100 to $130 per month. Women who breast-feed do need to add about 500 calories a day to their normal diet to cover the energy required for milk production. These calories are best added with extra servings from the five food groups of the Food Guide Pyramid. *For more about the Pyramid, see "The Food Guide Pyramid: Your Healthful Eating Guide" in chapter 10.*

There's less odor involved with breast-feeding. Diaper-changing odor is less offensive, and if a breast-fed infant spits up, there's very little smell, and it doesn't stain clothing.

An added benefit: with nursing, mother takes time to relax every few hours. That's often a welcome and needed change of pace from the added demands of being a new parent.

What about long-term benefits? Women who have breast-fed have a lower risk of developing premenopausal breast cancer, ovarian cancer, and osteoporosis.

To learn more about eating while breast-feeding, see "For Those Who Breast-Feed" in chapter 17.

Do Babies Need Extra Water?

Newborns need little or no extra water. Except for periods of hot weather when your baby perspires, breast milk or infant formula usually supply enough fluid. If water is needed, offer 1 to 2 ounces of plain water after a feeding; water shouldn't take the place of breast milk or formula. For safety's sake when your baby is less than four months of age, boil water first, then chill it, or offer sterilized bottled water. When babies begin eating solid food, offer plain water.

Your child needs water to replace fluids lost through diarrhea or vomiting. Diarrhea and vomiting can lead to dehydration—and its complications—if fluids aren't replaced. Rather than water or juice, your doctor or pediatric nurse may recommend an oral electrolyte maintenance solution, sold near baby foods in your grocery store, to prevent dehydration. Besides fluid, the solution contains glucose (a form of sugar) and minerals (sodium, chloride, and potassium) called electrolytes. Electrolytes help maintain fluid balance in your baby's body cells. These minerals are lost through body fluids.

Important: Consult your doctor or pediatric nurse before feeding an oral electrolyte maintenance solution to children under two years of age (or older children, too). Besides the risk of dehydration, diarrhea and vomiting signal possible illness that may require medical attention! If diarrhea, vomiting, or fever persists longer than twenty-four hours, consult your doctor or pediatric nurse. An electrolyte maintenance solution won't stop diarrhea or vomiting, but it does prevent dehydration.

Perfecting the Breast-Feeding Technique

While breast-feeding is nature's way of providing ideal nutrition for infants, the "art" of breast-feeding might not come as naturally! Like learning any new skill, the keys to success are knowledge, practice, and the support of family, friends, and perhaps coworkers and employers. Discuss your decision to breast-feed with your doctor before delivery and remind hospital staff when you arrive at the hospital.

Getting Started

● To build confidence and to help ensure an adequate milk supply, start nursing as soon after delivery as possible. The best time to start is within twenty to thirty minutes after your baby is born, perhaps right in the delivery room. The first feeding will be short, about ten minutes. "Rooming in" at the hospital may make your first days with nursing more successful.

● Relax and make yourself comfortable. These are important prerequisites. Find a comfortable chair with good arm and back support. Or lie down with pillows strategically positioned to help you support the baby. If you are comfortable and well supported, it's easy to hold your baby, and you won't feel much tension in your neck, back, and shoulders.

● Plan to nurse on demand—that is, whenever your baby says it's time to eat. Increased alertness or activity, rooting toward your breast, or mouthing are all signs that your baby is hungry. Typically, crying is a late signal of hunger. Trying to establish a schedule early on may frustrate you both. As reassurance, you can't "spoil" your baby by feeding him or her on demand. Most babies fall into their own schedule with time.

● Be prepared to nurse very frequently during the first months—about eight to twelve times every twenty-four hours. That's not only because a newborn's stomach is small, but also because nutrient needs are exceptional during this period of rapid growth and development.

Frequent nursing helps establish your milk supply and keeps your breasts from becoming hard and swollen. Breasts that feel full and heavy are your own signal that it's time to nurse. Then as the milk "lets down," or moves from the inner breast to the nipple, you may feel a tingling sensation.

Latching On

Some newborns instinctively start sucking the moment they're first put to their mother's breast. (Maybe they practiced sucking their thumb even before birth.) Others nuzzle first, just to get used to the feeling of warmth, security, and softness from their mother. Either way is normal.

● Help your baby latch on by stroking the cheek nearest your breast. As your baby turns toward your nipple, guide your baby's mouth so that he or she can take in

as much of the areola (dark area of the nipple) as possible, not just the nipple. Newborns have a "rooting reflex" at the breast; they open their mouths naturally.

● Try to offer both breasts at each feeding, and let your baby nurse as long as he or she wants (about ten to twenty minutes on each breast). The last portion of milk your baby drinks from each breast is called "hind milk." This milk is higher in fat and helps the baby feel full and satisfied after feeding.

● Release your baby from the breast by gently putting your finger into the corner of his or her mouth. (Wash your hands before starting to nurse.) This will ease the baby's grip and break the suction without discomfort. Wait until you feel the suction release before pulling away from your baby.

Breast-Feeding: About Your Baby

● Burp your baby when you change breasts and at the end of the feeding. This relieves any discomfort from air swallowed while nursing. To burp a baby, hold him or her upright on your shoulder, or lay your baby "tummy-side down" across your lap. Then gently rub or pat your baby's back. It's normal for a baby to spit up a bit of milk.

● Trust your baby to let you know when he or she has had enough to eat. When your baby feels full, he or she may close his or her lips, turn away, or even fall asleep. Sometimes babies take a rest during a feeding, too, making it hard to know when one feeding stops and the next begins! Is your baby getting enough milk? *See "Nursing: Reassuring Signs of Success" in this chapter.*

● Don't worry about your baby's loose stools. It's normal for a breast-fed baby to have loose, yellowish stools, which may resemble watery "mustard seeds."

Breast-Feeding: About You

● Because babies nurse more vigorously when they start feeding, alternate the breast you offer first. Clip a safety pin to your bra as a reminder. Alternating the breast has several benefits. It ensures that both breasts are emptied regularly, and it helps prevent breast tenderness. Vary the nursing position and allow your nipples to "air dry" after feedings to avoid breast tenderness.

● If your breasts are tender or reddened, or if you feel achy and feverish, contact your doctor. You may have a plugged duct or breast infection (mastitis). An antibiotic might be prescribed. Usually you can keep on nursing while an infection clears up.

● If your breasts feel tight and full, soften them with a warm shower, or express a small amount of milk. To express milk means to stimulate milk flow by hand or with a breast pump. Fullness and discomfort are signs of engorgement and may happen when your milk supply first comes in or if you've gone too long between feedings. Wearing undergarments with proper support helps, too. When breasts become too full, your baby won't be able to latch on correctly, which can cause nipple soreness.

● Don't be surprised if your milk "lets down" and leaks a bit when you hear your baby cry, or even when you think about him or her. It's natural. You might wear pads (without plastic liners) to protect from any leaking.

● If you get thirsty during breast-feeding, pour yourself some water or juice first.

Breast-Feeding Cautions

Use caution if you smoke, drink alcoholic beverages, use some herbal supplements, or take medication. These substances may affect milk production and the let-down reflex. But some pass into the mother's milk, too, at the same levels as in her bloodstream.

When you're nursing, avoid smoking and drinking alcoholic beverages. If you do, do so in moderation— and not right before breast-feeding. When mothers smoke, babies are more likely to get sinus infections, colic, or become fussy. Even secondhand smoke is harmful, so dads and other caregivers are wise to avoid smoking, too. Smoking around babies increases the risk for Sudden Infant Death Syndrome (SIDS).

Talk to your physician about taking medications, including over-the-counter medications, and herbal supplements during breast-feeding. Take your own

---

Some Steps in Breast-Feeding

1. *Snuggle "tummy to tummy."*
Cradle baby in your arms with his or her tummy against your tummy. Baby's head should rest in the bend of your elbow. Your forearm should support the baby's back, with your hand on his bottom.

2. *Place nipple directly in front of your baby's mouth.*
Your baby's head should be in a straight line with his or her body. If his or her head is tilted back or your baby has to turn to reach your nipple, your baby is in the wrong position.

3. *Keep a good position.*
Keep your baby well supported. Make sure your baby is facing straight on to the nipple and does not have his or her head back or neck turned. Make sure your back is straight and you are not leaning over your baby.

4. *Nurse as long as your baby wants.*
Try to use both breasts at each feeding. To take your baby off the breast, release the suction by putting your little finger in the corner of his or her mouth. Wait until you feel the suction release before removing your baby.

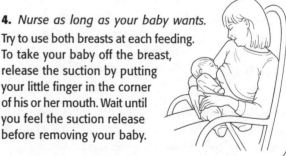

medications, even if they're safe for babies, after nursing, not before.

Getting Help for Breast-Feeding

Remember: you and your baby are learning about breast-feeding together. It's okay to ask for help with feeding techniques. Besides the delivery room nurse, certified lactation consultants in many hospitals teach breast-feeding techniques and answer parents' questions. Some may visit you and your baby later at home to help you perfect your skills.

Within the first one to two weeks, nursing mothers and their newborns should see their pediatrician or healthcare professional. That's another chance to check your feeding techniques. If you're discharged from the hospital less than forty-eight hours after delivery, your first checkup should be within two to four days after birth.

You can also seek help and get support and reassurance from the La Leche League, a registered dietitian (RD), a nurse midwife, or another health professional with experience in lactation counseling. Women who have been successful at breast-feeding, such as La Leche League volunteers, offer great support and practical advice to new mothers. *To find sound, reliable advice on infant feeding and breast-feeding, see "How to Find Nutrition Help . . ." in chapter 24.*

Nursing: Reassuring Signs of Success

Not knowing how much milk their infant consumes, some parents feel uncomfortable about breast-feeding. You probably don't need to worry about having enough milk. Your body is miraculous. If your baby needs and demands more, your body probably will make more milk to satisfy the demands of nursing—even when you try to lose extra pounds gained during pregnancy. Even mothers of twins and triplets can produce enough milk to nurse successfully.

Look for these signs that nursing is going well:

● Following the third or fourth day after birth, your baby has six or more wet diapers, soiled with light-colored urine, every twenty-four hours. Most newborns will wet fewer diapers while receiving only colostrum.

● Your baby nurses at least eight times every twenty-four hours, and maybe up to twelve times daily, in the first month. If your baby sleeps longer than a four-hour stretch, you may need to awaken him or her for a feeding. While nursing, you should feel sucking and hear the infant swallowing.

● The baby's weight steadily increases. Make certain your baby is weighed at the doctor's office within a week or two after delivery to monitor weight gain, and regularly thereafter. During checkups, your baby's weight and length will be measured and assessed. Doctors check a baby's measurements against reference growth curves. If your child doesn't gain weight properly, there may be a feeding problem or a medical problem.

Initially babies may lose a little weight right after their birth. That's normal. However, if your baby doesn't regain his or her birthweight by three weeks of age, your doctor or pediatric nurse will need to monitor him or her frequently to rule out any problems. From birth to six months, babies typically gain 4 to 8 ounces per week.

Have You Ever Wondered

. . . if you can breast-feed if you're sick? Yes—usually it's safe to continue breast-feeding. It even offers added protection for your baby, who already has been exposed to any "bug" before you experienced any symptoms. In breast milk you pass on some immunity through the antibodies your own body produces to fight the infection. If you're taking any medications to treat an illness, talk to your pediatrician to make sure they're compatible with breast-feeding. Severe illness may require weaning; again consult your doctor.

. . . how to successfully breast-feed twins? Wonder if you'll produce enough milk? Remember, your milk supply operates on the principle of supply and demand; with more breast-feeding, your body produces more breast milk. In the early weeks, you may be able to feed both infants simultaneously—an efficient use of time.

Talk to your pediatrician about the need for a supplemental bottle. If your babies are growing normally, it's probably not needed unless you need help from other caregivers. Seek help from a lactation counselor for any special guidance for successfully nursing "multiples," such as help with positioning for two infants.

Breast-Feeding Positions

If you're a nursing mom, you may want to experiment with these positions as you feed your baby:

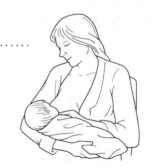

Cradle position. Sit up straight with your baby cradled in your arm. His or her head should be slightly elevated and resting in the crux of your elbow. You and your baby should be comfortably positioned "tummy to tummy," with baby's mouth level with your nipple. Be sure that your baby is facing straight toward you, without having his or her head, back, or neck turned.

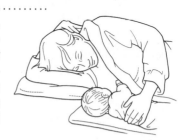

Lying down. Lie on your side with the baby on his or her side, too. Place pillows under your head and behind your back for comfort. Position your baby "tummy to tummy" so his or her mouth is next to your nipple. Use a folded towel or a pillow to elevate your baby to the correct height. This position is especially comfortable for women who've had a cesarean delivery. You can feed your baby from both breasts on one side, or turn onto your other side to nurse from your second breast.

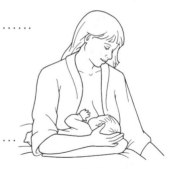

"Football" position. Hold your baby with the head facing your breast, and his or her body tucked under your arm at your side. Your forearm supports the baby's back, and his or her legs and feet should point toward your back. Rest the baby on a pillow near your elbow to give support and slightly raise his or her head.

Whatever the position, enjoy the eye contact with your baby. This helps build the mother-baby bond and helps your baby feel secure.

A Few Words for Dad . . .

A father can play a very important role in the success of breast-feeding. He can offer support, encouragement, and confidence to a new mother. Ways that fathers can get involved include attending prenatal breast-feeding classes with an expectant mother, reading a book on breast-feeding, arranging pillows, and bringing a snack or a beverage for mom when breast-feeding. A father also can burp the baby, change diapers, massage mom's neck and shoulders to encourage relaxation, and give baby a supplemental bottle. By sharing household responsibilities, caring for other children, shopping, and doing other tasks, he takes other pressures and interruptions away from mom.

What about Supplemental Bottles?

Breast-feeding abides by the law of supply and demand. Nursing stimulates the flow of milk—and increases its production as baby demands more to meet his or her needs. So supplemental bottles usually aren't needed—unless your pediatrician advises it, perhaps if your baby loses weight and doesn't regain it.

Although nursing may temporarily limit your independence, offering a supplemental bottle too soon may discourage your baby from nursing. Until your milk supply is established, stay close at hand for feeding.

If you choose to offer a supplemental bottle or a pacifier, wait about four weeks after birth, or until breast-feeding is well established. Because the nipple on a bottle or a pacifier is different from the breast, it can confuse a baby who is just learning to breast-feed.

Once the milk supply is constant—and both you and your baby are comfortable with nursing—a supplemental bottle lets dad, siblings, and other caregivers share in feeding. Expressed breast milk or commercially prepared infant formula may be offered in a supplemental bottle. *Note:* When nursing sessions are replaced regularly with supplemental bottles—without expressing milk—a mother's breasts will compensate by producing less milk.

For guidance on storing breast milk, see "Breast Milk: Safe Handling and Storage" in this chapter. For more about infant formula and bottle feeding, see "Another Healthful Option: Bottle-Feeding," also in this chapter.

Breast-Feeding for a Back-to-Work Schedule

To continue breast-feeding, changing from maternity leave to a back-to-work schedule takes adjustment. Some moms express milk during their workday. In that way, their baby can have bottles of mother's milk when mom's away. Other moms breast-feed when they can be with their baby; caregivers offer infant formula when mom can't. And some babies take both—bottles of expressed breast milk and of formula. Choose the option that works best for you and your baby.

If you're a back-to-work nursing mom (or need to be away from home regularly), consider these guidelines for breast-feeding success:

● Before you take maternity leave, work out a plan with your employer. Perhaps work at home for a while, or plan your schedule for short days, flextime, or longer breaks.

● Select a caregiver for your baby who is supportive of breast-feeding.

● Plan to nurse before you leave for work, soon after you return from work, and during the evening to keep your milk supply strong. A routine helps.

● If you plan to express milk during the workday, try

to make your plans before your maternity leave. If necessary, arrange for a private area to relax, free from interruptions. (You'll need fifteen to thirty minutes, usually twice a day.) Unoccupied offices or women's lounges may be options. And you'll need access to a refrigerator, or a small cooler with ice packs, to store breast milk. *For tips on safe handing of expressed milk, see "Breast Milk: Safe Handling and Storage" in this chapter.*

● Before you go back to work, help your baby learn to take expressed breast milk or infant formula from a bottle. Wait at least four weeks after delivery so your own milk supply is well established. If you wait too long, your baby may be less willing to take a bottle. Experiment with different types of bottle nipples to find one your baby likes. This may be the perfect chance to involve dad in feeding! *For more about the different types of bottle nipples, see "Bottles and Nipples: Baby Feeding Supplies" later in this chapter.*

● If your work schedule and the travel distance from work allow, schedule feeding visits with your baby during your breaks. Let the caregiver know when you'll arrive. In that way, your baby won't be fed too soon before your visits. To make it easier, choose a caregiver near your workplace.

● For the same reason, let the caregiver know when you'll pick up your baby after work. Together, schedule feedings so your baby won't eat too close to the end of your workday.

Vitamin and Mineral Supplements for Breast-Fed Babies

Until solid foods are introduced—at about four to six months of age—breast milk can be a complete source of nutrition for infants. However, three nutrients may warrant additional consideration. Ask your doctor for advice.

Iron. Iron is important for the manufacture of hemoglobin, the part of red blood cells that carry oxygen throughout the body. Iron also is essential for your baby's brain development and growth.

In the last trimester before birth, babies accumulate enough iron stores to last through their first four to six months of life. Breast milk also contains easily absorbed iron. After four to six months, however, most babies need more iron. Breast-fed babies may be at risk for being iron-deficient if another source of iron—usually iron-fortified cereal—isn't introduced. Talk to your dietitian or health professional about what is best for your baby.

Premature infants who breast-feed may need iron supplementation earlier. They had less time to build adequate iron reserves before birth.

Fluoride. Your baby's teeth started to develop even before you could see them. Fluoride, a mineral often found in tap water, helps develop strong teeth and prevent cavities later.

Breast milk contains little fluoride—even if the mother's drinking water is fluoridated. If your breast-fed infant takes supplemental formula made with fluoridated water—at least 0.3 ppm (parts per million) of fluoride—your baby may get enough fluoride. If your child is breast-fed only or drinks formula made with well water, distilled water, unfluoridated bottled water, or city unfluoridated water, your doctor may advise a fluoride supplement. Breast-fed infants who take supplemental ready-to-use formula also may need a fluoride supplement; these formulas usually are prepared with water low in fluoride.

If fluoride supplementation is needed, about six months of age usually is a good time to start. At your baby's six-month checkup, ask your doctor. A fluoride supplement may be prescribed.

Vitamin D. This vitamin helps your baby use calcium from breast milk (and infant formula) to help bones grow and develop. When skin is exposed to sunlight, the body can make vitamin D—but a little sunshine goes a long way! A baby doesn't need much sunlight to produce enough vitamin D.

Unlike infant formula and fortified cow milk, breast milk doesn't contain much vitamin D. For breast-fed babies who stay indoors (perhaps in winter) or dark-skinned babies, your baby's doctor may advise a supplement.

Other vitamins. Babies of strict vegetarian mothers may need a vitamin B_{12} supplement. *See "The Vegetarian Mom" in chapter 20 for more advice for vegetarian moms who breast-feed.*

Always get advice from your baby's healthcare provider or a registered dietitian before giving nutrient supplements to a baby, child, or teen of any age!

Weaning . . . When and How?

Weaning is the slow, gradual process that helps your baby eat and enjoy your family's foods. The time for weaning is an individual matter for mother and baby. Experts encourage moms to breast-feed for at least twelve months. Babies benefit from breast-feeding

Breast Milk: Safe Handling and Storage

- Wash your hands before expressing milk.
- If you use a breast pump, review the operation and cleaning instructions.
- Glass or plastic? Store refrigerated breast milk in plastic (made specifically for storing breast milk) or clean collection bottles. Plastic retains the protective properties of refrigerated breast milk better. You also can freeze breast milk in either plastic or glass containers.
- Use expressed breast milk stored in the refrigerator within eight days. Use milk kept at room temperature within six to ten hours, colostrum within twelve hours.
- If you work outside your home, or need to be away, consider stocking a milk supply in your freezer during maternity leave. Breast milk can be frozen:
  - In a freezer compartment inside the refrigerator for up to two weeks
  - In a refrigerator-freezer with a separate freezer door for three to four months
  - In a separate freezer at temperatures below 0° F for six months or longer.

  Date expressed milk kept in the refrigerator or freezer. Then rotate the milk—first in, first out.
- Store expressed milk in 2- to 4-ounce portions to avoid wasting unused milk after a feeding. Because bacteria from the baby's mouth can contaminate milk in the bottle, always discard milk that's left in the bottle after feeding.
- Thaw breast milk in the refrigerator, under warm, running water, or in a pan of water on the stove. Do not thaw or heat breast milk in a microwave oven. Before feeding thawed breast milk, gently shake the container to mix layers that may have become separated. Once thawed, use breast milk within 24 hours; avoid refreezing it.

for as long as it's mutually right for mother and baby.

No matter how long you choose to nurse, start complementary foods, too, when your baby's ready: when his or her birth weight has doubled *and* your baby is at least 13 pounds. Talk to your pediatrician about timing. When your baby eats other foods, too, you'll probably nurse less often: typically first thing in the morning, naptimes, and bedtime.

When you choose to wean your baby, introduce either infant formula or cow milk, depending on your baby's age. If your baby is under twelve months of age, wean from breast milk to iron-fortified infant formula. If your baby is twelve months or older, whole cow milk is appropriate.

Should you wean your baby to a bottle or a cup? That depends on his or her developmental readiness. Between four and six months, most infants will drink or suck small amounts of liquid from a cup or a glass when someone else holds it. Older babies and toddlers usually have the coordination to drink fluids from a cup or a straw. However, for infants under six months of age, a bottle is probably the best choice to ensure enough fluid.

Another Healthful Option: Bottle-Feeding

Breast-feeding may or may not be right for you. In rare cases, a woman may not be able to breast-feed for physical or health reasons. Some may feel uncomfortable. Others may take medications that wouldn't be safe if passed through their breast milk to the baby. Still others have cultural or work-related reasons. In all of these cases, parents can feel reassured that bottle-feeding is a healthful option.

Infant formula also is a good supplement for nursing moms when a mother chooses to skip a breast-feeding, or when the mother doesn't make enough breast milk for her baby.

If you choose bottle-feeding, feel assured: commercially prepared infant formulas are as similar to mother's milk as currently possible. Infant formulas have enough nutrients and food energy (calories) for your baby until you introduce solid foods—usually at about four to six months of age. And infant formulas

supply the right balanced of fats, carbohydrates, and proteins. Unlike breast milk, however, formulas lack protective factors such as antibodies to promote immunity.

Knowing When Your Baby's Had Enough

There's no exact science to bottle-feeding, but these are some signs that suggest that your baby's had enough:

- Your baby may close his or her mouth or turn away from the bottle.
- Your baby may fall asleep.
- Your baby may get fussy with your repeated attempts to offer the bottle.
- Your baby may bite or play with the bottle nipple.

With Baby . . . That's More than One!

Are you an experienced parent—with one or more other children? If so, feeding a newborn isn't new to you. Yet, every baby is different—so be prepared to learn new parenting skills. One child may be a fussy eater; another, ready and eager to eat. One may be ready for solid foods at four months; another, at six months. Observe, respect, and enjoy their unique differences.

Do you wish that you had handled infant or child feeding differently with your first child? That's normal, too, especially for a first-time parent. You were learning! It's okay to change your feeding approach with your next child.

Perhaps the biggest change is trying to do several things at once: trying to feed a baby, older children, and others in your family—including you. Enlist help from your preschooler or school-age child, without expecting too much. An older child can be your helper, but shouldn't be responsible for your baby. Tasks as simple as wiping baby's sticky hands, getting a bib, or picking up a bottle that falls to the floor make your older child feel helpful, "grown up," and important.

Remember, too: a new baby competes for your attention, which may lead to fussy eating from another child. Give your older child personal time at the table, too; include him or her in table talk. And try to keep mealtime calm and pleasant—despite all that's happening around the table.

Even after babies take solids, continue infant formula until your baby's first birthday. Similar to breast-feeding, cuddling a baby while he or she takes a bottle also builds a close, nurturing relationship with all those who share the responsibility of feeding: dad, siblings, grandparents, and other caregivers.

Formula: What Type?

Commercially prepared infant formulas are sold in powdered, liquid concentrate, or ready-to-feed forms. Before feeding, dilute powdered and liquid-concentrate formulas with water. Ready-to-feed formulas don't need to be diluted. Instead they're ready "as is" to feed your baby—packaged in cans or in bottles.

What's in a name? Regardless of which formula you use, commercially-prepared infant formulas are usually cow milk-based or soy-based. Formulas based on modified cow milk are appropriate for most babies. A soy-based or specialty formula might be best for the small number of babies who are sensitive to protein in cow milk or who have trouble digesting lactose, which is the sugar in milk. Vegetarian moms who don't choose to breast-feed may prefer a soy-based formula, too. For premature or low-birthweight babies, a soy-based formula probably won't be recommended. Ask your baby's healthcare provider.

Old-fashioned homemade formulas from canned evaporated milk and corn syrup may have nourished you or your mother, but they're nutritionally inferior to today's commercial formulas. And corn syrup may contain botulinum spores, which produce a harmful toxin that can be deadly. Your baby's better off with commercially prepared, iron-fortified infant formula.

Here are some things to consider when choosing a formula:

Iron. Many infant formulas are fortified with iron. Iron is a key mineral in forming hemoglobin, the part of red blood cells that carries oxygen to cells to make energy. Your baby also needs iron for brain development; an iron deficiency may cause irreversible delays in your baby's development. Full-term babies are born with enough iron stores to last four to six months. An iron-fortified formula right from the start helps keep a baby's iron stores adequate.

Choose an iron-fortified formula for your baby, or ask your baby's doctor, pediatric nurse, or a registered dietitian to recommend one. If your baby starts on a formula without iron, switch to an iron-fortified formula by four months. To clear up a common misperception, iron added to infant formula won't cause constipation or other feeding problems. Continue an iron-fortified formula until twelve months, when your baby is already eating a variety of foods, and starts cow milk.

Fluoride. The mineral fluoride helps your baby develop strong teeth and protects teeth from cavities. When you mix powdered or liquid concentrate formulas with water, you add fluoride, too—if your water supply is fluoridated. Ready-to-feed formulas aren't prepared with fluoridated water. If you regularly offer ready-to-feed formula or if your water supply isn't fluoridated to a level of 0.3 ppm (parts per million) of fluoride, ask your baby's doctor about fluoride supplementation.

Recipe for Success

For mixing infant formula, careful measuring, cleanliness, and refrigeration constitute the "recipe for suc-

Cow Milk: When? What Type?

As a great source of calcium and other nutrients, cow milk is an ideal food for toddlers, children, and adults. However, it isn't appropriate for infants younger than twelve months of age. While some infant formulas are made from cow milk, it's been modified to meet an infant's special needs.

Unmodified cow milk isn't the best food for young infants for several reasons. Its high protein content is hard for a baby's immature system to digest and process. The potassium and sodium contents also are higher than recommended for babies. Cow milk is low in iron; the iron it does contain isn't absorbed well. And it doesn't provide enough zinc, vitamins C and E, copper, and essential fatty acids—nutrients that babies need to grow and develop.

Goat milk isn't a suitable alternative either, for many of the same reasons as cow milk. If you choose to offer goat milk after age one, make sure it's vitamin D-fortified. To clear up a misconception, babies who are allergic to the protein in cow milk are probably allergic to the protein in goat milk, too.

cess." When properly mixed, powdered, concentrated, and ready-to-feed infant formulas are identical in their nutritional composition. The primary differences are price and how much time you need to prepare formula.

No matter what type of formula you choose, follow these guidelines:

● Wash your hands first. With an immature immune system, your baby is highly susceptible to foodborne illness.

● Pay careful attention to mixing instructions on the formula label. Adding too much water dilutes it. Then your baby may not get enough nutrients or food energy. Conversely, adding too little water concentrates the formula too much. Then it's hard for a baby to digest, and it supplies too much food energy at one feeding and not enough fluids to prevent dehydration.

Have You Ever Wondered

. . . if you can substitute vegetarian milk, such as soy milk or rice milk, for breast milk or formula? No, even if they're fortified with vitamins and minerals, they don't have enough proteins (except soy milk) and fats. Wait until after two years of age, but even then talk to your doctor, pediatric nurse, or registered dietitian first.

. . . if your baby needs formula fortified with DHA and ARA? Infant formulas with two fatty acids—docosahexaenoic acid (DHA) and arachidonic acid (ARA)—now are sold in the United States.

Found naturally in breast milk, DHA and ARA are important components of cell membranes in the brain and the retina. Infants also produce these fatty acids inside the body when adequate amounts of essential fatty acids—alpha-linolenic acid and linoleic acid—are present in infant formula. *See chapter 3, "Fat Facts."*

DHA and ARA added to infant formula may provide developmental benefits (brain and vision), especially for premature infants. As of 2002, these nutrients have been reviewed and are generally recognized as safe (GRAS) for full-term infants by the U.S. Food and Drug Administration (FDA), but not yet for preterm infants. The benefits of these formulas are still inconclusive. For more current information, check *www.FDA.gov.* Ask your physician before choosing these formulas for your infant. The formula label will indicate the presence of DHA and ARA.

Powdered and concentrated formulas are best mixed with water that's been brought to a rolling boil for at least one minute, and then allowed to cool. Bottled water that's labeled as "sterile" is also an option, unless otherwise advised by your baby's doctor. *For more on bottled waters, see "What about Bottled Water?" in chapter 8.*

● If your baby does well with one type and brand of infant formula, stick with it unless your baby's doctor advises otherwise. If you switch, check the label. The "recipe" for mixing the new formula may differ from the brand you used first.

● Always use clean bottles and baby-bottle nipples. *See the following "Bottles and Nipples: Baby Feeding Supplies" for cleaning tips.*

● For convenience, prepare a supply of bottles—enough for the day ahead. Date and refrigerate the prepared infant formula. Once opened, ready-to-feed formula and liquid concentrates must be refrigerated and used within forty-eight hours.

● Infant formula can be fed to a baby at a cold temperature, room temperature, or at a slightly warm temperature. Always test the temperature of the formula to avoid burning the baby. *To bring chilled bottles to room temperature or to slightly warm, see "Play It Safe: Warming Baby's Bottle and Food" later in this chapter.*

● Discard formula left in the bottle after feeding. Bacteria from your baby's mouth can contaminate formula and cause spoilage. To avoid too much leftover, fill the bottle with less. Make more as your baby's appetite dictates.

Bottles and Nipples: Baby Feeding Supplies

Baby bottles. Plastic or glass bottles, or disposable bottle bags? The choice is yours. Some parents keep a variety of baby-bottle sizes and styles on hand for different purposes. For example, disposable bottle bags are handy when you're on the go and when washing facilities are limited. For convenience, bottles with disposable liners let you toss away the used liner when the feeding is done. Small-size bottles are perfect for holding 2- or 3-ounce feedings during the first weeks after delivery. Be cautious of bottles with cute shapes; they're often hard to clean.

Baby-bottle nipples come in a variety of shapes and sizes, too. Choose nipples that correspond to your baby's mouth size and developmental needs. A baby's comfort and ease of sucking are the criteria to use when choosing a nipple.

There are four basic baby-bottle nipple types: a regular nipple with slow, medium, or fast flow (the number and size of the holes will determine flow); a nipple for very small or premature babies; an orthodontic nipple, which imitates the shape of a human nipple during breast-feeding; and a cleft-palate nipple. A cleft-palate nipple is meant for babies who have a lip or palate problem that keeps them from sucking properly.

Keep bottle-feeding equipment in good working order:

● Discard cracked or chipped bottles that could break and spill formula onto your baby.

● Replace nipples regularly as they can become "gummy" or cracked with age. Check them by pulling the tip before each use.

● Check the size of the opening on new nipples and then periodically as you use them. Formula should flow from the nipple in even drops—not a steady stream. If the milk flows too quickly, your baby could choke, so discard the nipple. If the milk flows too slowly for your baby, consider trying a nipple with more holes, designed for older babies.

When it comes to preparing infant formula and washing bottles, cleanliness is essential! Your baby's immune system isn't fully developed, so he or she is very susceptible to foodborne illness from improperly cleaned feeding equipment.

● Use plenty of hot, soapy water to wash your hands, work area, measuring utensils, bottles, and nipples. If possible, wash bottles right away when they're easier to clean.

● Thoroughly clean bottles and nipples by washing them with hot, soapy water and rinsing well. Sanitize nipples and bottles by placing them in boiling water for two minutes. Then let them air-dry. Or wash bottles, rings, and caps in the top rack of the dishwasher.

How Much Formula?

Your baby's appetite is a good guide to the amount of infant formula he or she needs—and how often. That depends in part on the stage of development. In addition, some babies drink a little more or less depending on when solid food is introduced. Use this chart *only* as a guide.

AGE	NUMBER OF FEEDINGS PER DAY	TOTAL AMOUNT OF FORMULA PER DAY (OZ.)
Birth to 4 months	6–8	18–32
4 to 6 months	4–6	28–45
6 to 9 months	3–5	24–32
9 to 12 months	2–4	24–32

Look for special dishwasher baskets designed to hold bottle parts, and keep them from falling to the bottom of the dishwasher.

● Remember that the outer "shell" of bottles with disposable bottle bags needs regular washing to destroy bacteria.

Bottle-Feeding Techniques: All in the Family!

Bottle-feeding gives the whole family warm, cozy moments with the baby. Nestled in the arms of a parent, sibling, grandparent, or other caregiver, babies feel safe and comfortable. Consider these tips for your bottle-feeding techniques:

● Find a comfortable place, perhaps a chair with an armrest. Hold your baby with his or her head slightly raised, resting on your elbow. That allows a baby to suck from the bottle and to swallow easily.

● Avoid propping your baby in bed or in an infant seat with a bottle. Babies can choke! And if they fall asleep with a bottle in their mouth, formula that bathes the teeth can promote baby-bottle tooth decay. Remove the bottle promptly if your baby falls asleep while eating.

● Angle the bottle to help prevent your baby from swallowing too much air. The nipple should stay full with formula when your baby is eating.

● To ease discomfort from air bubbles swallowed during feeding, burp your baby in the middle and at the end of feedings. Hold him or her upright at your shoulder, or lie your baby tummy down across your lap. Then gently pat or rub your baby's back.

● Keep a clean, damp washcloth handy. It's normal for babies to spit up some formula during burping.

● When your baby's done, take the nipple out of his or her mouth. Sucking on an empty bottle causes air bubbles in your baby's tummy and may make him or her uncomfortable.

Baby's Bottle-Feeding Routine

Newborns eat frequently in the first months after birth—perhaps every two hours! They need nutrients and food energy to fuel their rapid growth. Since their stomachs are small, just 2 ounces, or as many as 4 ounces of infant formula, may be enough for the early feedings. *See "How Much Formula?" on page 380 for guidelines during the first twelve months.*

Formula-fed babies usually need twenty to thirty minutes to finish a bottle. If it takes less than fifteen minutes for a newborn to finish a bottle, use a nipple with smaller holes. If it takes longer and if the baby is sucking actively, make sure the holes aren't clogged. Or try a nipple with more holes.

As with a breast-fed baby, plan to bottle-feed on demand—when a baby signals hunger. Trying to impose a feeding routine will frustrate you both. You can't spoil your baby by feeding on demand. A formula-fed baby may not eat as often; formula digests more slowly than breast milk.

Should formula be warm, cool, or at room temperature? That's up to you. Your baby will become accustomed to whatever temperature you usually provide. If you warm it, just be careful so your baby doesn't get burned. *For tips, see "Play It Safe: Warming Baby's Bottle and Food" later in this chapter.*

Let your baby decide how much to drink. Pay attention to his or her appetite; your baby doesn't need to finish a bottle. In fact, forcing your baby to finish it focuses too much on eating—which may lead to over- or underfeeding. To learn good eating habits, your baby needs to learn hunger and fullness cues.

Need more parenting tips for feeding your baby? Check here for "how-tos":

● Look ahead to toddler and preschool feeding—see chapter 16.

● Eat smart during pregnancy and breast-feeding—see chapter 17.

● Know signs of food allergies or intolerances—see chapter 21.

● Find a nutrition expert experienced in infant feeding—see chapter 24.

Physical Activity: Guidelines for Infants

Physical activity is important from the beginning of life! Sedentary activity can delay the start of rolling over, crawling, and walking as well as cognitive development, and can lead to a preference for inactive play and perhaps set the stage for childhood obesity. Rather than confine your baby to a stroller, playpen, or infant or car seat, start a habit of active living now. During this first year of life, find ways to help your child stay active:

● Spend part of each day with active baby games such as peekaboo and pat-a-cake.

● Find ways to help your infant safely and actively explore his or her surroundings.

● Avoid restricting your infant's movements for prolonged periods of time.

● Choose activities that encourage your infant to move large muscles (arms, legs, hands, and feet).

If your baby has six or more wet diapers a day, seems content between feedings, and if his or her weight increases steadily, your baby's probably getting enough. If not, check with your doctor or pediatric nurse. *For more signs that your baby has had enough to eat, see "Knowing When Your Baby's Had Enough" earlier in this chapter.*

Solid Advice on Solid Foods

Just when parents master breast-feeding routines or formula mixing, babies show that they're ready to join the high-chair crowd! Starting solid foods is just one more adventure in the journey of child feeding.

Throughout the first year, breast milk or iron-fortified infant formula continues to be your baby's most important source of nutrients and energy. (Wait until after twelve months for cow milk.) At four to six months, most infants are physically ready to begin solids. Typically they're added in this order:

- Iron-fortified, single-grain infant cereal (mixed with breast milk or formula), single strained fruits and vegetables—four to six months.

- Strained meats/poultry, unsweetened fruit juices (vitamin C-fortified) in a cup, plain toast, and teething biscuits—seven to nine months.

- Chopped soft fruits and vegetables; meats; unsweetened dry cereals; plain, soft bread; and pasta—ten to twelve months.

For more detailed guidelines for introducing foods during the first year, see "Infant Feeding Plan: A Basic Guideline" later in this chapter.

Ready, Willing, and Able

Although most babies are ready to start solid foods between four to six months of age, don't rely solely on the calendar! Babies must be physically and developmentally ready for solid foods. Remember, each baby is different. Age is just a point of reference. If babies aren't ready to eat solid food, it will likely end up on their lap—not in their tummy. Offering solids too soon only frustrates baby, parents, and other caregivers.

Until about four months, babies are unable to effectively coordinate their tongue to push food to the back of their mouth for swallowing. Well-meaning friends and family may tell you to start solid foods earlier to help your baby sleep through the night. However, babies sleep through the night only after their nervous system develops more fully. In fact, offering solids too soon stresses a baby's immature digestive system, and most passes right through to the diaper.

When is the right time to start solid foods? Usually, no sooner than four months of age. Then, if your baby weighs at least 13 pounds and has doubled his or her birthweight, it might be time. Let your baby be the judge. There's no one calendar date that's right for all babies. Watch for these milestones that suggest that he or she may be ready to join the league of solid-food eaters:

- *Baby can sit with little support.* Your baby can control his or her head and may even be able to lift up his or her chest, shoulders, and head when lying tummy down. By this time your baby also can turn away to signal "enough."

- *Baby has an appetite for more.* If your baby is hungry after eight to ten breast-feedings or drinks more than 32 ounces of formula, it may be time for solids.

Have You Ever Wondered

. . . if it's okay to offer solid foods in a bottle? No. For most babies, offering solid foods from a bottle isn't wise. One problem? Possible delay in learning feeding skills. Cereal or other foods from a bottle also can cause choking. This practice may encourage your baby to overeat (too much food energy, or calories). With spoon-feeding, resting between bites gives your baby time to feel full and so learn self-regulation. Cereal in a bottle also may take the place of breast milk or formula, along with the nutrients they supply.

To clarify a misconception, offering cereal in a bottle won't help baby sleep through the night or stop crying, either.

. . . what you can do to relieve the discomfort of teething? You might rub your baby's tender gums gently with your clean finger, perhaps with a little teething gel along the gumline. A chilled teething ring—kept in the refrigerator, not in the freezer—also can help. Chewing on textured solid foods, such as teething biscuits or bagel pieces, helps teething, too. Offer these foods when your baby is sitting up, and stay nearby. Chill baby foods, too; they may feel better than warm foods.

More drooling and swollen, tender gums signal teething. Be aware that a runny nose, diarrhea, fever, or rash probably are symptoms of illness, not teething.

Caring for Baby Teeth

Good dental care begins at birth—even before baby teeth appear! Healthy teeth let children chew food easier, learn to talk clearly, and smile with self-assurance.

Make cleaning your baby's teeth and gums part of the daily bathtub routine. Starting at birth, clean your baby's gums with a soft infant toothbrush and water, or use a clean, wet washcloth or gauze pad. Do this after every feeding. Skip toothpaste, which babies often swallow.

Schedule your baby's first visit to a pediatric dentist after the first tooth appears (at about six to twelve months).

Fluoride is a mineral that helps teeth develop and resist decay. In many places, fluoride is naturally present in local water supplies at various levels. If you live in an area that doesn't have fluoridated water, ask your baby's doctor if your baby or child needs a fluoride supplement. Unless your child's dentist advises otherwise, wait until after age two or three to start with fluoridated toothpaste. *For more information on fluoride, see "Vitamin and Mineral Supplements for Breast-Fed Babies" and "Formula: What Type?" earlier in this chapter. For more about fluoridated water, see "The Fluoride Connection" in chapter 8.*

To avoid tooth decay, do not put your infant, toddler, or young child to bed with a bottle of juice, formula, or milk. The liquid that bathes the teeth and gums from sucking on the bottle stays on teeth and can cause tooth decay. That happens even if a baby's teeth haven't yet erupted through the gums. If your child won't nap or go to bed at night without a bottle, fill it with plain water instead.

For more about dental care, see "Your Smile: Sugar and Oral Health" in chapter 5.

● *Baby shows interest in foods you're eating.* As the baby watches, he or she leans forward and may even open his or her mouth in anticipation. Take a trial run with appropriate solid foods. If your baby doesn't seem interested, wait a few weeks, then try again. Avoid forcing a child to eat solid foods.

● *Baby can move foods from the front to the back of the mouth.* Up to about four months of age, babies will try to push food out with their tongue. As they develop, the tongue becomes more coordinated and moves back and forth. This allows your baby to swallow foods from a spoon.

Something New: Eating from a Spoon!

Learning to eat the first solid food—usually iron-fortified cereal—from a spoon is a big transition in infant feeding. It's a step toward independence. And it encourages chewing and swallowing skills.

Spoon feeding has challenges. It's messier. At first, more food may end up on the bib and face than in the mouth. Try this to make the transition pleasant:

● Relax. This is a new eating adventure for both of you! Pick a time when your baby is relaxed and not ravenously hungry. Smile, and talk as you feed your baby. Your soothing voice will make new food experiences more pleasant—and talking helps with language development, too.

● Of course, wash your hands first. And keep baby food safe and clean.

● Use a small spoon with a long handle—and just a little bit of food on the tip of the spoon.

● Start with a teaspoon or two of food. Then work up to one to two tablespoons, two to three times a day.

● Let your baby set the pace for feeding. Don't try to go faster or slower.

● Seat your baby straight or propped upright, facing forward. This makes swallowing easier and helps prevent choking.

● Introduce new foods at the start of the meal. Once satisfied, your baby may be less willing to try a new taste. If he or she refuses a new food, that's okay; try it again in a few days or weeks.

Infant Cereal: Timing Is Everything

Your baby's first solid food should be a source of iron, such as iron-fortified infant cereal. With cereals, opt for ones developed for babies. They're easier to digest than varieties made for older children and adults. Iron-fortified infant cereals help babies maintain their iron stores.

● Start with rice cereal. It's often best as the first cereal because it's least likely to cause allergic reactions.

● When it comes to your baby's first cereal feedings, keep the cereal mixture thin. Start with just one part cereal to four parts of breast milk or infant formula. Once your baby develops eating skills—and a taste for cereal—mix in less liquid so it's thicker. Don't mix in honey or corn syrup, which may contain small amounts of bacteria (botulism) spores that can be harmful to infants.

● Be prepared if your baby refuses cereal at first. Try again in a few days. Infant cereal tastes different from the familiar breast milk or formula. The texture is different, too—not to mention the difference between a nipple and a spoon!

● Once your baby has eaten rice cereal for several days with no signs of intolerance or allergy, expand his or her tastes by offering barley or oat cereal. *To determine if a food may be causing a reaction, see "Food Sensitivities and Your Baby" on this page.* Hold off on wheat cereal until after your baby's first birthday. Some infants are sensitive to wheat before one year of age.

● Once your baby starts eating more cereal, he or she will take less breast milk or infant formula. Breast milk or iron-fortified formula still should be the mainstay of the diet during the first year.

Solid Foods: What Comes Next?

Once your baby accepts cereal, try strained vegetables and fruits; after that, meats and breads. It doesn't matter which you offer first: vegetables or fruits. Some parents opt for vegetables first. But it makes no difference.

● One by one, offer a variety of foods to your baby. This lays the groundwork for a healthful diet throughout life. *For more about the importance of eating many different foods, see "Variety: Good for You, Good for Baby!" on page 385.*

● Try single foods first: for example, fruits—apple-

sauce, pears, peaches, prunes (dried plums), bananas; vegetables—sweet potato, carrots, squash, peas, green beans; juice—apple, pear; meat—beef, chicken, turkey, ham; legumes or tofu (for vegetarian infants); and egg yolks. Juice fortified with vitamin C helps your baby absorb iron from food.

● Start with smooth foods that are easy to swallow. Babies can eat mashed or finely chopped foods when their teeth start to appear and when they start to make chewing motions. Foods with a bit of texture help with teething.

Food Sensitivities and Your Baby

Some babies are sensitive to certain foods. You know by their reaction—perhaps a rash, wheezing, diarrhea, or vomiting. Most babies outgrow these reactions once their digestive and immune systems mature. (To reassure you . . . a baby's stool often changes color and consistency when new foods are eaten. These changes don't necessarily indicate a food sensitivity.) To best monitor your baby for food-induced reactions:

● Keep track of the foods your baby eats. Choose single-grain infant cereals and plain fruits, vegetables, and meats instead of mixed varieties or "dinners" until you know what foods your baby can handle. If your baby has a reaction, stop that food for a while.

● As you introduce new foods, offer one new food at a time. Wait three to five days before offering the next new food. If your baby has trouble with a certain food, you'll more likely know what food causes the reaction.

● Save egg whites until after your baby's first birthday. Young babies may be sensitive to the protein in egg whites. Cooked egg yolks are okay—although the iron they contain isn't well absorbed.

● Be watchful of foods that contain common allergens, including peanuts, tree nuts, soy, eggs, fish, shellfish, wheat, and milk. Use the ingredient list on food labels to identify these ingredients.

● If any food causes a significant and ongoing reaction, talk to your baby's doctor, pediatric nurse, or registered dietitian about it. Together, you can establish an eating plan that's best for your baby.

For more about food intolerances and allergies, see chapter 21, "Sensitive about Food."

● Offer juice in a cup, not a bottle. Sucking juice too long from a bottle exposes a baby's teeth to natural sugars in fruit juice. Prolonged contact with sugars can promote tooth decay.

● At about six to nine months of age, most babies enjoy drinking from a cup—or at least trying to use it! Offer juice, water, or formula in a child-size unbreakable cup. A cup without handles may be easier for a young child to hold. Covered cups with a spout also are helpful at this stage. Babies are clumsy with a cup at first but usually catch on quickly.

● As your baby gets more teeth and gets interested in self-feeding—at about nine to twelve months of age—introduce finger foods. Soft, ripe fruit without peels or seeds and cooked vegetables are good for tiny fingers. Avoid foods a baby can choke on. *See "For Babies, Toddlers, and Preschoolers: How to Avoid Choking" in this chapter.*

● Teething biscuits, breadsticks, and rice cakes are good natural "teethers" for your baby, too. Chewing on these foods eases a baby's sore gums while offering a chance to eat a healthful snack—"all by myself"! *For more on self-feeding, see "'Feeding Myself'" in this chapter.*

● Remember, plain tastes best. Babies need the opportunity to develop a taste for the natural flavor of foods without added sugar, salt, or other flavorings. Seasonings are not added to many varieties of commercially prepared baby foods. Read the product label to find out.

● As you choose foods for your baby, don't restrict fat. Growing babies need the energy and essential fatty acids that fat provides. *See "Fat Facts for Kids" in chapter 16.*

● As your baby grows and develops a bigger appetite, offer more solid foods. *The chart "Infant Feeding Plan: A Basic Guideline" in this chapter suggests amounts.*

Variety: Good for You, Good for Baby!

Variety certainly is the spice of life—especially when it comes to forming good eating habits for your baby.

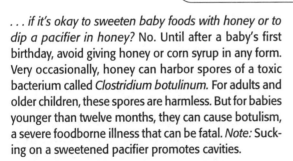

Have You Ever Wondered

. . . if it's okay to sweeten baby foods with honey or to dip a pacifier in honey? No. Until after a baby's first birthday, avoid giving honey or corn syrup in any form. Very occasionally, honey can harbor spores of a toxic bacterium called *Clostridium botulinum.* For adults and older children, these spores are harmless. But for babies younger than twelve months, they can cause botulism, a severe foodborne illness that can be fatal. *Note:* Sucking on a sweetened pacifier promotes cavities.

. . . when your baby can have fruit juice? Before six months fruit juice offers no nutritional benefits, advises the American Academy of Pediatrics. After six months pasteurized 100 percent fruit juice (not fruit drinks) is an option, as long as your baby doesn't drink too much of it. Four to 6 ounces of juice a day are more than enough.

Offer juice in a small cup at mealtime or snacktime—not from a bottle, covered cup, or juice box, which promotes sipping juice throughout the day. Juice shouldn't be given in a bedtime bottle, or to manage your baby's diarrhea. Remember, except that fruit has more fiber, fruit juice and fruit offer the same nutritional benefits for older babies.

. . . if a chubby baby is more likely to become an over-weight adult? Relax if you're concerned. Chubbiness during infancy generally doesn't lead to adult overweight. Rather than worry or restrict food, respect your baby's appetite. That helps your baby learn to eat the right amount of food, not over- or undereat. Restricting food may keep your baby from getting nutrients and energy needed to grow and develop, and may cause a failure to thrive.

. . . if your baby needs a vitamin supplement when he or she starts solid foods? Ask your pediatrician. A specially formulated infant supplement may be recommended if you're not sure if foods supply enough, if your family is vegetarian, or if your baby needs to restrict food for any reason.

Feeding Myself

As babies master spoon feeding, they're gradually ready to feed themselves. Watch for signals that suggest your baby is ready: perhaps trying to help you, or taking a cup away, or putting his or her hand on yours.

- Start with finger foods. It's easy because eating by hand is utensil-free.

- Give your baby a spoon to hold in one hand while you use another for feeding. This gives your baby practice grasping a utensil.

- Offer baby-friendly utensils: a small, rounded spoon with a straight, wide handle, and a dish with high, straight sides.

- Use the two-spoon approach. Give an empty one to your baby, and fill the other with baby food. Then switch so baby has a filled spoon for self-feeding.

- Be patient—and relaxed. Food will end up on the floor. Your baby will need lots of practice before being able to eat a whole meal without your help.

- Always stay with your baby when he or she is self-feeding. In that way you'll be around if he or she starts to choke.

Tip: Start a lifelong habit of family mealtime. Bring your baby's high chair to the family table, even if you need to feed your baby first.

Offering your baby a wide variety of foods with different flavors, colors, shapes, and textures helps ensure that his or her nutrition needs are met. Variety makes mealtime more fun, too! As an aside, babies perceive sweet tastes first; both amniotic fluid and breast milk are sweet. Other taste perceptions develop during a baby's first year.

Like you, your baby may like some foods better than others. That's normal. Likes and dislikes may change from week to week. Continue to offer food variety. You may offer a new food or flavor several times before a child accepts it—so keep trying. If not now, try again in a few days. Don't let your own food biases limit your baby's preferences. Your baby or toddler may like those foods!

Learning to enjoy a variety of solid foods helps establish a lifetime of good eating habits. This is why variety is so important, even in the early years.

Fruits and Vegetables

They're good sources of vitamin C, beta carotene, other nutrients, and phytonutrients. By offering these foods frequently at mealtime, children become familiar with fruit and vegetable flavors. That helps set the stage for accepting and enjoying them throughout life.

Breads, Cereals, and Other Grain Foods

Offer iron-fortified cereal to babies and toddlers. To enhance iron absorption, serve those that contain iron along with foods that contain vitamin C, such as fruits and fortified infant juices. Other grain products include soft, cooked pasta or rice, soft breads, dry cereals, crackers, and teething biscuits.

Caution with high-fiber foods: Some high-fiber cereals, such as bran, and raw vegetables are low in calories yet high in bulk. Avoid offering large amounts of these foods to infants; they fill a small stomach without providing many nutrients or calories. Infants and young children get enough fiber from a variety of foods.

Meats, Milk Products, and Other Protein Sources

These foods are valuable sources of protein, calcium, iron, zinc, and other minerals that your baby needs to develop bones and muscles, as well as for his or her blood supply and brain development.

Offer a variety of soft, pureed, or finely chopped meats such as chicken, turkey, or beef. By age seven to eight months, well-cooked, pureed legumes (perhaps strained) or mashed tofu are options for vegetarian infants; since tofu is made of soy, be watchful for potential food allergies. (Wait until after one year of age to offer smooth nut and seed butters, spread on bread or crackers.) After twelve months, if children no longer take breast milk or infant formula, whole milk is an important source of energy, calcium, proteins, essential fatty acids, and some other nutrients. Growing bones need an adequate supply of calcium from food. Good sources include cheese, milk, and calcium-fortified cottage cheese. Health experts don't advise feeding lower-fat dairy foods, such as low-fat or fat-free milk, to children under two years of age. If you offer yogurt (often sold as low-fat), make sure your child also consumes whole-milk dairy foods.

Have You Ever Wondered ?

. . . what foods help your baby avoid constipation? For one, offer a combination of foods to keep stools a consistency that's easier to pass. Some foods produce firmer stools: for example, bananas, rice, soy, and foods made from white flour. Others produce softer stools: for example, apricots, peas, peaches, pears, and prunes (dried plums). Drinking enough fluid helps soften stools, too.

If your baby gets constipated, offer apple juice twice a day, or prune juice for something stronger. Get advice from your pediatrician if this doesn't work.

Play It Safe: Warming Baby's Bottle and Food

Babies enjoy breast milk, infant formula, and baby foods either warm or cool. Unlike most adults, babies have no physical or emotional need for warmed liquids and warmed foods. However, like adults, they prefer foods that are familiar.

● If you want to serve foods at warm temperatures, play it safe so your baby won't get burned. Warm bottles of formula or breast milk in a pan of warm water or under a stream of warm tap water. You can do the same with frozen breast milk, or defrost it overnight in the refrigerator.

● Avoid heating milk to a boiling temperature. Boiling temperatures destroy some nutrients, and for breast milk, some protective properties.

● Shake the bottle during and after warming to evenly distribute the heat. And always test a few drops on the back of your hand, not your wrist; the back of your hand is more sensitive. The formula or milk should be tepid, or just slightly warm to the touch.

Microwave Warming: Be Very Cautious

Be very cautious if you heat formula or baby food in a microwave oven. Microwaving creates uneven heating, or "hot spots," that can burn a baby's mouth and skin. A bottle or food may feel cool on the outside while the inner contents reach scorching temperatures. And since food doesn't heat evenly, microwaving may not destroy bacteria that cause foodborne illness. Another problem: sometimes plastic bottle liners explode if their contents become too hot.

Avoid using the microwave oven to warm breast milk. Because microwave heating produces high temperatures quickly, some vitamins and protective factors in breast milk may be destroyed.

For warmed bottles . . . heat them only until the formula or milk is tepid.

● Warm chilled formula (portions of 4 ounces or more) in the microwave oven.

● Use clear, microwave-safe, plastic baby bottles. Avoid glass and colored plastic bottles, and plastic liners, which may crack, melt, or burst.

● Remove the bottletop (cap and ring) and nipple before warming the bottle in the microwave oven. The bottle shouldn't be covered when warming it.

● Warm a 4-ounce bottle on high power (100 percent) for no more than thirty seconds; forty-five seconds are tops for an 8-ounce bottle. Remember, you're only warming the bottle, not making it hot!

● After warming, replace the nipple and bottletop (ring and cap). Invert the bottle ten times to distribute the heat.

● Test the temperature of the formula or milk on the back of your hand. If the formula or milk barely feels warm, offer it right away. Don't allow the warmed bottle to sit out at room temperature. If the bottle was overheated, place in the refrigerator until cool enough to feed to your baby.

For solid foods . . . warm foods in the microwave oven until just lukewarm.

● Place food in a microwave-safe dish rather than leaving it in the jar. As in baby bottles, food in jars can develop hot spots.

● Heat only the amount you'll need. Less food heats faster than more food, and some ovens heat faster than others. Fifteen seconds on high (100 percent power) for 4 ounces of baby food are enough. Remember that higher-fat foods such as meat and eggs often heat faster, too.

● Read warming guidelines on baby food labels. And remember that baby foods can be served cold, at room temperature, or slightly warm.

INFANT FEEDING PLAN: A BASIC GUIDELINE

Babies differ in their size, appetite, and readiness for solid food. This guide offers a general time frame for introducing baby foods and table foods into an infant's eating pattern.

However, some babies may be ready for certain foods a little sooner; others, somewhat later. Your baby's doctor, pediatric nurse, or a registered dietitian will recommend an eating pattern to meet your baby's individual needs.

AGE AND DEVELOPMENT	SELF-FEEDING SKILLS	FOODS TO INTRODUCE/INFANT IS READY FOR . . .
Birth to 4 months		
Sucks and roots toward a nipple Sticks out tongue when solid food or a spoon is put in his or her mouth	Sees breast or bottle, and is eager to eat	Breast milk or iron-fortified infant formula is all infant needs; *note:* supplemental water is not required or recommended
4 to 6 months		
Sits up alone or with support Holds head up on own Indicates desire for food by watching a spoon, opening mouth for spoon, closing lips over spoon, and swallowing Indicates disinterest in food or a feeling of fullness by leaning back, closing mouth, and turning head away Can depress tongue and move semisolid food from spoon to back of mouth for swallowing Smacks lips	Pats or puts hands on breast or bottle	Iron-fortified infant cereal (introduces a supplementary source of iron)
6 to 9 months		
Starts teething Starts to move lips while chewing Begins chewing up and down Moves jaw and tongue up and down Can close lips to eat	Plays with spoon May help soon find mouth Holds bottle Feeds self crackers, toast, cookies, etc. Feeds from cup with help	Plain, cooked, pureed, or mashed vegetables (introduces new flavors and textures); *note:* avoid combination meat and vegetable dinners Plain, soft pureed, or mashed fruits; *note:* avoid fruit desserts Plain, pureed, minced, or finely chopped meat, poultry, fish, cooked egg yolk; *note:* avoid combination meat and vegetable or vegetable and meat dinners

AGE AND DEVELOPMENT	SELF-FEEDING SKILLS	FOODS TO INTRODUCE/INFANT IS READY FOR . . .
		Cooked mashed legumes, lentils, tofu, grains, toast, crackers, dry unsweetened cereals, zwieback
		Limited amounts of unsweetened fruit juices offered in a child-size cup; *note:* juice is not necessary but may provide variety
9 to 12 months		
Starts rotary chewing movement	Can hold own bottle well	Soft, bite-size pieces of vegetables, mashed potatoes, fruits, meats, and alternatives; soft breads such as bagels, rolls, plain muffins; rice noodles
Begins a biting rhythm	Can hold cup but may spill	
Licks food from lower lip	Picks up food in fingers or palms	
Improves small motor skills	Puts food in mouth	
		Finger foods: soft, cooked vegetables cut into bite-size pieces; soft, ripe, peeled, fresh fruit or canned fruits; strips of tender, lean meat; soft, whole legumes or lentils; diced tofu; peanut butter
		Yogurt, cheese, cottage cheese (as breast milk or formula intake starts to decrease)

Source: Adapted from The Chicago Dietetic Association, The South Suburban Dietetic Association, Dietitians of Canada, *Manual of Clinical Dietetics* (Chicago: American Dietetic Association, 2000).

● After microwaving, allow food to "rest"; food will continue to heat through. Stir the food to distribute the heat.

● Test the temperature of the food before feeding it to your baby; the food should be just lukewarm. Use a clean spoon to feed the baby.

For more about the safe use of a microwave oven, see "Play It Microwave-Safe" in chapter 12.

Baby Food—Make It Yourself?

In spite of the added work, some parents get satisfaction from preparing baby food themselves. However, that requires extra care to keep baby's food safe and to retain the nutrients from fresh foods.

Commercial baby foods are nutritious options for feeding baby, too. Today's commercial baby foods provide balance and variety with carefully controlled and consistent nutrient content.

Follow these guidelines if you choose to prepare homemade baby food:

● Wash your hands before preparing baby food.

● Always use clean cutting boards, utensils, and containers to cook, puree, and store homemade baby food.

● Wash, peel, and remove seeds or pits from produce. Take special care with fruits and vegetables that are grown close to the ground; they may contain spores for *Clostridium botulinum* that can cause foodborne illness.

Avoid Feeding
from the Baby Food Jar

Feeding directly from the jar introduces bacteria from your baby's mouth to the spoon and into the food. If you save the uneaten food, bacteria in leftovers can grow and may cause diarrhea, vomiting, and other symptoms of foodborne illness if used at a later feeding.

● Instead, spoon small amounts of baby food from the jar into a feeding dish, and feed from there. If your baby needs a second helping, just take more from the jar with a clean spoon.

● As soon as you finish feeding your baby, cap opened jars of baby food that haven't come in contact with your baby's saliva. You may then safely refrigerate them for up to three days.

Unopened jars of baby food have the same shelf life as other canned foods. Check the product dating on the label or lid, then use the baby food while it's still at its peak quality. *To learn how to read product dating, see "More Reading on the Food Label" in chapter 11.* Most jars of baby food have a safety button on top. If the button's indented, the food should be safe. As the vacuum is released on the seal, you'll hear a "pop" when you open the jar.

● Start with fresh or frozen vegetables. Cook them until tender by steaming or microwaving, then puree or mash. There's no need to add salt, other seasonings, or sweeteners. Remember, a baby's tastes aren't the same as yours.

● Puree or mash fresh fruit or fruit canned in its own juice. Never add honey or corn syrup.

● Avoid putting egg whites in homemade baby food until the baby's first birthday. Egg whites, more likely than egg yolks, may cause an allergic reaction. Cook any egg whites you feed your toddler.

● Cook meats, poultry, and egg yolks until well done. Babies are especially susceptible to foodborne illnesses caused by eating undercooked meats, poultry, and eggs. Again, there's no need for added flavorings.

● Prepare foods with a texture appropriate for the baby's feeding stage. Puree foods in a food processor,

blender, or baby food grinder, or mash them with a fork; or chop them well, so your baby won't choke.

● Cover, and refrigerate or freeze homemade baby food immediately after it's prepared. If refrigerated, keep homemade baby food in a covered container for no more than three days.

● For convenience, freeze prepared baby food for later use. Freeze it in small portions in a clean ice cube tray. Once frozen, put the cubes into clean, airtight, plastic bags for single-serve portions. As another method, use the "plop and freeze" technique: plop meal-size spoonfuls of pureed food onto a cookie sheet, freeze, then transfer the frozen baby food to clean plastic bags for continued freezing.

● Label and date homemade baby food. You can keep fruit and vegetable purees frozen for six to eight months; frozen, pureed cooked meat, poultry, and fish, for ten weeks.

Tips for Travel,
Tips for Day Care

● Pack unopened jars of commercial baby food. Even cereal comes in jars. Ready-to-feed formula in a prepackaged bottle is handy, especially since it doesn't require refrigeration. Or use powdered formula. Just premeasure water and powder into separate containers, then mix when it's needed.

● Keep perishable food, such as bottles of prepared infant formula or breast milk, well chilled. Pack them in an insulated container with frozen cold packs or buried in ice in a plastic bag. When you arrive at your destination, refrigerate.

Bottles, already cold from your refrigerator, can stay safe for up to eight hours in sterile sealed bottles in an insulated bottle bag, or for about four hours if they're stored in ice cubes in a plastic bag.

● Have everything handy: food, utensils, bib, and baby wipes or a clean, damp washcloth. If someone else is feeding your baby, provide feeding instructions, too, including the time and approximate amount to feed.

● Keep food separate from soiled diapers. And don't put food and bottles in a diaper bag that's frequently exposed to soiled diapers.

Food Labels: For Infants under Two Years

The Dietary Guidelines for Americans don't apply to children under age two—and neither do the Nutrition Facts on the labels of foods for adults.

Although they use the Nutrition Facts format, infant food labels are different from adult food labels—and supply different information. *This page shows a typical infant food label.* The label gives information that helps parents choose food with the kinds and amounts of nutrients that infants and toddlers need.

Serving size. For infant foods, serving sizes are based on average amounts that infants and toddlers under two years of age usually eat at one time. For example, for oatmeal, that's ¼ cup. On adult food labels, serving sizes are based on average amounts adults typically eat at one time; again for oatmeal, that may be given as ½ cup or 1 ounce of uncooked oatmeal.

Total fat. Infant food labels (foods for children under two years) list the total fat content in a single serving of food. But unlike adult food labels, they don't give the calories from fat or from saturated fat, nor the saturated fat or cholesterol content. These details aren't included because babies and toddlers under two years of age need fat as a concentrated energy source to fuel their rapid growth. Parents and other caregivers shouldn't try to limit an infant's fat intake.

% Daily Values (DVs). The % Daily Values for protein and some vitamins and minerals are listed on food labels for infants and children under four years of age. You won't find % DVs for fat, cholesterol, sodium, potassium, carbohydrates, and fiber, however; no Daily Values for them are set for children under age four.

For more about food labels, see "Today's Food Labels" in chapter 11, which includes more detail on the Nutrition Facts panel on adult food labels.

Nutrition Facts

Serving Size 1/4 cup (15g)
Servings Per Container About 30

Amount Per Serving

Calories 60

Total Fat	1g
Sodium	0mg
Potassium	50mg
Total Carbohydrate	10g
Fiber	1g
Sugars	0g
Protein	2g

	Infants	Children
% Daily Value	**0-1**	**1-4**
Protein	7%	6%
Vitamin A	0%	0%
Vitamin C	0%	0%
Calcium	15%	10%
Iron	45%	60%
Vitamin E	15%	8%
Thiamin	45%	30%
Riboflavin	45%	30%
Niacin	25%	20%
Phosphorus	15%	10%

For Babies, Toddlers, and Preschoolers: How to Avoid Choking

Having teeth doesn't mean children can handle all foods. Small, hard foods . . . slippery foods . . . and sticky foods can block the air passage, cutting off a child's supply of oxygen.

● Don't offer these foods to children younger than three or four years of age:

● *Small, hard foods*—nuts, seeds, popcorn, snack chips, pretzels, raw carrots, snack puffs, raisins. For toddlers and preschoolers, cut foods cut into slightly larger pieces that they can bite and chew, but not put whole into their mouths.

● *Slippery foods*—whole grapes; large pieces of meats, poultry, and frankfurter; and candy and cough drops, which may be swallowed before they're adequately chewed. Chop grapes, meat, poultry, hot dogs, and other foods in small pieces. Avoid offering chewing gum.

● Be careful with sticky foods, too, such as peanut butter. Spread only a thin layer on bread. Avoid giving your baby peanut butter from a spoon or finger. If it gets stuck in your baby's throat, he or she may have trouble breathing.

● Avoid propping your baby's bottle. Refrain from feeding your baby in the car, too; helping a choking baby is harder when the car's moving.

● Offer appropriate foods. Finger foods for older babies and toddlers are pieces of banana, graham crackers, strips of cheese, or bagels.

● Watch young children while they eat. That includes watching older brothers and sisters who may offer foods that younger children can't handle yet.

● Insist that children sit to eat or drink. They shouldn't eat when they're lying down or running around. As children develop eating skills, encourage them to take enough time to chew well.

● Be prepared to use the Heimlich maneuver quickly to dislodge solid foods that obstruct the air passage. Do this when a child is choking and can't breathe, cough, talk, or cry. The technique for infants and toddlers differs somewhat from that for adults. *See the illustrated description. For a description of the Heimlich maneuver for older children, teens, and adults, see chapter 12.*

● Always have your doctor see your child after a serious choking incident to be sure that the lungs and airway are clear.

When an Infant Is Choking . . .

Lay the child down, face up, on a firm surface and kneel or stand at victim's feel, or hold infant on your lap facing away from you. Place the middle and index fingers of both your hands below his rib cage and above his navel. Press into the victim's abdomen with a quick upward thrust. Be very gentle. Repeat until object is expelled.

If your baby isn't breathing: Clear any obstructions from the mouth. If there is no pulse, start CPR (two breaths followed by five gentle chest thrusts). Continue CPR until baby starts breathing or help arrives.

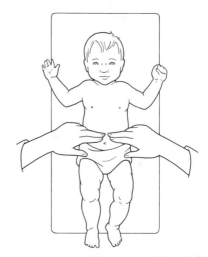

Source: Courtesy of the Heimlich Institute, Cincinnati, Ohio.

CHAPTER 16

Food to Grow On

Food nourishes at every age and stage in a child's life: infancy, the toddler and preschool years, school-age years, and adolescence. Careful food choices not only help ensure the physical nourishment of a child's growing body but also can nourish his or her social, emotional, and psychological development.

Whatever the age, children and teens need the same nutrients as adults. Only the amounts change. Like you, they need energy from food—but more relative to their body weight. They enjoy many of the same foods you like, but the form and combinations may differ.

Your challenge as a parent or a caregiver? First, be a good role model for healthful eating and active living for kids. After all, parents and other caregivers are a child's first and most influential teachers. And second, support your child's chances to make wise food choices. It's up to you to recognize and respect his or her unique needs, to make a variety of nourishing and appropriate foods available, and to set a routine (time and place) for eating. Your child has responsibilities, too: learning skills to make sound food choices, and listening to body cues to learn to eat the right amount.

Remember that you have more influence on your child or teen's food choices and daily living patterns than you may think. When you take care of yourself (eat smart and move more), you take care of your child and family, too!

Toddlers and Preschoolers: Food for the Early Years

Do young children seem like sponges, absorbing all the sights, sounds, and tastes of the world around them? Young children are impressionable and both ready and eager to learn. That makes the preschool years a great time to nurture positive attitudes toward eating and help children learn to eat and enjoy a variety of foods. Establishing good eating habits and active lifestyles now starts a pattern that can last a lifetime!

While toddlers and preschoolers grow at a slower rate than infants, toddlers and preschoolers need enough energy from food to fuel active play, learning, and the next stages of growth. They also need enough nutrients to promote their growth and health. Starting in the early years, good nutrition and healthful lifestyle habits can reduce the risks for overweight and obesity, diabetes, heart disease, cancer, and other chronic diseases later in life.

Food for Hungry Tummies

What's healthful eating for young children? A variety of foods with different textures, tastes, and colors—in adequate amounts—provides the nutrients and the food energy children need to thrive. Nourishment can come from a wide array of food.

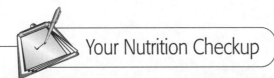

Your Nutrition Checkup

Eating and Activity: Family Matters

Family styles influence a child's eating and physical activity patterns and attitudes for life. What children eat and how much they move—and their attitude toward both—have lifelong implications for health.

Take a moment to assess your own family's eating and physical activity practices. As a parent, family member, or caregiver:

Do You . . .	Always	Usually	Sometimes	Never
Eat your meals as a family?	___	___	___	___
Serve meals and snacks on a regular schedule?	___	___	___	___
Give your youngster freedom to choose the foods he or she eats?	___	___	___	___
Respect a child's appetite when he or she has had enough?	___	___	___	___
Involve children in planning and preparing family food?	___	___	___	___
Make an effort to keep mealtimes pleasant?	___	___	___	___
Include snacks as part of the day's eating plan?	___	___	___	___
Attempt to keep eating to the kitchen, dining room, or another designated place?	___	___	___	___
Set a good role model with your food decisions?	___	___	___	___
Avoid rewarding or punishing a child with food?	___	___	___	___
Give kids enough time to eat?	___	___	___	___
Turn off the TV while you eat together?	___	___	___	___
Offer foods that appeal to children?	___	___	___	___
Serve a variety of foods for meals and snacks?	___	___	___	___
Offer new foods and new food combinations?	___	___	___	___
Avoid forcing a child to eat?	___	___	___	___
Set a good role model by being physically active?	___	___	___	___
Limit TV time to one to two hours daily?	___	___	___	___
Encourage children to play actively?	___	___	___	___
Enjoy physical activity regularly as a family?	___	___	___	___
Subtotal	___	___	___	___

Now score yourself:

Count the number of check marks in each column. Then multiply by these scores.

What's your total?

"Always":   3 points

"Usually":   2 points

"Sometimes": 1 points

"Never":   0 point

Your total score _____

What does your score suggest?

If you scored 40 to 60 points, you already apply what you know about nurturing positive eating and physical activity patterns. Read on for more ideas.

A score of 20 to 39 suggests you're on the right track for feeding and exercising with kids. But you still have room to make positive changes in your family's lifestyle. Check this chapter for more practical tips.

Less than 20, try to incorporate a few changes in your family's approach to food and physical activity. Read on for some steps to get you started.

394

What about nutrients? Carbohydrates should be children's main energy source. How much? Their energy needs depend on their growth rate, body size, and level of physical activity; most young children need 1,300 to 1,700 calories a day. They need enough protein for growing and for substances (hormones and enzymes) that stimulate body processes. Children need moderate amounts of fat, too, again for growth and to meet their energy needs; see *"Fat Facts for Kids" later in this chapter.* The food variety recommended by the Food Guide Pyramid also supplies the vitamins and minerals that young children need to thrive, although calcium and iron are two nutrients that may need your attention. *For specific nutrient amounts, see the Dietary Reference Intakes in the Appendices.*

For every nutrient, children have many choices. If your children won't touch sweet potatoes, offer a wedge of cantaloupe; both are good sources of vitamin A. Is milk rejected? Try chocolate or another flavored milk or offer other calcium-rich foods—such as cheese or yogurt. If you offer different kinds of healthful foods regularly, your child will learn to enjoy many of them—and reap their benefits. Remember that children often refuse foods the first time. Just keep trying! *Use the Food Guide Pyramid for Young Children later in this chapter as a guide for planning daily meals and snacks for kids.*

Whole milk, rather than low-fat varieties, is recommended for children twelve to twenty-four months of age. Whole milk supplies more fat and calories than low-fat or fat-free milk. As a concentrated source of energy, fat helps fuel this period of fairly rapid growth. And the extra cholesterol in whole milk helps a young child's brain develop properly. After the second birthday, any type of milk is okay to drink. Choose the type that matches your child's energy needs.

Enough to Eat, without Overfeeding

You can lead a young child to the table, but you can't make a child eat—nor should you! Let your child's appetite guide how much food is enough. Remember that a pattern of overeating can lead to overweight. And underfeeding also can lead to weight gain if your child sneaks food to satisfy hunger when you're not looking.

How much do toddlers and preschoolers need to eat? Although they're no longer babies, young

Have You Ever W

. . . what to do if your preschooler see. First discuss your concerns with your child's u. child's size may be normal. A growth chart, recor. regular health exams, will track your child's height anu weight and show how he or she fits within a healthy range. Some kids gain a little extra weight to support an upcoming growth spurt.

If your child is overweight, withholding food isn't healthful. Low-calorie diets often don't supply the food energy and nutrients he or she needs to grow, develop, and learn properly. Healthful eating habits, combined with plenty of active play, can help most overweight kids grow into their healthy weight—without a special diet. *See "Weighty Problems for Children—Overwieght" in this chapter.*

. . . if a vegetarian diet is okay for kids? A well-planned vegetarian diet—even a vegan diet—can supply all the nutrients that children need for their growth and energy needs. Calcium and iron need special attention. If your child doesn't eat any meat, poultry, fish, eggs, and dairy foods, be especially cautious about good sources of vitamin B_{12}, vitamin D, and zinc. *For more guidance, see chapter 20, "The Vegetarian Way."* A nutrient supplement might be a good idea; ask your healthcare provider.

. . . how to find out if your child is getting enough iron? For young children, iron deficiency anemia is the most common nutrition problem. That's why children are screened for anemia in regular checkups. Children need enough iron to support growth, replace normal iron loss, and produce energy for learning and play. *See chapter 4 for ways to include iron-rich foods in family meals.*

children aren't ready for adult-size portions. Adult servings can overwhelm small appetites. Children's stomachs aren't big enough to handle large portions. Judge how much your child needs to eat:

● Serve a toddler or a preschooler small helpings—certainly smaller than yours. Let the child ask for more. As a guide to portion size, some experts advise one tablespoon of every food served for every year in age.

For children ages two and over, use the Food Guide Pyramid for Young Children in this chapter as a guide for the total amount for the day.

"Do as I Do": Are You a Good Role Model?

Did *you* eat *your* vegetables today? Did *you* drink milk? Did *you* take a walk or do something physically active, not just sit by the TV or the computer? Did *you* eat just a handful of chips, or the whole bagful?

Children learn their habits, attitudes, and beliefs about eating and physical activity as they watch and interact with you: parent, older sibling, other caregiver. By mimicking you, they explore their world, try "grown-up" behavior, and hope to please you. Whether you intend to or not, role modeling probably is the most powerful, effective way to help your child to eat smart and move more.

Most kids want to do what others do! So the next time you order a drink to go with a fast food meal, eat when you're stressed or bored, or decide how you'll spend a leisure afternoon, think about the messages you send. The best way to help your child eat healthier is for you to do so!

● Respect your child's hunger and satiety cues. When he or she starts to play with food, becomes restless, or sends signals of "no more," remove the food. Or let your child leave the table. Knowing what it feels like to be full—and when to stop eating—help children learn to eat enough, but not to overeat.

● Do away with the "clean plate" club. This practice may encourage overeating or a food aversion—habits that could set up a child for weight or nutritional problems later. If your child always leaves food on his or her plate, you may be offering too much food. Offer smaller portions to smaller people!

Day-to-day and meal-to-meal appetite fluctuations are normal. Children's appetites often decrease after their first birthday as their growth slows. In fact, expect a child to pick at meals on occasion. Chances are that he or she will make up for it later. If your child is growing normally, seems healthy, and has energy to play, he or she probably is eating enough. Unsure? Talk to your child's doctor.

How often should young children eat? Try to keep to an eating schedule. Most children do best with a routine—when meals and snacks are served at about the same time each day. "Pacifier snacks" eaten while standing in line at the supermarket—or snacks just a half hour before a meal—may interfere with a child's eating routine.

Younger children may need to eat five to six times a day because their small stomachs don't hold much. Plan food-group snacks as part of the day's meal schedule, and space them between meals. *See "Snacks Equal Good Nutrition" in this chapter.*

For sample menus that meet the nutrient and energy needs of most young children, see "To Get Started: Sample Menus for Toddlers and Preschoolers" in this chapter.

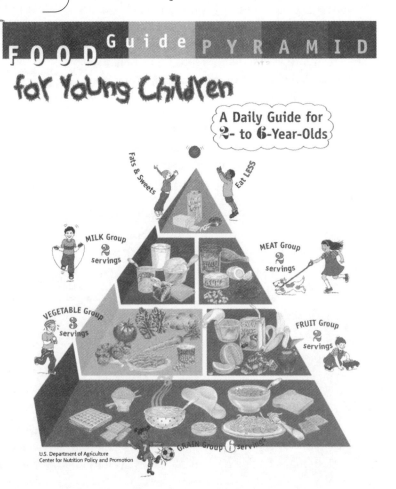

Food Guide PYRAMID for Young Children

A Daily Guide for 2- to 6-Year-Olds

Fats & Sweets — Eat LESS

MILK Group 2 servings

MEAT Group 2 servings

VEGETABLE Group 3 servings

FRUIT Group 2 servings

GRAIN Group 6 servings

U.S. Department of Agriculture
Center for Nutrition Policy and Promotion

Mealtime Tactics

Parents and caregivers supply the three _w_'s of meals and snacks: _what_ foods are offered, and _when_ and _where_ they're eaten. The child fills in the other _w_ and _h_: _which_ offered foods to eat and _how_ much.

- While physical activity promotes a healthy appetite, plan a quiet time before meals and snacks. Kids eat best when they're more relaxed.

- Remember that your child learns by watching you and older siblings. Eat together as a family. Set a good example by eating a variety of foods—including vegetables—yourself. Eating together also is a good chance to talk and to practice appropriate table manners.

- Even if you can't eat together, be there! Young children need supervision in case they start to choke. Someone who's choking may not be able to make sounds you can hear easily. _For foods that may cause choking or ways to safely handle a choking incident, see "For Babies, Toddlers, and Preschoolers: How to Avoid Choking" in chapter 15._

- Encourage kids to sit while they eat. Give youngsters a booster seat so they can reach their food easily. Discourage eating while standing, walking, or lying down.

- Reward children with affection and attention—not food. Using food as a reward or a punishment only promotes unhealthy attitudes about food and perhaps emotional overeating.

- Respect food preferences. Give young children the freedom to choose and reject foods, just as older children and adults do. Just encourage young children to politely say "No, thank you." Making food choices is a competency children need to master.

- Avoid the notion of "forbidden" foods. That may cause your child to want them more. All foods can be part of your child's healthful eating plan.

- Serve "designer dinners," featuring a variety of colors and textures. Cut food into interesting shapes, and arrange it attractively on the plate. Kids react to inviting foods just as you do!

- Get kids involved in preparing meals. Even young children can tear apart lettuce leaves for a salad or break up green beans into smaller pieces. Children are more likely to try foods that they have helped prepare.

- Offer foods with kid appeal. Many younger children prefer plain, unmixed foods. Foods with funny names—such as Monster Mash potatoes (mashed sweet potatoes) or Bugs on a Log (raisins and peanut butter on celery)—may help kids to try new foods. Kids often like finger foods, too. Offer raw vegetables to easily nibble in hand; be careful with foods that may cause choking. _For vegetables that taste good raw, see "Produce 'Package'" in chapter 10._

- Encourage children to practice serving themselves—for example, pouring milk from a pitcher, spreading peanut butter on bread, or spooning food from a serving bowl to their plate. Even though spills are messy, they're part of becoming independent.

- Make eating and family time the focus of meal and snack time—not TV watching. Use this chance to talk together and reinforce their good eating habits.

- Focus on the whole meal, not just on desserts. Avoid making desserts a reward.

- Stock your kitchen with child-size dishes and utensils that children can use with ease: cups they can get their hands around; broad, straight, short-handled utensils; spoons with a wide mouth; forks with blunt tines; and plates with a curved lip.

- Even in this fast-paced world, give kids enough time to eat. Remember, they're just learning to feed themselves. Time pressure puts stress on eating and takes the pleasure away.

- Toddlers and preschoolers live to play! Encourage a sense of fun and adventure by making family meals pleasant. Recall the day's events, share each other's company, and talk about the food: its colors, flavors, and textures.

To Get Started: Sample Menus for Toddlers and Preschoolers

Sample Menu for a Preschool Child, Ages One to Three Years	Sample Menu for a Preschool Child, Ages Four to Five Years
Breakfast	*Breakfast*
Cream of Wheat (¼ cup)	Cream of Wheat (½ cup)
Hard-cooked egg (½ to 1)	Hard-cooked egg (1)
Banana (½)	Banana (½)
Whole milk* (½ cup)	Low-fat milk (¾ cup)
Midmorning Snack	*Midmorning Snack*
Cheese (½ oz.)	Cheese (¾ oz.)
Crackers (3)	Crackers (4)
Orange juice (½ cup)	Orange juice (½ cup)
Lunch	*Lunch*
Vegetable soup (½ cup)	Vegetable soup (¾ cup)
Peanut butter (1 tbsp.)	Peanut butter (2 tbsp.)
Whole-wheat bread (1 slice)	Whole-wheat bread (1 slice)
Cooked carrots (¼ cup)	Cooked carrots (¼ cup)
Whole milk* (½ cup)	Low-fat milk (¾ cup)
Midafternoon Snack	*Midafternoon Snack*
Canned peaches (¼ cup)	Canned peaches (¼ cup)
Vanilla wafers (2)	Vanilla wafers (3)
Dinner	*Dinner*
Meat loaf (2 oz.)	Meat loaf (3 oz.)
Cooked spaghetti (¼ cup)	Cooked spaghetti (½ cup)
Broccoli (¼ cup)	Broccoli (½ cup)
Coleslaw (¼ cup)	Coleslaw (½ cup)
Margarine (1 tsp.)	Margarine (1 tsp.)
Dinner roll (½)	Dinner roll (1 medium)
Whole milk* (½ cup)	Low-fat milk (1 cup)

*Children older than two years can be given low-fat milk.

Feeding Choosy Eaters

Does your child refuse to eat green foods? Does he or she suddenly react to an all-time favorite food with an "I don't like this," or simply "no"? Are you concerned because your youngster won't eat vegetables?

Bouts of independence are part of being a toddler or a young child. "Choosy" eating may be your child's early attempts to make decisions and be assertive—a natural part of growing up. It may reflect a smaller appetite as his or her growth rate slows a bit, too. Or "no" may really mean "I want your attention."

Relax and be patient. And arm yourself with practical solutions for handling the "downs and ups" of child feeding:

● Avoid the "short order cook" routine. At mealtime, serve at least one food you know your child likes. But expect your tot to eat foods that the rest of the family enjoys.

● Offer choices, but not too many, rather than asking your child open-ended questions such as, "What do you want to eat?" Deciding between or among two or three foods gives your child a feeling of control. It's also good practice for learning how to make food decisions.

● Make food simple, plain, and recognizable. "Unmix" the food if it's an issue; put aside some ingredients for mixed dishes before assembling the recipe, even a salad or a sandwich. Then let your child put food together as he or she likes. *Tip:* Some kids don't like different foods to "touch" on their plates.

● Involve kids. Even choosy eaters eat foods they help plan, buy, or make. Together, plan a meal around foods your child likes. When you shop, ask your child to pick a new food for the family to try. Ask for a kitchen helper; for example, even small children can wash fresh fruit or put meat between bread slices for a sandwich.

● Allow hot food to cool down and cold food to warm up a little before serving it. Many children dislike extreme temperatures.

● If your child won't eat certain foods, perhaps spinach, don't worry. Just offer a similar food-group food, maybe broccoli. Or try carrots. Foods from the same food group supply similar nutrients.

● Moisten dry foods such as meat if they're hard to chew. A little cheese sauce or fruit or vegetable juice might help. Serve drier foods alongside "naturally" moist foods such as mashed potatoes or cottage cheese. Or offer "dipping" sauces with finger foods—kids love to dip!

● Trust your child's appetite. Forcing children to eat can start a lifelong habit of overeating. Instead, following hunger and satiety cues is part of learning to eat the right amount.

● Limit table time. Sitting at the table without eating for a long time doesn't teach good food habits. At the end of mealtime, quietly remove the plate.

Fat Facts for Kids

For a young child's eating plan, put away some adult notions about fat. A low-fat eating plan isn't advised for children under two years of age—and cutting way back on fat for older children isn't recommended either.

Fat is an important source of the energy, or calories, that support a young child's rapid growth, learning, and play. Two fatty acids—linoleic and alpha-linolenic acid—are essential for growing and brain development. Food must supply them because the body can't make them. Kids also need some fat from food to help their bodies use vitamins A, D, E, and K and to add flavor to food.

Starting at age two, advice for children mirrors the advice for their parents: eat a diet moderate in total fat and low in saturated fat.

● Moderate in total fat: on average, no more than 30 percent of calories from fat daily. For children who need about 1,600 calories a day, that's no more than 53 fat grams, or 480 calories from fat per day on average.

● Low in saturated fat: on average, no more than 10 percent of total calories from saturated fat daily. And go easy on "trans fats." *For more about guidelines for fat intake, see chapter 3.*

Grain products, fruits, vegetables, low-fat dairy foods, and other protein-rich foods (lean meat, poultry, fish, beans, and nuts) should supply most of a child's food energy. Remember that this guideline refers to your child's overall eating plan *and yours* for several days—not to one food, one meal, or even one day's intake.

If that's true, can your child eat French fries, chicken nuggets, cheese, and ice cream occasionally? Sure. Small amounts of higher-fat foods can fit in a child's healthful eating plan. Just be sure his or her overall choices are moderate in fat and low in "sat fats."

Going easy on fat is good family advice, too. Family meals and snacks, prepared with less fat, teach a lifelong habit of lower-fat eating. Later in life that habit reduces your child's risk for many health problems. Another benefit: eating too much fat may add excess calories and result in weight gain, even at an early age.

For more about fat in a healthful diet, see chapter 3, "Fat Facts"; chapter 13 offers ways to prepare family foods with less fat.

● Most of all, relax. And be a good role model (eat your veggies, drink your milk) yourself.

● Avoid conflict and criticism at mealtime; otherwise your child may use food for "table control." Focus your attention on the positives in your child's eating behavior, not on your child's food. And unless you're prepared for a self-fulfilling prophecy, skip labeling your child as a "picky eater."

● Remember, what your child eats over several days—not just one meal—is what really counts!

Tasting Something New!

Babies try one new food after another as they start solids, each time adding more food variety to their diet. The tasting adventure continues throughout childhood—and on into adulthood. More variety increases the chance for good nutrition and adds interest and fun to eating. And more variety can mean more vitamins, minerals, and phytonutrients.

Help children be willing food "tryers." It's part of the challenge and pleasure of learning about food. Be aware: young children typically have more tastebuds and may be more sensitive to flavors than you are.

● Offer new foods at the start of meals. That's when children are the most hungry. But make the rest of the meal familiar.

● Encourage children to taste at least one bite of a new food—or a food prepared in a different way. Don't force them. Just be matter-of-fact.

Food Jags

What do you do when youngsters get "stuck" on a food? If he or she keeps asking for the same food meal after meal, the child is on a "food jag." Food jags are common in the toddler years.

More frustrating for you than harmful for kids, you're smart to remain low key about food jags. The more you focus on them, the longer they may last.

Actually, it's okay to offer the food they want again and again and again! Just include other foods alongside to encourage variety. Most "monotonous diners" soon tire of eating the same food so often.

If your child rejects whole categories of food for more than two weeks, talk to your child's doctor or a registered dietitian.

● Keep quiet about foods you don't like. Try not to let your food dislikes keep your child from trying new foods.

● Before offering the new food, talk about it: color, texture, size, shape, aroma, not whether it tastes "good" or "bad." Let kids help you prepare it. They'll be more willing to taste!

● Serve the same food in different forms—for example, raw carrot sticks and cooked carrot coins. In that way they'll learn to enjoy a more varied eating style—the same food prepared in different ways.

● Keep trying! Kids may need to taste a food five to ten times before they learn to like it. And accept a fact of life: it's okay not to like every food.

Remember, whenever you expose children to some foods but limit others, you also limit the variety of foods they learn to eat and enjoy. That has an impact on the overall nutritional quality of their food pattern for life!

Snacks Equal Good Nutrition

Young children like to snack. That's good news! With their small stomachs, they may not meet their nutrition needs with just three meals a day. Snacks can fill in the nutrient and food-energy gaps from their meals.

If snacks conjure up images of high-calorie, low-nutrient foods—think again! Wise snack foods for people of all ages, including young children, come *mostly* from the Pyramid's five food groups. Milk (flavored or not) is a good snack drink; go easy on fruit juice. Make snacks a healthful part of your child's day:

● Let snacks supplement regular meals, not replace them. Plan for two to three food-group snacks plus three meals a day. Children age two to five usually need to eat every two to three hours. Younger children may need to eat more often.

● Plan ahead by keeping food-group snacks handy. *Check "Child-Friendly Snacks" on page 401.* An occasional piece of candy is okay, but avoid labeling it as a "special treat" to avoid undue emphasis. Just be matter-of-fact about it.

● Offer snacks two hours or more before meals. In that way youngsters are hungry at mealtime.

Hand-Washing Basics

Kids can't see them—but germs that cause illness are everywhere! For children, who have less immunity, proper hand washing and food safety are especially important.

Teach children good hand-washing habits—always before and after handling food and eating, and after using the bathroom, touching a pet, combing hair, blowing their nose, or coughing or sneezing into their hands:

● Wash hands with soap and warm water, rubbing hands for twenty seconds. (It's good counting practice, too.)

● Get a safe stool so your child can reach the sink, the faucet, and the soap.

● Practice with your child. Rub a little cinnamon and oil on your child's hands. Watch what happens if he or she doesn't wash hands well. Cinnamon that stays on hands represents germs.

● Be a good role model. *Always* wash your hands properly, too.

● Offer snacks when kids are hungry, not to calm tears or reward behavior. Otherwise you teach a pattern of emotional overeating. Maybe your child just needs attention, not food.

● Choose snacks to fill in the gaps from meals. If your child's meals come up short on vegetables or grain products, offer them at snacktime.

● Offer small snack portions. Let your child ask for more if he or she is still hungry.

● Think "fun" at snacktime. Children enjoy foods with sensory appeal: brightly colored fruits and vegetables; the aroma of baking bread or freshly cut watermelon; the texture differences of soft, creamy cheese with crisp, crunchy crackers.

● Encourage tooth brushing after snacks of any kind, not only after sweets.

Exploring More about Food

Food offers a world of experiences well suited to how children learn. Because food can become a "hands-on" activity, everyday tasks can get kids involved in food—and so promote healthful eating. Try these simple ways to explore food with young children:

● As you walk the supermarket aisles, encourage children to name the fruits and vegetables in the produce aisle or the canned food aisle, or to say the colors of foods they know. Find foods that are new to them, and talk about their color, shape, size, and feel.

● At home, as you take vegetables out of grocery bags, talk about the part of the plant each one grows on: leaf (cabbage, lettuce, greens), roots (carrot, potato), stalk (celery, asparagus), flower (broccoli, cauliflower, artichoke), and seed (peas, corn).

● Grow foods from seed in your backyard garden. Perhaps start the seeds in paper cups on your windowsill. Kids enjoy eating foods they grow themselves—and it's a great science lesson!

● Have children help decide what foods to serve. Perhaps show them pictures of vegetables and fruits. Have them pick the ones to make for family meals.

● As preschoolers are ready, give them simple tasks to help with family meals. They might wash fruit, arrange bread in a basket, put ready-to-eat cereal in bowls, or help set the table. Most children like to help. They feel good about themselves when they can say, for example, "I poured it!" Working together in the kitchen offers many chances to nurture children. *"Kids' Kitchen" later in this chapter provides more ideas.*

● Expand their world by reading books about food to children. Ask a librarian, preschool teacher, or head of the children's book department in a store to suggest titles. Prepare some foods from the stories.

For more about cooking with kids, including kitchen safety tips, see "Kids' Kitchen" later in this chapter.

Food in Child Care: Check It Out!

Warm and caring staff, a safe environment, opportunities for development and self-expression—that's what most parents look for when they choose child care. If you look for child care, rank good nutrition, food-safety standards, and active play high on your checklist, too. If your child has a food allergy or needs to avoid any food for religious or other reasons, find out how that's handled.

Child-Friendly Snacks

For children under age four, avoid popcorn, nuts, seeds, and other hard, small, whole foods to avoid choking. Chop raw carrots and grapes and cooked hot dogs in small pieces.

Grains Group
Animal crackers; cereal (dry or with milk); bagel; English muffin; graham crackers; pita (pocket) bread; rice cake; toast; tortilla; air-popped popcorn; pretzels. Go for whole-grain varieties whenever possible.

Milk Group
Cheese; cottage cheese; pudding; milk (including flavored milk); string cheese; yogurt; frozen yogurt

Vegetable Group
Any raw vegetable (cut in strips or circles); vegetable soup

Fruit Group
Any fresh fruit (sliced for finger food); canned or frozen fruit; fruit juice*; fruit leather; dried fruit

Meat and Beans Group
Bean soup; peanut butter; hard-cooked egg; turkey or meat cubes; tuna salad

* See advice about fruit juice in "Have You Ever Wondered . . . are fruit juices and fruit drinks good choices for kids?" in this chapter.

Consider the importance of the food served. A child may eat two or more meals and snacks in a child-care facility, so the nutritional quality must be high. Since a young child is developing eating skills and food attitudes that will affect long-term health, the overall eating environment is important, too.

A child-care setting offers many opportunities for spreading illness: food service, diapering, toileting, and close contact with others. For this reason, cleanliness and safe food handling are "musts." Infants and young children have immature immune systems; they're more vulnerable to catching a cold, flu, or other illness from others.

To help establish a lifelong habit of active living, children regularly involved in child care need a program with safe, fun, and developmentally appropriate ways to move more and sit less. Choose a program that makes active play a priority. Besides health, active living teaches social skills and helps develop body skills.

. . . what to do if you think your child can't drink milk?
Before you say "can't," know that milk sensitivity is often
a matter of degree. Lactose intolerance, or difficulty
digesting the sugar in milk, is more common than a milk
allergy. And it's easy to manage—often by giving the child
smaller, more frequent portions of milk. Also easier to
digest: chocolate milk; cheese, which has milk's nutrients; and milk itself enjoyed with an oatmeal cookie,
banana, or other snack.

   If you suspect a milk sensitivity, seek advice from
your child's doctor, pediatric nurse, or a registered dietitian. Don't simply give up milk! Your child depends on
you for calcium and other nutrients that milk provides
for proper growth. For tips on handling a child's sensitivity to milk, *see "Lactose Intolerance: A Matter of
Degree" in chapter 21.*

   *. . . what to do if your child has a phobia, or a fear, of
trying new foods?* Just relax, and give your child time to
outgrow it. Even kids who resist trying new foods can eat
in a healthful way, according to studies of kids' eating
behavior. In the meantime, offer a variety of foods, and
enjoy them yourself.

   As you look for child care, these factors suggest
high standards of cleanliness, nutrition, and active
play:

Food preparation and storage areas . . .

- Neat and very clean
- Properly labeled and well-covered foods
- Adequate refrigeration and heating equipment
- Perishable foods stored in the refrigerator

Hand-washing area . . .

- Child-size sinks, or safe stepping stools for
adult-size sinks
- Soap and paper towels

Mealtimes and snacktimes . . .

- Meals and snacks with a variety of foods from
the various groups of the Food Guide Pyramid.
(Most child-care settings have specific guidelines
and menus; ask to see them.)

- Tables and chairs appropriately sized for children's comfort, or high chairs, or booster seats
- Child-size utensils and covered cups with spouts
to help young children master their feeding skills
- Adult supervision at snacktimes and mealtimes
and adequate staffing for feeding infants and children with special needs

Diaper-changing and toilet areas . . .

- Very clean
- Located away from food, eating, and play areas
- Closed containers for soiled diapers, tissues, and
wipes
- Daily removal of soiled items

Other areas . . .

- Separate storage for each child's toothbrush,
comb, and clothing
- Ample space between cots, nap rugs, or cribs.

Observe what goes on in the child-care setting. You
should be able to answer "yes" to these questions:

- Do children, staff, and volunteers wash their
hands before and after eating or participating in
food activities?
- Do children wash their hands after outdoor play,
toileting, touching animals, sneezing, or wiping
their nose?
- Does each child have his or her own washcloth?
- Are child-care providers practicing appropriate
sanitation and food-handling techniques?
- Are bottles and foods brought from home refrigerated, and if necessary, heated safely? (*Hint:* When
you send food, always label it with your child's
name. Transport perishable foods in an insulated
sack with a cold pack.)
- Is food that's left on a child's plate discarded
properly?
- Do children each have their own dish, cup, and
utensils, rather than share?
- Does an adult eat with the children, serving as a
good role model? Can you volunteer from time to
time?
- Are menus posted, or are they sent home with
the children?

● Are the foods appropriate for the age of the children (e.g., no foods that may be choking hazards)?

● Are plates, cups, and utensils washed and sanitized after each use?

● Are toys that go into a child's mouth sanitized regularly?

● Do child-care providers and parents wash their hands thoroughly after every diaper check and change?

● Are food activities such as tasting parties, food preparation, growing food from seed, field trips, and circle time activities part of the child-care program? Can you be a parent volunteer?

● Is safe, physically active play part of the daily routine? Is it well supervised? Does it match the abilities of children?

Parents as Partners

For the many children in child care, feeding is a shared responsibility. Together, parents and child-care providers offer foods that nourish kids. And together they help children develop skills and a positive attitude about eating. Here's what you can do:

Physical Activity for Toddlers and Preschoolers

Toddlers and preschoolers: they like to run, jump, throw, and kick. Active living helps your child learn a variety of body skills, mental skills, and social skills, and begins a habit of lifelong active living and a healthy weight. And it's fun! Those skills develop when children have opportunities to move in their daily life. As a parent, it's up to you to encourage active play:

● Balance sedentary play (such as reading together) with plenty of active play.

● Choose day care that makes safe, active play a priority.

● Set aside time each day for active play together, perhaps tossing a ball, playing tag, or taking a family walk.

● Designate an inside and an outside area that's safe, where your child can freely jump, roll, and tumble.

● Pick toys that "move"—perhaps a ball or a tricycle.

● Join a play group together.

Have You Ever Wondered

. . . are fruit juices and fruit drinks good choices for kids? Actually, that takes a two-part answer.

Fruit juices: You know that kids need two to four fruit group servings daily. Fruit juice is one option, but be aware that too much juice can add up to a lot of calories, or crowd out other nourishing foods and beverages such as milk, and can spoil appetites. An excessive amount also can lead to diarrhea and intestinal discomfort. Sipping a lot of juice even promotes tooth decay. For children and teens, the American Academy of Pediatrics advises:

● *ages 1 to 6 years:* $1/2$ to $3/4$ cup (4 to 6 ounces) of fruit juice daily, maximum

● *ages 7 to 18 years:* 1 to $1^1/2$ cup (8 to 12 ounces) of fruit juice daily, maximum

For food safety sake, avoid unpasteurized juice.

Fruit drinks: They have some juice and perhaps added vitamin C or calcium, but they don't offer as many nutrients as fruit juice or milk. Read the Nutrition Facts and ingredient list to compare. *See "Juicy Story: Fruit Juice, Juice Drink, Fruit Drink . . . or Just Plain Water?" in chapter 8.*

. . . about iron poisoning—how does it happen? Iron poisoning from adult iron capsules or tablets—or from vitamin pills with iron—occurs when children accidentally swallow them. This can happen, too, if iron tablets meant for children aren't taken as directed, but instead at a higher dosage in a short period. If your doctor prescribes extra iron for your child, give it *only* as directed.

Iron poisoning can cause serious injury, even death. Call your doctor or a poison control center immediately if your child accidentally swallows a supplement with iron. Keep iron pills and all other pills in child-safe containers where your child can't reach them. *Note:* A healthful diet with iron-fortified foods won't cause iron poisoning!

● If your child has a feeding problem—perhaps a food sensitivity—address it together.

● Ask for a menu of meals and snacks. Identify new foods. Talk about and prepare these foods at home. Reinforce food tasting by serving foods your child first tries in day care.

● Practice hand washing before kids start child care.

Need more practical, easy ways to help your kids eat healthy? Check here for "how-tos":

- Help your child with proper dental care—see chapter 5.

- Help your child or teenager eat smart for sports—see chapter 19.

- Feed a vegetarian child or teen—see chapter 20.

- Deal with food allergies or intolerances at home, at day care, in school, or in a restaurant—see chapter 21.

- Find a nutrition expert experienced in issues for feeding kids—see chapter 24.

- If schedules allow, volunteer in a child-care setting to support the center's nutrition program. Offer to help with meal planning. Prepare a family food as a group activity for your child to share with classmates. Occasionally eat with children or help chaperon a food-related field trip. Or gather empty food packages and other kitchen supplies for play areas or for food activities. Early childhood educators appreciate this type of help!

Eating ABCs for School-Age Children

School-age youngsters—no longer preschoolers, not yet teens—are establishing habits that last a lifetime. For their good health and healthy weight, nutrition *and* physical activity should rank high as priorities.

During these years, children gain control of the world around them. They push for independence, associate more with their peers, and make more choices of their own. Because they're away from home more often, people other than family have a growing role in shaping their food decisions. A recent study showed that school-age children acknowledge teachers and schools, then parents as their main sources of nutrition information; television, books, then health professionals ranked next.

Keep these thoughts in mind as you help your school-age child develop healthful eating and active living habits to last a lifetime:

Nutrients. Children don't need any special foods for their growth, energy, and health, just enough food energy and nutrients. In fact, they need the same nutrients as their parents do, only in different amounts. However, two nutrients may need special attention: iron and calcium. Zinc, important for growth, may come up short, too.

Many different foods can provide the nutrients your child needs now—and prepare for the growth demands of adolescence. Eating at least the minimum number of servings from the Food Guide Pyramid supplies enough of the nutrients for most children. *See "Pyramid Power for Kids" in this chapter.* Adult guidelines for fat and cholesterol apply to school-age children, too; *see "Fat Facts for Kids" in this chapter. See "How Much Fiber: Just Add Five!" in this chapter for a fiber guideline.*

Growth. Children age six to twelve years grow about 2 inches per year. This represents a weight gain of about 5 pounds yearly. To look at it another way, children grow 1 to 2 feet and almost double their weight during these years.

Before you compare your child with another, remember that even in this period of steady growth, children's body sizes, shapes, and growth patterns vary. Most children grow in a pattern that's more like a parent than an unrelated friend. (Get out your family photo album for a visual memory.) *"BMIs for Kids: Tracking Their Growth" in this chapter offers a look at your child's growth pattern.*

A school-age child's appetite gradually increases; most eat more just before a growth spurt. During childhood, growth is gradual, accelerating most just prior to and during early adolescence: for girls, from ages ten through fourteen, and for boys, from ages twelve through sixteen. As long as a child is growing normally, he or she is getting enough calories.

Food Preferences and Habits. Children's appetites and food preferences are changeable. Eating small amounts or not eating certain foods may simply mean that your child is testing his or her tastes, or perhaps exerting independence.

BMIs for Kids: Tracking Their Growth

Growth charts—using the Body Mass Index (BMI) designed for children ages two and over, and teens—track growth, and a child's or a teen's weight in relation to height. These charts are used to assess whether a child *may be* underweight, at risk for overweight, or overweight. As importantly, the BMI charts assure parents and kids that there's a wide range of "normal." A muscular kid isn't necessarily fat, and a slim kid isn't necessarily underweight. They're simply different.

As children mature, it's normal for their body fat to change. Each child's growth clock, body size, and shape are individual; girls and boys differ, too. Some kids plump up before puberty to prepare for their next rapid growth spurt. Remember, your child will likely grow as one of his or her parents did at the same age.

As a parent, you can use these charts to help track your child's growth. Be aware that even the extremes—5th percentile or 95th percentile—don't necessarily mean your child is underweight or overweight. Let your physician make that determination, using additional measures. *See the Appendices for the Growth Charts with Body Mass Index for Age Percentiles for Boys and for Girls, 2 to 20 Years.*

Children learn their food habits by watching others—not just parents, but also friends, teachers, and media. For parents: your food choices and lifestyle habits help set their food decisions and behavior. How big are your portions? Do you eat a variety of foods? Try new foods? Skip the urge to eat to relieve stress? Fit in physical activity each day?

Set up chances for your child to make healthful choices and establish good eating habits. *See "Empower Your Kids: Seven How-tos for Smart Snacking" on this page.*

Nutrition Knowledge. Depending on their age, many children know the healthful eating basics. And most know that they need to eat smart and move their bodies to stay healthy. The challenge for parents, teachers, and other adults is to help kids link what they know and what they do.

Take time to help your child practice what's learned about healthful eating at school. For example, encourage your child to use the Food Guide Pyramid to choose or help plan a family meal or their own snack.

Physical Activity. For good health, children need to move! Yet today, many don't move enough. Among the reasons? Excess TV watching, too much leisure time at the computer or with video games, concern about safe outdoor play, riding instead of walking to school, and fewer opportunities for noncompetitive play in school. Inactivity is linked to the dramatic rise in childhood overweight.

How much physical activity? Children need at least sixty minutes of physical activity a day. Active play can provide enough.

Nutrition for Growing Up

School-age children love to measure their progress from year to year on a growth chart. They want energy to run and play—and the energy to do well in school.

Empower Your Kids: Seven How-tos for Smart Snacking

Here's the key to healthful food choices: very visible, convenient, effortless—great taste.

1. Ask your kids what food-group foods they'd like to have on hand. Buy them!

2. "Walk" your kids through the kitchen so they know where these foods are kept.

3. Keep fresh fruit on the counter where kids see it.

4. Wash and cut up veggies ahead, so they're ready to eat.

5. Use see-through containers, clear plastic bags, or containers covered with plastic wrap so kids can see what's inside.

6. Put food where kids can reach it, perhaps on lower shelves in your refrigerator, pantry, or cabinet. Keep "sometimes" foods such as cookies and chips away in cabinets where they're less convenient to reach, especially for impulse eaters.

7. Buy food in single-serve containers for grab-and-go eating—for example, milk, raisins, juice, fruit cups, pudding, baby carrots. "Single serve" is enough for one serving, not two or three.

Parents, teachers, and other caregivers have the same priorities. How can children eat to grow up healthy . . . and have energy to learn and play?

Pyramid Power for Kids

Meant for children age two or more, as well as for teens and adults, the Food Guide Pyramid guides healthful eating. It's flexible enough for everyone and any food—including foods youngsters like most.

Inside the Food Groups. Eating many different foods—both among and within the five food groups—provides the food energy and a variety of nutrients that growing, active children need:

- Milk, yogurt, and cheese provide calcium, vitamin D, and protein for their growing bones, teeth, and muscles.

- Meat, poultry, fish, eggs, beans, nuts, and seeds supply protein, iron, B vitamins, and some minerals to support growth of their body cells and healthy blood.

- Breads, cereals, pasta, and other grain products provide complex carbohydrates, B vitamins, iron, other minerals, and fiber. Complex "carbs" should be their main energy source. Try to have at least half the servings from this group come from whole-grain foods.

- Vegetables provide beta carotene (which forms vitamin A) and vitamin C, complex carbohydrates, and fiber. They also supply significant amounts of some B vitamins, potassium, calcium, and other minerals.

- Fruit supplies beta carotene and vitamin C, potassium, and some other minerals to keep their skin, eyes, and gums healthy. Fruit also supplies carbohydrate and fiber. Kids like fruit—a nutritious sweet snack with a natural supply of sugar!

How much is enough? *Check the information in "Pyramid Servings for School-Age Children" on this page.*

Variety: More than Burgers and Pizza. Your child can enjoy foods he or she likes: perhaps a hamburger, pizza, fries, and ice cream. Enjoying more variety—not too much of any one food or food group—is important, too. Teach your child how to enjoy other

---

Pyramid Servings for School-Age Children

Energy needs of school-age children vary, largely due to growth rate, activity level, and body size. Most school-age children need about 1,800 to 2,500 calories a day, assuming they include about sixty minutes of active play as well. Here's how children can meet that calorie target and get the nutrients they need:

FOOD GROUP	NUMBER OF SERVINGS
Grains	6 to 9
Vegetable	3 to 4
Fruit	2 to 3
Milk	2 to 3
Meat and Beans	2 to 3 (about 5 to 6 oz.)

For more about the Pyramid and serving sizes for each group, see "What's Inside the Pyramid?" in chapter 10. Children may prefer smaller portions. That's okay if their portions add up to the total recommended for the day.

For the "Fats, Oils, and Sweets" on the Pyramid tip, go easy—using small amounts to add flavor and enjoyment to your child's meals.

---

veggies besides fries; fruit as a sweet snack, not just ice cream; and other kinds of protein-rich sandwiches. *See "Foods to 'Chews'" in this chapter for other ideas.*

Go Easy on "Sometimes Foods." What about candy and soft drinks? If children eat enough food-group servings without overdoing on calories, they can enjoy foods from the Pyramid tip occasionally, as well as some food-group foods with more fat. Overall food choices, not just one food or one meal, are what counts.

Let's Learn about the Pyramid! Primary-grade children are ready to learn basic messages of the Food Guide Pyramid: where foods fit in the food groups, how to choose foods for variety, and how many food group servings they need each day. Older children are better able to learn about moderation and balance.

To help your child think about all the different foods in his or her meals and snacks, try this simple finger game. Name each finger and the thumb on one

How Much Fiber? Just Add Five!

You know you need fiber. Kids do, too. From childhood on, an eating pattern that's low in fat and cholesterol and high in fiber-containing foods, such as whole grains, legumes, vegetables, and fruits, helps reduce the risk of heart disease, diabetes, and some types of cancer later in life.

How much fiber do kids need? That depends on their age. As they grow and develop, they need more and more.

Adding five to your child's age is an easy-to-remember number for how much fiber your child needs. Use it for healthy kids from ages three to eighteen:

child's age + 5 = the grams of dietary fiber daily

For example, a 6-year-old child would need about 11 grams of fiber daily; 6 + 5 = 11. And a 12-year-old would be smart to eat about 17 fiber grams daily; 12 + 5 = 17.

Remember: Just add five!

● Offer raw finger-food veggies. Kids may prefer uncooked vegetables. They like to "dip," too. So offer salsa, bean dip, or herb-flavored plain yogurt.

● Kids like the bright color and crisp texture of vegetables. To keep them appealing, steam or microwave veggies in small amounts of water, or stir-fry.

● Start a "veggie club." Try to taste vegetables from A to Z, and check off letters of the alphabet as you go! As you shop, let kids pick a new vegetable as a family "adventure." Post a tasting chart on the refrigerator door to recognize family tasters.

● Grow veggies together. If you don't have a garden, plant a container garden. Most kids eat vegetables they grow!

● From your library, check out children's books about vegetables. Read the story, then taste the veggies together!

● Nothing works? Offer more fruit, which is another source of vitamins A and C.

Source: "Healthy Start: Food to Grow On," volume IV (Food Marketing Institute, American Dietetic Association, and American Academy of Pediatrics, 1995). Reprinted with permission by the Food Marketing Institute, ©1995.

hand for one of the five food groups. Then have your child count the food groups he or she ate—one food group per finger. Try this when you talk about choices on school menus. **Caution:** Experiencing and enjoying a variety of foods is appropriate for kids; they don't need to master the Pyramid!

Five-a-Day for Kids: The Challenge

Kids—and adults, too—are urged to eat at least "five a day"—three vegetable and two fruit servings—for plenty of health reasons! Yet American kids typically eat just half that much, and more than half their vegetable intake is potatoes (most often high-fat fries) or tomatoes. Studies show that snacks are much more likely to be cookies, chips, other salty snacks, candy, and dessert foods than either fruit or veggies.

What's a parent to do when vegetables are greeted with a chorus of "yuck"?

● Add veggies to kid favorites. Mix peas into macaroni and cheese. Add carrot shreds to spaghetti sauce, chili, lasagna, even peanut butter. Put zucchini shreds into burgers or mashed potatoes.

● "Fortify" ready-to-eat soup with extra vegetables or canned beans.

What about Nutrient Supplements?

Does your child eat a variety of foods? Do his or her meals and snacks follow Pyramid advice? If so, your child probably doesn't need a nutrient supplement. Meals and snacks likely supply enough vitamins and other nutrients for growth and health. Food is the best nutrient source, anyway.

If your child has a feeding problem that lasts for several weeks or if you're unsure about your child's nutrient intake, get expert advice. Before you give your child a supplement, talk to your child's doctor or a registered dietitian.

Beware of claims for supplements targeted to help children get over colds, depression, or attention deficit disorder, among others. These claims aren't supported by sound science, and such supplements may be harmful. An appropriate supplement may be recommended: (1) if your child avoids an entire food group due to a food dislike, allergy, or intolerance, or (2) if your child is a vegetarian. If your water supply isn't fluoridated, a fluoride supplement may be advised.

If your health provider recommends a nutrient supplement for your child:

● Buy what's advised, perhaps a children's supplement. Check with the pharmacist if you need help. It should have no more than 100 percent of the Daily Values (DV). Unless stated otherwise, the % Daily Values stated on the Supplement Facts panel are meant for children age four or older, as well as for adults. On supplements meant for younger children, look for the % DV for children under age four. **Beware:** *An adult iron supplement can be dangerous for children!*

● Choose a supplement with a childproof cap. Store it out of your child's reach.

● Give a supplement only in the safe, recommended dose. Too much can be harmful.

● Remember that supplements are just that—supplements. They are not an excuse to forgo good eating habits!

● Remind children that supplements aren't candy, even if they come in fun names, colors, shapes, and package designs.

● Remember that enriched and fortified foods may have the same added nutrients that the supplement has. Read labels to make sure your child doesn't get too much.

For more about dietary supplements, see chapter 23.

Eating Strategies for Children

How can you help your school-age child eat well? Many feeding strategies you used during the preschool

---

Foods to "Chews"

Chances are that some of your child's favorite foods are higher in fat and food energy. To get the most nutrition and to trim calories and fat, offer these foods:

MORE OFTEN . . .	LESS OFTEN . . .
Baked potato	French fries
Baked or grilled chicken	Fried chicken strips and nuggets
Bagels or English muffins	Doughnuts and breakfast pastries
Graham crackers, animal crackers, fig bars	Chocolate-chip cookies, cupcakes
Pretzels, plain popcorn	Potato chips
Milk, fruit juice	Soft drinks
Raw vegetable snacks, fruit	Candy
Frozen yogurt	Ice cream

---

years apply now, too. *See "Mealtime Tactics" earlier in this chapter.* Keep these ideas top-of-mind, too:

Most school-age children do best with a regular meal schedule. Like preschoolers, they can't compensate for hunger as adults can. When meals aren't regular or when meals are missed, children tend to snack more heavily throughout the day, so they're less hungry at mealtime.

For the same reason, breakfast skipping is a concern. Breakfast is a healthful and important start for a day of learning and active play. *See "Nutrition and Learning" and "Easy Breakfasts for Kids to Make" in this chapter.*

The family table offers nutrition benefits—and more! According to recent research, kids who eat frequent family dinners also eat more calcium, iron, fiber, and several vitamins, and less saturated fat and trans fats. They also eat one more fruit or vegetable serving daily. So the family table matters!

Telling kids to eat nutritious foods and have good table manners is one thing; showing them is the best teacher! The family table also promotes family bonding—a time to talk and listen and to create family memories.

Have You Ever Wondered

. . . if herbal supplements are good for kids? Although touted as "natural" remedies or "healthy" alternatives, herbal supplements should be used only under the guidance of a qualified healthcare provider. Their effects can be powerful, potentially harmful to your child, and perhaps ineffective for the advertised benefit.

● Eat as a family—if possible, at least once a day. If it's breakfast, set the table the night before for less effort in the morning.

● If your family is always "on the go," designate family dinner nights. Planning ahead makes it easier to fit family meals in.

● Cook fast, eat slowly. Spend your kitchen time together at the table rather than on making a fancy meal. *See "Quick-to-Fix-Meal Tips" in chapter 10.*

● Turn off the TV, and put the phone answering system on to make food and family important.

● Eat around a table, not side by side at the counter. That's better for conversation and eye contact.

● Keep family mealtime positive: pleasant talk, a chance for everyone (including your child) to share and get attention, a mealtime that's neither rushed nor prolonged.

Children need to make their own food decisions. They usually eat better when they feel in control of their own food choices. As an adult, provide a variety of nutrient-rich foods—new and familiar—from which your child can choose.

● Let your child choose what and how much to eat from what you offer. Respect his or her food preferences and appetite. And help your child to eat slowly and pay attention to feeling full. Give your child the freedom to politely refuse foods he or she doesn't want.

● Involve kids in planning meals and snacks. It's a chance to practice making food decisions. Children often eat foods that they help plan and prepare.

● Encourage your child to try new foods—without forcing or bribing them. Trying new foods is like a new hobby; it expands his or her food knowledge, experience, and skills. Include foods from cultures other than your own. Acknowledge that your child will like some, but not all, of those foods. That's okay.

Kids learn to like mostly foods they eat often. If you offer fruits and vegetables regularly—and if they see you eating them, too—the chances are that your child will learn to like them.

Snacks help children eat for health. Chosen carefully, they supply food group servings—and nutrients—that may be missing from the day's meals. Snacks can help supply food energy that growing, active children need. Kids who use up more energy in active play, organized sports, or after-school activities need more food energy—and more snacks—than kids who watch TV, play video games, or have a sedentary after-school routine. *For snacks kids can make, see "Kitchen Nutrition: Healthful, No-Cook Snacks for Kids" later in this chapter. For more about snacking, see "That Snack Attack!" in chapter 10.*

What children eat over several days counts—not what they eat for one meal or one day. There's no need for concern if your child occasionally skips food-group foods or doesn't eat much at a meal.

Children develop good eating habits when mealtimes and snacktimes are pleasant. Mealtime stress can lead to emotional overeating or undereating, so try to avoid fussing, nagging, arguing, or complaining at the table.

Nutrition and Learning

Why do kids need breakfast? Among other reasons, a well-nourished child is ready to learn. Fit kids more likely have the energy, stamina, and self-esteem that enhance their ability to learn. Healthful eating, along with regular physical activity, help kids get and stay fit.

Nutrition experts, other health professionals, and educators have long recognized that severe nutrient deficiencies—improper growth, retarded mental development, and very low energy levels—hinder learning. Studies show that iron deficiency among children leads to poor behavior, difficulty concentrating, and poor performance.

Mild undernutrition isn't as easily recognized. But it, too, may affect how children learn—for example, a mild iron deficiency can affect brain function. Mild undernutrition may not be an economic issue, but instead be a matter of poor food choices or meal skipping.

On a regular basis, breakfast skipping is linked to lower school achievement and performance. Conversely, a morning meal helps children succeed with learning. They have energy to learn. Studies show that breakfast eaters tend to have higher school attendance, less tardiness, and fewer hunger-induced stomach aches in the morning. Their overall test scores are better. And they concentrate better, solve problems more easily, and have better muscle coordination. Kids who eat breakfast are less likely to be overweight and more likely to get enough calcium, too. *For more about breakfast and learning and ways to fit breakfast in for your child, see "Why Breakfast?" in chapter 10 and "Easy Breakfasts for Kids to Make" in this chapter.*

For Kids Only—Today's School Meals

What's for school lunch? What's for school breakfast? For parents, school meals offer an inexpensive, convenient, and nutritious solution for one or two meals for their kids. For many children and teens, school meals contribute significantly to their overall nutrient and energy intake. For kids who aren't hungry first thing in the morning, school breakfast may offer the perfect solution.

In most school districts—probably yours—school meals are regulated through the U.S. Department of Agriculture (USDA). The USDA meal patterns are designed carefully to supply about one-quarter of a child's need for key nutrients and energy from School Breakfast, and about one-third of them from School Lunch, at five different age or grade groups.

The USDA's National School Food Service Program has taken a lead in a national effort to help children and teens make healthful food choices. The challenge? Serving meals that appeal to kids and support advice from the Food Guide Pyramid and the Dietary Guidelines for Americans. Local school meal programs are charged with planning and serving meals that help children expand the variety of foods in their diet; add more fruits, vegetables, and grains, preferably whole-grains, to the foods they already eat; and construct a diet lower in fat.

For that reason, many schools have modified their menus—for example, serving leaner beef, oven-baked fries, sandwiches served on whole-grain bread, dried and fresh fruit, salad bars, and reduced-fat and fat-free milk along with whole milk.

Because most school meals have federal financial support, children and teens of all income levels have access to nutritious meals during the school day at a low cost. Some kids qualify for free or reduced-price meals.

If your child buys school meals, he or she may have choices on the cafeteria line, perhaps more than one

vegetable or several types of milk. In many schools, students can select three to five items from the school lunch menu for the same price. Other schools provide up to seven items, including more fruits and vegetables. Having choices helps students build smart eating skills—and it helps ensure that children eat healthful meals. It's part of "eating right" education!

As a parent volunteer, you can be involved in and support school meals in your community—and help your child or teen choose healthful meals at school:

● Get familiar with the menu. Keep a current school lunch menu and perhaps a breakfast menu in your kitchen. Find them in school mailings or in your local newspaper. You can ask for nutrition information about the menus from the school food service director.

● Go over the menu with your child; especially talk about new foods. Talk about making choices on the cafeteria line; practice at home.

● If your child has a food allergy, restricts food for any reason (perhaps for religious, cultural, or health reasons), or chooses to be a vegetarian, talk to a school administrator and school food service staff. Most schools can prepare meals that match your child's unique needs—if they know ahead.

● Get involved. Join the parent advisory committee for the school food service program. If none exists, take the lead and work with the school to set one up.

● Have lunch—or breakfast—with kids occasionally. Parents usually are welcome to eat a meal at school. That gives you a chance to become more familiar with the school food program, the types of foods served, and the overall atmosphere in the school cafeteria.

● Get to know the school food service staff. Volunteer to help with special meal events, with new food tastings, or at regular meal hours. Express your support. As you build relationships, pass along constructive suggestions.

● Support school nutrition education. Find out what your children are learning, and help them apply it at home.

● In the upper grades, school menus often offer burgers, pizza, and tacos. Encourage your child to choose a salad, fresh fruit, yogurt, and/or milk to go with them.

● Encourage school clubs and parent associations to serve food-group food and drinks for fund-raising events, school parties, and in school vending machines.

Another school-related tip: Be an advocate for physical activity as part of every school day. More and more schools and communities are recognizing that active play is a lifelong habit that children need to learn and practice now!

Brown-Bagging It!

Often, the older the children are, the more they want to join classmates in the cafeteria line. But some children prefer to carry a bag lunch. If that's true for your child, pack meals that please—foods that are easy to prepare and fun to eat as well as healthful, safe, and nutritious.

● What tote will your child choose: brown bag, insulated bag, or lunch box? Ask what your child prefers. For most kids, having the "right" container is important. A lunch box is easier to clean, and it may keep food cool longer. Just be sure to wash it after every use! If a brown bag is preferred, always use a new one.

● If you send perishable foods, such as a sandwich with meat, include a small, frozen cold pack. And remind the child to bring it back home! A frozen can or box of juice also keeps food cool.

● Plan easy-to-eat foods—for example, sandwiches, raw vegetable pieces (carrots, red or green bell peppers, cucumbers, cherry tomatoes), crackers, cheese slices or cubes, string cheese, whole fruit, individual containers of pudding, or an oatmeal cookie. *See "Produce 'Package'" in chapter 10 for easy-to-pack raw veggies.* If you pack an orange, score the rind so it's easy to peel—or tuck in a tangerine instead! It's okay to pack a brownie or a small bag of chips as part of a healthful bag lunch. Kids may need the extra energy they supply.

● Remember milk money. Kids need the calcium in dairy foods for their growing bones!

● Expect children to help plan and prepare their school lunches. When they're involved, they'll probably eat every morsel—rather than trade their raw veggies for someone else's cookie.

● Remind kids to store their carried meals at school in a clean, safe place—away from sunlight and the heat vent in the classroom and not in a dirty gym bag!

Easy Breakfasts for Kids to Make

Breakfast—with food from the Milk, Grains, Fruit, and/or Meat and Beans Groups—can set your child in a healthful nutrition direction for the day. What's for breakfast? Even if kids are on their own in the morning, most can make these easy breakfasts. For at least three food groups, they go down even "healthier" with juice or milk!

G = Grains , **V** = Vegetable, **F** = Fruit, **M** = Milk, **MB** = Meat and Beans

● Cheese slices served with—or melted on—toast	**M** **G**
● Iron-fortified cereal and milk, with banana slices	**G** **M** **F**
● Peanut butter spread on toasted whole grain bread or a waffle, or rolled inside a wheat tortilla	**MB** **G**
● Fruit—bananas, strawberries, raisins—and milk on instant oatmeal	**F** **M** **G**
● Cold pizza	**G** **M** **V**
● Leftover spaghetti or macaroni and cheese	**G** **M**
● Apple and cheese slices between whole-wheat or graham crackers	**F** **M** **G**
● Breakfast cereal topped with fresh fruit and a scoop of frozen yogurt	**G** **F** **M**

● *Hint:* Add extra pleasure to a carried meal with an occasional surprise tucked inside—a riddle, a comic, or a note that says, "You're somebody special!" Knowing that someone cares is "nourishing" in its own way.

For more about carried meals and food safety, see "Carry It Safe" in chapter 12.

Weighty Problems for Children—Overweight

Over the past thirty years, the number of overweight children in the United States has about tripled, with about 13 percent of kids ages six to eleven considered overweight, and 14 percent of teens ages twelve to nineteen overweight, according to the Centers for Disease Control and Prevention. Obesity rates have risen, too. In fact, overweight has been described as the most common nutrition problem among American children today.

Excess weight during these early years can have long-term physical and psychological consequences.

Have You Ever Wondered?

... how you know if your child is eating right? Start by asking: Is my child growing well? Does he or she have energy to play and learn? If so, he or she probably is eating enough. Your child's doctor, pediatric nurse, or a registered dietitian can help you monitor your child's growth and development by plotting his or her progress on a growth chart. The other question to ask: Is your child eating a variety of foods and enough servings from the Food Guide Pyramid? If so, he or she probably is getting enough nutrients to grow well.

... if your child gets enough to drink? Active children need eight or more cups of water during the day, as you do. Children perspire with active play, even outside in cold weather when they're bundled up. Just plain water is great for replenishing fluids; bring some along if you plan to be out for longer than an hour, or go on an extended car trip. Kids may drink more water if it's offered in appealing "sports bottles." *Check chapter 19 if your child is involved in strenuous sports.*

... if sugar causes kids to be hyperactive? No. There's no scientific evidence linking sugar to behavior. *For more about hyperactivity and eating, see "Does Food Cause Childhood Hyperactivity?" in chapter 21.*

Compared with normal-weight peers, overweight children more likely become obese adults, and so more prone to health problems later in life—for example, diabetes, heart disease, high blood pressure, stroke, osteoarthritis, gallbladder disease, and some forms of cancer. Research shows that 60 percent of overweight children, ages five to ten, have at least one heart disease risk factor.

Of concern, obese children are about 50 percent more likely to develop insulin resistance, which often precedes adult-onset Type 2 diabetes. Type 2 diabetes, usually seen in overweight adults, now is being seen in children and teens as well! And complications from diabetes are appearing sooner, too. *See "Children and Diabetes" in chapter 22 for more on diabetes.*

There are psychological prices, too: overweight children may lose their self-esteem, have a poor body image, feel emotionally stressed, and perhaps isolate themselves from their peers.

Why do children become overweight? There's no one reason. Family history, inactivity, and poor food habits all contribute to childhood weight problems. A child with one or two overweight parents has a higher risk, but there's a debate whether the reasons are genetic, behavioral, or both. Such a recent epidemic of obesity means it's probably not limited to genetic factors alone. It's true, however, that children often mimic the food and lifestyle habits they observe at home. Heavy snacking, irregular meals, inactivity, and eating a lot of high-fat foods can contribute to weight problems, too. It's highly unlikely that a child's weight problem is caused by a hormone imbalance.

A family history doesn't destine children to being overweight adults. Often children shed extra "kid" fat during the rapid growth spurt of puberty. Overweight kids won't necessarily be overweight adults, either. However, the risk goes up as children get older if they still carry excess weight. Increased physical activity and balanced, healthful eating are key to helping prevent a child from becoming overweight. Addressing weight problems early is important.

How do you know if your child is overweight? Adults should never assess a child's body weight by their own standards. BMI charts for adults aren't meant for kids! *Instead see "BMIs for Kids: Tracking Their Growth" earlier in this chapter.* At each stage of development, children have different amounts of body fat.

Children of the same age aren't necessarily the same shape either. Your child's doctor should make the assessment.

How can adults help overweight children achieve a healthy weight—without giving up good nutrition? Because their bodies are growing and developing, weight loss isn't the best approach for most children. Instead, for most kids, slowing or stopping weight gain so a child grows into his or her weight is usually best. In other words, let a child's height catch up with his or her weight. A diet that's too restrictive—with too few calories—may not supply the food energy and nutrients a child needs for normal growth and development and can trigger unhealthy binge eating if the child feels too deprived.

Weight problems aren't just about food. Many other factors, such as emotions, family problems, lifestyle, and self-image, intertwine with eating behavior. Address the whole child—emotionally, socially, mentally, and physically—as you seek approaches to weight management.

In many cases, lifestyle changes—often for the whole family—offer the best approach for helping an overweight child manage his or her weight. *"Eating Strategies for Children" earlier in this chapter also apply to every child—overweight, normal weight, or underweight.*

If Your Child or Teen Has a Weight Problem . . .

● Seek professional advice. Your child needs a medical evaluation first. A registered dietitian, your doctor, or the school nurse can help you find an approach that's right for the nutritional and developmental needs of your child. Keep in mind that weight loss approaches for adults aren't right for children. *See "How to Find Nutrition Help . . ." in chapter 24.*

● Encourage physical activities your child enjoys. Besides burning calories, physical activity indirectly affects eating—for example, appetite control, stress release, and mental diversion from eating. Make physical activity a family affair. When parents are physically active, the chances are that their kids are active, too.

● Be aware that overweight children are often self-conscious in organized or competitive games. Instead, encourage activities such as walking the dog or biking, where skill and an audience are less important. *For more about physical activity, see "Get Up and Move, Turn Off the Tube!" later in this chapter.*

● Give your child more control over how much to eat. That may seem counterintuitive; however, when parents put pressure or restrictions on food choices too much, kids don't learn self-regulation. They may overeat if they can't read their own body signals for hunger and satiety.

● Consider other reasons to avoid restricting food. An overly restricted eating approach may keep your child from getting nutrients he or she needs. Restrictions also may lead to sneaking food, perhaps at someone else's home, and then feeling guilty or bad about themselves.

● Involve your whole family in healthful eating. In that way your overweight child won't feel singled out—and everybody benefits!

● Tailor portion sizes for your child. Large portions may encourage overeating. Use smaller plates so less looks like more. A hungry child can always ask for more.

● Avoid undue attention to eating. For example, forget rewarding or punishing a child with food. In that way you won't reinforce an emotional link to eating.

● Stock your kitchen with lower-calorie snack choices such as raw vegetables, fruit, juice, milk, or vanilla wafers. Instead of heavy snacking, count on meals to provide most of your child's nutrients and food energy.

● Avoid labeling food choices as "good" or "bad." Instead, help your child see how any food can fit in an eating pattern that's healthful. Even kids who need to trim extra pounds of body fat can have an occasional cookie or a piece of candy. In fact, they probably need a high-calorie snack from time to time to meet their energy needs. Labeling food as "good" or "bad" puts inappropriate significance on food. Anyway, the body doesn't see food in black-and-white terms. It's the whole eating plan that counts.

● Store food out of sight, and be careful about bringing a lot of higher-calorie foods into the house. When food sits on the kitchen counter, grabbing a cookie or a handful of chips may be more habit than hunger. For many people—kids, too—just seeing food stimulates the appetite.

● Set time limits on watching television—no more than one or two hours daily. Limit video games and computer time, too. All three keep kids away from outside play. Inactivity often leads to weight problems. Children who watch four or more hours of television a day are twice as likely to be overweight as youngsters who don't.

● Make a household practice for everyone: eat only in the kitchen or dining room. Kids probably won't eat as much—and they'll be more conscious about eating. High-calorie snacks that may go along with TV watching or homework can add to any problem.

● Refrain from eating meals in front of the TV, too. It's easy to eat more when attention is shifted away from the meal and satiety cues, and instead to a TV show.

● Take time to talk to your child about his or her feelings. Observe emotions and subsequent behavior. Together look for ways other than eating to address emotions. Help your child understand: even though eating may feel good for a while, food can't solve problems!

Have You Ever Wondered

... if foods grown with pesticides are safe for kids? With more than a hundred required tests directly relevant to children and infants, there's no evidence that children are being harmed from pesticide residues in food, water, or the environment. Any residue is hundreds to thousands of times lower than what might potentially pose a health risk. The safety evaluation takes children's diets, body weight, and rapid growth into account. And the Food Quality Assurance Act of 1996 includes additional provisions aimed at protecting children from pesticides. The health benefits of eating fruits and vegetables far outweigh any potential risk.

As a precaution, rinse vegetables to remove any residues. *For more answers to questions about foods grown with pesticides see "Pesticides: Carefully Controlled" in chapter 9.*

... if lead in drinking water is harmful to children? Infants and children are at higher risk for lead poisoning than others. Among other problems, lead that builds up in the body over time can cause brain damage. *To learn how to detect and deal with lead in drinking water see "Get the Lead Out!" in chapter 8.*

● Be aware that sometimes kids say they're hungry when they're really bored or want your attention. Probe a little. Offer a snack, perhaps a cracker or an apple. If neither one sounds right to the child, he or she is probably bored, not hungry.

For more on childhood obesity, see "Obesity and Kids: A Heavy Burden" in chapter 2.

More Weighty Problems for Children— Fear of Weight Gain

A desire to be overly thin, prompted both by media messages and by what parents say and do, is reaching down to school-age children. Children, mostly girls, as young as age six or seven express concerns about their body image and gaining weight. Among other things, inappropriate weight loss at this age can interfere with a child's growth—and may lead to eating disorders down the road.

Parents may play an even bigger role than media, according to some research, in shaping a child's body image. Here's what you can do now, even before your child hits adolescence:

● Quit worrying about your child's weight. Instead, strive for a positive eating relationship with your child. Teach healthful eating habits.

● Refrain from negative comments about your own weight or anyone else's weight. Avoid pressuring your child to conform to any particular body size or shape.

● Set a good example in the way you manage your own weight and in the way you feel about your own body image. Skip the lure of fad dieting for yourself.

● Encourage physical activity to build muscles and coordination. And work to develop your child's social skills, self-confidence, and self-esteem.

See "Disordered Eating: Problems, Signs, and Help" in chapter 2 and "Mainly for Girls: Pressure to Be Thin" later in this chapter.

Eating Out with Kids

Eating out with kids? It may be a necessity in your busy lifestyle—or perhaps a special treat for your family. To make restaurant meals a healthful and pleasant experience for the whole family, and a chance to teach kids how to behave away from home:

● Choose a restaurant that caters to children. A place that serves food quickly probably is best; waiting too long at the table is hard for kids. If you have a toddler and preschooler, ask for a high chair or a booster seat.

Should You Have Your Child's Cholesterol Level Checked?

Perhaps, but it's not routinely recommended for all children. Do so if your own total count is 240 mg/dL (milligrams per deciliter of blood) or higher, or if you or your spouse has suffered a heart attack before age fifty-five, or if you have a family history of heart disease before age fifty-five. Then your child may be at risk for high blood cholesterol levels.

If your child has a higher than normal blood cholesterol level, don't panic. High cholesterol levels among children don't necessarily predict high levels in adulthood. But when children come from high-risk families, you're prudent to check with your doctor and work with a registered dietitian to bring the level down. It may be good advice for the whole family!

For young people ages two through nineteen years with a parent with high blood cholesterol or a family history of early heart disease, these blood cholesterol levels should be noted for children and teens:

LEVELS	TOTAL CHOLESTEROL (MG/DL)	LDL CHOLESTEROL (MG/DL)
High	200 or greater	130 or greater
Borderline	170 to 199	110 to 129
Acceptable	Less than 170	Less than 110

Compelling research suggests that the process of atherosclerosis starts in childhood. For that reason, the American Heart Association notes that children and teens with these risk factors for heart disease need attention:

● Cigarette smoking: discourage it.

● High blood pressure: identify and treat it.

● Obesity: prevent it or reduce weight.

● Diabetes: diagnose and treat it.

● Inactivity: encourage regular aerobic exercise (thirty to sixty minutes three to four days a week).

For more about blood cholesterol levels see "Heart Disease: The Blood Lipid Connection" in chapter 22.

Save upscale table service for older children, teens, and adults.

● Match your eating-out schedule to a child's needs. When meals are delayed, kids can't compensate for hunger pangs as adults can. You'll only end up with a cranky meal companion! Offer a small snack ahead if you need to.

● Ask for a children's menu or look for simply prepared foods on the regular menu. Skip the urge to just order fries or fried chicken nuggets for your child. Most restaurants can prepare simple "kid foods" such as a hamburger or a grilled cheese sandwich or pasta.

● Before ordering, ask about the preparation. Most young and school-age children like plain foods with the sauce or the dressing on the side. In that way they have a choice.

● Choose two or three suitable menu items. Then let your child pick—and even place the order if he or she wants to. (Avoid pressuring your child.) Making choices encourages independence and gives kids control over their eating.

● Let kids order familiar favorites when they eat out. For new foods offer a bite or two from your order.

● If regular portions are too big for children, ask for appetizer portions. Or share an order . . . perhaps between two kids or with you. Kids shouldn't be expected to "polish" their plate. Instead, consider bringing leftovers home safely.

What if . . . Your Child Gets Fussy in a Restaurant?

● Excuse yourselves from the table. Take a short walk.

● Talk in a calm, quiet, and positive way. This isn't the place for loud discipline.

● Avoid forcing your child to eat. Instead, have the meal packed to take home.

● Ask if the restaurant has a paper place mat to color or draw on. Think ahead. Bring your own crayons, too—just in case.

● Bring along a stuffed animal to "share" the fun.

Source: Duyff, R.L. *Nibbles for Health* (Washington, D.C.: U.S. Department of Agriculture, 2002).

● Curb your child's appetite while you wait for the order. Ask for a small portion of raw vegetables or bread—just enough to take the edge off hunger, but not enough to interfere with a meal. Ask for water *with* the meal, not before, so your child doesn't fill up on liquids.

● Make eating out a pleasant experience for kids. Engage them in table talk as you wait for your meal.

For more about ordering in a restaurant, see "Have It Your Way!" in chapter 14.

Ten Things for Kids to Do Instead of Watching TV

1. Encourage kids to set up a jump rope contest. If they're older, go "double dutch" with two ropes. (A Hula Hoop contest is fun, too.)

2. Take the dog for a brisk walk together. Don't have a dog? Have kids take their teddy bears for a stroll instead. Walking as a family is good talking time!

3. Give kids colored chalk to create a sidewalk mural. Or draw a hopscotch game—fun to play alone or with friends.

4. Don't let rainy days put a damper on fun! Turn up the radio and dance inside.

5. Start a "hundred" walking club. Who's first in your family to walk a hundred times up and down the sidewalk or the stairs in your house?

6. Play a game of tag or kickball in the playground, park, or backyard.

7. If there's snow, make a snowman or go sledding. Or take the family ice skating at any time of year at an ice rink—even in July!

8. On warm days, go in-line skating or ride bikes (remember the helmet and pads), or run through sprinkler "rain."

9. Enjoy a hike together in a nearby park or forest preserve. Have kids find ten points of natural interest to enjoy as you hike.

10. Host a neighborhood bicycle wash outside—or a dog wash instead!

Source: Adapted from *"Healthy Start: Food to Grow On,"* vol. IV (Food Marketing Institute, American Dietetic Association, and American Academy of Pediatrics, 1995). Reprinted with permission by the Food Marketing Institute, ©1995.

Get Up and Move, Turn Off the Tube!

Smart eating is just part of a healthy start on life. Kids need to be physically active, too!

Today's children often watch TV during their "prime time" for play. In fact, by first grade, many kids have watched five thousand hours of TV. According to health experts, children who watch too much TV may not get enough physical exercise or creative activity. That's why health experts recommend limiting TV time—no more than one to two hours per day. To prevent your "tater tots" from becoming the next generation of "couch potatoes," make physical activity fun and part of your family's routine.

Active Play: Good Moves for Children

Just what makes physical activity so important for kids of all ages? Good physical health and fitness are obvious reasons. Through active and safe play, children also can develop social skills, build a positive self-image, enhance their ability to learn, and even help protect themselves from danger. An active child is also more likely be an active adult!

● Regular physical activity helps with a child's physical development. It builds muscular strength, including a strong heart muscle. Strong muscles promote good posture, which, in turn, affects a child's health and self-image. Weight-bearing activities such as running and skating help strengthen growing bones. Being active also helps build stamina, a quality that promotes learning and play.

● Can children quickly run in case of danger? Although each circumstance requires different physical demands, strong, physically fit children deal better with many emergencies. Regular physical activity offers better protection from danger!

● Active kids are more likely to keep their bodies lean and avoid the growing problem of overweight. Health experts recommend increased physical activity as one of the best ways for kids to trim extra body fat.

● Regular physical activity supports the learning process in other ways. Many activities develop a child's coordination. Playing catch, for example, develops eye-hand coordination. Jumping rope or hopscotch helps teach spatial relationships, while soccer helps develop manipulative skills.

● As children play actively with others, they also develop and practice social skills. With games of all kinds, they can share, cooperate, communicate, support each other, and act as a team.

● Being on a winning team isn't the only way to build self-esteem. Succeeding at any physical activity—riding a bike, swimming a lap, or catching a ball—helps build self-confidence and a positive self-image.

● Active play can be part of the joy of childhood! When physical activity is pleasant, it more likely becomes a lifelong habit. In the long run, a lifestyle that includes regular physical activity lowers the risk of many chronic diseases.

Kids, Go for It!

For good health, children need at least sixty minutes of physical activity each day. Kids don't need a structured activity program to meet this goal. And competitive sports may not be appropriate for some kids; they can create unnecessary pressure and take the fun away.

Active play—biking, in-line skating, playing tag, jump-roping, swimming, or tossing a Frisbee, among others—can offer enough exercise for most children. Besides, it can be fun! *Hint:* Be sure that children have appropriate safety gear such as helmets, knee pads, or life jackets, as well as sunscreen (even in cold weather) and appropriate clothing.

Next time your kids say they don't know what to do besides watch TV, suggest something active. *See "Ten Things for Kids to Do Instead of Watching TV" on page 416.*

To promote an active lifestyle you need to make your moves, too. Join kids in active play—perhaps hike together as a weekend outing, ride bikes after dinner, play a quick game of catch or hopscotch after work, clean up a local nature trail, knead a loaf of bread, or take an active vacation (perhaps with hiking, swimming, or skiing). Plan for family activities, perhaps after dinner or every Saturday morning so that exercise happens!

Until the teen years, avoid the urge to compete with your kids in organized games such as tennis; usually a child is no match for adult strength and skill. Physical activity needs to feel good to the body and the mind!

Do you need after-school care for your kids? Look for programs that include physical activity: perhaps in Scout groups, outdoor centers, recreational and community centers, or your child's school. Or sign them up for gymnastics, dance, or swim classes.

For more ideas on putting physical activity into your whole family's lifestyle, see "Twenty Everyday Ways to Get Moving" in chapter 2.

Kids' Kitchen

Your kitchen can be a learning laboratory! Just like learning to read and write, becoming self-sufficient with food preparation is a life skill your child or teen needs to accomplish. The kitchen is one place where kids learn about food and become health-wise consumers of food.

If you're a single parent or in a dual-career household, your child also may share responsibility for family nutrition and be expected to feed himself or herself sometimes. Depending on age, your child may help with family food shopping, preparation, and cleanup. Becoming skilled in the kitchen is more than fun. Even for kids, it may be a necessity!

Let's Cook!

Prepare food with your child—and explore a wide variety of foods. At the same time, your child can learn how to handle and prepare foods in a safe, healthful way.

When kids cook, they practice all kinds of other skills—besides how to handle and prepare foods to nourish themselves and keep food safe to eat. By reading a recipe, children learn new words and practice reading. They identify foods and learn their qualities as they gather ingredients. By preparing a recipe, they practice measuring, counting, timing, sequencing, and following directions. Slicing, pouring, rolling dough, and shaping meat patties are among the food preparation activities that develop small-muscle movement and eye-hand coordination. Food preparation is practical science, too. Children might watch dough rise, see eggs coagulate, or observe how sugar dissolves in water.

Preparing food also promotes your child's social and emotional development. Children feel good about themselves when they successfully prepare foods they

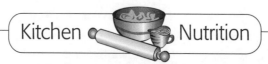

Kitchen Nutrition

Healthful, No-Cook Snacks for Kids

Kids have a case of the after-school munchies? Try these healthful, no-cook snacks. They're easy and fun to make—and depending on your child's age, require little or no adult supervision.

G = Grains, **F** = Fruit, **V** = Vegetable, **MB** = Meat and Beans, **M** = Milk

- *Snack Kebobs.* Cut raw vegetables and fruit into chunks. Skewer them onto thin pretzel sticks. (*Note:* To prevent discoloration, dip cut apples, bananas, or pears in orange juice.) **V** **F** **G**

- *Veggies with Dip.* Cut celery, zucchini, cucumbers, or carrots into sticks or coins. Then dip them into prepared salsa. **V**

- *Banana Pops.* Peel a banana. Dip it in yogurt, then roll in crushed breakfast cereal; freeze. **F** **M** **G**

- *Fruit Slices and PB.* Spread peanut butter on apple or banana slices. **F** **MB**

- *Fruit Shake-ups.* Put ½ cup low-fat fruit yogurt and ½ cup cold fruit juice in a nonbreakable, covered container. Make sure the lid is tight. Then shake it up, and pour into a cup. **M** **F**

- *Pudding Shakes.* Use the same technique for making fruit shake-ups, but instead mix ½ cup milk with 3 tablespoons of instant pudding mix. **M**

- *Sandwich Cutouts.* Using cookie cutters with fun shapes like dinosaurs, stars, and hearts, cut slices of cheese, meat, and whole-grain bread. Then put them together to make fun sandwiches. Eat the edges, too. **M** **MB** **G**

- *Peanut Butter Balls.* Mix peanut butter and bran or cornflakes in a bowl. Shape the mixture into balls with clean hands. Then roll them in crushed graham crackers. **M** **G**

- *Salsa Quesadillas.* Fill a soft tortilla with cheese and salsa, fold over, and grill. **G** **M** **V**

- *Ice Cream–Wiches.* Put a small scoop of ice cream or frozen yogurt between two oatmeal cookies or frozen waffles. Make a batch of these sandwiches ahead, and freeze them. **M** **G**

- *Ants on a Log.* Fill celery with peanut butter. Arrange raisins along the top. **V** **MB** **F**

---

can eat—and share with others. And it's an opportunity to explore foods of other cultures and respect the similarities and the differences. Most important, preparing food together can be a nice time for your child to spend with you.

To get started, consider these guidelines for kitchen success with kids:

- Choose foods and recipes that match your child's abilities. With foods a child might prepare alone, first make them together.

- For young cooks, choose illustrated children's cookbooks that show the foods, measurements, and steps along the way. Go over the safety and sanitation tips at the front of a child's cookbook.

- Ask your child to suggest foods he or she would like to make. Make it a total experience by shopping for ingredients together, too.

- Before you start, wash your hands! And review safety precautions. Supervise children as they learn to work with knives, the stove, and other potentially dangerous equipment. Follow good cleanliness habits, too. *See "Kitchen Safety Alert" on page 419.*

- Besides cooking together, have your child help you store food properly for food safety.

- Use this chance to show your child how to handle food to keep it clean and safe from spoilage and foodborne illness. Among the things to learn and practice: hand washing, using clean utensils for different foods, and using a meat thermometer. *For more guidance, see chapter 12.*

For easy recipes that children can prepare for snacks—or any meal of the day—see "Kitchen Nutrition: Healthful, No-Cook Snacks for Kids" on page 418.

Kitchen Safety Alert

With all that goes on in a kitchen, food preparation sends some "red flags" for kids' safety. Cooking is safe—if your child learns to be careful. Make the kitchen a fun, rewarding place for kids; teach the basics of kitchen safety.

Microwave Oven Safety for Kids

Because burns are a common hazard related to microwave oven use, make sure children know how to use a microwave oven safely.

- Make sure the microwave oven is on a sturdy stand—one that's low enough for kids. If children need to reach too high, they may pull a hot dish down on themselves.

- Teach children to read the controls on the microwave oven—the time, the power level, and the "start" and "stop" controls. If kids can't read them, they're too young to operate a microwave oven alone.

- Keep microwave-safe containers in one place—within a child's reach. Have them use only these containers.

- Always have a child use potholders to remove heated food from the microwave oven—whether the food is hot or not. In that way it becomes a habit. Keep potholders handy for kids.

- Teach children to stir heated food before tasting. That distributes the heat and avoids hot spots that can cause burns.

- Show them how to open containers so that steam escapes away from their face. That includes packages of popped microwave popcorn.

- Until you're sure that children have mastered the art of microwaving, provide supervision.

For more tips on using a microwave oven safely, see "Play It Microwave-Safe" in chapter 12.

- Remind children to always wash their hands with soap and water before and after they handle food. Because children practice what they see, you'll probably get the message across easily—by always washing your own hands.

- Supervise your child when preparing food . . . always when he or she handles hot liquids, knives, appliances, and other potentially dangerous equipment.

- As your child is ready, teach kitchen safety tips: to use potholders when handling hot pans, pots, and dishes . . . to handle knives safely . . . to be very careful with hot liquids . . . and to use appliances safely. *See "Microwave Oven Safety for Kids" on this page.*

- Set limits on what your child can—and can't—do without proper supervision. For example, your child can't use the oven if he or she is home alone.

- Remind your child to be aware of his or her hair and clothes before using the stove. Large, loose-fitting garments and long hair can catch fire.

- Practice what you preach. Your child will take his or her kitchen-safety cues from you.

- Practice what to do in case of fire. That includes "drop and roll" to smother the flames in case his or her clothes catch fire. Keep a fire extinguisher in view and teach your child how to use it.

- Try to keep food and utensils your child will use within easy reach. Keep a sturdy stool handy if he or she needs to reach higher. Remind your child not to climb on the counters or on a wobbling stool!

- Teach kids—even preschoolers—to call 911 (or emergency numbers such as those for the fire department, poison control center, or police in your area). Post the phone numbers in your kitchen where children can see them easily. Include the phone numbers of your doctor, a neighbor, and a relative.

- Practice the Heimlich maneuver with children. Like you, they can save the life of someone who's choking—if they know how. *See "How to Avoid Choking" in chapter 12. For infants, see "For Babies, Toddlers, and Preschoolers: How to Avoid Choking" in chapter 15.*

● Keep a first-aid kit handy and well stocked. Teach your child how to use it in case of a minor injury while cooking.

For more on preventing injuries, see "Quick Tips for Injury Prevention" in chapter 12.

Feeding the Teen Machine

By adolescence, many kids make most of their own decisions about their food choices. Other than filling the refrigerator and kitchen shelves with food and preparing family meals, parents have far less control over what their adolescent child eats. Teenagers themselves exert stronger influence over family eating than before, perhaps sharing the shopping and food preparation. Compared with their childhood years, they probably consume more food and beverages away from home.

Chances are that teenagers know the basics of nutrition and healthful eating. However, peer pressure, school and work schedules, a sense of independence, lack of personal discipline, unrealistic notions about

Teens, Did You Know

... unhealthy dieting can stop you from growing to your full height? Your body needs calories and other nutrients to grow and develop fully. Most teens shouldn't "diet."

... your bones take in the most calcium during your teen years and early twenties? Calcium gives your bones strength. The best sources are milk, yogurt, and cheese, and most teens need four servings of dairy foods daily.

... if you don't eat breakfast, your body is like a computer without power?

... eating cookies, candy, or other sweet foods before an athletic event won't give you an energy boost?

... for girls, when you have a menstrual period you lose iron? If you don't eat iron-rich foods to replace this loss, you may feel weak and tired.

... pizza and hamburgers are healthful food choices, especially if you know which toppings to choose—and you eat sensible amounts?

... eating smart and moving more help you feel good, look good, and do your best!

body weight, and a poor self-image are among the barriers to healthful eating. Food choices may not reflect what teens know about eating for fitness—much to their parents' dismay!

The same holds true for physical activity. Kids know why they should move more, but doing so has barriers, too.

Sound familiar? In a nutshell, adolescents often don't connect their immediate food and physical activity patterns to their long- or short-term health. Many teens live in a wonderful world of invulnerability. Others follow misguided advice: supplements for muscle building, unsafe dieting for weight loss, energy drinks—for energy! Read on for a few "teen-friendly" fitness strategies.

Many nutrition issues that concern adults also apply to your teenager: for example, high-fat eating, fast foods, meal skipping, fad diets and weight control, eating too few fruits and vegetables, energy drinks, sports nutrition. Throughout the book, you'll find strategies your teen can use to address these issues.

Food, Nutrients, and the Teen Years

Second only to infancy, adolescence is the fastest growth stage in life! Even when teens reach their adult height (for girls sooner than for boys), their bodies are still growing and developing.

Puberty marks the start of the teenage growth spurt. That time differs for each child. For girls, puberty typically begins at about age twelve or thirteen, about two years younger than for boys. From the school-age years through the teens, the average youngster grows to be 20 percent taller and 50 percent heavier. Body changes that happen as children mature are stressful for some, and may affect their self-image and perhaps the choices they make about eating and physical activity. (Some overweight children may develop sooner, but for now, there are too many unanswered questions to know why.)

How your teenage child grows—when, how, and how much—has more to do with genes than with food choices. However, smart eating does help determine if your child grows to his or her maximum height potential—with strong bones and a fit body.

All teens need enough calcium for bone growth and strength; protein for every body cell including muscles; carbohydrates and fats for energy; and vitamins and minerals for the "sparks" that make it all happen. Energy and nutrient needs increase to meet the growth demands of adolescence. Teens need understanding parents who appreciate that their adolescent's growth pattern, although different from a friend's, is perfectly normal.

Food Energy: How Much?

Teenage boys have high energy needs: on average, 2,500 calories a day if they're eleven to fourteen years old, and 2,800 calories a day if they're fifteen to eighteen years of age. That's up from 2,000 calories a day for a seven- to ten-year-old child. Teenage girls need more, too: about 2,200 calories a day if they're eleven to eighteen years old, compared to 2,000 calories a day when they were a bit younger. Depending on their size, growth rate, and activity level, some may need less, others more. Those involved in strenuous physical activity such as soccer, basketball, football, or other sports may need 3,500 calories (more or less) daily.

Nutrients: For Some, An All-Time High

Many nutrient recommendations go up during adolescence. *Check the Dietary Reference Intakes in the Appendices to see how much.* As teens consume more food-group foods, they also get a nutrient and food energy boost to meet the demands of growth, health, and perhaps more physical activity. Typically, teens need to eat more fiber-rich foods, too. *For advice about fiber, see "How Much Fiber? Just Add Five!" in this chapter.*

Three nutrients are typically short in a teenager's food choices: calcium, iron, and perhaps zinc. That's usually due to poor food choices, or for girls especially, simply not eating enough. Read on to learn more about these minerals.

Pregnancy affects a teenage girl's nutrition needs. Like any pregnancy, the need for nutrients and energy goes up; for teens, the recommendations are higher than for adult women, for their own growth and development, and for the developing fetus. *For more on the nutrition needs of a teenage pregnancy, see "For Pregnant Teens: Good Nutrition" in chapter 17.*

Calcium: A Growing Issue. "I'm sixteen, and I've stopped growing. So why do I need milk?" Actually,

bones keep on growing into the adult years. Even when teenagers reach their adult height, bones continue to grow stronger as they become more dense. In fact, almost half of an adult's bone mass forms during the teen years. The stronger bones become during adolescence, the lower the risk of osteoporosis later on. Yet, only about 14 percent of girls and about 36 percent of boys ages twelve to nineteen in the United States consume the recommended amount of calcium!

Some experts say that osteoporosis is really an adolescent health problem that manifests itself in later years. Teenagers—children, too—who don't consume enough calcium put their bones at risk for the long term. They may start their adult years with a calcium deficit in their bones. With bone loss that comes as a natural part of aging, they have less to draw on, and their risk for osteoporosis, or brittle bone disease, goes up.

Teens are advised to consume enough calcium-rich foods so their bones become as strong as they can be. For children and teens ages nine through eighteen, three to four servings of calcium-rich foods each day provide enough calcium for growing bones. According to the Dietary Reference Intakes, 1,300 milligrams of calcium daily is considered an Adequate Intake (AI). An 8-ounce glass of milk has about 300 milligrams of calcium.

What foods are teens' best calcium sources? Milk Group foods—including milk, yogurt, and cheese—have the most per serving, although a variety of foods have smaller amounts of calcium. Milk also contains other nutrients essential to healthy bone and tooth development: vitamins D, A, and B_{12}, potassium, magnesium, and protein. Canned salmon and sardines with bones, as well as some vegetables (such as mustard greens, collard greens, okra, broccoli, and bok choy), supply calcium. And some prepared foods are calcium-fortified, including some juice, soy drinks, breads, and breakfast cereal. *For more on calcium and a list of calcium-rich foods, see "Calcium: A Closer Look" in chapter 4.*

Why don't many teens consume enough calcium-rich dairy foods? Perhaps there's no milk on hand at home, or perhaps they don't like it. Maybe kids haven't made a habit of drinking milk with fast food. Or perhaps soft drinks compete. If milk is cold, convenient, and "cool," your teen more likely will drink it. *Tip:*

Fill the fridge with flavored milk or yogurt drinks sold in "cool," single-serving containers.

Many teenage girls misguidedly link milk drinking to their fear of getting fat, including teens on fad diets or those with eating disorders. Yet those who watch calories can consume low-fat or fat-free dairy foods. One 8-ounce serving of fat-free milk supplies fewer calories than 8 ounces of a soft drink or juice: only 86 calories and almost no fat, yet fat-free milk has as much calcium as whole milk!

Vegan eating patterns and lactose intolerance may be barriers, too. In either case, teens have plenty of practical ways to get enough calcium. *See chapter 20 for more about vegetarian eating, and chapter 21 for more about lactose intolerance.*

For more about bone health during adulthood, see "Osteoporosis: Reduce the Risks" in chapter 22.

Iron: The Fatigue Connection. Does your teenager seem chronically tired? Fatigue may come from too little sleep, an exhausting schedule, strenuous activity (a good kind of fatigue), or the emotional ups and downs of adolescence. But feeling tired also may be a symptom of a health problem or low iron levels in the blood.

Iron is part of blood's hemoglobin, which carries oxygen to body cells. Once there, oxygen helps cells produce energy. When iron is in short supply, there's less oxygen available to produce energy—hence fatigue.

Have You Ever Wondered

... besides drinking milk, how can teens keep their bones healthy? Like milk, yogurt, cheese, and pudding are all calcium-rich, bone-building foods. In addition, calcium-fortified soy milk and tofu, as well as calcium-fortified and dark green vegetables, provide calcium, too. Regular weight-bearing activities such as dancing, soccer, running, weight lifting, tennis, and volleyball are important since they trigger bone tissue to form. Going easy on soft drinks if they edge out calcium-rich milk is smart advice. Smoking also may have a negative effect on bone formation; teens who smoke are smart to kick the habit.

Iron needs go up dramatically in the teen years. During childhood (ages nine to thirteen) both boys and girls need about 8 milligrams of iron daily, according to the Dietary Reference Intakes. For adolescence, more muscle mass and a greater blood supply demand more iron, so the recommendation jumps to 15 milligrams of iron daily for girls ages fourteen to eighteen, and 11 milligrams daily for boys that age. Girls need more to replace iron losses from their menstrual flow. *See "Menstrual Cycle: More Iron for Women" in chapter 17.*

Many teens—girls especially—don't consume enough iron. Poor food choices or restricting food to lose weight are two common reasons. Kids who don't eat meat regularly may not consume enough either. Unlike calcium, the effects of low iron intake can be apparent during the teenage years.

Iron comes from a variety of foods: meat, poultry, and seafood as well as legumes, enriched grain products, and some vegetables. For example, the iron in some common foods is:

- 3-ounce hamburger—2 milligrams
- ½ cup of baked beans or refried beans—2 milligrams
- 1 slice of enriched bread—1 milligram
- 1 cup of iron-fortified breakfast cereal—4 milligrams (more or less). For cereal, check the Nutrition Facts on food labels for the specific amount. *For information on reading labels, see "What's on the Label?" in chapter 11.*

Teens who drink orange juice with their morning toast or cereal get an iron boost, too. Its vitamin C content makes iron from plant sources and eggs more usable by the body. Kids who just grab toast to eat at the bus stop, but skip the juice, don't get the full benefit of the iron in bread. For some teens, vitamin C is a problem nutrient, too.

For more on iron in a healthful diet, see "Iron: A Closer Look" in chapter 4.

Zinc: Another Essential Mineral. Although it gets less attention, zinc often comes up short for teens, too. Besides its other functions, zinc is essential for growth and sexual maturation. For teens who don't eat meat and other animal-based foods, a lack of zinc may affect development.

The Pyramid for Teens

The Food Guide Pyramid truly is a family guideline—meant for teens, too. Since teens need more food energy (calories) than children do, teens need more food-group servings.

The goal if you're a teen? Choose enough servings toward or at the top of the serving ranges if you need 2,500 calories a day or more (many teen boys), and midrange if you need about 2,200 calories daily (many teen girls). The extra energy should come mainly from foods high in complex carbohydrates—and not from a high-fat eating pattern or from too many foods in the Pyramid tip. *As a guide to serving amounts for teens, see "How Many Servings a Day for You?" in chapter 10.*

A simple way to help teens think about the Pyramid guidelines:

● Fats, oils and sweets—*eat less* because they add extra calories but little or no nutrients.

● Milk Group and Meat and Beans Group—*eat enough* low-fat dairy foods for calcium and enough lean meat or beans for iron.

● Vegetable Group and Fruit Group—*eat more* fruits and vegetables than you're used to eating.

● Grains Group—*eat plenty* of breads, cereals, rice and pasta as your best foods for energy.

Source: yourSELF: Team Nutrition (Washington, D.C.: U.S. Department of Agriculture, 1998).

Smart choices at school meals can add many food-group servings to a teen's personal Pyramid. How? Eat school lunch—at least three of the menu options, and preferably not fries and a burger or pizza each day. Fitness-conscious teens can still eat chips, candy, and soft drinks with lunch if they've eaten food group foods and if they need the extra calories. *For more about school meals see "For Kids Only—Today's School Meals" earlier in this chapter.*

Great Snacking!

With their high energy and nutrient needs, especially during their growth spurt, teens often need snacks as a "refueling stop." Boys especially may need snacks to fill their bottomless pit. Snacks help to fill in nutrient gaps that meal choices miss: yogurt as a snack, for

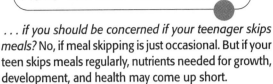

Have You Ever Wondered

... if you should be concerned if your teenager skips meals? No, if meal skipping is just occasional. But if your teen skips meals regularly, nutrients needed for growth, development, and health may come up short.

Teenage girls often skip breakfast or lunch to save on calories, then perhaps miss out on foods that supply nutrients (calcium, iron). Of special concern: high-calcium foods such as milk; iron-fortified cereals; and vitamin C-rich fruits and juices. Later teens may satisfy their hunger with high-calorie, high-fat snack foods. The net result: more calories, fewer nutrients. *For more on meal skipping see "Meal Skipping: Poor Option!" in chapter 10.*

example, if a teen doesn't drink milk for lunch. To teens, snacking is even more: part of a social pattern and something to do when teenagers get together!

The real issue with teen snacking isn't whether they do—or don't. Instead, these are among the nutrition issues: (1) high-calorie snacks replacing nutrient-rich meals; (2) mindless or emotional snacking that adds to excess calories; (3) large, even super-size, portions that add up on calories, and perhaps fat and added sugars; and (4) overdoing on soft drinks and other snacks from the Pyramid tip.

Since teens will snack, support their ability to snack smart: juice or milk from a vending machine; a small burger with milk at a fast-food restaurant; or fruit, raw vegetables, yogurt, or cereal with milk from the kitchen at home. *For more about healthful snacking—and easy, nutritious snack ideas—see "That Snack Attack!" in chapter 10.*

Your Teen's Food Choices: What You Can Do

Bigger appetites, busy lifestyles, emotional swings, struggles for independence, peer pressure: they challenge how and what teens eat. As a parent you can influence the eating habits of a teenager—subtly, of course! Try this:

● Stock the kitchen with easy-to-grab nutrition. Foods that take little or no effort—for example, whole fruit, yogurt, hummus, cut-up veggie sticks, string cheese, and bagels—are most likely eaten. (Ease is one reason why kids reach for chips.) *See "Empower Your Kids: Seven How-tos for Smart Eating" earlier in this chapter for more ideas.*

● Still . . . make time for family meals, even if you need to schedule around after-school activities and jobs, and put family meals on the calendar days in advance. It's a good time to get connected. (Save stressful conversations for later.) What's more, research suggests nutritional benefits! For teens, eating family meals is linked to eating more fruit and vegetables and less soft drinks and less fried, high-fat, and sugar-laden foods.

● Encourage an elective class in foods, nutrition and wellness, or consumer health. That's a great way for teens to learn practical basics of sound nutrition and healthful eating. These classes are also full of applied science, math, and social studies!

● Help teens build skills. Let your teenager plan, shop for, and then cook family meals. The kitchen is a great place to practice what's learned in a foods class. *Some of the tips in "Kids' Kitchen" in this chapter might help younger teens.*

● Talk through the options at fast-food restaurants. Your teen may be clueless about all the choices out there. There's more than burgers, fries, and soft drinks.

● Help kids tune into portion size. A small bag of chips can be as much fun to eat as a bigger bag, with far fewer calories! The same goes for soft drinks. *See "Portion Distortion?" in chapter 10.*

● Set a good example for wellness and lifestyle—for example, with regular physical activity, lower-fat eating, sensible portions, and not smoking. Kids notice when adults "walk their talk." Not surprisingly, research suggests that boys tend to follow their dad's lifestyles; girls, their mother's.

● Help your teen deal with peer pressure. In that way he or she will have strategies to follow personal goals for smart eating, rather than simply going with the crowd.

● In your talk, tie smart eating and active living to what matters to your teen—growing normally; feeling good; looking good; and doing well in school, sports, or a personal interest (music, drama, art, whatever).

Even when teens seem to disregard what you suggest, they likely "hear" your encouragement, concern, and example.

If Your Teen Decides to Become a Vegetarian. Support the decision by helping him or her make food choices that continue to promote growth and health. It's not uncommon for teenagers to opt for an eating style that reflects their independence and emerging beliefs. Regardless, a vegetarian eating style can supply all the nutrients and energy teenagers need if they know how to do so.

A strict vegetarian diet with no animal foods, if not planned properly, may not supply all the nutrients an adolescent needs to grow. It's easiest to meet nutrient needs of growing teens with an eating plan that includes dairy foods and eggs, plenty of legumes, and small amounts of meat, seafood, and chicken. *For more about a healthful vegetarian eating style see chapter 20, "The Vegetarian Way."*

Move Your "Bod"

Does your teen move in high gear on a "24/7" schedule—school to after-school activities and perhaps to a job? Do homework, time with friends, and seemingly hours on the phone or the Internet fit in between? Remember, a busy schedule may not translate to an active lifestyle!

Moving more promotes all the benefits that are near and dear to the teenage heart: looking good, being in shape, being strong, feeling energetic, being self-confident, doing well in school, and having an overall good outlook on life.

There's more. Being active now helps reduce the risk for some chronic health problems later, including diabetes, heart disease, obesity, and osteoporosis—especially if teens make it a lifelong habit.

The physical activity guideline for teens? Try to stay physically active. Research shows that physical activity drops dramatically when kids hit the teen years. Yet the general guideline is at least thirty minutes of moderate and vigorous activity five or more times weekly. Use the Activity Pyramid here to get a good balance of activities that stretch, strengthen, and give your heart a workout. Kids of every ability, shape, and size benefit with regular physical activity. *For*

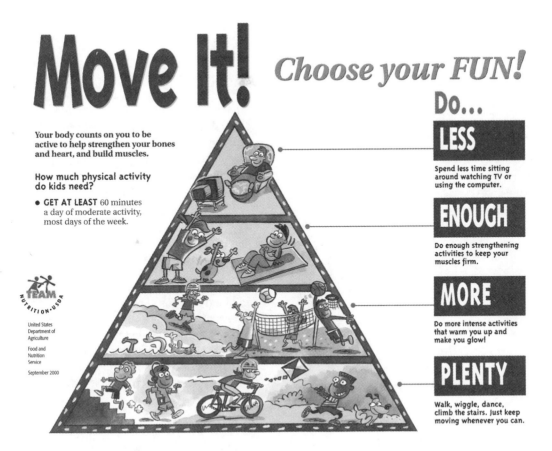

Move It!

Your body counts on you to be active to help strengthen your bones and heart, and build muscles.

How much physical activity do kids need?

- **GET AT LEAST** 60 minutes a day of moderate activity, most days of the week.

United States
Department of
Agriculture

Food and
Nutrition
Service

September 2000

Choose your FUN!

Do...

LESS

Spend less time sitting around watching TV or using the computer.

ENOUGH

Do enough strengthening activities to keep your muscles firm.

MORE

Do more intense activities that warm you up and make you glow!

PLENTY

Walk, wiggle, dance, climb the stairs. Just keep moving whenever you can.

more about guidelines and benefits of physical activity, see "Get Physical!" in chapter 2.

Kids on the Move: Overcoming the Barriers

Why are more and more teenagers less and less active? Perhaps it's the family pattern they "inherited." But for every reason teens give, there's an easy, often fun solution. Offer these tips as starters to teens:

Reason: "I'd rather watch TV." Teenagers watch on average twenty hours of television a week, which burns little energy.

Solution: Get some self-discipline: limit your TV time to fit in other types of fun. Or multitask: watch TV while you do something active, perhaps lift weights, do push-ups or sit-ups, or dance in front of the TV. (Kids: it's not weird to move more.)

Reason: "It's too far to walk there." So kids ride in or drive cars to school, the store, friends' homes, the library, or work.

Solution: Skip the school bus or car if you can. Walk or use a bike, scooter, or in-line skates. (Remember a helmet and perhaps knee pads, for safety.)

Reason: "I'd rather play video games or get on the computer."

Solution: Mental exercise is great, but—take an active break from sitting. It's good for your eyes and your head. In fact, your brain's synapses may work faster with some physical activity!

Reason: "I don't have time." Perhaps leisure time for active fun is limited.

Solution: Fit physical activity into what you need to do anyway. Perhaps wash the family car. Volunteer for your share of the household chores—the ones that make you move more, like raking leaves or sweeping sidewalks.

Reason: "My school doesn't require me to take more PE."

Solution: Sign up for PE at school anyway, not just during the summer. (For parents, support efforts for more physical education at school.) Or take a community aerobics, dance, or martial arts class.

Reason: "I'm self-conscious." Some kids feel that way, perhaps if they're less adept at sports or overweight.

Solution: Try anyway. Other kids may feel the same way, and they probably aren't looking at you. Focus on individual sports such as biking and in-line skating, where the emphasis is on fun, not performance.

Reason: "I don't want to sweat or mess up my hair." That's probably more true for teenage girls than boys.

Solution: Do everyday activities, such as walking to school or doing household tasks, that don't work up a sweat. Even if you do sweat, fitness is more important anyway.

Get Fit with a Friend

Is your teenager looking for something to do? You might suggest these active ways to get fit with a friend—and have fun, too.

- Do something active: play tennis, go in-line skating, go hiking, or enjoy dancing at a school function. *Hint:* You don't need a date for line dancing.

- Instead of talking on the phone, walk and talk with your friends.

- Sign up for a school or community sports team. You don't need to "play varsity" for health benefits.

- Join the marching band if you play a musical instrument. Try out for cheerleading, majorettes, or the pom-pom squad.

- Volunteer as a stagehand for school plays. You'll get plenty of activity doing stage chores.

- Do some community service—for example, at a community garden, home-building project, children's day camp, community clean-up, or animal center.

- Baby-sit! Play actively with children.

- Get a neighborhood job: mow lawns, shovel snow, wash cars, do yardwork.

For more physical activity ideas for teens, see "Twenty Everyday Ways to Get Moving" in chapter 2.

Have You Ever Wondered

... what to eat to control acne? Although all kinds of foods get blamed, teenage acne is linked to hormonal changes, rarely to food choices. The best approach to healthy skin is to eat an overall varied and balanced diet, keep skin clean, get enough rest—and wait. After the body matures, most acne clears up. If problems are severe or persist, talk to a dermatologist. Sometimes a skin application that contains a derivative of vitamin A is prescribed; simply taking a vitamin A tablet won't clear the skin.

Caution: If the doctor prescribes Accutane (isotretinoin) to treat severe acne, avoid supplements with vitamin A. Together, Accutane and vitamin A have toxic effects. Taking Accutane can also raise cholesterol and blood lipid (fat) levels until the treatment stops. Because of the many potential psychological (depression, lack of concentration, irritability, and suicidal thoughts, among others) and physical (including unusual fatigue and appetite loss) side effects of Accutane, make sure your teen follows dosage directions carefully, *under close supervision of a physician.*

... if kids who wear braces should avoid eating raw vegetables and fruits? No! It's true that hard, crunchy, or sticky foods can damage braces. But kids don't need to give up vegetables and fruits. Instead they might choose softer types: perhaps a ripe peach or a banana rather than a crisp apple, or cucumber sticks rather than a whole, raw carrot. Or they might cut these foods into bite-size pieces instead of eating them whole. Consult your child's orthodontist for a list of foods that might damage braces.

Weight: Right-Sized?

Eager for acceptance, yet self-conscious about body changes, most teens view their body image as a big issue. Even though their bodies come in different sizes, shapes, and stages of growth, most weigh in within a healthy range. In growing numbers, some deal with overweight. Others use misguided approaches for trying to achieve an unrealistic weight or body size. Still others are victims of disordered eating. Remember, the right weight is a range, not a single number; and it's about health, not just looks.

If Your Teen Is Overweight

Teens who truly are overweight—or at risk for over-weight—need a healthful, realistic, safe way to manage their weight. That includes both physical activity and a smart eating plan, not "dieting." Adult diets aren't meant for teens. Unless a doctor advises it, the teen years aren't a time for a weight loss diet. For many, growing into an appropriate weight is healthier; dieting may deprive a growing teen of needed nutrients.

Weight is a sensitive issue for everyone, especially kids. The best approach is positive—no nagging, forbidden foods, or criticism; a negative approach is sure-fire defeat. Instead, understanding, love, and support go a long way in helping teens and children cope with and address weight issues.

● Help eliminate whatever triggers eating, such as the sight of high-calorie snacks on the kitchen counter.

● Reassess the family's eating style. Make gradual improvements together. Gradual changes often become permanent ones.

● Do fun, active things together. You both benefit!

● Talk, listen, and offer support and alternatives for emotional issues that trigger eating.

● Gather the resources your teen needs. Keep nutritious, lower-calorie foods, including vegetables and fruits, on hand and convenient. Prepare family meals that support your teen's strategies for managing weight.

● Most of all, be accepting. Your love doesn't depend on your teen's weight loss. Unconditional acceptance goes a long way in promoting a positive self-image, which helps promote a healthy weight.

For more tips see "Weighty Problems for Children—Overweight" earlier in this chapter.

Mainly for Girls: Pressure to Be Thin

To many teens, looks are almost everything! As their bodies develop and take on adult curves, it's normal to focus on body image. Often, however, teens have unrealistic notions about their own weight. Many girls especially—about 50 percent of nine- to fifteen-year-olds—see themselves as overweight. And about 23 percent of boys in the same age group do, too. In reality, about 25 percent of twelve- to nineteen-year-olds are overweight, or at risk for overweight.

Pressure to be thin is closely linked to pressure to fit in and to be accepted by peers. Thin people are viewed as successful, popular, and attractive. This message gets reinforced by media images and celebrities—and by parents and friends. However, even celebrities they try to emulate may not have a "perfect look" in reality; computers can manipulate their photo images.

Teenage girls tend to diet, often poorly, as their main approach to an attractive body, while boys often put more emphasis on exercise. For girls, the pursuit of thinness often leads to fad dieting—usually ineffective, often dangerous. These diets are especially risky during adolescence, when teenagers' nutrient needs for growth and energy are high. Trying to lose weight fast to "look good" for a dance or a swim party is neither realistic nor healthful. *For more on fad diets see "'Diets' That Don't Work!" in chapter 2.*

Teens who truly are overweight—or at risk for over-weight—need a realistic, safe way to manage their weight. That includes both physical activity and a smart eating plan, not "dieting."

Disordered Eating. Sometimes a teen's pursuit of thinness leads to obsession—a more serious health concern—perhaps caused by trauma or a life change. Although not overweight, and perhaps even under-weight, some teenagers see themselves as fat. Sometimes a distorted body image begins as teens develop sexual characteristics.

A distorted body image may lead to disordered eating. Teens, whose nutrient needs are high, instead may eat very little, or purge with self-induced vomiting or laxative abuse. Disordered eating can result in extreme undernourishment and weight loss—even death. Because eating disorders are linked to psychological problems, attention from a mental health professional, as well as your child's physician, is essential.

Most victims of eating disorders are teenage girls and young women. For example, one percent of girls age twelve to eighteen has anorexia nervosa. Although less common, teenage boys, in increasing numbers, have eating disorders, too. *To learn more, see "Disordered Eating: Problems, Signs, and Help" in chapter 2.*

Mostly for Boys: Bodybuilding

Most teenage boys want to build muscle (have great "abs"), not lose weight, to look good. Many know the value of weight training for bodybuilding. But for some, the size and shape of their muscles become obsessions that lead to seemingly constant weight lifting and workouts. They may also have the misguided notion that eating more protein builds muscle mass, too. Some opt for more meat portions, perhaps at the expense of foods high in complex carbohydrates; others take protein supplements and "bulk-up" drugs such as steroids. Muscle-building steroids are dangerous; *see "Ergogenic Aids: No Substitute for Training" in chapter 19.*

Although protein needs go up from childhood, an extra amount has no bodybuilding benefits. Following the recommendations of the Food Guide Pyramid supplies all the protein that teenage boys need—whether they're involved in weight training or not. Like extra carbohydrate or dietary fat, extra protein is deposited in the body as fat, not muscle.

A high-protein diet also may contribute a high percentage of calories from fat. That's especially true when teenage boys opt for fewer foods high in complex carbohydrates, such as bread, pasta, rice, and cereal. The best advice for teenage bodybuilders? Follow the guidelines of the Food Guide Pyramid and be sensible with a weight-training program.

The key to building muscle is an overall good exercise program and plenty of carbohydrates to fuel longer workouts. Through exercise, which creates a demand for more muscle, protein enters the muscles and makes them larger. *See "Muscle Myths" in chapter 19.*

What about making weight for wrestling or football? Offer this advice to teenage boys: Cutting down on food or beverages to "make weight" won't promote physical performance. Instead, muscles may get weaker and smaller, even if you consume protein. If you don't eat enough calories, your body burns some protein in your muscles for energy. Drinking too little water can make you dehydrated, which may hinder physical performance, too. As for girls, crash dieting for sports and body image, along with a poor self-image, are factors that can lead to disordered eating.

For more on food for sports and making weight, see "Making Weight" in chapter 19.

CHAPTER 17

For Women Only

Women—this chapter is meant especially for you and your unique nutrition needs! Only in the past ten to fifteen years have women's unique health needs received much attention in medical research. Until then, women's health needs were projected in studies done mostly with men! Except for pregnancy and breast-feeding, health concerns related to the female reproductive system were largely ignored. Today medical research, health promotion, and healthcare address gender differences. And nutrition often is center stage in initiatives for women's health.

Consider briefly a few gender-related nutrition differences. Of course, you need the same nutrients that men do—perhaps more of some, depending on your age. Yet, if you're physically smaller, you likely need fewer calories, or food energy, to deliver those nutrients.

Unless men shift their physical activity level, the nutrition needs of healthy males don't change much over a lifetime. That's not true for women. Complexities of the reproductive system, the ups and downs of female hormones, and the physical demands of childbearing affect nutrition needs and healthcare. Menstruation, pregnancy, breast-feeding, and menopause all have nutrition implications.

● *If you're in your reproductive years,* check the beginning of the chapter for healthful eating advice specific to women's health.

● *For nutrition advice during pregnancy and breast-feeding,* go to the middle of the chapter.

● *If you're near or dealing with menopause,* turn to the chapter end, where you'll find nutrition guidance for your continued health and well-being.

For nutrition issues related to breast cancer, see "Breast Cancer: Do Food Choices Make a Difference?" in this chapter.

Childbearing Years: Nutrition, Menstruation, and Prepregnancy

The choice is yours! Healthful eating, active living, and hormones are intertwined in the unique and complex issues of women's health. Whether or not you choose to have children, the choices you make now, during your childbearing years, affect the quality and length of your life for the long run. Many of those choices are uniquely female.

Menstrual Cycle: More Iron for Women

In your childbearing years you need more iron than men do. Why? To replace iron loss from menstrual flow. On average, women lose about ¼ cup of blood with each menstrual period. Those with a heavy flow may lose more. For women who don't replace that iron, menstrual loss—combined with low iron intake, frequent dieting, and a low vitamin C intake—contribute to iron deficiency and perhaps to anemia.

For women ages nineteen to fifty, the Recommended Dietary Allowance (RDA) for iron is 18 milligrams of iron daily. During pregnancy, the recommendation increases to 27 milligrams daily. To compare, adult men need only 8 milligrams of iron daily. With menopause, a woman's need for iron drops and equals that of men.

To get enough iron from food, eat iron-rich foods such as meat, poultry, fortified cereal, enriched rice, and legumes. Remember that iron from grain products, legumes, and eggs isn't absorbed as well. So enjoy these foods with vitamin C-rich foods: perhaps citrus fruit with your morning cereal or scrambled egg. Consult your healthcare provider about an iron supplement, too. *For more about iron and food sources see "Iron: A Closer Look" in chapter 4. See chapter 22 for "Anemia: 'Tired Blood'" and "Iron Supplements: Enhancing the Benefit" in chapter 23.*

Food Choices: Control for PMS?

Do you experience the uncomfortable symptoms of premenstrual syndrome (PMS)? Women have described as many as two hundred different symptoms: physical symptoms such as acne, backaches, bloating, tender breasts, and headaches; food cravings; and psychological symptoms such as anxiety, irritability, and insomnia.

PMS—a condition, not a disease—starts as many as fourteen days before a woman's period, then stops when menstrual flow starts. Shifts in hormone levels are the likely cause. Because body water fluctuates during the menstrual cycle, your body may retain fluids prior to your period. Fluid retention usually disappears soon after it's over.

PMS gets plenty of attention in women's media, yet there's little consensus on its causes or treatment, and little conclusive research on links between nutrition and its symptoms. Despite claims, there's no evidence of any link between PMS and nutritional deficiencies. Here's what's known—and unknown—about "headlines" about PMS:

● *Calcium* may help reduce fluid retention and regulate mood-related brain chemicals, but research isn't conclusive. Regardless, there's good reason to boost your calcium intake. Calcium is essential for lifelong bone health, yet most women don't get enough!

● *Phytoestrogens* are weak, naturally occurring plant estrogens that may help relieve some PMS symptoms. Science hasn't yet determined how much is adequate, or the interaction between phytoestrogens and other hormones. Still, foods with phytoestrogens such as tofu, tempeh, soy milk, and many other soy foods are worth enjoying for their potential health benefits.

● *Salt.* If you retain a lot of water (five pounds or more) before your period, try cutting down on salt for a week to ten days before your period, or ask your doctor about a diuretic. Research suggests that higher progesterone levels before your period cause your body to excrete sodium naturally. The general guideline is to limit sodium intake to 2,400 milligrams per day; for most women there's no need for further limits. Do not limit fluids!

● What about dietary supplements? Despite anecdotal claims, no conclusive research indicates that vitamin B_6, vitamin E, or magnesium alleviate PMS symptoms—and megadoses of vitamin B_6 can cause nerve damage. Except for the psychological effect, large doses of other vitamins, herbals, or botanicals such as evening primrose oil don't alleviate the symptoms either, and they may be harmful. *For more about supplements, see chapter 23.*

Until more is known, general guidelines for good health may help you cope with PMS, if it's a problem. Eat an overall healthful diet. Live an active lifestyle. Relax, learn to alleviate stress, and cope with mood swings. And get plenty of rest.

Physical activity, too, may offer some real benefits! First, a good workout stimulates the release of brain endorphins, which can help relieve PMS moodiness such as anxiety or depression. Just before your period, endorphin levels are low. Second, if you tend to eat more before your period, exercise can also help you keep your weight stable. And third, sweating may help reduce bloating if you retain less fluid.

Consult your doctor if PMS symptoms incapacitate you. Before you attribute ongoing symptoms to PMS, talk to your healthcare provider. Diabetes, pelvic

Have You Ever Wondered ?

. . . if you need extra vitamins if you use oral contraceptives? No. An overall eating plan that's varied and balanced can supply enough nutrients if you're on the pill. However, taking an oral contraceptive over a period of time may exacerbate symptoms of a nutrient deficiency. For example, vitamin B_6—found in whole grains, legumes, meat, poultry, and fish—helps the body produce serotonin, which helps regulate mood and pain. A vitamin B_6 deficiency may trigger mood-related side effects related to oral contraceptives.

. . . if drinking cranberry juice helps protect you from urinary tract infections? Maybe. It appears that substances in cranberries may prevent certain bacteria that cause infection from sticking to the urinary tract wall. Many women suffer from urinary tract infections sometime in their lives. Although urine is normally bacteria-free, bacteria can travel from the rectum, across the skin surface, and into the bladder and cause infection. Studies are investigating the role of drinking cranberry juice in reducing urinary tract bacteria.

If you feel the symptoms—frequent and urgent need to urinate, painful urination, cloudy or bloody urine, or lower back or abdominal pain—seek advice for proper treatment from your doctor.

. . . can food choices reduce the symptoms of fibromyalgia? A syndrome more common in women in their twenties and thirties than in men, fibromyalgia results in chronic pain in fibrous tissues, muscles, tendons, and other connective tissues, and often sleeplessness. Although there's no known cure, a healthy weight helps keep pain in check by putting less pressure on muscles and tissues around joints. Relieving stress, staying physically active, and avoiding caffeine six to eight hours before sleeptime helps. *For more sleep-promoting tips see "Drink Smart—and Get Your Zzzzzzzs!" in chapter 8.* Some herbal supplements are touted for relief, but research isn't conclusive; some may be harmful.

---

infections, depression, and other health problems may be misdiagnosed as PMS.

Other Health Issues: A Nutrition Link?

Vaginal Yeast Infections

Do food choices either promote or prevent vaginal "yeast infections," or *Candida vulvovaginitis?* ("Vulvo" means the external female genitals.) *Candida* is a fungus that commonly lives in the mouth, intestinal tract, vagina, and other moist, warm, and dark body areas. For teenage girls and women, *Candida* may cause vaginal "yeast infections" with several symptoms: vaginal itching, redness, or pain; a thick, white, "cheesy" vaginal discharge; discomfort during urination; and perhaps white or yellow skin patches around the vaginal area. Recent use of antibiotics, uncontrolled diabetes, pregnancy, high-estrogen contraceptives, immunosuppression, thyroid or endocrine disorders, and corticosteroid therapy are among the risk factors linked to yeast infections.

Does eating yogurt prevent it? Eating a cup of yogurt with *active cultures* each day may offer some protection from vaginal "yeast infections." However, the evidence isn't conclusive. Regardless, that same cup of yogurt does supply 300 to 450 milligrams of calcium, which is good for bone health!

To refute a commonly heard myth, there's no scientific evidence that eating sugary foods contributes to "yeast infections." Neither do processed foods, fruit, or milk. Avoiding these foods or taking certain dietary supplements or antifungal drugs doesn't appear to prevent it.

Be aware that *Candida* isn't the only cause of vaginitis. Bacteria, viruses, and chemical irritants are among other causes. The best way to proper treatment is accurate diagnosis from your healthcare provider. If you're prone to "yeast infections," lower your risk with good hygiene, avoiding vaginal sprays and douches, and wearing cotton garments that don't hold in moisture and heat.

Fibrocystic Breast Disease

Between 10 and 20 percent of women experience fibrocystic breast disease (FBD), benign but often painful breast lumps. Despite anecdotal claims, no carefully controlled research evidence links non-cancerous breast lumps to caffeine intake. In fact, both the National Cancer Institute and the American Medical Association's Council on Scientific Affairs report that FBD isn't associated with caffeine intake. The use of vitamin E as a treatment is controversial.

Because fibrocystic breast disease is linked to hormone levels, it usually subsides with menopause—unless a woman receives hormone replacement therapy.

As a safety check for breast health, examine your breasts carefully each month. Get regular mammograms and professional examinations yearly after age forty. And consult your doctor about any breast lumps that appear.

Polycystic Ovary Syndrome

Are you aware of polycystic ovary syndrome (PCOS)? It's an often undiagnosed hormonal problem with a cluster of symptoms, including ovarian cysts, irregular menstrual cycles, acne, excess facial hair, obesity, fertility problems, and male pattern hair thinning. The concerns extend even farther. PCOS increases the risk of several health problems: diabetes, heart disease, high blood pressure, and uterine and breast cancer.

Although the causes of PCOS aren't known, it's a lifelong problem that may run in families and begin in adolescence. Insulin resistance (which affects the way your body uses blood sugar) and a high level of male hormones such as testosterone may explain some symptoms. PCOS isn't easy to diagnose; however, blood tests for hormone levels and ultrasound exams for ovarian cysts reveal clues.

Because of the short- and long-term health implications, talk to your healthcare provider if you suspect PCOS or have its symptoms. Some women with PCOS have no signs. Treatment may include weight loss and hormone therapy. Some women also need treatment for diabetes or high blood pressure.

Before Pregnancy

Thinking about pregnancy? If so, inventory your health and nutrition habits now. Initiating good health and nutrition habits before pregnancy—or simply nudging healthful eating and active living back into your lifestyle—promotes your health and establishes the healthy environment your baby needs to develop normally during pregnancy. And you'll be fit and ready! Your baby develops rapidly during the first weeks of pregnancy, perhaps before you even know you're expecting.

Whether you're preparing for pregnancy or not, advice for all healthy women is the same: To get enough of the forty or so nutrients essential for your good health—and your baby's health, too—*use the Food Guide Pyramid, explained in chapter 10, as your "before, during, and after" pregnancy guide to healthful eating.*

Fertility: Nutrition Links

Healthful eating not only prepares your body for pregnancy but also can affect fertility in ways that aren't yet clear. A few guidelines are worth noting if you're trying to get pregnant:

● Aim for your healthy weight. Either extreme underweight or extreme overweight may affect the menstrual cycle and ovulation and so reduce fertility. How? The body produces estrogen in the ovaries and in fat cells. Being very thin, the body won't produce as much estrogen in fat cells. With obesity, the body's fat cells produce too much. Either way throws off the delicate hormonal balance that promotes fertility.

● Take caution with dietary supplements touted to enhance fertility. Not enough is known about the risks or the benefits of extra vitamins, minerals, or herbals and how they might affect the unborn baby.

● If you're having difficulty getting pregnant, explore the reasons and a sound approach to infertility with your doctor. In that way you'll also eliminate any health problems that you or your spouse may have. *See "Polycystic Ovary Syndrome" on this page.*

Folic Acid: Take Note!

To prepare for pregnancy, all nutrients are essential. One merits special consideration: folate, or folic acid (a B vitamin). Folic acid is the form of folate in fortified foods and supplements. Folate is essential to good

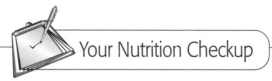

Your Nutrition Checkup

Ironing Out the Differences, for Calcium and Folate, Too!

How do your food choices stack up for three nutrients of concern to women: calcium, iron, and folate? In each pair, which food would you choose?

For more calcium . . .

COLUMN A

_____ ½ cup frozen yogurt
_____ 1 oz. Cheddar cheese
_____ 3 oz. canned tuna
_____ 1 cup milk
_____ 1 slice cheesecake
_____ 2 tbsp. yogurt cheese*
_____ ½ cup lettuce
_____ ½ cup tofu (with calcium sulfate)

COLUMN B

_____ ½ cup ice cream
_____ ½ cup cottage cheese
_____ 3 oz. canned salmon with bones
_____ 1 cup apple juice
_____ ½ cup pudding
_____ 2 tbsp. cream cheese
_____ ½ cup turnip greens
_____ ½ cup pinto beans

See "Kitchen Nutrition: Yogurt Cheese" in chapter 3 for a recipe.

For more iron . . .

COLUMN A

_____ 1 cup fortified breakfast cereal
_____ 3 oz. broiled sirloin steak
_____ ½ cup cooked green beans
_____ ½ cup cooked zucchini
_____ 1 egg yolk
_____ ⅓ cup grapes
_____ 2 tbsp. peanut butter
_____ 1 oz. pumpkin seeds

COLUMN B

_____ 1 slice whole-wheat toast
_____ 3 oz. broiled cod
_____ ½ cup cooked kidney beans
_____ ½ cup boiled spinach
_____ 1 egg white
_____ ⅓ cup raisins
_____ 3 oz. broiled chicken breast
_____ 1 oz. pretzels

For more folate . . .

COLUMN A

_____ 1 cup fortified breakfast cereal
_____ ½ cup mashed potatoes
_____ 6 oz. apple juice
_____ 1 cup raw spinach

COLUMN B

_____ 1 bread slice
_____ ½ cup pasta
_____ 6 oz. orange juice
_____ 1 cup iceberg lettuce

Now score yourself:

For each pair, these foods contain:

● *More calcium*—frozen yogurt, Cheddar cheese, canned salmon with bones, milk, pudding, yogurt cheese, turnip greens, tofu (with calcium sulfate)

● *More iron*—fortified breakfast cereal, sirloin steak, kidney beans, spinach, egg yolk, raisins, chicken breast, pumpkin seeds

● *More folate*—fortified breakfast cereal, pasta,* orange juice, spinach

*Most grain products are fortified with folic acid by law.

Give yourself 5 points for each selection you got right—perfect score, 40 points for calcium, 40 points for iron, and 20 points for folate. The higher your score, the more calcium, iron, and folate you likely consume—*if* these foods really are your "picks" for the day. *Tip:* Partner plant sources of iron with meat, poultry, or fish, or with a vitamin C-rich food to enhance its absorption.

To check specific calcium and iron content in these food pairs, see "Counting Up Calcium" and "Counting Up Iron" in chapter 4. Fruits and vegetables are among your best folate sources; *assess your fruit and vegetable intake using "Can You Count Up to 'Five a Day'?" in chapter 4.* Fortified grain products, whole grains, nuts, legumes, and liver are good folate sources, too.

health, and your body needs it to manufacture new cells and genetic material. Soon after conception, folate helps develop the neural tube, which becomes your baby's spinal cord and brain.

Women who consume enough folate, particularly in the weeks prior to conception and during the first three months of pregnancy, may reduce the risk of neural tube defects, which occur when the neural tube does not close completely. In fact, as many as 75 percent of serious birth defects in the spine and neural tube (spina bifida) and brain (anencephaly) might be prevented if women consumed enough folic acid in the critical time before and in the early weeks of pregnancy.

About twenty-five hundred newborns in the United States are born each year with neural tube defects. Since 1998, when grain products became fortified by law with folic acid (a form of folate), the incidence has gone down significantly. A diet with insufficient folic acid is one cause of neural tube defects.

Even a varied, well-balanced eating plan may not supply enough folate to protect against birth defects. For that reason, nutrition experts advise that all women of childbearing age consume 400 micrograms of folic acid daily from fortified foods, vitamin supplements, or a combination of the two . . . in addition to the folate naturally found in food.

● Eat a variety of foods with naturally occurring folate—for example, citrus fruits and juices; dark-green leafy vegetables; nuts; legumes; and liver.

● Read food labels to identify foods fortified with folic acid—for example, most breads, flour, crackers,

---

EVERY AGE AND STAGE OF LIFE: WHY A HEALTHY WEIGHT?

For girls . . . A healthy weight—not overweight—during childhood offers protection for the long term: protecting them from adult obesity and helping blood cholesterol and triglyceride levels stay at healthy levels. During the growing-up years, a healthy weight boosts self-esteem, important for emotional and social development.

For teen and young-adult women . . . As with girls, a healthy weight—not overweight—reduces the chances of adult obesity later. Beyond that, maintaining a healthy weight promotes physical health in other ways: lower risk for high blood cholesterol levels, for diabetes, and for high blood pressure; less arthritis risk in later life; and perhaps easier breast cancer detection. On the flipside, a healthy weight—not underweight—helps teens and young women develop and maintain strong bones for peak bone mass. For emotional health, a healthy weight feels good and boosts self-esteem.

For women in their child-bearing years . . . The benefits of a healthy weight throughout the child-bearing years mirror those of the teen and young-adult years. In addition, a healthy weight promotes fertility and helps reduce the risk for gallbladder disease.

For pregnant and breast-feeding women . . . Most important, keeping a healthy weight (not dieting) helps ensure a healthy pregnancy outcome: promotes normal fetal development and improves the chances of a healthy, full-term birth. When maternal weight is healthy, childbirth is both easier and safer. During breast-feeding, a healthy weight helps maintain the quality and volume of breast milk. And keeping a healthy weight during pregnancy and breast-feeding lowers a woman's risk for obesity later.

For women after menopause . . . As before, a healthy weight offers protection from some health problems, including breast cancer, some other cancers, heart disease, and diabetes. Among other benefits, helping to prevent the tendency for risky abdominal weight gain, as body weight shifts after menopause. As always, a healthy weight feels good!

For older women . . . A healthy weight continues to offer protection from some cancers, heart disease, and diabetes. What's more, a healthy weight—not underweight—helps bones remain strong, cushions bones and organs from fracture and other injury (in case of fall), and protects against body wasting that can come with serious illness.

See "Weighing the Risks" in chapter 2 for more reasons to maintain a healthy weight.

cornmeal, farina, pasta, and rice. If folic acid is added to breakfast cereals, it's listed on the label's Nutrition Facts. For fortified foods, the label may carry a health claim—that adequate folate intake may decrease the risk for neural tube defects.

● Consult your doctor or a registered dietitian (RD) about appropriate levels of supplements with folic acid. Taking in too much folate—more than 1,000 micrograms a day—can mask the symptoms of pernicious anemia, a condition that can cause nerve damage. (Pernicious anemia may result from a vitamin B_{12} deficiency.) Taking large doses from vitamin pills, not from food sources, is the usual reason why symptoms are masked.

For more on folate, see chapter 4.

More Prepregnancy Advice

● Even before pregnancy, refrain from any practices that may harm your developing baby: cigarette smoking, drinking alcoholic beverages, and inappropriate drug use. Important stages in your baby's development start right after conception. Before you know you're pregnant, potentially harmful substances already may have effects.

● Discuss any over-the-counter and prescription medications you take with your doctor. They, too, may be harmful to your developing baby. If necessary, other medications may be substituted.

● Stay physically active or initiate moderate physical activity in your daily lifestyle. That will help prepare you to be "fit" for a healthy pregnancy.

Congratulations! You're Expecting!

Being a nurturing parent begins at the moment of conception. Although you can't change your age or genetic traits, there's plenty you can do during the nine months of pregnancy to ensure your well-being and that of your unborn baby: eat wisely, stay physically active, and get plenty of rest. There's more good advice to follow: see your doctor regularly, stop smoking (if that's a habit), and avoid alcoholic drinks and inap-

propriate drugs. Women who follow this advice tend to have fewer complications during pregnancy, labor, and delivery, and deliver larger, healthier babies.

"Weighting" for Your New Arrival

"How much weight should I gain?" That's one of the top questions expectant mothers ask. In the last twenty-six weeks of pregnancy, your baby will grow fast, gaining about 1 ounce every day. Besides "baby weight," the weight you gain supports changes in your body and helps prepare you for breast-feeding.

Appropriate weight gain helps ensure a healthy outcome. In fact, your baby's birthweight depends on your weight gain during pregnancy. If you don't gain enough, your chance for delivering a low-birthweight infant goes up. Babies who weigh less than $5\frac{1}{2}$ pounds at birth are at greater risk for developmental difficulties and health problems. The problems of gaining too much? Both delivery and returning to your prepregnancy weight may be more difficult. In fact, excessive weight gain during pregnancy has been linked to rising obesity rates among women.

If you were dieting for weight loss before pregnancy, put that regimen aside for these nine months. Pregnancy is *not* a good time to skimp on calories, follow a weight-loss diet, or restrict weight gain!

How much should you expect to gain during pregnancy? Because every woman is unique, your doctor will advise you about the weight-gain range that's right for you. That advice depends on several factors:

● *Your weight before pregnancy.* Women at a healthy weight for their height (BMI 19.8 to 26) are advised to gain 25 to 35 pounds during pregnancy. Underweight women (BMI < 19.8) are advised to gain a little more, 28 to 40 pounds. Overweight women (BMI 26 to 29) may be advised to gain less, 15 to 25 pounds. Obese women (BMI > 29) are urged to gain at least 15 pounds. A healthcare professional can help calculate your Body Mass Index. *For more about healthy prepregnancy weight see "Body Basics: What's Your Healthy Weight?" in chapter 2.*

● *Your height.* Because all women are different, a range of weight gain is recommended—not just one targeted weight. For instance, very short women (62 inches or less) should aim for the lower end of the range for weight gain.

● *Your age.* Young teens (until age eighteen), who are at greater risk for delivering low-birthweight babies, are encouraged to gain at the higher end of the weight-gain range. Pregnancy puts greater demands on their own growing, developing bodies. *For more on teenage pregnancy see "For Pregnant Teens: Good Nutrition" in this chapter.*

● *Your race.* Black women are encouraged to gain at the higher end of their weight-gain range, too. That's because African American women are at greater risk for delivering low-birthweight infants.

● *Expecting twins or triplets?* Regardless of your BMI, your doctor may recommend a 35- to -45-pound weight gain for twins, and a 50-pound weight gain for triplets.

Where Does Weight Gain Go?

Your baby may weigh about 7 to 8 pounds at birth—but you'll gain more. Why? Many parts of your body support pregnancy. For example, your blood volume expands by about 50 percent. Your breasts increase in size. Your body also stores fat to sustain the baby's rapid growth and to provide energy for labor, delivery, and breast-feeding. Here's where pregnancy weight gain typically goes:

	Average Weight Gain (in pounds)
Baby	7 to 8
Placenta	1 to 2
Amniotic fluid	2
Mother	
Breasts	1
Uterus	2
Increase in blood volume	3
Body fat	5 or more
Increased muscle tissue and fluid	4 to 7
Total	At least 25 pounds

Weight Gain and Loss: Slow and Steady

Your rate of weight gain during pregnancy is as important as the amount. Expect 2 to 4 pounds of weight gain during your first three months; for teens, 4 to 6 pounds. After that, you'll probably gain ¾ to 1 pound per week. From month to month, you may gain a little more or a little less.

If you gain weight faster, here's how you might cut calories without depriving yourself or your baby of nutrients:

● Substitute fat-free or lower-fat milk, yogurt, and cheese for whole-milk products. And choose lean meats, poultry, and fish.

● Broil, bake, grill, or stir-fry foods instead of frying them.

● Eat smaller portions—enough to match Pyramid serving guidelines. *See chapter 10 for Pyramid advice and tips on serving sizes.*

● Cut down on foods high in fat and calories and low in nutrients, such as candy, cake, pastries, and rich desserts.

● Increase your physical activity within your doctor's guidelines.

Delivering your baby may be the fastest weight you ever lose! Between the baby and fluid loss, some new moms lose up to 10 pounds right after delivery, and another 5 pounds within the first month or so. For others, weight comes off more gradually, over a longer time period. Most women continue to lose weight slowly and steadily for six to twelve months after delivery. How fast you shed "baby weight" depends on how physically active you are, your calorie intake, and whether you breast-feed.

Returning to your prepregnancy weight—slowly and steadily—is important for your continued health. Yet that's not always easy. Why? It may be the shift in your lifestyle. In fact, studies suggest that lifestyle changes, not physical changes related to pregnancy, are likely reasons for postpregnancy weight gain. *For guidance on healthy weight loss see "Weight Management: Strategies That Work!" in chapter 2.*

Pregnancy: A Meal Ticket for Two

Did you know that it takes about 80,000 calories (about 300 extra calories a day after the first trimester) over nine months for a healthy baby to develop? An additional 300 calories a day during pregnancy do not sound like much. And they really aren't! You'll see that eating for two doesn't need to be much different than eating for one. The key is to "choose your calories by the company they keep"—in other words, choose nutrient-rich foods for extra calories.

The Food Guide Pyramid provides the guidelines for the nutrients and the energy needed for your "meal ticket for two." A few more Pyramid servings can supply all you need. *See chapter 10 for more about the Pyramid.*

How do 300 calories translate into "real food"? Try these nutrient-rich food combinations. They also supply more than 10 grams of protein, the extra amount needed during pregnancy:

- 1 ounce of cold cereal, a banana, and 1 cup of fat-free milk, or

- 1 baked potato with skin, topped with ½ cup each of broccoli and cauliflower, and 1 ounce of low-fat cheese, or

- 2 ounces of turkey on 2 slices of whole-grain or enriched bread, topped with lettuce, tomato, and sprouts.

Nutrients: For You and Baby, Too!

During pregnancy, your need for most nutrients and food energy goes up somewhat. Eating a variety of foods from all five food groups is the best way to get what you need. What if you don't follow the Pyramid guideline? An inadequate diet may impair your baby's development, and he or she may be underweight at birth. *See "The Food Guide Pyramid: Your Healthful Eating Guide" in chapter 10.*

Caution: If you've been pregnant recently, or if you've breast-fed within the past year, your body's nutritional reserves may be low. Problems during a previous pregnancy are another reason to make a special effort to eat wisely for a healthy pregnancy.

For specific nutrient recommendations during pregnancy see the Appendices. If you're vegetarian, see "The Vegetarian Mom" in chapter 20.

Baby-Building Protein

The structural components of body cells—your baby's and yours—are mostly protein. Changes in your own body, particularly the placenta, also require protein. An eating plan that matches the Food Guide Pyramid provides enough protein for a healthy pregnancy.

When you're pregnant, you need somewhat more protein than before pregnancy: about 10 *more* grams of protein a day. That adds up to 60 grams of protein daily, compared with 50 grams advised for nonpregnant women. To put those extra 10 grams of protein in perspective, a 3-ounce meat patty has about 20 grams of protein, and 8 ounces of milk supply about 8 grams of protein. Most nonpregnant women easily consume more than 60 grams of protein daily.

If you're a vegetarian and consume plenty of legumes, grain products, vegetables, and fruits, you won't have a problem consuming enough protein. If you're concerned, consult a registered dietitian to make sure you're getting enough. *See "Protein Power" in chapter 20.*

Fuel for Your Unborn Baby

Your baby needs a constant supply of energy . . . every minute for about 280 days . . . to grow! For protein to build body cells, your body needs an adequate energy supply. Otherwise your body uses protein for energy instead of cell building.

Keep in mind: eating for two (or more!) doesn't mean your calorie need doubles. After the first trimester you need about 300 calories a day more. If you're moderately active and need about 2,200 calories daily before pregnancy to maintain your weight, about 2,500 calories a day are right for now. Ask your doctor about your calorie need if you're pregnant with more than one baby.

Carbohydrates, your body's main energy source, quickly and efficiently convert to energy. "Carbs" come from fruits, vegetables, legumes, and grain products. Although fats in food supply calories, most food energy should come from carbohydrates.

Another note about fat: Your baby needs linoleic acid—an essential fatty acid—for the development of the central nervous system, including brain cells. Restricting fat too much isn't advised.

To fuel a healthy pregnancy, make your extra

calories count! Choose mostly nutrient-rich foods from the Pyramid's five food groups. They provide you and your baby with a healthful dose of nutrients, too. *For ways to "spend" 300 extra calories, see "Pregnancy: A Meal Ticket for Two" in this chapter.*

Vital Vitamins

If carbohydrates are the fuel of human life, vitamins are sparks that make body processes happen! Although all vitamins are important during pregnancy, some need special attention, including those important for cell division and the formation of new life.

A varied and balanced approach to eating is the best way to get vitamins you and your unborn baby need. Your doctor may prescribe a prenatal vitamin/mineral supplement, too. *For more about choosing a supplement see "Vitamin/Mineral Supplements: Benefits and Risks" in chapter 23.*

Have You Ever Wondered

...if nonnutritive sweeteners are safe to consume during pregnancy? Current research shows no reason to avoid foods and beverages with nonnutritive, or intense sweeteners: aspartame, saccharin, acesulfame potassium, and sucralose. Instead of calorie-free soft drinks and candies, more nutritious foods and beverages may be better choices for mothers-to-be. Drink milk, juice, and water.

Exception: Pregnant women with the rare genetic disorder called phenylketonuria (PKU) should avoid foods sweetened with aspartame. People with PKU cannot break down phenylalanine, which is an amino acid in aspartame. Then phenylalanine can reach high levels in the mother's blood and may affect the developing baby. Studies show that women with the PKU gene, but not the disease, metabolize aspartame well enough to protect their unborn baby from abnormal phenylalanine levels. If you have PKU or carry the gene, talk to your doctor.

Nonnutritive sweeteners can be useful to pregnant women with diabetes, who need to control their caloric intake, or to pregnant women who enjoy sweet flavors. Since most women need more energy during pregnancy, calorie restriction usually is discouraged. *For more about intense sweeteners and about aspartame and PKU, see "Intense Sweeteners: Flavor without Calories" in chapter 5.*

Vitamin A. Vitamin A, for example, promotes the growth and the health of cells and tissues throughout the body—yours and your baby's. There's no need for any extra from a supplement. Your everyday food choices can provide enough vitamin A for pregnancy.

What about supplements? Some contain Vitamin A levels that far exceed the Recommended Dietary Allowance. In fact, research suggests that excessive amounts from supplements (10,000 IU of vitamin A daily) increase the risk of birth defects. Take supplements only in amounts recommended by your doctor. Check the Supplement Facts panel on the label, and choose one with no more than 100 percent of the Daily Value for vitamin A.

Eating plenty of fruits and vegetables high in beta carotene (which forms vitamin A) isn't a problem. Beta carotene does not convert to vitamin A when blood levels of vitamin A are normal.

Folate and Other B Vitamins. By consuming an extra 300 calories a day, you'll likely consume enough extra of most B vitamins. During pregnancy you need more thiamin, riboflavin, and niacin to use the extra energy from food. And you need more vitamin B_6 to help protein make new body cells.

The need for folate, another B vitamin, increases during pregnancy—from 400 micrograms daily before pregnancy to 600 micrograms daily. Get 400 micrograms from fortified foods or supplements, and the remaining 200 micrograms from foods with naturally occurring folate. Consuming enough during the first three months is especially critical for lowering a newborn's risk for neural tube, or spinal cord, damage. *For more about folate prior to and during pregnancy see "Before Pregnancy" earlier in this chapter.*

The need for vitamin B_{12} also goes up during pregnancy. This vitamin is found in foods of animal origin such as milk, eggs, cheese, and meats. Vegetarian women who don't consume any foods of animal origin need a reliable source of vitamin B_{12}—perhaps a fortified breakfast cereal or a vitamin B_{12} supplement.

Vitamin C. The need for vitamin C goes up a bit, too. But a ¾-cup serving of orange juice supplies enough for a day! Besides its other functions, vitamin C helps your body absorb iron from plant sources of food. That's important because your iron needs increase by about 50 percent during pregnancy.

Vitamin D. To help your body absorb the calcium needed for pregnancy, consume enough vitamin D. Vitamin D-fortified milk is a good source. If you're a vegetarian who doesn't consume dairy foods, you may need a vitamin D supplement—especially if you aren't exposed to direct sunlight. Your body produces vitamin D when your skin comes in contact with sunlight.

For more about vitamins, see "Vitamins: The Basics" in chapter 4.

Minerals—Giving Body Structure

Minerals are part of a baby's bones and teeth. Along with protein and vitamins, minerals make blood cells and other body tissues, too. Minerals also take part in many body processes that support pregnancy. A few minerals require special attention during pregnancy: calcium, iron, and sometimes zinc.

Calcium. You need enough calcium now for two reasons: your baby's developing bones, and preserving your own bone mass. Without enough calcium, your body will withdraw calcium from your bones to build your baby's bones. You can't afford the loss! Research suggests that you also may reduce the chances of developing toxemia and high blood pressure if you consume enough calcium.

The calcium recommendation doesn't change for pregnancy: 1,000 milligrams of calcium daily for adult women, and 1,300 milligrams daily for pregnant teens. Yet before, during, and after pregnancy, many women don't get enough—often not enough calcium to protect against osteoporosis later in life. *See "Osteoporosis: Reduce the Risks" in chapter 22.*

Three servings (four servings for teens) from the MIlk Group supply nearly all the calcium you need daily. An 8-ounce serving of milk or yogurt provides about 300 milligrams of calcium. Leafy, green vegetables; canned fish (with bones); tofu processed with calcium; and calcium-fortified soy milk, juice, cereal, and bread also are good calcium sources. *For more about calcium and ways to include calcium-rich foods in your meals and snacks see "Calcium: A Closer Look" in chapter 4 and "Calcium Supplements: A Bone-Builder" in chapter 23.*

Doctors may prescribe a calcium supplement for women who don't consume enough calcium-rich foods.

Have You Ever Wondered

... if you need a multivitamin/mineral supplement during pregnancy? Check with your doctor. A balanced diet with a variety of foods can provide healthy women with enough nutrients for pregnancy. Your doctor or registered dietitian may recommend a prenatal multivitamin/mineral supplement to help ensure that you get enough iron, folic acid, and other nutrients.

If you follow a strict vegetarian diet (no foods of animal origin), if you're pregnant with more than one baby, or if your diet lacks critical nutrients, your doctor may prescribe a supplement, too. *See chapter 23, "Supplements: Use and Abuse."*

Iron. Why do you need so much more iron during pregnancy—up from 18 to 27 milligrams daily for adult women? Iron is essential for making hemoglobin, a component of blood. During pregnancy your blood volume increases by about 50 percent. Hemoglobin carries oxygen throughout your body, including to the placenta for your unborn baby.

For enough iron, consume good iron sources every day: lean meat; poultry; legumes; eggs; iron-fortified grain products; and green, leafy vegetables. Eat good sources of vitamin C such as citrus fruits and juices, broccoli, tomatoes, and kiwi, with iron-rich foods since vitamin C helps your body absorb iron.

Besides an iron-rich diet your doctor probably will prescribe a low-dose (30 milligrams per day) iron supplement or a prenatal vitamin supplement with iron. Why? Iron deficiency, the most common nutritional deficiency during pregnancy, increases the risk for a premature delivery or the delivery of a low-birthweight baby. Although widely available in food, iron isn't always well absorbed. Many women start pregnancy with marginal iron stores, which increases the chance for becoming anemic. If you have iron-deficiency anemia, your doctor may prescribe a higher dosage.

Your body absorbs iron from a supplement best on an empty stomach or with vitamin C-rich juice but not with meals. Conversely, taking an iron supplement with coffee or tea may decrease its absorption.

Sometimes taking iron supplements during pregnancy causes side effects such as nausea, constipation, and appetite loss. If that happens, try taking the supplement with meals even though the iron may not be absorbed as well. Then make sure you eat more food sources of iron. A lower dosage might help, too; talk to your doctor.

For more about iron in a healthful diet see "Iron: A Closer Look" in chapter 4 and "Iron Supplements: Enhancing the Benefit" in chapter 23.

Zinc. The need for zinc, essential for cell growth and brain development, increases by 50 percent during pregnancy. Zinc comes in a variety of foods, but it's most available from foods of animal origin such as meat, seafood, and poultry. Whole-grain products have zinc, too, but it's not absorbed as well. Most women, except perhaps some vegetarian women, get enough zinc during pregnancy from their everyday food choices, especially from protein-rich foods. **Caution:** Take an iron supplement according to the recommended dosage; too much iron can interfere with zinc absorption.

Sodium. You don't need to restrict sodium during pregnancy—unless your doctor advises you to do so. And if you limited your sodium intake before pregnancy, continue to do so as your doctor recommends. Pregnant or not, choosing and preparing food with less salt and sodium still is good advice. *See chapter 7, "Sodium: A Salty Subject."*

For more about minerals in a healthful eating plan see "Minerals—Not 'Heavy Metal'" in chapter 4.

And Water, Too

Remember, water is a nutrient. As part of your body's transportation system it carries nutrients to body cells and carries waste products away. That includes nourishment that passes through the placenta to your baby. You need fluids—at least 8 to 12 cups daily—for your own and your baby's increased blood volume. When you feel thirsty, drink more!

For Pregnant Teens: Good Nutrition

School, activities, and frantic social schedules often take good nutrition off a teen's "top ten" list. Still growing, a pregnant teen's need for food energy,

protein, and some vitamins and minerals often exceeds that of adult women, however. What a pregnant teen eats today affects her own short- and long-term health and her baby's future.

Figure-conscious teens may be reluctant to gain weight during pregnancy. However, teens need to understand that pregnancy isn't the time to restrict calories or follow a weight-control diet! Pregnancy is just a temporary body change, and extra pounds aren't just the fetus or mother's body fat. *See "Where Does Weight Gain Go?" earlier in this chapter.*

Until age eighteen, pregnant teens need to gain more weight than adult women do. Most healthy young mothers gain about 35 pounds by the end of their pregnancy. Gaining at the upper end of the suggested range helps the mother deliver a healthier, normal-birthweight baby. *See advice for weight gain earlier in this chapter.*

A baby grows "around the clock." Yet, typical teenage food habits—meal-skipping, high-calorie/low-nutrient foods and drinks—often don't provide the ongoing supply of nutrients an unborn baby needs. A pattern of three meals and three nutritious snacks daily, which follow Pyramid guidelines, can provide enough nourishment for a teenage pregnancy. *Use the Food Guide Pyramid, explained in chapter 10, as a guide.*

A varied, balanced eating plan is the only way to provide enough nutrients and food energy during pregnancy and to "feed" an unborn baby! Although doctors often prescribe a multivitamin/mineral supplement for pregnant teens, it's meant to supplement, not replace, meals or snacks.

Adolescent pregnancy is considered high risk. A teenager's body is still growing, perhaps competing with the unborn baby for nutrients. With poor food choices and an inadequate nutrient intake, a teenage mom more likely delivers a low-birthweight baby. The chances of anemia and pre-eclampsia (or toxemia) are higher, too. Untreated pre-eclampsia is dangerous and potentially life-threatening for the mother and the baby. Symptoms include sudden weight gain, abdominal pain, and high blood pressure. For these reasons, prenatal care with nutrition counseling is essential

For more about nutrition during adolescence see "Feeding the Teen Machine" in chapter 16.

Discomforts of Pregnancy

With so many changes taking place in your body, occasional discomforts during pregnancy really aren't surprising. A few changes in what—and how—you eat may relieve vomiting and nausea, constipation, heartburn, and swelling.

Dealing with Nausea and Vomiting

Often referred to as "morning sickness," nausea or vomiting is experienced by 50 to 90 percent of moms-to-be. Hormonal changes, particularly rising estrogen levels, are likely responsible.

Somewhat of a misnomer, "morning sickness" may occur at any time—day or night. And it may continue past the first three months of pregnancy.

Some women complain about just minor queasiness. Persistent, severe nausea with spells of vomiting can leave other pregnant women at risk for dehydration and weight loss.

If you're pregnant, these suggestions might keep nausea at bay:

● Skip foods with strong flavors (perhaps spicy foods) or aromas if they trigger nausea. Pregnant women often have an exaggerated sense of smell, making a common aroma seem unappealing.

● Before getting out of bed, eat starchy foods such as crackers, plain toast, or dry cereal. That helps remove stomach acid. Get out of bed slowly.

● Enjoy small meals every two to three hours to prevent an empty stomach. Drink beverages between, not with, meals, and be sure you're well hydrated!

● Eat easy-to-digest carbohydrate foods, such as plain pasta, crackers, potatoes, rice, fruits, and vegetables, and low-fat protein foods such as lean meat, fish, poultry, and eggs. Limit fried and other high-fat foods if they cause discomfort.

● Savor every bite! Eat meals slowly. In fact, try to make your surroundings stress-free.

● Before bedtime eat a small snack such as peanut butter on crackers and a glass of milk, or cereal and milk.

● Experiment with beverages that may calm a queasy stomach: lemon or ginger tea, lemonade, ginger ale, or water flavored with a slice of lemon or ginger.

● Choose those foods that appeal and that "stay down." Even if your food choices aren't "nutritionally perfect," that's okay if queasiness doesn't last longer than a few days. If the problem persists, talk to your doctor or a registered dietitian.

● Consult your doctor if you vomit more than twice daily.

Constipation during Pregnancy

Since becoming pregnant, do you occasionally feel constipated? Many women do. Hormonal changes relax muscles to accommodate your expanding uterus, and that slows the action in your intestine. Taking an iron supplement can aggravate constipation, too.

For some women, constipation, along with pressure from the baby, leads to hemorrhoids. Hemorrhoids are large, swollen veins in the rectum.

Try these ways to prevent or ease constipation and the discomfort of hemorrhoids:

● Drink 8 to 12 cups of fluid daily. Besides water, include milk, fruit juice, and perhaps broth in your fluid allowance. *For more about fluids in a healthful eating plan, see chapter 8.*

● Eat high-fiber foods: whole-grain foods, bran, vegetables, fruits, and legumes.

● Enjoy the natural laxative effect of dried plums (prunes), prune juice, and figs.

● Be physically active every day. Like swimming and prenatal exercise classes, walking is good exercise during pregnancy. Regular activity stimulates normal bowel function.

● Unless your doctor prescribes them, don't take laxatives. For hemorrhoids, ask your doctor to recommend a safe suppository or ointment.

Just Heartburn

Especially during the last three months, you may complain about heartburn. That may happen as your baby puts pressure on your digestive organs. To relieve your discomfort:

● Eat small meals frequently—every two to three hours.

● Cut down on caffeinated and carbonated beverages.

● Eat slowly in relaxed surroundings.

● Walk after you eat to help gastric, or stomach, juices go down, not up. If you don't walk, at least remain seated for an hour or two after eating, rather than lie down.

● Avoid large meals before bedtime.

● Sleep with your head elevated.

● Wear comfortable, loose-fitting clothes.

● Consult your doctor before taking antacids. Some contain sodium bicarbonate (baking soda), which can interfere with the absorption of vitamins and minerals.

Pregnancy and Alcoholic Beverages Don't Mix!

Your blood passes through every organ in your body, through the placenta, and into the circulatory system of your unborn baby. Your baby will be exposed to any alcohol or drugs in your blood.

Even at moderate levels (one drink a day), women who regularly consume alcohol during pregnancy increase their risk for miscarriage or delivering low-birthweight babies. A condition called fetal alcohol syndrome (FAS) is associated with excessive drinking. Infants with FAS may be born with birth defects: retarded growth, mental impairment, or physical malformations.

If you're trying to conceive or you're already pregnant, health experts advise to avoid beer, wine, or other alcoholic beverages completely. A safe level for alcohol intake during pregnancy is unknown. Health experts don't know if babies differ in their sensitivity to alcohol. As a reminder, alcoholic beverages carry a label warning about the dangers of drinking during pregnancy and its relation to birth defects.

> GOVERNMENT WARNING:
>
> (1) ACCORDING TO THE SURGEON GENERAL, WOMEN SHOULD NOT DRINK ALCOHOLIC BEVERAGES DURING PREGNANCY BECAUSE OF THE RISK OF BIRTH DEFECTS. (2) CONSUMPTION OF ALCOHOLIC BEVERAGES IMPAIRS YOUR ABILITY TO DRIVE A CAR OR OPERATE MACHINERY, AND MAY CAUSE HEALTH PROBLEMS.

Swelling—Part of Pregnancy

Swelling is normal, especially in the last three months of pregnancy. Water retained in your ankles, hands, and wrists is a reservoir for your expanded blood volume. It offsets the water lost during delivery, and it's used later for breast milk. Even with swelling, drink plenty of water!

Unless your doctor advises otherwise, avoid diuretics, or medications that increase water loss through urination. There's no need to limit salt to prevent swelling, either; use iodized salt—just enough to match your taste. Iodine is a mineral essential for you and your baby.

To relieve the discomfort of moderate swelling, use these techniques:

● Put your feet up. And when you sit, get up to stretch to improve your circulation. Try not to stand for a long period of time.

● Rest on your left side to aid circulation.

● Wear comfortable shoes, perhaps a larger size.

● Avoid tight clothes, tight stockings, tight-fitting rings, and anything else that restricts circulation.

● If swelling is excessive, this may be a sign of pre-eclampsia, or toxemia. Other signs include high blood pressure, a sudden weight gain, headaches, and abdominal pain. Advise your doctor right away if you develop these symptoms. Untreated, pre-eclampsia can be dangerous later in pregnancy, even life-threatening for both mother and baby. *Note:* Pre-eclampsia has been linked to low calcium and low protein intake during pregnancy.

Pregnancy and Diabetes

Gestational diabetes—which usually starts around the middle of pregnancy and ends after delivery—is a health problem for some pregnant women. Who's at risk? Women with a family history of diabetes, obese women, those who've had a problem pregnancy, and women over age forty. As a safeguard, most women are routinely tested for gestational diabetes at about twenty-four to twenty-eight weeks.

Diabetes during pregnancy increases the risk for high blood pressure and toxemia. Toxemia, accompanied by swelling, high blood pressure, and excess protein in urine, is dangerous. Women with gestational diabetes often have big babies, who may be difficult to deliver, and they may need a cesarean delivery. The risk for getting diabetes later in life is higher among women who develop gestational diabetes.

If you have gestational diabetes, you can deliver a healthy baby. However, it's important for your doctor to monitor gestational diabetes carefully and prescribe treatment, typically a combination of diet and physical activity. A registered dietitian can help you develop an eating plan to control your blood sugar

levels. *See "Diabetes: A Growing Health Concern" in chapter 22.*

Pregnancy: More Reasons for Food Safety

At any time of life, handling food properly to avoid foodborne illness is important. Pregnancy is no exception. Besides the general cautions, several food safety issues are of special concern now:

● *Listeria,* a bacterium that may contaminate soft cheese, unpasteurized milk, hot dogs, and deli meats, can cause miscarriage in the first trimester and serious illness or stillbirth later.

● *Toxoplasmosis,* a parasite linked to undercooked meat or poultry, can be passed from mother to unborn baby, causing severe symptoms. Because cat feces carry this parasite, avoid cat litter, limit your contact with cats, and always wash your hands with soap and water after handling them.

● *E. coli 0157:H7*, a bacterium associated with raw and undercooked meat and unpasteurized milk, is highly toxic. This life-threatening strain, which can cause severe kidney, intestinal, and brain damage, can pass to your unborn baby.

● *Lead* exposure during pregnancy is linked to miscarriage and stillbirth, low-birthweight babies, and damage to a baby's nervous system. Among the sources of lead: water from lead pipes or pipes with lead solder, food served on ceramic plates with improperly applied lead glaze, and beverages kept and served in lead crystal decanters or glasses.

● *Methyl mercury and PCBs (polychlorinated biphenyls)*, chemical pollutants found in some fish, are especially harmful to unborn babies and young children, whose bodies are just developing. Mercury poisoning, for example, may damage the nervous system. Since you may pass these contaminants on, pregnancy and breast-feeding are not the time to eat long-lived fish (shark, swordfish, king mackerel, and tilefish), which contain the highest levels of methyl mercury.

See chapter 12 for specific precautions for these foodborne illnesses, as well as for general food safety guidance. Chapter 8 addresses lead poisoning and water.

Have You Ever Wondered ?

. . . if pregnant and nursing women can eat fish? Yes—but not long-lived fish such as shark, swordfish, king mackerel, and tilefish. No matter how you prepare or cook fish, you can't get rid of the methyl mercury they may carry. Especially during pregnancy, avoid raw fish and seafood, too, to reduce your risk of viral and bacterial infection. Enjoy other kinds of fish: shellfish, canned fish, smaller ocean fish, or farm-raised fish. You can safely eat 12 ounces of cooked fish each week.

. . . if herbal supplements are safe during pregnancy and nursing? There's not enough scientific evidence yet to recommend safe levels for herbal supplements for pregnant or nursing moms. However, some are known to be harmful to a baby—for example, comfrey may cause liver damage, blue cohosh may cause heart defects, and pennyroyal may cause spontaneous abortions. Other herbs identified as potentially harmful include aloe, barberry, buckthorn, burdock, cascara, chamomile, coltsfoot, cornsilk, devil's claw root, Dong Quai, ephedra, goldenseal, hawthorne, horseradish, licorice, lily of the valley, lobelia, rue, sassafras, senna, St. John's wort, uva ursi, and yarrow.

. . . if herbal teas are okay to drink during pregnancy? Some, but not all, are considered safe if you enjoy no more than two to three cups a day. Blackberry, citrus peel, ginger, lemon balm, orange peel, and rose-hip teas are among those considered safe if they've been processed according to government safety standards.

Stay Active!

For most pregnancies, mild to moderate physical activity benefits the mom—and won't affect the unborn child. Consider the unique benefits of staying active during pregnancy!

- Helps you look and feel good as your body changes
- Promotes your muscle tone, stamina, and strength
- Helps reduce leg and back pain, constipation, swelling, and bloating
- Promotes blood circulation and may help prevent varicose veins
- Helps your posture and balance—important as your center of gravity shifts
- Helps you sleep better
- Prepares your body for labor and childbirth
- After your baby's born, helps your body get back in shape!

Caution: Pregnancy isn't the time to exercise to lose or keep from gaining weight.

Healthcare professionals advise moderate activity for most pregnant women: perhaps walking, swimming, modified low-impact aerobics, or stationary cycling. The right level of physical activity depends on your health and how active you've always been.

Caution: Avoid strenuous activity during your first trimester. Overexertion, which may cause your unborn baby to become overheated at a critical time of development, increases the risk for birth defects.

With minor changes you may be able to continue your regular physical activity routine. Just remember, as your body shape changes and you gain weight, your center of gravity shifts, too. That puts more stress on your muscles and joints, particularly in your lower back and pelvis. Some activities get harder to do, especially during the last three months. Injury is more likely, too, as changes in your hormones cause ligaments in your joints to stretch. Exercise with care. Avoid jerky, bouncy movements—and don't overdo.

Keep these pointers in mind:

- Talk with your doctor about your approach to physical activity during pregnancy—including any new activities you plan to do. Your doctor may advise against exercise if you have a high-risk pregnancy: high blood pressure induced by pregnancy, symptoms or a history of early contractions (preterm labor), vaginal bleeding, or early rupture of membranes. Other health conditions, such as heart or lung disease, may limit your physical activity, too.

- With your doctor, choose an activity plan that keeps you fit, matches your health needs and lifestyle, and prepares you for delivery. Find out if your hospital, clinic, or health club offers an exercise program for pregnant women. These programs usually include exercises to help with labor, including deep breathing and stretching.

- Start slowly. If you haven't been active, start with low-intensity activity—according to your doctor's advice.

- Stick with a routine—at least three times a week. This isn't the time to stop and start with spurts of heavy exercise.

- Enjoy a variety of activities that build strength and that condition your heart and lungs. Remember to stretch your muscles before and afterward.

- After the first twenty weeks, avoid any exercises you do while lying on your back. In that position it may be harder for your blood to circulate.

- Drink plenty of water—before, during and after physical activity—and wear appropriate clothing to avoid getting overheated and dehydrated.

- Wear a supportive bra to protect your breasts.

- If you feel tired, stop before you feel exhausted. If you can talk as you move, your level of physical activity is right.

- If you experience any problems, stop your activity and consult your doctor right away. These are warning signs: pain (in general, or in your back or pubic area), dizziness or feeling faint, vaginal bleeding, shortness of breath, rapid or irregular heartbeat, discomfort when you walk, uterine contractions and chest pain, and fluid leaking from your vagina.

- After delivery, resume your prepregnancy routine gradually, as you're physically able. Start with walking; use a stroller or a front/back carrier so you and your baby can walk together. Another option: Check in your community for a postpartum exercise class.

For Those Who Breast-Feed

The decision to breast-feed is personal, dependent on many factors. If you decide it's right for you and your baby, make smart eating a priority. Your needs for energy and some nutrients are higher now than during pregnancy.

If you're able, breast-feeding is good for your baby—and good for you. Besides the physical benefits to your baby and the emotional nurturing you share, breast-feeding can help you return to your prepregnancy shape and weight, and reduce blood loss after pregnancy. Although not conclusive, recent research suggests that breast-feeding may offer health benefits later in your life: reduced risk of breast cancer, ovarian cancer, and osteoporosis. *For more about the benefits of and techniques for breast-feeding see "Breast-Feeding Your Baby" in chapter 15.*

Your Energy Sources

Your fuel supply for milk production comes from two sources: energy stored as body fat during pregnancy, and extra energy from food choices. To produce breast milk, your body uses about 100 to 150 calories a day from the fat you stored during pregnancy. That's why breast-feeding helps many new mothers lose pregnancy weight —often without trying!

While breast-feeding, you also need to eat about 500 extra calories a day. If you needed about 2,200 calories to maintain your weight before your pregnancy, you may need about 2,700 calories a day now.

Pass the Pickles: Cravings and Food Aversions

Whether it's pickles and ice cream or other foods, cravings, as well as food aversions, are common during pregnancy. Although the exact cause is unknown, taste perceptions may change with hormonal changes. Usually taste buds "realign" after the first trimester, or sometimes not until after the baby's birth.

Unless you avoid an entire food group, food aversions are harmless. Just substitute nutritionally similar foods. For instance, if broccoli loses its appeal, substitute another vegetable that you enjoy and tolerate. Most cravings are harmless unless foods you crave replace more nutritious foods.

Caution: Cravings for nonfood substances, a condition called pica, can be dangerous. The cultural practice of craving cornstarch, ashes, laundry starch, clay, or other odd substances comes from folklore that started hundreds of years ago. It was believed that eating a particular substance might decrease nausea, promote a healthy baby, or ease delivery. There's no evidence that this practice works—and it can be harmful for you and your baby.

Get those added calories by enjoying more nutrient-rich foods from the Pyramid's five food groups. Adding an extra serving or so from each food group during the day provides enough extra energy and nutrients for breast-feeding. *See "How Many Servings a Day for You?" in chapter 10.*

After you've established your breast-feeding routine, evaluate your energy intake. Consider your activity level, your weight gain during pregnancy, and your weight loss since delivery. Do you need more or less than 500 extra calories a day? Ask your lactation counselor or a registered dietitian for guidance.

While you're nursing, steer away from restrictive weight-loss regimens. Dipping below 1,800 calories daily may decrease your milk volume and compromise your own nutritional status. Losing 2 to 4 pounds a month, however, probably won't affect your milk supply; gradual weight loss is healthier for you anyway. Losing more than 4 to 5 pounds a month after the first month isn't advised.

Now about Nutrients

The need for most nutrients increases during breast-feeding. A few need special attention, especially if you breast-feed longer than two or three months:

Protein. Your everyday food choices supply enough protein while breast-feeding. For example, the protein from an extra serving or two of milk supplies the extra protein and calcium you need.

Calcium. Your calcium needs don't change when you're breast-feeding. Still, make sure you consume

enough. If you come up short, your body may draw from calcium in your bones so the calcium content in breast milk remains adequate. Calcium losses in your bones may put you at greater risk for osteoporosis later in life. Periodontal problems also may crop up after pregnancy and nursing, perhaps related to calcium drain. Enjoy at least three calcium-rich dairy foods daily. And eat vegetables, and fish with edible bones; they're both good calcium sources. *See "Osteoporosis: Reduce the Risks" in chapter 22.*

Zinc. Nursing increases the need for zinc. Zinc that your body uses easily comes from foods of animal origin. Pay special attention to zinc, especially if you're a vegetarian.

Vitamin B_{12} and Vitamin D. Make sure you consume enough to ensure an optimal amount of these vitamins in breast milk. Because vitamin B_{12} is found only in foods of animal origin, some vegetarians may need a vitamin B_{12} supplement. If you eat meat, poultry, fish, eggs, and dairy products, you're likely getting enough.

Breast milk doesn't have much vitamin D. If your diet is low in vitamin D or if you aren't exposed to sunlight, your breast milk may have even less. Milk is fortified with vitamin D, and sunlight helps your body produce vitamin D. Some vegetarians may need a vitamin D supplement.

Folate. Especially if you're considering another pregnancy soon, consume the recommended 500 micrograms daily of folate—from fortified grain products and supplements as well as from fruits and vegetables—while breast-feeding. *For more about folate see "Before Pregnancy" earlier in this chapter.*

Vitamin B_6. The need for this B vitamin goes up, yet nursing mothers often don't consume enough. Chicken, fish, and pork are the best sources, followed by whole grain products and legumes.

Multivitamin/mineral Supplement. If you took a prenatal vitamin/mineral supplement during pregnancy, your doctor may recommend that you continue. You can get enough nutrients from food—if you choose wisely. If your own food choices come up short on calories or nutrients, in most cases your breast milk still will be sufficient to support your baby's growth and development—but at the expense of your own

---

(Have You Ever Wondered ❓)

... if your food choices affect the flavor of your breast milk? Eating strongly flavored foods such as onions, garlic, broccoli, cabbage, cauliflower, garlic, "hot" spicy food, or beans may give your breast milk an off-flavor. These flavors make some babies fussy; other babies don't notice. If some foods seem to upset your baby, eat less of them, less often. What you eat may cause a harmless color change, too. Breast milk usually is white or bluish-white.

nutrient reserves! *To choose an appropriate supplement see "Vitamin/Mineral Supplements: Benefits and Risks" in chapter 23.*

For more about vitamins and minerals see chapter 4, and for specific Dietary Reference Intakes during breast-feeding see the Appendices.

Remember Fluids!

To ensure an adequate milk supply and to prevent dehydration, drink enough fluids to satisfy your thirst. That's the amount to keep your urine pale yellow or nearly colorless. As during pregnancy, you need at least 8 to 12 cups of fluids daily—more if you're thirsty. If you're constipated or if your urine is concentrated, drink more fluids! *Tip:* Keep water, milk, or fruit juice handy to sip as you nurse. Milk and juice supply other nutrients you need in extra amounts for nursing: calcium from milk and vitamin C from most fruit juices.

Nonfoods: Effect on Breast Milk?

While you breast-feed, take the same precautions you did during pregnancy. Whether it's food, beverages, or other substances, what you consume may be passed to your baby.

Alcoholic Beverages

The alcohol you drink passes into breast milk, so steer away from wine or beer for relaxation. Contrary to popular belief, no scientific evidence suggests that an alcoholic drink promotes the "letdown" reflex anyway.

An occasional alcoholic drink probably won't affect your baby or interfere with nursing, but heavy drinking may inhibit your "letdown" reflex. Alcohol in breast milk may cause your baby to be less alert. In excess, it may affect brain development.

There's no guideline on how much is safe—another reason to avoid alcoholic beverages when you're nursing. If you want an occasional drink, do so after breast-feeding, or postpone nursing for at least an hour for each drink you ingest. That gives your body time to break down alcohol before you nurse again.

Smoking

Nicotine passes into breast milk. If you're a smoker and quit during pregnancy, breast-feeding isn't the

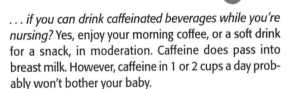

Have You Ever Wondered

. . . if you can drink caffeinated beverages while you're nursing? Yes, enjoy your morning coffee, or a soft drink for a snack, in moderation. Caffeine does pass into breast milk. However, caffeine in 1 or 2 cups a day probably won't bother your baby.

. . . if vegetarian eating supplies adequate nutrition for breast-feeding? A vegetarian mom who consumes dairy products, and perhaps eggs, can easily get enough nutrients. For vegans, who avoid all foods of animal origin, calcium, vitamin D, iron, and vitamin B$_{12}$ need special attention. *For more on vegetarian eating see "The Vegetarian Mom" in chapter 20.*

. . . if you can pass food allergens through breast milk to your baby? For starters, it's highly unlikely that your baby can't tolerate breast milk; allergic reactions from human milk are extremely rare.

Although uncommon, some babies react to allergens passed through breast milk—for example, an allergy to cow milk protein or to the protein in peanuts. If you suspect an allergy, never make the diagnosis yourself! Talk to your doctor for a qualified diagnosis. Then get help from a registered dietitian to help you manage any allergy. With guidance you probably can continue breast-feeding. *See "Food Allergies: Commonly Uncommon" in chapter 21.*

. . . if exercise affects your breast milk? Being active probably won't affect the amount or the composition of your breast milk. If you're highly active, your milk may have more lactic acid right after you exercise. Lactic acid may affect the flavor, but it doesn't appear to be harmful to infants.

time to take up the habit again. Nicotine can reduce your milk supply, and increase your baby's chance for colic, a sinus infection, or fussiness. Smoking near your baby is risky, too, exposing him or her to secondhand smoke and possibly getting burned. Too close to a nursing session, smoking even may inhibit your "letdown" reflex.

If you still choose to smoke, don't smoke near your baby—not even in the same room. Try to avoid smoking for 2½ hours before nursing, and never smoke as you nurse!

Medications

Consult your doctor about any prescription and over-the-counter medication you're taking, even an aspirin! Most pass into breast milk in concentrations that pose no harm to your infant. But there are some exceptions.

Recreational drugs—which pass into breast milk—are never considered safe for you or your baby!

For more about nursing see "Breast-Feeding Your Baby" in chapter 15.

Breast Cancer: Do Food Choices Make a Difference?

Breast cancer: it's a common fear among women for good reason. Breast cancer is the most common cancer among North American women, striking nearly two hundred thousand women annually. And it's the second most common cause of cancer death for women, killing nearly fifty thousand women a year.

All women are vulnerable to breast cancer—eventually. What's your risk? Among the probable risk factors: family history of breast cancer, early menstruation, late menopause (after age fifty-five), older-age pregnancy of a first child, some forms of benign breast disease, obesity after menopause, ovarian and endometrial cancer, exposure to ionizing radiation, and simply getting older.

The causes of breast cancer aren't understood. Yet, healthful eating—plenty of fiber, fruits and vegetables, and a diet low in fat—may help protect you from breast lesions and cancer. Although the reasons aren't clear, dietary fiber, beta carotene, and vitamin C (found in fruits and vegetables) may lower breast cancer risk. That's one more reason to enjoy at least five fruit and vegetable servings daily—and whole-grain foods for their fiber, too!

Eating a low-fat diet may lower your risk for breast cancer, although research results aren't conclusive. Some scientists theorize a link between fat intake and estrogen. As dietary fat goes up, estrogen levels in breast tissue do, too, which may promote cancer growth. Researchers also are investigating a protective role from omega-3 fatty acids and monounsaturated fats; little research has yet been done on the effects of trans fatty acids. Stay tuned!

Are you a "pear" or an "apple"? The place where extra pounds of body fat settle on your body may make a difference. Early research suggests that women who carry excess body fat around the abdomen (apple shape) may have an increased breast cancer risk. After menopause, more excess weight is often distributed around the midsection. After menopause, weight gain is associated with increased cancer risk, perhaps related to estrogens formed in the body's fat tissues. Being physically active helps you keep your healthy weight, so move more, too!

Another possible link: excessive alcoholic beverage consumption may increase the chances of breast cancer. A daily limit of 5 ounces of wine, 12 ounces of beer, or 1½ ounces of 80-proof distilled spirits is recommended for all women. If you're at high risk for breast cancer, you may be better off enjoying non-alcoholic drinks instead.

If you are considering hormone replacement therapy (HRT) or estrogen replacement therapy (ERT), weigh the benefits and the risks. Although HRT or ERT may reduce discomforts of menopause and the risk of osteoporosis, each is linked to increased breast cancer risk. Talk to your doctor about the best approach for you.

Are foods with phytoestrogens—for example, soy with the isoflavone genistein—an appropriate alternative to HRT if you're at high risk for breast cancer? On one hand, the estrogenlike effects in isoflavones may be harmful for women already at high risk for breast cancer. New research also suggests that phytoestrogens in soy are selective and don't have much effect on breast tissue. Since the jury's still out, talk to your physician before adding soy to your meals and snacks if you have breast cancer, if you're at high risk for breast cancer, or if you're taking tamoxifen, a hormone-blocking drug related to estrogen. Dietary soy supplements aren't advised, either. Research is under way to explore another food that may protect against hormone-sensitive cancers: flaxseed, which contains a type of phytoestrogen called lignan.

The bottom-line nutrition advice to protect against breast cancer: Make your overall food choices lower in fat and full of fruits, vegetables, and whole-grain foods. Aim for your healthy weight. And make early detection a habit: monthly self-examination, yearly mammograms, and routine breast examination. *See chapter 22 for more about nutrition and cancer.*

Have You Ever Wondered

. . . if foods designed for women are worth it? "Feminine foods," or those nutritionally designed for women's needs, may offer health benefits—for example, soy milk products, cereals fully fortified with folic acid, and juice with added calcium. Read food labels to know what you're buying, then decide if you need the extra nutrients or phytonutrients they provide. These foods often cost more. If you already consume enough from other food sources, you probably don't need them.

. . . if feeling tired could be a thyroid problem? Perhaps. Symptoms of hypothyroidism include fatigue and mood swings. However, with mild hypothyroidism, you may feel fine. Cold intolerance; dry, brittle hair and skin; hoarseness; difficulty swallowing; and forgetfulness are other symptoms, usually associated with more severe hypothyroidism. Of the eleven million people in the United States with hypothryroidism, most are women and elderly people. *For more about a thyroid problem and its potential consequences see chapter 22.*

Now for Menopause

Menopause, when hormone levels slowly drop, is a natural passage in a woman's life cycle—and not a health problem. So relax, and accept the changes as normal. Once symptoms such as hot flashes, mood swings, and sleeplessness disappear, postmenopausal women are free of discomforts that came with their monthly menstrual cycle.

The menopausal years are gradual. Menopausal changes are closely linked to hormone levels, most specifically to estrogen. Perimenopause typically starts in a woman's midforties and lasts for four to six years as the body gradually produces less estrogen and progesterone. Menopause is twelve months after the last period, on average—at age fifty-one; postmenopause follows.

As always, an overall healthful diet—with enough servings from the Food Guide Pyramid—is important advice for menopause. Healthful eating promotes good health, and good health minimizes the discomforts of menopause. *See "The Food Guide Pyramid: Your Healthful Eating Guide" in chapter 10.*

At this stage of life, physical activity remains a priority. You're well aware of the benefits to weight management; to heart and bone health; and to lower risks for heart disease, diabetes, and cancer. An active lifestyle also can reduce the discomforts of menopause. *For ways to add physical activity to your lifestyle see "Get Physical!" in chapter 2.*

Iron Needs Drop

On the "up" side, your iron need drops with menopause—from 18 to 8 milligrams of iron a day— since you no longer have menstrual loss, so your risk for iron deficiency also goes down. Unless your doctor advises otherwise, stop taking iron supplements. Consuming too much iron, typically from a supplement, can be harmful—especially if you have a genetic disorder called hemochromatosis.

Weight Gain: A New Problem?

On the "down" side, some menopausal women gain weight—some having weight problems for the first time in their life! Why? It's partly age. Metabolic rate, or the speed at which the body uses energy, often slows as hormone levels change. There's often another reason. In midlife, many women shift to more sedentary living, using less food energy as they get older. That promotes weight problems if eating habits remain unchanged. As an aside, research doesn't support the perception that hormone replacement causes weight gain.

Besides going up in dress size, what are the risks? Being overweight increases the chances for many health problems that start to appear after menopause. Changing hormone levels affect body fat distribution as more fat gets stored around the abdomen. Central body fat appears to be riskier for heart disease, higher cholesterol levels, high blood pressure, and insulin resistance than lower body fat.

You don't need be resigned to gain weight after menopause! To maintain your weight or to drop a few pounds if you need to, adjust your food choices. Follow the Pyramid guidelines and choose mostly lean and lower-fat foods. Move more, too—that includes strength training to maintain muscle and to keep your bones healthy! *See chapter 2, "Your Healthy Weight."*

Calcium Needs Go Up

Bone loss is part of aging. With a drop in estrogen levels during menopause, women lose bone faster, so calcium needs increase. Boosting your calcium intake and getting more weight-bearing exercise help slow bone loss and reduce the risk for osteoporosis.

The National Institutes of Health advises 1,500 milligrams of calcium a day after menopause for women who don't take estrogen, and 1,000 milligrams of calcium for those who do. After age fifty, 1,200 milligrams of calcium daily is considered an Adequate Intake, according to Dietary Reference Intakes. As a reference, one 8-ounce glass of milk supplies about 300 milligrams of calcium. *For more about calcium and bone health see "Calcium: A Closer Look" in chapter 4 and "Osteoporosis: Reducing the Risks" in chapter 22.*

Heart Disease: A Woman's Issue, Too!

As estrogen levels drop with menopause, women no longer have the same protection that estrogen gives from heart disease and high blood pressure. HDL levels drop, and triglyceride levels increase. That's true whether menopause is natural or surgical. As a result, women's risks for heart disease parallel those of men—but seven to ten years later in life! Their death rate is higher, perhaps due to increased age or more risk factors. In fact, heart disease (not breast cancer) is the number-one killer and disabler of American women; a woman is three times more likely to get cardiovascular disease than breast cancer. About two-thirds of women who die of heart disease had no previous symptoms.

Have You Ever Wondered

... if extra magnesium will ward off hot flashes? There's no evidence that dietary supplements—including extra magnesium—effectively treat the discomforts of menopause. However, adequate magnesium from food does help promote bone health after menopause by helping the body use calcium properly.

The signs of heart disease for women often differ from those of men—and may go unrecognized or ignored. Women often have angina first, rather than a heart attack. A woman's symptoms may be intermittent: unexplained heartburn, profound fatigue, nausea, shortness of breath, and pain that comes and goes. Treadmill stress tests for diagnosis are less reliable for women than for men, too.

Women—if you haven't done so already, make heart-healthy choices. Start with small steps, then work up. This book is full of practical advice:

● Eat a diet that's low in saturated fat and cholesterol and moderate in total fat. Enjoy plenty of grain products, vegetables, and fruits.

● Stay physically active (or get started).

● Keep a healthy weight. Your risk for heart disease is higher if most of your body fat is around your abdomen rather than your hips and thighs.

● Control diabetes if you have it. Keep your healthy weight to lower your risk of type 2 diabetes. Diabetes increases heart disease risk, for women even more than for men.

● Lower your blood pressure if it's too high. Choose and prepare foods with less salt in case your blood pressure is sodium-sensitive.

● Control stress in your daily life, especially if it leads to overeating, smoking, or other risky behaviors.

● If you smoke, quit. If you don't, don't start.

● Consult with your doctor about hormone replacement therapy. Be aware that the research isn't conclusive about its link to heart health. *See "ERT or HRT: For Some Women" on this page.*

ERT or HRT: For Some Women

Many women live almost a third of their lives, about thirty years, with normally low estrogen levels. As their reproductive hormones diminish, every body cell—particularly in the cardiovascular, skeletal, and reproductive systems—is affected. For that reason, estrogen replacement therapy (ERT) or hormone replacement therapy (HRT), which combines estrogen and progestin, are options to consider. (Women who've had a hysterectomy need only estrogen, not the combination.)

Need more tips specific to women's health? Check here for "how-tos":

- Help an adolescent girl address some nutrition issues that start during puberty—see chapter 16.
- Follow a safe, effective strategy for reaching and keeping your healthy weight after pregnancy, menopause, or at any other time of life—see chapter 2.
- Protect yourself from—or deal with—chronic health problems that afflict women: heart disease, diabetes, cancer (including breast cancer), osteoporosis, and anemia—see chapter 22.
- Choose a supplement ("multi," calcium, iron) if you need it—see chapter 23.
- Find a nutrition expert experienced in women's health issues—see chapter 24.

ERT or HRT may ease hot flashes and other menopausal discomforts and may help reduce the risk for osteoporosis. For women with premature menopause, hormone replacement may be especially important. *For more about hormone replacement therapy and bone health see "Protect Your 'Support System'" in chapter 22.*

HRT or ERT isn't right for every woman—for example, those who already have cardiovascular disease or breast cancer, and those with a greater risk for breast cancer. Women with a history of migraine headaches, diabetes, history of stroke, abnormally high blood pressure, history of blood clots in veins, severe obesity, and some other health problems are advised against it, too. *See "Breast Cancer: Do Food Choices Make a Difference?" in this chapter.*

Although hormone replacement has been advised over the past decade as protection from heart disease, new research is reexamining the cardioprotective benefits and risks. The American Heart Association doesn't advise HRT for postmenopausal women with heart disease; protection for women without heart disease is unclear.

If you're approaching or experiencing menopause, talk to your doctor to see if the benefits of hormone replacement outweigh your personal risks. If you choose to use it, see your healthcare professional regularly.

If HRT or ERT isn't right for you, foods with estrogenlike compounds may be the answer. Phytoestrogens in soy called isoflavones (genistein and daidzein) are getting a great deal of attention from researchers. It's thought that these substances, found in many soy products (tofu, tempeh, soy drinks—not soy oil), may help offset the effects of reduced estrogen production by the ovaries, helping to decrease the symptoms of menopause. They also may play a role in reducing the risk for osteoporosis. Even though science doesn't have the whole story on soy yet, enjoying more soy from food probably can't hurt. *For more about soy foods see "What's 'Soy' Good?" in chapter 11.*

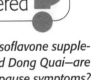

Have You Ever Wondered

. . . if these supplements—soy and isoflavone supplements, black cohosh, wild yam, and Dong Quai—are safe, effective treatments for menopause symptoms? Even though they're "natural," herbal and botanical supplements may not be safe or effective. Here's what the American College of Obstetricians and Gynececologists advises for menopausal symptoms:

- *Soy and isoflavones* in amounts found in food are safe and perhaps helpful in the short run (two years or less). Products with isoflavone extracts haven't been proven safe or effective. Large doses in supplements may interact with estrogen; they may be harmful, especially for women with a history of estrogen-dependent cancer such as breast cancer.
- In the very short term (six months or less), *black cohosh* may relieve hot flashes and night sweats. It's okay to try it—but not for long.
- For *Dong Quai* there's no sound evidence to support its use. On the contrary, it's potentially toxic and may increase the risk of skin cancer related to sun exposure. So skip this one.
- Because the hormones in *wild and Mexican yam* aren't bioavailable, they have no effect. No published reports show that wild yam cream is effective. Again, probably not worth the money.

CHAPTER 18

For Mature Adults
Healthful Eating!

Are you catching the age wave—or how about an older relative or a friend? Are you in the "sandwich generation"—in between caring for kids and older parents?

Due to better healthcare, longer life expectancy, and the aging of the baby boom generation, the number of mature American adults is on the rise. By 2010 ninety million Americans may be a "fifty plus" mature adult, according to projections, with only seventy-four million age eighteen or under. And by 2030, people aged sixty-five or older are expected to make up 20 percent (compared to 12 percent in the mid-1990s) of the U.S. population, with the eighty-five-plus group projected to grow the fastest!

What is a "mature adult"? Actually, there's no one concise category to describe the diversity of "mature adults" whose ages span a half century—from their fifties into their hundreds. Many live a full, active lifestyle that differs little from life in their thirties or forties. Others are limited by health and lifestyle challenges that began at a younger age. Except for a few shifts in nutrient needs, overall health and attitude define aging more than calendar age does.

So, with what you know now, do you wish you were sixteen again? If so, would you make smarter food choices? Fit more activity into your life? Deal with stress better? Try to sleep more?

You can't change the past—or stop the clock. "Anti-aging" is impossible, but the choices made now or at any age and health condition can slow the changes and the challenges that come with getting older, and perhaps even extend youth. The results? Feeling good longer, and enjoying life now and in years to come. Sound good? Start now—to eat smarter and move more!

Aged to Perfection!

It's no secret: how you eat—and how active you are—have plenty to do with your biological age. *For healthy, mature adults, the Dietary Guidelines, described in chapter 1, and the Food Guide Pyramid, described in chapter 10, still serve as sound, credible advice for healthful eating.* And thirty minutes of moderate physical activity each day continues to be a smart lifestyle choice.

Smart food choices and active living today may help you feel younger, stay healthier, more productive and self-sufficient, enjoy a higher quality of life—and even prevent, or at least delay, health problems that often come with aging. *See "How 'Old' Are You? Biomarkers of Age" on page 453.*

Of course, life and health change gradually as the years go by. Yet for each of us, getting older differs. And diversity describes every decade of the mature years: "fifty plus," "seventy plus," even "ninety plus"!

Eating for Healthy Aging

Whether you're over fifty or seventy, you (or an older relative or friend) need the same nutrients—proteins,

How "Old" Are You? Biomarkers of Age

Eager to slow the physical changes of aging? Want to feel as young as you are? Rather than wait until you notice signs of aging, a fitness routine—healthful eating and regular physical activity—can help slow or reverse "biomarkers," or changes, that come with getting older.

- *Your muscle mass and strength.* Stamina, ease of movement, ability to handle heavy objects, feeling energetic, and even physical appearance depend on muscle strength and flexibility. Yet, with age, muscle size and strength decrease naturally; for each decade of adult life, people lose about six to seven pounds of muscle. That rate hastens after age forty-five. Regular physical activity helps you maintain muscle size, strength, and other qualities of youth.

- *The rate your body uses energy.* The rate your body uses energy declines with age: about 2 percent for every decade. Body composition, along with hormone changes, is part of the reason. You can't fool Mother Nature entirely. But if you're physically active and keep your muscle mass, your body burns energy a little faster; muscle burns more energy than body fat.

- *Your percentage of body fat.* With age, body fat gradually replaces muscle—even if your eating and activity patterns stay the same. Besides losing that firm, muscular shape of youth, any extra body fat increases your risk for high blood pressure, heart disease, stroke, some cancers, diabetes, arthritis, and breathing problems. "Midriff bulge" is a sure sign that you're probably not twenty-five anymore! The bottom line: try to keep lean.

- *Your bone density.* Healthy bones let you enjoy physical activity as you age with less risk of fractures. Yet bone loss is a natural part of aging. If you keep your bones strong, you may avoid a "dowager's hump," which often appears with osteoporosis. *See "Osteoporosis: Reduce the Risks" in chapter 22 for ways to slow bone loss.*

- *Your cholesterol/HDL levels.* Age is one reason why total and LDL cholesterol rise. As a heart-healthy strategy, losing weight, regular physical activity, and smart eating can help bring down your total and your LDL blood cholesterol levels and raise your "good" HDL blood cholesterol levels. *See "Heart Disease: The Blood Lipid Connection" in chapter 22.*

- *Your blood sugar tolerance.* With age, blood sugar levels may rise for several reasons. In part, your body may not produce as much insulin with age. Physical activity, along with keeping a healthy weight, can help keep blood sugar levels within normal and help you avoid type 2 diabetes.

- *Your body's "thermostat."* Fluids are your body's natural cooling system. As you get older, your sense of thirst may diminish, putting you at greater risk for dehydration. Still, your body needs at least 6 to 8 cups of fluid daily from water, juice, milk, other beverages, and food. Physical activity helps your body regulate its internal temperature.

- *Your aerobic capacity.* With age, your body's ability to use the oxygen you breathe efficiently declines. With continued vigorous physical activity, your body pumps more oxygen to your muscles.

---

carbohydrates, fats, vitamins, minerals, and water—as always, but perhaps in slightly different amounts. When health or lifestyle problems limit food choices, or when meals and medications need careful coordination, consuming enough may be a challenge!

After age fifty, a few nutrients may need special attention: proteins, calcium, vitamin D, vitamin C, iron, vitamin A, folate, vitamin B_6, vitamin B_{12}, zinc, and water. Among the reasons? Physical changes with aging affect how your body digests food,

absorbs its nutrients, and excretes wastes. Eating enough fiber-rich foods aids digestion and helps prevent the discomfort of constipation—two problems that may come with aging.

What's the nutrient advice? Dietary Reference Intakes (DRIs) provide nutrient guidance for two groups of mature, healthy adults: those age fifty-one or over, and those age seventy-one or over. *For specific amounts see the chart in the Appendices. Nutrient advice may differ for people with health problems; see chapter 22.*

Energy: Spending Calories Wisely

As people get older, most use less energy, or calories, than they did in their younger years. In fact, calorie needs may decrease by as much as 25 percent for two reasons. First, basic body processes use energy at a slower rate. Most adults lose about 2 to 3 percent of their lean body mass, or muscle, each decade of their adult life; the body uses less energy to maintain body fat than to maintain muscle. Second, many mature adults need fewer calories for their less physically active lifestyles. Yet nutrient needs don't change much; in some cases they're somewhat higher.

How many calories? Although calorie needs vary depending on activity level and age, many mature adults need about 1,600 calories daily, perhaps 25 percent less than during younger adult years. Don't seem like much? Chosen carefully; those 1,600 calories can be nutrient-packed.

Here's the challenge for mature adults: Get about the same amount of nutrients, but with fewer calories! Here's how: choose mostly lean and low-fat foods from the five food groups on the three lower levels of the Food Guide Pyramid; eat the minimum number of food group recommended servings; and go easy on foods from the Pyramid tip. With that approach you'll likely consume enough protein, vitamins, and minerals for health. Here's how:

Grains Group	6 servings
Vegetable Group	3 servings
Fruit Group	2 servings
Milk Group	2 servings
Meat and Beans Group	2 servings (or a total of 5 oz.)

To learn about serving sizes (and how to avoid oversizing your portions) and foods in each food group see "The Food Guide Pyramid: Your Healthful Eating Guide" in chapter 10. Chapter 13, "Kitchen Nutrition," offers easy, practical ways to add nutrients to food without having to eat more food.

As in younger years, mature, healthy adults are urged to keep their overall food choices low in saturated fat and cholesterol, and to moderate their fat intake (no more than 30 percent of total calories from fat). Remember that a gram of fat supplies more than twice the calories that a gram of either carbohydrate or

---

Eat Your Fruits and Vegetables!

The advice you've likely given kids applies to you, too: Eat your fruits and vegetables! Fruits and vegetables are your best sources of beta-carotene (which forms vitamin A), vitamin C, and folate, as well as an array of antioxidants and other phytonutrients. *See "Antioxidant Vitamins: A Closer Look" in chapter 4 for more about the potential health-promoting benefits of antioxidants.* They also can supply fiber, important for health-promoting benefits and overcoming constipation.

Have chewing problems? That's no reason to give up fruits or vegetables. Just make "softer" choices: perhaps ripe bananas, baked or steamed winter squash, cooked peas, sliced peaches, baked sweet or baking potatoes, cooked spinach, stewed tomatoes, or steamed cauliflower.

Concerned that fresh produce might take a bite out of your pocketbook? Look for seasonal fruits and vegetables, when they typically cost less. And stock up on canned and frozen fruits and vegetables, and dried fruits, when they're specially priced. Canned and frozen fruits and vegetables offer convenience, especially for housebound adults. If you or someone you're caring for needs a special diet, talk to a registered dietitian about buying these foods. Use the Nutrition Facts on food labels, too. Some canned vegetables and frozen vegetables with sauces contain added salt. Plain, frozen vegetables and no-salt-added canned vegetables may be better choices for a low-sodium diet.

---

protein does, so watching your fat intake is one approach to calorie control, too. Limiting fat, saturated fat, and cholesterol may also be part of managing risk factors for heart disease and other chronic health problems.

Get most of your food energy from carbohydrates. Foods with complex carbohydrates such as bread, cereal, pasta, rice, vegetables, and beans, supply many nutrients and fiber, too. Fruit, with naturally occurring sugars, also supplies vitamins A and C, and fiber. *If you're managing "carbs" for diabetes, see "Diabetes: A Growing Health Concern" in chapter 22.*

Protein: An Issue for Some

Protein: you're certainly not growing, but you still need it! If you eat two servings, or a total of 5 ounces, from the Meat and Beans Group of the Food Guide Pyramid, you're likely consuming enough protein. So what's the issue?

Some older adults don't consume enough protein-rich foods. Sometimes meat or poultry are hard to chew and swallow, so they may be left on the plate. Other people may have trouble digesting milk, another good protein source. Those with limited finances might avoid meat, poultry, or fish because they often cost more than many other foods.

How can you be sure to get enough high-quality protein?

● If you're on a budget, keep meat, poultry, and fish portions small. Or combine meat, poultry, and fish with other ingredients in casserole dishes so a small amount goes farther. Consider less expensive protein sources, too, such as eggs, legumes, and peanut butter. Remember, you need only an equivalent of about 5 ounces a day.

● Chop your meat or poultry well if you need to.

● If you have trouble chewing, have your teeth and gums (and perhaps dentures) checked. *See "Chewing Problems?" in this chapter.*

● Include dairy products. Milk, cheese, and yogurt—and foods made with these ingredients—supply protein, too. If milk disagrees with you, enjoy cheese or yogurt. *See chapter 21 for ways to enjoy milk if you're lactose-sensitive.*

● Consult a registered dietitian for other ways to ensure enough high-quality protein in your day's food choices.

Have You Ever Wondered

. . . why milk doesn't seem to agree with you anymore? Some older adults have trouble digesting milk, even though they had no problem in younger years. The reason? The small intestine may no longer produce as much lactase. Lactase, an enzyme, digests the natural sugar, called lactose, in milk.

To continue to enjoy milk and reap its calcium and vitamin D benefits, try this. Drink milk in small amounts; usually your body can handle a little at a time. Try buttermilk, yogurt, cheese, or a special lactose-reduced milk. Custard, pudding, and cream soup may be tolerated better, too. Try other foods that supply calcium, including some dark-green leafy vegetables and canned fish (sardines and salmon) with bones. *For more tips see "Lactose Intolerance: A Matter of Degree" in chapter 21.*

. . . if you should avoid animal-based foods (meat, eggs, milk, cheese) with fat and cholesterol to protect yourself from heart disease? There's no reason for "fat phobia." Thinking that you need to avoid meat, dairy foods, and eggs to protect against heart disease is unfounded—especially if that means missing out on these nutrient-dense foods. They supply other nutrients that often end up short in the diets of older adults: calcium, iron, zinc, and vitamins B_6 and B_{12}.

If you don't have heart disease, and if your blood cholesterol levels are within a healthful range, be sensible—and enjoy these foods in moderation, using guidelines from the Food Guide Pyramid.

. . . if extra vitamin E will keep you young? We all dream of the fountain of youth. Many claims made for vitamin E are really distortions of research done with animals that shouldn't be applied to humans. Taking vitamin E supplements won't stop or reverse the aging process. And in the bigger picture, they won't cure sterility, premenstrual syndrome for younger women, or ulcers, to name a few.

Research is being done to explore the potential benefits of taking extra amounts of vitamin E, however. As an antioxidant it may play a protective role against some health problems including atherosclerosis, cataract formation, and Alzheimer's and Parkinson's diseases. It's too soon to advise levels higher than the Recommended Dietary Allowance of 15 milligrams of alpha-tocopherol a day; *see chapter 4 for more about vitamin E.*

Until more is known, make food choices that supply enough vitamin E. If you take a supplement, choose one with no more than 100 percent of the Daily Value for vitamin E. And talk to a registered dietitian to help you sort through the current facts about vitamin E.

For more about protein see "Protein Power" in chapter 20.

Calcium: As Important As Ever

Why is calcium still so important? Calcium plays a primary role in keeping your bones healthy and so helps reduce the risks of osteoporosis, or brittle-bone disease. That's true for both men and women!

For mature adults, calcium needs are higher. To help maintain bone mass, calcium recommendations increase by 20 percent. For both men and women over age fifty, the Adequate Intake level from the Dietary Reference Intakes is 1,200 milligrams of calcium daily. That's almost as much as growing children and teens need daily.

The risk for osteoporosis goes up with age. By age seventy, between 30 and 40 percent of all women have had at least one fracture linked to osteoporosis. The percent continues to climb, even for men who develop bone disease later in life. *See "Osteoporosis: Reduce the Risks" in chapter 22.*

Age is only one reason why older adults have a higher risk for bone disease. Many don't consume enough calcium-rich foods, especially if dairy foods aren't a regular part of their meals or snacks. With age, the body doesn't absorb calcium from food as well, either. In addition, many older adults don't get enough weight-bearing exercise, which helps to keep bones stronger. Vitamin D, which helps the body use calcium, may be limited in food choices, too.

There's good news if you're an older adult: Even if you haven't been consuming enough calcium all along, it's not too late to consume more now. You still can reduce your risk of bone fractures as you get older. At the same time, consume enough vitamin D and do some weight-bearing exercise, such as walking. Aim for a total of thirty minutes of activity each day, taken all at once or split into shorter segments throughout the day.

Which foods supply calcium? Milk, yogurt, and cheese are the best sources. For example, an 8-ounce glass of milk supplies about 300 milligrams of calcium, so two or three servings put you well on your way. Milk is a good source of vitamin D and potassium, too, which might come up short for many mature adults. In addition, some dark-green leafy vegetables, fish with edible bones (such as canned salmon), calcium-fortified soy beverages, tofu made with calcium sulfate, and other fortified foods also have significant amounts of calcium.

Hint: Calcium in food is more bioavailable than in a supplement. But if you do take a calcium supplement, choose one with vitamin D, and take it between meals. Calcium can hinder the absorption of iron from your meals. *See "Calcium Supplements: A Bone Builder?" in chapter 23.*

Vitamin D: The Sunshine Vitamin

To keep bones strong as you age, your body needs calcium—along with its partner vitamin D. Vitamin D helps deposit calcium in your bones and helps protect you from bone disease by keeping them stronger.

Vitamin D is unique. It's known as the "sunshine vitamin" because your body makes it after sunlight, or ultraviolet light, hits your skin. For adequate vitamin D production you need about twenty to thirty minutes of sun (without sunscreen) on your hands and face two to three times per week. If you stay indoors, your body may lack vitamin D, especially if you don't drink milk fortified with vitamin D.

With age, the body doesn't make vitamin D from sunlight as easily. Adding to the risk, many older adults are housebound or they're covered up outside, especially in northern climates, so their exposure to sunshine is limited.

Like calcium, the need for vitamin D goes up after age fifty. In fact, it doubles to 400 International Units (IUs), or 10 micrograms, daily. And after age seventy, the recommended daily intake level goes up again, to 600 IUs for both men and women.

Vitamin D is added to most milk, and it may be added to other foods such as cereals. You'll find vitamin D listed on the Nutrition Facts on food packages if it's been added. If you drink milk regularly, though, you probably consume enough—even if you can't get outdoors. Otherwise you may need a vitamin D supplement, but consult your doctor or registered dietitian first. Taking high doses from a dietary supplement can be harmful. Kidney damage, weak bones or muscles, and excessive bleeding are all associated with taking too much over time.

The Iron–Vitamin C Connection

Most people who follow guidelines of the Food Guide Pyramid consume enough iron and vitamin C. Yet, for older adults, a poor diet may lead to a deficiency in one or both of these nutrients. Iron deficiency causes anemia, which can make you feel weak, tired, and irritable, or lose concentration. *See "Anemia: 'Tired Blood'" in chapter 22.* Iron deficiency may have other causes: reduced iron absorption as the body secretes less digestive juices or when antacids interfere; blood loss from ulcers, hemorrhoids, or other health problems; and medications (perhaps taking too many aspirins) that cause blood loss.

Although iron and vitamin C come from very different foods, their role in health is quite connected. Vitamin C helps your body absorb iron from eggs and from plant sources of food. Vitamin C is especially important if you rely heavily on beans, whole grains, and iron-enriched cereals as iron sources.

A few tips to avoid iron deficiency:

● Choose economical sources of iron, including iron-enriched cereals; beans; whole grains; lean, ground meat; eggs; and liver.

● Enjoy a vitamin C-rich fruit or fruit juice such as citrus fruit, melon, or berries, with your meal to boost your absorption of iron. It's easy to get enough vitamin C if fruits are a regular part of your meals and snacks.

● Add a little meat, poultry, or fish to grain-based meals. Their iron content will help your body absorb the iron in the grains.

Vitamin C may offer some other health-promoting benefits. As an antioxidant it may help lower the risk for cataracts and some cancers, for example. For any nutrient, including vitamin C, try to get enough from food first, not a supplement. Besides, vitamin C-rich foods have other nutrients, such as potassium, and phytonutrients that promote health. Insufficient intake of vitamin C is linked to memory loss, and the excessively high amounts obtained from supplements can cause diarrhea, kidney damage, and bladder problems.

For iron, the recommendation for adults ages fifty-one on is 8 milligrams a day; that's less than half of what women need before menopause. Consult with your doctor before taking an iron supplement. A sup-plement with too much iron for you can be harmful. For some people with a genetic illness called hemochromatosis, iron is absorbed more readily and can build up in various body organs, causing irreparable damage.

Other Nutrients

Besides those just mentioned, a few others may come up short in the eating patterns of mature Americans. Not getting enough of any single nutrient on one day or even for several days isn't a cause for concern. But for those who don't consume a balanced diet with enough nutrients over a longer period—several weeks or months—a nutrient supplement may be prescribed, especially for elderly people.

Miracles? Dream On!

All too often, charlatans prey on mature adults with promises of easy cures or ways to stay young. Many products they peddle are foods, substances from food, or dietary supplements. And typically there's no evidence that their claims or products offer any benefit for treating arthritis, heart disease, cancer, Alzheimer's disease, or other maladies—or for helping people live longer.

Many "miracle" products are costly. Money used to buy them is better spent on healthful, flavorful foods.

Their harm may go farther than the pocketbook. These remedies may mask symptoms, offer false hope, or worse yet, keep people from seeking reliable healthcare that can make a difference to health. And these products may interfere with the action of prescribed medications—or perhaps with the absorption of nutrients in food.

Always be cautious of promises that seem too good to be true. *To learn how to judge what you read and hear about nutrition and health, see chapter 24.* And always consult your doctor or a registered dietitian before trying these products—or any type of alternative healthcare. *Chapter 23 explores what's known and unknown about many supplements, some promoted as "antiaging."* Be aware that many people claim to be nutrition experts, but some aren't qualified. *To find a registered dietitian, other qualified expert, or resources in your community, see chapter 24.*

Vitamin A. Vitamin A (and beta carotene, which turns into vitamin A) helps eyes adjust to dim light and protects skin and other body tissues. Consuming enough vitamin A won't cure poor eyesight, but too little could make it worse. The best sources: food—deep-green leafy and deep-yellow vegetables and fruits. Since the liver can't handle excess vitamin A as well with age, too much vitamin A from supplements can be especially harmful for older adults.

A Day of Good Nutrition

Here's an easy-to-make, easy-to-digest, low-cost menu for a whole day of good nutrition. If you count up the servings, you'll see it supplies enough from all five food groups of the Food Guide Pyramid. It's a menu that adds up to about 1,600 to 1,700 calories.

Breakfast:

   2 grapefruit or ¾ cup orange juice (perhaps calcium-fortified)
   ¾ cup bran flakes with ½ cup low-fat or fat-free milk
   1 slice toast with 1 teaspoon margarine or jam
   Coffee, tea, or water

Snack:

   2 graham crackers
   1 cup low-fat fruit yogurt

Lunch:

   1 cup lentil or split-pea soup
   ½ cup coleslaw
   1 corn muffin
   ½ cup canned, juice-packed fruit
   Coffee, tea, or water

Dinner:

   3 ounces skinless chicken breast, baked with Italian seasoning
   1 baked sweet potato with 1 teaspoon margarine
   ½ cup creamed spinach
   1 dinner roll
   ½ cup low-fat ice cream
   Coffee, tea, or water

Snack:

   ½ whole-wheat English muffin with 1 tablespoon apple butter
   1 cup low-fat or fat-free milk

Folate. Folate, a B vitamin, helps your body make red blood cells. Not consuming enough over a period of time may lead to anemia and age-related hearing loss. Along with other B vitamins, folate may play a role in heart health, too, by removing homocysteine from the bloodstream; high homocysteine levels are a potential risk factor for heart disease. Good sources include leafy green vegetables, some fruits, legumes, liver, fortified cereals and other grain products, and wheat germ.

Vitamin B_{12}. Vitamin B_{12}, or cobalamin, works with folate to make red blood cells. Not getting enough also can lead to anemia and high levels of homocysteine. Among older adults, low levels of vitamins B_{12} and B_6 are linked to memory loss, and low levels of B_{12}, to age-related hearing loss. With coexisting conditions, other symptoms of vitamin B_{12} deficiency may go unrecognized. Meat, poultry, fish, eggs, and dairy foods are all good sources. To avoid deficiency, mature adults are urged to eat vitamin B_{12}-fortified foods and to take a supplement with vitamin B_{12}. Some health problems impair the body's ability to absorb vitamin B_{12}.

Vitamin B_6. Vitamin B_6 often comes up short for older adults, too. The recommendation for vitamin B_6 goes up slightly after age fifty, from 1.3 milligrams per day for men and women to 1.5 milligrams daily for women and 1.7 milligrams daily for men. Among the good sources: chicken, fish, and pork, and to a lesser degree, whole grains, nuts, and legumes.

Zinc. Zinc from foods such as beef, whole grains, and milk helps your body fight infections and repair body tissue. Yet absorption decreases with age. Even a marginal deficiency may affect the ability to taste, heal wounds, and provide immunity.

   To learn more about these vitamins and minerals and more, see chapter 4, "Vitamins, Minerals, and Phytonutrients: Variety on Your Plate!"

Thirst Quenchers: Drink Fluids

Thirsty? The average healthy adult uses up about 2½ quarts of fluid daily by urinating, perspiring, breathing, and eliminating other body wastes. To keep from getting dehydrated, your body needs to have fluids replaced. Thirst is the body's signal to drink more.

With age come changes that affect fluid intake. The sense of thirst often diminishes, so mature adults may not be able to count on thirst as their primary reminder to drink fluids. Kidneys may not conserve fluids as they once did either, so the body holds on to less water. Those who have trouble getting around may deliberately limit fluid intake to avoid bathroom trips; fear of incontinence also keeps some people from drinking enough.

Dehydration is a health concern during the mature years, especially in warmer weather and for those who don't drink enough fluid. And adequate fluid intake is linked to other health issues:

- Everyone needs enough water to help rid the body of wastes. With less fluid, the chances of constipation rise.

- While fluid helps keep kidneys healthy, dehydration can cause kidney problems.

- Many older adults have less saliva to help with chewing and swallowing. Drinking water or other liquids at meals makes eating easier.

- Some medications need to be taken with water. And some medications, such as diuretics, cause the body to lose water.

- In older adults, dehydration may cause symptoms that seem like dementia, or impaired mental function, or might worsen existing dementia.

- In extreme cases dehydration can lead to death.

Mature adults need plenty of fluids. Food provides some water, but drinking a minimum of 6 to 8 cups daily is advised. Any beverage—juice, milk, soup, tea, coffee, soft drinks—supplies water. Plain water is great, too! Remember that juice, milk, and soup offer other nutrients as well.

Caffeinated beverages such as regular coffee, tea, and colas are best consumed in moderation. Caffeine has a diuretic effect, increasing the need to urinate and, as a result, promotes some fluid loss.

If you have trouble remembering how much water you drank during the day, try this: Fill a jug or a jar with 8 cups (64 ounces) of water each morning. Place it in your refrigerator. Use that water for drinking and for making juice, lemonade, soup, tea, and coffee.

When the water is gone, you probably met your fluid goal for the day.

For more about water as an essential nutrient and the risks of dehydration see "A Fluid Asset" in chapter 8.

Never Too Late for Exercise

No matter what your age, it's never too late to get moving. Whether you're pushing sixty, seventy, eighty, or perhaps even ninety, you can strengthen your muscles, improve agility and balance, and get other benefits from moving more, even if you haven't been physically active for a long time. Regardless of overall health, most people can participate in some form of enjoyable physical activity.

The Reasons Are Many

What are the benefits of physical activity for mature adults? For the most part, they're the same as for anyone else. Among them:

- Moving your body burns energy. That's an aid to keeping a healthy weight.

- Activities that put weight on your bones, such as walking, help preserve your bone density. The benefit? Helping to reduce your risk for bone disease.

- Regular physical activity of all kinds helps keep your heart and lungs healthier. Aim for a total of thirty minutes of moderate activity each day. Do some aerobic activity if you can; ask your doctor first.

- Being active helps keep your blood pressure, blood cholesterol, and blood sugar normal. That reduces the risks related to several health problems, such as high blood pressure, heart disease, and diabetes.

- Many activities help minimize muscle loss and keep muscles strong. When you stay stronger, you often have better balance and may be able to remain independent. And you're less likely to fall and fracture your bones.

- Being active often helps your digestion and

appetite—a benefit if food seems to be losing its appeal.

● For those with trouble sleeping, a problem that often comes with getting older, physical activity helps promote sleep.

Health Alert: Foodborne Illness

Keep food safe! Mature adults are at greater risk for foodborne illness than their younger counterparts. The reason? The immune system can't always fight back as easily with age, especially for those battling other health problems, such as diabetes or kidney disease, or for those dealing with some cancer treatments. With age, stomach acids, which help reduce intestinal bacteria, decrease. Even mild foodborne illness can have a serious health effect.

Although the kitchen seems clean, poor eyesight or inadequate lighting may keep people from noticing food spills or visual signs of food spoilage. And for those with less energy, proper cleaning may be hard to do.

The following tips are useful to people of any age, and especially to adults as they get older:

● If you need glasses, wear them as you handle and prepare food.

● Turn up the lights. Mature adults may have more trouble with glare from one light source.

● Label perishable food with a date. Use a dark marker that's easy to read. Don't count on memory alone to know your own "use by" date.

● Don't rely on your senses of sight, smell, or taste to determine if food is safe to eat. Contaminated food may not have an off-flavor or off-smell. With impaired vision, cross-contamination of salad vegetables and raw meat juices may not be obvious.

● Cook simply to save your energy for cleanup, too. Frozen and canned foods are quick, nutritious, and easy to cook.

● Feeling short on energy? Feel comfortable about asking a younger family member or a friend to help occasionally with kitchen tasks.

● Portions too big when you eat out? If you bring food home in a "doggie bag," refrigerate it right away, and reheat it to steaming or boiling before you eat it— within a few days.

Follow the general steps for food safety described in chapter 12, "The Safe Kitchen."

● If you're feeling depressed, being active—especially if you enjoy group activities—can be just the antidote!

● Being active has a way of boosting your feeling of overall well-being.

You Can Do It!

For healthy older adults, like their younger counterparts, health experts advise a total of thirty minutes of moderate activity every day, if possible. If you walk, that's about two miles. You don't need to do all your activity at one time, however. Instead try three ten-minute spurts of activities that you enjoy.

The key to fitting physical activity into your everyday routine is to make it fun! Choose activities that improve endurance, strength, and flexibility. Here are some ideas:

● Try walking—around the block or around the mall. Walk a dog or invite a friend if you'd like companionship. If you don't have a sidewalk, mall walking is safe—especially in bad weather.

● Do some gardening without electric tools.

● Go swimming. Or try a variety of aqua exercises, such as stretching, walking, dancing, or doing aerobics in the water. These are great activities, especially if you're not steady on your feet. They may help relieve some of the joint pain that accompanies arthritis.

● If you golf, "go the course"—without the golf cart.

● Go dancing. Even a moderate two-step is good exercise—and a great way to be with other people.

● Take a class in t'ai chi, a series of slow, controlled movements.

● To keep your arms strong, lift "weights." Use canned foods from your kitchen shelves, bean bags, or 1- to 5-pound hand or ankle weights.

● Learn some chair exercises—good for people who aren't steady on their feet or who have degenerative joint disease. You can "sit and be fit" even if you're confined to a wheelchair or need a walker.

● Want to keep up with everyday tasks such as bending for a newspaper, reaching an upper shelf, or making a bed? Fit in some stretching activities that increase the range of motion in your ankles, knees, hips, shoulders, neck, and back.

● Sign up for an exercise class or an individual fitness program especially designed for mature adults. If needed, check with your community center or area hospital for special classes meant for people with special needs.

For more ideas see "Twenty Everyday Ways to Get Moving" in chapter 2.

If you haven't been physically active, talk to your doctor before getting started. Together plan activities and a sensible approach that's safe, effective, and right for you. Most important, start slowly, work toward your goal gradually, and enjoy!

Tip: No matter what activity you're involved in, drink plenty of water before, during, and afterward.

When Lifestyles Change

Lifestyle changes accompany each stage in your life. Think about the independence that came with becoming an adult, the responsibility that comes with parenthood, or the freedom of having kids finally leave the "nest." At some point the mature years also bring new lifestyles and health conditions that impact what, where, when, and even with whom you eat. And losing a spouse, moving away from a lifelong community of friends, even retiring can change social interaction that revolves around food.

Eating Alone—Special, Too!

The kitchen table: for many, eating provides a time to enjoy the company of others. That's especially true for those who've spent their adult life cooking for a family. However, the pleasure of preparing food, even eating, may diminish when eating alone. Eating alone can feel boring or depressing. If you're in that position, or know someone who is, you can help spark a tired appetite.

Making Meals Special: Solo or Not

If you're a "single," you don't need to always dine alone. Eat with friends occasionally:

● Set a standing date with a friend, a relative, or a grandchild for lunch or dinner at your home.

● If you're still "into cooking" but need someone to cook for, organize a dining club of like-minded friends.

● Cut down on the effort. Get together with other mature adults for weekly or monthly potluck suppers. Take turns acting as host.

● Take advantage of meals offered at the local senior citizens' center. Many serve a full midday meal on weekdays. Usually the price is right. In some communities, local churches and schools serve meals for older adults.

Added benefits: Senior citizen meals offer a place to meet old and new friends. And you can enjoy a meal that takes more work to prepare than you'd likely do for yourself. Take advantage of an exercise class when you go!

● When eating out, enjoy early-bird specials, when the portions are usually smaller and the prices are right. Consider splitting an order or take home half for another meal if restaurant portions seem too large. Eat out for breakfast or lunch, when portions are smaller and prices are lower. Some restaurants also have senior citizen prices—just ask. *For more tips on eating out see chapter 14, "Your Food Away from Home."*

When you do dine solo, make eating a special event. Looking forward to mealtime can offer a boost to both your appetite and your morale!

● Set your place at the table, perhaps with a place mat, napkin, candles, and centerpiece. You'll feel more like you've had a meal—and with more enjoyment—than if you had eaten right from the cooking pot!

● For a change of pace, enjoy eating in different places: the kitchen, patio or deck, dining room, or perhaps on a tray by the fireplace.

● Create some atmosphere or interest. Turn on the radio. Play a favorite music tape or CD. Or watch your favorite television show as you eat.

● Make food preparation easy, especially when you cook for one.

See "Have You Ever Wondered . . . how to feel comfortable when you dine alone?" in chapter 14.

Meals–Fast, Simple, Nutritious

Some mature adults say they have no time to cook. They're too busy living life to its fullest. For others, lack of inclination or energy or perhaps less mobility require quick and easy solutions for nutritious eating.

Whatever the reason, try these tasty "meals in minutes" for starters:

● For a quick breakfast, add hot milk to instant hot cereal. It's just as fast to prepare as ready-to-eat cereals.

● Keep frozen dinners and entrées on hand for quick cooking and easy cleanup. For the most nutrition, buy frozen meals with meat, poultry, or fish; a starchy food (such as rice, pasta, or potato); and a vegetable. Team

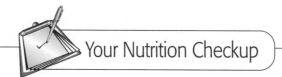 Your Nutrition Checkup

Mature Adults: Nutritionally Healthy?

I f you're a mature adult, use this checklist for insight into your nutritional health. If you care for an older adult, perhaps a parent, use it to be a better caregiver.

Read each statement. If a statement applies to you or someone you know, circle the number in the "yes" column. Then tally up the nutritional score of "yes" answers.

	YES
I have an illness or a condition that made me change the kind and/or amount of food I eat.	2 points
I eat fewer than two meals per day.	3 points
I eat few fruits or vegetables, or milk products.	2 points
I have three or more drinks of beer, liquor, or wine almost every day.	2 points
I have tooth or mouth problems that make it hard for me to eat.	2 points
I don't always have enough money to buy the food I need.	4 points
I eat alone most of the time.	1 point
I take three or more different prescribed or over-the-counter drugs a day.	1 point
Without wanting to, I have lost or gained 10 pounds in the past six months.	2 points
I am not always physically able to shop, cook, and/or feed myself.	2 points
Total _____ points	

What's your nutritional score? If it's . . .

0–2 . . . Good! But check again in six months.

3–5 . . . You're at moderate nutritional risk. Try to make some changes—suggested here—that improve your eating habits and lifestyle. Get advice from a registered dietitian or another qualified nutrition professional . . . or if you're older, from a local senior citizens' center, state or area Agency on Aging, health department, or senior nutrition program. And check again in three months.

6 or more . . . You're at high nutritional risk. The next time you see your doctor, registered dietitian, or other qualified health or social service professional, share your answers to this checklist. Talk about any problems, and ask for assistance. Read on for practical ways to follow their advice.

Source: Reprinted with permission by the Nutrition Screening Initiative, a project of the American Academy of Family Physicians, the American Dietetic Association, and the National Council on Aging, Inc., and funded in part by a grant from Ross Products Division, Abbott Laboratories Inc. Go to *http://www.aafp.org/nsi/* for a copy of this checklist.

them with a salad, a roll, a piece of fruit, and milk for a hearty meal that takes little effort.

● Trying to lose weight? You might choose from one of the many lower-calorie frozen dinners available.

● Watching your salt intake to help control high blood pressure? Check the sodium on frozen meals and canned ones (stews, soups, and chilies). Many have more sodium; look for those with less. Use MSG instead of salt; it offers flavor with one-third less sodium.

● Prepare food ahead for later in the week, or to freeze as leftovers. For instance, make lower-fat meat-balls with lean, ground turkey or beef. Brown the meatballs, drain any grease, then combine with tomato sauce. Serve over pasta on one day, over rice the next, and freeze the rest for later.

DETERMINE the Warning Signs of Poor Nutrition

If you're a mature adult, or if you care for someone older, be alert for these warning signs of poor nutrition. They spell the word "determine." Anyone with three or more of these risk factors should consult a doctor, a registered dietitian (RD), or other healthcare professional:

Disease

Eating poorly

Tooth loss or mouth pain

Economic hardship

Reduced social contact

Many medicines

Involuntary weight loss or gain

Needs assistance in self-care

Elder years above age eighty

Source: Reprinted with permission by the Nutrition Screening Initiative, a project of the American Academy of Family Physicians, the American Dietetic Association, and the National Council on Aging, Inc., and funded in part by a grant from Ross Products Division, Abbott Laboratories Inc.

These warning signs suggest risk but don't diagnose any health condition.

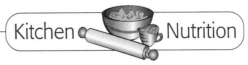

Meals in Minutes

Check the clock. You can prepare this nutritious, flavorful supper without much effort!

● Place a sliced red or white potato into a small baking dish sprayed with vegetable oil spray. Toss with 2 teaspoons of olive oil and $\frac{1}{2}$ teaspoon of crushed rosemary or basil, or your favorite herbs. Bake at 400° F for about forty minutes, until they're tender.

● In another small baking dish, place a chicken breast or two smaller pieces of chicken. Sprinkle the chicken with lemon juice or Italian salad dressing before popping it into the oven to bake.

● Set the table. Relax with a book or television for about thirty-five minutes.

● Spoon canned apricot halves into a dish.

● Take out a dinner roll.

● Pour a tall glass of refreshing milk.

● Enjoy your dinner!

● Freeze homemade soups, stews, lasagna, and other casserole dishes in single-serving containers. Then thaw enough for one or two meals at a time. Label and date your packages to keep track of what you have in the freezer.

● For easy-to-prepare salads, wash, tear, and dry salad greens. Then store them in a plastic container for three or four days. Or purchase washed, cut salad greens in a bag. So when you want a salad, put a handful of greens in a bowl and add your favorite toppings, perhaps sliced tomatoes, grated carrots, sliced deli meat or cheese, or canned kidney beans. Serve with milk, bread, and canned fruit.

● Visit the supermarket salad bar for single servings of washed and chopped fruits and vegetables.

"Maxing Out" Your Food Dollar

Another adjustment may affect food decisions: learning to live and eat on a fixed income. If medical and prescription costs go up at the same time, there may not be much money to spare. For many older adults, economic challenges can get in the way of healthful eating.

By shopping wisely, you can maximize your food dollar and get the most nutrition for your money.

Depending on income, many older adults qualify for food stamps, a program of the U.S. Department of Health and Human Services. Food stamps are used like cash in food stores, giving people access to a healthful diet. Usually food stamps aren't meant for dining out, although for older adults, some restaurants are authorized to accept them in exchange for low-cost meals; check before you order.

To find out if you—or someone you know—qualifies for food stamps, talk to a registered dietitian, social worker, or your local senior center. Or check the government pages in your phone book for your local food stamp office. *Also see "Nutrition $ense" in chapter 11 for more ways to maximize your food dollar on a fixed income.*

Hassle-Free Shopping

As people get a little older, popping in and out of the supermarket may take a little more effort. But there's no reason to let your kitchen shelves get bare. Learn to shop without the hassles:

● Start your shopping trip before you get to the store. Plan ahead. Make a grocery list. In that way you won't need to repeat your steps through the store.

● Shop at quiet times, such as weekday mornings, when stores aren't crowded. Daytime shopping, when it's easier to see curbs and potholes, is safer anyway. If you must shop at night, pick a store with a well-lit parking lot, or ask someone to go with you.

● Ask for help with carrying your groceries. Besides the assistance, it's extra security for you in the parking lot.

● Feeling less stable on your feet? Use the shopping cart for balance—even if you have just a few items to buy.

● If you're less mobile, shop in stores with a battery-powered, sit-down grocery cart. It's a courtesy service that your supermarket may offer.

● If you have trouble with night vision, shop during daylight hours.

● Don't drive or use public transportation? Check with your local area Agency on Aging for shopping assistance. Your community may offer shopping transportation for senior citizens.

● Keep an emergency supply of nonperishable foods on the shelf: nonfat dry milk or boxed milk, dried fruit, canned foods (fruit, vegetables, juice, tuna, soup, stew, beans), peanut butter, and cereal. In that way you won't need to head to the store when it's raining or snowing.

● If you have ideas that could make shopping more convenient for older shoppers, talk with the store manager. With the growing numbers of senior citizens as customers, they'll likely listen to your thoughts.

● If you qualify, get a sticker for your car that lets you park in spots for the handicapped.

● Ask about special services from your supermarket: home delivery or telephone ordering. If you're computer-savvy, you might be able to order food online.

When Cooking Is Too Much

Can't cook anymore? That doesn't necessarily mean giving up living on your own. Many communities offer services for older adults to assure access to nutritious meals. Look for these services where you live:

● Meals on Wheels brings food to people who are housebound.

● Home healthcare aides help by shopping and preparing meals for older disabled people.

● Community centers offer hot meals. Some are part of adult day-care programs. Minivans may be available to transfer people to the center. *See "Food in Adult Day and Nursing Care: Questions to Ask!" on page 465.*

● Many churches, synagogues, and other community groups provide volunteers who help older adults with shopping and food preparation.

For assistance, talk to a registered dietitian or a social worker. Or call your local area Agency on Aging. *Or see "How to Find Nutrition Help . . ." in chapter 24.*

Food in Adult Day and Residential Care: Questions to Ask!

Meals offer more than nourishment to daily life. That's especially true for many older adults, who look forward to meals as a time to be with others and as "mileposts" in their day.

As you look for adult day or residential care for yourself, or for any older friend or family member,

find out about the food service. Look for "yes" answers to these questions:

Facilities:

- Is the dining area clean and attractive?
- Are menus printed with lettering that's big enough for older people to read?
- Is the dining area well lit throughout, not just with "mood" lighting or single lights that cause glare?
- Does the dining area encourage socializing?

Food:

- Are people given choices from a variety of foods?
- Are plenty of beverages available throughout the day?
- Is the menu changed often, so the menu cycle doesn't get monotonous?
- Are fresh fruits and vegetables served often?
- Is food served attractively?
- Are religious and cultural food restrictions honored and respected? How about special food preferences?
- Are holidays and special events celebrated with special menus?
- Are special meals, such as low-sodium or soft meals, provided to those who need them?
- Are people offered a chance to make food requests that aren't on the menu?

Staff:

- Is mealtime viewed as important to daily life at the facility?
- Is a full- or part-time registered dietitian on staff?
- Are people encouraged to eat in a common dining room? Are they assisted to get there if needed?
- Do staff or volunteers help those with any eating difficulties, perhaps cutting food or helping them eat?
- Do staff or volunteers wear sanitary gloves when they're helping people eat so they don't spread infection?
- Are people given enough time to eat, and not rushed?

Sandwiched In?

Are you among the many adults who fit in the "sandwich generation": with children or teens yet to raise and an elderly parent to care for? If so, learn to cope without becoming overly stressed:

- Start by taking care of you: eat smart, fit regular physical activity in, and try to stay rested. Overcome stress or lack of time so they don't become barriers! You'll be more effective in all your family roles as parent, son or daughter, or perhaps spouse—and perhaps in the workforce or your volunteer work.

- Plan openly with your whole family, including kids and an elder parent(s), so that goals, responsibilities, and expectations are clear. That includes activities that surround eating: shopping, food preparation and cleanup, eating schedules, and family meals.

- Share responsibilities as a family rather than attempt to do everything yourself. Try to avoid neglecting one family member to care for another.

- Gather a support network that may include adult day care, home-delivered meals if you work all day, and other senior citizen services for your parent. Ask for help, and accept when it's offered.

- Accept the fact that you'll be tired and perhaps angry sometimes. That's okay, so discard any feelings of guilt. Instead, get help so you can have a break, even if it's just for a few hours. Maybe it's a good time to do something physically active. If negative feelings trigger eating, find another emotional outlet.

- Respect everyone's privacy, dignity, and independence.

● For those who can't leave their rooms, is food brought to them on attractive trays?

● If they need help, is it given promptly so food doesn't get cold? Are trays also removed promptly?

● For a nursing home, does the staff keep track of each person's weight, and how much they eat and drink?

● Are special food and nutrition needs given individual attention?

Changes That Challenge

What's changed? That depends. If you've inherited a great set of genes, and taken care of yourself throughout life, you have a better chance of living a long, vital life. You may feel "fit as a fiddle" without many apparent physical signs of aging. Wrinkles and gray hairs hardly seem to count. In fact, they make you look wise and distinguished.

In the long run, some physical changes are inevitable. The reasons that the human body ages—and the rate of change—are still scientific speculation. But genetics, nutrition, lifestyle, disease, and environment are among the reasons. Many physical and lifestyle changes affect food choices and nutrition.

Medications used to manage many health problems also may have side effects related to food or nutrition. *To learn about interactions among food, nutrients, and medications, see "Food and Medicine" in chapter 22.*

Aging with "Taste"

"That recipe just doesn't have the flavor that I always remembered!" You might hear that comment from an older adult. Maybe you've said it yourself! The truth is that the senses of smell, taste, and touch decline gradually, with acuity loss starting at about age sixty; some people notice the effects more than others. And medications or health conditions might alter your flavor perceptions. Fortunately, there are ways to boost the flavor and the appeal of food.

Less Sense-Able

You've probably given it little thought, but throughout your life, smell and taste have affected the quality of your life, your overall health, and your personal safety. Think about simple pleasures: the variety of flavors in a holiday meal, the aromas of bread baking or turkey roasting in the oven, the sounds of popping popcorn, or the sizzle of food on the grill. Food's wonderful flavors encourage a healthy appetite and help stimulate digestion.

Your senses also provide clues to the off-flavor or appearance of deteriorating food, or perhaps to a kitchen fire or a gas leak in the kitchen stove. All these sensory experiences with food may change with age and health problems.

Consider this. Flavor is really several perceptions: the senses of smell and taste, as well as touch (temperature and mouth feel). With aging, taste buds and smell receptors may not be quite as sensitive or as numerous. The ability to sense sweet and salty tastes may wane sooner than bitter and sour tastes. That's why many foods may seem bitter, and why some older people reach for the salt shaker or the sugar bowl. Differences in saliva—composition and amount—may affect flavor, too. *For more about food and flavor see "'Flavor' the Difference" in chapter 13.*

Have You Ever Wondered

. . . if taking lecithin or gingko biloba can help prevent memory loss? No, but it's a common wish, especially for those who constantly misplace eyeglasses or shoes! In fact, no conclusive studies show that taking lecithin (a type of fat) or gingko biloba improves memory, thinking, or learning. Under a doctor's supervision, gingko biloba may be used to help treat the symptoms of age-related memory loss and dementia.

. . . if taking a multivitamin/mineral supplement is a good idea? Consuming a wide variety of food, in sufficient amounts, is the best approach to adequate nutrition, no matter what your age, if you're healthy. However, your physician may suggest a multivitamin/mineral supplement meant for older adults, especially if you limit your food choices. For older adults, supplements with vitamin B$_{12}$, vitamin D, and calcium may be recommended. Talk to your doctor about any supplement before you take it.

Age isn't the only reason for changes in taste and smell. Medications and health problems may interfere, too. Some medicines leave a bitter flavor that affects saliva and, as a result, the flavor of food. Some cause nausea, resulting in appetite loss, or dry mouth. Medicines also may suppress taste and smell. And health problems such as diabetes, high blood pressure, cancer, and liver disease, all common among older people, may alter taste and smell.

Fortunately, you can overcome, or at least accommodate to, many sensory changes that affect your food experiences and your personal nutrition. For example:

● Can't easily read food labels, an oven thermometer, or medication instructions? Get glasses for the first time, change your eyeglasses or contact lens prescription, or keep a magnifying glass handy. Large-print cookbooks are useful, too.

● Have trouble hearing a kitchen timer, food bubbling over on the stove, or a faucet you forgot to turn off? Find out if you need a hearing aid.

● Paying attention to losses of smell and taste—and their effects on nutrition and the pleasure of eating—are just as important. When food "just doesn't taste as good as it used to," some older adults lose interest in eating. Small appetites and skipped meals can result in poor nutrition. Read on for ways to compensate.

"Sage" Advice for a Flavor Boost

Compensating for diminished taste or smell is within your control. Just intensify the taste and the aroma of food. Vary the temperature and the texture—-and make it more visually appealing. Despite a common myth, older adults can tolerate spicy foods.

● Perk up flavors by using more herbs, spices, and lemon juice. To compensate for age-related taste loss, you might need twice as much herb or spice. For example, accent roasted poultry, poultry stew, or stuffing with sage. Carrots, acorn squash, and creamed spinach taste good with a dash of nutmeg. Simmer a bay leaf in soups and stews. Add a pinch of thyme or cumin to peas, lima beans, or other legumes. Or try dill weed or seed in potato soup, cooked cabbage, or coleslaw. *See "A Pinch of Flavor: How to Cook with Herbs and Spices" in chapter 13. Hint:* If any spices cause stomach irritation, stick with herbs.

● Add crunch to lunch—and dinner, too! Texture adds to the mouth feel and flavor of food. A variety of textures helps make up for a loss of taste and smell. What's easy? Crushed crackers on soup, chopped nuts on vegetables or in rice dishes, coleslaw as a salad, or crushed cornflakes on ice cream or pudding.

● Use strong-flavored ingredients: garlic, onion, sharp cheese, flavored vinegars and oils, concentrated fruit sauce, and jam. Use fats that add flavor: olive oil, nut oils, peanut butter, and butter.

● For less fat, impart flavor with herb rubs instead of marinades, gravy, or sauces.

● Enjoy food variety with different flavors.

● Include foods of different temperatures at each meal to perk up your sensations of flavor. Serve hot foods hot, not lukewarm, to enhance flavor. Extreme hot or cold temperatures, however, tend to lessen flavors.

● Serve yourself colorful, attractive food. A simple sprig of parsley or a tomato slice on the plate can add to its appeal.

● Take time to enjoy the foods' full flavors. Chew well.

● If you smoke, stop. Smoking reduces the ability to perceive flavors.

● Avoid overexposing your taste buds to strong or bitter flavors, such as coffee, which can temporarily deaden sensitivity to other flavors.

● If you've lost interest in eating, talk to your doctor, and consult a registered dietitian about other ways to make food more appealing.

For more about flavor see "'Resetting' Your Table . . . for Taste and Health" in chapter 13.

A Few Words about Constipation

Constipation is a persistent problem for many people as they get older. The reason? The digestive system may get a little sluggish. Not getting enough fluid or fiber and being inactive may compound the problem. With constipation, stools get hard and can't be passed out of the body without straining. And the body's normal elimination schedule may change.

Being physically active, drinking enough fluids, and eating enough fiber are ways to stay regular—and avoid constipation. If these remedies don't work, ask a registered dietitian or your doctor for more advice.

● Drink at least 6 to 8 cups of water or other fluids daily. Fluids help your stools stay softer, bulkier, and easier to eliminate.

● Consume plenty of fiber-rich foods: legumes, whole-grain breads and cereals, vegetables, and fruits. Fiber gives bulk to stools, making them easier to pass through the colon. *For more about fiber for health, including fiber pills and powders, see chapter 6, "Fiber: Your Body's Broom."*

● Listen to nature's call! The longer waste remains in your large intestine, the more difficult it is to eliminate. The body continues to draw out water, so stools get harder.

● Keep physically active and get enough rest. Both help keep your body regular.

● Avoid taking laxatives, as well as fiber pills and powders, unless your doctor recommends them. Food may pass through your intestinal tract faster than vitamins and minerals can be absorbed. And some may cause your body to lose fluids and potassium. A cup of tea or warm water with lemon, taken first thing in the morning, can act as a gentle, natural laxative.

For more about dealing with constipation see "Gastrointestinal Conditions" in chapter 22.

Not Hungry?

While many older adults say they just don't have an appetite, there's no single cause for that complaint. Some have digestive problems that cause appetite loss. And medication or health problems also may be a cause. For some, the problem is psychological: loneliness, depression, or anxiety, among others.

Regardless, people who don't eat adequately increase their chances for poor nutrition and its nega-

tive consequences. Try these tips to perk up a tired appetite:

● Try to identify the problem. If certain foods cause discomfort, such as heartburn or gas, find alternatives. Talk to your doctor about your medication; if it's causing a problem, something else might be prescribed.

● Eat four to six smaller meals and keep portions small. You may always take seconds if you're hungry for more. And smaller meals may be easier to digest.

● Give yourself enough time to eat. Rushing through a meal can cause discomfort.

● To get your digestive juices flowing, serve foods hot. Heat brings out the aroma of food, usually making it more enticing.

● Make your overall meal look appealing. Food that's attractively arranged and served may help bring your appetite back!

● If possible, increase your physical activity. That may promote a healthier appetite.

● If you're confined to bed, ask someone to help keep your room pleasant. Remove bedpans and other unpleasant things. Enjoy a plant, and turn on some music!

Chewing Problems?

For many mature adults, poor appetite isn't much of a nutrition problem. Instead, tooth loss or mouth pain may be. An astounding number of people lose all their teeth by age sixty-five. And many have poorly fitting dentures that cause chewing problems and mouth sores.

What's at the root of oral health problems? Cavities may come to mind first. Yet gum, or periodontal, disease is the most common cause of tooth loss among older adults. As a result, many have missing, loose, or diseased teeth and sore, diseased gums. People with dentures may be able to eat all the foods they've always enjoyed if dentures fit right. If not, the resulting discomfort and mouth pain may keep them from eating a well-balanced diet. And osteoarthritis may hinder chewing if it affects the lower jaw.

A dry mouth is another problem that may cause

Need more practical, easy ways to eat smart as the years go by? Check here for "how-tos":

- Boost your appetite if you don't feel hungry—see chapter 2.

- Find smart ways to lose, gain, or maintain your weight—see chapter 2.

- Make quick, simple meals if you don't have a lot of energy—see chapter 10.

- Get more for your food dollar on a fixed income—see chapter 11.

- Protect yourself from foodborne illness—see chapter 12.

- Get more nutrition for fewer calories—see chapter 13.

- Perk up food's flavor with herbs and spices if food no longer tastes as good. Improve food's look, too—see chapter 13.

- Eat out, yet still match your health needs—see chapter 14.

- Eat to manage health problems—see chapter 22.

- Get easy, personalized tips from a nutrition expert—see chapter 24.

chewing and swallowing difficulties, especially if food is dry and hard to chew. As people get older, they may not have as much saliva flow to help soften food and wash it down. Medications, some health problems, and treatment such as chemotherapy also may decrease saliva flow or cause chewing and swallowing problems. *See "Cancer Treatment: Handling Side Effects" in chapter 22.*

If you have chewing problems, make sure oral problems don't become a barrier to good nutrition.

- See your dentist, or go to a dentist who specializes in care for older adults. Many oral health problems can be treated. And dentures that don't fit properly should be adjusted.

- Choose softer foods that are easier to chew. Chop foods well to reduce your risk of choking. All five food groups of the Food Guide Pyramid have foods that are softer and easier to eat. *See "The Food Guide Pyramid: Your Healthful Eating Guide" in chapter 10.*

- *Grains Group:* cooked cereal, cooked rice, cooked pasta, soft bread or rolls, softer crackers
- *Fruit Group:* fruit juice, cooked or canned fruit, avocados, bananas, grapefruit and orange sections, soft fruit
- *Vegetable Group:* vegetable juice, cooked vegetables, mashed potatoes, salads with soft vegetables, chopped lettuce
- *Milk Group:* milk, cheese, yogurt, pudding, ice cream, milk shakes
- *Meat and Beans Group:* chopped, lean meat, chopped chicken or turkey, canned fish, tender cooked fish, eggs, tofu, hummus, creamy peanut butter

- Drink water or other fluids with meals and snacks to make swallowing easier.

- Consult a registered dietitian. Together you can plan for foods that you can eat comfortably without compromising your nutrient intake.

There's good news: Tooth loss and chewing difficulty aren't inevitable parts of aging. Good oral care—starting now, whatever your age—can help you keep the teeth you were born with. *See "Keep Teeth and Gums Healthy" in chapter 5.*

Gum disease is highly preventable. Proper brushing, daily flossing, and regular cleaning by a dentist or a hygienist can keep gum disease at bay. If you can, have your teeth cleaned twice a year, and perhaps more often if you have gum disease. *For more about gum disease see "Keep Smiling: Prevent Gum Disease" in chapter 22.*

Weight Loss—or Gain?

Have you lost weight as a result of a poor appetite or health problems? Or have extra pounds crept on over the years? Maintaining or improving your weight may be a health step you need to take. Talk to your doctor or a registered dietitian about the weight that's healthy for you.

Whether you need to keep weight on, or take it off, eat in a healthful way and remain as physically active as you can. *See "Never Too Late for Exercise" earlier in this chapter.*

Weight Loss: A Concern

Weight loss may be a health problem, especially if you haven't tried to lose. If that happens, first and foremost, find out why! Perhaps the reason is poor oral health or immobility that makes grocery shopping or food preparation difficult. Weight loss may signal an emotional problem, perhaps depression and/or bereavement, or social isolation. Unexpected weight loss also is a symptom for some serious health problems, including cancer. Talk to your doctor!

Besides other health implications, weight loss may be linked to physical weakness when muscle mass, not just body fat, is lost. Loss of physical strength increases the risk for falls, and as a result, bone fractures. Being underweight also may slow recovery from sickness or surgery.

To gain or to maintain weight:

● Eat enough. Use the Food Guide Pyramid as your guide for consuming enough servings and enough variety among its five food groups.

● Eat five or six small meals a day if you fill up quickly at meals.

● Stick to a regular meal schedule so you don't forget to eat.

● Keep healthful and easy foods handy for snacking: milk, yogurt, fruit, vegetables, crackers, whole-wheat bread, cereal, and peanut butter.

● Eat with someone else to spark your appetite.

● Instead of coffee or tea, which supplies few calories, drink cocoa, milk, soup, or juice.

● Make casseroles, soups, stews, and side dishes heartier by adding whole milk, cheese, beans, rice, or pasta.

● Talk to a registered dietitian (RD) or your doctor about ways to boost calories and nutrients in your meals and snacks. An RD can provide you with ideas for high-calorie meals and drinks, and if necessary, can help you select the right canned nutrition supplement drink or dietary supplement. Find an appropriate way to stay physically active so you maintain your body's muscle mass—and, as a result, your strength. Again talk to your doctor, and perhaps a trained physical therapist.

Be aware that some medications, including low-dose antidepressant drugs, may enhance appetite.

Weight Gain: An Issue, Too

As you get older, you need fewer calories to maintain your weight. It's not surprising, then, to gain a few pounds—especially if you're more sedentary and still eat as you always have. The concern is that being overweight increases the risks for high blood pressure, heart disease, diabetes, and certain cancers. If you have one of these problems already, dropping just a few pounds may lower your blood pressure, total blood cholesterol level, or blood sugar level.

Before you start trying to lose weight, talk to your physician about an effective and safe approach that matches your health needs. These strategies may work for you:

To lose weight:

● Use the Food Guide Pyramid as your daily eating guide. Choose mostly lean and low-fat or fat-free foods. Eat the least amount from the recommended serving ranges for the five food groups. And go easy on foods from the Pyramid tip.

● Eat regular meals. Meal-skipping often leads to snacking and possibly overeating.

● Choose snacks carefully: fruits, vegetables, low-fat yogurt, fat-free or low-fat milk, breakfast cereal, and frozen yogurt.

● Trim fat from food choices. Remove skin from turkey or chicken before eating it. Choose lean meats and trim visible fat. Bake, broil, microwave, or steam foods instead of frying them. Use low-fat or fat-free milk, yogurt, and cheese. Switch to low-calorie or fat-free salad dressings. Go easy on butter, margarine, cream, and sour cream. *For more ways to trim fat in food preparation, see "Fat and Cholesterol Trimmers" in chapter 13.*

● Eat smaller portions—and still meet Pyramid guidelines.

● If you drink alcoholic beverages, do so in moderation: no more than one drink a day for women, and two for men. If you're taking medication, you might need to avoid alcoholic drinks altogether.

● Keep active and busy to prevent eating from boredom or loneliness. And learn to recognize signals for hunger and satiety.

● Find safe and appropriate ways to move more and sit less. You'll get more health-promoting benefits than weight control alone!

● Beware of weight-loss plans with unrealistic promises. *See "'Diets' That Don't Work!" in chapter 2.*

"Moving Ideas" for Physical Limitations

Some older adults move with the same grace, stamina, and dexterity of their earlier years. For others, health problems limit physical abilities: for example, arthritis, diabetes, osteoporosis, Parkinson's disease, respiratory diseases, and strokes. Even healthy, mature adults may become gradually less active, so they have less strength and stamina for everyday tasks.

For those who enjoy independent living, some general tips can make food preparation and eating easier:

● Does your tile or wooden floor seem slippery? Wear flat, rubber-soled shoes in the kitchen. And wipe up spills immediately so you don't slip!

● Be careful of loose rugs by the sink or other places in your kitchen. They may feel good underfoot, but they're easy to trip or slip on.

● If you're unsteady or need a cane, use a rolling tea cart to move food, dishes, and kitchen equipment from place to place.

● A wheelchair or a walker with a flat seat can be used to move things, too; check with a medical supply store to find them.

● Sit while you work. Use the kitchen table for food preparation, or get a stable chair or stool that's high enough for working at the counter or the stove.

● Give yourself time. Things may take a little longer to do as you get older.

● Get a loud kitchen timer if you have trouble hearing. Especially if you're forgetful, using a timer when you cook can avoid burned food and kitchen fires.

● Cooking for just one? Use a microwave or toaster oven rather than the conventional oven.

● Organize your kitchen for efficiency—everything within easy reach. Keep mixers, blenders, and other heavy, small appliances on the counter. Keep heavy pots and pans on lower shelves, too.

● If you have vision problems, keep a magnifying glass handy, and have your eyes checked and fitted for glasses. That makes it easier to read expiration dates and small type on food labels.

● Use a cutting board with contrasting colors if you have trouble with vision; for example, it may be hard to safely cut an onion on a white plastic cutting board.

● Have trouble with manual tasks such as opening jars and cans, or perhaps cutting? Kitchen devices are sold to make food preparation easier for people with arthritis or other problems, and for those partly paralyzed by a stroke. Again, check a medical supply store to find these devices. *See "Have You Ever Wondered . . . if you can eat anything to relieve arthritis?" in chapter 22.*

● Get a cordless phone. You won't need to dash to the phone while you're cooking. Just keep it near you. It's a good safety measure, too, in case you fall.

● If you use a walker or a wheelchair, talk to a registered dietitian or a physical therapist about ways to change your kitchen for independent living.

● Another kitchen safety tip: Avoid using your oven as a room heater. It can be dangerous! If heating is a problem where you live, let someone know—a relative, landlord, building manager, or social worker, among others. *For other kitchen safety tips see "Quick Tips for Injury Prevention" in chapter 12.*

● Use an all-in-one fork and spoon if you have trouble with one hand. Check with a medical supply store or catalog to find one.

● Drink soup from a mug. It's easier than using a soup spoon—and there's one less utensil to wash.

● Get dishes with a higher rim and a rubber, no-slip back. The rim helps you push food onto your spoon or fork.

● Set your table with plastic placemats. They're easy to clean. And dishes won't slide on them, as they might on the table surface.

● Shaky with a cup? Get a covered cup with a drinking spout or place for a straw.

● If you use a wheelchair, buy an oven with front controls and a side-hinged door. Install it next to the sink or your work area, not across the kitchen. Put in low countertops and "pull-outs," such as cutting boards, in your kitchen, too. Talk to a physical therapist or a registered dietitian about other kitchen design solutions.

● Rather than avoid certain categories of foods, accept help if you need it. You need nourishment from a variety of foods.

Meals and Snacks: When You Need a Special Diet

Many health problems—physical and emotional—that arise with aging require major changes in what and how people eat. Discuss that with your doctor during your regular checkups—annually or more often as your doctor advises. Never self-diagnose an ongoing disease, or prescribe your own special diet or dietary supplement to treat it. And be careful of so-called miracle cures. *See "Miracles? Dream On!" earlier in this chapter.*

For any health condition, there's no one recommended diet. Each person needs individual nutrition advice because needs differ so much. And sometimes more than one health problem needs to be treated at the same time. If a special (therapeutic) diet is prescribed for you, consult your doctor or a registered dietitian for guidance. And have your progress monitored, as he or she advises. *For more tips see "If Your Doctor Prescribes a Special Eating Plan . . . " in chapter 22.*

To manage your health, your food choices may need as much of your attention as following directions for medications. It's all for your good health! To find a registered dietitian, ask your doctor. *See "How to Find Nutrition Help" in chapter 24.*

Give a Helping Hand!

To people who are sick, weak, or injured, good nutrition is often the best medicine! Regardless of age, those with difficulty feeding themselves may need a caring, helping hand.

If you offer help, make mealtime pleasant:

● Help with hand washing before and after eating. Use a wet, soapy washcloth or premoistened towels or a hand sanitizer if the person can't get to the sink.

● Make sure that the food is the right consistency. You might need to chop or puree it if chewing is difficult.

● Let the person decide what foods to eat first, next, and so on. Even when people can't feed themselves, most want to feel in control of their lives.

● For dignity's sake, provide a napkin or an apron to help him or her keep clean.

● Offer some finger foods to eat independently. For example, try banana slices, orange sections, bread (cut in quarters), a soft roll, cheese sticks, or meat (sliced in strips).

● Offer a drink between bites to help with chewing and swallowing. Provide a straw and a cup that's not too big. You can always pour more.

● Consider how far the person can reach for a cup or a dish. Arrange the place setting for easy reach.

● Sit together at the same level as you offer food. Share pleasant conversation in a normal tone, even if you need to do all the talking. To be sure you understand a response, repeat or rephrase it.

● Relax and be patient. Encourage self-expression of any kind. The meal should not feel rushed, especially if the person has trouble chewing or swallowing.

● Offer small bites, and suggest a spoon rather than a fork. It's easier for holding food and less likely to jab his or her mouth.

● If you can, eat your meal at the same time to continue the joy and the normalcy of social interaction at mealtime.

● Clean any spills right away. You might keep a clean cloth handy.

● Most important, respect the person's needs and desires. Expect frustration, and handle it without a negative reaction. Counting on others for personal care can be emotionally difficult.

● Let the nurse or other caregivers know what and how much the person has eaten. In that way other meals and snacks can be adjusted accordingly.

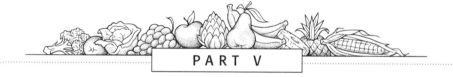

Healthful Eating

Special Issues

PART V

CHAPTER 19

Athlete's Guide
Winning Nutrition

On your mark . . . get set . . . go! Whether you train for competitive sports, or work out for your own good health or just for fun, what you eat and drink—and when—is part of your formula for athletic success. Good nutrition can't replace training, effort, talent, and personal drive. But there's no question that what you eat and drink over time make a difference when your goal is peak performance.

Whether competitive or recreational, physical activity puts extra demands on your body. As an athlete, you use more energy, lose more body fluids, and put extra stress on your muscles, joints, and bones. Fortunately, your "training table" can increase your endurance and help prevent dehydration and injury. Most important, healthful eating helps you feel good and stay fit overall.

Nutrients for Active Living

Whether you're a world-class athlete or just enthusiastically active, nutrition is fundamental to your peak physical performance. To put in your best effort, you need the same nutrients as nonathletes: carbohydrates, proteins, fats, vitamins, minerals, and water. If you're highly active, however, you may need slightly more of some nutrients.

What are the major differences in your nutrient needs? To replace fluid losses, athletes need more fluids to stay hydrated during high activity. And working muscles need more energy-supplying nutrients, especially carbohydrates.

Thirst for Success!

Do you drink plenty of water? Athletes and nonathletes often overlook fluids; yet physical endurance and strength depend on them.

When you're physically active, you lose fluids as sweat evaporates from your skin. As you breathe, often heavily, you exhale moisture, too. A 150-pound athlete can lose 1½ quarts, or 3 pounds, of fluid in just one hour. That equals six 8-ounce glasses of water. With heavy training, fluid loss can be higher. You need to replace the fluids you lose.

Fluids for Peak Performance

What's the risk if you begin physical activity even slightly dehydrated, or lose too much fluid while you're active? Even small losses of 1 to 2 percent of

Did You Know

. . . heat stroke, caused by severe dehydration, ranks second among the reported cases of death among high school athletes?

. . . taking extra vitamins or minerals (beyond the Recommended Dietary Allowances) offers no added advantage to athletic performance?

. . . a high-carbohydrate diet can boost your endurance?

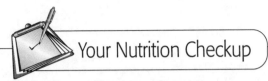

Your Nutrition Checkup

Eat to Compete

Sports nutrition is filled with misconceptions—all based on the drive for top performance. As an athlete, are you tuned into the facts, or the myths?

TRUE OR FALSE?

T	F	
____	____	**1.** If you train properly for sports, you don't need to worry as much about replacing fluids.
____	____	**2.** Vitamin supplements supply extra energy for heavy workouts.
____	____	**3.** A steak dinner is the best precompetition meal.
____	____	**4.** Fasting is a good approach for "making weight."
____	____	**5.** Except for football and other contact sports, the leaner you are, the better.
____	____	**6.** Drinking milk before a heavy workout causes stomach cramps.
____	____	**7.** Salt tablets prevent muscle cramps.
____	____	**8.** If you eat a lot of protein, you'll build a lot of muscle.
____	____	**9.** Creatine supplements are necessary to build muscle and give you energy to train.

Now score yourself:

Do you eat smart to compete? Be aware that *every statement above is false.* For each true-false statement, these are the facts:

1. *Fact:* To avoid dehydration, everyone—even well-trained athletes—needs to stay hydrated before, during, and after physical activity. Besides water, sports drinks are an option; read on for more about fluids for athletes. Training won't protect you from dehydration!

2. *Fact:* Vitamins don't supply energy; carbohydrates, fats, and proteins do. If you're already following the advice of the Food Guide Pyramid and eating enough servings to meet your energy needs, there's no reason for vitamin supplements. The small amount of extra vitamins—for example, B vitamins—you need to produce extra energy from carbohydrates, fats, and proteins comes from extra servings of food-group foods.

3. *Fact:* A high-carbohydrate meal is the best precompetition meal. It supplies the best fuel for working muscles. A steak dinner may taste great, but it's typically high in proteins and fats instead.

   If steak gives you a "mental edge," enjoy a small portion. And eat plenty of carbohydrate-rich foods with it: perhaps baked potato, pasta, or rice; carrots; a dinner roll; a fruit salad; and frozen yogurt for dessert.

4. *Fact:* Fasting is never advised for athletes! It often causes fatigue, reduced glycogen stores, the potential for muscle loss, dehydration, and decreased performance. For young athletes, fasting keeps them from consuming nutrients essential to their growth and development.

5. *Fact:* Yes, a lean, muscular body performs better. And being lean is healthier, too. But you can be too lean. Among its many functions, fat cushions body organs, providing protection from injury. For endurance sports, fat converts to energy after the body's glycogen stores are used. If you're too lean, you may tire too quickly. And restricting energy intake too much to avoid body fat may create a nutrient deficiency.

6. *Fact:* Contrary to popular myth, drinking milk before physical exertion doesn't cause stomach discomfort or digestive problems. Over time, not consuming enough calcium—a key nutrient in milk—may contribute to muscle cramps instead. Whether you choose to drink milk before a heavy workout is a personal matter.

   If you have trouble digesting milk, the problem might be lactose intolerance. If so, you can still drink milk as part of your training diet. *For guidance see "Lactose Intolerance: A Matter of Degree" in chapter 21.*

7. *Fact:* Many things can contribute to cramping—fluid, sodium, potassium, and calcium losses. Most often,

muscle cramps are a sign of dehydration. You don't need salt tablets to replace the small amount of sodium you lose when you sweat. Your normal diet supplies enough.

8. *Fact:* Exercise, not a lot of extra protein, builds muscle mass. To build muscles, you need to work them more and gradually increase their workload. You may think of muscles as all protein. But actually 15 to 20 percent is protein; 70 to 75 percent is water; and 5 to 7 percent is fat, glycogen, and minerals.

   Most recreational exercisers need about 0.5 to 0.75 gram of protein each day for every pound of body weight. Weight lifters need more for strength training: 0.7 to 0.9 gram of protein daily per pound

of body weight. That amount can be provided easily by food (meat, poultry, fish, dairy foods, eggs, grain products), without the need for protein supplements.

9. *Fact:* Creatine supplements are not needed to build muscle. Good food choices and plenty of hard work in the weight room are the only things that build muscle. Some college and professional athletes use creatine to help store this energy source in their muscles for extra fuel, but creatine use is not recommended for any athletes under age eighteen.

   Missed any? Read on for more about the facts of eating for peak physical performance.

---

your body weight can hinder your physical performance, particularly during warm weather. (That's about 2 or 3 pounds for a 150-pound person.) Dehydration can affect your strength, endurance, and aerobic capacity. How does fluid promote performance?

For energy production. Fluids are part of the cycle of energy production. As part of blood, water helps carry oxygen and glucose to your muscle cells. There, oxygen and glucose help produce energy. Blood removes waste by-products as muscle cells generate energy and passes them to urine. Fluid losses decrease blood volume, so your heart must work harder to deliver enough oxygen to your cells.

For cooling down. Exercise generates heat as a by-product of energy production. Sweat helps cool you down.

As you move your muscles, your body's overall temperature goes up, and you sweat. As sweat evaporates, your skin and the blood just under your skin cool. Cooler blood that flows throughout your body helps protect you from overheating. If you don't replace fluids lost through perspiration, your body's fluid balance is thrown off—a bigger problem as working muscles continue to generate more heat.

For transporting other nutrients. Water in your bloodstream carries other nutrients for performance, including electrolytes.

As a cushion. The water around your body's tissues and organs offers protection from all the jostles and jolts that go along with exercise.

Protection from dehydration. Continued fluid loss—beyond the early stages of dehydration—increases your chances of heat injury, such as heat cramps, heat exhaustion, and heat stroke. *Severe dehydration can even be life-threatening. See "Dehydration Alert!" later in this chapter.*

For more about water in a healthful eating plan see "A Fluid Asset" in chapter 8.

Fluids: Tips to Avoid Dehydration and Overheating

No matter what your sport—running, bicycling, swimming, tennis, even walking and golfing—or rigorous activity, drink enough fluid to avoid dehydration. Getting enough isn't always easy.

● Drink plenty of fluids—before, during, and after physical activity. Carry a water bottle, especially if you have no available water source. Or find out where you can get fluids: store, water fountain, others; bring money. Rehydrating yourself after activity helps you recover faster, both physically and mentally.

● Drink fluids by schedule (every fifteen minutes during activity)—even when you don't feel thirsty. Your thirst mechanism may not send thirst signals when you're exercising. In fact, thirst is a symptom of dehydration, so drink fluids before that happens. *Follow the schedule recommended in this chapter, "For Rigorous Activity: How Much Fluid?"*

● Wear lightweight clothes in warm weather. Be aware that fabrics that hold heat—such as tights, body

For Rigorous Activity: How Much Fluid?

For rigorous activity, make a point of drinking fluids at all times during the day—not just after your workout or competition. How much fluid is enough? Here's a schedule that can keep you from becoming dehydrated:

WHEN TO DRINK	ABOUT HOW MUCH (One medium mouthful of fluid = about 1 ounce; 1 cup = 8 ounces.)
2 hours before activity	2 cups (and drink plenty with meals)
15 minutes before activity	1 to 2 cups
Every 15 minutes during activity	½ to 1 cup
After activity	3 cups for each pound of body weight lost

Source: Christine A. Rosenbloom, ed., *Sports Nutrition: A Guide for the Professional Working with Active People* (Chicago: American Dietetic Association, 2000).

suits, heavy gear—as well as helmets and other protective gear, won't let sweat evaporate.

● Replace water weight. Weigh yourself before and after a heavy workout. Your nude weight is best. Or make sure you're wearing the same clothing when you weigh yourself—before and after. Replace each pound of weight you lose with 3 cups of water, carbohydrate drink, or other fluid to bring your fluid balance back to normal.

● Check the color of your urine. Dark-colored urine indicates dehydration. Increase your fluid intake so your urine is pale and nearly colorless before you start exercising again.

● Be especially careful if you exercise intensely in warm, humid weather. Consider how much hotter you feel on humid days. Sweat doesn't evaporate from your skin quickly, so you don't get the cooling benefits. That's why on humid days it's easier to get hyperthermia, or overheated, as you exercise. Hyperthermia can lead to heat stroke, which can be fatal!

● Know the signs of dehydration. Some early signs are flushed skin, fatigue, increased body temperature, and increased breathing and pulse rate, followed by dizziness, increased weakness, and labored breathing with exercise. Replace fluids before symptoms get too serious. *See "Dehydration: Look for Body Signals!" in chapter 8.*

● Drink, rather than simply pour water over your head. Drinking is the only way to rehydrate and cool your body from the inside out.

For more about fluids and active children see "Fluids: Caution for Kids" later in this chapter.

Which Fluids?

What should you drink before, during, and after rigorous activity? Try water, fruit juices, sports drinks, or other beverages. For workouts of less than thirty minutes of continuous activity and recreational walking, sports drinks, juices, and water are all good choices. For fluid replacers for other sports, keep reading.

Water: The Best Choice. Cool water is preferred by most exercisers; in fact, water has been described as an athlete's best ergogenic aid!

Water helps lower and normalize your body's core temperature from inside when you're hot, and it moves quickly from your digestive tract to your tissues.

Cold water is a fine choice. Contrary to popular myth, drinking cold water during exercise doesn't cause stomach cramps for most athletes; stomach

Have You Ever Wondered

... if swimmers need to worry about dehydration? Like any athlete, swimmers perspire to keep from overheating. However, swimmers probably don't notice their sweat—at least not while they're in the water. Like other athletes, they need to drink plenty of fluids before, during, and after rigorous swimming.

... if dehydration is a concern with cold-weather sports such as ice skating or skiing? Even in a cool or cold environment, you lose fluids. An added reason: attire for some cold weather sports doesn't "breathe" or allow the body to cool down.

cramps may come from dehydration, but not drinking cold water. For outside activity in cold weather, drink water that's warm or at room temperature to help protect you from hypothermia, or low body temperature.

Sports Drinks?

Often marketed as "power drinks," sports drinks can benefit some athletes under a variety of circumstances, especially in hot, humid conditions. In fact, sports drinks with 6 to 8 percent carbohydrate (14 to 19 grams of carbohydrate per 8 ounces) may be better than water or diluted fruit juice for fluid replacement.

For activities lasting longer than an hour, try sports drinks. If you're a long-distance runner or long-distance bicyclist, or involved in other endurance events (longer than ninety minutes), sports drinks may offer some performance benefits. New research shows a benefit for high-intensity activity (perhaps sprinting or playing hockey) lasting thirty minutes or more.

The simple form of carbohydrate, called glucose, in sports drinks is a more immediate fuel, or energy, source for working muscles. It may help prevent muscle glycogen from being depleted too fast and so help lengthen performance time. (Muscle glycogen is carbohydrate that's stored in muscle.) Glucose in sports drinks also helps the fluid get out of the gut and into the bloodstream.

Compared to juice or soft drinks, sports drinks are more diluted. This means that the fluid and glucose supplied by a sports drink can be absorbed and used more readily by the body. If you'd like to see if a drink falls in the 6 to 8 percent carbohydrate range, use this formula:

- Find the grams of carbohydrate and the serving size (in milliliters—mL) on the label (8 ounces is about 240 mL).

- Divide the grams of carbohydrate by the serving size (in mL) and multiply by 100 to determine the percent of carbohydrate.

- Example: 14 grams carbohydrate/240 mL × 100 = 6%

Besides fluid and energy, sports drinks supply electrolytes. As you perspire, your body loses very small amounts of sodium and other electrolytes. For most athletes, a normal diet replaces what's lost. But endurance athletes perspire much more, so they're at greater risk for sodium depletion. Sodium and other electrolytes in sports drinks may be beneficial. During exercise that's longer than 60 minutes, or for exercise performed in high heat or humidity, drinks with electrolytes help to enhance fluid absorption. *For more about electrolytes see "Electrolytes: Sweat 'Em!" later in this chapter.*

You don't lose vitamins when you sweat, so you don't need sports drinks with extra vitamins. The extra food you eat for more food energy also provides any extra B vitamins you need for energy production.

If you're an endurance athlete, experiment with sports drinks and other fluids during practices and low-key competition. Drink them early enough so you

---

Have You Ever Wondered ?

. . . if caffeine can boost your physical performance? Maybe—and maybe not. People react to caffeine in different ways. Caffeine does stimulate the central nervous system, so it may help you feel more alert and attentive. And it may enhance your performance.

For caffeine-sensitive athletes, caffeine may exacerbate pre-event anxiety. And it may promote headaches, stomach upset, or diarrhea. Be aware that caffeine is a diuretic, which stimulates water loss—a greater problem in hot weather and for endurance athletes.

If you enjoy coffee, tea, or soft drinks with caffeine, experiment during training, not competition. A single cup may help—or at least not hinder—your performance. But avoid caffeine tablets or several cups of caffeinated drinks. High levels of caffeine in urine—comparable to the amount from drinking three to five large cups of coffee an hour before competition—are banned by the International Olympic Committee (IOC) and the National Collegiate Athletic Association (NCAA). To screen athletes, caffeine concentration in urine is measured; to compete, it must not exceed 12 micrograms (by the IOC) or 15 micrograms (by the NCAA) per milliliter of urine.

If you drink caffeinated beverages, drink enough other fluids, too, to replace fluids lost through sweat. Caffeinated beverages are made with water. Despite the diuretic effects of caffeine, drinking these beverages still leaves you with a positive intake of water. *For more about caffeine see "Drinks: With or without Caffeine?" in chapter 8.*

don't get dehydrated. Then any fluid may upset your stomach.

If the appealing flavor of sports drinks encourages you to drink more fluids—or if they give you a psychological boost—enjoy them, but don't overdo. If you're watching your weight, remember that they supply calories.

Fruit Juice or Soft Drinks? Compared with sports drinks, sugars in soft drinks and fruit juice are more concentrated: 10 to 15 percent carbohydrate. They aren't recommended during exercise because of their high sugar content and, for soft drinks, their carbonation. Drinks with a lot of sugar take longer to be absorbed, and they may cause cramps, diarrhea, or nausea. Carbonation can make you feel full and make your throat burn, so you drink less fluid.

You can dilute fruit juice—if you like the flavor. Unlike sports drinks, diluted fruit juice doesn't provide any sodium; depending on how much it's diluted, it may not contain enough carbohydrates to help the athlete.

Alcoholic Drinks: Not Now! Alcoholic beverages can impair, not enhance, your physical performance. Consider all the reasons to skip alcoholic drinks—at least until after you replenish the fluids you lose in your workout:

● If you're looking for a carbohydrate source, look elsewhere. A 12-ounce can of beer has less than a third of the "carbs" provided by a 12-ounce serving of orange juice. Calories from alcohol don't fuel muscle work.

● Alcohol is a diuretic, which promotes water loss and dehydration. It works as a depressant, affecting your brain's ability to reason and make judgments and perhaps your reaction time. And it may impair your coordination, balance, muscle reflexes, and visual perception.

● For the endurance athlete it has another effect: When you drink a beer, wine, or mixed drink, your liver works to detoxify and metabolize the alcohol. This process can interfere with the liver's job of forming extra blood glucose for prolonged physical activity. The possible result? Early fatigue.

If you want a beer or a wine cooler *after* a workout, first replenish the fluids you lost with water. Then enjoy your drink.

Dehydration Alert!

As you exercise, be alert for conditions that increase your fluid loss through sweat. With more perspiration, your body dehydrates faster.

● *Temperature.* The higher the temperature, the greater your sweat losses.

● *Intensity.* The harder you work out, the greater your sweat losses.

● *Body size.* The larger the athlete, the greater the sweat losses. Males generally sweat more than females.

● *Duration.* The longer the workout, the greater your fluid losses.

● *Fitness.* Well-trained athletes sweat more, starting to sweat at a lower body temperature. Why? The function of sweating is to cool the body. The well-trained athlete cools his or her body more efficiently than an untrained person.

Source: Debbi Sowell Jennings and Suzanne Nelson Steen, *Play Hard, Eat Right* (Minneapolis: American Dietetic Association, Chronimed Publishing, 1995).

Energy to Burn

Athletes: The only way to have enough energy for physical activity is to consume enough energy. How much energy, or calories, should you consume per day? That's a very individual matter. A 200-pound body builder has very different needs than an 80-pound gymnast. A physical training program may use 2,000 to 6,000 or more calories daily—a huge range.

● The amount of energy you need for sports depends partly on your body composition, body weight, and level of fitness. Body size (consider a male football player and a female gymnast) also makes a big difference. When two people ski together at the same intensity, the person weighing more would likely burn more calories.

● The harder, the longer, and the more often you work out, the more energy you require for your muscles' work. Any activity such as cycling, power walking, or swimming is a bigger energy burner if done more vigorously.

● Not surprisingly, some sports burn more energy than others. That's simply because they're more intense or their duration is longer. Both a golf game and downhill skiing may last several hours. But skiing uses more energy since it's more physically demanding for larger muscle groups.

What nutrients supply energy? Carbohydrates for activities that take high-intensity, short bursts of energy, and both carbohydrates and fats for longer activity.

For the energy costs of several sports see "Burning Calories with Activity" in chapter 2. To estimate your own energy needs see "Your 'Weigh': Figuring Your Energy Needs" in chapter 2. Or have a registered dietitian (RD) help you.

Carbohydrate Power

For sports and everyday living, carbohydrates are your body's foremost energy source—and the main fuel for working muscles. Nutrition experts advise athletes to consume 6 to 10 grams of carbohydrate for every kilogram of body weight. For an athlete who weighs 120 pounds (55 kilograms), that's 330 to 550 grams of carbohydrate; for a 175-pound (80-kilogram) athlete, that's 480 to 800 grams of "carbs." (One pound equals 2.2 kilograms.)

Along with training, a high-carbohydrate eating plan promotes overall fitness and offers a competitive edge. With "carbs" (not fats or proteins) as the main fuel, you can maintain rigorous activity longer. Training helps your body use carbohydrates efficiently and store more as muscle glycogen. Stored in muscles, glycogen is fuel ready to power your physical activity.

WHAT'S YOUR "CARB" GOAL?

IF YOUR DAY'S FOOD CHOICES PROVIDE . . .	YOUR CARBOHYDRATE GOAL IS ABOUT . . . (65% OF TOTAL ENERGY)
2,000 calories	320 grams*
2,500 calories	410 grams*
3,000 calories	490 grams*
3,500 calories	570 grams*
4,000 calories	650 grams*

*How does that translate to food? *See the chart "Carbohydrates in Food: Quick Rule of Thumb" in this chapter.*

For Working Muscles

To power working muscles, stored energy comes mostly from muscle or liver glycogen, and from blood sugar (also known as blood glucose). Glycogen is your body's storage form of carbohydrate. Depending on the intensity and the duration of exercise, fat and, for endurance athletes, even a small amount of protein supply energy, too.

Carbohydrates are broken down during digestion and changed to blood sugar, or glucose. Some blood sugar, which is circulated in your bloodstream, is used immediately for energy. The rest is stored as muscle and liver glycogen, or it's converted to fat if excess calories are consumed. The more muscle glycogen you can store, the more you have to power physical activity.

Your body's glycogen stores are continually used and replenished. When you need more energy, your body fuels muscles with a mix of both carbohydrate (glycogen) and fat. The higher the immediate intensity of an activity, the greater the use of glycogen. Lower-intensity and longer activities use more fat and less glycogen.

● For sports that require short, intense energy spurts (anaerobic activities), muscle glycogen is the main energy source used. That includes tennis, volleyball, baseball, weight lifting, sprinting, and even bowling.

● Sports that require both intensity and endurance also use mostly muscle glycogen. Basketball and football are two examples.

● For endurance activities (aerobic activities) such as long-distance running or long-distance bicycling, your body first uses some glycogen, then relies mostly on its fat stores for fuel.

See "Carbohydrates: Your 'Power' Source" in chapter 5.

Fuel Up!

"Carbs" are an athlete's best energy source. (Eat enough every day to keep your muscle and liver glycogen stores up.) Carbohydrates in food are complex sugars (starches) and simple sugars (sucrose, lactose, fructose, and glucose). Both supply energy and replenish your muscle glycogen. For energy, the main difference is that simple sugars in food are digested and absorbed into your bloodstream faster. Complex carbohydrates must be broken down first.

What foods contain carbohydrates? Complex carbohydrates come from cereals, breads, rice, pasta, vegetables, and legumes (beans and peas). Sugars (both naturally occurring and added) are in fruit, fruit juice, milk, cookies, cakes, candy, and soft drinks, among other foods.

Get your "carbs" from individual foods or in a variety of mixed dishes:

● *Made with breads, grains, cereals, and pastas:* wild rice pilaf; salads made with different types of pasta, such as spinach pasta; whole-wheat or buckwheat pancakes; sandwiches made with every kind of bread, including a bagel or pita bread; animal crackers, gingersnaps, graham crackers, or oatmeal-raisin cookies; homemade fruit and nut breads.

● *Made with fruits or vegetables:* dried fruit mixes; stuffed spuds such as a baked potato stuffed with broccoli; fresh fruit salad; and raw vegetables with yogurt dip.

● *Made with legumes* (chickpeas, kidney beans, split peas, pinto beans, black beans, lentils, and other dried peas and beans): bean enchiladas; black bean and split pea soups; vegetarian baked beans; and chili.

For the specific carbohydrate content of many foods see "'Carbo' Foods" in the Appendices.

"CARBOHYDRATES" IN FOOD: QUICK RULE OF THUMB	
FOOD	**CARBOHYDRATES**
Bread and cereal serving (l slice bread, or ½ cup rice or pasta, or 1 ounce dry cereal)	About 15 grams
Starchy vegetable serving (½ cup)	About 15 grams
Fruit serving (½ cup, or 1 small to medium whole fruit)	About 10 to 15 grams
Vegetable serving (½ cup cooked or raw)	About 5 grams
Milk serving (l cup)	About 12 grams

Have You Ever Wondered

. . . how you can avoid "hitting the wall"? When endurance athletes run out of glucose, they're too tired to continue exerting themselves. To maintain your supply for as long as possible for endurance sports, follow an eating regimen that's high in carbohydrates. Have a sports drink if your workout lasts an hour or more. Eat a carbohydrate-rich snack right afterward when your body can store glycogen at a faster rate. Regular physical training also helps; your muscles adapt, gradually storing more glycogen for intense workouts.

Carbohydrate Loading

Your muscles and liver store glycogen—but only a limited amount—which must be replaced after each bout of exercise. Endurance athletes worry that they may "hit the wall," or feel extremely fatigued, before finishing. When this happens they've run out of glycogen.

The more glycogen you store, the longer it lasts. Carbohydrate loading (or glycogen loading) may help you "stockpile" two to three times more glycogen in your muscles for extended activity. Carbohydrate loading won't make you pedal harder or run faster. But it may help you perform longer before getting tired.

How do you "load up" your muscles? Combine rest and eating extra carbohydrates.

● For several days before an endurance event, gradually decrease training. By tapering off on your exercise, your muscles rest, so they can "stock up" glycogen.

● For three days before the event, gradually increase your carbohydrate calories, mostly complex carbohydrates, to 65 to 70 percent of your energy intake *without* increasing your total calorie intake.

Until recently, some endurance athletes followed a week-long regimen of carbohydrate loading. But three days of rest and extra carbohydrates are simpler and just as effective for most athletes.

Reminders: In your normal training diet, 60 to 65 percent of your energy should come from carbohydrates. Whole grains, cereal, legumes, and starchy vegetables are good sources of complex carbohydrates.

You should also know that carbohydrate loading is most effective with trained athletes. Generally having more muscle, their bodies have more capacity to store extra glycogen. "Occasional" or "weekend" athletes shouldn't expect the same results.

What sports should you "carb load" for? If you're a trained athlete, try it for either endurance events such as marathons and triathlons that last longer than ninety minutes, or for all-day events such as swim meets, a series of tennis matches, distance bicycling, or soccer games. For shorter events, a normal, carbohydrate-rich approach to eating supplies enough glycogen.

Caution: Carbohydrate loading is not advised for school-age children or teens. If you have diabetes or high blood triglycerides, talk to your doctor and a registered dietitian before trying this regimen.

Low-Fat Eating, Still Best!

Fat also fuels working muscles. In fact, it's a more concentrated energy source. And it performs other body functions, such as transporting fat-soluble vitamins and providing essential fatty acids. For good health, consume fat as one source of fuel. Rather than try to eat almost "fat-free," be smart: low in saturated fat and moderate in your fat intake.

Fat as Fuel

As an energy source, fat helps power activities of longer duration such as hiking or marathon running. Because fat doesn't convert to energy as fast as carbohydrates, fat doesn't power quick energy spurts such as returning a tennis serve or running a 100-yard dash.

Unlike glycogen, fat needs oxygen for energy metabolism. That's why endurance sports, fueled in part by fat, are called aerobic activities. "Aerobic" means with oxygen, and aerobic activities require a continuous intake of oxygen. The more you train, the more easily you breathe during longer activity; the oxygen you take in helps convert fat to energy.

No matter where it comes from—carbohydrates, proteins, or fats—your body stores extra energy as body fat. These fat stores supply energy for aerobic activity. Even if you're lean, you likely have enough fat

stores to fuel prolonged or endurance activity. You don't need to eat more fat!

For Athletes: How Much Fat?

Advice for athletes is the same as that for all healthy people: eat a diet low in saturated fat and cholesterol and moderate in total fat. To get enough calories for sports, yet not too much fat, 20 to 30 percent of your total calories from fat is a good guideline. Most of your food energy—60 to 65 percent—should come from carbohydrates. With a high-fat diet your carbohydrate or protein intake may come up short.

Athletes who consume too little fat, often to keep weight and body fat down, may risk a shortfall in food energy; young athletes may not consume enough essential fatty acids for normal growth and development. Among female athletes—often dancers, gymnasts, and skaters—a very-low-fat diet may interfere with menstrual cycles and pose lifelong health implications.

Do you burn a lot of energy? Since your calorie needs are higher, your total fat intake is probably higher, too. That's often true for football linemen and weight lifters, who may use 4,000 calories or more a day. Still, fats shouldn't contribute more than 30 percent of your total energy.

Have You Ever Wondered

. . . if eating a candy bar right before rigorous activity supercharges your body? No; even though carbohydrates supply energy, a candy bar won't supply extra energy right away. A high-carbohydrate diet for *several days before* physical activity makes the real difference.

For endurance activities of ninety minutes or longer, a sugary snack or drink before exercise (or even during an event) may enhance your stamina. It slowly makes its way to your muscles as your glycogen stores get used up.

Keep your snack or drink small: no more than about 200 calories. Too much sugar may slow the time it takes water to leave your stomach, so your body won't replace fluids as quickly. Your best approach? Enjoy a sports drink. You'll consume a little sugar to fuel your muscles—but not too much to impair rehydration.

Action plan. Do you need to cut back on fat? If so, get more food energy from carbohydrates. Remember that fat isn't stored as muscle glycogen; "carbs" are. Here's one strategy for cutting fat and boosting carbohydrates: Eat a baked potato more often than fries. Replace the fat calories you didn't eat from fries with a slice of bread, a good source of "carbs."

For more about fat in a healthful eating plan, and for ways to moderate fat in your food choices, see chapter 3, "Fat Facts."

Protein—More Is Not Necessarily Better

Athlete or not, you need protein. But what's enough? Is more protein better? This nutrient needs no special attention just because you're physically active or building muscle. When it comes to overall fitness or strength building, extra protein—beyond the amount recommended—offers no added performance benefits.

Your body uses protein for a wide range of purposes: to build and repair body tissues; to make enzymes, hormones, and other body chemicals; to transport nutrients; to make your muscles contract; and to regulate body processes such as water balance. If you don't consume enough carbohydrates for your high-energy demands, your body uses protein for energy instead. That's counterproductive to your physical goals!

Although protein supplies energy, extra amounts aren't your best fuel. Extra protein is stored as fat anyway, and not used for energy—if you've already consumed enough food energy. For anyone, protein should supply only 12 to 15 percent of overall energy intake.

Most athletes need just slightly more protein than nonathletes do. Because athletes usually eat more, they easily get what they need.

How Much Protein?

How much protein do you need for sports? Base the amount on your body weight, not your energy need.

● Nonathletes need slightly less than 0.5 gram of protein per pound of body weight.

● For most recreational exercisers, 0.5 to 0.75 gram of protein per pound of body weight is enough. (The upper end of the range is recommended for athletes involved in strength or speed training.) For a 150-pound athlete that adds up to about 75 to 115 grams of protein each day . . . and just 2 to 4 ounces more meat, chicken, or fish a day than recommended for nonathletes. As a point of reference, 3 ounces of lean beef supply about 30 grams of protein; 8 ounces of milk supply 8 grams of protein; and even a slice of bread has 2 grams of protein or more. (*Note:* More than 1 gram of protein per pound of body weight isn't advised.)

● Adult competitive athletes need 0.6 to 0.9 gram of protein per pound of body weight. Adults building muscle mass, including weight lifters and football players, may need more: 0.7 to 0.9 gram of protein daily per pound. Teen athletes need enough for growth and muscle building: 0.9 to 1 gram of protein per pound.

Source for protein needs: N. Clark, *Nancy Clark's Sport Nutrition Guidebook,* 2nd ed. (Champaign, Ill.: Human Kinetics, 1997).

Muscle Myths

You've likely heard the long-held myth that extra protein builds more muscle. In truth, only athletic training builds muscle strength and size. Consuming more protein—from food or dietary supplements—won't make any difference. You've got to work your muscles!

Can amino acid supplements build muscle? Despite claims, amino acid supplements won't increase your muscle size or strength. By definition, amino acids are the building blocks of protein. Twenty different amino acids link together to make proteins in food and in body tissue. Food supplies amino acids in proportions your body needs. To your body, amino acids in supplements are no different from those in foods you already enjoy. And in food they "taste" better and likely cost much less.

Most athletes get enough protein—and enough amino acids—from food. Protein-rich foods supply other nutrients, too, while amino acid supplements supply only amino acids.

Caution about excess protein. Extra protein is *not* stored in your body for future use as protein. Instead, it's either used as energy or stored as body fat. A high-protein diet also may be high in fat.

Too much protein or amino acids can be harmful. Side effects include metabolic imbalance, toxicity, nervous system disorders, and perhaps kidney problems. No research supports any benefits from the amino acids arginine or lysine for muscle growth.

When you consume excess protein, you need more water to excrete the urea, a waste product formed when protein turns to body fat. So excess protein increases the chances of dehydration—and increases the need to urinate. That's an inconvenience during a workout.

Bottom line: To build muscle, consume enough calories from "carbs," follow advice for protein from food (no need for extra), and train regularly.

For more about substances touted for high performance see "Ergogenic Aids: No Substitute for Training" at the end of this chapter.

Protein-Rich Foods: How Much?

The average American diet supplies more than enough protein. Two or three servings (just 6 to 7 ounces total) of lean meat, poultry, fish, eggs, beans, nuts, or seeds daily, along with protein from dairy foods and grain products, supply enough for most athletes. Athletes involved in endurance sports and weight lifters need somewhat more: three to four servings of lean meat or alternatives daily; remember, a serving is just about 3 ounces!

Good protein sources include lean meat, poultry, and fish; milk, cheese, and yogurt; eggs; beans and tofu; and nuts, seeds, and peanut butter. Cereal, breads, and vegetables also contain smaller amounts of protein—about 2 to 3 grams of protein per Pyramid serving; *check chapter 10 for serving sizes.* If you're a vegetarian, you can consume enough protein for rigorous activity; just choose foods carefully.

For more about protein and amino acids see "Protein Power" in chapter 20.

Vitamins and Minerals: Sense and Nonsense

Vitamins and minerals trigger body processes for physical performance. Although not an energy source, some help produce energy from carbohydrates, fats, and proteins. Some help your muscles relax and contract. Others are part of hemoglobin in blood that carries oxygen to cells to power aerobic activity. *For more about their role in health see chapter 4, "Vitamins, Minerals, and Phytonutrients: Variety on Your Plate!"*

If you burn more energy, you need more of some vitamins and minerals. Just eating more food probably provides the extra. In fact, an athlete with a hearty appetite has a better chance of consuming enough vitamins and minerals than someone who's less active and so eats less. However, athletes who try to lose weight by consuming too few calories or eliminating whole food groups are at greater risk for vitamin and mineral deficiencies.

For enough vitamins and minerals, eat a wide variety of foods from all five food groups of the Food Guide Pyramid in chapter 10.

Electrolytes? Sweat 'Em!

Your sweat is made of water along with three minerals known as electrolytes: sodium, chloride, and potassium. Among their many functions, electrolytes help maintain your body's water balance—a critical function for athletes. They also help your muscles, including your heart muscle, contract and relax. And they help transmit nerve impulses.

Taste the sweat on your upper lip. You know how salty it can be! As you perspire during a physical workout, your body loses small amounts of electrolytes, mostly sodium. Most athletes replace sodium and other electrolytes just through foods they normally eat. Be assured that the average American consumes more than enough sodium to replace losses from perspiration—no need for extra sodium or salt tablets. When you perspire heavily, focus your attention on extra fluids instead.

Have You Ever Wondered ?

. . . if athletes benefit from extra chromium? No, but misleading claims about chromium picolinate, which is a dietary supplement, have raised the question. No scientific evidence shows that taking a chromium supplement improves physical performance, builds muscle, burns body fat, or prolongs youth. For that matter, the role of chromium in your overall health isn't well understood, although early research suggests benefits to some people with diabetes or glucose intolerance.

Whole-grain foods, ready-to-eat cereals, beans, apples, and peanuts are some food sources of chromium; most people get enough from their normal diet. Supplements aren't advised; chromium supplements, for example, may interfere with the work of iron in the blood.

Endurance athletes, who sweat heavily for long periods, may need to replace sodium and other electrolytes. Again, salt tablets aren't advised; they may cause stomach irritation, promote dehydration, and affect performance. Instead, a sports drink with electrolytes, or salty foods, such as crackers and cheese, probably offer enough. Sodium from those sources helps speed rehydration. *See "Sports Drinks?" earlier in this chapter.*

For more about electrolytes see "Sodium: You Need Some!" in chapter 7.

About Iron

Athletes: your muscle cells need iron to produce energy! Iron is part of hemoglobin, the part of red blood cells that carries oxygen to your body cells. Oxygen is used in energy metabolism, specifically for aerobic activities where fat converts to energy. An iron shortfall, even if it's small, can affect your physical performance.

The Recommended Dietary Allowance (RDA) for iron is 18 milligrams daily for premenopausal women and 8 milligrams daily for men. Premenopausal women have a higher iron need because of iron losses in monthly menstrual periods. For teens it's 15 milligrams of iron a day for females and 11 milligrams of iron for males. How much is too much? The Tolerable Upper Intake Level (UL) is 45 milligrams of iron per day for ages fourteen and over.

Getting enough iron may be an issue—especially if you're female, or if most of your iron comes from foods of plant origin such as legumes and grains. Plant sources of iron aren't absorbed as efficiently as iron from animal sources. To improve its absorption, eat these foods with a vitamin C-rich food such as citrus fruit.

Even if you consume enough iron, you may be iron-depleted if you're involved in endurance sports. Prolonged exercise such as marathon running and long-distance bicycling promotes iron loss. With more exercise you sweat more, losing some iron through perspiration. Endurance athletes may lose iron through urine, feces, and intestinal bleeding. If you're an endurance athlete, have your iron status checked periodically.

All experts agree that athletes need plenty of iron-containing foods. Good sources include lean red meat, dark poultry meat, iron-fortified cereals, and legumes.

Talk to your doctor or a registered dietitian about taking a multivitamin supplement with iron, especially if you're involved in rigorous, prolonged activity. That's especially important for women. *Be aware that taking large doses of an iron supplement can be harmful to those with a rare genetic disorder called hemochromatosis; see "Iron" in chapter 4.*

For more about iron and its food sources see "Iron: A Closer Look" in chapter 4 and "Menstrual Cycle: More Iron for Women" in chapter 17.

Calcium and Weight-Bearing Exercise: Bone-Building Duo

Calcium and weight-bearing exercise: they're a winning combination for building and maintaining strong, healthy bones. Your goal? To maximize your calcium stores early in life, then maintain that level to later minimize the loss that comes with age.

Consuming enough calcium, at least 1,000 to 1,300 milligrams a day, depending on your age, offers protection against bone loss. Weight-bearing activity such as running, cross-country skiing, tennis, and soccer promotes the deposit of calcium into the matrix, or structure, of bones. While swimming and cycling offer many benefits of physical activity, they aren't weight-bearing, so they don't build bone.

Have You Ever Wondered

. . . if heavy training causes "sports anemia"? Perhaps, in the early stages of training. "Sports anemia" isn't really anemia. Instead it's often caused by increased blood volume in the early weeks of training. Iron concentration in blood dilutes slightly as your body adapts to more physical activity.

If you develop sports anemia, that's normal. It will disappear once your training program is off and running. Sports anemia probably won't affect performance or your blood's ability to carry oxygen to cells. Taking iron supplements won't make a difference.

Feeling tired may result from other aspects of training. If fatigue persists, or if you think you're at risk for other types of anemia, including iron-deficiency anemia, check with your doctor. *See "Anemia: 'Tired Blood'" in chapter 22.*

Calcium and Female Athletes. For female athletes (including teens), calcium is an issue. Why? To start with, many don't consume enough calcium for bone health.

High levels of physical activity, along with low levels of body fat and perhaps eating disorders, may cause menstrual periods to stop. For teens and young women this hinders the deposit of calcium into bones at a time when bones should be developing at their maximum rate. Female athletes who've stopped menstruating are at special risk for bone problems later in life.

Women: For your bones' sake, pay attention if your periods stop. Talk to your doctor. This is *not* a normal outcome of physical activity. Stress fractures caused by weakened bones may seriously affect your physical performance. And the long-range impact on bone health: increased osteoporosis risk. For bone health, your doctor may recommend a higher calcium intake, or perhaps a calcium supplement. *See "Osteoporosis: Reduce the Risks" in chapter 22.*

Supplements: Not "Energy-Charged"

Contrary to unscientific claims, there's no need for vitamin or mineral supplements for sports if you're already well nourished. The "extra" won't offer you an energy boost or added physical benefits—immediately or over the long run. Even if you are deficient in one or more nutrients, popping a supplement pill right before physical activity has no immediate effect.

Although B vitamins help your body use energy from food, no vitamin supplies energy. Since you likely eat more when you're physically active, you'll get the extra B vitamins you need from food—if your food choices are nutrient-dense. Just choose from the Pyramid's five food groups.

If you decide to take a supplement, choose a multivitamin/mineral supplement with no more than 100 percent of the Daily Values (DVs) for vitamins and minerals—unless your doctor prescribes more for special health reasons. *See "Dietary Supplements: What Are They?" in chapter 23.*

A High-Performance Diet

Training that includes healthful eating prepares you to achieve and maintain your strength, flexibility, and endurance. What's the best training diet? One that's

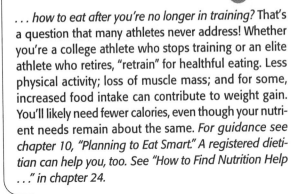

Have You Ever Wondered

... how to eat after you're no longer in training? That's a question that many athletes never address! Whether you're a college athlete who stops training or an elite athlete who retires, "retrain" for healthful eating. Less physical activity; loss of muscle mass; and for some, increased food intake can contribute to weight gain. You'll likely need fewer calories, even though your nutrient needs remain about the same. *For guidance see chapter 10, "Planning to Eat Smart." A registered dietitian can help you, too. See "How to Find Nutrition Help . . ." in chapter 24.*

varied, moderate, and balanced. Sound familiar? It's high in carbohydrates, with enough proteins, vitamins, minerals, and not too much fat. High-performance eating is appropriate for all physically active people, not just those training for sports.

The Athlete's Pyramid

Except for food energy, healthful eating for athletics and for rigorous active living doesn't differ much from advice for nonathletes. Both on- and off-season, the Food Guide Pyramid offers the best eating guidelines. Because it's flexible, it works, no matter how much energy you need or what sport you choose. There's no single eating plan for sports.

From chapter 10, you're well aware that the Pyramid categorizes foods into five groups, each with a serving range. Fats, oils, and sweets fit in the Pyramid tip, with the advice to eat sparingly. From the bottom to the top of the serving ranges, food choices from the Pyramid can supply 1,600 to 2,800 calories, depending on your energy needs.

For many athletes, energy needs are higher—as many as 6,000 calories a day, for example, for some football players. To meet higher energy demands, choose more servings of nutrient-dense, carbohydrate-rich foods, mostly from the Grains Group and the Vegetable and Fruit Groups of the Food Guide Pyramid. In contrast, although a high-fat diet offers plenty of concentrated energy (from fat), it carries risks for heart disease—even for highly active people. *For more about the Pyramid, serving amounts, and serving sizes see "The Food Guide Pyramid: Your Healthful Eating Guide" in chapter 10.*

An added reminder: Drink enough fluids during training. It's a good time to practice drinking "on schedule," not just for thirst.

Especially for Children

You've heard that today's kids don't move enough. Yet many do enjoy vigorous play or competitive sports. And their food and beverage choices power all they do: first and foremost, for growth and development, and second, for the added demands of physical activity.

Nutrients for active kids. The Food Guide Pyramid applies to food choices for all kids. Except for calories and fluids, the nutrient needs for child athletes are about the same as for child nonathletes.

Food energy for active kids. Energy needs depend on the child's age, body size, and the sport. Estimated energy needs for children ages seven to ten are 2,000 calories a day. For kids ages eleven to fourteen, it's more: 2,500 calories a day for boys and 2,200 calories a day for girls. Active kids may need more to fuel activity.

Does your highly active child consume enough food energy? Here's a clue: Watch his or her performance. Children who tire easily may not be eating enough. Another clue: Monitor your child's growth with your physician. If your child is growing normally, his or her energy (caloric) intake is likely okay. If you're still unsure, ask your doctor to refer you to a registered dietitian who can help you create an eating plan that matches your child's energy needs.

Have You Ever Wondered

. . . where to get nutrition advice for athletic performance—or to find out if your current food choices help or hinder your training? Talk to a registered dietitian, perhaps with a specialty in sports nutrition, or other qualified expert for help in determining your energy needs, evaluating your eating plan, and strategizing ways to eat for peak performance. Be aware that "personal trainer" isn't a regulated professional specialty. Some trainers are highly qualified exercise specialists; others aren't.

Weight: For Child Athletes

For all children, normal growth and development should be the top priority. Their weight should never be manipulated to meet goals required for sports!

Remember, child athletes aren't the same as teen and adult athletes. Because they're growing and because their growth spurts aren't always predictable, their body composition can't be judged in the same way. At certain times—for example, before puberty—a child's body naturally stores more body fat to prepare for the next growth spurt. And each child matures at his or her own time and rate.

An eating approach for sports can't change the genetic "body clock" and so speed up physical changes that enhance athletic performance. Supplements and ergogenic aids that are promoted to build muscle, prevent fat gain, or improve performance are never appropriate for children and teens! *For more about healthful eating during the childhood years see "Eating ABCs for School-Age Children" in chapter 16.*

Always talk to your doctor about the best weight for your child. An inaccurate assessment may result in a weight goal that isn't healthy.

For more information about body weight see "Compete in a Weight Category?" later in this chapter.

Fluids: caution for kids. Children are more likely to get overheated from strenuous activity. As a result, they're at greater risk for dehydration than teens and adults. Even when children play actively in the backyard, they need plenty of fluids.

Why is the risk for dehydration higher? Because kids don't perspire as much as teens and adults; a kid's body's "air conditioning" system is less effective. Kids generate more body heat with exercise, too. A child's "thermostat" doesn't adjust as quickly during exercise in hot weather. Protective gear used in many sports, such as hockey and football, hinders their bodies' ability to cool off, too.

To protect children from becoming dehydrated:

● Encourage them to drink plenty of cool fluids before, during, and after physical activities.

● Offer regular fluid breaks (every fifteen minutes) and ensure that fluids are readily available. Perhaps give them a water bottle. Once they're thirsty, they're already on the way to dehydration.

● Weigh them before and after exercise, then replace fluids: 2 to 3 cups per pound of weight loss.

● Supervise them carefully when they're active, especially on hot days, when fluid needs are even greater.

During Pregnancy and Breast-feeding

Pregnancy. With their doctor's approval, active women may continue their sport—at least in the earlier part of pregnancy. Less active women may initiate low-level activities gradually—again with their doctor's approval. Being physically active during pregnancy offers many benefits, among them a psychological lift, optimal weight gain, better aerobic fitness, and an easier labor and delivery

If you're a pregnant woman, or planning for pregnancy, ask your doctor about precautions. Overheating your body early in pregnancy can affect the development of your unborn baby. (**Caution:** If you use a hot tub after exercise to relax—a fetus can be overheated in the hot tub, too, without you knowing.) If you have anemia, hypertension, diabetes, and other health problems, rigorous activity during pregnancy may not be advised.

All the nutritional issues that relate to a healthy pregnancy apply to female athletes, too. The guidelines? Eat a varied and balanced diet—with enough energy to support your pregnancy, your own needs, and the demands of physical activity. If your energy intake is too low, you may not gain enough weight and your baby may not grow adequately.

Fluid replacement, always important, has even more health implications now. During pregnancy you need more fluids as your own and your baby's blood volume increases. If you don't drink enough, you're at greater risk for dehydration and overheating.

Breast-feeding. With a doctor's guidance, most women can engage in sports or some other form of regular physically activity if they're breast-feeding.

Breast-feeding itself requires an additional 500 calories for milk production. With more physical activity, you need more; the actual amount depends on the duration and the intensity of your workout.

The Food Guide Pyramid offers guidance for planning a varied, balanced, and moderate eating plan during breast-feeding—whether you're an athlete or not.

Your needs for fluids increase during breast-feeding, too. Without exercise, you need about 3 cups more, or at least 11 cups daily. When you work out, drink even more fluids to avoid dehydration.

For more about healthful eating and physical activity during pregnancy and breast-feeding see "Congratulations! You're Expecting!" and "For Those Who Breast-feed" in chapter 17. Talk to a registered dietitian, too, for guidance when you're physically active or involved in sports.

For Vegetarians

Are you among the athletes and physically active people who choose a vegetarian eating style? Vegetarian eating can provide enough fuel and nutrients for peak athletic performance—if you choose meals and snacks carefully.

As with any high-performance diet, carbohydrate-rich foods should be the focal point of an eating plan—usually not a problem for vegetarians. Follow the advice from the Food Guide Pyramid (vegetarian-style). And focus on a varied and balanced diet, not on avoiding fat.

If you're a vegetarian who consumes dairy foods and perhaps eggs, getting enough of most nutrients, including protein, poses little challenge. If you're a vegan who eats no foods of animal origin, choose carefully to ensure adequate intake of protein, vitamin B_{12}, iron, zinc, calcium, and perhaps energy (for muscular athletes, who use more energy).

For some vegetarian athletes, consuming enough energy—from an eating plan of bulky, plant-based foods—is a challenge. Eating six to eight meals or snacks a day might be a practical solution.

For guidance on healthful vegetarian eating see chapter 20, "The Vegetarian Way."

Different Sports, Different Approaches to Eating?

No matter what sport you choose, the Food Guide Pyramid is your guide for high-performance eating. Choose enough servings for the food energy you need.

The most significant nutrition difference from sport to sport relates to energy. The duration and intensity of activity, as well as body size, make the difference.

● A 200-pound football player probably uses more energy than a 90-pound gymnast.

● A baseball player uses less energy than a soccer player, who's almost constantly in motion.

● A cross-country skier or a long-distance runner likely uses more energy overall (taken from glycogen stores) than a tennis player or a golfer, who uses spurts of energy (powered mostly by glucose).

Every sport demands adequate fluids to replace perspiration and breathing losses, too. In sports with prolonged, intense activity, athletes may perspire more—especially during hot weather.

Endurance Sports

Both in training and in competition, endurance sports—cross-country and marathon running, cross-country skiing, distance bicycling, field hockey, long-distance swimming, and soccer—require more energy. Activity that lasts longer than an hour depletes glycogen stores. Fortunately, for a well-trained athlete, the energy source shifts, as the body burns stored fat efficiently. In addition, endurance athletes may use some protein for energy. However, endurance athletes do not need to consume more protein than strength-training athletes; endurance athletes should aim for 0.6 to 0.8 gram of protein per pound of body weight.

Energy needed for endurance sports depends on body size, duration of activity, and overall effort. For the elite athlete that may be as high as 4,000 to 6,000 calories daily, chosen from a high-carbohydrate diet, with 60 to 65 percent energy from "carbs." Best sources: foods in the Grains Group and in the Vegetable and Fruit Groups of the Food Guide Pyramid.

Nonendurance Sports

Nonendurance sports—baseball, bowling, golf, martial arts, softball, speed skating, sprint swimming, tennis, track and field, volleyball, and weight lifting—are fueled by short bursts of energy, perhaps just for two or three minutes or even several seconds. While these sports take an intense, all-out effort, they don't use as much energy overall, simply because their duration is shorter.

Still, nonendurance sports might be of high or moderate intensity. The overall energy demand depends not only on the duration but also on the intensity and the athlete's body size.

Except for calories, nutrient needs for athletes

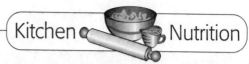

Food for Your Training Table

For training meals that are high in carbohydrates, adequate in protein, and moderate in fat, try these mealtime combinations:

● Chili made with kidney beans and lean beef.

● Vegetable stir-fry with lean pork cubes, chicken, shrimp, or tofu served over rice (go easy on the added oil).

● Soft corn tortillas filled with vegetarian refried beans and topped with tomato sauce or salsa, and cheese. (On a can of refried beans, check the fat content on the label's Nutrition Facts.)

● Grilled fish kebobs (chunks of fresh fish alternating with cherry tomatoes, green peppers, and pineapple on a skewer) served on brown rice.

● Lentils (alone or mixed with lean ground beef) in spaghetti sauce on whole-wheat pasta.

● Green peppers stuffed with a mixture of lean ground turkey and brown rice. Add a mixed green salad, and finish the meal with angel food cake topped with strawberries.

● Strips of lean roast sirloin served with a baked potato, steamed carrots and cauliflower, and whole-wheat rolls.

● Chicken salad (made with reduced-calorie mayonnaise, grated lemon peel, and tarragon) on rye bread with tomato slices and sprouts. Serve with vegetable soup, whole-wheat crackers, and cantaloupe slices.

involved in endurance and nonendurance sports are about the same. Again, the Pyramid offers a healthful eating guideline. And 60 to 65 percent of overall energy should come from carbohydrate-rich foods.

Making Weight

Most athletes are concerned about their weight. For example, in football, extra weight may be an advantage for a defensive lineman. For swimmers, some body fat may offer buoyancy. And for gymnasts and skaters, a slim body may add to the aesthetics of performance.

For some athletes, weight cycling is an issue. Those who weigh more during their off-season may need to drop a few pounds for training and competition. Others need to "bulk up," perhaps to train and compete in contact sports. Either way, what's the healthful, most effective approach to your best competitive weight?

Whatever your sport, for your peak performance, enter the competitive season at your best weight. Instead of trying to "make weight" quickly to train and compete, stay at your best weight year-'round.

Body Composition: Fit, Not Fat

For athletic performance, your body composition is more important than your weight—even if you compete in a weight category. (That's true for nonathletes, too.) Health risks go up as the proportion of body fat increases beyond "healthy." A lean, muscular body has benefits beyond athletics and good looks, to overall fitness for life.

What's healthy for athletes? Male athletes typically have body fat values of 5 to 12 percent; female athletes, 10 to 20 percent. The difference depends on the sport and even differences within a sport. For nonathletes, body fat levels of 15 to 18 percent for men and 20 to 25 percent for women are considered acceptable. Body fat levels that dip below 4 percent for men and 10 percent for women suggest an eating disorder. *See "Body Fat Varies by Sport!" on this page.*

You can't measure your body fat or composition accurately on your own. Instead, seek a trained health expert who uses professional methods for measurement, such as skinfold measurements, underwater weighing, and bioelectrical impedance (done with a computer). A registered dietitian or an exercise physiologist also can target the goals for a healthy weight and body composition (percent body fat) for your best physical performance. *See "How to Find Nutrition Help" in chapter 24. For more about body composition see "Body Weight, Body Fat" in chapter 2.*

Lose Fat, Not Muscle

Do you need to lose weight? Choose an approach that helps you lose fat, not muscle. Start your weight loss strategies ahead—well before training and competition. Then maintain your healthy weight so you have energy and strength when you need them most.

Body Fat Varies by Sport!*

What's the right body composition for sports? That depends. Body fat ranges vary from athlete to athlete, sport to sport, and even for specific positions or events on a team. For elite, or skilled, athletes, these are average percentages of body fat. These averages aren't necessarily goals or desirable levels of body fat for you as an athlete involved in one of these sports.

ATHLETES	% BODY FAT MALE	% BODY FAT FEMALE
Baseball/softball players	8–14	12–18
Basketball players	6–12	10–16
Body builders	5–8	6–12
Cyclers	5–11	8–15
Football players	6–18	——
Gymnasts	5–12	8–16
Skaters	5–12	8–16
Skiers	7–15	10–18
Soccer players	6–14	10–18
Swimmers	6–12	10–18
Tennis players	6–14	10–20
Volleyball players	7–15	10–18
Wrestlers	5–16	——

*For elite, or the most skilled, athletes.

Source: Reprinted by permission from J. H. Wilmore and D. L. Costill, *Physiology of Sport and Exercise* 2nd ed. (1999).

Getting the Lean Advantage

Most important, set a weight goal that's realistic and healthy for you—one that considers your body composition and that offers the best competitive edge for your sport. If you need to drop a few pounds, make your weight loss gradual: ½ to 1 pound a week. To lose about 1 pound a week, cut back on your day's energy intake by about 250 calories and boost your training to burn 250 calories more. (*Hint:* 1 pound of body fat equals 3,500 calories.) To cut back on calories, follow guidelines of the Food Guide Pyramid, but eat fewer servings within the recommended range. *See "The Athlete's Pyramid" earlier in this chapter.*

Remember that carbohydrates are the fuel that your working muscles need. Get most of your energy from complex carbohydrates: grain products, legumes, vegetables, and fruits. Cut back on higher-fat foods.

For weight loss, physical activity does more than burn calories. Exercise boosts your metabolic rate, or the rate at which your body uses energy. Muscles you build with more activity use more energy than body fat does, too.

Be aware that a quick weight-loss regimen that's low in calories may interfere with your physical performance, first by shorting your energy supply. With many quick regimens you'll likely lose muscle, along with body fat, and deplete your stores of muscle glycogen. Depending on your approach, your weight loss may be partly water loss—a problem for athletes, who need to keep adequately hydrated.

In your off-season training program, learn to maintain weight so you stay at the best weight for your sport. *To lose weight in a healthful way see "Weight Management: Strategies That Work!" in chapter 2.*

"Leanest" Isn't Always Better!

The notion that you can never be too thin or too lean may compromise your physical performance! Athletes obsessed with a lean, thin body risk eating disorders and all the dangers (some life-threatening) that accompany severe weight loss. Among the other concerns, for athletes, a body that's too lean may not sweat and cool down properly. The chance for dehydration goes up, and physical endurance is reduced.

If you, someone you train with, or your child shows signs of an eating disorder, seek help. Talk to the person about your concern, as well as the family, friends, or the coach. A registered dietitian also can offer an expert perspective on eating disorders. *For more insight and guidance see "Disordered Eating: Problems, Signs, and Help" in chapter 2.*

Compete in a Weight Category?

If you're a wrestler, weight lifter, oarsman, boxer, or body builder who competes in a weight category, body weight may be critically important. Being the heaviest competitor in a lower weight class often is believed to provide a competitive edge. Even an extra pound or two may make a difference in weight class or performance.

For good health, endurance, strength, and best performance, the better advice is to compete in a weight class that's realistic for your body composition. And maintain your optimal weight throughout the competitive season, rather than cycle to "make weight" in unhealthful ways for competition.

Water weight is *not* unnecessary body weight, so sweating off pounds to make weight for wrestling—or any other sport—only hinders performance. Because it leads to dehydration, losing as little as 2 to 3 percent of body weight from sweat (e.g., 3 or 4 pounds, or 6 to 8 cups of fluid, in a 150-pound athlete) can be very dangerous. Even a 1 percent weight loss from fluid loss makes a difference!

Fasting, or drastically cutting back on food, isn't healthy or performance-enhancing, either! And feeling hungry is distracting. More importantly, with fasting, your body won't store the muscle glycogen you need as energy for training and competition. A careful healthful eating plan—that starts well before "weigh in"—is the smartest way to reach and stay in your weight class. Without ongoing, sensible weight management you might continue with the same weight dilemma and "weight cycle" for the next competition—and the next and the next!

Gain Muscle, Not Fat

Hockey and football are among the sports where extra body weight aids performance. Trying to "bulk up" too fast, however, may put more fat on your body than muscle—especially if you eat extra calories without enough exercise. If you're already involved in strenuous training, gaining weight may not be as easy as it sounds. You may use energy faster than you consume it!

To build muscle, engage in strength-building activity and consume enough energy from food. Contrary to popular myth, you don't need more protein, just more energy from a variety of nutritious foods. *See "Muscle Myths" earlier in this chapter.*

As with weight loss, the key to weight gain is "gradual and steady": about ½ to 1 pound a week. To get the extra energy to fuel exercise and build muscle:

- Eat frequent minimeals.

- Increase portions at mealtime.

- Snack between meals.

- Get most of your extra energy from nutrient-dense, high-carbohydrate foods—for example, granola or muesli topped with nuts or dried fruit.

● As an extra meal or snack, try liquid meal supplements for convenient, high-carbohydrate nourishment.

For guidance on healthy weight gain see "When You Want to Gain" in chapter 2.

The Game Plan

It's the day of the big event. You're excited and perhaps a bit anxious. You've trained hard. What should you eat to maximize your performance? Your game plan now—what you eat before, during, and after competition or a heavy workout—makes a difference.

For endurance events, think farther ahead—before your pre-event meal. Several days beforehand, you might eat more carbohydrates and gradually rest your muscles. In that way, you'll store extra muscle glycogen and won't tire as quickly during the event. *See "Carbohydrate Loading" in this chapter.*

In fact, for any sport, eat for peak performance well ahead. Most energy for competition comes from foods you ate earlier in the week, not from your pre-event meal. For training, eat plenty of carbohydrates, moderate amounts of protein, not much fat, and drink plenty of fluids.

Remember that on competition day, even carefully planned meals can't make up for a poor training diet. Eat with fitness in mind all along the way.

Before You Compete

Before competition? Choose a pre-event meal or snack—light, easy to digest, high-carbohydrate—that matches your physical performance goals. In that way you can perform to your ability without tiring too soon. Eating helps prevent the distraction of hunger pangs. Although eating won't provide immediate energy, it can supply energy for exercise that lasts an hour or more. Drink enough, too, to fully hydrate your body before strenuous exercise.

The "right" pre-event meal or snack differs from athlete to athlete, event to event, and time of day. During your training, experiment with different foods, food combinations, amounts, and timing. And keep these guidelines in mind:

Timing. Finish eating one to four hours before your workout or competition. That allows enough time for food to digest so your stomach doesn't feel full or uncomfortable.

What about morning competition? Eat a hearty, high-carbohydrate dinner and bedtime snack the night before. Then in the morning, eat a light, high-carbohydrate meal or snack. Eating two hours before exercise helps replenish your liver glycogen and satisfy hunger.

Small meals. Choose a small meal or snack. The amount depends on what makes you feel comfortable.

High "carbs." Enjoy a high-"carb" meal or snack that's moderate in protein and low in fat. It gets digested and

Have You Ever Wondered

. . . if it's okay to compete on an empty stomach? You're better off eating. Research shows that food consumed within four hours of physical activity is used as fuel for working muscles. For morning events, eating is especially important for endurance. It replenishes liver glycogen and helps maintain your blood sugar level. So don't skip breakfast, just eat something light!

. . . what to eat before competition if you feel too nervous to eat? If you get pre-event jitters, drinking a liquid meal supplement or a fruit milkshake you make yourself might help. It provides the nutrients and the fluids needed for competition. And it might be more easily digested and absorbed than a full meal. Liquid meals also contribute fluids.

. . . if fructose tablets during prolonged exercise are a good energy source? Fructose isn't converted to energy as fast as glucose is; fructose converts to liver glycogen first. You're better off with a drink that offers glucose or sucrose. Fructose also can cause gastrointestinal distress (bloating, cramping, or diarrhea).

. . . if a "complete nutrition supplement," perhaps an energy bar or drink, or a power gel, will aid performance? Although certainly not "complete nutrition," energy bars and drinks may be an energy source, but not a meal replacement, for physical activity. Power gels supply "carbs," too, but usually few vitamins or minerals. A quick check of the Nutrition Facts on the label reveals their calorie and nutrient contribution. Although energy bars, drinks, or gels may be convenient during an endurance event, eat fruit or a starchy snack such as a bagel afterward instead.

Pre-Event Meals—for Starters

There's no single menu prescribed for pre-event eating, but these three high-carbohydrate menus show what you might eat before you compete:

MEAL 1	MEAL 2	MEAL 3
● 1 cup cereal	● 2 cups beef noodle soup	● 2 pancakes with 2 tbsp. syrup
● 1 banana	● 6 crackers	● 1 cup fat-free yogurt
● 8 oz. fat-free milk	● 1 medium baked potato	● ½ cup strawberries
● 1 bagel with 1 tbsp. jelly	● 1 cup vegetable juice	● 1 cup apple juice
● ¾ cup cranberry juice drink		

Calories

630	620	625

Carbohydrates

136 g	116 g	110 g

absorbed faster. (Consuming about ½ gram to 2 grams of carbohydrate per pound of body weight is about right.)

Make pasta, rice, potatoes, or bread the "center" of your plate. A high-fat meal may cause indigestion or nausea with heavy exercise. *See "Pre-Event Meals—for Starters" on this page and "'Carbo' Foods" in the Appendices.*

Contrary to common belief, eating small amounts of fat won't keep your body from storing muscle glycogen. You don't need to totally avoid fat. Just a little may make your food taste better.

No discomfort. Skip foods that may cause intestinal discomfort during competition: gas-causing foods such as beans, cabbage, onions, cauliflower, and turnips, and bulky, high-fiber foods such as raw fruits and vegetables with seeds and tough skin, bran, nuts, and seeds.

Familiar foods. Enjoy familiar foods and beverages. This isn't the time to try something new that may disagree with you.

Enough fluids. About two hours ahead, drink at least 2 cups of fluid. Then about fifteen minutes ahead, drink another 1 to 2 cups of fluids. Milk's okay before strenuous exercise. Stress and loss of body fluids—not milk—often slow saliva flow, causing "cotton mouth," or a dry mouth.

"Feel-good" foods. If a certain food or meal seems to enhance your performance, enjoy it—if you can fit it into your pre-event eating strategy.

During Competition

Nourishment during physical activity depends on your sport.

● *During most activities,* drinking plenty of fluids is the only real issue. Every fifteen or so minutes, you're wise to drink ½ to 1 cup of fluids.

● *During endurance sports of sixty minutes or more,* a slightly sweetened carbohydrate drink (sports drink) or snack may help maintain your blood sugar levels, boost your stamina, and enhance your performance. Thirty to 60 grams of carbohydrates an hour are advised.

Often sports drinks are easy to digest, especially if you're involved in intense activity. And they count as fluids, too. Their flavor may encourage their consumption as well, especially among children. Whether you choose a sports drink or a solid snack, perhaps orange slices, remember to also drink ½ to 1 cup of fluids every fifteen or so minutes!

● *During day-long events or regional tournaments,* snack on high-carbohydrate, low-fat foods. Between matches, sets, or other competitive events, these foods are among the many good choices: crackers, bagels, rice cakes, orange slices, apples, bananas, and fruit bars. Bring snacks along so you don't need to rely on a concessions stand. Consuming fluids all day long remains important.

After You Compete

From an exercise standpoint, your cool-down routine is just as important as your warm-up. And what you eat and drink after a workout is as important as your pre-event eating routine. Protect your health, recover physically and mentally from your activity—and build your endurance for next time.

Make fluids your first priority! First and foremost, after competition or a heavy workout, replace your fluid loss. The amount depends on how much weight you lose through exercise. Simply weigh yourself before and afterward; the difference is your water weight. For every pound you lose, drink at least 2 cups of fluid. And continue to drink fluids throughout the day until you return to your pre-exercise weight.

What fluids are best? Drink fluids with carbohydrates, such as juice or sports drinks. They replace fluids and help your body replenish muscle glycogen. You might try plain water, milk, and watery foods such a soup or watermelon, too. *See "Food: A Water Source" in chapter 8.*

Refuel your muscles with carbohydrates. Within the first several hours after competition or a heavy workout, eat a meal or a snack high in carbohydrates and low in fats and proteins. For muscle glycogen recovery, the sooner you eat, the better.

For every pound of body weight, strive for about ½ gram of carbohydrates. For example, if you weigh 150 pounds, eat at least 75 grams of carbohydrates. That's easy to do with a high-carbohydrate snack or meal. For strenuous exercise that lasts ninety minutes or longer, consume that much in carbohydrates within thirty minutes after exercise, then again about two hours later. *For some high-carbohydrate foods see "'Carbo' Foods" in the Appendices.*

If you aren't hungry right away, drink juice or a sports drink for fluids and "carbs." Because sports drinks are a diluted source of "carbs," you need to double the amount of sports drink to get the same amount of carbohydrates—for example, 32 ounces of a sports drink and 16 ounces of juice each supply about 50 grams of carbohydrates. When your hunger returns, enjoy a carbohydrate-rich meal or snack.

How about electrolytes? Through perspiration, you lose electrolytes such as sodium. Because the average American diet supplies more than enough, enjoy your meal—and perhaps a sports drink—after endurance sports. You'll get enough sodium and other electrolytes to replace your losses.

You don't need a salt tablet. It may cause cramping, dehydration, and stomach irritation. Concentrated amounts of salt cause the stomach to draw fluids from other parts of the body as they dilute the salt.

Ergogenic Aids: No Substitute for Training

"Blast your body with energy!". . . "Best muscle cell volumizers!" . . . "Guaranteed for fresh new muscle growth!". . . "Nutrition for faster muscle recovery and longer endurance!"

Of course, you want to make the most of every workout and increase your competitive edge. But do you take supplements without questioning their merits? It's easy to be lured by advertising claims that ergogenic aids (both dietary and hormonal supplements) improve strength, endurance, or recovery time, especially when anatomical graphics and charts make those claims appear so credible. Adding to the confusion, valid and invalid advice often appear side by side in fitness magazines.

"Ergogenic" means the potential to increase work output. Despite slick advertising and marketing, only proper training and all-out effort can do that.

So what about the "proven results"? Perceived performance benefits of ergogenic aids often come from individual reports or a misunderstanding of physiology itself, or from claims taken out of scientific context, rather than valid research findings. Their purported claims may be more psychological than physical. It's well documented that the side effects of many ergogenic aids ultimately may hinder performance and may cause harm, especially in the long run!

Dietary Supplements

A slew of dietary supplements—amino acid supplements, bee pollen, carnitine, chromium picolinate, creatine, ephedra, glutamine, HMB (beta-hydroxy beta methylbutyrate), and whey protein, among others, as well as many herbs—are promoted for better physical performance. Yet, they're effectiveness and safety are undetermined.

● *Amino acids.* Amino acid supplements such as arginine, branched-chain amino acids (BCAAs), and ornithine are often promoted to build muscle and increase fat loss among athletes. But most athletes consume more than enough amino acids from food, so these products are an unnecessary expense. *See "Muscle Myths" in this chapter.*

● *Carnitine.* Carnitine is a body chemical composed of two essential amino acids, lysine and methionine. As an ergogenic aid, carnitine has been promoted for more energy, aerobic power, and body fat reduction. However, the human body produces adequate amounts, and foods of animal origin are good sources. There's no need to take extra. *For more on amino acids see "Protein Power" in chapter 20.*

● *Chromium picolinate.* Chromium picolinate is promoted as an ergogenic aid for athletes, as well as an aid to weight loss. Because chromium is part of insulin, it plays a role in energy production. Deficiencies of chromium from food choices are rare, however. When chromium levels are normal, there doesn't appear to be any benefit from taking a supplement. In supplements, chromium levels are significantly higher than the Recommended Dietary Allowance (RDA). Excess levels may have adverse effects—and offer no benefits.

● *Creatine phosphate.* This ergogenic aid is promoted to increase muscle mass and strength, enhance energy, and delay fatigue. In fact, creatine is an amino acid that's made in the liver from other amino acids; the body makes an adequate supply. Research suggests that creatine supplements may increase muscle strength for anaerobic exercise; yet there's no research on its long-term effects. In addition, athletes tend to take larger doses than manufacturers recommend. Creatine is not advised for teenage athletes!

● *Pangamic acid.* Touted as vitamin B_{15}, it's not a vitamin at all. Instead it's an inconsistent mixture of substances, including some that are potentially hazardous. Although extolled as an energy enhancer for athletes, it has no proven benefits.

● *Spirulina.* Spirulina, a blue-green alga, is often touted as a high-energy food. It can offer nutrients to the diet, but it has no energy-producing qualities. Spirulina is high in protein and contains small amounts of vitamin B_{12}. However, much of its vitamin B_{12} is inactive and cannot be absorbed by humans.

● *Wheat germ and wheat germ oil.* Both products are promoted as ergogenic aids. Although no proven ben-

When You're on the Road

Planes, trains, and automobiles get you where you're going. But how do you keep physically active—or perhaps keep up a training regimen—when you travel? Plan ahead!

- Pack comfortable clothes and footwear, including workout clothes or a bathing suit. Take a jump rope, running or walking shoes, or plastic dumbbells you can fill with water. In that way you won't need special facilities to work out.

- Choose a hotel with exercise equipment, then make time to use it. Before you make your reservation, ask about the facilities: an indoor or outdoor pool; tennis courts; bicycle rentals; and gym equipment such as a treadmill, step machine, or rowing machine.

- If you belong to a health club at home, check ahead for membership benefits elsewhere.

- At the airport, wait for your flight by walking the concourse; skip people movers. On a long train or plane trip, walk up and down the aisle several times. Ask for an aisle seat so you won't have to climb over your fellow passengers. Do simple stretching exercises to avoid feeling stiff.

- Ask for an early wake-up call so you can get a jump start on your day with a thirty-minute walk or jog. Get a guidebook to map out your way—or the hotel's front desk may have a walking map.

- Skip the taxicab. If it's a safe, reasonable distance, walk to your business meeting, museums, shops, or restaurants in comfortable walking shoes.

- If you're driving, take regular breaks. Your passengers—including kids—will ride more comfortably after some physical activity.

- Check the local television guide for a televised workout or yoga stretching class. Or take along a tape player and exercise tape.

efits exist, there aren't any known side effects or adverse reactions from ingesting them. In fact, wheat germ supplies nutrients such as proteins, B vitamins, and vitamin E.

In addition to being costly, these supplements often are sold on the same shelf as vitamin/mineral supplements in dosages recommended by physicians— another point of confusion. *See chapter 23 for a discussion of other dietary supplements, including those described above.*

Hormonal Supplements

Hormonal supplements such as steroids and dehydroepiandrosterone (DHEA) are another type of dietary supplement. Why the concern about them? As a category of ergogenic aid, they're powerful drugs!

Teens should *never* use steroids. Contrary to many a young adolescent boy's wish, steroids won't bulk up muscles if he hasn't gone through puberty. And adolescents who use them may not grow to their normal height.

● *Muscle-building (or anabolic) steroids* are synthesized to act like testosterone, a male sex hormone. Steroids can help build bigger muscles—often at a physical price—and don't ensure physical performance.

Their use can have dangerous and often permanent side effects. For example, in men, steroids may cause acne, testicular damage, enlarged breasts, and a lower sperm count. Used by women, steroids may cause masculine qualities: a lower voice, facial hair, smaller breasts, and loss of (or irregular) menstrual cycle. Other potential risks: increased risk for injury, blood clots, and gastrointestinal problems as well as liver damage, heart disease, and cancer. Steroid use is banned by the International Olympic Committee and condemned by the American Academy of Pediatrics and the American College of Sports Medicine.

● *Dehydroepiandrosterone (DHEA),* sold as a safe alternative to anabolic steroids, is still an androgenic steroid, banned by the International Olympic Committee and the National Collegiate Athletic Association. Evidence doesn't back up the claims: to increase energy, decrease body fat, counteract stress, and slow aging. In the short run, DHEA also can have unpleasant side effects, including facial hair growth, acne, enlarged liver, rapid heartbeat, and testicular damage. With its potential effect on testosterone and estradiol (a female steroid produced in the ovaries) levels, its use may be risky for people with a family history of prostate or breast cancer.

Building muscle gradually through physical activity is still the healthful, time-honored, most effective, and fair approach! *For more information see "Muscle Myths" earlier in this chapter.*

Need more tips specific to eating for active living? Check here for "how-tos":

● Manage weight for sports sensibly—see chapter 2.

● Spot the signs of eating disorders in athletes—see chapter 2.

● Exercise safely during pregnancy—see chapter 17.

● Sort through claims for ergogenic dietary supplements—see chapter 23.

● Find a nutrition expert experienced in sports nutrition, especially if you're an elite or professional athlete, or if you have a health condition—see chapter 24.

CHAPTER 20

The Vegetarian Way

Pasta salad with vegetables. Polenta topped with homemade tomato sauce and freshly grated Parmesan cheese. Bean burritos. Portobello mushroom sandwich layered with stir-fried onions and peppers. Split-pea soup with rye bread. Veggie-cheese pizza. Barley-cheese stuffed peppers. Lentil curry. Bean curd lo mein.

Today's cookbooks, magazines, and restaurant menus are full of vegetarian dishes created with nutritious, flavorful food combinations. Whether you choose a vegetarian eating style or not, these dishes add food variety, interest, and flavor experiences to smart eating.

A plant-based diet isn't new. Yet today vegetarian eating styles and dishes are capturing more attention among consumers, health professionals, and the food industry. Have you noticed how many vegetarian products have hit the market, among them nut loafs, tofuburgers, veggie cheese, soyburgers, and sausage made from textured vegetable protein? Among the many reasons for a vegetarian way of eating: potential health benefits.

Being Vegetarian

What does it mean to be a vegetarian? For some, it's a way of eating; for others, a whole lifestyle. And nonvegetarians simply may enjoy the flavors and food variety in plant-based dishes—regularly or as an occasional switch from their everyday fare.

Why Vegetarian?

Vegetarian eating styles differ, as do the many reasons why people choose to become vegetarians. With today's focus on fitness, many cite health reasons. Others express concerns about the environment, compassion for animals, or their belief in nonviolence. For some, religious, spiritual, or ethical reasons define their strict vegetarian lifestyle. Several religions advocate vegetarian eating—for example, Hinduism and the Seventh-Day Adventist Church. For some, being a vegetarian reflects their ethical approach to addressing world hunger. Still others simply prefer the flavors and food mixtures of vegetarian dishes, and may recognize that a plant-based diet often costs less.

Health Benefits

Either choice—vegetarian or nonvegetarian eating—can supply enough nutrients and food substances to nourish you, promote your health, and help prevent health problems. No matter what your approach, the nutrition bottom line depends on your food choices over time. In fact, eating a vegetarian diet can be an easy way to follow the advice of the Dietary Guidelines for Americans.

Studies show a positive link between vegetarian eating and health. In general, the incidence of, or the death rate from, some health problems—heart disease, high blood pressure, type 2 diabetes, and some forms of cancer—tends to be lower among vegetarians.

Body mass index, an indication of overweight and obesity, is typically less, too. Among vegetarians, total blood cholesterol and LDL ("bad") cholesterol are usually lower; however, HDL ("good") cholesterol and triglyceride levels may or may not be.

Potential health-promoting benefits of vegetarian eating may come from the nutrients and phytonutrients (or plant substances) in the overall food choices. A vegetarian approach to eating tends to be low in saturated fat, cholesterol, and animal protein, and higher in complex carbohydrates, fiber, folate, carotenoids, and other phytonutrients. Those same qualities can come from a carefully chosen nonvegetarian diet.

Food choices may not be the only reason for the health benefits, however. Vegetarians often make other lifestyle choices that promote health, such as regular physical exercise, not smoking, and moderating ingestion of or avoiding alcoholic beverages.

Being vegetarian doesn't necessarily ensure a healthful eating style, however. Poorly planned, the chance for some nutritional deficiencies goes up. And like any way of eating, a vegetarian eating style also can be high in fat and cholesterol, low in fiber, or both. The nutritional content of a vegetarian style of eating depends on overall food choices over several days.

What Type?

In its broadest definition, being "vegetarian" means avoiding foods from animal sources. Instead, plant sources of food—grains, legumes, nuts, vegetables, and fruits—form the basis of the diet. That's what vegetarians have in common.

As a matter of choice, many vegetarians eat dairy products, and perhaps eggs. Others avoid meat, but eat fish or poultry, at least occasionally, or eat meat, fish, or poultry simply as they would a condiment or a side dish. Among today's "new vegetarians," only a small percent completely avoid foods of animal origin.

If you're a vegetarian, you may describe yourself in one of these ways:

- *Lacto-ovo-vegetarian,* who chooses an eating approach with eggs and dairy products but no meat, poultry, and fish. The prefix "lacto" refers to milk; "ovo" refers to eggs. Most vegetarians in the United States fit within this category.

- *Lacto-vegetarian,* who avoids meat, poultry, fish, and eggs (and egg derivatives such as albumin or egg whites) but eats dairy products.

- *Strict vegetarian, or vegan* (VEE-gahn or VEHJ-ahn), who follows an eating plan with no animal products: no meat, poultry, fish, eggs, milk, cheese, or other dairy products.

Vegans may avoid foods with animal products as ingredients, too: for example, *no* refried beans made with lard; *no* fries cooked in beef tallow; baked goods made *without* butter, eggs, or albumin (from eggs); *no* margarine made with whey or casein (from milk); *no* foods flavored with meat extracts; and no foods with gelatin (from animal bones and hooves). Some avoid honey, which is made by bees.

- *Semivegetarian,* who usually follows a vegetarian eating pattern but occasionally eats meat, poultry, or fish.

Have You Ever Wondered

. . . if "vegetarian" on a food label means "low-fat," too? No, it doesn't. Foods labeled as "vegetarian" on their package labeling—and on restaurant menus—may contain high-fat ingredients. Foods that can be higher in fat include textured soy patties and hot dogs, soy cheese, refried beans, and snack bars. Even tofu may have more fat than you'd think: 4 ounces (about ½ cup) has about 95 calories and 6 fat grams, mostly from polyunsaturated fats, compared with about 150 calories and 5 fat grams in 4 ounces of uncooked beef round steak. Read the Nutrition Facts panel on food labels to compare the calories and the nutrients in food.

. . . if a macrobiotic diet is healthful? No. A macrobiotic diet—an extremely restrictive diet with some grains, and perhaps a few vegetables, followed for spiritual beliefs and not for health reasons—doesn't follow basic principles of healthful eating: food variety and balance. It gradually eliminates food categories and restricts fluids. Ultimately a macrobiotic diet supplies only certain grains and small amounts of fluid. As a result, this eating style is deficient in many essential nutrients and can lead to dehydration, which may be life-threatening. To dispel a myth, a macrobiotic diet won't cure cancer.

Not Just for Vegetarians: Quick and Healthful Snacks

Popcorn

Dairy or soy yogurt

Pretzels

Cottage cheese

Crackers

Muffins

Oatmeal cookies

Sunflower and pumpkin seeds

Fresh or canned fruit

Dried fruit

Peanuts or soy nuts

Fruit shakes

Fruit juice

Raw vegetables (carrots, broccoli, zucchini)

Fruit leather

Tomato juice

Crackers and cheese

Trail mix

Bean tacos or burritos

Cheese and veggie pizza (or cheeseless pizza)

Bagels and peanut butter

Focaccia bread (with or without cheese)

Hummus (mashed chickpea dip) with pita points

Nut butter and crackers

Fruit/cereal bars

Milk or calcium-fortified soy milk or rice milk

Fig cookies

Tofu dip

Smoothies made with milk, or with soy or rice milk

Vegetarian Diets: Nutritionally Speaking

Can vegetarian eating supply your body with enough nutrients? Yes. As with any eating style, you need to choose foods carefully—and consume enough food energy, or calories, yet not too many.

For vegetarians who consume dairy products and perhaps eggs, nutrition issues don't differ much from those of nonvegetarians. Consume enough, but not too many calories—still smart advice. Go easy on saturated fat, trans fats, and cholesterol—as well as total fat, added sugars, and salt, too. If you choose mostly lower-fat or fat-free dairy products, along with plenty of grains (especially whole grains), vegetables, and fruits, a typical lacto-ovo-vegetarian diet can be high in fiber, low in saturated fat and cholesterol, and moderate in total fat: nutrition goals for all healthy people!

For vegans, the nutrition issues differ somewhat. Without any foods of animal origin, getting enough calories to maintain a healthy weight can be a challenge, especially for growing children and teens. And nutrients that may come up short need special attention: vitamin B_{12}, vitamin D, calcium, iron, and zinc. Nonetheless, planned wisely, a vegan diet can provide enough nutrients for overall good health, too.

Protein Power

With vegetarian eating, the issue of protein often arises. Why? Because vegetarians eat less—or perhaps no—foods of animal origin; meat, poultry, fish, eggs, and dairy foods are all sources of concentrated protein. For most vegetarians, adequate protein isn't a concern, however. Except for fruit, almost every food of plant origin contains protein—at least a small amount. And legumes, nuts, and seeds are good sources.

Is the protein sufficient? Yes—even though a vegetarian diet may be slightly lower in total protein than a nonvegetarian diet. And if protein quality is lower, vegetarians may need somewhat more protein. Yet a plant-based diet, chosen wisely with plenty of food variety and sufficient food energy, likely provides more than enough protein for most vegetarians. Here's why—and how!

More about Proteins

We often think of protein as a single nutrient. Yet, proteins in both food and your body cells are made up of building blocks, or amino acids, each with a somewhat different structure. Although many more appear in nature, your body uses only about twenty amino acids to make body proteins. Like carbohydrates and fats, amino acids are unique combinations of carbon, hydrogen, and oxygen. However, amino acids also have nitrogen, which makes their physiological structure and functions uniquely their own.

How proteins are made. Of the twenty or so amino acids your body uses, nine are considered essential. Because your body can't make them, your food choices must supply them. Their names may sound familiar: histidine (essential for infants but perhaps not for healthy adults), isoleucine, leucine, lysine, methionine, phenylalanine, threonine, tryptophan, and valine. You might see some—perhaps phenylalanine and tryptophan—on food labels.

Other amino acids are nonessential. Your body makes them—if you consume enough essential amino acids and enough calories during the day. Just eat many different foods with protein throughout the day to get the full variety of amino acids.

Amino acids are described as protein's "building blocks." Like notes in a music scale or letters of the alphabet, they're arranged in countless ways. The same music notes create symphonies, jazz, and pop hits. And the same twenty-six letters of the alphabet form thousands of words in many languages, each word with its own meaning. It's the same for amino acids. In a single cell in your body, ten thousand different proteins may exist—each with a different arrangement of amino acids.

To get their meaning, words must be spelled correctly. And amino acids in proteins must be arranged in a precise order to function normally. The genetic code in every cell—called DNA, or deoxyribonucleic acid—carries the instructions for "spelling" each protein.

What proteins do. As nutrients, proteins perform many functions. For one, proteins are part of every body cell. Your body's different tissues—skin, muscles, bone, and organs, for example—are unique because the amino acid patterns in their proteins differ. Your body needs a constant supply of proteins to repair body cells as they wear out. During times of growth—infancy, childhood, adolescence, and pregnancy—the body also needs proteins to make new body tissues.

Beyond that, proteins help regulate body processes. As enzymes and hormones, they make various chemical reactions happen—for example, a nonessen-

tial amino acid, L-arginine, may play a role in heart health by helping to keep blood vessels open. As antibodies, amino acids help protect you from disease-carrying bacteria and viruses.

Proteins also supply your body with energy if you don't consume enough from carbohydrates and fats. Otherwise, proteins can be saved for their unique function: to build and repair body tissue. When you consume more protein than you need, it's broken down and stored as body fat, not as a reserve supply of protein.

Where proteins come from. Meat, poultry, fish, eggs, milk, cheese, yogurt, and soy provide all nine essential amino acids. For that reason they're often referred to as "complete" proteins.

Legumes (beans and peas), seeds, and nuts supply plenty of nearly complete proteins with almost all nine essential amino acids. Grain products and many vegetables supply proteins, too, in smaller amounts and "incomplete," meaning they're missing several essential amino acids.

Consider this: a 1-cup serving of rice and beans (half rice, half beans) supplies about 10 grams of protein. Add 1 cup of milk or soy milk for, respectively, 8 or 6 grams of protein; a green vegetable side dish for 1 gram or 2 grams of protein; one whole-wheat roll, about 4 more grams of protein. That adds up to at least 21 grams of protein. The Recommended Dietary Allowance for adults is 0.8 gram per kilogram of weight; a kilogram is 2.2 pounds. For an average adult man that's about 63 grams of protein a day; for an average woman, 53 grams of protein daily.

Have You Ever Wondered

. . . what wheat gluten is, and how it's used in cooking? Wheat gluten, also known as seitan, is wheat protein. It has a chewy, meaty texture, making it a good, protein-rich ingredient in casseroles, soups, pasta sauces, and other recipes calling for chopped or ground meat or poultry. Look for wheat gluten in specialty stores. **Caution:** People with gluten intolerance should avoid wheat gluten. *See "Gluten Intolerance: Often a Lifelong Condition" in chapter 21.*

Completing the Equation

For the body to make its many proteins, your food choices must supply essential amino acids—in sufficient amounts. Animal proteins supply them all, in proportions needed to make new body proteins. Except for soybeans, plant proteins lack one or more of the essential amino acids. That's why their protein is often called "incomplete." When your meals and snacks provide a variety of plant-based foods and your food energy needs are met, you get all the amino acids your body needs.

To obtain complete protein, there's no need to combine specific foods at each meal, as once thought. Your body makes its own complete proteins if you eat a variety of plant foods—legumes, nuts, seeds, grains, vegetables, and fruits—and enough calories throughout the day. Whatever amino acid one food lacks can come from other foods you eat during the day. *The general guideline is to follow the advice of the "Daily Food Guide for Vegetarians" later in this chapter.*

Vitamin B_{12}: A Challenge for Vegans

Like other B vitamins, vitamin B_{12}, also called cobalamin, fulfills many functions in health. For one, it helps your body make red blood cells and use fats and amino acids, and it's part of the structure of every body cell. A deficiency of vitamin B_{12} isn't likely in the short run for two reasons: vitamin B_{12} needs are small, and it's a nutrient that's stored and recycled in your body. Over time, however, a vitamin B_{12} deficiency can result in anemia and severe, irreversible nerve damage.

Unlike some nutrients, vitamin B_{12} doesn't make the health news much, perhaps because it's so widely available in foods of animal origin. With some exceptions, getting enough isn't a concern for most vegetarians—at least those who consume dairy products or eggs.

For vegans, however, vitamin B_{12} is a nutrition concern. Plants only supply this nutrient when soil with vitamin B_{12}-producing microorganisms clings to fruits and vegetables and isn't removed completely before eating. In the United States, fruits and vegetables are scrubbed clean; they usually have no soil with these microorganisms on them. So most vegans need to look elsewhere for a reliable source of vitamin B_{12}.

For those who limit or avoid foods from animal sources, a vitamin B_{12} supplement or foods fortified with vitamin B_{12} are advised. Since vitamin B_{12} isn't absorbed as well with age, older vegetarians may benefit by taking a supplement as well.

● Look for breakfast cereals, soy milk or rice milk products, or vegetarian burger patties that are fortified with vitamin B_{12}. Or consider a vitamin B_{12} supplement. Read the Nutrition Facts panel on food and supplement labels to check the vitamin B_{12} content. And know that "cyanocobalamin" is its most bioavailable form. In other words, it's the form the body absorbs easily.

● If you choose a supplement, don't take more than 100 percent of the Daily Value (DV) for vitamin B_{12}. Check the Supplement Facts.

● Be aware that seaweed, algae, spirulina, and fermented plant foods such as tempeh and miso aren't good sources of vitamin B_{12}—even if the package says so. The vitamin B_{12} is inactive, so it's not in a form that the human body can use. Vitamin B_{12} in beer and other fermented foods isn't reliable, either.

● Nutritional yeast can be a source of vitamin B_{12} if it's grown on a medium that's enriched with vitamin B_{12}—for example, Red Star Nutrition Yeast T6635. However, the yeast typically used in baking doesn't supply any. Check the label to find out. Don't count on yeast to supply any vitamin B_{12} unless you've checked it out.

For more about vitamin B_{12} see chapter 4.

Fatty Acid: An Essential

Somewhat like the amino acids that make up proteins, fats are made up of fatty acids. Among them, alpha-linolenic acid (ALA) is considered essential, since your body can't make it. In your body, alpha-linolenic acid converts to an omega-3 fatty acid (DHA, or docosahexaenoic acid), which keeps your brain, central nervous system, and membranes throughout your body healthy; omega-3s also may offer protection against some ongoing health problems such as heart disease.

Vegetarians are urged to consume alpha-linolenic acid from plant-based ingredients, since they convert to other omega-3s—for example, canola oil, soy oil, walnuts, ground flaxseed, soybeans, and other nuts and seeds. Fatty fish and eggs supply omega-3 fatty acids for some. (*Another tip for fat:* choose vegetable oil and tub margarine more often than stick margarine, which is high in trans fatty acids.)

Research hasn't identified the implications of low levels of omega-3s (DHA) in health. And there's no Dietary Reference Intake, or recommendation, yet set for omega-3 fatty acids. However, some studies suggest that about 0.5 percent of calories—about 10 calories—from omega-3s in a 2,000-calorie daily eating plan probably are enough. Ten calories are just a little more than 1 gram of fat.

Vitamin D: Not Just from Sunshine!

Vitamin D works as a nutrient partner, helping your body absorb calcium and phosphorus, then depositing them in bones and teeth.

Your body also makes its own vitamin D when your skin is exposed to sunlight. About five to fifteen minutes per day (or twenty to forty minutes of sun three times a week) on your hands, arms, and face without sunscreen are ample time for your body to produce enough vitamin D. If you're darker-skinned or live in a cloudy or smoggy area, you may need more sun exposure; just don't overdo!

Few foods are naturally high in vitamin D, so in the United States, most milk is vitamin D-fortified; some flavored milks are not vitamin D-fortified. Egg yolks also supply smaller amounts.

Vitamin D isn't an issue if you drink milk or if you're regularly exposed to sunlight. Just 8 ounces of milk provide 100 International Units of vitamin D, or about half the amount that adults age fifty or under need daily.

However, vegans—or anyone who doesn't drink milk—need to be careful to get enough vitamin D, especially during the winter in northern climates and if housebound. That's true, too, for older adults, who don't synthesize their own vitamin D as efficiently. Infants who breast-feed longer than six months without consuming a vitamin D supplement or who aren't exposed to sunlight are at risk, too.

● If you're a vegan, check the Nutrition Facts on food labels—some breakfast cereals, some soy beverages, and some calcium-fortified juices are fortified with vitamin D.

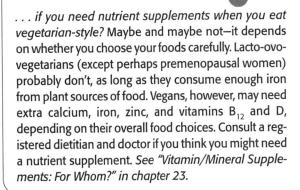

Have You Ever Wondered

. . . if you need nutrient supplements when you eat vegetarian-style? Maybe and maybe not—it depends on whether you choose your foods carefully. Lacto-ovo-vegetarians (except perhaps premenopausal women) probably don't, as long as they consume enough iron from plant sources of food. Vegans, however, may need extra calcium, iron, zinc, and vitamins B$_{12}$ and D, depending on their overall food choices. Consult a registered dietitian and doctor if you think you might need a nutrient supplement. *See "Vitamin/Mineral Supplements: For Whom?" in chapter 23.*

● If you're in doubt, talk to your doctor or a registered dietitian (RD) about taking a vitamin D supplement. Choose a supplement with no more than 100 percent of the Daily Values (DVs) per day. Larger doses can be dangerous and should be avoided.

For more about vitamin D see chapter 4. For more about vitamin D and older adults see "Vitamin D: The Sunshine Vitamin" in chapter 18.

Calcium: Getting Enough

Calcium—you know it best as a bone builder. But calcium also helps your muscles contract; transfers nerve impulses; helps your blood clot; helps your heart beat; and for kids, builds healthy teeth. If you're a vegetarian, how can you consume enough?

Vegetarians who consume dairy products have excellent calcium sources built into their daily eating plan: milk, cheese, and yogurt. Two to three servings from the Milk Group daily contribute much of the calcium advised by the Dietary Reference Intakes—at least for many.

Vegans, too, can get enough calcium from plant foods alone. But it may take more planning. Vegans may not need quite as much calcium, as some studies suggest. This may be because vegetarians seem to absorb and retain more calcium from food. The typically high-protein diet of nonvegetarians may actually decrease calcium absorption and increase its excretion through urine; in contrast, soy protein may decrease calcium excretion, perhaps due to its lower sulfur amino acid content. Vegetarians also have lower rates of osteoporosis, or brittle bone disease. Factors besides calcium in their food choices, including regular weight-bearing activity, may play a part. *See "Osteoporosis: Reduce the Risks" in chapter 22.*

If you're a vegan, what's the calcium advice? Currently, consume the level established in the DRI for your age group—for example, 1,000 milligrams of calcium per day is an Adequate Intake if you're age nineteen to fifty (more if you're a teenager or over age fifty). You'll need enough vitamin D to help your body absorb and use the calcium you consume effectively. If you can't consume enough calcium from food, a supplement probably makes sense for you.

Which foods of plant origin supply calcium?

● Try tofu processed with calcium, calcium-fortified soy or rice beverages, broccoli, seeds (sunflower seeds), nuts, legumes, some greens (kale, collards, mustard greens), okra, rutabaga, bok choy, dried figs, tortillas (made from lime-processed corn), and calcium-fortified orange juice and breakfast cereal.

● Beet greens, rhubarb, spinach, Swiss chard, and a grain called amaranth supply calcium, but your body cannot use it. These foods contain oxalates that bind calcium, blocking its absorption. Some grain products also contain small amounts of calcium, but they may contain phytates that block calcium absorption.

For more about calcium for health and food sources of calcium see "Calcium: A Closer Look" in chapter 4. And for food preparation tips, see "Calcium Boosters" in chapter 13.

Iron—Make the Most of It!

Because it often comes up short, iron needs special attention, especially by growing children and women of childbearing age. That's true whether you're a vegetarian or not. Among other reasons, your body needs iron as part of the complex process of energy production. Not consuming enough may result in fatigue and perhaps iron-deficiency anemia.

What are the iron-related issues for vegetarians? Foods of plant origin certainly contain iron, called nonheme iron, which isn't absorbed as well as heme iron in meat and other foods of animal origin. So the challenge for vegetarians is this: Improve the absorption of nonheme iron from food—easy, if you know how.

● Start by consuming plant sources of food that contain nonheme iron: legumes; iron-fortified cereals and breads, especially whole-wheat breads; whole-grain products; tofu; some dark-green leafy vegetables (such as spinach or beet greens); seeds; tempeh; prune juice; dried fruits; and blackstrap molasses. For lacto-ovo-vegetarians, eggs also supply nonheme iron.

● Include a vitamin C-rich food at every meal. Vitamin C-rich foods such as citrus fruits or juices, broccoli, tomatoes, and green or red peppers, help your body absorb iron from plant sources of food and from eggs. *For a list of vitamin C-rich fruits and vegetables see chapter 4.*

● If you're a semivegetarian, eating a little meat, poultry, and fish helps your body absorb nonheme iron from plant sources of food, and perhaps from eggs.

● If you cook foods in iron pots or skillets, some iron from the pots or skillets may pass into food. That's especially true when ingredients are high in acid, such as tomatoes, and when you simmer foods (such as soups and stews) for a while.

See "Iron: A Closer Look" in chapter 4.

Zinc: Not to Overlook

Zinc, a mineral, is essential for growth, repairing body cells, and energy production. And it's associated with more than two hundred enzymes that control your body processes. Without meat, poultry, and seafood, zinc may come up short in a vegetarian diet.

For lacto-ovo-vegetarians, milk, cheese, yogurt, and eggs all supply zinc. In addition, many foods of plant origin contain zinc—but its bioavailability (availability to your body) is less than from animal foods. Most vegetarian diets supply enough zinc to keep blood levels within a normal range.

Science hasn't yet clarified the effect of marginal zinc status. However, even mild deficiencies may impair mental performance, according to recent studies; that's an issue not only for adults but for children and teens as well.

To make sure you consume enough zinc, follow these tips if you're a vegetarian:

● Eat a variety of foods with zinc: whole-wheat bread; whole grains, especially the germ and bran; legumes; tofu; seeds; and nuts in amounts recommended for health. Be aware that grains lose zinc when they're processed to make refined flour. And substances in plant sources such as fiber and phytates can inhibit zinc absorption. Phytates, however, are broken down during the process of yeast fermentation called leavening in baking yeast breads.

● Be cautious of zinc supplements, which can have harmful side effects in high dosages. If your doctor or registered dietitian recommends a supplement, stick with a vitamin-mineral combination with 100 percent or less of the Daily Value (DV) for zinc.

For more about zinc see chapter 4.

Throughout the Life Cycle

People at any age can follow a vegetarian way of eating—and get the nourishment they need for health. The nutrition issues differ somewhat, depending on the stage in life.

If you or someone in your family becomes a vegetarian, consult a registered dietitian for help in planning a nutritious vegetarian eating plan. Some dietitians specialize in vegetarian nutrition. Getting sound nutrition advice is especially important during pregnancy, breast-feeding, recovery from illness, and for times of growth (infancy, childhood, and adolescence). *See "How to Find Nutrition Help . . ." in chapter 24.*

The Vegetarian Mom

For pregnancy and breast-feeding: either a lacto-ovo-vegetarian eating plan or a vegan eating plan can supply the nutrients and the food energy needed to support the increased needs of both mother and baby.

If you've already mastered the skills of vegetarian eating, adjusting your food choices for pregnancy and breast-feeding won't require much extra effort. However, if vegetarian eating is new to you, seek nutrition advice from a registered dietitian, or perhaps wait, at least until after your baby is born.

You know that good nutrition during pregnancy and breast-feeding is important for both mother and baby. When a mom puts herself at nutritional risk, her baby's development may be affected, too.

If you're pregnant or nursing, follow these tips if you choose a vegetarian approach to eating:

● Keep tabs on your weight gain during pregnancy. For vegetarian and nonvegetarian women, pregnancy requires about 300 extra calories a day; breast-feeding, about 500 calories more than needed before pregnancy. Healthy weight gain for a full-term pregnancy is 25 to 35 pounds for most women. *See " 'Weighting' for Your New Arrival" in chapter 17.*

Research shows that babies born to vegetarian moms are similar in birthweight to babies born to nonvegetarian women—as long as the mother is well nourished during pregnancy. That's good news. **Caution:** if you don't consume enough food energy (calories) during pregnancy, your weight gain may be too low to sustain the normal development of the fetus. As a result, your baby may be born with a low birthweight. And if your calorie intake is less than needed while nursing, your body may not produce enough breast milk.

● For enough calcium during pregnancy and breast-feeding, you need 1,000 milligrams daily if you're age 19 or over, and 1,300 milligrams daily for teens. If you consume dairy products, getting enough calcium for pregnancy and breast-feeding is easy. Just follow the guidelines from the Food Guide Pyramid: two to three Milk Group servings daily. *If you're a vegan, see "Calcium: Getting Enough" earlier in this chapter for more about plant sources of calcium.* A calcium supplement may be advised for you, too; check with your healthcare provider.

Babies need calcium for developing bones and teeth. If you don't consume enough calcium during pregnancy and breast-feeding, your body will give up some calcium stores in your bones. That may put you at greater risk for bone disease as you get older.

● During pregnancy and breast-feeding, your need for vitamin D is the same as before—but you still need enough to help absorb calcium. If you're lacto-vegetarian, drink milk fortified with vitamin D. If you're a vegan, you may need a vitamin D supplement, especially if your exposure to sunlight is limited.

● Consult your doctor or a registered dietitian about an iron supplement. Most pregnant women—vegetarians and nonvegetarians—are advised to take an iron supplement. If you take one, follow the recommended dosage. Too much iron can interfere with zinc absorption, putting your newborn at risk for a zinc deficiency.

● For vegans, consume a reliable source of vitamin B_{12}—perhaps fortified breakfast cereals or a vitamin B_{12} supplement. During pregnancy, you need more for the developing fetus and your own increased blood supply. For women age nineteen and over, the need for vitamin B_{12} goes from 2.4 micrograms daily before pregnancy, to 2.6 micrograms daily during pregnancy and 2.8 micrograms daily during breast-feeding. Without enough vitamin B_{12} during pregnancy and nursing, your baby may be at risk for anemia and nerve damage.

● With a vegetarian diet you probably consume enough folate, also known as folic acid. Still, as a precaution, get enough folic acid prior to and during pregnancy to avoid neural tube (spinal cord) defects in the fetus. Many plant sources of food are good sources of this B vitamin: leafy vegetables, legumes, some fruits, wheat germ, and grains products fortified with folic acid. A folate (folic acid) supplement still may be advised. Consult your doctor or a registered dietitian.

● If you're a vegan and breast-feeding, make sure you consume sources of linolenic acid (ground flaxseed and flaxseed, canola, or soy oil) to help increase the linolenic acid in breast milk.

● The need for zinc increases by 50 percent during pregnancy. Vegetarian women may need a zinc supplement if they don't consume enough from food.

For more about nutrition during pregnancy and breast-feeding see chapter 17.

Feeding Vegetarian Kids

Are your kids vegetarians? That's okay—as long as their overall food choices are healthful. Simply avoiding animal-based foods isn't enough. Like all children and teens, they need enough food variety and energy (calories) for growth, energy, and health. Chosen carefully, either a lacto-ovo-vegetarian or a vegan eating style can provide for the relatively high nutrient needs of kids. They also need skills for making smart choices

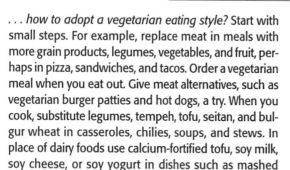

Have You Ever Wondered

. . . how to adopt a vegetarian eating style? Start with small steps. For example, replace meat in meals with more grain products, legumes, vegetables, and fruit, perhaps in pizza, sandwiches, and tacos. Order a vegetarian meal when you eat out. Give meat alternatives, such as vegetarian burger patties and hot dogs, a try. When you cook, substitute legumes, tempeh, tofu, seitan, and bulgur wheat in casseroles, chilies, soups, and stews. In place of dairy foods use calcium-fortified tofu, soy milk, soy cheese, or soy yogurt in dishes such as mashed potatoes, casseroles, and lasagna.

. . . if soy milk is a good substitute for cow milk for children and adults? Check the Nutrition Facts on the food label. The calcium content of soy milks varies. Some are fortified with calcium and vitamin D, but not all. If the cost of fluid soy milk is an issue, look for powdered soy milk. Cow milk also supplies other nutrients, including vitamin A, riboflavin (vitamin B_2), vitamin B_{12}, and phosphorus—nutrients needed by adults and growing children alike. Make sure other food choices supply enough of these nutrients, too.

As an aside, fortified rice milk is another option, but it doesn't provide as much protein as soy milk does. It doesn't offer all the nutrients that cow milk does.

. . . if it's okay for your teenager to control weight with a vegetarian diet? Yes, if your teen's food choices are varied and balanced—and if your teen keeps a healthy weight. Vegetarian eating doesn't lead to eating disorders. However, if a vegetarian approach to eating results in too much weight loss, it may signal an eating disorder. Eating disorders can be harmful, even life-threatening. If that happens, seek professional help. And help your teen understand that vegetarian eating isn't always low-calorie; energy, or calorie, content depends on your teen's overall food choices. *See "Eating Disorders: Problems, Signs, and Help" in chapter 2.*

. . . if a vegetarian athlete can consume enough protein without using special foods or supplements? Yes— *just follow the "Daily Food Guide for Vegetarians" in this chapter.* If you want a "safety net," enjoy another meat alternate from the Meat and Beans Group. *For more on vegetarian eating for athletes see chapter 19, "Athlete's Guide: Winning Nutrition."*

from the array of foods that fit in their vegetarian diets.

For the voracious appetites of many children and teens, getting enough calories may seem easy enough. Yet many vegetarian meals are low in fat and high in fiber, so they fill up kids without supplying enough calories. Vegan diets especially can be "bulky," yet low in energy.

What happens when children and teens don't consume enough calories? Their bodies use protein from food for energy, not for growing new body cells. An energy deficiency can retard growth and impair brain function. Under the guidance of your healthcare provider, monitor your child's growth.

To meet the demands of growth, include higher-calorie foods in meals and snacks for older children and teens. Provide some foods with more fat, especially foods higher in unsaturated fats such as nuts, seeds, and nut butters. Foods with some added sugars, such as oatmeal cookies and ice cream, may provide food energy, but go easy. Encourage frequent snacks that provide plenty of nutrients as well as food energy—for example, a peanut butter sandwich and milk, raw vegetables with hummus or tofu dip, ready-to-eat breakfast cereal, fruit, or finger-food veggies. *For snack ideas see "Not Just for Vegetarians . . . Quick and Healthful Snacks" earlier in this chapter.*

Lacto-ovo-vegetarians generally can get enough nutrients from well-chosen foods alone. But for vegan infants, children, and teens, some nutrients may need special attention: calcium, iron, zinc, vitamin B_{12}, and vitamin D. If your child is a vegan, offer a variety of foods with adequate amounts of these nutrients. Poor choices can put vegetarian kids at greater risk for nutrient inadequacies and their health consequences than nonvegetarian kids. *For guidance see "Vegetarian Diets: Nutritionally Speaking" in this chapter.*

Especially for Babies

Breast milk is the best "first food" for babies. When breast-feeding isn't chosen, commercial infant formulas, including soy formulas, are a healthful option. **Caution:** Neither cow milk nor regular soy milk or rice milk are suitable substitutes for infant formula!

Infants breast-fed for longer than four to six months are at risk for iron and vitamin D deficiencies. That's true whether the mom is a vegetarian or not. As a guideline for all infants at this time: Healthcare providers may advise an iron-fortified cereal or an iron supplement, and perhaps a vitamin D supplement if the baby's exposure to sunlight is limited. For breast-fed vegan infants a vitamin B_{12} supplement may be recommended, too, if the mother doesn't consume vitamin B_{12}-fortified foods.

Time to introduce protein-rich solid foods? Offer pureed tofu, cottage cheese, and pureed or strained legumes to vegetarian babies. Before age two, babies need enough fat to develop a healthy nervous system; this isn't the time to restrict fat in food!

Health advice. If your infant, child, or teen follows a vegetarian eating style, consult a registered dietitian, your doctor, or a pediatric nurse for support and

If Your Teen Decides to Become a Vegetarian

Many teens today equate being vegetarian with being "cool." If your teen chooses to be a vegetarian for any reason, support a smart approach:

- Make a shopping list together of food group foods that fit your teen's vegetarian "style"—and keep those foods on hand: perhaps hummus, cheese, and crackers; cow milk; calcium-fortified soy milk; trail mix with nuts; fruit; raw veggies; yogurt; and other quick, portable vegetarian snacks.

- Plan vegetarian main dishes that your whole family can enjoy, such as chili with beans, vegetarian pizza, or bean tacos. In that way, you won't need to feel like a short-order cook.

- For some dishes, prepare them two ways with just a simple substitution: a veggieburger for your teen and beefburgers for the rest of the family.

- Prepare vegetarian foods that can be the main dish for your teen and a side dish for others—for example, rice and beans, or pasta primavera. Offer milk.

- Encourage your vegetarian teen to share in food preparation. It's great practice for applying the basics of healthful vegetarian eating.

- Talk about eating-out options so your teen is prepared to make wise choices with peers.

- Whether you're a vegetarian or not, be a role model for healthful eating and healthful living.

- Most of all, be supportive and learn about smart vegetarian eating together.

nutrition counseling. For vegans, ask about nutrient supplements.

For more about feeding infants, children, and teens, see chapters 15 and 16.

Vegetarian Fare for Older Adults

Are you an older adult who prefers a vegetarian eating style? If so, your overall nutrition needs and concerns are similar to those of other older adults and other vegetarians.

Two nutrients need special attention for older vegetarians: vitamin D and vitamin B_{12}. Those confined to the house without exposure to sunlight may be deficient in vitamin D unless they drink milk. With age, the body may not absorb vitamin B_{12} efficiently, either. That's especially a concern for vegetarians who don't have a reliable food source of vitamin B_{12}. Eating foods fortified with vitamin B_{12} or taking a supplement can prevent vitamin B_{12} deficiency.

In later years, people are at greater risk for some health problems if they don't get the variety of nutrients they need. *Use the "Daily Food Guide for Vegetarians" in this chapter as a guide for healthful eating.* Older adults, especially those recovering from illness, need to be cautious if they follow a vegan diet. *See chapter 18, "For Mature Adults: Healthful Eating!"*

"Vegging Out" the Healthful Way!

Planned carefully, a vegetarian eating style can provide what you need for growth (if you're a teen) and good health. That takes commitment. But once you understand it, being a smart vegetarian takes no more effort than any other approach to smart eating. Start here:

● Get enough calories, without overdoing, to meet energy needs. This is especially important during childhood, the teen years, pregnancy, and breast-feeding.

What's on the Menu?

Vegetarian menus can be easy to prepare. To make food preparation fast and easier, choose dishes that everyone—vegetarians and nonvegetarians—around your dinner table will enjoy.

Breakfast

1 cup oatmeal* (made with milk or calcium- and vitamin D-fortified soy milk) with
   2 tablespoons sliced almonds and
   2 tablespoons raisins
2 slices whole-wheat toast with jelly
¾ cup orange juice
Coffee or tea
*or ready-to-eat breakfast cereal fortified with vitamins B_{12} and D

Lunch

1½ cups hearty lentil soup
Mixed garden salad with 2 tablespoons sunflower seeds and low-fat dressing
Carrot and green pepper sticks with salsa
1 whole-grain muffin
1 cup fat-free milk or calcium- and vitamin D-fortified soy milk

Snack

Bagel with 2 tablespoons peanut butter
Iced tea with fresh lemon

Dinner

1½ cups tomato and herb-seasoned rice with kidney beans
¾ cup steamed broccoli with lemon juice and sesame seeds
½ cup fresh fruit salad
1 slice Italian foccacia bread
½ cup fresh fruit salad
1 cup fat-free milk or calcium- and vitamin D-fortified soy milk
½ cup fruit sorbet topped with 1 tablespoon chopped nuts

Snack

1 slice nut or raisin bread
Sparkling water

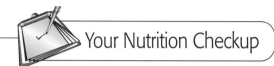

Your Nutrition Checkup: For Vegetarians

You've chosen to follow a vegetarian diet—perhaps with health in mind. But are you making smart choices? Take this ten-question survey as a quick check.

Do you eat:

YES No

1. A wide variety of grain products (including whole grains), legumes, nuts, vegetables, and fruits?
2. At least six servings of bread, rice, pasta, and other grain products daily, of which at least three daily servings are whole grain?
3. Three to five vegetable servings daily?
4. Two to four fruit servings daily?
5. A vitamin C-rich food with meals whenever you can?
6. Enough calories to maintain a healthy weight?
7. Mostly nutrient-dense foods and go easy on fats, oils, and sugars?
8. Two to three servings (5 to 7 ounces) of legumes and other meat alternates each day?

Just for lacto- and lacto-ovo-vegetarians (if you're a vegan, skip ahead):

9. Two to three servings of milk, yogurt, or cheese daily?
10. Eggs occasionally (so you stay under 300 milligrams of cholesterol a day)? *(Skip this question if you're a lacto-vegetarian.)*

Just for vegans (if you're a lacto- or lacto-ovo-vegetarian, skip these two questions):

9. Foods of plant origin that are high in calcium?
10. Foods that are fortified with vitamins B_{12} and D (or take a supplement that provides no more than 100 percent of the Daily Value)?

Now score yourself. Give yourself a point for every "yes."

If you scored a perfect "10," your food choices do promote your good health. If you scored "9" and only answered nine questions, the same applies—your food choices probably supply enough nutrients and perhaps offer other health benefits.

If you said "no" to any item, read on, then make changes to eat smarter and healthier—the vegetarian way!

● *Consume a variety from the five food groups of the Food Guide Pyramid, or use the "Daily Food Guide for Vegetarians" in this chapter.* Try meat alternatives from the Meat and Beans Group. If you're a vegan, try calcium-fortified soy milk from the Milk Group. For lacto-ovo-vegetarians, choose mostly lower-fat and fat-free dairy foods.

● Enjoy a variety of fruits, vegetables, and grain products (especially whole grains) for their nutrient, fiber, and phytonutrient benefits.

● Go easy on high-fat foods, including those from the Pyramid tip (fats, oils, and sweets)—even if they do come from plant sources.

● For vegans, consume reliable sources of vitamin B_{12} such as fortified breakfast cereal or soy milk and vitamin D, especially if your exposure to sunlight is limited.

Follow the Food Guide

For your good health, follow the advice of the Dietary Guidelines for Americans, meant for vegetarians and nonvegetarians alike. *To put these guidelines in action see the "Food Guide for Vegetarian Meal Planning" later in this chapter.*

Vegetarian Way: Bread, Cereal, Rice, and Pasta

As for nonvegetarians, eat at least six servings of breads, cereals, rice, or pasta each day. Choose whole-grain products whenever you can—at least three servings per day. That includes whole-wheat bread, breakfast cereal, and pasta; brown rice; and other whole-grain products. *See "What Is a Whole Grain?" in chapter 6.* Besides the complex carbohydrates, iron, fiber, and phytonutrients they provide, whole grains supply zinc, too, which may be inadequate in food patterns of vegetarians.

● Make grain dishes the centerpiece of your menu—perhaps tabouli, barley, rice pilaf, risotto, rice or noodle dishes, gnocchi, or polenta. Add interest to vegetarian meals with a greater variety of breads, including focaccia, bagels, tortillas, pita bread, chapatis, and naan. And try breads made with a variety of grains: oats, rye, and cornmeal, to name a few. *Tip:* Because of their processing method, some corn tortillas supply calcium. Check the label.

● Add cooked grains to all kinds of foods. For example, stuff vegetables (eggplant, bell peppers, cabbage, and zucchini) with cooked grain mixtures: rice, oats, and barley, among others. Blend cooked grains with shredded vegetables and perhaps tofu for vegetable patties or croquettes. Toss cooked grains (not just rice or noodles) with stir-fried vegetables. And add bulgur, barley, and other cooked grains to soups, stews, and chilies.

● Choose fortified breakfast cereals. Read the Nutrition Facts panel on food labels for added nutrients, including iron, vitamin B_{12}, and zinc.

Vegetarian Way: Vegetables

Aim for three to five servings of vegetables a day. For everyone—especially vegans—choose vegetables that are good sources of calcium: dark-green leafy vegetables (such as kale, mustard, collard, or turnip greens), bok choy, and broccoli. Dark-green leafy vegetables also supply iron.

● Choose vegetables that are high in vitamin C—for example, broccoli, tomatoes, and green and red peppers. Vitamin C helps your body absorb iron in eggs and in plant sources of food. *For the vitamin C content of some vegetables see "Vitamin C: More than Citrus" in chapter 4.*

● Plan meals with several different vegetables, not just garden salads, baked potatoes, and fries. In that way you get the nutrient and phytonutrient benefits of variety.

Vegetarian Way: Fruits

Include two to four servings of fruit each day.

● Enjoy a variety of fruits, including a good food source of vitamin C, such as citrus fruits, melons, and berries. *For the amount of vitamin C in various fruits see "Vitamin C: More than Citrus" in chapter 4.*

● To get enough fruit, enjoy it for dessert and snacks—either as fresh, whole, or sliced fruit; prepared in cobblers; ice-cream toppers; or in thick, fruity smoothies.

● Look for calcium-fortified juice as an added source of calcium, especially if you're a vegan.

Vegetarian Way: Legumes and Other Meat Alternates

Include two to three servings of legumes and other meat alternates every day. These foods supply protein and iron, as meat, poultry, and fish do for nonvegetarians. Except for eggs, most meat alternates are low in total fat and saturated fat and have no cholesterol.

● Make legumes a mealtime regular—eat them most days of the week. They contribute proteins and are good sources of complex carbohydrates, fiber, and phytonutrients. *For a description of the variety of legumes and tips for cooking them see chapter 6.*

● Use soybean products—tofu, tempeh, textured soy protein, and soy milk—in your food preparation. Try them in stir-fry dishes, casseroles, lasagna, soups, and burger patties. *See "What's 'Soy' Good?" in chapter 11.*

Stocking the Vegetarian Kitchen

Today's supermarkets sell all the foods you need for a healthful, vegetarian diet—even vegetarian convenience foods. You don't need to shop elsewhere, but specialty stores may carry less common items (such as textured soy protein, quinoa, kosher gelatin, and wheat gluten).

No matter where you shop, plan ahead. Shop with a list. Read food labels to find foods with ingredients that match your needs. The ingredient list helps identify animal-derived ingredients. Check the grocery aisle for shelf-stable foods such as boxed soy milk. For your vegetarian kitchen, stock up on foods such as these:

Breads, Cereals, Rice, Pasta, and Other Grain Products

- Ready-to-eat, fortified, and whole-grain breakfast cereals
- Quick-cooking whole-grain and enriched cereals such as oatmeal and muesli
- Whole-grain and enriched breads, bagels, rolls, and crackers such as rye and whole wheat, and mixed grain rice such as brown, wild, basmati, white, and others
- Pastas such as macaroni, spaghetti, fettuccini, and couscous (perhaps made without eggs)
- Corn or flour tortillas, pita bread, bagels, and other breads*
- Popcorn
- Wheat germ, bran, and wheat gluten (seitan)
- Other grains such as barley, bulgur, millet, and quinoa
- Flour—whole wheat, rye, cornmeal

*Read labels if you're vegan; some breads have ingredients derived from eggs, or they're brushed with eggs to make them shine.

Legumes and Meat Substitutes

- Canned, frozen, and fresh legumes such as pintos, black beans, split peas, soybeans, and garbanzos
- Dried legumes
- Vegetarian refried beans
- Dried legume mixes such as refried beans, falafel, and hummus (mashed chickpeas)
- Tofu and tempeh
- Miso
- Soy-protein patties, soy bacon, soy sausages

- Soy milk, soy cheese, soy yogurt
- Soynuts
- Soy flour, soy grits
- Textured soy protein
- Myco-protein (Quorn) meat alternatives sold as patties, sausages, and cold cuts
- Peanut butter
- Nut and seed spreads such as almond butter and tahini (sesame seed spread)
- Nuts such as pecans, almonds, walnuts, hazelnuts, and cashews
- Seeds such as sesame, pumpkin, and sunflower
- Eggs or egg substitute*

*For vegans, egg replacer powder, made from tapioca starch and leavenings (not a meat alternative)

Fruits and Vegetables

- Frozen and canned fruit, vegetables, and juice
- Fresh fruits and vegetables
- Tomato sauce
- Frozen and boxed (shelf-stable) fruit juice concentrate
- Dried fruits such as raisins, dried plums (prunes), dried cranberries, dates, and dried apricots

Dairy and Dairy Alternatives

- Vitamin D-fortified milk
- Calcium-fortified soy milk
- Cheese (dairy or soy-based)
- Yogurt (dairy or soy-based)
- Dry milk powder
- Ice cream, frozen yogurt, or nondairy ice cream

Combination Foods

- Canned and frozen vegetarian soups
- Frozen vegetarian entrées such as bean burritos or vegetable potstickers
- Canned vegetarian dishes such as chili without meat
- Vegetable pizza

Fats and Sugars

- Vegetable oil, plain and flavor-infused
- Margarine (perhaps soy margarine) or butter

Stocking the Vegetarian Kitchen *(continued)*

- Salad dressing (perhaps made without eggs), tofu-based mayonnaise
- Vegetarian gravy and sauce mixes
- Syrup, jam, jelly, and molasses
- Refined sugar, brown sugar, honey, and other sweeteners

Condiments, Seasonings, and Other Flavorings

- Herbs and spices
- Vinegar, plain and flavored
- Sauces such as chutney, salsa, soy sauce, teriyaki sauce
- Canned vegetable broth and broth mix
- Vegetable bouillon

● If you eat eggs, watch how much you eat. For your cardiovascular health, try to limit your cholesterol intake to 300 milligrams or less a day; one egg yolk has about 215 milligrams of cholesterol. Make egg-based dishes lower in fat by substituting egg whites for some of the whole eggs. Examples of egg-based dishes include quiche, omelettes, frittata, scrambled eggs, French toast, egg salad, and egg foo yung.

● Include nuts, nut butters (almond butter, cashew butter, peanut butter), seeds, and seed spread (tahini, or sesame seed spread). They, too, supply protein and an array of phytonutrients. Since they're fairly high in fat, go easy; most fat from nuts is unsaturated.

Vegetarian Way: Milk, Yogurt, and Cheese

The advice: eat two to three servings from the Milk Group daily. Lacto-vegetarians can enjoy milk, yogurt, and cheese—choose mostly lower-fat and fat-free dairy products for less fat.

For vegans—in fact, all vegetarians—calcium-fortified soy milk offers an alternative; look for soy milk that's also fortified with vitamin D. Read the Nutrition Facts on food labels to compare soy beverages. Milk supplies about 300 milligrams of calcium per serving; choose soy milk with at least this much. If soy-based products aren't calcium-fortified, they can't count as an alternative to milk. Especially if you're vegan, look for other calcium-rich food in other food groups. Find adequate sources of cow milk's other nutrients.

Vegetarian Way: Fats, Oils, and Sweets

As with any approach to eating, go easy on high-fat foods such as salad dressings, cooking oils, and spreads. The same goes for sweets such as candies and soft drinks, including fruit-flavored drinks.

Reminder: Just because they're derived from plant sources doesn't mean they're low in fat, added sugars, or calories!

Food Guide for Vegetarian Meal Planning

To eat the vegetarian way, use the Food Guide Pyramid guidelines—with a few easy changes. For each food group, only the suggested amounts and variety of choices differ slightly. *See "Daily Food Guide for Vegetarians" on page 513.*

Adapting Your Recipes

Looking for vegetarian recipes? Check the bookstore and magazine racks for many flavor-filled dishes from vegetarian cookbooks and publications. Go online! Or with just a few changes, adapt recipes from almost any cookbook or magazine for vegetarian-style eating—even if you choose to avoid eggs and dairy products. Try these recipe hints for adjusting recipes.

Instead of meat, poultry, or fish . . .

● *In casseroles, stews, soups, lasagna, and chili,* substitute cooked or canned legumes for meat: perhaps kidney beans in chili or stew, or red lentils in spaghetti sauce or stuffed cabbage rolls, or refried beans in burritos, tacos, and enchiladas. Or add textured soy protein, often sold in granular form.

● *In stir-fry dishes,* use firm tofu, tempeh, soyburgers, or sausage, cooked beans, nuts, or sesame seeds in place of meat, poultry, or seafood. *Hint:* For more flavor, marinate tofu before adding it to dishes.

● *For grilling,* cube and skewer firm tofu and tempeh with vegetables.

Daily Food Guide for Vegetarians

Fats, oils, sweets: use sparingly—candy, butter, margarine, salad dressing, cooking oil

MILK AND MILK ALTERNATIVES GROUP*
6–8 servings daily

½ cup milk, yogurt, fortified soymilk, or calcium-fortified orange juice

¾ oz. natural cheese

½ to 1 cup cottage cheese

¼ cup calcium-set tofu

1 cup cooked dry beans (soy, white, navy, great northern, kidney)

¼ cup almonds

3 tbsp. sesame tahini or almond butter

1 cup cooked or 2 cups raw bok choy, Chinese cabbage, broccoli, collards, kale, okra

1 tbsp. blackstrap molasses

5 figs

VEGETABLE GROUP
3–5 servings daily

½ cup cooked or chopped raw vegetables

1 cup raw, leafy vegetables

¾ cup vegetable juice

DRY BEANS, NUTS, SEEDS, EGGS, AND MEAT SUBSTITUTES GROUP
2–3 servings daily

1 cup cooked dry beans, lentils, or peas

2 cups soy milk

½ cup tofu or tempeh

2 oz. vegetarian "meats" or soy cheese

2 eggs or 4 egg whites

¼ cup nuts or seeds

3 tbsp. nut or seed butters

FRUIT GROUP
2–4 servings daily

¾ cup juice

¼ cup dried fruit

½ cup chopped, raw fruit

½ cup canned fruit

1 medium-size piece of fruit such as banana, apple, or orange

BREAD, CEREAL, RICE, AND PASTA GROUP
6–11 servings daily

1 slice bread

½ bagel, bun, or English muffin

1 oz. ready-to-eat cereal

2 tbsp. wheat germ

½ cup cooked grains, cereal, rice, or pasta

*Many milk alternatives double as servings from the Vegetable Group or Beans Group. To count as a milk alternative serving, fortified foods or beverages should provide at least 15 percent of the Daily Value for calcium, or 100 to 150 milligrams of calcium per serving.

Other essentials for those who consume little or no animal products:

Vitamin B_{12}—fortified foods or a supplement

Vitamin D—fortified foods or a supplement

Omega-3 fats—1 to 2 daily servings; 1 teaspoon flaxseed oil, 3 tablespoons walnuts, 4 teaspoons canola or soybean oil

Source: American Dietetic Association.

● *On pizza, hot sandwiches, sloppy Joes, and other dishes that typically call for meat,* use soy-protein patties, bacon, or sausages.

● Prepare pasta sauces, pizza toppings, soups, stews, and other mixed dishes as you always do—but skip the meat and add more chopped vegetables. If you eat dairy products, sprinkle cheese on top for more protein and calcium.

Instead of eggs . . .

Eggs offer functional qualities to recipes—for example, thickening, binding ingredients together, clarifying stock, coating breaded foods, and leavening. A leavener lightens the texture and increases the volume of baked goods. Without eggs, the qualities of food often change. So experiment!

● Try these ingredients in place of eggs—but know that the results may differ from the original recipe. In place of one egg:
  ● ½ mashed banana (in breads, muffins, or pancakes)
  ● 2 tablespoons of cornstarch or arrowroot
  ● ¼ cup of tofu (Blend it with liquid ingredients until smooth; then add it to dry ingredients.)
  ● ¼ cup of pureed fruit, applesauce, or canned pumpkin
  ● Egg replacer powder, or vegetarian egg replacement (often sold in specialty stores)
  ● ¼ cup of cooked oatmeal or mashed potatoes (in vegetarian burgers or loaves)

● Try scrambled tofu—flavored with herbs—for breakfast!

Instead of dairy foods . . .

● For vegans, use soy margarine in place of butter or other margarines. Most margarine contains some ingredients derived from milk, such as whey or casein. Cookies, pastries, and other baked goods made with margarine may have a different texture than those made with butter. Remember that lard is another fat of animal origin and that stick margarine contains trans fatty acids.

● Enjoy thick, creamy fruit shakes? If you're a lacto-vegetarian, make them with milk, ice cream, or frozen yogurt. If you're a vegan, blend fruit instead with soft tofu, soy milk, or nondairy ice cream—or make all-fruit smoothies!

● Use tofu, soy milk, soy cheese, and soy yogurt in recipes that call for dairy products. Crumbled tofu, for example, can take the place of ricotta cheese in lasagna. Soft tofu makes a great dip or sauce; blend it with other ingredients. And in baked foods, 1 cup of soy milk plus 1 tablespoon of vinegar may take the place of 1 cup of buttermilk.

● For dessert enjoy fruit sorbet in place of sherbet and ice cream.

Instead of gelatin . . .

● Use kosher gelatin, made from a sea vegetable. Find it in a specialty food shop.

Now for Eating Out

What choices do you have when you eat out? Plenty! More and more traditional restaurants and cafeterias cater to "all the time" or "sometime" vegetarians. Fast-food restaurants offer meatless salads that are big enough to enjoy as an entrée—as well as vegetarian deli sandwiches, pita pockets, pizzas, and tacos. In many ethnic restaurants—for example, Indo-Pakistani, other Asian, and Middle Eastern—vegetarian dishes are among their specialties.

Need more strategies for healthful vegetarian eating? Check here for "how-tos":

● Get a great list of interesting fruits, vegetables, and grains—see chapter 9.

● Check your menu options from all five food groups—see chapter 10.

● Scout for soy and other plant-based foods when you shop—see chapter 11.

● Lock vitamins in and boost calcium when you prepare food—see chapter 13.

● Ask questions about vegetarian options when you eat out—see chapter 14.

● Use dietary supplements appropriately to fill in any nutrient gaps—see chapter 23.

Whether you're a vegetarian or simply enjoy an occasional vegetarian meal, be savvy.

● Before you order, talk to your server about ingredients in the dish. Ask about ingredients in vegetarian dishes prepared without eggs, dairy products, or other ingredients from animal sources, if that's your choice. For chain restaurants, contact the company to ask about ingredients if you frequently dine there.

● If the menu doesn't offer a vegetarian entrée, order a salad with vegetable soup and perhaps bread, or several vegetable appetizers. A fruit plate—with or without cheese or yogurt—can make an appealing entrée.

● If you choose the salad bar, "toss" your salad with kidney beans, chickpeas, and a few sunflower seeds . . . as well as vegetables that have more vitamin C. (Remember that vitamin C helps your body absorb iron from plant sources of food.) If you're a lacto-ovo-vegetarian, you might spoon on some cottage cheese, shredded cheese, and chopped or sliced hard-cooked eggs. (*Hint:* Go easy on high-fat salad dressing, or choose a low-fat dressing. If you're vegan, find out if the dressing has ingredients derived from egg; if so, vinegar and oil is great!)

● Choose an ethnic restaurant that's likely to have vegetarian options. Perhaps try the cuisines of the Middle East, Greece, India, China, Mexico, or parts of Africa. (*Tip for vegans:* Ghee, used in many dishes from India, is melted, clarified butter.) *Also see "Vegetarian Dishes in the Global Kitchen" on this page.*

● For airline meals ask for a vegetarian meal when you book your flight. If you need to, find out ahead if the meal is egg- and dairy-free. For airlines that don't offer vegetarian meals, request a fruit plate or pack your own snacks. *See "Dining at 35,000 Feet!" in chapter 14.*

● For organized meal functions, request a vegetarian meal ahead.

School Meals for Vegetarian Kids

● Review school menus with your child, and practice what he or she might order. If the school doesn't provide menus to parents, ask the school staff to provide them.

● Suggest the salad bar as a nutritious option—if it's available. A salad bar can be a good place to go for fresh vegetables and possibly for other nutrient-packed choices, including fruits, beans, sunflower seeds, cheese, or hard-cooked eggs.

● When the menu doesn't offer an option for your child, pack a lunch. A peanut butter sandwich is always popular. For the child who doesn't want to appear different, it's the food that almost all kids eat—vegetarian or not!

Vegetarian Dishes in the Global Kitchen

Delicious and nutritious—vegetarian dishes are typical fare in many parts of the world. As you flip the pages of ethnic cookbooks or glance through the menu of an ethnic restaurant, try to build your meal around dishes like these. They're typically made without meat, poultry, or fish—but check to be sure. Internationally, rice and beans—a high-protein food combination—also comes to the table nearly everywhere uniquely prepared and seasoned.

Caribbean
  Callaloo: one-pot meal (stew) made with dark-green leafy vegetables, a variety of other vegetables, peppers, and seasonings
  Black-eyed pea patties: black-eyed peas mashed with eggs and seasonings, then quickly pan-fried in a small amount of oil
  Pois et ris: kidney beans and rice flavored with smoked meat and seasonings
  Gunga: pigeon peas and rice

China
  Vegetable-tofu stir-fry: variety of thinly sliced vegetables and cubed bean curd stir-fried with soy sauce and perhaps vegetable broth
  Egg foo yung: frittatalike dish made by combining slightly whipped eggs with sliced vegetables, then frying in a skillet until browned; also may be prepared with meat or poultry
  Hot and sour soup: hot soup with tofu
  Vegetable potstickers: steamed vegetable dumplings
  Soybean cakes: stir-fried tofu with steamed rice

Vegetarian Dishes in the Global Kitchen *(continued)*

East Africa

Kunde (bean and groundnut stew): stew made of black-eyed peas, peanuts (groundnuts), tomatoes, and onions; a similar stew is made in West Africa, often without peanuts

Injera and lentil stew: flat bread served with cooked lentils; this is an Ethiopian dish

France

Vegetable quiche: pie made with a custard of egg and cheese mixed with chopped vegetables such as leeks, spinach, asparagus, and mushrooms

Ratatouille: soup or stew made of eggplant, tomatoes, onions, green peppers, and other vegetables; enjoy with crusty French bread

Greece

Tzatziki (cucumber-yogurt salad): plain yogurt mixed with shredded cucumber, garlic, and perhaps black olives; served with crusty bread

Vegetable-stuffed eggplant: eggplants hollowed and filled with chopped vegetables, cooked grains, and sometimes nuts

Spanakopita (spinach pie): pita made with a phyllo-dough crust and filled with a mixture of spinach, feta cheese, and eggs

India

Dohkla: steamed cakes made of rice and beans

Vegetable curry dishes: combination of chopped vegetables and lentils flavored with a curry mix and perhaps served with basmati rice

Idli or dhoka: steamed bean and rice cakes

Indonesia

Gado-gado: cooked vegetable salad with a peanut sauce; often seasoned with chilies

Italy

Pasta primavera: cooked pasta tossed with lightly cooked vegetables, with or without Parmesan cheese

Vegetable risotto: arborio rice, cooked in vegetable broth and combined with cooked vegetables and perhaps cooked beans or nuts, with or without grated cheese

Eggplant parmesan: sliced eggplant prepared by dipping it into a mixture of eggs and milk, coating it with breadcrumbs and Parmesan cheese,

and sautéeing it; to serve, it's topped with tomato sauce

Pasta e fagioli: pasta and white bean "stew" seasoned with herbs; usually prepared without meat

Mexico

Bean burrito: vegetarian refried beans wrapped in a soft tortilla, with or without cheese topping

Chiles rellenos: poblano peppers stuffed with cheese, dipped in an egg batter, and baked or fried; if they're fried, they're high in fat

Huevos rancheros (Mexican eggs): scrambled eggs prepared with onions, and served with tomato salsa, vegetarian refried beans, and tortillas

Vegetable fajitas: stir-fried vegetables and perhaps tofu rolled in a soft tortilla; often served with guacamole

Middle East

Falafel sandwich: ground chickpea patties (fried), tucked in pita bread with lettuce shreds and chopped tomato, topped with tahini (sesame seed spread)

Tabouli: salad made with bulgur, tomatoes, parsley, mint or chives, lemon juice, and perhaps cooked white beans

Ful: brown bean casserole made with tomatoes, lemons, parsley, and eggs

Mujadarah: lentils and rice seasoned with cumin, onions, and lemon

Native American Southwest

Maricopa bean stew: stew made of corn, beans, and cholla buds

South America

Ochos rios: kidney beans and rice flavored with shredded coconut

Spain

Tortilla à la española (Spanish omelette): egg omelette, made with potatoes, onions, and other vegetables

Vegetable paella: saffron-flavored rice dish with tomatoes and other vegetables

Switzerland

Cheese fondue: cheese melted with wine and served with chunks of crusty bread

Raclette: cheese "scraped" from a melted piece of hard cheese, then spread on a boiled potato or dark bread

CHAPTER 21

Sensitive about Food

Sensitive to certain foods? Maybe and maybe not. A queasy stomach, itchy skin, or diarrhea might be a reaction to something you ate. But it may or may not be what you think. So avoid the urge to give foods a bum rap without exploring the cause!

A food sensitivity, or adverse reaction to food, can't be overlooked as a health issue. It can seriously affect and disrupt the quality of life. The causes of discomfort are more numerous, and perhaps more complex, than you may think. Among the types of food sensitivities:

● *Food intolerances.* For metabolic reasons, people with a food intolerance can't digest part of certain foods or a food component. Food intolerances have other causes as well.

● *Food allergies.* A food allergy rallies the body's disease-fighting (immune) system to action, creating unpleasant, sometimes serious, symptoms. In other words, the immune system starts to work even though the person isn't sick. That's why symptoms appear.

● *Other adverse reactions to food.* Infectious organisms such as bacteria, parasites, or viruses, which cause foodborne illness, or contaminants such as chemicals in water where seafood is harvested, can cause an adverse body reaction.

● *Psychological reasons.* Feelings of discomfort after eating can also be wrapped up with many emotions. Even though there's no physical reason, just thinking about a certain food that may be associated with an unpleasant experience can make some people feel sick!

If a certain food seems to bother you, skip the temptation to self-diagnose. Instead, check with your physician. For example, a reaction to milk is more likely an intolerance than a food allergy; let your doctor diagnose your symptoms. This chapter can help you get familiar with possible causes. Be aware that an adverse reaction may be a foodborne illness; *see chapter 12, "The Safe Kitchen," for a closer look at identifying and preventing foodborne illnesses.*

Food Intolerances and Other Adverse Food Reactions: Copycat Symptoms

If your body reacts to food or a food component, you may have a food intolerance, not an allergy. Unlike food allergies, food intolerances don't involve the immune system. However, because they prompt many of the same symptoms—nausea, diarrhea, and abdominal cramps—food intolerances are often mislabeled as "allergies."

With a food intolerance, physical reactions to a food often result from faulty metabolism. The body can't adequately digest a certain component of a particular food—perhaps because a digestive enzyme is deficient. Substances that are part of a food's natural chemistry—such as theobromine in coffee or tea, or serotonin in bananas or tomatoes—may cause reactions, too.

Depending on the type of food intolerance, most people can eat small servings of the problem food without unpleasant side effects. (People with gluten intolerance and those with sulfite sensitivity are exceptions.) In contrast, people with food allergies usually need to eliminate the problem food from their diet altogether.

Lactose Intolerance: A Matter of Degree

Do you like milk but think that milk doesn't like you? Then you may be lactose-intolerant—and not allergic to milk. The good news is: A serving of milk may be "friendlier" than you think!

Lactose is a natural sugar in milk and milk products. During digestion, an intestinal enzyme called lactase breaks down lactose into smaller, more easily digested sugars. People with lactose intolerance produce too little lactase to adequately digest the amount of lactose in foods and beverages containing milk. Left undigested, lactose is fermented by "healthy" bacteria in the intestinal tract. This fermentation produces uncomfortable symptoms—for example, nausea, cramping, bloating, abdominal pain, gas, and diarrhea.

For people with lactose intolerance, symptoms may begin from fifteen minutes to several hours after consuming foods or drinks containing lactose. The severity of symptoms varies from person to person—and how much and when lactose is consumed in relation to other foods.

A milk allergy is quite different. It's an allergic reaction to the protein components, such as casein, in milk. People who have a milk allergy usually must avoid all milk products. People with lactose intolerance can eat dairy products in varying amounts; that's because lactose intolerance is a matter of degree. If you suspect lactose intolerance, avoid self-diagnosis. Instead, see your doctor for a medical diagnosis; the symptoms might be caused by another condition. Lactose intolerance is diagnosed with one of several tests: a blood test, a hydrogen breath test, or a stool acidity test (used for infants and young children).

Who's Likely to Be Lactose-Intolerant?

Anyone can be lactose-intolerant. From birth, most infants produce the lactase enzyme. With age, however, the body may produce less lactase. It's an inherited condition that doesn't happen to everybody.

How many people have low levels of lactase? About thirty million American adults; however, a large proportion of them have few if any symptoms. And many

HOW MUCH LACTOSE?

PRODUCT	SERVING SIZE (APPROXIMATE)	LACTOSE (GM)
Milk: whole, reduced-fat, low-fat, fat-free, sweet acidophilus milk, or buttermilk	1 cup	10–12
Goat milk	1 cup	9
Lactose-reduced milk	1 cup	2–4
Nonfat dry milk	1/3 cup	12
Half-and-half	1/2 cup	5
Whipping cream	1/2 cup	3
Sour cream	1/2 cup	4
Sweetened condensed milk	1 cup	30
Evaporated milk	1 cup	24
Butter, margarine	1 tsp.	Trace
Cottage cheese	1/2 cup	2–3
Yogurt, low-fat	1 cup	5
Cheese: American, Swiss, blue, Cheddar, Parmesan, or cream cheese	1 oz.	1–2
Ice cream, regular and low-fat	1/2 cup	6–9
Sherbet, orange	1/2 cup	2

Lactose-free foods include:
- Broth-based soups
- Plain meat, fish, and poultry
- Fruits and vegetables, plain
- Tofu and tofu products
- Soy and rice beverages
- Breads, cereal, crackers, and desserts made without milk, dry milk, or whey

people who think they're lactose-intolerant really aren't. In the United States, Asians and Native Americans (about 80 percent of them) tend to be the most lactose-intolerant groups. An estimated 75 percent of African Americans, 50 percent of Hispanic Americans, and 20 percent of Caucasian Americans have varying degrees of lactose intolerance. People whose ancestors come from northern or western Europe tend to maintain adequate lactose levels throughout their lives.

Lactose intolerance is sometimes linked to other issues. For example, some medications lower lactase production in the body. Lactose intolerance can be a side effect of certain medical conditions, such as intestinal disease or gastric (stomach) surgery. Depending on the cause, lactose intolerance may be short-term.

Lactose in Food: Which "Whey"?

Lactose usually comes from foods containing milk or milk solids. *The chart "How Much Lactose?" on page 518 suggests how much.* Prepared foods, even those labeled "nondairy," may contain lactose, too. If you're *very* lactose-intolerant, you may need to check labels carefully.

● Look for label ingredient terms that suggest lactose: milk, dry milk solids (including nonfat milk solids), buttermilk, lactose, malted milk, sour or sweet cream, margarine, whey, whey protein concentrate, and cheese.

● Recognize baked and processed foods that often contain small amounts of lactose: bread, candy and cookies, cold cuts and hot dogs, salad dressings, drink mixes, commercial sauces and gravies, cream soups, drink mixes, dry cereals, prepared foods (such as frozen pizza, lasagna, and waffles), salad dressings made with milk or cheese, and sugar substitutes.

● Be aware that some medications also contain lactose. If you're lactose-intolerant, consult with your physician or pharmacist about appropriate medications.

Dairy Foods: Don't Give 'Em Up!

So you've been diagnosed as lactose-intolerant. That's not a reason to give up dairy foods! Lactose intolerance isn't an "all or nothing" condition. Instead, it's a matter of degree. Most people with difficulty digesting lactose can still consume foods with lactose. It's

For Those with Lactose Intolerance: Another Option

As another option, food products have been developed for people with lactose intolerance. Some products are lactose-reduced. Others contain lactase, the enzyme that digests milk sugar and that's deficient to some degree in people with lactose intolerance. *If you're lactose-intolerant and if "Lactose: Tips for Tolerance" in this chapter isn't enough:*

● Look for lactose-reduced or lactose-free milk and other dairy foods at the supermarket. Lactose-reduced milk has 70 percent less lactose than regular milk, and lactose-free milk is virtually free of any lactose.

● Add lactase enzyme, available in tablets or in drops, to fluid milk before drinking it. You'll find instructions on the package. Your milk will taste slightly sweeter because added lactase breaks down the lactose in milk into simpler, sweeter sugars.

● As another option, look for a lactase supplement to chew or swallow before eating lactose-rich foods. With a supplemental supply of lactase, you can eat without discomfort. Read the timing and dosage instructions on the package label.

just a matter of knowing which foods contain lactose—and knowing your personal tolerance level.

Needlessly eliminating milk and other dairy foods from your diet may pose nutritional risks. They're important sources of calcium, protein, riboflavin, vitamins A and D, magnesium, phosphorus, and many other nutrients.

Calcium, for example, is especially important because of its role in growing and maintaining strong bones. An adequate amount of calcium helps children and teens grow strong, healthy bones and helps prevent the bone-thinning disease called osteoporosis. Milk and other dairy foods supply 75 percent of the calcium in the American food supply. Without these foods, meeting your calcium requirement can be challenging. *For more about calcium in a healthful diet see "Calcium: A Closer Look" in chapter 4.*

If you're lactose-intolerant, consult a registered dietitian (RD) for help with planning a diet that's adequate in calcium while controlling the lactose in your meals and snacks. In extreme cases or for children or pregnant women with lactose intolerance, a physician or a registered dietitian also may recommend a calcium supplement.

Lactose: Tips for Tolerance

Lactose intolerance is easy to manage. Most people with difficulty digesting lactose can include some dairy and other lactose-containing foods in their meals and snacks. In fact, 80 percent of people with lower levels of lactase can drink a cup of milk without discomfort.

If you—or someone in your family—has trouble digesting lactose, try these tips to comfortably include lactose-containing foods in meals and snacks:

● Experiment! Start with small amounts of lactose-containing foods. Then gradually increase the portion size to determine your personal tolerance level.

● Enjoy lactose-containing foods as part of a meal or a snack, rather than alone. Try a milk-fruit smoothie, or milk and fruit on your morning cereal. The mix of foods slows release of lactose into the digestive system, making it easier to digest. Think of this as "diluting" the lactose.

Have You Ever Wondered

... if goat milk is a good substitute for cow milk for someone with lactose intolerance? Goat milk has slightly less lactose: 9 grams of lactose per cup, compared with 11 grams of lactose in one cup of cow milk.

... if a nondairy creamer can replace milk for someone who's lactose-intolerant? How about nonfat dry milk? No. Nondairy creamers may contain lactose. Check the label. The nutrient content of the creamer and the milk is different. In a nondairy creamer, the protein quality and the amounts of calcium and vitamins A and C are lower than in milk. Regarding nonfat dry milk, remember that fat, not lactose, has been removed from milk.

... if a/B milk offers unique health benefits? From a nutritional standpoint, milk with added a/B cultures (acidophilus and bifidobacteria cultures) is similar to the milk it's made from. Although research isn't conclusive, these cultures may help improve lactose digestion, promote healthy bacteria in the GI tract, and help lower blood pressure.

● Eat smaller, more frequent portions of lactose-rich foods. For example, drink 1/2- or 3/4-cup servings of milk several times throughout the day instead of 1-cup servings one, two, or three times daily.

● Choose calcium-rich foods that are naturally lower in lactose, such as aged cheese. When cheese is made, curds (or solids) are separated from the whey (or watery liquid); most lactose is in the whey. Aged cheeses such as Swiss, colby, Parmesan, and Cheddar lose most of their lactose during processing and aging. Much of the lactose is removed with the whey.

● Try dairy foods (yogurt and buttermilk) made with active cultures. They're easier to digest because their "friendly" bacteria help digest the lactose. Not all cultured dairy foods contain live cultures. Look for the National Yogurt Association's seal "Live and Active Cultures" on the yogurt carton.

● Opt for whole-milk dairy products. The higher fat content of whole-milk dairy products may help to slow the rate of digestion, allowing a gradual release of lactose. Then in your overall food choices, choose other foods with less fat.

● Even if you're sensitive to lactose, include a variety of calcium-rich foods in your diet every day. In addition to dairy foods, enjoy these other calcium sources: dark-green leafy vegetables such as broccoli and greens; calcium-fortified products such as juice, bread, and cereal; and canned sardines and salmon with bones. For canned fish you need to eat the bones to get the calcium!

● Become a label sleuth. Check the ingredient list on the food label for words that may indicate lactose. *See "Lactose in Food: Which 'Whey'?" in this chapter.*

● Don't be fooled by lactobacillus or sweet acidophilus milks. Most are no lower in lactose. They're tolerated about the same as other forms of milk.

Gluten Intolerance: Often a Lifelong Condition

Pasta, tortillas, bagels, whole-wheat bread: all great sources of complex "carbs," nutrients, and perhaps fiber for most people. Yet, those with gluten intolerance need to build their healthful eating plan with other grain products.

Gluten intolerance—also referred to as gluten-sensitive enteropathy or celiac disease—is an intes-

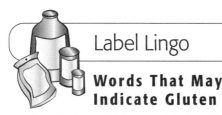

Label Lingo

Words That May Indicate Gluten

For people with gluten intolerance, label reading is very important! These are among the ingredients that indicate the presence of gluten:

- Emulsifiers
- Stabilizers
- Thickeners
- Barley
- Cereals: wheat, rye, triticale, barley, kamut, and oat
- Flour, self-rising flour, enriched flour, graham flour, durum flour
- Food starch and modified food starch
- Gluten flour
- Hydrolyzed vegetable protein (HVP)
- Malt or cereal extracts
- Malt flavoring
- Oat bran
- Oats
- Rye
- Soy sauce (made from wheat; look for gluten-free soy sauce)
- Wheat (spelt, triticale, bulgur, farina, kamut)
- Wheat-based semolina
- Wheat germ and bran
- Wheat starch

Source: The Chicago Dietetic Association, The South Shore Suburban Dietetic Association, and Dietitians of Canada, *Manual of Clinical Dietetics,* 6th ed. (Chicago, American Dietetic Association, 2000).

tinal disorder and not a true food intolerance. For those who have it, the body can't tolerate gluten (a form of protein) in wheat, rye, barley, and perhaps oats.

For people with gluten intolerance, consuming gluten damages the lining of the small intestine. As a result, the damaged intestine has an impaired ability to absorb nutrients, including carbohydrates, proteins, fats, and fat-soluble vitamins. For someone with gluten intolerance, the risk for malnutrition is high. The potential risks extend farther: premature osteoporosis, colon cancer, autoimmune disorders (including thyroid disease and type 1 diabetes), arthritis, miscarriage, and birth defects.

Who's at risk? As a genetic disorder, gluten intolerance is more common among people with European roots. The actual incidence in the United States is unknown but may run as high as 1 in every 150 Americans. The challenge is: Gluten intolerance is often misdiagnosed, and its varying symptoms often imitate other health problems. Often it goes undetected until triggered by other body stresses: perhaps surgery, a viral infection, or pregnancy.

What are the symptoms? They vary. Weakness, appetite loss, weight loss, chronic diarrhea, and abdominal cramps and bloating are common; some experience a painful rash, muscle cramps, or joint pain. Among women, gluten intolerance may interfere with the menstrual cycle. For children, gluten intolerance is especially risky. Unless the condition is well managed, gluten intolerance can affect a child's behavior and ability to grow and learn. Chronic irritability is a warning sign. For growth and development, a child's high energy and nutrient needs require adequate nourishment.

Gluten intolerance can occur at any age. Symptoms may appear first during infancy when cereal is started. But most cases are diagnosed in the adult years, often ten years after the first symptoms. Temporary lactose intolerance may accompany gluten intolerance, happening at least until the condition is under control and the small intestine heals. The healing may take months or years.

The primary treatment for gluten intolerance is a lifelong, strict eating regimen; *a gluten-free diet is a "must."* Once gluten is eliminated from the diet, the small intestine can heal itself. Nutrient absorption then improves, and the symptoms disappear. Those with gluten intolerance can live a long, healthy life. If you think you have gluten intolerance, consult your physician for a diagnosis.

Which Foods for Gluten Intolerance?

Gluten in four grains—wheat, rye, barley, and perhaps oats—is damaging. To manage gluten intolerance, these four grains, and any food or food component made from them, must be avoided. Although not technically a grain, buckwheat, which is a seed, should be avoided, too. Even trace amounts of gluten in the diet can damage the small intestine.

Avoiding wheat is probably the biggest challenge for people with gluten intolerance. That's because wheat is the main ingredient in so many foods: baked foods, bread, breakfast cereal, breaded foods, crackers, pretzels, and pasta, among others. Gluten-containing ingredients show up as additives (thickeners, fillers, and stabilizers) in many other products, too, including batter-dipped vegetables, scalloped potatoes, canned soup, lunch meat, pudding, beer, salad dressing, canned tuna—and even some medications, toothpastes, and mouthwashes.

Gluten-containing ingredients may be hard to detect because they may appear under a different name as part of another ingredient. *See "Label Lingo: Words That May Indicate Gluten" in this chapter.*

Knowing how to identify gluten is important when you're asking for ingredients information from food manufacturers. Technically, "gluten" is a generic term that describes the protein component of grain. Although rice and corn contain gluten, it's in a different form, so it's not harmful. Gluten from barley, rye, wheat, and perhaps oats needs to be avoided.

Eating Gluten-Free!

Coping with gluten intolerance requires a strict eating regimen. While it's hard to follow at first, this condition can be managed with food choices, not medication. If you—or someone you know—deals with gluten intolerance, these are some guidelines to follow:

● Consult a registered dietitian. He or she can help you learn how to live with gluten intolerance—and enjoy eating! *See "How to Find Nutrition Help . . ." in chapter 24 for tips on finding a qualified nutrition expert.*

● Enjoy what you can eat. Corn and rice are two readily available safe grains. Skip oats, since they may be produced and harvested in equipment used for handling wheat. As a result, cross-contamination may be a problem.

● Look for gluten-free grains, flour, and food products in local food stores. Can't find them in your grocery store? Check specialty or health food stores. Mail-order outlets also can be a source of alternate flours for baking, as well as prepared foods, mixes, grains, and specialty ingredients.

● Read food labels carefully! Many commercially prepared foods—baked, frozen, and canned—have gluten-containing ingredients. Even though they seem okay, these are among the many foods that may or may not be a problem: flavored and frozen yogurt, rice crackers, luncheon meats, egg substitutes, French fries (especially in restaurants), salad dressings, pudding mixes, canned soups, flavored teas, candies, seasoning mixes, tortilla chips, and Worcestershire sauce. Spotting ingredients and additives with gluten *must* become second nature. Check the ingredient list for terms such as those in *"Label Lingo: Words That May Indicate Gluten" in this chapter.*

● Get to know the origin, composition, and production of ingredients. For example, flavored chips may be dusted with an ingredient made with wheat. Since the amount is less than 2 percent by weight, the ingredient may not be listed on the label. Another example: vinegars, which are distilled from grain, are okay except for malt vinegar in the United States. Malt vinegar is a problem because malt by definition in the United States is barley; it may be added to or used as the starting mash to produce malt vinegar. Ingredients used in prepared foods, such as marinades and barbecue sauce, may have malt vinegar, too.

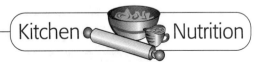

Gluten-Free Substitutions for Flour

● *1 tablespoon wheat flour equals*

    1½ teaspoons cornstarch, arrowroot, white rice flour, *or* potato starch

    2 teaspoons tapioca *or* uncooked rice

● *1 cup wheat flour equals*

    2 cups brown rice flour *or* sweet rice flour

    1 cup fine cornmeal *or* corn flour

    ⅞ cup white *or* brown rice flour

    ⅝ cup potato starch

    1 cup soy flour plus ¼ cup potato starch flour

    ¾ cup rice flour plus ¼ cup cornstarch

Source: The Chicago Dietetic Association, The South Shore Suburban Dietetic Association, and Dietitians of Canada, *Manual of Clinical Dietetics,* 6th ed. (Chicago: American Dietetic Association, 2000).

... if a wheat allergy is the same as gluten intolerance (celiac disease or gluten-sensitive enteropathy)? No, they're two different conditions: different physiological responses, treated in different ways. With a wheat allergy, wheat products and foods made with wheat products must be avoided. If you're allergic to wheat, you can consume wheat substitutes, including oats, rye, and barley. *See "Gluten Intolerance: Often a Lifelong Condition" in this chapter for ways to cope with gluten intolerance.*

● Substitute gluten-free flour for wheat flour in food preparation. Use corn, rice, soy, arrowroot, tapioca, or potato flours, or perhaps a mixture, instead of wheat flour in recipes. These flours are gluten-free. Because they give a different flavor and texture to the baked foods, using these flours takes practice and experimentation.

● Keep up-to-date with food products so you can choose gluten-free foods. Contact food manufacturers for their current ingredient lists. As you know, recipes for prepared foods change. You'll find the company name, address, and perhaps a toll-free consumer information service number on the food label.

● Eating away from home? If you're on the road, pack gluten-free foods. For long flights, order a gluten-free meal when you make your airline reservation. Read restaurant menus carefully and ask questions. If you're a guest in someone's home, tell him or her about your special food needs ahead, and offer to bring food. *For more tips on ordering from a menu see "Restaurant Eater's Tip List" in chapter 14.*

● Seek out local and national support groups. It's a great way to share information and recipes with others who have the same condition. Many support groups publish lists of acceptable food products by brand name. That makes shopping and following a gluten-free diet easier. A registered dietitian can help you find a support group.

Sensitive to Additives? Maybe, Maybe Not

Do you wonder about the functions of those hard-to-pronounce ingredients listed on the label of your favorite foods? You probably know most are additives, but you may not know exactly why they are added to foods.

Additives serve a number of important functions in food. For instance, they may improve the nutritional value of food, just as B vitamins and iron are added to flour. Some additives, such as spices and colors, enhance the taste and the appearance of food products. Others prevent spoilage or give foods the consistency you expect. Without them our food supply likely would be far more limited. *See "Additives: Safe at the Plate" in chapter 9 for more on food additives.*

Except on rare occasions, we consume many food additives without side effects. For those who do experience adverse reactions, the response is commonly an intolerance—not a true allergy—to the additive.

In the United States, the Food and Drug Administration (FDA) regulates food additives; food intolerances and allergies are considered as part of their approval process. Certain food additives—preservatives, colors, and flavors—are linked more commonly to food sensitivities than others. But just how strong is the link? Read on.

For the Sulfite-Sensitive

Have you ever wondered why dried apricots and dehydrated potatoes list "sulfites" on the ingredient list of

Where Might You Find Sulfites?

● Dried fruits such as apricots
● Frozen or prepackaged avocado dip
● Instant and frozen potatoes such as French fries, potato chips, dried potatoes, and potato flakes
● Wine, beer
● Cider
● Fruit juices
● Wine vinegar
● Gelatin
● Maraschino cherries
● Lemon juice
● Salad dressings and sauces from dry mixes
● Shrimp, canned seafood soups
● Pickled products
● Canned or dried soups

a food label? Sulfites are used to prevent certain foods from browning, such as light-colored fruits, dried fruits, and vegetables. Added to beer, wine, and other fermented foods, sulfites slow the growth of bacteria.

The term "sulfites" is a catchall, referring to a variety of additives commonly used in food. Usually they have "sulf" in their names. Sulfites may be listed on food labels as sulfur dioxide, sodium sulfite, sodium or potassium bisulfite, and sodium or potassium metabisulfite.

Sulfites, as part of a varied diet, pose no risk of side effects for most of us. However, for 5 to 10 percent of the population, sulfites may provoke an adverse reaction. About 1.7 percent of asthmatics more often react to sulfites than others do, and the reaction may be severe.

For those who are sulfite-sensitive, reactions may include wheezing, diarrhea, stomach ache, hives, or swelling. Fortunately, side effects are mild for most people. However, reactions may become life-threatening for those who are very sensitive to sulfite. *In rare cases these individuals may experience anaphylactic shock.* As with other food intolerances and allergies, consult a doctor if you think you're sulfite-sensitive. Don't self-diagnose.

Because sulfites can trigger intense reactions in sulfite-sensitive asthmatics, the U.S. Food and Drug Administration prohibits the use of sulfites on fruits and vegetables (except potatoes) intended to be served or sold raw. In the past, sulfites were sometimes used to keep fruits and vegetables fresh longer on restaurant salad bars, but that's no longer allowed.

Sulfites also can destroy the B vitamin called thiamin. For that reason they're not allowed in foods such as enriched bread and flour. These foods are major sources of thiamin in the American diet.

If you're among those rare individuals who are sulfite-sensitive, follow these guidelines:

● Check food labels, and choose foods without sulfite-containing additives. Be aware that they're used in varying amounts in many packaged foods—not just dried fruit, dehydrated potatoes, and fruit juices. By law, when sulfites are present in detectable amounts, the label must indicate it has sulfites. *See "Where Might You Find Sulfites?" in this chapter for a list of foods that might contain sulfites.*

Does Food Cause Childhood Hyperactivity?

The commonly held notion linking sugar or other food additives to hyperactive behavior or attention deficit hyperactivity disorder (ADHD) in children has never been scientifically proven. Although the exact cause of ADHD isn't known, factors such as genetics and environmental influences have been suggested.

The Feingold diet, popularized for its claimed ability to manage ADHD, has been touted as an approach for treating hyperactive children. The eating plan restricts foods containing salicylates, which are present in almonds, certain fruits and vegetables, artificial flavors and colors, and preservatives. However, the reported success is based on anecdotal data, not scientifically proven methods of research. The extra attention given to children on the Feingold diet may be the reason for the child's behavior change, not the change in food choices. Although many other studies have been conducted attempting to link eating with hyperactivity, the Feingold results haven't been replicated.

Until researchers learn more, the best management of ADHD includes behavioral modification and medication, if warranted by a doctor.

For more about the misconceptions between sugar and behavior see "Sugar Myths" in chapter 5.

● Be careful of alcoholic beverages. Since 1988, labels on beer and wine must state "Contains Sulfites" if applicable.

● Ask questions in restaurants before you order. For example, ask if canned foods, vegetables, or potato products contain—or were treated with—sulfites.

Coloring . . . by Any Other Name!

Although the incidence is rare, a very small number of people are sensitive to a coloring added to food. FD&C Yellow No. 5, also called tartrazine, is a dye used to color foods, beverages, and medications. Research indicates that FD&C Yellow No. 5 may trigger hives, itching, and nasal congestion. But the incidence is limited to just one or two of every ten thousand people. Yellow No. 5 is the only food coloring known to cause such reactions.

... if you can be sensitive to MSG? Perhaps, but not likely. Some people describe varying symptoms, including body tingling or warmth, and chest pain after eating foods containing monosodium glutamate (MSG). The symptoms, usually mild, often last less than an hour. Collectively the symptoms have been referred to as "Chinese restaurant syndrome" because MSG is so common in Chinese cuisine.

Actually, research hasn't found a definitive link between MSG or Chinese food, and any adverse side effects. Other components in those foods, perhaps a common allergen such as soy, could be the culprits if you have an adverse reaction.

If you want to moderate your MSG intake—or if you seem sensitive to it—see if you can order food without added MSG in Asian restaurants. If the menu says "No MSG" it likely means no added MSG. MSG is likely in other ingredients, such as soy sauce; glutamate itself is naturally in virtually all protein-containing foods. Check food labels to guide your food selection, too. Glutamate that naturally occurs in food won't be on the ingredient list, so you may want to consult a registered dietitian for guidance. *To learn more see "MSG—Another Flavor Enhancer" in chapter 7.*

Whenever added to a food or a medication, FD&C Yellow No. 5 must be listed on the label or package insert. If you're sensitive to this coloring, read labels carefully. Foods and beverages likely to contain tartrazine include soft drinks; ice cream and sherbets; gelatins; salad dressings; cheese dishes; seasoned salts; candies; flavor extracts; and pudding, cake, and frosting mixes.

Aspartame: PKU Warning

Since their discovery, intense or low-calorie sweeteners—aspartame, saccharin, acesulfame K, sucralose, and tagatose—have been thoroughly investigated by regulatory agencies around the globe as well as by leading scientific organizations. Evidence indicates that their long-term intake is safe and not associated with adverse health effects. *"Quintet of Sweet Options" in chapter 5 looks at these sweeteners.* With one exception, low-calorie sweeteners do not cause symptoms of food sensitivity. *However, people with*

the rare genetic disorder phenylketonuria (PKU) should avoid foods sweetened with aspartame.

Aspartame is made from two amino acids (aspartic acid and phenylalanine) and methanol. The same amino acids are found naturally in foods such as meat, milk, fruit, and vegetables. Regardless of the source, people with PKU cannot metabolize phenylalanine properly, so they can consume only limited amounts. Unmanaged, PKU can cause tissue damage, and in infants, brain damage. As a precaution, all babies are screened for PKU at birth.

For those who suffer from this disorder, foods and beverages containing aspartame carry a label warning stating "Phenylketonurics: Contains Phenylalanine." One of the most widely accepted food additives, aspartame is found in many products, including carbonated and powdered soft drinks, yogurt, pudding and gelatins, frozen desserts, hot beverage mixes, and candy. You'll find aspartame listed in the ingredient

My Aching Head

Two to 20 percent of Americans suffer migraines (severe head pain plus a range of other symptoms such as nausea, vomiting, or increased sensitivity to light, sound, and smells). Migraine headaches can affect anyone, but women are three times more likely than men to suffer. Certain foods are blamed, but there's little agreement about the link between foods and headaches.

The causes of migraine headaches are complicated and not well understood. Certain components of food—natural or added—have been suspected, but not proven, to be causes of headaches in some people. Tyrosine (in cheese and chocolate), histamine (in red wine), caffeine (in coffee and cola), benzoic acid (a preservative), and alcohol may be food-related triggers. Susceptible individuals may be affected by a combination of factors, not just food.

If you experience chronic headaches, check with your physician for a medical diagnosis. To determine which foods, if any, trigger migraine attacks, keep a diary of what you eat. Depending on how often your attacks occur, you may need to keep the diary for several weeks.

If you're diagnosed with migraine headaches and you feel you're susceptible to food triggers, a registered dietitian can recommend appropriate substitutes for suspected food triggers.

list of the food label—and the PKU warning also lets you know it's there.

Food Allergies: Commonly Uncommon

Have you ever heard parents say that their child is allergic to milk, then remark that he or she has no adverse reactions to chocolate milk? Or maybe you avoid a particular food yourself, believing you have an allergy to it? Although food allergies are not to be taken lightly, you may be surprised at just how infrequently true food allergies occur. Consider that:

● One in three adults believes that he or she is allergic to milk. However, only 2 to 2.5 percent of adults (about 6 million Americans) suffer from true food allergies of any kind!

● An estimated 4 to 6 percent of infants and 1 to 2 percent of children are diagnosed with food allergies. Infants usually outgrow them by the time they become adults.

If food allergies are so uncommon, why do millions claim they're allergic? Because food allergies are often self-diagnosed and because the symptoms can mimic other food-induced ailments such as foodborne illness and food intolerances. People often use the term "allergy" loosely to describe almost any physical reaction to food—even if it's psychological!

Who is likely to develop a food allergy? Anyone. However, most occur among people with a family history of allergies. Nonfood allergies are more common than food allergies. Food allergies are often inherited, and almost all are identified early in life. Infants are much more likely to have food allergies than adults, although many allergies are outgrown. A milk allergy, for example, is usually outgrown by age three.

Food Allergies: What Are They?

A true food allergy, sometimes called food hypersensitivity, causes the body's immune system to react even though the person isn't sick. The body reacts to a usually harmless food substance, thinking it's harmful. An allergen, which is usually a protein in the troublesome food, sets off a chain of immune system reactions.

When an allergy-prone person eats a food that causes an allergic reaction, his or her body scrambles to protect itself by making immunoglubulin E (IgE) antibodies. These antibodies trigger the release of body chemicals such as histamine. In turn, these body chemicals cause uncomfortable symptoms associated with food allergies, such as a runny nose, itchy skin, nausea, even a rapid heartbeat, or in severe cases, anaphylaxis.

Something You Ate?

It's lunchtime. You make your toddler his or her first peanut butter and jelly sandwich. An hour later you notice the child has broken out with an itchy rash. You've heard that peanuts commonly contain food allergens. Is your child allergic to the peanut butter in the sandwich? Maybe . . . or maybe not! In any case, a call to the child's doctor is certainly in order.

Actually, any food can cause an allergic reaction in a susceptible person. However, some foods are more likely than others to set off a reaction. Milk, eggs, wheat, and soy, as well as fish, crustacea (especially shrimp), peanuts, and tree nuts (such as walnuts) are the most common foods with allergens, causing 90 percent of allergic reactions. Raw soybeans and sprouts tend to be more allergenic than tofu, tempeh, and miso. An allergy to egg, milk, soy, or wheat often is outgrown. A peanut allergy lasts for life.

Symptoms? Something to Sneeze About

What are the symptoms of a food allergy? Different people react to the same allergen in different ways. Even if a food contains a common allergen, you can't predict whether you may have an allergic reaction. Symptoms may appear within seconds or up to several

---

What Food Allergies Are Most Common?

● *Adults:* peanuts, crustacea (crab, crawfish, lobster, shrimp), tree nuts (almonds, Brazil nuts, hazelnuts, pecans, walnuts, others), fish

● *Children:* milk, eggs, peanuts, soybeans, tree nuts, wheat, fish, shellfish

hours after eating the food that triggers the reaction. In exceptionally sensitive people, just the touch or the smell of the food can provoke a reaction!

What's the Sign?

The most common symptoms include swelling, sneezing, and nausea. Most symptoms affect the skin, respiratory system, stomach, or intestines:

Skin reactions:

- Swelling of the lips, tongue, and face
- Itchy eyes
- Hives
- Rash (eczema)

Respiratory tract reactions:

- Itching and/or tightness in the throat
- Shortness of breath
- Dry or raspy cough
- Runny nose
- Wheezing (asthma)

Digestive tract reactions:

- Abdominal pain
- Nausea
- Vomiting
- Diarrhea

Source: Celide Barnes Koerner and Anne Muoz-Furlong, *Food Allergies* (New York: John Wiley & Sons, 1998).

A severe allergic reaction also can cause a drop in blood pressure, loss of consciousness, and death.

Keep in mind that these symptoms may be caused by other food- or nonfood-related conditions. For an accurate diagnosis you need a complete medical evaluation by a board-certified allergist.

Emotions associated with food experiences, and not the food itself, can even cause a reaction. Just the appearance, smell, or taste of food might trigger an emotional reaction resulting in symptoms that mimic a food allergy or food intolerance. Or someone might get these symptoms by believing the food is harmful. Even if you suspect that emotions are at the root of an adverse reaction to food, check with your physician. Symptoms may stem from a more serious physical condition.

To date there's no known scientific link between food allergies and arthritis, migraine headaches,

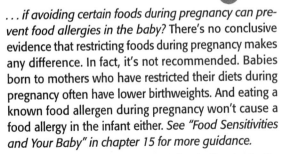

Have You Ever Wondered

. . . if avoiding certain foods during pregnancy can prevent food allergies in the baby? There's no conclusive evidence that restricting foods during pregnancy makes any difference. In fact, it's not recommended. Babies born to mothers who have restricted their diets during pregnancy often have lower birthweights. And eating a known food allergen during pregnancy won't cause a food allergy in the infant either. *See "Food Sensitivities and Your Baby" in chapter 15 for more guidance.*

. . . if breast-feeding can prevent food allergies in the baby? Perhaps so. For those with a family history of allergies, breast-fed babies are less likely to have food allergies. As a precaution against potential allergens in breast milk, the American Academy of Pediatrics suggests that nursing mothers of susceptible infants (with a family history of allergies) are wise to skip peanuts and peanut-containing foods. *See "Breast-Feeding Your Baby" in chapter 15 for more information.*

behavioral problems, ear infections, and urinary tract infections, although research in these areas is under way.

Food Allergies: The Dangerous Side

For most people with food allergies, the reactions are more uncomfortable than dangerous. In rare cases, however, an anaphylactic reaction can occur. When many different body systems react at the same time, this allergic response to food can be severe and even life-threatening. Even a touch, whiff, or tiny bite of a food allergen can be harmful.

With an anaphylactic reaction, symptoms often develop quickly—within a few seconds or minutes after eating—and progress quickly from mild to severe. They may include extreme itching, a swelling of the throat that makes breathing difficult, sweating, rapid or irregular heartbeat, low blood pressure, nausea, diarrhea, loss of consciousness, and cardiac arrest and shock. Without immediate medical attention the affected person may die. What foods may cause a severe reaction? *Although the cases are rare, any food allergen can cause anaphylaxis; of the incidences, most are caused by allergens in tree nuts, eggs, peanuts, or shellfish (crustacea).*

Is the reaction the same every time? Perhaps not. Its severity depends on two things: how allergic a person is and how much allergen is consumed.

Warning! If you—or a family member—experience severe food reactions, plan in advance how you would handle accidental ingestion of the "trigger" allergen. The person should wear an identification bracelet or necklace to alert others. And he or she should carry epinephrine (adrenaline) that can be injected quickly to counter the allergen. Because the body's responses can be life-threatening, call 911 or an ambulance immediately if someone has severe allergic reactions.

Itching for a Cause?

If you have symptoms, a doctor can help you "scratch" the surface to find the cause with a medical diagnosis.

A board-certified allergist (certified by the American Academy of Allergy, Asthma, and Immunology) is best equipped to diagnose food allergies. Never try to self-diagnose. Someone with a food allergy should be under a doctor's care.

True food allergies can be measured and evaluated clinically—with no need for "hunches." In that way unrelated medical conditions are eliminated. Typically the diagnosis includes a medical history, a physical exam, and possibly a food diary, elimination diet, and laboratory tests. As an initial screening your doctor may use a skin test; an allergist will confirm a food allergy with more definitive tests. *Check "Pass the Test?" later in this chapter.*

Keeping track of how your body reacts to a specific food one time after another may help you detect a food allergy or intolerance on your own. But be careful about self-diagnosis. The cause may be a more

---

Helping Kids Deal with Food Allergies

Whether your child—or his or her pal—has a food allergy, kids need to learn how to deal with food allergies. Banning allergenic foods from schools or other child-focused environments doesn't teach self-care. Instead it creates a false sense of security about the safety of the real world of food.

If your child has a food allergy, help him or her develop coping skills:

● Educate the day-care facility, school, camp director, or bus driver about your child's food allergy. Bring a signed letter from your child's healthcare provider. Together develop an individualized approach for avoiding allergens without making your child feel "different" or isolated.

● Include all the food-related events in your approach: parties, birthday treats, in-class food activities, recess, field trips, and food that your child and classmates bring from home.

● With your healthcare provider, other responsible adults, and your child, make a plan for epinephrine administration (for severe reactions) or antihistamine (for milder reactions). Come up with a way your child can signal for help—fast!

● Go over the menu to identify foods to avoid. Plan for substitutes—with the food service staff—or for home-prepared food.

● Teach your children why and how to avoid "food swapping"—and foods that could cause a reaction.

For more parenting tips on school meals see "For Kids Only—Today's School Meals" in chapter 16.

● Equip your child. When old enough to be responsible, children and teens who have severe reactions should carry an EpiPen or other form of epinephrine, a personal emergency card (perhaps in a fun backpack), a medical-alert necklace or bracelet, and a parent's phone number. An antihistamine may be enough for milder reactions.

With these skills help your child be a friend to a friend:

● Take friends seriously if they say they have a food allergy. Ask questions. Help them at school, with foods you offer at home, and with party foods.

● Don't swap or share food—even if you think it's safe to eat.

● Wash your hands after you eat so you don't transfer food to other things your friend may touch.

● Get immediate help if your friend gets sick.

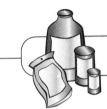

Label Lingo

Some Terms for Common Allergens

FOOD ALLERGY	INGREDIENTS WITH ALLERGEN	MAY CONTAIN ALLERGENS
Egg	Albumin (or albumen) Egg (dried, powdered, solids, white, yolk) Eggnog Lysozyme (used in Europe) Mayonnaise Meringue (meringue powder) Surimi	Flavoring (natural and artificial) Lecithin Macaroni Marzipan Marshmallows Nougat Pasta
Milk	Artificial butter flavor Butter, butter fat, butter oil Buttermilk Casein (casein hydrolysate) Caseinates (in all forms) Cheese Cottage cheese Curds Custard Ghee Half-and-half Lactalbumin, lactalbumin phosphate Lactoglobulin Lactulose Milk (all forms: condensed, derivative, dry, evaporated, goat milk, low-fat, malted, milkfat, nonfat, powder, protein, skim, solids, whole) Nougat Pudding Rennet casein Sour cream, sour cream solids Sour milk solids Whey Yogurt	Caramel candies Chocolate Favorings (natural and artificial) High-protein flour Lactic acid starter culture Lactose Luncheon meat, hot dogs, sausages Margarine Nondairy products
Peanuts	Artificial nuts Beer nuts Cold, pressed, expelled, or extruded peanut oil Ground nuts Goobers Mandelonas Mixed nuts Monkey nuts Nu-Nuts flavored nuts Nut meat Nut pieces Peanut Peanut butter Peanut flour	African, Chinese, Indonesian, Mexican, Thai, Vietnamese dishes Baked goods Candy Chili Egg rolls Enchilada sauce Flavorings (natural, artificial) Marzipan Nougat Sunflower seeds (*Note:* Studies show that most individuals with allergy can safely eat peanut oil—not cold-pressed, expelled, or extruded peanut oil. Arachis oil is peanut oil. Experts advise peanut-allergic people to avoid tree nuts as well.)

Some Terms for Common Allergens *(continued)*

FOOD ALLERGY	INGREDIENTS WITH ALLERGEN	MAY CONTAIN ALLERGENS
Shellfish	Abalone Clams (cherrystone, littleneck, pismo, quahog) Cockle (periwinkle, sea urchin) Crab Crawfish (crayfish, ecrevisse) Lobster (langouste, langoustine, scampo, coral, tomalley) Mollusks Mussels Octopus Oysters Prawns Scallops Shrimp (crevette) Snails (escargot) Squid (calamiri)	Bouillabaisse Fish stock Flavoring (natural, artificial) Seafood flavoring (i.e., crab or clam extract) Surimi
Soy	Edamame Hydrolyzed soy protein Miso Natto Shoyu sauce Soy (soy albumin, soy fiber, soy grits, soy milk, soy nuts, soy sprouts) Soya Soybean (curd, granules) Soy protein (concentrate, isolate) Soy sauce Tamari Tempeh Tofu TVP (textured vegetable protein)	Asian cuisine Flavoring (natural, artificial) Vegetable broth Vegetable gum Vegetable starch (*Note:* Studies show that most soy-allergic individuals may safely eat soy lecithin and soybean oil.)
Tree nuts	Almonds Artificial nuts Brazil nuts Caponata Cashews Chestnuts Filbert/hazelnuts Gianduja (nut mixture in some chocolate) Hickory nuts Macadamia nuts Mandelonas Marzipan/almond paste Nan-gai nuts Nougat Nut butters (i.e., cashew butter) Nut meat Natural nut extract (i.e., almond, walnut) Nutmeal Nut oil Nut paste (i.e., almond paste) Nut pieces Pecans (Masuga nuts)	Flavoring (natural, artificial) Mortadella (may contain pistachios) (*Note:* Experts advise tree nut-allergic people to avoid peanuts as well.)

FOOD ALLERGY	INGREDIENTS WITH ALLERGEN	MAY CONTAIN ALLERGENS
	Pesto	
	Pine nuts (Indian, piñon, pinyon, pignoli, pigñolia, and pignon nuts)	
	Pistachios	
	Pralines	
	Walnuts	
Wheat	Bran	Flavoring (natural, artificial)
	Bread crumbs	Hydrolyzed protein
	Bulgur	Soy sauce
	Couscous	Starch (gelatinzed starch, modified starch, modified food starch, vegetable starch)
	Cracker meal	Surimi
	Durum	
	Farina	
	Flour (all-purpose, bread, durum, enriched, graham, high-gluten, high-protein, instant, pastry, self-rising, soft-wheat, steel-ground, stone-ground, whole-wheat)	
	Gluten	
	Kamut	
	Matzoh, matzoh meal (matzo)	
	Pasta	
	Seitan	
	Semolina	
	Spelt	
	Vital gluten	
	Wheat (bran, germ, malt, starch)	
	Whole wheat berries	

Source: © The Food Allergy and Anaphylaxis Network (Fairfax, Va., 2001).

serious medical problem. Eliminating groups of foods from your eating pattern because you suspect a food allergy is not a smart idea. Sweeping dietary changes based only on a "hunch" may keep you from getting the nutrients needed for good health!

For the Record

Suspect a food allergy? During a medical exam you'll likely need to describe your symptoms and give some medical history to unravel the mystery. Be prepared to answer such questions as:

- What are your symptoms?

- How long does it take for symptoms to appear after eating the food in question?

- How much of the food must you eat before you get a reaction?

- Do the symptoms occur every time you eat the food?

- Do other factors, such as physical activity or drinking alcoholic beverages, bring on symptoms?

- Does anyone in your family have allergies? Food allergies?

You may be asked to keep a food diary, too, with all the foods, beverages (including alcoholic beverages), and medications you consume over a determined period. That includes brand names of commercially prepared foods. You'll also keep track of your reactions and how soon after eating they appeared. By itself, the diary can't confirm a cause-and-effect relationship between a food and symptoms. But the information can suggest a connection to investigate further.

An elimination diet offers another way to uncover a cause. Your doctor may instruct you to eliminate the suspicious food from your diet for a while. If the symptoms go away, then reappear when you eat the food again, you may be allergic to it.

Keeping a food diary or following an elimination diet on your own may seem easy. However, detecting ingredients in prepared foods that cause allergic reactions may not be so easy. A registered dietitian has the expertise to help you.

Pass the Test?

Various medical tests can help diagnose food allergies.

● The *skin-prick* test uses small amounts of diluted food extracts "pricked" into the skin. If the skin reacts to the extracts with a mosquito-bite-like bump, you may have a food allergy.

● *Blood tests* are done by checking for antibodies. Remember, the presence of antibodies, released by your immune system, signals a reaction to an allergen. For example, a test called a radioallergosorbent test (RAST) uses a sample of blood to determine the presence of IgE antibodies.

● In a *challenge test,* likely given in a doctor's office, the patient gets a sample that's either the suspected food allergen or a placebo. The placebo won't produce an allergic reaction. The response is watched carefully. If there are no symptoms, the challenge gets repeated with higher doses. This test must be done under the supervision of a physician—never on your own.

● *Tests using a food extract* are considered unreliable and quite costly.

"How-Tos" for Coping with Food Allergies

If you're diagnosed with a true food allergy, what's next? You'll likely need to avoid the troublesome food—and prepare and choose meals and snacks with

Have You Ever Wondered

. . . if peanut, soy, or nut oils can cause an allergic response? Most peanut and soy oils are highly refined, making them free of the protein allergen. Research shows that people with peanut or soy allergies don't have reactions to these commonly used oils; extremely sensitive people are still wise to be cautious. Cold-pressed peanut and tree nut oils are processed differently and may contain small amounts of protein allergens that can trigger a reaction.

. . . if chocolate really causes acne? No; chocolate doesn't cause acne or make acne worse. Hormones and hygiene, rather than an allergy to chocolate, are more likely the culprits. A true food allergy to chocolate is rare. Instead, a reaction to eating a chocolate bar may come from other ingredients mixed in, such as nuts or milk.

. . . if foods modified by biotechnology contain allergens? It's possible. But scientists don't know yet what specific substances in any food cause an allergic reaction. Until more is known, the U.S. Food and Drug Administration policy states that any protein taken from a food causing a known allergic reaction should be considered allergenic, too. And it must be listed on the label of a food produced by biotechnology. See *"Food Biotechnology: The Future Is Today!"* in chapter 9.

. . . if food allergies trigger asthma? Only in very rare cases. The usual triggers are allergens in dust, molds, pollen, and animals; pollutants in the air; respiratory infections; some medications; physical activity; and perhaps weather changes. If food appears to be a trigger, consult your doctor.

. . . if there's a cure for food allergies? Research is under way to find a vaccine that may reduce or eliminate the symptoms of severe food allergies. At this time there's no known cure, however. Avoiding foods with allergens is the only protective approach.

. . . if soy is a good substitute for people with other allergies? Yes, if the person isn't allergic to soy, too. Calcium-fortified soy milk can substitute for cow milk—if you get milk's other nutrients elsewhere. Soy nuts can be used in place of peanuts or tree nuts.

. . . if foods labeled as "nondairy" are okay for people with milk allergies? You need to read the label to find out. For most people with a milk allergy, a key protein in milk called casein causes a reaction. Casein or caseinates are common additives.

. . . why macaroni is excluded from an egg-free diet? Like egg noodles, it may contain eggs. Read the ingredient list.

care! If you must eliminate a food, or a category of food, plan carefully to ensure that your eating plan is nutritionally adequate and fits your food preferences and lifestyle.

Start by seeking professional help. A registered dietitian can help you learn to manage a food allergy while eating a varied and balanced diet. For example, ask about making food substitutions, reading food labels, and dining away from home. Ask about nutrient supplements, too, in case you need to make up for any vitamins or minerals missed in an allergen-free diet. *See chapter 23 for more on supplements.*

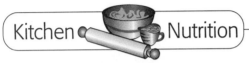

Handy Substitutions for Allergen-Free Cooking

Egg-free recipes: to substitute for 1 egg, mix one of these:

- 1 teaspoon baking powder, 1 tablespoon liquid, 1 tablespoon vinegar
- 2 tablespoons flour + 1 ½ tablespoons shortening + ½ teaspoon baking powder + 2 tablespoons liquid (appropriate for recipe: water, vinegar, juice, broth)
- 1 teaspoon yeast dissolved in ¼ cup warm water
- 1 ½ tablespoons water, 1 ½ tablespoons oil, 1 teaspoon baking powder
- 1 packet plain gelatin, 1 tablespoon warm water (use immediately)

Wheat-free recipes: to substitute for 1 cup wheat flour, try one of these:

- ¾ cup rice flour
- ½ cup potato starch flour and ½ cup soy flour
- 1 cup corn flour
- ⅔ cup brown rice flour and ⅓ cup potato flour

Milk-free recipes: to substitute for an equal amount of milk, try one of these:

- Fruit juice
- Rice milk or soy milk
- Water

Source: © The Food Allergy and Anaphylaxis Network (Fairfax, Va., 2001).

Always prepare for emergencies! Carry injectable epinephrine, or for less severe reactions, antihistamine and bronchodilators, in case you accidentally consume a food allergen. Wear an identification necklace or bracelet that identifies your allergy.

Eating Allergen-Free at Home

Whether for yourself or a family member, here's how to buy, prepare, and serve food to cope with a food allergy. By the way, simply cooking a food or scraping the allergenic food (e.g., peanuts) off the plate won't make it safe for food allergy sufferers.

- Read food labels for "undercover" allergens every time you buy or use food. If, for example, you're allergic to eggs, you'd need to know that eggs are common ingredients in mayonnaise, many salad dressings, and ice cream. Food labels list the ingredients in the food inside the package. The chart *"Label Lingo: Some Terms for Common Allergens"* in this chapter gives *some ingredients to watch for on ingredient lists of food labels if you have a food allergy.*

The food industry and the U.S. Food and Drug Administration are working on ways to make food ingredient labeling more clear and useful for those with food allergies. Many (but not all) manufacturers voluntarily identify ingredients with the eight most common food allergens near the ingredient list, using plain language that consumers can understand. For example, you might see an asterisk by an ingredient with a nearby statement, "Contains milk and eggs." Or you might see voluntary information like this on a package.

> ALLERGY INFORMATION: MANUFACTURED ON EQUIPMENT THAT PROCESSES PRODUCTS CONTAINING PEANUTS AND OTHER NUTS.

Source: FDA Consumer (2001).

Some ingredients language is still confusing, however; for example, the phrase "may contain" is often overused.

- Keep up-to-date on ingredients in food products. Periodically, food manufacturers change the ingredients; the same food from different manufacturers may have a different "recipe." So even if you're a longtime customer of a certain food, check the ingredient list on the label every time you buy it.

● If you have a milk or a casein allergy, look for kosher foods that display the word "pareve" or "parve" on the label. These foods are milk-free, or perhaps have only a very small amount of milk (not a problem for lactose intolerance, but perhaps for a milk allergy). However, if a "D" appears next to the kosher symbol, it does have an ingredient derived from milk. "DE" means that it was produced in equipment for foods with dairy ingredients; consider avoiding these foods, too. *See chapter 11 for kosher symbols.*

● Contact food manufacturers for their current ingredient lists or for answers to your questions. You'll find the company name, address, and perhaps a toll-free consumer information service number on the food label.

● Practice new ways of cooking. In time, substituting one food for another in food preparation will become second nature. Find a cookbook or online source of allergen-free recipes. You may need to experiment to find substitutions that work.

● Be careful with cooking and serving to avoid any cross-contact between the food allergen and foods prepared without the allergenic ingredient. See *"Allergen-Free: Sharpen Your Cooking Skills" on this page.* The same rule applies elsewhere—for example, for a milk allergy, avoid deli meats, since cheese and meat may be cut with the same slicer.

Eating Allergen-Free away from Home

For food allergy sufferers, eating away from home can be the greatest challenge. You're not in control of the ingredients or the food preparation:

● Be "ingredient-savvy" when you eat out. Keep restaurant menus handy to review ahead.

● Explain your needs to your food server. Ask about the menu—ingredients and preparation—before you order. The same dish prepared in different restaurants may not have the same ingredients. Play it safe by ordering plain foods such as grilled meats, steamed vegetables, and fresh fruits.

● **Caution!** Avoid these situations:

● Buffet-style or family-style service—since the same serving utensils may be used for different dishes.

Allergen-Free: Sharpen Your Cooking Skills

Preparing dishes without allergenic foods seems obvious: Just leave the ingredient out of the recipe or off the plate! However, a few other "how-tos" can help ensure a reaction-free meal or snack:

● Use *different and clean* utensils (including knives and spatulas), containers, cutting boards, and serving utensils for foods prepared *without* the food allergen.

> *For example, for a peanut allergy:* Just wiping off a knife used to spread peanut butter isn't enough. Use a clean, separate knife for the next ingredient, perhaps jelly, you plan on spreading. The same holds true for cleaning a blender after making an ice cream shake with peanut ingredients.

● Use different cooking oils to cook allergenic and nonallergenic foods. Deep-frying doesn't destroy allergens.

> *For example, for a seafood allergy:* Use different cooking oil in a clean frying pan to deep-fry shrimp rather than what you used to make French fries or other foods. Serve them on a separate plate with different utensils, too.

● Be careful with "hidden," allergenic ingredients in a dish.

> *For example, for a tree nut allergy:* Ground nuts added to a muffin batter or a breading mix may go unnoticed by an unsuspecting allergy sufferer. Even a bottle of gourmet barbecue sauce may have nuts!

> *For a fish allergy:* Bottled fish sauce in a stir-fry sauce or a salad dressing could be an undetected problem, too.

> *For an egg allergy:* Sometimes eggs are used to hold meatballs and fish croquettes together.

> *For a soy allergy:* Soy flours and soy protein are used in increasingly more baked goods and other prepared foods.

● Fried foods—since the same oil may be used for many different foods.

● Seafood restaurants if you have a fish allergy—since cooking utensils may contact fish protein.

● Many Asian or African foods if you have a tree nut or peanut allergy—since nuts and peanuts are common in these ethnic cuisines.

● Breaded foods—since the problem protein may transfer if the same breading mix is used for different types of food.

● Scooped ice cream—since the scooper for several flavors may be kept in the same tub of water.

● Baked goods if you're allergic to soy or wheat. Today more breads, pizza crusts, and other doughs are made with soy flour; wheat is often added to rye bread.

● Carry your own food on airlines. Ask for the peanut-free snack if you have a peanut allergy.

● Not sure about the food when you eat out? Ask about the ingredients, or brown-bag your own food. If you're a guest in someone's home, offer to bring your own food or to help with food preparation.

● Be a sensitive host. As you invite your guests, ask about any special food needs—in case they feel uncomfortable telling you. Adjust the menu or prepare some foods differently if you need to.

For more education about food allergies, and a cookbook, newsletters, and other support, contact the Food Allergy and Anaphylaxis Network. *See "Resources You Can Use" at the back of this book for contact information.*

Need more strategies for handling food sensitivities? Check here for "how-tos":

● Sharpen up on ingredient detection as you shop—see chapter 11.

● Ask the right menu questions when you eat out—see chapter 14.

● Monitor an infant's food-induced reactions—see chapter 15.

● Get more help from a registered dietitian—see chapter 24.

● Find organizations that offer additional help—see "Resources You Can Use."

CHAPTER 22

Smart Eating to Prevent and Treat Disease

A healthful eating pattern and lifestyle from the start are your best approaches for staying healthy and preventing disease, or at least slowing its course. Most health problems don't start with a single event in your life. Instead, they're a combination of factors. Some you can't control, such as your family history, gender, or age; but many you can.

This chapter addresses several common health problems that concern Americans: (1) their prevention and risk reduction and (2) the treatment of health problems or their symptoms. This overview may or may not apply to your unique needs. For advice specific to you or to someone you care for, consult with your doctor, a registered dietitian, and other members of your personal healthcare team.

Your Healthy Heart

We've all heard the statistics. Heart disease is America's number one killer. Although its onset is slightly postponed for women, it's a disease that affects both genders. More than 60 million of the nation's more than 300 million people have some form of cardiovascular disease, and it accounts for about 950,000, or about 40 percent, of deaths annually in the United States. The truth is, many deaths from either heart attacks or strokes are preventable. That's especially true for people with total cholesterol levels between 180 and 250 mg/dL, which is the majority of adult Americans.

DAMAGE CONTROL

Of the fifteen leading causes of death in the United States, six are associated directly with diet, and seven with excessive intake of alcoholic beverages. Paying attention to what you eat and drink can pay off in good health and longevity.

RANK AND CAUSE*	RISK FACTORS DIET-RELATED	RISK FACTORS ALCOHOL-RELATED
1. Heart disease	X	X
2. Cancers	X	X
3. Strokes	X	
4. Chronic lower respiratory diseases		
5. Accidents and injuries		X
6. Diabetes	X	
7. Influenza and pneumonia		
8. Alzheimer's disease		
9. Kidney diseases	X	X
10. Septicemia (bacterial infection in the blood)		
11. Suicide		X
12. Liver disease and cirrhosis		X
13. Hypertension	X	
14. Homicide		X
15. Aortic aneurysm		

*Source: National Vital Statistics Reports 49, no. 3 (June 26, 2001) (reflecting 1999 data).

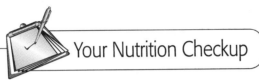

Do It for You!

Take care of you for you—and all those in your life! You can't control your age, gender, or family history, but there's plenty you can do to stay fit. For many health problems, the risk factors are the same, so the same smart living patterns may protect you from several chronic diseases.

How well are you protecting your health? If you can answer "yes" to the following questions, check to the left; fill in your own numbers in the blanks on the right.

Your Body's "Maintenance" Program

_____ Does your body mass index (BMI) fit within a range that's healthy? _____ BMI*

_____ Have you had a recent physical exam?

If you know your numbers, are they within a normal/optimal range?

_____ Total blood cholesterol (below 200 mg/dL): _____ mg/dL

_____ HDL blood cholesterol (more than 60 mg/dL): _____ mg/dL

_____ LDL blood cholesterol (below 100 mg/dL): _____ mg/dL

_____ Triglycerides (below 150 mg/dL): _____ mg/dL

_____ Blood pressure (below 140/90 mm Hg): __/__ mm Hg

_____ Fasting blood sugar (below 110 mg/dL): _____ mg/dL

*See "Body Mass Index: Fit or Fat?" in chapter 2 to figure your BMI.

Eat—for the Health of It!

_____ Do you try to consume at least six servings* of breads, cereals, rice, pasta, and other grain products daily?

_____ Of these grain products, do you eat at least three whole-grain† products each day?

_____ Do you try to eat at least five servings* of fruits and vegetables with a colorful variety each day?

_____ Do you consume enough calcium-rich dairy foods daily: at least two servings,* and perhaps more, if you're a teen, a woman going through menopause, or age fifty plus?

_____ Do you try to eat protein-rich foods that add up to 5 to 7 ounces daily (e.g., meat, poultry, fish, eggs, beans, and nuts)?

_____ Do you choose foods low in saturated fat and cholesterol, and moderate in total fat, most of the time (e.g., lean meat, skinless poultry, fish, low-fat or fat-free dairy foods)?

_____ Do you try to eat legumes (beans) several times a week? (Besides being low in fat, they're high in protein, iron, and fiber.)

_____ Do you go easy on foods that deliver energy, or calories, but few nutrients (e.g., fats and sweets)?

_____ Do you choose and prepare food with less salt?

*Check chapter 10 for serving sizes.
†See "What Is a Whole Grain? in chapter 6.

Do It for You! *(continued)*

Now . . . Your Lifestyle

_____ Do you get at least thirty minutes of moderate physical activity most, if not all days, of the week?

_____ Are some of your physical activities weight-bearing (e.g., walking, dancing, tennis)?

_____ If you drink alcoholic beverages, do you do so in moderation (no more than one drink daily for women, or two for men)?

Now count up all your "yes" answers:

For each checkmark, give yourself five points. What's your total score? _____

Of course, these twenty eating and active living factors aren't the only ways to promote your good health. But the more often you said "yes," the better your chances are for a long, healthy life.

What does your score suggest? It only indicates how many different ways you may already be protecting yourself from health problems. And it suggests where you might improve.

Having a score of 50 compared with a perfect 100 doesn't mean you're twice as likely to develop heart disease, cancer, diabetes, or some other health problem. And this quick checkup is not meant for diagnosis, either. That's the role of your doctor in your regular physical checkups. However, your responses might point to risk factors that may contribute to health problems later. Read on to explore the role of nutrition in common health conditions.

What Is Heart Disease?

"Heart disease" describes several health problems that relate to the heart and blood vessels. Heart attacks and strokes may come to your mind first. However, high blood pressure, angina (chest pain), poor circulation, and abnormal heartbeats are among the other forms of heart disease, too.

Heart Disease: Are You at Risk?

What increases your risk for heart disease or high blood cholesterol levels? Two risk factors aren't within your control: age and genetic tendency. Yet many other risk factors are. Do any apply to you?

Risk factors you can't control:

● Family history of early heart disease (father or brother with heart disease before age fifty-five; mother or sister, before age sixty-five). African Americans, who more likely have high blood pressure, are at higher risk. So are Mexican Americans, Native Americans, Native Hawaiians, and some Asian Americans.

● Getting older (men over age forty-five; women over age fifty-five). Before menopause, women usually have lower cholesterol than men their age; after menopause, women's LDL cholesterol often rises.

Major risk factors:

● Cigarette smoking, which is a significant risk factor for heart disease. Cigar and pipe smoking, as well as secondhand smoke, are risk factors, too.

● High blood pressure, which causes the heart to work harder and so enlarge and weaken.

● High or borderline-high blood cholesterol levels (over 200 milligrams per deciliter).

● Lack of exercise.

● Overweight and obesity, especially with excess abdominal fat. The excess puts strain on the heart, raises blood pressure, raises both cholesterol and tricylceride levels, and lowers the HDL cholesterol level.

● Diabetes, even if under control. People with diabetes have an especially high risk of dying from a heart attack.

Other risk factors:

● Too much alcohol intake, which can raise blood pressure, cause heart failure, and lead to a stroke. And it can contribute to high trigylcerides and irregular heartbeat.

● Taking birth control pills (if you smoke or have other risk factors).

● Stress, perhaps due to other factors, such as overeating or smoking more.

Having a high risk doesn't mean you're sure to have a heart attack or a stroke. That's good news! However, the more risks for heart disease you have, the greater your statistical chances. Using data from the long-term Framingham Heart Study, an interactive tool has been created to measure your ten-year statistical risk for a heart attack. Check out the Web site *http://hin.nhlbi.nih.gov/atpiii/calculator.asp?usertype=prof* for your risk score. Changes in your food choices and lifestyle, and perhaps weight reduction and medication, can lower your risk score.

Insulin Resistance Syndrome, or "Syndrome X"

Insulin resistance syndrome, often called "syndrome X" or metabolic syndrome, is a quartet of health conditions: diabetes, abnormal lipid levels, high blood pressure, and obesity. When all these problems exist together, the risk for heart disease, a heart attack, and a stroke is many times higher. Two factors are among those that play a key role in the development of insulin resistance: inactivity and overeating. The Centers for Disease Control and Prevention estimates that 22 percent of all U.S. adults have insulin resistance syndrome, with significantly higher rates for older populations of adults.

With insulin resistance syndrome, body cells don't respond normally to insulin. The pancreas produces more insulin to overcome this insensitivity; however, insulin instead builds up in blood, contributing to high blood pressure, glucose intolerance, and abnormal levels of cholesterol and triglycerides. Upper body obesity adds to the problem, too.

The treatment? Address all four conditions at the same time; the recommendations for dealing with them are consistent. This includes increased physical activity, achieving a healthy weight, and a diet that's low in saturated fat (less than 10 percent of total calories), more *moderate* in total fat content (30 to 35 percent of total calories), and *moderate* in carbohydrates. To the contrary, a high-carbohydrate, low-fat diet may aggravate the effects of this syndrome. Along with diet therapy, medications also may be prescribed to help control diabetes, hypertension, and high blood lipids (cholesterol and triglycerides). *See "Diabetes: A Growing Health Concern" in this chapter.*

See "Heart Disease: A Woman's Issue, Too!" in chapter 17.

Heart Disease: The Blood Lipid Connection

High total and LDL cholesterol levels are major risk factors for heart disease. Conversely, lowering these cholesterol numbers and raising HDL cholesterol levels reduce the risk. What's the link?

Cholesterol, a fatlike substance produced in your liver, is found in everyone's bloodstream. As part of every body cell, it's essential to human health and cell-building. There's no Recommended Dietary Allowance for consuming enough cholesterol because your body makes it, too.

Blood cholesterol is a problem only if your total or LDL blood cholesterol gets too high and your HDL too low. When total and LDL blood cholesterol levels are elevated, deposits of cholesterol, called plaque, collect on arterial and other blood vessel walls. This condition is called atherosclerosis, or hardening of the arteries. As fatty plaques build up, arteries gradually become more narrow and may slow or block the flow of oxygen-rich blood. Chest pain may result without enough oxygen to the heart.

Plaque buildup happens silently, usually without symptoms. Warnings in the form of chest pains may not occur until vessels are about 75 percent blocked. Often a heart attack or a stroke strikes with no warning at all. A clot in a narrowed artery blocks blood flow to the heart, causing a heart attack. With a stroke, blood can't flow to the brain. The higher the blood cholesterol level, the greater the risk. When abnormally high total and LDL blood cholesterol levels go down, so does the risk for heart attack and stroke.

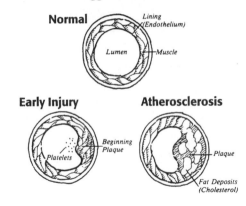

Clogged Arteries

For good health, aim to fit your blood cholesterol level within a normal range. *Check "Strive for Desirable Blood Lipid Levels" in this chapter.* Remember that high total blood cholesterol isn't the only risk factor for heart disease, and even a total of 200 or less won't automatically keep you safe.

Why Do Blood Cholesterol Levels Rise and Fall?

That's a complex question. Usually there's no single reason. For some people, high or low blood cholesterol is an inherited tendency; in part, genetics affects how much cholesterol your body makes. Families with heart disease share more than their genetic makeup. People also grow up with similar lifestyle habits that may raise cholesterol levels—perhaps high-fat eating, excessive calories, inactivity, excessive alcohol intake, or smoking.

From a nutrition standpoint, a diet high in fat, especially saturated fat, is a factor for high blood cholesterol levels—in fact, compared to other dietary components, "sat fats" have the most significant cholesterol-raising effect for most of us. Obesity, which tends to increase cholesterol levels, is a key factor. Some people are cholesterol-sensitive—that is, a high-cholesterol diet significantly boosts their total blood cholesterol level and LDL blood cholesterol level. *For more on dietary fat and cholesterol see chapter 3.*

HDLs and LDLs: The Ups and the Downs. Lipoproteins—both HDLs and LDLs—transport "packages" of cholesterol through your blood. Here's how they work:

● High-density lipoproteins (HDLs), or good blood cholesterol, act like waste removal vehicles. They take cholesterol from blood and artery walls to your liver for removal from the body. According to the National Heart, Lung, and Blood Institute, a level of 60 mg/dL or more protects from heart disease. *Tip:* Remember "H" stands for HDLs and "healthy."

● Low-density lipoproteins (LDLs), or bad blood cholesterol, work like delivery vehicles. They keep blood cholesterol circulating in your bloodstream, depositing plaque on artery walls along the way. As plaque builds up, the risk for atherosclerosis goes up, too. For optimal health, keep LDLs at less than 100 mg/dL. *Tip:* Remember "L" stands for LDLs and "lousy."

With these in mind, the heart-smart goal is obvious: high levels of HDLs and low levels of LDLs (both within normal guidelines).

The next questions: How do you boost your HDLs? How do you lower your LDLs?

● *To increase HDL blood cholesterol:* Stay physically active and trim any extra pounds of body fat if you're not at your healthy weight. Reduce fat intake to no more than 30 percent calories from fat in your overall diet. Replace some saturated fats with monounsaturates. If you smoke, quit.

● *To decrease LDL blood cholesterol:* Substitute unsaturated fats for saturated fats, while keeping total fat and dietary cholesterol low, and cut back on trans fatty acids (found in partly hydrogenated vegetable oils). Soluble fiber and soy protein also may help lower LDL cholesterol. Keeping excess body weight off may help, too.

"Strive for Desirable Blood Lipid Levels" in this chapter shows target levels for HDLs and LDLs. For more about them see "The 'Good' and the 'Bad'" in chapter 3.

Prevention: Cholesterol Countdown. A heart-healthy eating pattern—a diet low in saturated fat and dietary cholesterol with more foods high in complex carbohydrates—helps reduce or maintain blood cholesterol levels. *For more about fat and cholesterol in food and health see chapter 3, "Fat Facts."*

● Be moderate in the total fat you consume—no more than 30 percent of your total calories a day *(see chapter 3)*—rather than attempt to cut fat out of your diet entirely. You need some fat to keep you healthy. And many foods with fat also contain other nutrients your body needs. *Tip:* In the Nutrition Facts on food labels, 100% Daily Value (for 2,000 calories daily) is 65 fat grams, which is 30 percent of total calories.

● Follow an eating pattern that's low in saturated fat—less than 10 percent of your total daily calories *(see chapter 3),* or not more than a third of your total fat intake. "Sat fats" boost blood cholesterol levels more than anything else you consume. You probably won't need to track "sat fats." By keeping your total fat intake moderate, you'll likely consume less saturated fat at the same time. Substitute unsaturated fats for saturated fats, without increasing your total fat intake.

● Go easy on trans fatty acids, too—the kind in partially hydrogenated margarines and some snack foods. They, too, are cholesterol-raising. *See chapter 3 for more on trans fatty acids.*

● Follow an eating plan that's low in cholesterol—less than 300 milligrams a day. Although not as significant as cutting back on saturated fat, reducing your dietary cholesterol may help lower your blood cholesterol level. You don't need to eliminate foods with cholesterol. These same foods—milk, cheese, eggs, poultry, fish, and meat—supply plenty of nutrients your body needs.

● If you're already at your healthy weight, enjoy foods with more complex "carbs" as you cut back on fat. Otherwise you'll lose weight. Grain products, beans, and vegetables all contain complex carbohydrates. *See "From Complex to Simple . . ." in chapter 5, and "Too Much of a Good Thing?" in chapter 3 for more guidance on fat and cholesterol.*

● Eat more fiber. Fiber-rich foods may help lower blood cholesterol levels. That's because soluble fiber—for example, in oats—may bind with cholesterol before it can be absorbed into your bloodstream, eliminating it with waste. *See chapter 6 for ways to boost your fiber intake.*

● Eat more fruits and vegetables, which are mostly low in fat. Besides their fiber content, emerging research also suggests a link to high intakes of antioxidant vitamins: beta carotene and vitamin C, which may be heart-protective.

On the Cutting Edge of Science. Other substances in food also may be cholesterol-lowering; hence the interest in functional foods. *See "Functional Foods for Heart Health!" in this chapter.* For some, research evidence is strong; for others, it's preliminary but promising. Here are some new areas of scientific investigation.

● *Fiber.* Fiber may help lower blood cholesterol, especially for those with high levels, offering some protection from heart disease. It also may improve the ratio between LDL and HDL cholesterol. However, not all fiber—just soluble fiber—has this effect. In the intestine, soluble fiber binds to cholesterol-rich bile acids, passing them out of the body as waste rather than reabsorbing them. Soluble fiber—fiber that

dissolves in water—is found in oatmeal, oat bran, rice, wheat bran, barley, canned or cooked dried beans (such as kidney and pinto beans), and many fruits and vegetables. *For more on soluble fiber see "Fiber: Heart Healthy, Too!" in chapter 6.*

For the record, no long-term studies show heart-healthy benefits from fiber supplements. At least for now, they're not recommended as an approach for reducing heart disease risk.

● *Soybean products.* Soybeans and soy products such as soy milk, tofu, tempeh, and soyburgers (but not soybean oil) may contain several phytonutrients that promote heart health. Soy protein and isoflavones get the most consumer attention for their ability to help lower total cholesterol and LDLs. In fact, the U.S. Food and Drug Administration has approved a health claim for labeling: 25 grams of soy protein per day, as part of a diet low in saturated fat and cholesterol, can reduce the risk of heart disease. With so many soy products on the market today, it's easier to consume 25 grams of soy protein daily.

SOY PROTEIN: HOW MUCH?

FOODS WITH SOY PROTEIN (EXAMPLES)	AMOUNT OF SOY PROTEIN (GRAMS)
½ cup tempeh	19.5
¼ cup roasted soy nuts	19
4 oz. firm tofu	13
1 soy protein bar	14
1 soyburger	10 to 12
8 oz. plain soy milk	10
1 soy sausage link	6

Source: FDA Consumer (May-June 2000).

● *Plant stanols and sterols.* Plant stanols and sterols, found naturally in fruits, vegetables, and plant oils, have a cholesterol-lowering effect. They work by inhibiting the absorption of cholesterol (from food and bile acids) in the intestine; instead, cholesterol passes out of the body through waste.

Some spreads are formulated to be high in plant sterol esters (Take Control) and plant stanol esters (Benecol). These can be effective for lowering cholesterol for those with elevated levels. To be effective, you need to consume enough: two servings of a spread that contains plant stanol or sterol esters daily—with meals—as part of an eating plan that's low in saturated fat and cholesterol. *See "Functional Nutrition: Stanol- and Sterol-Based Ingredients" in chapter 3.*

● *Omega-3 fatty acids.* "Omega-3s" from fatty fish may reduce the risk of heart disease, although the data aren't conclusive. That's why the American Heart Association recommends eating two weekly servings of fatty fish, such as tuna or salmon. It's not known if omega-3 fatty acids from other sources—for example canola, soy, and flaxseed oil—have a similar effect. *See "Eat Your Omega-3s and -6s" in chapter 3.*

● *Folic acid.* The fact that today's grain products are fortified with folic acid (a form of folate) to prevent neural tube defects also may benefit heart health (another reason to enjoy grain products). Here's why: A high level of homocysteine, an amino acid (a protein) in the blood, may indicate heart disease. Although the reasons aren't clear, homocysteine may promote buildup of plaque in the arteries. Folic acid

(a B vitamin), and perhaps vitamins B_6 and B_{12}, appear to lower an elevated level of homocysteine in blood, helping to protect against heart disease. (A physician can order a lab test to check your homocysteine level.)

Besides getting folate from grain products, vegetables, and fruits, you can also take a multivitamin supplement with 100% of the Daily Value for folic acid (400 micrograms). Check with your physician before taking more than that.

● *Antioxidant nutrients.* Antioxidant nutrients in food may benefit the heart. Vitamin E may offer protection from blood clots and atherosclerosis, and vitamin C may help keep blood vessels flexible. The evidence is too weak to recommend vitamin supplements; instead, enjoy a variety of nutrient-rich, plant-based foods that supply antioxidant nutrients.

● *Arginine.* The amino acid arginine may protect against atherosclerosis. However, studies haven't yet determined how much is either safe or effective. Not enough is known yet to advise any benefits from extra arginine.

Functional Foods for Heart Health!

FOODS WITH POTENTIAL FUNCTIONAL BENEFITS	FUNCTIONAL SIGNIFICANCE
Beans, peas, barley	Soluble fiber, saponins
Soybeans, other soy-based foods (not oil)	Soy protein, isoflavones, saponins, plant sterols, perhaps fiber
Oats, flaxseed (ground), psyllium	Soluble fiber, lignan
Citrus fruit	Flavonoids, ferulic acid, caffeic acid
Salmon, tuna, sardines, mackerel	Omega-3 fatty acids
Eggs with omega-3 fatty acids	Omega-3-fatty acids
Onions, scallions, shallots, garlic, leeks	Allyl sulfides
Red grapes, purple grape juice, red wine	Phenols, resveratrol, ellagic acid
Vegetables	Plant sterols, ferulic acid, antioxidant vitamins, fiber
Nuts (almonds, walnuts, pecans, hazelnuts, others)	Phytic acid, arginine, plant sterols
Tea (green or black)	Catechins
Fermented dairy products	Probiotics
Some cholesterol-lowering spreads	Plant sterol and stanol esters

See "Phytonutrients—a 'Crop' for Good Health" in chapter 4 and "Functional Foods: A New Wave" in chapter 9 for more about phytonutrients and functional foods.

Eating for Your Heart

What should you eat for heart health? Here's what the American Heart Association (AHA) advises. The AHA's dietary guidelines are parallel to the USDA's Dietary Guidelines for Americans; *see chapter 1.*

AHA DIETARY GUIDELINES

Achieve an overall healthy eating pattern.	● Consume a variety of fruits, vegetables, and grain products, including whole grains.
	● Include fat-free and low-fat dairy products, fish,* legumes, poultry, and lean meats.
	*At least two servings (6 oz.) of fish per week.
Achieve a healthy body weight.	● Match intake of energy (calories) to overall energy needs; limit consumption of foods with a high caloric density and/or low nutritional quality, including those with a high sugar content.
	● Maintain a level of physical activity that achieves fitness and balances energy expenditure with energy intake; for weight reduction, expenditure should exceed intake.
Achieve a desirable cholesterol and lipoprotein profile.	● Limit the intake of foods with a high content of saturated fatty acids and cholesterol.*
	● Substitute grains and unsaturated fatty acids from vegetables, fish, legumes, and nuts.
	*Also limit trans fatty acids.
Achieve a desirable blood pressure level.	● Limit the intake of salt (sodium chloride) to less than 6 grams* a day.
	● Limit alcohol consumption (no more than 1 drink per day for women, and 2 drinks per day for men).
	● Maintain a healthy body weight and dietary pattern that emphasizes vegetables, fruits, and low-fat or fat-free dairy products.
	*Six grams of sodium chloride contain 2,400 milligrams of sodium.

Source: Reproduced with permission. *Scientific Statement AHA Dietary Guidelines Revision 2000.* ©2000, American Heart Association.

Triglycerides: Another Health Issue

High blood triglycerides get much less attention than cholesterol, yet they're significantly linked to heart disease. As with cholesterol, high blood triglyceride levels don't mean you'll develop heart disease; but the chance goes up if you have other risk factors.

Triglycerides are the main form of fat in foods, whether they're saturated, polyunsaturated, or monounsaturated. Once consumed, your liver processes them. Excess calories from any source—carbohydrates, proteins, or fats—change to triglycerides for storage as body fat. Alcohol also can boost the liver's production of triglycerides.

Your blood triglyceride level normally goes up after eating. It's also affected by alcohol intake, medication, hormones, diet, menstrual cycle, time of day, and recent exercise.

Because of the risk for heart disease, the National Heart, Lung, and Blood Institute recommends treating people with borderline-high and high triglyceride levels. If your blood triglyceride level consistently exceeds normal, weight control, physical activity, and perhaps medication may bring it down. (Normal is below 150mg/dL.) In fact, the advice for lowering total blood cholesterol levels also applies to reducing triglyceride levels. Of specific dietary and lifestyle importance:

● Maintain or improve your weight. Weight loss alone may significantly lower triglyceride levels.

● Live an active lifestyle. Along with maintaining a healthy weight, regular exercise can lower triglyceride levels. It also raises HDL cholesterol in the blood.

● Go easy on sugary foods, especially if you're diagnosed with insulin resistance.

● If you drink alcoholic beverages, consume just moderate amounts or skip them entirely. Check with your doctor and a registered dietitian.

● Eat fatty fish, since their omega-3 fatty acids may help lower triglycerides.

Testing, Testing: Know Your Numbers!

Numbers don't tell the whole story of heart health, but they're good predictors. Know your blood lipid numbers—total cholesterol, LDL and HDL and triglyceride levels—whether or not you're at risk for heart disease.

Unless you're screened regularly, high lipid levels usually go unnoticed because symptoms aren't obvious. If you're age twenty or older, have your cholesterol level checked at least every five years—and more often if you're considerably older or at risk for heart disease. If your first results are high, your doctor may advise another test soon. Rather than self-diagnose, let your physician or a registered dietitian (RD) interpret your test results—and guide you to achieve and maintain your cholesterol numbers at healthy levels. *For children, see "Should You Have Your Child's Cholesterol Level Checked?" in chapter 16.*

Blood lipid levels are measured from a blood sample. What about cholesterol screenings at a shopping mall or a health fair? As an initial screening, these finger stick tests for cholesterol may be good indicators. If your cholesterol number is borderline high or high—or if you have other risk factors for heart disease—have it rechecked with your healthcare provider to verify the results. Depending on the techniques and the equipment, a finger stick screening may be less accurate than tests done in your doctor's office or a health center.

For a complete picture, your physician likely will order a lipoprotein profile: LDL, total, and HDL cholesterol levels as well as blood triglycerides. Triglyceride levels are especially important if you have other risk factors—for example, high total blood cholesterol; two or more risk factors for heart disease, such as smoking and obesity; or health problems related to triglycerides, such as diabetes, high blood pressure, obesity, chronic kidney disease, or circulatory disease.

What about over-the-counter cholesterol tests? Done properly, according to package instructions, they can be relatively accurate. However, home tests measure only total blood cholesterol levels, not HDLs, LDLs, and triglycerides. Like any finger stick test, verify the results with your healthcare provider—especially if your results are 200 mg/dL or more for total blood cholesterol and if you have other risk factors, such as a family history of heart disease.

STRIVE FOR DESIRABLE BLOOD LIPID LEVELS

To lower your heart disease risk, strive to keep your blood lipid levels at desirable levels for life. If you don't know your blood cholesterol numbers, check soon as your first step to heart-health care. Then act on the results!

LEVEL	CATEGORY
Total Cholesterol	
● Less than 200 mg/dL	Desirable
● 200-239 mg/dL	Borderline high
● 240 mg/dL and above	High
LDL Cholesterol (lower is better)	
● Less than 100 mg/dL	Optimal
● 100-129 mg/dL	Near optimal/above optimal
● 130-159 mg/dL	Borderline high
● 160-189 mg/dL	High
● 190 mg/dL and above	Very high
Triglyceride	
● Less than 150 mg/dL	Normal
● 150-199 mg/dL	Borderline high
● 200-499 mg/dL	High
● 500 mg/dL or more	Very high
HDL Cholesterol (higher is better)	
● Less than 40 mg/dL	Low
● 60 mg/dL or more	High

Source: National Heart, Lung, and Blood Institute, National Institutes of Health (2001).

If You're Dealing with High Lipid Levels

You can bring your numbers down. However, it takes effort and commitment, changes in your eating and lifestyle, and perhaps medication. Here's what you need to do. If you have diabetes, you may need more aggressive treatment for high LDL and total cholesterol levels. Other heart-disease-related problems may require other dietary changes; get advice from your doctor or a registered dietitian.

TLC for Heart Health

If you have high cholesterol, especially high LDLs, give your heart some "TLC": Therapeutic Lifestyle Changes. This guidance from the National Heart, Lung, and Blood Institute has three parts: a cholesterol-lowering eating plan, weight management, and plenty of physical activity.

Eating for TLC. If you're among the many Americans with high or borderline high total blood cholesterol or LDL cholesterol levels, a few changes in your food choices and lifestyle may bring your numbers down . . . and boost your HDLs. Even if your levels are normal, these guidelines make sense. Your risk for heart disease goes down!

- Less than 7 percent of your calories from saturated fat. *See chapter 3 for figuring percent of calories from fat.*

- Less than 200 mg of cholesterol a day.

- Enough calories to maintain your weight, without gaining.

- More soluble fiber if reducing "sat fats" and cholesterol aren't enough.

- Cholesterol-lowering, butterlike spreads (with plant stanol or sterol esters) for more LDL-lowering benefits

Weight Management. Maintain or improve your weight. The more excess body fat you have, the greater your risk for heart disease. Where your body stores extra body fat also makes a difference to heart health. Those who carry a "spare tire" around their abdomen have a higher cardiac risk than those with extra padding around their hips and thighs. *See chapter 2, "Your Healthy Weight."*

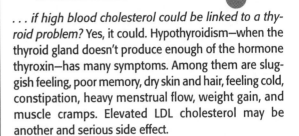

Have You Ever Wondered

. . . if high blood cholesterol could be linked to a thyroid problem? Yes, it could. Hypothyroidism—when the thyroid gland doesn't produce enough of the hormone thyroxin—has many symptoms. Among them are sluggish feeling, poor memory, dry skin and hair, feeling cold, constipation, heavy menstrual flow, weight gain, and muscle cramps. Elevated LDL cholesterol may be another and serious side effect.

Treating hypothyroidism with medication—thyroid hormone—also helps reduce high LDL cholesterol levels associated with this condition. Untreated, hypothyroidism can damage the cardiovascular system permanently.

As part of a routine physical exam, have your physician check for thyroid problems. Hypothyroidism is much more common among women than among men.

Lifestyle Changes. Diet alone and weight management aren't the only ways to lower blood cholesterol levels. A few other lifestyle changes, including active living, also can reduce your risk for heart disease.

- Keep moving! Regular, moderate activity helps keep your blood cholesterol and triglyceride levels normal. It helps boost your HDLs and lower your LDLs, helps reduce blood pressure, helps your body control stress, and helps control body weight as you burn energy. More vigorous aerobic activity gives your heart muscle a good workout and ultimately helps your whole cardiovascular system work more efficiently. *For more benefits see "Ten Reasons to Make the 'Right Moves'" in chapter 1. "Get Physical!" in chapter 2 offers ways to fit physical activity into your life.*

- If you have high blood pressure, get it under control. High blood pressure, or hypertension, is a key risk factor for heart attack and stroke. *See "Blood Pressure: Under Control?" in this chapter for more on high blood pressure.*

- If you smoke, give up the habit. It's a key factor in sudden death from cardiovascular disease. Smoking seems to raise blood pressure levels and heart rate. It may lower HDL cholesterol levels, too. And smoking may increase the tendency of blood to clot and so lead to a heart attack. The good news is: For those who stop smoking, the risk for heart disease goes down over the years, even for longtime smokers.

● If you have diabetes, keep it under control. African Americans have a greater risk for diabetes, mainly because they have a higher risk for high blood pressure.

● Reduce stress. Although the evidence linking stress and cardiovascular disease is weak, you're still wise to learn how to control stress, especially if you eat or smoke to relieve stress.

Cholesterol-Lowering Medication

Depending on your numbers, your doctor may recommend cholesterol-lowering medication. By reducing your total and LDL cholesterol with eating and lifestyle choices, you may need a lower dose of medication.

For women, hormone replacement therapy (HRT) isn't an alternative for cholesterol-lowering medication. According to the National Heart, Lung, and Blood Institute, research indicates that HRT doesn't reduce the risk for heart disease, stroke, or death after menopause, and it may increase the chances for gallbladder disease and the blockage of blood vessels (perhaps to the heart or brain) by a blood clot. In contrast, if prescribed, cholesterol-lowering drugs reduce heart attacks and stroke among women.

Blood Pressure: Under Control?

Do you know your blood pressure reading? High blood pressure, or hypertension, often creeps up slowly and quietly. Until it's advanced, there usually are no symptoms. But undetected and uncontrolled, high blood pressure may cause damage to the heart, brain, and kidneys for years without you knowing. Sometimes the first sign of high blood pressure is a heart attack or a stroke.

Why the concern? High blood pressure is a main risk factor for heart attack, strokes, and kidney disease. In fact, more than a million heart attacks and half a million strokes yearly are caused in part by high blood pressure. By putting pressure on blood vessels in the eye, it may damage the retina, impair vision, and even cause blindness. Fortunately, high blood pressure is treatable.

About 23 percent of Americans (one in four adults) have high blood pressure, according to 2001 data, yet only about half are being treated for it. Far fewer have their blood pressure under control. And 13 percent of Americans have high-normal blood pressure.

What Is High Blood Pressure?

You've heard the term "high blood pressure" many times. But do you know what it really is? And how

---

WARNING SIGNS: HEART ATTACK AND STROKE

HEART ATTACK*

● Chest discomfort or pain: uncomfortable pressure, squeezing, fullness, or pain, usually in the center of the chest, that lasts more than a few minutes or that goes away and comes back

● Discomfort or pain in other areas of the upper body—for example, one or both arms, the back, neck, jaw, or stomach

● Shortness of breath

● Other signs: perhaps breaking out in a cold sweat, nausea, or light-headedness

STROKE

● Sudden numbness or weakness of the face, arm, or leg, especially on one side of the body

● Sudden confusion, trouble speaking or understanding

● Sudden trouble seeing in one or both eyes

● Sudden trouble walking; dizziness; loss of balance or coordination

● Sudden, severe headache with no known cause

*Warning signs for men and women may differ. Women may not feel chest pain but may experience other symptoms, such as jaw ache, nausea, or extreme fatigue.

Sources: American Heart Association, American Stroke Association.

Have You Ever Wondered

. . . how many eggs you can eat for heart health? In the past, the guideline was no more than three egg yolks a week, including those in cooked foods. Unless your physician advises less, today's advice is more liberal—even one egg yolk daily—if you limit your overall cholesterol intake to 300 milligrams daily; one egg yolk has about 215 milligrams of cholesterol. To check the cholesterol content per serving in any packaged food, check the Nutrition Facts on the label or displayed near fresh produce, meat, poultry, and seafood.

. . . if eating more olive oil will help prevent heart disease? Perhaps, but not if you end up eating a diet that's high in total fat. An eating plan that's low in saturated fat and cholesterol and moderate in total fat is still recommended for heart health. In your quest for a heart-healthy eating plan, substitute some monounsaturated fats for some saturated fats in your food choices. Olive, canola, and peanut oils are all high in monounsaturated fats.

. . . if garlic is good for your heart? Perhaps, but the research is preliminary. The benefits of large amounts are untested. Best advice: Enjoy the flavor of garlic, but don't count on it for heart-healthy benefits. Fol-

low accepted methods to keep your blood cholesterol under control: Stay physically active and eat a diet that's low in fat, saturated fat, and cholesterol.

Although you can buy garlic pills and extracts, supplements may lack the phytonutrients that impart potential cholesterol-lowering benefits. And garlic supplements may cause stomach irritation and nausea.

. . . if fish oil supplements can protect your heart? Fish oil supplements are promoted for their omega-3 fatty acids and their potential for lowering the risk for blocked blood vessels and heart attacks. However, proper dosage has not been determined, and they can't cancel out the effects of a high-fat diet. Best guideline: Enjoy fatty fish instead, and follow an overall low-fat eating plan.

. . . if fat replacers offer heart-healthy benefits? Perhaps—if you use them to replace full-fat foods and avoid consuming too many calories overall. In part because these products are relatively new, no research shows long-term benefits. Until more is known, use them to give you flexibility in a healthful eating plan with fat control. *See "About Fat Replacers" in chapter 3.*

does hypertension start? For reasons that aren't completely clear, the system that regulates blood flow in the body malfunctions.

Blood pressure is the force of blood against the walls of the arteries. It's normal for blood pressure to rise and fall during the day. High blood pressure, or hypertension, means consistently higher-than-normal pressure on blood vessel walls. It happens over time as blood gets pushed with more tension through arterioles, or small blood vessels, that become stiff and constricted. High blood pressure also damages artery walls and speeds plaque formation, narrowing the passage for blood. As plaque builds up in the arteries and blood flow is restricted, blood pressure goes up even higher.

High blood pressure causes the heart to work harder; the higher the pressure, the greater the work and the greater the risk of heart attack and stroke. High blood pressure also can cause other problems, such as heart failure, kidney disease, and blindness. These problems are the result of damage that high blood

pressure causes in the blood vessels of the heart, kidneys, and eyes.

Hypertension isn't emotional tension or stress, although stress may raise blood pressure levels temporarily. Even people who are calm and relaxed can have high blood pressure. For some people, stress may be a factor, although the evidence isn't clear-cut. Just in case—and for the overall quality of your life—learn to relieve stress.

High Blood Pressure: Are You at Risk?

High blood pressure appears to be a complex problem, and in most cases its causes are still unknown. Only about 5 to 10 percent of cases can be attributed to known health problems, such as kidney disease. Yet health experts can identify people with increased risk. Check to see if you're at risk.

● *Family history of high blood pressure?* People appear to have a genetic tendency for high blood pressure. If there's been a woman under age sixty-five or

A Toast to Heart Health

Does moderate drinking reduce the risk for heart disease? Maybe, although people who don't drink aren't advised to start. Moderate drinking (red or white wine, beer, or distilled spirits) may offer heart-health benefits for some people. Moderate drinking also may raise HDL levels and keep some LDL cholesterol from forming, according to recent research. Resveratrol, a phytonutrient in the skins and seeds of grapes, may function as an antioxidant, promoting heart health; it also may help keep blood platelets from sticking together. Eating plenty of fruits and vegetables may give a bigger antioxidant boost. There's a fine line between how much alcohol is protective, though, and how much instead may promote heart disease, high blood pressure, and strokes. Remember, alcohol also can raise triglyceride levels.

There's reason for caution. Research linking alcoholic beverages and heart health isn't conclusive. Among unanswered questions, we don't yet know who may benefit. Even if a minor benefit exists, moderate drinking is only one factor related to heart health. Other lifestyle factors may play a role—for example, wine drinkers may be more physically active, and they may drink wine with meals, which may help affect blood lipid (fat) levels. *See "Red Wine: Heart-Healthy?" in chapter 8.*

Excessive and binge drinking is risky. Besides potentially leading to high blood pressure, heart failure, and excess calories, too much drinking can lead to other cardiovascular conditions, including stroke, irregular heartbeat, and sudden cardiac death. For pregnant women, excessive drinking can lead to fetal alcohol syndrome.

Until we know more, moderation is advised. No more than one drink a day for women, or no more than two drinks a day for men may lower the risk for heart disease. A drink is 12 ounces of regular beer, or 5 ounces of wine, or 1.5 ounces of distilled spirits.

Alcoholic beverages also supply extra calories, so if you're trying to control weight for heart health, control calories from alcoholic beverages, too.

The U.S. Food and Drug Administration offers another warning. If you take aspirin regularly for heart health, avoid drinking. Talk to your doctor if you choose to start aspirin therapy.

For more about alcoholic beverages in a healthful eating plan see "Alcoholic Beverages: In Moderation" in chapter 8.

FUNCTIONAL FOODS: HOW MUCH FOR BENEFITS?

To get the *potential* health-promoting benefits of functional foods, you must consume enough!

FUNCTIONAL FOOD	AMOUNT PER DAY	LINKED TO
Fructooligosaccharides	3–10 g	● Lower blood pressure ● Lower total cholesterol ● Improved GI health
Fish rich in omega-3 fatty acids	> 6 oz. a week	● Lower risk of heart disease
Garlic	600–900 mg (about 1 fresh clove)	● Lower blood pressure ● Lower total cholesterol
Grape juice	8–16 oz.	● Less clumping of red blood cells
Red wine	8 oz.	● Less clumping of red blood cells
Soy protein	25 g	● Lower LDL cholesterol
Tea, green or black	4–6 cups	● Lower risk for cancer of the stomach and esophagus
Vegetables and fruit	5–9 servings	● Lower risk for colon, breast, and prostate cancers

Source: C. Thomson, A.S. Bloch, and C.M. Hasler, "Functional Food—Position of the ADA," © American Dietetic Association. Reprinted with permission from *Journal of the American Dietetic Association,* 99: 1278 (1999).

a man under age fifty-five related to you in your family with hypertension or heart disease, your chances are higher.

● *Race?* African Americans have higher average blood pressure levels, and they tend to be more sodium-sensitive than European Americans. Typically African Americans develop hypertension earlier in life. As a result, they're at significantly greater risk for kidney disease as hypertension progresses and for death from strokes and heart disease. Some Asians also are at greater risk.

● *Overweight?* Extra body fat, especially around the waist and midriff, increases the risk for high blood pressure. And excessive weight puts more strain on the heart.

● *Your age?* For many people, blood pressure goes up as they get older. For men it's sooner, perhaps starting by ages forty-five to fifty. Women often are protected through menopause; for them, high blood pressure often starts about seven to ten years later. Just because you're older doesn't mean you'll develop high blood pressure, however.

● *Sodium-sensitive?* For up to 30 percent of the American population, an eating plan that's high in sodium may contribute to high blood pressure. And cutting back on sodium may help lower blood pressure. There's no way to predict whose blood pressure may be sodium-sensitive. Just in case, healthy normal adults are advised to limit sodium to no more than 2,400 milligrams daily.

● *Smoker?* Smoking makes your heart work harder and raises your blood pressure.

● *Too much drinking?* Heavy drinking may increase the risk for high blood pressure, too.

● *Diabetes?* People with diabetes may develop high blood pressure if their condition isn't managed carefully—another reason to keep diabetes under control from the time it's first diagnosed. Up to 65 percent of people with diabetes have it. *See "Diabetes: A Growing Health Concern" in this chapter.*

● *High blood lipids?* If your blood lipids are high, they contribute to hypertension as well as to atherosclerosis. *See "Strive for Desirable Blood Lipid Levels" earlier in this chapter.*

Testing, Testing: Know Your Blood Pressure Reading

The measurement of blood pressure is really two readings that look like a fraction. For example, an optimal reading is 120/80 mm Hg, expressed as "120 over 80" (mm Hg is millimeters of mercury). If it's less, that's okay.

● The number on top, which is higher, is called the systolic pressure. That's the pressure when your heart (actually the ventricle) contracts, pumping blood out to your arteries.

● The number on the bottom is called diastolic pressure, which is the pressure on your arteries between heartbeats, when your heart is at rest.

To find out if you have high blood pressure, have it checked at least every two years. If it's high normal (130–139 mm Hg over 85-89 mm Hg) or high, have it checked more often. Even children should be checked as part of their regular physical exams.

Blood pressure may fluctuate a bit during the day. Often the doctor's visit itself makes the number rise slightly; that's sometimes called "white-coat hypertension," which refers to white medical lab coats. To diagnose high blood pressure you need two higher-than-normal readings taken one to several weeks apart.

Whether you suspect high blood pressure or not, have your blood pressure checked regularly. If either your systolic or your diastolic number, or both, are consistently at or above 140/90 mm Hg, there's cause for concern. Take steps to bring your blood pressure down. Usually high blood pressure is managed by a combination of medication, diet, and lifestyle changes. For those with diabetes, a yet lower blood pressure goal might be advised.

Note: Your local pharmacist may offer blood pressure readings as a free service. Or you can buy an electronic blood pressure measuring device to use at home. To check its accuracy, bring it to your next doctor's visit.

Not Too "Pressured"

Having a family history of high blood pressure doesn't necessarily mean you'll get it. And you can take preventive steps to lower your odds. In fact, many of the Dietary Guidelines promote blood pressure control

BLOOD PRESSURE: FOR ADULTS*

CATEGORY		SYSTOLIC[†]		DIASTOLIC[†]
Optimal		<120 mm Hg	and	<80 mm Hg
Normal		<130 mm Hg	and	<85 mm Hg
High Normal		130-139 mm Hg	or	85-89 mm Hg
High[‡]	Stage 1	140-159 mm Hg	or	90-99 mm Hg
	Stage 2	160-179 mm Hg	or	100-109 mm Hg
	Stage 3	≥180 mm Hg	or	≥110 mm Hg

*These categories are for people age eighteen or over. The categories are for those not on a high blood pressure medication and who have no short-term serious illness.

[†]If your systolic and diastolic fall into different categories, your overall status is the higher category. For example, 160/80 mm Hg would be stage 2 hypertension (high blood pressure).

[‡]These levels are based on the average of two or more readings, taken at two or more times, after initial screening.

Source: Sixth Report of the Joint National Committee on Prevention, Detection, Evaluation, and Treatment of High Blood Pressure, National Institutes of Health/National Heart, Lung, and Blood Institute (1997).

and protect against hypertension! *See "What's Smart Eating? Guidelines for Americans" in chapter 1.*

● If you have a few pounds to shed, do so. Losing even 10 pounds, through smart eating and physical activity, may bring your blood pressure down—perhaps enough to avoid medication. As part of your weight loss plan, low-fat eating lowers blood lipid levels, too—a benefit to heart health and diabetes management. *See chapter 2, "Your Healthy Weight."*

Have You Ever Wondered

... what to do if you have a high-normal blood pressure reading? Even high-normal blood pressure appears to increase cardiovascular risk significantly. If you fit into this category, you're smart to monitor your blood pressure regularly—and to make lifestyle and dietary changes now to bring your blood pressure down to a healthier level. That's equally important if you have high cholesterol levels, diabetes, or other cardiovascular risk factors, or if you're an older adult.

● Fit in regular physical activity. Sedentary living doesn't cause high blood pressure, but regular aerobic activity such as brisk walking, swimming, or biking may help bring it down. Moreover, physical activity can help you maintain a healthy weight.

● Eat less salt, to help limit your sodium intake to 2,400 milligrams a day. Put the salt shaker away. Use Nutrition Facts on food labels to find processed foods with less sodium. Ask restaurants to go easy on the salt in the foods you order. For more about sodium *see "Link to High Blood Pressure," "About Salt Substitutes," and "Flavor . . . with Less Salt and Sodium" in chapter 7.*

● Put dairy foods and other calcium-rich foods on the "menu." Three minerals—calcium, magnesium, and potassium—help regulate blood pressure. Calcium, and perhaps magnesium and potassium, which are all found in dairy foods, appear to be protective. *See "Counting Up Calcium" in chapter 4.* No conclusive evidence shows that calcium and magnesium supplements offer extra benefits.

● Eat plenty of fruits and vegetables—at least five servings a day. More is even better! The potassium and magnesium found in many fruits and vegetables may help control your blood pressure. *For more about potassium and magnesium and their food sources see "Minerals—Not 'Heavy Metal'" in chapter 4.*

● Follow the DASH eating plan, established by the National Heart, Lung, and Blood Institute of the National Institutes of Health in the mid-1990s. The DASH (Dietary Approaches to Stop Hypertension) diet emphasizes food rather than nutrients for lowering blood pressure. Similar to the Food Guide Pyramid, it puts more emphasis on fruits and vegetables; like the Pyramid, it also advises low-fat and fat-free dairy foods and lean meat, poultry, and fish.

The DASH diet has been shown to lower blood pressure: down 6 to 11 mm Hg for systolic blood pressure and down 3 to 6 mm Hg for diastolic blood pressure. That's enough to lower hypertension risk significantly. In research studies, the DASH plan worked quickly—lowering blood pressure within two weeks. The benefits of the DASH diet were even better when combined with less sodium (down to 1,500 milligrams daily) in the DASH-Sodium study; blood pressure dropped even more, especially for those with hypertension. *See "DASH to Health" on this page for a meal plan.*

● Go easy on alcoholic beverages—if you drink. No more than one drink a day for women, and two for men, appear safe. Be aware that alcoholic beverages may interfere with medication for hypertension.

If You Have High Blood Pressure . . .

Relax. Although it's a lifelong condition, you can control high blood pressure and live a long, healthy life.

Have You Ever Wondered

... if caffeine causes high blood pressure? Since caffeine is a mild stimulant, you may think so. However, studies show that caffeine may result in only a very slight, temporary rise in blood pressure level.

The key is following your physician's advice faithfully. Treatment will likely include a shift in your eating approach, weight loss (if you're overweight), more physical activity, smoking cessation (if you smoke), and perhaps blood pressure medication.

● Make a plan of action with your healthcare provider, *following the advice in "Not Too 'Pressured'" in this chapter. Get help for adopting the DASH diet.*

DASH to Health

Good news about DASH: it's a taste-appealing switch from just no-salt-added eating—and it makes a difference in lowering blood pressure. It may even be an alternative to medication.

The DASH diet is similar to the Food Guide Pyramid plan but recommends more fruits and vegetables. Its guidelines are based on 2,000 calories a day, compared with 1,600 to 2,800 calories daily for the Pyramid.

Depending on your energy needs, your number of daily servings in a food group for the DASH diet may differ from these.

To follow the DASH diet, add more fruits and vegetables to your plate gradually—that's easier. Make fruits, vegetables, and grain products the main foci of your meal; enjoy smaller amounts of meat, poultry, or fish.

DASH EATING PLAN: BUILDING ON THE PYRAMID

FOOD GROUP	DASH DIET		FOOD GUIDE PYRAMID*
	DAILY SERVINGS*	SIGNIFICANCE	DAILY SERVINGS*
Grains and grain products	7 to 8	Carbohydrates (major source of energy), fiber	6 to 11
Vegetables	4 to 5	Potassium, magnesium, fiber	3 to 5
Fruits	4 to 5	Potassium, magnesium, fiber	2 to 4
Low-fat or fat-free dairy foods	2 to 3	Calcium, protein, potassium, magnesium	2 to 3 (mostly low-fat and fat-free foods)
Meats, poultry, and fish	2 or less	Protein, magnesium	2 to 3
Nuts, seeds, and legumes	4 to 5 per week	Magnesium, potassium, protein, fiber	(Part of meat group)
Fats and oils	2 to 3		Use sparingly
Sweets	5 per week		Use sparingly

For more about serving sizes and the Food Guide Pyramid see chapter 10.

● If your doctor prescribes antihypertensive medication, take it faithfully. If other tactics, like weight loss, lower your blood pressure level, taking medication may not be forever. Follow directions for medications carefully. Different blood pressure medications work in different ways; some may interact with other medications—for example, for diabetes or kidney disease.

● If your doctor prescribes a sodium-modified diet, a registered dietitian can help you plan, follow through, and monitor your sodium intake.

Cancer Connection

After heart disease, cancer is the second leading cause of illness and death in the United States, currently accounting for one in four deaths. According to 2002 data, cancer will strike about one in three adults. Among men, the incidence of prostate cancer is highest, followed by lung and bronchial cancer, then colorectal cancer. And for women, the prevalence of breast cancer is highest, followed by lung, then colorectal cancer. The overall death rate follows a similar order except that lung cancer for both men and women leaps to the top.

Almost half of all cancer deaths can be prevented with early detection and treatment. In fact, cancer has become a chronic disease for many, as cancer survivors are living longer. At every stage of this disease—before, during, and after treatment, during remission, during recurrence, and during palliative and hospice care—good nutrition is important to dealing with and surviving cancer. (Palliative care eases the effects that accompany terminal stages of cancer.)

What Is Cancer?

Cancer is an assortment of diseases characterized by abnormal cell growth that can spread and destroy other organs and body tissue. Cancers are classified by the body tissues where the cancer starts, such as the colon, breast, or skin.

Cancer starts with a single cell that has divided abnormally and does not function as it should. An altered body cell multiplies at an abnormally fast rate. These abnormal cells continue to use the body's resources, including nutrients, to multiply. In the process, they disrupt and eventually destroy the normal

function of the tissue or organ where they grow. These cancerous cells can metastasize, or spread through the bloodstream or the lymphatic system to other parts of the body, invading and destroying healthy body tissues and organs far from the original tumor.

The causes of cancer are varied and not always clear. Some cancers appear to be genetic and run in families. However, most cancers are caused by environmental and lifestyle factors. Cancer promoters, called carcinogens, include viruses, chemicals, and lifestyle and environmental factors.

Reducing Your Cancer Risk

Since some risk factors are controllable, the best prevention is to keep cancer from starting in the first place. Among the risk factors within your control: the use of tobacco; your dietary intake; exposure to sunlight (ultraviolet radiation); and exposure to carcinogens, or cancer-causing agents. In fact, 60 to 70 percent of all cancer cases are directly related to daily food and lifestyle choices; according to 2002 data from the American Cancer Society, one-third of cancer deaths were related to nutrition, physical inactivity, obesity, and other lifestyle factors. Taking a few small steps may be enough to significantly reduce your cancer risk.

Eat Smart: Reduce Your Cancer Risk

Dietary guidelines for cancer prevention are similar to those for preventing other health problems, including heart disease, diabetes, and high blood pressure. This same eating approach promotes overall well-being. *Throughout this book you'll find practical tips for eating to prevent cancer.* Keep in mind that no single food or nutrient causes or prevents cancer.

● Enjoy a variety of plant-based foods: vegetables, fruits, legumes (beans), and whole grains. A high-fiber diet, typically low in fat, too, may protect you from colon and rectal cancer. The reasons? Fiber helps move waste through your digestive tract faster, so harmful substances don't have much contact time with your intestinal walls. And because fiber makes stools bulkier, potentially harmful substances are diluted. *For tips on boosting your fiber intake see "For Fiber—Variety!" in chapter 6.* As important, plant-based foods contain a complex mixture of cancer-fighting nutrients and phytonutrients.

● Eat your veggies—and fruits! Vegetables and fruits have a complex composition of vitamins, minerals, fiber, and phytonutrients, which appear to protect against various cancers—from the esophagus through the GI (gastrointestinal) tract to the rectum. What's more, they're low in fat. These foods also may protect you from breast, bladder, pancreatic, lung, and larynx cancer. The American Institute for Cancer Research estimates 20 percent fewer cancer cases if Americans ate at least five servings of fruits and vegetables daily! *See "Antioxidant Nutrients: A Closer Look" and "Phytonutrients—a 'Crop' for Good Health" in chapter 4.*

Could dietary supplements offer similar benefits? That's a question that science has not yet answered. Foods are likely more effective than supplements because they provide a full array of substances in a safe and effective mix.

● Maintain your own healthy weight—and stay physically active. Obesity is linked to cancer of the uterus and perhaps breast, colorectal, prostate, and kidney cancers. The best approach to weight management is twofold: (1) stay physically active with thirty minutes or more of moderate activity on most if not all days of the week and (2) avoid eating more calories (food energy) than your body uses. *See chapter 2, "Your Healthy Weight."*

Besides weight management, physical activity may help protect against cancer by affecting hormone levels and helping to stimulate your colon to eliminate waste. In fact, regular physical activity is linked to lower risk of colon cancer, and perhaps lung and breast cancers. *For more about benefits of physical activity see chapter 1.*

● Go easy on alcoholic beverages, if you drink at all. Excessive drinking increases your chances for liver, mouth, throat, pharynx, larynx, and esophagus cancers—and even more if you smoke. As with other health problems, moderation is the key—no more than one drink daily for women, and two for men. Some studies suggest that breast cancer risk may go up even with moderate drinking. Drinking also may increase colorectal cancer.

● Limit fat and salt. When it comes to health risks related to high-fat eating, heart disease is "top of mind" for many people. Yet a high-fat approach to eating, especially animal fat, also is linked to some types of cancer, including lung, colon, rectum, breast, uterus, and prostate cancers. An eating plan that's low in saturated fat and trans fatty acids is advised.

Why limit salt, salt-cured, salt-pickled, smoked, and salty foods? They probably increase the risk for stomach cancer, especially among people and cultures who eat a lot of salt-preserved foods.

See chapters 3 and 7 for tips on eating less fat and salt.

● Avoid eating charred foods. Be aware that high-temperature cooking, such as grilling, broiling, and pan-frying, of meat, poultry, and fish cause heterocyclic amines (HCAs) to form. When fat from these foods drips onto fire, smoke and flames leave another substance, polycyclic aromatic hydrocarbons (PAHs),

---

Guidelines for Nutrition and Cancer Prevention

Guidelines for Nutrition and Cancer Prevention from the American Cancer Society offer sound, science-based advice for reducing your cancer risk. They mirror the Dietary Guidelines for Americans of the U.S. Department of Agriculture, *described in chapter 1.*

1. Choose most of the foods you eat from plant sources.
   ● Eat five or more servings of fruits and vegetables each day.
   ● Eat other foods from plant sources, such as breads, cereals, grain products, rice, pasta, or beans several times each day.

2. Limit your intake of high-fat foods, particularly from animal sources.
   ● Choose foods low in fat.
   ● Limit consumption of meats, especially high-fat meats.

3. Be physically active: achieve and maintain a healthy weight.
   ● Be at least moderately active for 30 minutes or more on most days of the week.
   ● Stay within your healthy weight range.

4. Limit consumption of alcoholic beverages, if you drink at all.

Source: American Cancer Society's Guidelines for Nutrition and Cancer Prevention, 2001. Reprinted with permission.

behind. Both HCAs and PAHs are potential carcinogens. Occasional high-heat cooking and eating of darkened foods is no cause for concern. However, a lot of high-heat cooking may possibly increase the chances of stomach and colorectal cancers. *See chapter 13 for tips on smart grilling.*

Smart Living for Reducing Cancer Risk

● Make your life a "nonsmoking" zone. Smoking, chewing tobacco, and secondhand smoke are linked to most cancer deaths in the United States. Although women fear breast cancer, more die annually of lung cancer linked to cigarette smoking. Smoking also lowers blood levels of some protective nutrients. In fact, smoking increases the chances of many other cancers, including oral, throat, esophageal, stomach, liver, prostate, and colorectal cancers. By quitting, the risk gradually declines.

● Limit your exposure to the sun, as well as sunlamps and tanning booths, to reduce your skin cancer risk. As part of your daily routine, wear protective clothing, UV-absorbing sunglasses, and use sunblock to protect your skin. A sunscreen with an SPF of 12 to 29 offers moderate protection; an SPF of 30 or more offers more production, advised if you're highly sensitive to the sun. Many moisturizing creams come with built-in sunscreen. Try to avoid peak sun exposure: 10:00 A.M. to 3:00 P.M. (when your shadow is shorter than you are).

Testing, Testing: Cancer Screening for Early Detection

Cancer develops gradually. The best cure: Stop cancer as soon as possible. That's why early detection is so important! On a monthly basis, perform self-exams: breast, testicular, skin. And make sure your regular physical checkups include routine cancer screening:

● Breast cancer—mammogram for women in their forties or older, every one to two years.

● Colorectal cancer—sigmoidoscopy (rectum and lower colon), colonoscopy (entire colon and rectum), fecal occult blood (blood in the stool), and digital rectal exam.

● Cervical cancer—annual Pap smear or as advised by your doctor for women.

● Skin cancer—a yearly all-over skin examination.

● Other screening—for prostate and testicular cancer for men, ovarian cancer for women, oral cancer, and lung cancer, as advised by your doctor.

In addition to cancer screening, be alert to symptoms of cancer: thickening or a lump in the breast or elsewhere, obvious change in a wart or a mole, a sore that doesn't heal, a nagging cough or hoarseness, changes in bowel or bladder habits, indigestion or difficulty swallowing, unexplained changes in weight, and unusual bleeding or discharge. See your doctor; the symptoms can indicate other things besides cancer.

Functional Foods to Lower Cancer Risk

Some Foods with *Potential* Functional Benefits	Functional Significance
Vegetables and fruits	Antioxidant vitamins, phytonutrients (allyl sulfides, anthocynanins, catechins, ellagic acid, isoflavones, lignan, limonoids, lutein, lycopene, saponins, sulphoraphane, fiber)
Beef, dairy foods, lamb	Conjugated linoleic acid (CLA)
Fermented dairy foods (e.g., yogurt, cultured buttermilk)	Probiotics
Low-fat foods (e.g., cheese, snack foods, meats, fish, dairy) as part of a low-fat diet	Low in total fat or saturated fat
Tea (green or black)	Catechins
Flaxseed (ground)	Lignans, fiber
Soybeans	Isoflavones (genistein)

See "Phytonutrients—a 'Crop' for Good Health" in chapter 4 and "Functional Foods: A New Wave" in chapter 9 for more about phytonutrients and functional foods.

If You're Dealing with a Cancer Diagnosis . . .

Good nutrition: it's essential if you've been diagnosed with cancer. The goals? To maintain weight and keep up your energy level and strength. To do that, you may need high-calorie foods and more proteins. That may be a change from the way you've been eating—and a challenge when you don't feel well. Your nutrition needs are unique to your cancer, the treatment, and your personal preferences. *For tips on boosting calories see chapter 2.* However, some cancer treatments can cause weight gain. For those individuals it is important to maintain a healthy weight.

Besides helping you feel stronger and better, good nutrition helps you handle the side effects of cancer treatment, reduce your chance of infection, and assist with your recovery from treatment or surgery.

Safe food handling takes on even more importance, since your immune response may not function as well as normal. With a low white blood cell count (common during chemotherapy and radiation) your body may not be able to fight infection or harmful foodborne bacteria effectively. *For guidance on food safety see chapter 12.*

A registered dietitian can help you with a plan for managing food choices if you're dealing with cancer. Ask your physician or healthcare professional for a referral to a registered dietitian.

Before Treatment or Surgery

Prepare—make good nutrition part of your pretreatment approach to cancer recovery. Start with a positive mind-set. Eat for health; being well nourished is a strategy for building your strength and reserves before surgery or treatment begins. Plan ahead by stocking your kitchen with foods you can eat while you're dealing with the possible side effects of treatment. Have nutritious snacks on hand; you may not have the energy to prepare food, or the appetite to eat. Gather your support team so you'll have help if and when you need it for food shopping, food preparation, and companionship. A support group dealing with cancer also is helpful for both psychological support and practical tips. Ask your physician, nurse, social worker, or other healthcare professional for support group information.

During "Chemo" and Radiation

Cancer treatment requires powerful medication or radiation that not only kills cancer cells but also can damage healthy body cells, resulting in possibly uncomfortable side effects. Careful food choices can help control some of the side effects that result from treatment. Most side effects go away once treatment is over.

To deal with side effects of chemotherapy or radiation that affect your ability to eat, try the strategies described here to stay well nourished. Frequent minimeals, for example, might help. If you feel tired, ask your family or a friend to help you with meals—or arrange for home-delivered meals to preserve your strength. *See "Cancer Treatment: Handling Side Effects" in this chapter.* For more advice, especially if side effects persist, talk to a registered dietitian.

Caution: talk to your doctor about any alternative or complementary therapies, such as herbal products, vitamins, or minerals, before you try them to relieve symptoms or to promote the quality of your life. Although some are safe and harmless, others can interfere with the effects of radiation or chemotherapy, or with your recovery from surgery. Some may have harmful side effects.

Chemotherapy. Chemotherapy uses oral or injected medications to stop or slow the progress of cancer cell growth. Among its common side effects are fatigue, diarrhea or constipation, nausea and vomiting, mouth tenderness or sores, and changes in the way food tastes and smells. To help you cope with the unpleasant effects of chemotherapy:

- Eat before your treatment. If your treatment takes several hours, bring a light snack along unless a light snack is offered during your treatment.

- When your appetite is good between treatments, nourish yourself well.

- As important, cut yourself some slack. Do your best when it's challenging to eat, and know that the side effects of chemotherapy usually go away once treatment is over.

See "Cancer Treatment: Handling Side Effects" in this chapter.

CANCER TREATMENT: HANDLING SIDE EFFECTS

Treatment and cancer itself often result in uncomfortable side effects that affect the desire and the ability to eat. If you experience these problems, these tips might make eating easier and more appealing. Remember, good nutrition is part of your treatment and your feeling of well-being.

IF YOU...	YOU CAN...
Have changes in your sense of taste and smell	• Try changing the temperature at which you eat certain foods. Hot foods may smell and taste stronger, so serving at a cool temperature may help. As cold foods get warmer, a sweet taste may get more pronounced, which may or may not be desirable. • Season foods with tart flavors (lemon, other citrus fruit, vinegar) or sweet flavors (sugar, honey, syrup) depending on the taste problem. • Chew lemon drops, mints, or gum to remove lingering taste. (Avoid sugarless gums if you have diarrhea.) • If a food tastes too sweet, add salt or a sour taste to counteract the sweetness. If a food is too sour, adding sugar may help. • Rinse your mouth with tea, ginger ale, salted water, or water with baking soda before eating to clear your taste buds. • Rinse your mouth and brush your teeth frequently to help with a bad taste in your mouth.
Have a poor appetite	• Eat five or six small meals instead of three larger meals. • Make the meal more enjoyable with flowers and nice dishes. Play music or watch your favorite TV show. Eat with family or friends. • Keep snacks handy to eat when you're hungry: hard-cooked eggs, luncheon meats, peanut butter, cheese, ice cream, granola bars, nutritional drinks and puddings, crackers, pretzels. • Eat high-calorie, high-protein foods at meals and snacktime. • Ask your doctor about medications to help relieve constipation, nausea, or pain if these problems are causing your poor appetite.
Feel constipated	• Try to stick to regular routines: eat at the same times each day, and try to be regular with bowel movements. • Drink 8 to 10 cups of liquid daily. Try water, prune juice, warm juice, tea, and hot lemonade. • If you feel gassy, limit gas-producing foods such as carbonated drinks, broccoli, cabbage, cauliflower, cucumbers, legumes (beans), and onions. To keep from swallowing air, drink through a straw, limit talking while you eat, and avoid chewing gum. • Eat high-fiber bulky foods, such as whole grain products, fruits and vegetables (skins on), popcorn, and legumes. • Eat breakfast with a hot drink and high-fiber breads and cereals. • Talk to your dietetics professional about a high-calorie, high-protein, fiber-containing liquid supplement. • Use laxatives only with your doctor's advice. Check with your doctor if you haven't had a bowel movement for three days or more.
Have diarrhea	• Drink plenty of mild, clear liquids throughout the day to prevent dehydration. Drink them at room temperature. • Eat small, frequent meals and snacks during the day. • Avoid high-fiber, high-fat (greasy, fried), spicy, or very sweet foods. When diarrhea is over, gradually eat foods with more fiber. • Limit milk products if you seem to have problems with milk during the period of diarrhea. • Avoid gas-producing foods. *(See tips for dealing with constipation.)* • Drink and eat foods high in sodium and potassium. *(See chapter 4.)* • Eat foods high in pectin (a type of fiber) such as applesauce, potatoes, oatmeal, rice, and bananas. • Call your doctor if diarrhea persists or increases, or if your stools have an unusual color or odor. • Drink at least one cup of liquid after each loose bowel movement. • Limit sugar-free gums and candies with sorbitol.
Have mouth sores or throat irritation	• Avoid tart, acidic, or salty beverages and foods. • Avoid rough-textured foods such as dry toast, crackers, granola, and raw fruits and vegetables.

IF YOU . . .	YOU CAN . . .
Have mouth sores or throat irritation *(continued)*	● Choose cool or lukewarm foods. ● Avoid alcohol, caffeine, carbonated beverages, and tobacco. ● Skip irritating spices such as chili powder, cloves, curry, hot sauces, nutmeg, and pepper. Season with herbs instead. ● Eat soft, bland, creamy foods such as cream soups, cheese, yogurt, mashed potatoes, cooked cereals, casseroles, milk shakes, and commercial liquid supplements. ● Blend and moisten dry or solid foods. ● Puree or liquefy foods in a blender to make them easier to swallow. ● Tilt your head back and forth to help foods and liquids flow to the back of your throat for easier swallowing. ● Drink through a straw to bypass mouth sores. ● Eat high-protein, high-calorie foods to speed healing. ● Rinse your mouth often with baking soda mouthwash (l quart of water and 1 tablespoon of baking soda) to remove food and germs.
Feel nauseous or queasy	● Eat six to eight small meals a day instead of three larger ones. ● Eat dry foods such as crackers or dry cereals when you awaken and every few hours. ● Choose foods that don't have a strong odor; eat foods that are cool, not icy cold or hot. ● Avoid foods that are overly sweet, fatty, fried, or spicy. ● Sit up or recline your head slightly for an hour after eating. ● Sip clear fluids—water, juice, flat soda, weak tea—throughout the day. ● Talk to your doctor about antinausea medication. ● Try bland, soft, easy-to-digest foods on treatment day: perhaps chicken noodle soup with saltines. ● Eat in a cool room without cooking odors or other aromas. Perhaps grill outside or cook in boilable bags. ● Rinse your mouth before and after meals. ● Suck on hard candy to remove any bad tastes in your mouth. ● Drink eight or more cups of fluids daily if you can, and an additional $1/2$ to 1 cup for each vomiting episode. Sip fluids thirty to sixty minutes after eating solid food.
Have a dry mouth or thick saliva	● Drink 8 to 12 cups of liquid daily to loosen mucus. Take a water bottle with you when away from home. ● Drink liquids through a straw. ● Eat soft, bland foods cold or at room temperature. Try blenderized fruits and vegetables; soft, cooked chicken and fish; well-thinned cereals; Popsicles; and slushies. ● Moisten foods with broth, soup, sauce, gravy, butter, or margarine. ● Suck on sour lemon drops, frozen grapes, Popsicles, or ice chips. Avoid chewing ice cubes that can damage your teeth. ● Keep your mouth clean with a soft-bristle toothbrush. Rinse your mouth before and after eating with water or a mild mouth rinse (made with 1 quart of water, $1/4$ teaspoon of salt, and 1 teaspoon of baking soda). Floss regularly. ● Avoid commercial mouthwashes, alcoholic and acidic beverages, and tobacco. ● Limit caffeinated drinks and foods that have a diuretic effect: coffee, tea, cola, chocolate. ● Moisten room air with a cool mist humidifier. Keep it clean to avoid the spread of bacteria.
Have trouble swallowing	● Get advice from your healthcare provider on special eating techniques. ● Drink 6 to 8 cups of fluid daily, thickened to a consistency right for you. ● Report any coughing or choking while eating to your doctor right away, especially if you have a fever. ● Eat small, frequent meals. ● Use liquid nutritional supplements if you can't eat enough food. ● Ask a registered dietitian to recommend thickening products and help you know how to use them: gelatin, tapioca or flour, commercial thickeners, pureed vegetables, instant potatoes, baby rice cereal.

Source: Adapted from M. S. Walker and K. Masino, eds., *Oncology Nutrition: Patient Education Materials* (Chicago: American Dietetic Association, 1998).

Radiation. This form of therapy damages cancer cells with a series of daily treatments of radiation. Side effects depend on the area of the body being treated, the dosage, and the frequency of treatment. These can be nausea, vomiting, sore throat or mouth, loss of taste, dry mouth, difficulty swallowing, diarrhea, or loss of appetite. Many side effects contribute to eating problems, yet good nutrition is important during and after what may be several weeks of treatment. To help you cope with the side effects of radiation:

- Eat before your daily treatment.

- If it takes time to get to a treatment center, bring along food to eat before and afterward. If you need to stay overnight, make plans beforehand for convenient, easy, and nutritious meals and snacks.

- Give your body some time to get over any side effects. Often side effects don't appear right away, but they can last two or three weeks after radiation treatments are over.

See "Cancer Treatment: Handling Side Effects" in this chapter.

Cancer Survival: After Treatment Ends

No special diet after cancer diagnosis and treatment can prevent the recurrence of cancer. However, healthful eating strategies and lifestyle habits can make a difference! Being well nourished can help you gradually rebuild your strength after treatment.

Try to follow guidance from the Food Guide Pyramid. Consult with a registered dietitian about any side effects that persist. *See "Resources You Can Use" for resources for cancer treatment and cancer survival.*

Diabetes: A Growing Health Concern

Diabetes has become an epidemic, affecting about seventeen million Americans. Yet about six million of them—*perhaps you or someone in your family*—don't know they have it! And nearly one million more each year are predicted to get it.

In 2002 the U.S. Department of Health and Human Services and the American Diabetes Association estimated that nearly 16 million Americans are affected by pre-diabetes, which sharply raises the risk for developing type 2 diabetes and increases the risk of heart disease by 50 percent. Most people with pre-diabetes are apt to develop diabetes within a decade unless they make modest changes in both their diet and their physical activity level.

If it's not managed properly, diabetes can have serious, even life-threatening, effects on health: eye problems including blindness, circulatory problems, nerve disease, and kidney disease and failure, among others. In fact, diabetes is the leading cause of blindness, leg and foot amputations, and kidney disease, and the sixth-leading cause of death in the United States. Diabetes also is a major risk factor for heart attacks and stroke. Damage can add up, even before you know you have it. The best way to reduce the risks for these problems is to keep your blood sugar level near the normal range.

Have You Ever Wondered

. . . if your diet can protect you from breast cancer? Scientists don't yet know the answer, but the question is under investigation. Until we learn more, women are advised to eat a low-fat diet, eat plenty of fruits and vegetables, maintain a healthy weight, and get regular physical activity. Be aware that men can develop breast cancer, too. *See "Breast Cancer: Do Food Choices Make a Difference?" in chapter 17.*

. . . if shark cartilage is effective against cancer? Touted as an anticancer agent, the active components in shark cartilage have not been identified. Limited scientific research doesn't support its use in blocking tumor formation. Because it may affect the development of blood vessels, taking shark cartilage could be risky for pregnant women and for those recovering from wounds, surgery, or heart ailments. Beyond that, shark cartilage taken as an oral supplement may not be absorbed by the body—and it may not be pure shark cartilage.

. . . if laetrile is an appropriate supplement for cancer treatment? Promoted as vitamin B_{17}, laetrile (also called amygdalin) isn't a vitamin. Instead it's a substance derived from the pits of apricots and other fruits. Although proposed as a treatment for cancer, laetrile contains cyanide, which can be lethal. Laetrile is neither approved by the FDA nor legal to import into the United States.

What Is Diabetes?

Simply defined, diabetes is a physiological condition that affects the way the body uses energy from sugar, starch, and other foods. Carbohydrates (sugars and starches) don't cause diabetes. The problem is that insulin, a hormone produced by the pancreas, isn't being produced or doesn't work correctly in the body and therefore, can't be used properly for energy metabolism.

How does insulin work for healthy people? During digestion, glucose is released from carbohydrates and absorbed to circulate as blood glucose, or blood sugar, to body cells. Among healthy people, insulin regulates blood sugar levels. It allows glucose to pass from blood into body cells for energy production. Insulin also helps the body use amino acids and fatty acids from food. For people without diabetes, insulin helps blood sugar levels stay in a normal range so eating has little effect on blood sugar.

With diabetes, the body can't control blood sugar levels normally. Too little or no insulin, or the inability to use insulin properly, hinders the body's ability to use energy nutrients—carbohydrates, proteins, and fats. Instead of "feeding" cells, glucose accumulates in blood, causing blood sugar levels to rise. Since it can't be used for energy, blood glucose spills into urine and gets excreted. That makes extra work for the kidneys, causing frequent urination and excessive thirst. Over time, high blood glucose levels can cause damage to kidneys, eyes, nerves, and the heart. As a key energy source, glucose is lost.

Diabetes belongs in three main categories: type 1, type 2, and gestational diabetes.

Type 1 (Insulin-Dependent) Diabetes. Type 1 diabetes, an autoimmune disease, accounts for 5 to 10 percent of diabetes cases. In this form of diabetes, the pancreas can't make insulin. Pancreatic beta cells that produce insulin have been destroyed, perhaps due to heredity or to damage prompted by a virus. The causes aren't clear. Why is it an autoimmune disease? "Auto" refers to "self"; the immune system, which normally protects the body from disease, instead attacks the beta cells that produce insulin.

The symptoms of type 1 diabetes often begin in childhood or the young adult years. However, people of any age can develop type 1 diabetes. Daily insulin injections or a continuous insulin pump, along with a careful eating and physical activity plan, are required to manage type 1 diabetes. Type 1 diabetes also requires regular self-monitoring of blood glucose levels.

Type 2 (Non-Insulin-Dependent) Diabetes. Type 2 diabetes, a metabolic disorder, accounts for 90 to 95 percent of diabetes cases, with the incidence rising along with obesity rates, sedentary lifestyles, and an aging population, as well as better or early detection. In fact, in the 1990s, the number of cases jumped by 30 percent. About 80 percent of those with type 2 diabetes are overweight. With type 2 diabetes, pancreatic cells don't produce enough insulin or don't respond to insulin normally (insulin resistance), even though the pancreas produces insulin.

Type 2 diabetes develops slowly and usually becomes evident after age forty; however, obese children are increasingly at risk, too. In type 2 diabetes, blood sugar levels often can be controlled through food choices, weight control, and physical activity alone. Taking oral hypoglycemic medicines may help the body produce more insulin or better use the insulin the body makes. Sometimes insulin injections are needed, too. Type 2 diabetes also requires regular self-monitoring of blood glucose levels.

Gestational Diabetes. Gestational diabetes occurs in 2 to 5 percent of pregnancies, resulting from changes in hormone levels. The risk is higher among obese and older women. Although it usually disappears after delivery, gestational diabetes needs careful control during pregnancy. Women with gestational diabetes often develop type 2 diabetes later in life, and usually in later pregnancies. *See "Pregnancy and Diabetes" in chapter 17 for more information on gestational diabetes.*

Early Detection

Early detection of diabetes is important. The longer the body is exposed to high blood sugar levels, the greater the damage to the nervous and circulatory systems and to the blood vessels in the eyes, kidneys, heart, and feet. The early years of diabetes offer an opportunity. If you have diabetes, that's when you can do the most to prevent or reduce its long-term consequences—and so live a longer life with fewer health problems.

According to the American Diabetes Association, many people don't know they have diabetes—despite the harmful consequences, especially when diabetes goes undetected for several years.

How would you know if you have it? These are common symptoms: frequent urination, unusual thirst, extreme hunger, unusual weight loss, extreme fatigue, and irritability. In addition, those with type 2 diabetes also may experience frequent infections; cuts and bruises that heal slowly; blurred vision; numb or tingling hands or feet; or recurring skin, gum, or bladder infections. Some people with type 2 diabetes have no outward signs associated with high blood sugar levels.

At Risk for Type 2?

With this growing epidemic, what puts someone at risk for type 2 diabetes? The odds go up with these risk factors:

● *Being over age forty-five.* With age, the pancreas is less efficient at producing insulin.

● *Having a close family member with diabetes.* You may have an inherited tendency or share circumstances that increase your risk.

● *Being in some racial or ethnic groups.* If you're of African American, Hispanic, Asian American, Pacific Islander, or Native American descent, your diabetes risk is higher.

● *Being overweight or obese.* With more body fat, body cells become more insulin-resistant.

● *Being physically inactive.*

● *Having low HDL cholesterol levels or high triglycerides.*

● *Having had gestational diabetes, or delivering a baby weighing 9 pounds or more.*

Even if you're at risk for type 2 diabetes, there's good news: With regular moderate exercise and weight reduction, if you're overweight, your odds drop.

Testing, Testing: Blood Sugar Tests

Diabetes may be detected first by a urine test, given as a routine part of most physical exams. However, blood glucose readings are much more accurate. Everyone age forty-five or over should have a blood glucose test every three years. If you're at high risk, blood glucose testing should start sooner and be more frequent. Be aware that screening tests, often done at community health events, aren't diagnostic, yet they can identify those at high risk who need further testing.

Done during a checkup, a blood glucose reading is done after an eight-hour fast. A fasting plasma glucose (blood glucose) of less than 110 milligrams/deciliter (mg/dL) is considered normal. Two readings over 125 mg/dL, taken on different days, are criteria for a diabetes diagnosis. Even if your reading is slightly lower—110 to 125 mg/dL—you need careful monitoring; that level is considered impaired fasting glucose, indicating a high risk for type 2 diabetes.

If you're diagnosed with diabetes, you may need to self-monitor, or test your own blood glucose. Without testing you won't know your blood glucose level unless it's very high or very low. Your doctor will set realistic target blood glucose levels for you—for example, before meals and bedtime. Before meals, a blood glucose level of 70 to 150 mg/dL is considered normal; about two hours after a meal, it should be less than 200. Your doctor, dietitian, or diabetes educator will show you how to self-monitor. Be aware that target levels for young children and older adults may differ.

Checking your blood glucose is easy once you get used to pricking your finger: just a drop of blood from a finger stick on a test strip, read by a blood glucose meter. Log the results, the time, and the date. Use the information to see if your diabetes care plan (eating, exercise, and medication) is working. Share your log with your physician.

Once you become adept at self-monitoring, you can use your blood glucose reading to know if you need to eat something or take medication. If your blood glucose is too low (perhaps below 70 mg/dL) or too high (perhaps above 240 mg/dL), you'll need to do something. Ask your doctor for your personal targets.

There's one more blood glucose test: glycosylated hemoglobin, or hemoglobin A1c. Done every two or three months during your visit to your doctor, this test measures the average glucose in your blood over the past two to three months, and whether your blood sugar levels are under control. It may be used as a diagnostic test, too.

To control blood sugar levels and diabetes-related complications, ongoing monitoring means testing your "ABCs": A for hemoglobin A1C, B for blood pressure, and C for cholesterol levels.

If you have type 1 diabetes, your doctor also may advise you to take a urine test for ketones, which are acids that build up in urine to toxic levels. When there is no insulin available, your body cells can't use glucose for energy and turn to burning fat, not carbohydrates, for energy. Without carbohydrates, or glucose, body cells can't burn fat completely, and ketones form as a by-product of fat burning. When ketones build up, a condition called ketoacidosis can occur and, if left untreated, can lead to a diabetic coma and even death. Talk to your doctor about the early symptoms; get immediate medical help if ketoacidosis develops.

If You Have Diabetes . . .

The goal for diabetes management is this: controlling your blood sugar levels so they stay as near to normal as possible. Like a teeter-totter, blood sugar levels go up (hyperglycemia) and down (hypoglycemia); that's part of dealing with diabetes. Those swings can be dangerous when diet, exercise, and medication such as insulin aren't balanced properly.

- *Too much food or too little insulin?* Your blood sugar level can soar, affecting your health now and very seriously down the road.

- *Too much exercise or too much insulin?* Blood sugar drops, and your body can't use blood glucose to produce enough energy.

To control "the ups and the downs," carefully manage what you eat, how much, and when—*no matter what type of diabetes you have.* Eating raises your blood sugar level; physical activity and medication lower it. For example, in case of low blood sugar, consume a *small amount* of a quick-acting carbohydrate, such as ½ cup of fruit juice, followed by a small amount of protein food, perhaps a cheese cube on a cracker.

Your doctor will likely advise a regular physical activity plan to help control your blood sugar levels and prevent weight gain, too—and sensible weight loss if you're overweight. In fact, for many people, smart eating, weight loss, and active living are enough to control their blood sugar level and to maintain good health. Others need diabetes medication to keep blood sugar under control.

Here's some general advice about managing diabetes and preventing its symptoms. For individualized guidance that matches your needs, consult your doctor and a registered dietitian (RD). Some dietitians, as well as some nurses, are also certified diabetes educators (CDEs).

Be aware: If you've just found out that you have diabetes, you may feel healthy. Even if it's hard to remember to stick with your eating and physical activity program, the long-term benefits are well worth the effort!

Manage Your Meals and Snacks

The game plan for smart eating with diabetes follows this general strategy: *Eat about the same amount of food, in the right balance, at about the same time daily; to avoid weight gain, balance your day's food choices with regular physical activity.* In the big picture, eating with diabetes follows principles of healthful eating for anybody—in fact, for your whole family. *See the Dietary Guidelines in chapter 1.* That can make meal management simpler.

What is the "right balance"? It's *food variety* with a balance of different types of food . . . *portion savvy* to eat the right amount of food . . . and *control of energy-producing nutrients* (carbohydrates, fats, and proteins).

For diabetes, there's no single eating plan; the guidelines have built-in flexibility. The amount and proportions of carbohydrates, proteins, and fats—the energy nutrients—you consume depend on you and your weight, blood cholesterol levels, and medical needs. Specific food choices are up to you, too, and what foods you enjoy. Your doctor, along with a registered dietitian, can help you plan what's right for you—portion sizes, types of food, and overall timing.

Portion savvy is important in diabetes management. Get out your measuring cups and spoons, and the kitchen scale. Measure your portions, as well as your cups, bowls, and dishes, until you get familiar with serving sizes.

Another tip: People with diabetes often have high blood pressure and risks for heart disease, or they may acquire these conditions down the line. As precautions, eat for heart health and control your sodium intake, too, if you have diabetes. Talk to your healthcare provider about guidance. *See "Your Healthy Heart" and "Blood Pressure: Under Control?" in this chapter.*

Food Pyramid for Diabetes. The Food Pyramid for Diabetes is a starting point to plan meals and snacks for diabetes management. *It's similar to the Food Guide Pyramid shown in chapter 10,* but adjusted to help people with diabetes manage carbohydrates and other energy nutrients more easily. As you look at this Pyramid, notice how it differs:

- The base of the Pyramid has "Starches" with grain products, as well as starchy vegetables (potatoes, legumes, corn).
- "Protein" foods include fish, poultry, meat, and tofu, as well as cheese. Despite their protein content, legumes (beans) fit with "Starches."
- The "Milk and Yogurt" group doesn't include cheese.
- "Sugary Foods" and "Fats and Oils" belong in two separate groups at the Pyramid tip.

It's long been known that sugar doesn't cause diabetes; neither do any carbohydrates. Sugar doesn't cause blood sugar levels to rise any more rapidly than starches do. Starches (pasta, rice, bread, fruits and vegetables, and other starchy foods) and sugars have a similar effect on blood sugar levels. People with diabetes can fit small amounts of sugary foods into their eating plan as carbohydrate foods. For diabetes management, the issue is the total amount of carbohydrates consumed, not just how much is sugar. The caution is that many sugary foods are low in nutrients and high in fat.

If you like sweet flavors, intense sweeteners (acesulfame potassium, aspartame, saccharin, and sucralose) offer some choices without increasing your blood sugar level or adding calories. For example, look for diet soft drinks, sugar-free candy, and ice cream sweetened with aspartame. These foods may allow you to fit other foods in. For example, by choosing yogurt sweetened with aspartame instead of sugared fruit, you might fit toast, a muffin, or crackers into your eating plan, too. **Warning:** If you have the disorder phenylketonuria (PKU), avoid foods sweetened with aspartame. *See "Aspartame: PKU Warning" in chapter 21.*

Polyols (sorbitol, mannitol, and xylitol) are sweeteners with fewer calories than sugar. They affect blood sugar level, but not as much as sugar and other nutritive sweeteners do. *See "Intense Sweeteners: Flavor without Calories" and "Polyols: Sugar Replacers" in chapter 5.*

A few more tips: As you make your choices, choose mostly lean, low-fat, and fat-free foods, not only for diabetes management but also to help keep blood lipid levels within a healthy range. Enjoy deep-yellow and orange vegetables and fruits; besides their other benefits, their beta carotene content may reduce problems related to type 2 diabetes.

How about fiber? Follow the same guidelines as for those who don't have diabetes: 20 to 35 grams of fiber a day from whole grains, legumes (beans), vegetables, and fruits. Besides the overall benefits, soluble fiber slows digestion and may slow glucose absorption during digestion. And both soluble and insoluble fiber help you feel full after eating—an aid to weight control. Extra amounts, perhaps from fiber supplements, won't offer significant added benefits. *See chapter 6, "Fiber: Your Body's Broom."*

Exchanges or Carbohydrate Counting? For more control of energy nutrients (carbohydrates, fats, proteins), your dietitian or diabetes educator can help you work out an eating plan using exchange lists or carbohydrate counting.

Exchanges are like food groups in the Pyramid. They're lists of foods

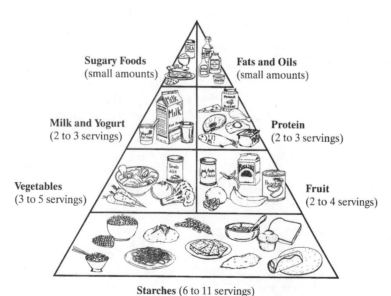

Sugary Foods
(small amounts)

Fats and Oils
(small amounts)

Milk and Yogurt
(2 to 3 servings)

Protein
(2 to 3 servings)

Vegetables
(3 to 5 servings)

Fruit
(2 to 4 servings)

Starches (6 to 11 servings)

FOOD PYRAMID FOR DIABETES: A GUIDE TO SERVINGS

The Food Pyramid for Diabetes can be your daily eating plan, especially for type 2 diabetes. Follow this serving guide, based on your day's calorie needs.

CATEGORIES	SERVINGS FOR 1,600 TO 2,000 CALORIES	SERVINGS FOR 2,000 TO TO 2,400 CALORIES	A SERVING IS*
Starchy foods (bread, cereal, rice, pasta, and starchy vegetables)	8	10	1 slice bread $\frac{1}{3}$ cup rice $\frac{1}{2}$ cup cooked cereal $\frac{3}{4}$ cup dry cereal flakes 1 small baked potato $\frac{1}{2}$ cup cooked legumes (beans)
Vegetables (except for starchy vegetables)	4	4	$\frac{1}{2}$ cup tomato juice $\frac{1}{2}$ cup cooked green or deep yellow vegetables 1 cup raw, leafy greens
Fruit	3	3	1 small apple $\frac{1}{2}$ cup fruit juice 2 tbsp. dry fruit $\frac{1}{2}$ cup canned fruit
Milk and yogurt	2	2	1 cup fat-free milk 1 cup nonfat yogurt
Protein (meat, poultry, fish, eggs, cheese)	2	2	2 to 3 oz. cooked fish, chicken, or lean meat 2 oz. cheese $\frac{1}{2}$ cup tofu
Fats	6 to 8	8 to 10	1 tbsp. regular salad dressing 1 tsp. regular margarine or oil 2 tbsp. light salad dressing 1 tbsp. light mayonnaise 1 bacon strip 6 whole peanuts
Sugary foods	0 to 1	0 to 1	1 plain cake doughnut $\frac{1}{12}$ of angel food cake 1 3-in.-diameter cookie 1 tbsp. maple syrup 4 chocolate Kisses

*Ask a registered dietitian or a certified diabetes educator where other foods fit.

Source: National Institute of Diabetes and Digestive and Kidney Diseases.

grouped together because they're alike; they're similar in carbohydrate, protein, fat, and calorie content. For that reason, foods within each list can be exchanged for other foods. Exchange lists fit within three overall groups: Carbohydrate Group (starch, fruit, milk, other carbohydrates, and vegetables lists), Meat and Meat Substitutes (very lean, lean, medium-fat, and high-fat meat and substitutes lists), and Fat Group (monunsaturated, polyunsaturated, and saturated fat lists). (Alcohol counts as fat exchanges.)

With specific numbers of exchanges from each list, you plan meals and snacks to get enough food variety and to spread out calories and energy-producing nutrients throughout the day. That helps you maintain your blood sugar level near normal, and balance food with exercise and diabetes medicines. Exchanges are published in *Exchange Lists for Meal Planning* from the American Dietetic Association and the American Diabetes Association.

Carbohydrate counting is another tool for managing your food intake and for keeping your blood glucose level in check. It allows you to more precisely match your food and insulin intake. It's an approach that's good for people who need tight control and are willing to make the effort.

With this approach, you keep track of the total carbohydrate grams you eat and drink for a day, trying to eat about the same number of carbohydrates, at the same time, each day. Remember, carbohydrates have more effect on blood sugar than any other nutrient. (*Tip:* For any meal or snack, try to keep within 5 grams of your target. The more "carbs" you consume, the higher your blood glucose level.) You need to take your fat and protein intake into account, too, since they also increase blood sugar level to some degree.

With carbohydrate counting, your "carbs" can come from any food source. Nutrient-rich foods (grain products, fruits, vegetables, legumes, and milk) are best, since together they supply vitamins, minerals, fiber, and phytonutrients. Sugary foods are often low in vitamins and nutrients, and perhaps high in fat.

Whatever approach to meal and snack planning you use:

● Get advice from a registered dietitian or a diabetes educator for an eating plan that's right for you— including how many exchanges from each exchange list, or how many carbohydrate grams, to strive for

daily. Plan how you'll spread out your eating during the day, too.

● Choose a variety of nutrient-rich foods that supply at least 60 percent of calories from carbohydrates. In a 2,000-calorie daily plan, that's 1,200 calories from total "carbs," or 300 carbohydrate grams. (One carbohydrate gram supplies 4 calories.) Your calorie needs depend on your age, activity level, body size, and perhaps a weight-loss plan.

● Check Nutrition Facts on food labels to know total carbohydrate grams, as well as fat and protein grams, in a single serving. Serving sizes on labels also can help with meal planning using exchange lists or the Food Pyramid for Diabetes. *To learn how to use food labels see chapter 11.*

● If you're counting "carbs" for unpackaged or restaurant foods, *check "'Carbo' Foods" in the Appendices.* For a more extensive list, find a book or a Web site source of carbohydrate facts; ask for nutrition information for restaurant menus when you eat out. Counting "carbs" in mixed foods takes a little know-how.

● To stick to your plan, be careful about portion sizes. Even for carbohydrate counting, learn serving sizes for exchanges—for example, one carbohydrate exchange provides about 15 grams of carbohydrates.

Check Your Clock. Keep to a regular meal and snack schedule—about the same amount of food, at about the same time daily—to keep your blood sugar level steady. Skipping meals or following an irregular eating pattern puts your blood sugar level out of kilter. To compound the problem, meal skipping may lead to overeating later and to an eating pattern that won't match your plan for managing diabetes.

● *Advice:* Stick to a regular meal and snack schedule. Carry an emergency snack in case you must change your regular eating routine. Consider several small meals, often better for blood sugar control than three big meals. A registered dietitian can help you pick the best food choices for snacking. If you need insulin or other diabetes medicine, take it on schedule, too.

Go Easy: Alcoholic Drinks. Can you enjoy alcoholic drinks now and then? That's a question to discuss with your doctor *before* you drink alcoholic beverages. Some people with diabetes are wise not to drink at all.

What are some risks? Drinking can worsen some

diabetes-related health problems such as high blood pressure, nerve damage from diabetes, and high triglyceride levels. Heavy drinking causes liver damage, which makes diabetes control harder. And alcoholic drinks contribute calories when you're trying to keep your weight under control. Alcoholic beverages also interfere with some diabetes medications.

If your blood glucose levels are under control and if your doctor indicates that alcoholic beverages in moderation are okay, a registered dietitian or a certified diabetes educator can help you work them into your meal plan. Keep these guidelines in mind:

● At most, limit alcoholic drinks: no more than one serving a day for women, and two for men—the same limits as for people without diabetes. A serving of alcohol is 5 ounces of wine, 12 ounces of beer, or 1½ ounces of distilled spirits. Discuss your individual limits with your doctor and registered dietitian.

● *Always* eat when you have an alcoholic drink to reduce the chance for hypoglycemia, or low blood sugar. When your liver is detoxifying alcohol, it doesn't produce as much glucose. Blood glucose that drops too low from drinking can be dangerous.

● As an alternative, choose low-alcohol wine or beer. They have fewer calories and less alcohol and carbohydrates than regular beer or sweet wine. Ask how they fit into your plan.

● Recognize that some wine coolers and mixed drinks (made with regular soda and juice) contain sugars. Count them as part of your eating plan (as fat and carbohydrate servings/exchanges) for diabetes management. Mix drinks or spritzers with sugar-free mixers such as club soda, diet soft drinks, diet tonic, seltzer, or water. Or try "virgin" drinks (no distilled spirits).

See "Taking Control: Drinking Responsibly!" in chapter 8.

Get Moving

Get moving! Active living is important in managing diabetes for several reasons. For one, regular physical activity increases insulin sensitivity, moving glucose out of blood more effectively. Second, being active can lower blood sugar as your muscles use glucose for energy. Third, physical activity burns energy, making weight management easier; your body controls your

blood sugar level better at a lower body weight. And fourth, regular physical activity helps reduce your risk for heart disease and high blood pressure, both linked to diabetes.

● Before you start a physical activity plan, talk with your doctor, along with a registered dietitian or a certified diabetes educator. Balance exercise with eating to keep your blood sugar level within a target range. If you take insulin, planning for exercise is a little more tricky.

● Before you start your physical activity, check your blood glucose level. If it's low (below 70 mg/dL or less), eat a snack with about 15 carbohydrate grams (a medium apple or bread slice); wait about a half hour, then check again. If it's 70 to 100 mg/dL, enjoy the same snack, then get moving. If your blood sugar is 100 to 150, it's okay to start, but eat a light snack if you plan to be active for thirty minutes or more. If your blood sugar is 240 mg/dL or more, wait, and get your blood sugar level down first.

● Take a carbohydrate-rich snack along when you're physically active—just in case you start feeling lightheaded. If that happens, stop moving and eat it. Too much exercise and not enough food can lead to hypoglycemia, or low blood sugar.

● Get a partner. Besides being more fun, it's safer. Let your partner know about your diabetes, and what to do if you need help.

● Wear a tag, a necklace, or a bracelet with diabetes identification. And wear proper footwear.

● Keep well hydrated when you're active. Water is a fine choice. Check with your doctor or a registered dietitian about beverage choices if you need a fast-acting carbohydrate source; fruit juice, regular soda, or a sports drink may be advised.

Control Your Weight

Whether you're overweight or not, manage your body weight as part of your personal approach for diabetes management. If you're overweight, losing 10 to 20 pounds may make blood sugar easier to control if you have type 2, non-insulin-dependent diabetes. Why? A lower weight helps lower insulin resistance, so you may no longer need diabetes medication. Other potential benefits of weight loss: lower blood lipid levels and lower blood pressure. Remember, with diabetes your risks for heart disease are higher! (Check with your doctor to see if weight loss is right for you.)

Consult a registered dietitian about losing or maintaining weight: how much you need to lose, over what time frame, and how to eat for weight loss and diabetes management. Limit weight loss to 1 pound weekly. *A few good tips for starters:* Choose mostly lean and low-fat foods. Rather than skip meals, eat smaller portions to consume fewer calories. And move more to use up calories! *See chapter 2, "Your Healthy Weight."*

Team Up for Health!

To manage diabetes properly, seek advice from your healthcare team, whose specialties help you deal with the complexities of diabetes: your physician, a registered dietitian, a certified diabetes educator, a nurse, an eye doctor, a podiatrist, and a pharmacist, among others. Follow through on your care plan.

Remember, you're the most important team member! For the team to work well:

● Set your target blood glucose levels with your doctor. For people with diabetes, near normal is generally

Have You Ever Wondered

. . . if people with diabetes should make food choices based on a food's glycemic index? First the definition: Glycemic index shows a food's potential for raising blood glucose level—how fast, how much, and how soon glucose level returns to normal. When eating a food with a glycemic index of less than 100, glucose is released more slowly; above 100, it's faster. Although it may surprise you, the glycemic index for sugar (92) is less than for mashed potatoes or white bread (100).

Whether there's any health benefit to selecting foods according to their glycemic index is controversial. On one hand, some research suggests that an overall eating plan with a lower glycemic index may reduce insulin response and so help lower the chances of heart disease, diabetes, and obesity. On the other hand, a glycemic index has been established for only a limited number of foods, and not for food combinations in meals and snacks or for the size of a meal. Having a low glycemic index doesn't mean a food is high in nutrients either. And individuals may respond differently. For now, stick to well-accepted approaches for diabetes management.

. . . if eating sugar or a carbohydrate-rich diet causes insulin resistance that results in weight gain? No, but some popular weight-loss book authors say so. Consuming carbohydrate-rich foods doesn't cause insulin resistance; excessive calories do. People who are overweight and sedentary may have symptoms of insulin resistance, a condition often diminished with moderate physical activity and weight loss.

. . . how you take insulin? Insulin needs to go directly into the bloodstream, either by injection or insulin pump.

Currently oral ingestion isn't effective because insulin would be broken down by digestion. Although not ready in the near future, new and easier ways to take insulin are under study: powdered in an inhaler, an insulin spray in the mouth, and a pill that gets past the stomach undigested, getting insulin directly to the liver.

. . . if drinking cow milk during infancy causes type 1 diabetes? There's no scientific evidence that milk protein from cow milk promotes type 1 diabetes in infants with an inherited tendency for diabetes. Regardless, the American Academy of Pediatrics (AAP) encourages breast-feeding for the first year of life, for all babies, including those with a strong family history of type 1 diabetes. For children age one year or older with diabetes, AAP recommends no restriction for cow milk.

. . . if you can stop taking insulin if you take chromium supplements? No. For type 1 diabetes, chromium supplements aren't an alternative to insulin. Chromium may help control blood sugar level for type 2 diabetes, but research evidence is still preliminary. If you have type 2 diabetes, talk to your doctor before taking any supplements. Enjoy foods with chromium—meat, eggs, whole-grain products, cheese—to get what you need. *See chapter 4 for more on chromium.*

. . . if any herbal products have a glucose-lowering ability? Despite claims, no conclusive research shows that herbal products offer benefits for managing diabetes. In fact, some may interact with diabetes medication. Talk to your doctor first, if you choose to try them—and never use them in place of insulin or other prescribed medicine.

Children and Diabetes

Type 1 diabetes is the most common form of diabetes among children. With the parallel rise in childhood obesity, more and more children are at risk for or diagnosed with type 2 diabetes. Dealing with diabetes during childhood and teenage years adds to the challenges of growing up. Most kids don't want to be different.

The first guideline—help your child maintain or grow into a healthy weight to reduce the chance of type 2 diabetes. If your child is overweight, ask your doctor about testing for diabetes at about age ten or at puberty if your child has other risk factors.

If your child is diagnosed with diabetes, accept and manage it together in a calm, careful, and positive way.

- Work closely with your child's healthcare team to manage diabetes and help your child grow normally—physically, mentally, and emotionally.

- Gradually involve your child in taking responsibility for his or her diabetes. Encourage rather than nag, even when things aren't perfect. Help your child learn when, how, and where to get help. Learning lifelong skills for diabetes management—and making them a habit—is part of growing up. Diabetes won't go away.

- Get advice from your healthcare team about handling special eating events such as birthday parties, sleepovers, field trips, and active play or sports.

- Be matter-of-fact, sensitive, and supportive as you help your child or teen learn about diabetes. A support group or diabetes camp for kids can help. Find a reliable Web site for kids about diabetes.

- Help teachers, baby-sitters, coaches, and others who supervise your child understand your child's diabetes and how they can support the diabetes care plan. Meet with them. Write instructions, list symptoms, and provide phone numbers for your doctor and other responsible adults. Provide appropriate snacks. Teach a sitter how to do blood sugar checks and give diabetes medication, if needed. Ensure that your child has the time and the privacy for diabetes care without discrimination.

- Help your child or teen feel comfortable about asking to leave class or play to monitor blood sugar and take insulin.

- Make diabetes management part of your parenting responsibility, but not the sole focus. Keep the joys of growing up and a healthy family life.

For more parenting tips see chapter 16, "Food to Grow On."

---

70 to 150 mg/dL. Be realistic; you can't avoid some "ups and downs." Numbers that are mostly within a safe range reduce your risks for complications.

- Keep all appointments for checkups, counseling, and laboratory tests. If your blood glucose levels are under control, see your doctor two to four times a year; if not under control, go in more often. Can't make it? Change your appointment—don't skip it!

- Take diabetes medications as directed, even if you're sick. Tell your doctor or pharmacist about all other medicine and dietary supplements (including herbal products) you take, both prescriptions and over-the-counter medications. Also tell your team about any side effects or problems you have with any medicine or supplement. Plan ahead, and call for new prescriptions or refills well before you run out. If you take insulin, ask about an insulin pump, which gives a constant, small dose. **Caution:** Diabetes medicines can't substitute for healthful eating and exercise.

- Learn to check your own blood glucose level. Self-monitoring, perhaps several times daily, is wise for anyone with diabetes, especially if you're taking diabetes medication, if you're pregnant, or if your blood glucose levels are low or out of control. For adults, ask about a noninvasive blood glucose monitoring device. It can check your blood glucose level every 20 minutes without puncturing your skin for a blood sample. Use it with conventional blood glucose monitoring.

- Learn how to detect and safely treat an insulin reaction, hypoglycemia, and hyperglycemia—before you get into severe danger. Immediate, appropriate treatment, perhaps medical assistance, is essential! Wear a medical alert tag or carry a card to let others know what to do in case you pass out.

● Consult a registered dietitian to create a healthful eating plan (Food Pyramid for Diabetes, exchange lists, or carbohydrate counting) specific to you, including an approach to managing weight. The dietitian also can offer specific advice on shopping, label reading, eating out, and using alcoholic beverages.

● Get help with stress control if needed. Under stress, it's harder to be diligent about diabetes care: staying active, eating smart, checking your blood sugar level, and perhaps controlling alcoholic beverages. Besides that, stress may affect your blood glucose level.

● Know that you don't need to struggle with diabetes alone. If your medications, eating plan, or physical activity program cause problems or concerns, make an appointment to explore new strategies with your health team members. Managing diabetes can be complex—but your health now and later depends on it!

Osteoporosis: Reduce the Risks

Although the signs of osteoporosis don't show up until later (usually age sixty or older), keeping your bones healthy is a lifelong process. From childhood and adolescence on, your eating and lifestyle habits can protect you from this debilitating disease later in life. No matter what your age now, it's not too late to start caring for your bones.

Osteoporosis Is . . .

Osteoporosis is a condition of gradually weakening, brittle bones. As bones lose calcium and other minerals, they become more fragile and porous. They may break under normal use or from just a minor fall. Because it progresses slowly and silently, people often don't realize they have osteoporosis until they fracture a bone. The spine, hip, and wrist are the most common fracture sites.

Among older adults, a "dowager's hump" is an obvious sign of osteoporosis. Vertebrae in the spine collapse as a result of bone loss. Collapse of several vertabrae leads to a loss of height, back pain, and increasing disability.

Osteoporosis affects most Americans over age seventy, especially women. But men get it, too. In fact, even if you add up all the cases of heart disease, stroke,

and diabetes in a year, osteoporosis is more common. In the United States alone, 1.5 million bone fractures annually are attributed to this bone disease each year. About 10 million Americans have osteoporosis; about 18 million more have low bone mass, making them at higher risk for osteoporosis. Of those with osteoporosis, about 80 percent are women. In fact, by the time women go through menopause, nearly one in three has developed osteoporosis. Looking at this disease another way, half of women and about 13 percent of men over age fifty will have a fracture related to osteoporosis in their lifetime.

Many hip fractures, common among older adults, are linked to bone disease. Besides pain, fractures cause changes in lifestyle and loss of independence. A person may no longer be able to dress alone or walk across a room. Hip fractures also can be fatal. An average of 24 percent of people age fifty or over with hip fractures die from complications within a year after their fracture.

To keep your bones healthy, help them become strong and dense while you can (until your early thirties). After that, help keep them strong by slowing the natural loss that comes with age. *For more about building bones see "Bone Up on Calcium" in chapter 4.*

You can't control some risk factors for osteoporosis: genetics, family history, gender, hormonal status, race/ethnic heritage, age, and body frame/weight. You can control other risk factors: what you eat, physical activity, cigarette smoking, alcohol intake, and using medications to help protect against osteoporosis.

Now, how bone-healthy are you?

● *Gender.* If you're female, you're about four times more likely than males to develop osteoporosis, for three reasons: (1) On average, most women have less bone mass to start with—and they lose it faster as they get older. (2) In young women, the hormone estrogen helps deposit calcium in bones. But as estrogen levels drop with menopause, bones are no longer protected. For the first five years after menopause, usually starting at age fifty, they lose bone faster. (3) From the teen years on, women typically eat fewer calcium-rich foods than men do.

● *Low body weight or small body frame.* If you're underweight, you likely have less bone mass than people with a healthy weight. Bone health is one of the

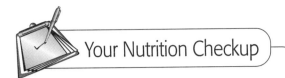

Your Nutrition Checkup

Osteoporosis: Are You at Risk?

While bone loss is a natural part of aging, osteoporosis and fractures don't need to be, according to the National Osteoporosis Foundation. As with any health problem, some women and men are at greater risk than others.

What's your risk? Check all those that apply to you.

Risk factors you can't control. Are you:

_____ **1.** Female?

_____ **2.** Underweight for your height? Or small-boned, with a slight body frame?

_____ **3.** Caucasian or Asian?

_____ **4.** Over age fifty-five?

_____ **5.** From a family with osteoporosis?

Risk factors you can control. Are you:

_____ **6.** Physically inactive?

_____ **7.** Consuming an overall eating plan that's low in calcium?

_____ **8.** Taking high doses of thyroid medication, or high or prolonged doses of cortisonelike medication for asthma, arthritis, or other diseases?

_____ **9.** A smoker?

_____ **10.** A heavy drinker of alcoholic beverages?

Adapted from: National Osteoporosis Foundation.

● *Age.* Bone is dynamic with an ongoing process of bone tissue replacement called remodeling. Until your early 30s, more bone tissue is re-formed than lost. After that, that equation flips. More bone is lost than is formed—up to 1 percent of bone loss per year, depending on individual differences. For women, during the first few years of menopause, there is more rapid bone loss.

● *Family history.* Osteoporosis runs in families. Not only do people inherit a genetic tendency toward bone disease, but also families often live similar lifestyles that may increase their risk.

● *Physical activity.* Being inactive—perhaps with a desk job, sedentary leisure time, driving—for a long time weakens bones. On the other hand, regular weight-bearing activities such as walking, strength training, and dancing trigger your body to deposit calcium in your bones. That makes them stronger and more dense.

● *Calcium intake.* Throughout life, calcium is a bone builder. If your calcium supply consistently has come up short before ages thirty to thirty-five, your bones may not be as dense as they could be. Lower calcium intake means that less bone was built. After age thirty-five or so, adults may lose bone faster when their food choices don't supply enough calcium.

● *Some medications.* The use of some medications is linked significantly to increased risk for osteoporosis: ongoing use of steroids, thyroid medicine, and cortisonelike medications.

● *Smoking.* For both men and women, smoking promotes bone loss. Among women, smoking lowers estrogen levels in blood, which further contributes to bone loss. If you're a smoker, that's another good reason to quit.

● *Heavy drinking.* Heavy drinking is linked to weaker bones. But reasons aren't clear—perhaps because heavy drinkers also make poor food choices.

benefits of keeping your weight within a healthy range for your height.

Women with eating disorders and those who exercise very strenuously increase their risk, too, because they may stop menstruating. Changes in their hormone levels may speed bone loss. Women with eating disorders may not consume enough calcium-rich foods either. *See "Disordered Eating: Problems, Signs, and Help" in chapter 2.*

● *Race/ethnic heritage.* Caucasians and Asians are at higher risk than Hispanics and African Americans, though people in these ethnic groups develop osteoporosis, too. Their bones usually are stronger and more dense throughout their lives, although all races and ethnic groups need the same amount of calcium.

Protect Your "Support System"

Good health is more than skin deep. Moisturizers and sunscreens may help keep your skin looking young. But to truly prolong the qualities of youth, bones also need your loving care.

Which Bone Is Healthy?

The dense structure of healthy bone depends largely on its calcium stores. As your body withdraws calcium, bone dissolves, leaving a void where calcium was once deposited. Gradually, bones become more porous and fragile. Once the structure of bone disappears, there's no place to redeposit calcium and new bone tissue. Bone loss from osteoporosis appears to be irreversible.

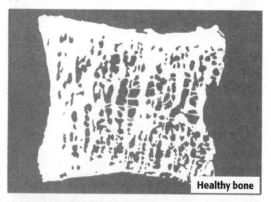

Healthy bone

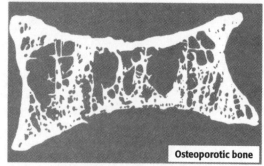

Osteoporotic bone

Source: Build Better Bone Now. Courtesy of National Dairy Council.

You can't control all factors that keep your "support system," or your skeleton, healthy. But regardless of age, gender, or body build, you can help reduce your risk for osteoporosis with smart eating and lifestyle choices.

Never Too Young—or Too Old—to Start

Osteoporosis is often described as a disease of youth that manifests itself in the senior years. Ideally, your bone health strategies began in your childhood and have continued throughout adulthood; in fact, almost 50 percent of bone formation occurs during the adolescent growth years. Even in your early adult years, bones get stronger and more dense. By the early thirties, bones are as dense as they'll ever be. The denser your bones are before middle age, the better able

they'll withstand bone loss that naturally goes with aging.

No matter what your age now, you're still young enough to make a difference in your bone health. Even though you can't replace lost bone as you age, your food choices and lifestyle patterns can slow the natural process of bone loss. *For more about caring for bones in the mature adult years, see "Calcium: As Important As Ever" in chapter 18.*

The Calcium Gap

By now you're well aware of the link between calcium and bone health. So if your food choices come up short, now's the time to close the calcium gap!

As an adult you still need plenty of calcium; 1,000 milligrams daily is considered an Adequate Intake (AI) for ages nineteen to fifty; 1,200 milligrams daily for ages fifty and over. Remember, an 8-ounce serving of milk or yogurt or 1½ ounces of cheese each supply about 300 milligrams of calcium. *For calcium-rich foods see "Calcium: A Closer Look" in chapter 4.* Teens need plenty of calcium, too; yet during this critical time of bone building, many switch from calcium-rich milk to soft drinks.

Consider other links to calcium. Caffeine can increase urinary loss of calcium, but moderate caffeine intake has little influence on bone health. One cup of regular coffee prevents the absorption of the calcium found in one teaspoon of milk. If your caffeine intake is high, you may cut back on caffeinated drinks, since this effect can add up—or enjoy latte (coffee with steamed milk) or tea with milk to make up the difference. Actually, sodium has a greater effect on calcium absorption than caffeine does; however, neither is significant if calcium intake is adequate.

Alcohol and smoking also can block calcium absorption. Smoking can speed bone loss; in fact, for women, a lifelong habit of smoking a pack of cigarettes a day may lower bone density by menopause an extra 5 to 10 percent. If you smoke, consider the bone-healthy benefits of quitting. Among other factors, excessive alcohol intake may inhibit some bone remodeling, increase calcium excretion, and increase the chance of falling. If you drink alcoholic beverages, drink only in moderation—for women, no more than one drink a day, and no more than two drinks daily for men.

The Vitamin D Connection

Vitamin D promotes calcium absorption. If you drink vitamin D-fortified milk, you probably consume enough to protect against bone disease. But if your calcium comes from other sources, get a little sunshine. Your body makes vitamin D when ultraviolet light touches your skin. If you can't go outdoors or if you cover up, pay special attention to getting enough vitamin D from food, or you might need a vitamin D supplement, particularly if you're over age seventy. *See "Vitamins: The Basics" in chapter 4 and "Vitamin D: The Sunshine Vitamin" in chapter 18.*

Move Those Bones!

Weight-bearing activity helps maintain bone density—if you consume enough calcium. If you're swimming, bicycling, or riding a stationary bike regularly, that's great. But these activities don't promote bone health because they aren't weight-bearing.

Add activities such as these to your "activity repertoire": walking, jogging, aerobic dancing, volleyball, tennis, dancing, or weight lifting—even mowing the grass or shoveling snow. You don't need expensive equipment or a fitness club to lift weights. To build arm and shoulder strength, use things you have around your house, such as canned goods.

For anyone, including teens and young adults in their bone-growing years, eating calcium-rich foods along with regular weight-bearing physical activity offers a great "combo" for long-term bone health!

Hormone Replacement Therapy (HRT)

Going through menopause? Consult your doctor about hormone replacement therapy. A low dose of estrogen, typically given with progestin (a form of progesterone), helps slow bone loss and may protect against other side effects of menopause, including hot flashes. Estrogen therapy also may be advised for younger women with amenorrhea (cessation of menstrual cycles) or who've had a hysterectomy.

If you decide to take estrogen, remember that it's just one strategy for your continued bone health. Consuming enough calcium and regular weight-bearing activity are important! *See "ERT or HRT: For Some Women" in chapter 17.*

Calcium Supplements

For many women, supplements help ensure an adequate calcium intake and offer protection from osteoporosis. However, the main nourishment for healthy bones should come from food, not pills. Food supplies other nutrients that your bones (and your whole body) need.

If you take calcium pills, use them to supplement, not replace, calcium-rich foods. *See "Calcium Supplements: A Bone Builder" in chapter 23.*

Testing, Testing: A Bone Density Scan

For women: If you're at high risk for osteoporosis, a bone-density test may be advised—especially if you've experienced early menopause, amenorrhea, a fracture from a minor strain, or if you have a family history of osteoporosis. Not at risk? Still, a bone density test at menopause offers a baseline for later, especially if you're contemplating estrogen therapy. Consult your doctor.

Bone density tests aren't invasive. Instead, they scan your spine, hip, and wrist like other X rays do. Your bone density scans are compared to standards of people like you in gender and size: someone age-matched to you and someone younger at peak bone mass. Bone density scanning is now covered by Medicare.

If You Have Osteoporosis . . .

Preventing and treating osteoporosis is often compared to balancing a three-legged stool: (1) enough calcium, (2) weight-bearing physical activity, and (3) estrogen. The best guidance: protect your bones from further deterioration. *Besides the sound advice in "Protect Your 'Support System'" in this chapter, remember this:*

● Protect yourself from slips and falls, when you might easily fracture a bone.

● Consult with your physician about osteoporosis medication such as aldendronate, which may help restore some bone. Equally important, talk to your doctor about other medications and supplements you take. Thyroid hormones and steroids may promote bone loss.

● Enjoy plenty of calcium-rich foods. They provide more for bone health (calcium, phosphorus, vitamin D)—and overall health—than supplements do. And a varied, well-balanced eating plan offers other nutrients that appear to promote bone density, including magnesium, potassium, and vitamin K.

● If you are not able to meet your calcium recommendation with foods—ones naturally rich in calcium as well as calcium-fortified foods—you may need a calcium supplement. Ask a dietitian or your physician about the right dosage and type. And enhance its absorption by taking it with food.

Gastrointestinal Conditions

Stomach ache? Diarrhea? Constipation? Heartburn? It's no surprise that discomfort and diseases of the gastrointestinal (GI) tract are linked to nutrition. If you don't feel like eating, or if a health problem interferes with the digestion of food or the absorption of nutrients, GI problems can affect your nutritional status.

Here's how you might deal with some GI problems. As always, see a doctor for a diagnosis if problems persist, and seek guidance from a dietetics professional for eating advice.

Gastric Reflux Disease

Is it heartburn—or gastric reflux disease? Heartburn is a main symptom of gastric reflux disease; however, gastric reflux disease is a more serious health problem. In gastric reflux disease, contents of the stomach flow backward into the esophagus. The symptoms? Besides heartburn, symptoms include pain that feels like an ulcer, difficulty swallowing, and regurgitating stomach acid. If you have these ongoing symptoms, check with your physician.

Gastric reflux disease is associated with several health conditions, such as hiatal hernia, abdominal pressure from obesity, and the heartburn of pregnancy.

If You Have Gastric Reflux Disease . . .

As part of your treatment, your doctor may recommend an eating plan that eliminates or reduces foods that irritate your esophagus or that cause reflux of stomach acids. Among the common food offenders: chocolate, alcoholic drinks, carbonated drinks, citrus juice, tomato products, coffee (with and without caffeine), and mint. High-fat foods and large meals may cause problems, too. Since obesity increases the risk, your doctor may advise weight loss.

A registered dietitian can provide guidelines for meals and snack planning. These eating-related tips also can help you treat gastric reflux disease:

● Eat small, more frequent meals.

● Sit up while you eat, and sit or stand for forty-five to sixty minutes after you eat.

● Eat at least two to three hours before bedtime. Skip late-night meals or bedtime snacks.

● Limit or avoid foods and beverages that cause discomfort, including chocolate, coffee, tea, cola, and alcoholic drinks. If other foods, such as tomatoes or oranges, give you trouble, try just small amounts, eaten with other foods.

● Wear loose-fitting clothes that don't put pressure on your abdomen.

● Achieve and keep your healthy weight.

● Sleep with your head slightly propped up on a pillow.

Your physician also may suggest changes in your lifestyle, medication, and perhaps surgery.

Diverticular Disease

Diverticular disease is really two conditions. *Diverticulosis* is a condition in which pouches, called diverticula, develop in the weakened walls of the

---

Have You Ever Wondered

. . . if you can get kidney stones by drinking milk? That's a common myth. Research doesn't support this misperception. In fact, drinking milk may reduce the risk. A high-calcium diet may decrease the absorption of oxalate, a substance in some plant-based foods that can form calcium oxalate kidney stones.

. . . if phytoestrogens in soybeans protect your bones? Maybe, since they act much like mild estrogens in the body. After menopause, as natural estrogen declines, phytoestrogens in soy products may help prevent bone some loss. *For more about soy foods see "What's 'Soy' Good?" in chapter 11.*

Have You Ever Wondered

... what causes heartburn? The discomfort of heartburn, or indigestion, occurs when digestive juices (hydrochloric acid) and food from your stomach back up into your esophagus. Your stomach lining is protected from acids that form during digestion, but the lining of your esophagus is sensitive to the burning sensation of stomach acids. That's why you feel discomfort or pain.

Foods themselves don't cause heartburn, but they may aggravate the condition by stimulating acid production. A problem with the esophageal sphincter may be involved, too. Foods high in acids, such as citrus fruit, as well as fatty or highly seasoned foods, may also cause problems for some people.

Heartburn isn't dangerous, just uncomfortable. And it can be treated with antacids. Consult your doctor about the best type for you; antacids can interfere with other medications. The danger can come if you ignore a heart attack, thinking it's simply heartburn. If the pain continues or if it happens an hour or more after eating, call your doctor immediately!

intestine, most often the colon. Diverticulosis is linked to an overall eating approach that's low in fiber. Constipation makes the problem worse. These pouches can become inflamed and infected from bacteria in feces that get trapped there—a health problem called *diverticulitis*. The majority (about 50 percent) of Americans ages sixty to eighty have diverticulosis; just about everybody does after age eighty.

If You Have Diverticular Disease . . .

● For diverticulosis eat plenty of high-fiber foods; keep waste moving through the intestines to avoid constipation. A high-fiber diet is likely the only treatment you need. You may not need to avoid nuts and seeds, as once believed. Studies don't support an association between inflammation of the diverticula and eating nuts and seeds. *See chapter 6 for more about dietary fiber.*

● For diverticulitis you need to clear up the infection and the inflammation. Treatment often includes antibiotics; perhaps a short-term liquid diet; bed rest; and, if the problem is severe, surgery.

Irritable Bowel Syndrome

Irritable bowel syndrome (IBS), an intestinal problem, doesn't have a clear cause; however, abnormal contractions in the intestine, stress, and food intolerance all may play a role. Symptoms might be abdominal pain or cramps as well as diarrhea, constipation, bloating, and gassiness. IBS also is known as colitis and spastic colon.

If you have these symptoms, check with your physician. They may be a sign of other serious diseases or disorders. Several tests are used to rule out other problems: complete blood count, stool examination, and sigmoidoscopy or colonoscopy.

Irritable bowel syndrome is different from inflammatory bowel disease (IBD)—Crohn's disease and ulcerative colitis—which requires careful medical treatment. With IBD a registered dietitian helps a patient create an individualized approach to eating that not only helps manage gastrointestinal (GI) symptoms but also helps to prevent malnutrition and helps the GI tract function normally.

If You Have Irritable Bowel Syndrome . . .

Many of the recommendations are good guidance for anyone: a high-fiber, low-fat approach to eating. In addition:

● Eat small, frequent meals. Chew your food well to aid digestion. And eat slowly so you don't swallow a lot of air, which may make you feel gassy.

● To prevent constipation, eat plenty of fiber-rich foods—20 to 35 grams of fiber per day.

● If a food irritates or causes too much gas, avoid it.

● Limit any substance that makes symptoms worse: perhaps caffeine; alcoholic drinks; fat; or sorbitol, a sugar alcohol. Sometimes fructose, the sugar in fruit and fruit drinks, isn't well tolerated; talk to your doctor before avoiding fruit if you suspect a problem.

● Drink more fluids—8 to 10 cups daily—to help prevent constipation.

● Learn to manage stress. Anxiety may affect the speed at which food residues pass through your GI tract.

● If you're lactose-intolerant, restrict lactose. *See "Lactose Intolerance: A Matter of Degree" in chapter 21.*

● Talk to your doctor about your medications. Some, such as antacids, may make symptoms worse. And some dietary supplements can have side effects that affect your GI tract—for example, aloe, black cohosh, garlic, gingko biloba, goldenseal, and saw palmetto, among others.

Ulcers

"Stress is giving me an ulcer!" In truth, it's not, although your body may secrete more stomach acid if you're under emotional strain. Most ulcers in the esophagus, stomach, and small intestine are caused by bacteria called *Heliobactor pylori;* in addition, the use of some anti-inflammatory medications and too much stomach acid, resulting from other health problems, are other causes. When the lining of the gastrointestinal tract is impaired for any number of reasons, the cells underneath can't protect themselves from stomach acids. If the damage goes deep enough, the ulcer may bleed and cause pain.

To refute another common myth, eating spicy foods doesn't cause ulcers either. In fact, no food choices cause or cure ulcers.

If You Have an Ulcer . . .

Antibiotics or antacids usually are prescribed to treat stomach ulcers: antibiotics to destroy the bacteria, or antacids to suppress stomach acids. In addition, your doctor may recommend dietary treatment. To heal an ulcer, you don't need to eat bland foods, as once thought. Instead, this advice is generally given:

Have You Ever Wondered

. . . how you can relieve hemorrhoids or constipation? Plenty of fiber-rich foods, plenty of fluids, and a physically active lifestyle all help prevent constipation and hemorrhoids. Equally important, pay attention to your body's signals. Delaying a bowel movement can lead to constipation and hard, dry stools, which are difficult to pass. For travelers, lack of access to a safe, reliable source of water, sweat loss in a hot climate, or a dry airplane cabin may contribute to drinking insufficient fluids that lead to constipation.

What's the benefit of physical activity? Being active helps maintain muscle tone throughout your body, including your intestinal tract.

If constipation is a chronic or a painful problem, talk to your physician. It might signal a more serious problem or an interaction with medication.

See "Avoiding the Trio: Constipation, Hemorrhoids, and Diverticulosis" in chapter 6. For tips for easing the problems see "Constipation during Pregnancy" in chapter 17 and the chart "Cancer Treatment: Handling Side Effects" in this chapter.

. . . how you should deal with diarrhea and vomiting? Both are symptoms of other health problems, some more serious than others. In either case, your body loses fluids that need replacing; these conditions can lead to dehydration and electrolyte imbalance.

What causes watery, loose stools, or diarrhea? Perhaps foodborne illness, infection, or medication. With diarrhea, waste passes through the intestine before fluids can be absorbed, or body fluids may pass from the cells into intestinal contents. For mild diarrhea, drink plenty of fluids and rest. For more severe or persistent diarrhea, see your physician.

Vomiting may result from motion imbalance, from a normal reaction to an irritating substance, or it may be symptomatic of many different health problems. When you vomit, the normal rhythmic movements of digestion reverse their direction, expelling your stomach, and perhaps intestinal, contents. Usually the best "medicine" is to drink fluids (in small, frequent amounts) and rest. For severe, persistent, or projectile vomiting, check with your physician immediately. You'll need proper rehydration, perhaps with electrolytes, and diagnosis and treatment of the underlying cause. *For more tips on dealing with diarrhea and vomiting see the chart "Cancer Treatment: Handling Side Effects" in this chapter.*

Both diarrhea and vomiting can be especially dangerous for infants. If they persist, call your healthcare provider immediately!

● Follow an overall, well-balanced eating plan. Sound familiar?

● Limit foods and seasonings that stimulate the flow of gastric juices: black pepper, chili powder, cloves, garlic, and caffeinated drinks. Decaffeinated coffee or tea may be a problem, too.

● Limit frequent snacking so your body secretes less stomach acids.

● Skip alcoholic beverages, smoking, and aspirin.

● Unless a certain food causes repeated discomfort, enjoy any food you choose—as long as it fits within your healthful approach to eating.

Keep Smiling: Prevent Gum Disease

From an oral health standpoint, a cavity-free mouth doesn't get you home free! Gum, or periodontal, disease, which affects about three-quarters of American adults, is the main cause of tooth loss, which, in turn, can affect food choices. As with tooth decay, bacteria in plaque (the gummy film that forms on teeth) and calculus are at the root of gum disease. In fact, these bacteria may thrive right along the gumline.

● Help prevent tooth loss by protecting your teeth from gum disease. Brush and floss regularly. By removing plaque along the gumline, bacteria in plaque are less able to irritate your gums. Plaque that isn't removed turns into calculus, or hard deposits, which you can't remove with brushing or flossing.

● Choose an overall eating plan with food variety and balance. Good nutrition makes your gums more resistant to infections caused by oral bacteria. And your gums need nutrients to stay healthy.

● Have regular dental checkups. Besides checking for gum problems, the dentist or dental hygienist will remove calculus buildup between teeth and along the gumline.

Anemia: "Tired Blood"

Have that "run-down" feeling? Perhaps you're overworked and underrested. More sleep and relaxation may be what you need to feel energetic again. Or perhaps your fatigue is a symptom of anemia.

Actually, anemia isn't a disease, but instead a symptom of other health problems. With anemia, you may—or may not—feel fatigued. Often there's a nutrition connection.

With anemia, the body doesn't have enough red blood cells, or they're not big enough, to transport oxygen from your lungs to your body cells. Hemoglobin, made with iron, is the part of red blood cells that carries oxygen to other tissues. Without enough oxygen, body cells can't produce enough energy. Then fatigue, pale skin, headache, weakness, lack of concentration, or irritability, among other symptoms, may set in. To produce enough healthy red blood cells, you need enough iron in your diet, as well as enough folate and vitamin B_{12}.

Is It an Iron Deficiency?

Anemia isn't a symptom of just one health problem. A form often described as "iron-poor blood" might come to mind first. In fact, iron deficiency, with its effect on hemoglobin, is the most common form of anemia, more likely affecting adult women of childbearing age, infants and children, and teenage girls. Anemia is a health problem that develops over time. If iron intake comes up short for an extended time, your body can't make enough hemoglobin.

Be aware that having an iron deficiency doesn't necessarily mean you're anemic. For anemia to occur you need a severe depletion of iron stored in your body, with low levels of hemoglobin in your blood.

Before menopause, women need more iron than men do, so women are at higher risk for anemia. Why?

● For starters, women need more iron due to monthly blood loss from menstruation.

● During pregnancy, women need 50 percent more iron: 27 milligrams a day, compared to 18 milligrams daily prior to pregnancy. The extra is needed for increased blood volume—at least three more pints of blood! Often a woman's stored iron gets used up to meet the demands of pregnancy.

● Women often don't consume enough iron-rich foods in their everyday food choices, perhaps because they restrict their food intake to their control weight.

Have You Ever Wondered

...why fair-skinned people often become pale with anemia? Hemoglobin gives blood its bright red color. With less hemoglobin in circulation, skin is paler. For people with darker skin, check the lining of the eye, which may become pale with anemia.

● Vegetarian women may come up short on iron. Plant sources of iron aren't absorbed as well as iron from meat, poultry, and fish.

Infants are at risk if their mothers had low iron status during pregnancy, or, if they bottle-feed, they take formula that's not iron-fortified.

For children, teens, and adults, an iron-rich eating plan can prevent this most common type of anemia. For some, especially pregnant women, iron supplements might be recommended, too.

For more, see "Iron: A Closer Look" in chapter 4.

Anemia: More than One Cause

Although most common, iron deficiency isn't the only cause of anemia. Deficiencies in vitamin B_{12} or folate are other nutrition-related causes. Anemia also may result from large blood loss, hereditary defects in blood cells (sickle-cell anemia), liver disease that affects body processes that use iron, or infections. "Sports anemia" isn't really anemia; *see "Have You Ever Wondered . . . if heavy training causes 'sports anemia'?" in chapter 19.*

Anemia: Linked to Vitamin B_{12}

Anemia from a vitamin B_{12} deficiency doesn't have a single cause; it's not just poor eating. Although uncommon, the problem might be a low intake of vitamin B_{12}. More often, however, it's pernicious anemia, caused by poor vitamin B_{12} absorption—perhaps due to lack of intrinsic factor, atrophic gastritis, or the surgical removal of part of the stomach or small intestine.

What's intrinsic factor? It's a body chemical, produced in the stomach, that helps your body absorb vitamin B_{12} in the intestine. If gastric juices lack intrinsic factor, perhaps for genetic reasons, or if the secretion of stomach juices is impaired, vitamin B_{12} can't be properly absorbed. With age (typically over age sixty), atrophic gastritis, a condition that causes the acid content of stomach secretions to decrease, can affect vitamin B_{12} absorption. Injury or surgical removal of part of the stomach also affects gastric juices and nutrient absorption. Your doctor will diagnose these problems and offer advice.

Because vitamin B_{12} comes only from animal sources of food (meat, fish, poultry, eggs, milk, and milk products), strict vegetarians, or vegans, can be at higher risk. They need a reliable source of vitamin B_{12}, perhaps a fortified breakfast cereal or a supplement, to protect against anemia. *See "Vitamin B_{12}: A Challenge for Vegans" in chapter 20.*

Anemia: Short on Folate

A folate deficiency can lead to anemia. Why? Folate is essential for cell growth and development. Without enough folate, red blood cells become enlarged but don't develop normally, so they can't carry oxygen to body cells as efficiently. Today most grain products are folic acid-fortified in the United States, so most people consume enough to avoid anemia. Folate also comes from leafy vegetables, some fruits, legumes (beans), and liver.

For women, a folate deficiency may show up later in pregnancy when folate needs are high. Early in pregnancy, a shortage of folate may lead to birth defects of the spinal cord. Whether or not you're at risk for anemia caused by folate deficiency, consume enough, especially if you're planning to get pregnant—or if you already are pregnant. *For more about folate and pregnancy see "Before Pregnancy" in chapter 17.*

Testing, Testing: Do You Have Anemia?

Before you self-diagnose your fatigue as anemia and then pop a pill, consult your doctor about your symptoms. And ask for a blood test.

A hemoglobin test or a hematocrit test is a simple, inexpensive blood test to screen for the possibility of anemia; however, many conditions can affect the results. If the test results are positive, your doctor may conduct more specific tests, for example: *for iron-deficiency anemia*—serum ferritin or total iron-binding capacity (TIBC); *for folate deficiency anemia*—serum folate; or *for vitamin B_{12} deficiency*—serum vitamin B_{12} or a Schilling test.

Proper diagnosis is essential for getting the right treatment for various types of anemia; their potentially harmful effects differ. For example, a folate supplement may "cure" blood-related symptoms of pernicious anemia but mask irreversible, potentially severe damage to the nervous system.

If You Have Anemia . . .

● Consult your physician or a registered dietitian about appropriate treatment for the type of anemia you have. Follow prescribed treatment or professional advice, not self-prescribed supplements.

● Keep any supplements in a safe place, where children can't reach them.

● Enjoy good food sources of all three nutrients: iron, vitamin B$_{12}$, and folate.

● Follow up with your physician, perhaps with appropriate blood tests to monitor your status.

● For more guidance, check here:

● *Iron—"Menstrual Cycle: More Iron for Women" in chapter 17, "Iron: A Closer Look" in chapter 4, and "Iron: The Fatigue Connection" for teenage girls in chapter 16.*
● *Vitamin B$_{12}$—"Vitamins: The Basics" in chapter 4.*
● *Folate—"Vitamins: The Basics" in chapter 4.*

Food and Medicine

Do you take over-the-counter medications, prescription medications, or both? Their safe, effective use is your responsibility—and an important part of medical treatment. Talk to your doctor, pharmacist, and perhaps a registered dietitian for the guidance you need.

Some Don't Mix

Taking medications may not seem like a nutrition issue. Yet, when food and medicines are taken

Have You Ever Wondered

. . . if you can eat anything to relieve arthritis? To date, no conclusive research shows that any food or nutrient can relieve the pain that comes with arthritis. Be wary of lures for products, including vitamin supplements, magnets, and copper bracelets, that claim to help, or of taking too many aspirins to relieve pain. Over time aspirin can irritate your stomach, causing bleeding you may not be aware of. That can lead to an iron deficiency. Talk to your doctor about a safe dosage.

Can glucosamine relieve arthritis pain? Perhaps, although research is still preliminary. Studies so far suggest that glucosamine may relieve the symptoms of osteoarthritis, the form of arthritis that occurs when cartilage that cushions joints breaks down. Glucosamine is a natural component of tendons, ligaments, and cartilage.

Research suggests that, like aspirin and ibuprofen, glucosamine may help dull the pain of stiffening joints. Early findings indicate that it also may help slow the progression of osteoarthritis; however, not enough is known to confirm its safety or effectiveness. A large, long-term study is under way in the United States to investigate the effectiveness, dosage, and safety of both glucosamine and chondroitin as treatments for

osteoarthritis. Neither supplement is recommended by the Arthritis Foundation for treating arthritis.

People with diabetes, shellfish allergies, and those taking blood-thinning medication or daily aspirin need to be especially cautious about taking glucosamine. Talk to your physician first before trying glucosamine.

The best nutritional advice for arthritis is: Follow a healthful eating plan and maintain a healthy weight. In that way you won't put too much strain on arthritic joints. The medically accepted advice also may include moderate physical activity, prescribed medication, protection of joints, and hot and cold applications.

. . . if antioxidants can protect your eyes from cataracts or macular degeneration? Maybe. Early research suggests that vitamins A and E, zinc, as well as lutein, zeaxanthin, and some fats may help prevent or slow (not restore) some eye changes that come with aging. Vitamin C may offer protection from cataracts. *See "Functional Nutrition: A Quick Look at Key Phytonutrients" in chapter 4 for lutein and zeaxanthin sources; chapter 4 also gives food sources of nutrients.* Talk to your eye care professional about whether an antioxidant supplement is right for you.

For other health conditions and problems, see these chapters:

- Breast cancer—chapter 17.
- Celiac disease (gluten intolerance)—chapter 21.
- Choking (Heimlich maneuver)—chapters 12 and 15 (infants and children).
- Constipation, hemorrhoids, and diverticulosis—chapters 6 and 17.
- Dehydration and heat stroke—chapter 8.
- Dental cavities—chapters 5 and 15 (infants).
- Eating disorders—chapters 2 and 16 (teens).
- Fibrocystic breast disease—chapter 17.
- Fibromylagia—chapter 17.
- Food allergies and intolerances—chapters 15 (infants) and 21.
- Foodborne illness—chapter 12.
- Lactose intolerance—chapter 21.
- Migraine headaches—chapter 21.
- Overweight and obesity—chapters 2 and 16 (children and teens).
- Polycystic ovary syndrome—chapter 17.
- Reactive hypoglycemia—chapter 5.
- Vaginal yeast infections—chapter 17.

together, they often interact. That's not surprising, since the chemistry of the stomach and the intestine differs before and several hours after eating. Food and the substances released in your body during digestion may either enhance or hinder the effectiveness of some medications. Some medications alter appetite, taste, or smell, and may cause mouth sores or a dry mouth, making swallowing difficult. Others may induce nausea or irritate the GI tract. Medications also can improve or interfere with nutrient absorption or use.

Your goal? To get the full benefits of both food and medicine. To do that, all medications, even aspirin, should be taken as directed:

- Some medications should be taken with meals. With food, they're less likely to irritate the stomach. Aspirin and ibuprofen are two examples.

- Some medications should be taken on an empty stomach, perhaps an hour before or three hours after eating. Food may slow their absorption and action. That's true of some antibiotics, for example.

- Some food and medications shouldn't be consumed within several hours of each other. For example, fruit juice (including grapefruit juice) and other high-acid foods can destroy one type of penicillin. And calcium in dairy foods and calcium supplements binds with tetracycline, so it passes through the body without being absorbed.

- Some medications should be taken with plenty of water. That's true of most cholesterol-lowering medications.

If Your Doctor Prescribes a Special Eating Plan . . .

Like your medication, a physician-prescribed eating plan—perhaps sodium-modified, high-fiber, gluten-free, or blenderized liquid—is essential to healthcare and disease management. In the world of medicine, a special meal plan is part of medical nutrition therapy. If your physician prescribes a special eating plan as part of your treatment for whatever conditions you might have:

- Get enough guidance so you can successfully comply. Ask for a referral to a registered dietitian for help in planning and monitoring your nutrition needs. You need an approach that matches your physical and personal needs and your food preferences. **Caution:** Let your doctor or dietitian know about any supplements you take.

- Follow the special nutrition plan faithfully. Record what you eat, your challenges, and successes to share later with your healthcare provider or dietitian. That's especially important if this is a long-term change in your eating regimen.

- Use Nutrition Facts and ingredient lists on food labels as information aids. A dietitian can help you learn to use label facts effectively.

- Get family support. Their encouragement and help in food shopping and preparation make any special eating plan easier to follow. Try to dovetail your meal plans; serve the same foods to the whole family whenever you can. For example, if you're on a fat-restricted diet, almost everyone can benefit from cutting back on fatty foods.

For more on getting the most from nutrition counseling see " When You Consult an Expert . . ." in chapter 24.

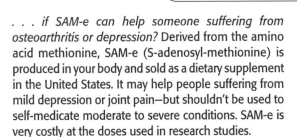

Have You Ever Wondered

. . . if SAM-e can help someone suffering from osteoarthritis or depression? Derived from the amino acid methionine, SAM-e (S-adenosyl-methionine) is produced in your body and sold as a dietary supplement in the United States. It may help people suffering from mild depression or joint pain—but shouldn't be used to self-medicate moderate to severe conditions. SAM-e is very costly at the doses used in research studies.

. . . if you can treat chronic fatigue with a special eating plan? Maybe. Research suggests that chronic fatigue syndrome may be linked with a disorder called neurally mediated hypotension, or low blood pressure. Treatment involves boosting salt and fluid intake to help regulate blood pressure, combined with medication. While this treatment holds promise for some, additional studies are under way to determine the best treatment regimen for most sufferers. Of course, an overall healthful eating plan that provides the nutrients and the calories you need to feel energetic, combined with adequate rest, physical activity, and stress management, also can make a difference. And for most people, moderate intakes of sodium still are advised.

. . . if you should heed the advice "Starve a cold and feed a fever"? Illness is no time to "starve" your body of nutrients. To fight infection, your body needs a supply of nutrients to build and maintain your natural defenses, so you still need balance and variety in your food choices. Extra rest helps, too. With a fever, drink plenty of fluids: juice, milk, soup, or water. If you don't have much appetite, eat bland, simple foods, perhaps more often. How about vitamin C? Well, it won't cure the common cold. No scientific evidence proves that a large dose, perhaps from a vitamin supplement, boosts immunity; however, it may shorten the duration of a cold and decrease the severity of cold symptoms.

. . . if lecithin can keep you healthy? Lecithin is a phospholipid, or a type of fat. Promoters make many claims for lecithin, for example, as a cure or prevention for arthritis, skin problems, gallstones, and nervous disorders, as well as memory problems and improved endurance. Others claim it dissolves cholesterol that's deposited in arteries. Because your body makes lecithin, taking it as a supplement doesn't appear to offer added benefits. Synthetic lecithin isn't well absorbed.

. . . if other healthcare treatments, such as acupuncture or herbal medicines, are safe and effective? Despite consumer attention to alternative treatments, little research backs up their safety or effectiveness. Although some have been used as traditional medicines for centuries, their success is shared mostly in individual reports, not scientific research. To gather sound research evidence to either support or dissuade their use, the Office of Complementary and Alternative Medicine recently was established within the National Institutes of Health. Some treatments may offer promise in certain circumstances.

Until more is known, alternative approaches to healthcare shouldn't replace treatment that's known to be safe and effective. If you do choose to try alternative or complementary care, talk to your doctor first. Some alternative approaches may interfere with the effectiveness of your doctor's prescribed treatment.

● Medications shouldn't be taken with alcoholic beverages. Alcohol can block the effects of some medications, and amplify the effects of others to potentially harmful levels. Medication also can intensify the effects of alcohol in your body.

How do you know to take medicine with a meal or on an empty stomach? Read the directions printed on the container or on an accompanying information sheet. You'll find information about when, how much per dose, and how long to take the medication. The directions also may state what to do if you miss a dose. Ask the doctor or the pharmacist if you don't fully understand. You can ask that directions be printed in large type. *Note:* With the long-term use of some medications, your doctor also may prescribe a dietary supplement.

You can't know about the potential interactions between all medicines and food. That's where the advice of your doctor, a pharmacist, or a registered dietitian comes in. *For a quick reference see "Common Interactions between Food and Some Medications" in this chapter.*

Medication: For Safety's Sake

● Talk to your doctor or pharmacist about all medications you're taking, including over-the-counter

COMMON INTERACTIONS BETWEEN FOOD AND SOME MEDICATIONS

MEDICINE CABINET PRESCRIPTION DRUGS AND OVER-THE-COUNTER PRODUCTS	KITCHEN CABINET: COMMON FOOD AND DRUG INTERACTIONS* (FOR SPECIFIC INFORMATION ABOUT YOUR MEDICATIONS, ASK YOUR DOCTOR OR YOUR PHARMACIST.)
Pain relievers ● Aspirin (e.g., Anacin, Bayer) ● Ibuprofen (e.g., Advil, Motrin, Nuprin)	Take these with food to avoid irritating your stomach. Also limit other stomach irritants, such as alcohol and caffeine.
Antibiotics ● Tetracycline (e.g., Achromycin, Sumycin) ● Penicillin (e.g., Pen-Vee K)	The calcium in dairy foods and in calcium and iron supplements can block the absorption of tetracycline-based products. Take these medications one hour or more before or after consuming dairy products or calcium supplements. When taken together, citrus fruits and fruit juices can destroy a type of penicillin.
Blood-thinning medication/anticoagulants ● Warfarin (e.g., Coumadin, Dicoumerol)	Eat in moderation foods with vitamin K, such as dark-green leafy greens; spinach; kale; turnip greens; green tea; and cauliflower. Too much vitamin K can make your blood clot faster.
Antidepressants ● MAO inhibitors (e.g., Marplan, Parnate)	When taken with foods high in tyramine (an amino acid found in protein foods), these medications may lead to increased blood pressure, fever, headache, vomiting, and possible death. Ask your doctor or a registered dietitian for a list of foods to avoid, such as beer, cheese, red wine, cured meats, aged cheese, avocados, sour cream, and yeast products.
Antacids containing ● Aluminum (e.g., Maalox, Amphojel) ● Calcium (e.g., Tums) ● Sodium (e.g., Alka-Seltzer)	Wait two to three hours after taking an aluminum-containing antacid before you drink or eat citrus fruits. Citrus fruits can increase the amount of aluminum your body absorbs. Antacids with aluminum also can cause a loss of bone-building calcium. Some antacids can weaken the absorption of heart-regulating medications such as digoxin (e.g., Lanoxin). Some antacids can weaken the effect of antiulcer medication (e.g., Tagamet) or drugs that treat high blood pressure (such as Inderal). Be sure to read all the alerts on the labels. If you have high blood pressure, read the label of antacids for the amount of sodium present.
Garlic pills	It is important for your blood to clot if you suffer a cut or undergo surgery. Substances in garlic appear to thin the blood. If you are already taking aspirin or other blood-thinning medications, taking garlic supplements may thin the blood too much.
Corticosteroids (Prednisone, Solumedrol, Hydrocortisone)	Because these medications increase sodium and water retention, which may lead to edema, go easy on foods high in sodium, such as cured meats, pickled vegetables, processed foods, cheese, salty snacks, and salt added at the table.
Medications for cancer treatment (tamoxifen, methotrexate)	Flavonoids in citrus fruits can help tamoxifen inhibit cancer cell growth. Methotrexate promotes folate deficiency; a folate supplement may be prescribed.

*Many supplements including herbal products may interact with medications, too. *See "Warning: Supplement Interactions!" in chapter 23.*

Source: To Your Health! Food & Activity Tips for Older Adults (National Council on Aging, National Institute on Aging, President's Council on Physical Fitness and Sports, and Food Marketing Institute, 1995). Used with permission.

medications and dietary supplements such as herbal products. Some medications and supplements have harmful interactions.

● Always take the medication as prescribed in the directions. If you don't take enough, or stop too soon, the medication may not work. Taking too much, too often can be dangerous. Depending on the medication, excessive amounts also may keep your body from absorbing essential nutrients or deplete your supply.

● Always take medicine in a well-lighted place. And put on your glasses if you wear them! Otherwise you might take the wrong medication or the wrong amount.

● Keep medicines in their original containers with the directions intact.

● Only take medicines prescribed for you, even if your symptoms seem similar to someone else's.

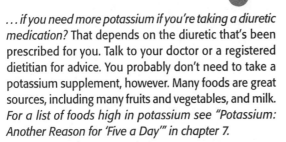

... *if you need more potassium if you're taking a diuretic medication?* That depends on the diuretic that's been prescribed for you. Talk to your doctor or a registered dietitian for advice. You probably don't need to take a potassium supplement, however. Many foods are great sources, including many fruits and vegetables, and milk. *For a list of foods high in potassium see "Potassium: Another Reason for 'Five a Day'" in chapter 7.*

. . . *if antacids are okay for ongoing indigestion?* Although your body may produce less stomach acid with age, you still may suffer from indigestion as you get older. Antacids, taken as directed, can help. However, excess amounts can deplete your body's phosphorus reserves, which may lead to softening of the bones, called osteomalacia.

Another caution: Taking antacids with calcium at mealtime may prevent your body from fully absorbing iron in food. Talk to your doctor about taking antacids. Symptoms that seem like indigestion could be something more serious.

. . . *what the term "medical foods" means?* They're not functional foods. Medical foods are meant for managing a disease or a health problem. Under a physician's supervision, they're either consumed or given in a tube feeding directly to the stomach.

● Flush unused or expired medicines down the toilet.

● With each checkup, review your medication plan with your doctor to make sure it's still right for you.

Medications: Sodium Alert

Are you on a sodium-modified eating plan? If so, talk to your doctor or pharmacist about medications. Some contain sodium, including some antacids and alkalizers, headache remedies, laxatives, sedatives, and others.

If you're taking medication prescribed for high blood pressure, eating less sodium may let your medication work more effectively. If sodium reduction helps control your blood pressure, you may be able to reduce the dosage of antihypertensive medication.

Need more tips for preventing or managing many health problems? Check here for "how-tos":

● Put more physical activity in your lifestyle —see chapters 1 and 2.

● Manage your weight sensibly and effectively—see chapter 2.

● Manage alcoholic drinks for health—see chapter 8.

● Follow overall eating guidelines for health promotion—see chapter 10.

● Shop smart to match your health needs—see chapter 11.

● Prepare foods to manage your health conditions—see chapter 13.

● Stick to your eating plan when you eat out—see chapter 14.

● Use supplements appropriately to avoid or manage health problems—see chapter 23.

● Find a nutrition expert trained to help with your health problems—see chapter 24.

● Identify resources to help deal with specific health conditions—see "Resources You Can Use."

Supplements
Use and Abuse

C ould a pill, a drink, or a supplement bar replace your dinner? For all those who enjoy the pleasure of eating, there's good news. The answer is unequivocally "no"!

Only food can provide the ideal mixture of vitamins, minerals, and other substances for health—qualities that can't be duplicated with dietary supplements. Fortunately for most Americans, there's plenty of quality, quantity, and variety in the food marketplace.

Despite this fact, more than half of Americans take dietary supplements of one kind or another, making it a business of $17 billion per year in 2002—and growing! Some people are prudent with their use, limiting the potency of their supplement to 100 percent or less of the Daily Values (DVs) and taking just the recommended dose. However, others self-prescribe high dosages of supplements, often at the advice of a friend or the media—not their healthcare provider. This practice is potentially dangerous.

Why do so many consumers take dietary supplements? The reasons are varied—sometimes medically valid, sometimes not. In low or appropriate dosages, *some* supplements offer health benefits under *some* circumstances. Some people use supplements with good intention: perhaps in search of protection from or a remedy for health problems such as depression, aging skin, cancer, or arthritis. Still others seek added benefits: perhaps better athletic performance or sexual prowess. Too often, supplement use is based on scientifically unfounded marketing promises

Supplement use is still largely a "world of the unknown": *unknown* benefits . . . *unknown* interactions with food, medicines, and other supplements . . . *undetermined* standards . . . *unknown* levels of safety and effectiveness, making dosages on package labels confusing. Fortunately, steps are under way to gather scientific evidence that answers questions about their safety and effectiveness.

Regardless, no supplements provide a quick, easy road to health—a way that appears easier than making wise food choices or staying physically active. Good nutrition depends on overall healthful eating and active living, not on the use of dietary supplements. And good health requires much more than a supplement or two, or more.

What, then, is appropriate—and inappropriate—use of dietary supplements?

Dietary Supplements: What Are They?

Dietary supplements are neither food nor drugs. Instead, they're products taken orally that contain a "dietary ingredient" meant to supplement the diet, not substitute for healthful foods. According to the Dietary Supplement Health and Education Act (DSHEA), approved in 1994, the term "dietary supplements" refers to a broad range of products: vitamins, minerals, herbs or other botanicals, and amino

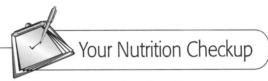

Your Nutrition Checkup

Supplements—Truth or Myth?

Many misconceptions surround dietary supplements. What do you think about using them?

FACT OR MYTH?

_____ _____ **1.** Nutrient supplements can make up for my poor food choices.

_____ _____ **2.** Taking supplements can prevent, treat, or cure disease.

_____ _____ **3.** Supplements boost my energy.

_____ _____ **4.** If it's herbal, it's not harmful.

_____ _____ **5.** "Stress" vitamins help me cope better with a lot of emotional stress.

_____ _____ **6.** A supplement can help me build muscle or get more from my physical performance.

_____ _____ **7.** A vitamin pill could protect my body from the harmful effects of smoking or alcohol.

_____ _____ **8.** Supplements make up for foods grown in depleted soil.

_____ _____ **9.** Popping a supplement pill can offer immediate benefits.

Here are the facts:

Misconceptions about dietary supplements are rampant. Even though consumers with these beliefs buy supplements, every statement is false!

1. _Fact:_ No dietary supplement can fix an ongoing pattern of poor food choices. Supplements may supply some vitamins and minerals, but not all the substances that food supplies for your optimal health. Only a varied and balanced eating pattern provides enough nutrient variety, phytonutrients, and other substances for health. If you eat right, you probably don't need a daily supplement.

2. _Fact:_ No scientific evidence in humans proves that a very high dosage of vitamin and mineral supplements prevents, treats, or cures cancer or other chronic illnesses. An extra amount of vitamin C won't prevent colds and flu, although it may reduce the symptoms. Some antioxidant nutrients, taken in higher dosages, may have protective effects, but research is still preliminary. _See "Antioxidant Vitamins: A Closer Look" in chapter 4._

3. _Fact:_ It would be great, but boosting your nutrient intake won't cause your cells to produce extra energy or more brain power. Only three nutrients—carbohydrates, fats, and proteins—supply energy or calories. Vitamins don't. Although B vitamins do _help_ body cells produce energy from the three energy nutrients, they don't produce energy themselves.

4. _Fact:_ Many powerful drugs and toxic chemicals are plant-based. Varieties of mushrooms can be classified as "culinary delicious" or "deadly dangerous." In the same vein, herbal supplements should be used with caution!

5. _Fact:_ Emotional stress doesn't increase nutrient needs. Any claims promoting dietary supplements to "destress" your life are misleading, too. The best dietary advice to meet the physical demands of stress: a varied, balanced eating plan. More "destressing" advice: stay active, get enough rest, and take some personal time out to relax.

6. _Fact:_ Athletes and other physically active people need about the same amount of nutrients as others do—just more energy, or calories, for the increased demands of exercise. The extra amount of food that active people eat supplies the very small amount of extra vitamins for energy production, too. Although protein needs are somewhat higher for some athletes, especially for those in strength-training sports, food can easily provide the extra. On another note, physical activity, not extra amino acids (protein), builds muscle. _For more on nutrition for athletes and ergogenic aids see chapter 19, "Athlete's Guide: Winning Nutrition."_

7. _Fact:_ Dietary supplements won't protect you from the harmful effects of smoking or alcohol abuse. Here's the real scoop: Smoking does increase the body's need for vitamin C; drinking excessive

Supplements—Truth or Myth? *(continued)*

amounts of alcoholic beverages can interfere with the body's use of most nutrients.

8. *Fact:* If soil can grow crops, the food produced is nutritious. When soil lacks minerals, plants don't grow properly and may not produce their potential yield. Scientific evidence doesn't show that crops grown in depleted soil have fewer nutrients than those grown in fertilized soil. Growing area does affect a food's iodine and selenium contents.

9. *Fact:* Usually not. Supplements won't give you instant results. For vitamins and minerals to do their work, they need several hours or several days to interact and do their work in your body. For any benefits from other dietary supplements, you likely need to take them even longer.

Read on to unravel the fiction and explore the facts about dietary supplements.

---

acids, as well as substances such as enzymes, hormones, concentrates, extracts, and metabolites.

Supplements are easy to spot. By law, they must be labeled "dietary supplements." About thirty thousand products are marketed in the United States as dietary supplements, with multivitamin/mineral supplements having the biggest market share—and with many new products launched each year. They're sold in many forms—for example, tablets, capsules, softgels, gelcaps, liquids, powders, and bars.

Vitamin/Mineral Supplements: Benefits and Risks

Do you take a vitamin and mineral supplement? Maybe you need to, maybe not. Many vitamins and minerals are sold as single supplements—for example, vitamins C and E, beta carotene, calcium, and iron. Often they're sold in large doses, perhaps more than you need. Others are "combos," sold as multivitamin/mineral supplements. What's right for you?

Vitamin/Mineral Supplements: For Whom?

Do you consume a varied, balanced diet? Supplements usually aren't necessary—*if* you're healthy and *if* you're able and willing to eat a balanced, varied diet. You probably can get all the vitamins and minerals you need from smart food choices. According to national studies, most Americans have enough healthful foods available to do that. Yet, under some circumstances, vitamin/mineral supplements do offer benefits.

If you fit in one of these categories, your doctor or a registered dietitian (RD) may recommend a dietary supplement. Are you . . .

● *A woman with heavy menstrual bleeding?* You may

need an iron supplement to replace iron from blood loss. To enhance absorption, take iron supplements with water or juice on an empty stomach. If nausea or constipation are problems, take iron supplements with food. Absorption may be decreased by as much as 50 percent when taken with a meal or a snack.

● *A woman who's pregnant or breast-feeding?* You need more of some nutrients, especially folate and iron—and perhaps calcium if you don't consume enough calcium-rich foods. Check the Supplement Facts on the label to make sure you're getting enough for a healthy pregnancy. Ask about a prenatal vitamin/mineral supplement. *See "Before Pregnancy" in chapter 17.*

● *A woman capable of becoming pregnant?* Consume 400 micrograms of folic acid (the synthetic form of folate) daily from fortified foods, vitamin supplements, or a combination of the two—*in addition to* folate found naturally in some fruits, vegetables, and legumes. The extra folic acid offers a safeguard against spinal cord defects in a developing fetus. Synthetic folic acid is better absorbed than food folate.

Foods fortified with folic acid include enriched grains such as flour, breads, cereals, pasta, and rice. If you take a supplement, choose one with a dosage of no more than 1,000 micrograms of folic acid daily.

● *A menopausal woman?* You might benefit from a calcium supplement, in addition to a calcium-rich diet, to slow calcium loss from bones. *See "Calcium Supplements: A Bone Builder" in this chapter.*

● *Someone on a highly restrictive weight loss regimen (<1,200 calories a day)?* You may not consume enough food to meet all your nutrient needs. Your doctor or a registered dietitian may recommend a multivitamin/mineral supplement. **Caution:** Unless under a doctor's supervision, very-low-calorie eating plans aren't advised. *See "'Diets' That Don't Work!" in chapter 2.*

● *A vegetarian?* You may need extra calcium, iron, zinc, and vitamins B$_{12}$ and D—if your regular eating pattern doesn't supply much, if any, meat, dairy, and other animal products. *For more about nutrition and the vegetarian style of eating see chapter 20, "The Vegetarian Way."*

● *Someone with limited milk intake and sunlight exposure?* If you have lactose intolerance, a milk allergy, or simply don't consume enough dairy foods, you may need a calcium supplement to slow calcium loss from your bones.

You may be advised to take a vitamin D supplement, too. (Older adults often need supplements.) Remember, fortified milk is the best source of vitamin D. Still, you need only a little sunlight for your body to make enough vitamin D: ten to fifteen minutes on your hands and face, two to three times a week. *See "Vitamin D: The Sunshine Vitamin" in chapter 18.*

● *Someone with a health condition that affects nutrient use?* Doctors often prescribe supplements for those with health problems that affect appetite or eating, or how nutrients are absorbed, used, or excreted—for example, digestive or liver problems. Surgery or injuries may increase the body's need for some nutrients. Some medications, such as antacids, antibiotics, laxatives, and diuretics, may interfere with the way the body uses nutrients.

Ten to 30 percent of adults over age fifty have atrophic gastritis, a condition that causes damage to stomach cells and so reduces the body's ability to absorb vitamin B$_{12}$. For that reason, adults in this age group are urged to get extra vitamin B$_{12}$ from a supplement or from fortified food.

● *Someone unable—or unwilling—to regularly consume a healthful diet?* You likely need a dietary supplement to fill in the nutrient gaps. However, eating smarter would be better! Take a supplement with the advice of a doctor or a registered dietitian. For example, premenopausal women who don't consume enough calcium from food likely need a calcium supplement—unless they're willing to improve their diet.

● *Some babies* may need a fluoride supplement—and perhaps iron or vitamin D. *See "Vitamin and Mineral Supplements for Breast-Fed Babies" in chapter 15.*

How do you know if you have a healthful eating plan—and if you likely consume enough nutrients? *Give yourself a "nutrition checkup," "How Did You Build Your Pyramid?" in chapter 10.*

If you have any questions about your own nutrient needs—or need for a supplement—talk to a registered dietitian or your doctor. *See "How to Find Nutrition Help . . ." in chapter 24 for help in finding a qualified nutrition expert.*

More Isn't Always Better!

A little is good, but a lot may *not* be healthier. As with other nutrients, such as fat, sugars, and sodium, moderation is your smart guideline for vitamins and minerals: enough, but not too much.

Supplements carry nutrition labeling; you know the amounts of vitamins and minerals in a single dosage. If you already eat a healthful diet, you probably don't need any more than a low-dose supplement. Taking a multivitamin/mineral supplement, with no more than 100 percent of the Daily Values (DVs) as a safety net, is generally considered safe. Most nutrient supplements are produced in low dosages.

Supplements that boast "high potency"—a much higher dosage than you may need—also are sold over the counter in pharmacies, grocery stores, health food stores, and through Internet and mail-order outlets. Either as single-nutrient supplements or vitamin-mineral combinations, high-potency supplements (significantly in excess of the Daily Values) can be harmful. Why can they be sold if you don't need so much? Currently no law limits supplement potency, except for potassium. Being prudent is up to you.

Risks. Consumed in excessive amounts, nutrients in some supplements can have undesirable side effects such as fatigue, diarrhea, and hair loss. Others may pose more serious risks—for example, kidney stones, liver or nerve damage, birth defects, or even death.

Because fat-soluble vitamins are stored in the body, taking high levels of some for a prolonged time can be toxic. For example, excess amounts of vitamin D can cause kidney damage and reduced bone density. Too much vitamin A, taken over time, can cause bone and liver damage, headaches, diarrhea, and birth defects.

Have You Ever Wondered

. . . why a nutrient supplement label may list the percent of vitamin A from beta carotene? The supplement may contain beta carotene but not vitamin A itself. However, the body converts beta carotene to vitamin A.

. . . if ridges or white marks on your fingernails suggest a vitamin deficiency? No, but it's a common misconception. Instead, they're often caused by a slight injury to the nail. Although they may have other causes, too, a nutrient deficiency isn't one of them.

Appearance-conscious teens often hear that taking gelatin pills strengthens nails, but there's no magic nutritional cure for nails that break and split. Fingernails are mainly dead protein cells that get their strength from amino acids. Gelatin doesn't contain these amino acids.

. . . if supplements with "phytonutrients" are a good choice? From *phyto,* Greek for plant, these botanical substances are extracted from vegetables and other plant foods. There's not enough scientific evidence to know if supplement manufacturers have picked the right active substance from plant sources for any benefit.

Plants have thousands of phytonutrients to choose from. And science hasn't yet revealed which one, if any, or what amount in a supplement might offer any health benefits. Better advice: Get your "phytos" from food. Any health-promoting benefit might come from the interaction of many phytonutrients provided naturally in food.

. . . if dietary supplements can protect against biological threats? No, although some supplement promoters may make this claim. According to the Centers for Disease Control and Prevention and the U.S. Food and Drug Administration (FDA), no current and credible scientific evidence suggests that supplements on the market today offer protection from or treatment for biological contaminants such as anthrax.

In the same vein, FDA advises against taking antibiotics for protection from foodborne illnesses caused by bacteria, unless they're prescribed by a doctor. Antibiotics can't protect against viruses or chemicals that contaminate food.

Water-soluble vitamin and mineral supplements can be risky if taken in excess, over time. For example, taking extra vitamin B_6 has been suggested to help relieve premenstrual tension. Yet there's limited evidence to support large vitamin B_6 doses for relief of premenstrual syndrome (PMS). Many women have viewed large vitamin B_6 doses as harmless, since they are water-soluble. Instead, they may cause irreversible nerve damage when taken in doses above the Tolerable Upper Intake Level (UL): 100 mg. per day.

As other examples, very high doses of vitamin C can cause diarrhea, kidney stones in people with kidney disease, and bladder problems. Liver damage may be caused by high doses of niacin (as time-released nicotinic acid); sometimes a physician will prescribe high doses of niacin to help lower an elevated blood cholesterol level. Excessive amounts of folic acid can hide symptoms of pernicious anemia, so the disease gets worse without being detected.

Children are more vulnerable to overdoses of vitamins and minerals than adults. In fact, excessive iron—perhaps from iron supplements intended for their mother—can be fatal to children.

The way your body handles large nutrient doses from dietary supplements depends on many factors. Your body size, supplement dose (amount and frequency), and how long you take them influence whether a megadose will be toxic for you.

See the Appendices to find out the Tolerable Upper Intake Level (UL) for many nutrients. The UL is the maximum amount that appears safe for most healthy people. Consuming more than that may increase your risk for some health problems.

Nutrient-Nutrient Interactions. High doses of some nutrients may result in deficiencies of others. For example: high calcium intake may inhibit the absorption of iron and other trace nutrients. High doses of vitamin E can interfere with the action of vitamin K and make anticoagulant drugs such as Coumadin (warfarin) more powerful.

Even low levels of dietary supplements may contribute to health problems for some people. For example, those at risk for hemochromatosis need to be careful of taking extra iron. Folic acid can mask a vitamin B_{12} deficiency, which may cause neurological damage. And zinc supplements in excess of the UL can decrease levels of "good" cholesterol (high-density lipoprotein blood cholesterol), impair immunity, and reduce copper status.

Any Benefits? Emerging research is exploring the link between higher levels of some antioxidant nutrients (vitamin C, vitamin E, and selenium) and reduced risk for some health problems. However, the jury's still out. Currently available research doesn't show that levels higher than the Recommended Dietary Allowance are effective in cancer or heart disease prevention. Until more is known, be cautious about taking supplements to protect against disease. *See "Antioxidant Nutrients: Enough, or Too Much?" in this chapter.*

Except for those few people with rare medical conditions, few people need more than 100 percent of their Recommended Dietary Allowances (RDAs) of any nutrient. Large doses of vitamins or minerals are prescribed only for certain medically diagnosed health problems. Even then, their use should be monitored carefully by a doctor.

That said, can you overdose on vitamins or minerals naturally occurring in food? That's highly unlikely. As we mentioned, taking very high doses of dietary supplements—or taking too many, too often—can be dangerous. But the vitamin and mineral content of food is much more balanced. In amounts normally consumed, even if you enjoy extra helpings, you won't consume toxic levels of nutrients. So eat a variety of foods—and enjoy! *Note:* Nutrient amounts can add up if you consume *a lot* of highly fortified foods.

Other Cautions

You may take dietary supplements for potential health benefits. It's not uncommon for people diagnosed with cancer, AIDS, or other life-threatening health problems, who are desperate for a cure, to put their hopes and healthcare dollars in alternative treatments, including dietary supplements. However, supplements may offer a false sense of security—and a serious problem if you neglect well-proven approaches to health or delay medical attention.

If you choose to take a dietary supplement, ask your healthcare provider. Seek medical attention and proven treatment for health problems first. Even if you're healthy, get regular medical checkups, eat wisely, and live a healthful lifestyle rather than rely on the "security" of supplements.

What We Know About . . .

Calcium Supplements: A Bone Builder. For people of every age, food choices can supply an adequate amount of calcium. As an extra safeguard, many doctors also recommend calcium supplements, especially for menopausal and postmenopausal women and for women who simply don't consume enough calcium. The reason? To help stave off bone loss that comes with hormonal changes.

If you're advised to take a calcium supplement, keep these pointers in mind:

● Read the label. Calcium in over-the-counter supplements isn't the same. First, the calcium amount differs. Multivitamin/mineral supplements don't have as much calcium as calcium supplements do.

Second, some forms of calcium are absorbed better than others. Calcium carbonate and oyster shell calcium, for example, aren't absorbed as well as calcium phosphate, citrate, or gluconate. *Bottom line:* Taking any calcium supplement with food makes the calcium more available.

● Avoid calcium supplements with dolomite or bonemeal, which might contain small amounts of hazardous contaminants: lead, arsenic, mercury, or cadmium. What's dolomite? A mineral compound found in marble and limestone.

● Take calcium supplements as intended—as a supplement, not as your only important calcium source. Although calcium supplements may boost calcium intake, they don't provide other nutrients your bones and body need: vitamin D, magnesium, phosphorus, and boron. Milk, for example, provides vitamin D, a nutrient that helps deposit calcium in your bones.

● If you take both calcium and iron supplements, take them at different times of the day. They'll each be better absorbed when taken on their own.

● If you take two or three low-dose tablets daily, space them throughout the day for better absorption. Calcium in supplements is absorbed best in doses of 500 milligrams or less, and when consumed with food.

● Follow the dosage recommended by your healthcare provider. The Tolerable Upper Intake Level for calcium is 2,500 milligrams daily, from food and supplements.

● Drink plenty of fluids with calcium supplements

to avoid constipation. In fact, if you take your calcium supplement with milk, the lactose and vitamin D in the milk can help to enhance absorption of the calcium.

● If you take medications or other nutrient supplements, ask your doctor or registered dietitian about interactions. For example, calcium and tetracycline bind together; neither one is adequately absorbed as a result. Calcium also inhibits magnesium, phosphorus, and zinc absorption.

● If you don't drink milk and want an alternative to calcium pills, consider calcium-fortified juice. One cup of calcium-fortified juice contains about 300 milligrams of calcium, the same amount as in a cup of milk, and provides vitamin C, folate, and other nutrients. Still, you need a vitamin D source to aid absorption; some calcium-fortified juices are also fortified with vitamin D.

● Calcium supplements—to protect against osteoporosis, or brittle-bone disease—can't make up for your lifestyle choices or for overall poor health habits, either. Regular weight-bearing physical activity is important for healthy bones. For healthy bones, avoid smoking, too.

Are calcium supplements right for everyone? For people with kidney damage or urinary tract stones, calcium supplements pose risks. If you have a history of kidney stones, the best advice is to take calcium supplements under your doctor's care. *For more about calcium and osteoporosis see "Osteoporosis: Reduce the Risks" in chapter 22.*

Iron Supplements: Enhancing the Benefit. Physicians often advise iron supplements for premenopausal and pregnant women, and for some children and teens. If you're advised to take an iron supplement, remember:

● Choose a form of iron, such as ferrous sulfate, that's better absorbed.

● Check the dosage when choosing an iron supplement. Dosages of 15 to 30 milligrams per day are likely adequate. Higher amounts should be taken only if prescribed by your healthcare provider.

● Take iron supplements on an empty stomach—between meals or before bedtime—to enhance absorption.

● Take them with water or juice, not with milk, coffee, or tea, which can inhibit absorption. As an aside,

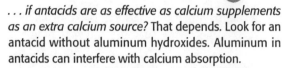

Have You Ever Wondered

. . . if antacids are as effective as calcium supplements as an extra calcium source? That depends. Look for an antacid without aluminum hydroxides. Aluminum in antacids can interfere with calcium absorption.

. . . if vitamin nasal sprays or patches are effective? No research evidence says so, even though they're promoted for faster, more efficient absorption. In fact, they may not be absorbed at all. Here's the reality check: Fat-soluble vitamins need fat from food to aid absorption. Vitamin C in your intestine aids iron absorption—a problem if vitamin C comes from a spray. Vitamin B_{12} binds with intrinsic factor made in the stomach during digestion. That cannot happen with a spray or a patch!

drinking vitamin C-rich juice with an iron supplement isn't necessary. Unlike nonheme iron in plant sources of food, the iron in supplements is already in a form that your body can absorb.

● Drink plenty of water to help avoid constipation, a common side effect from taking iron supplements.

● Store them where children can't reach them. Excess iron by children mistakenly taking adult supplements can be extremely toxic to children!

Herbals and Other Botanicals: Help or Harm?

Herbal and other botanical supplements may seem safe enough. After all, they're made from natural, fresh herbs or other parts of plants: flowers, leaves, roots, and seeds. And many have been used for centuries. In reality, there's nothing inherently harmless about botanical supplements, just because they're "natural." Despite the remarkable array of claims, scientific research is lacking for many herbal remedies.

Indeed, herbals and other botanicals have known medicinal qualities; 30 percent of today's drugs come from plants. Yet, herbals and other botanical supplements are also sold as dietary supplements rather than regulated as drugs. Like many plant-derived pharmaceuticals, these supplements can offer both positive health benefits and harmful side effects.

On the up side, enough scientific evidence has been collected on a handful of supplements to support their limited use. For example, under a doctor's guidance, gingko biloba may be used to help treat the symptoms of age-related memory loss and dementia (including Alzheimer's disease), and standardized saw palmetto extracts may help treat some urinary tract symptoms. A growing body of research evidence is being gathered about their safety and effectiveness, as well as their limitations and dangers.

On the down side, unlike pharmaceuticals, herbal and other botanical supplements aren't well regulated. Neither are other types of supplements, so you aren't as protected from misleading claims about herbals and other botanicals as you might think. *See "Quality and Effectiveness: Who's in Control"? in this chapter.*

According to current regulation, herbal remedies and other dietary supplements can enter the marketplace without U.S. Food and Drug Administration (FDA) approval—and without years of safety testing. Only those known to be truly dangerous are forbidden. Currently dosages of herbal remedies aren't standardized, so dosages vary among products.

Although packaging can't claim that a supplement cures or prevents disease, it may carry claims for its purported health role. Many claims have only scant backup evidence and don't require FDA approval.

Although Dietary Reference Intakes, with recommended intakes, exist for vitamins and minerals, no recommendation or safe dosage exists for herbals and other botanicals and for other nonnutrient supplements.

Herbal Ingredients: Hazardous to Health!

The FDA warns against the use of botanical supplements with these active ingredients, due to their serious, *even deadly,* side effects:

● *Aristolochic acid.* A substance in some traditional Chinese herbal products, aristolochic acid causes kidney damage and is a potent carcinogen. It's known or suspected to be in many products, including those with guan mu tong, ma dou ling, birthwort, Indian ginger, wild ginger, colic root, and many types of snakeroot.

ANTIOXIDANT NUTRIENTS: ENOUGH, OR TOO MUCH?

Antioxidant supplements are "hot" supplements—even though there's no conclusive evidence that taking daily amounts of antioxidant nutrients beyond their Recommended Dietary Allowance (RDA) prevents disease. If you choose to take them for their potential benefits, talk to your doctor first. Then avoid exceeding the Tolerable Upper Intake Level (UL) set for safety. To use Supplement Facts on labels, be aware that the %DVs for one serving, or dosage, are based on the Daily Values (DVs) used in labeling. *See "Antioxidants in Supplements" in chapter 4.*

ANTIOXIDANT NUTRIENT	RDA FOR WOMEN	RDA FOR MEN	DAILY VALUE (FOR LABELING)	UL FOR WOMEN AND MEN	ALSO NOTE
Vitamin C	75 mg	90 mg	60 mg	2,000 mg	Smokers need 35 mg more per day than nonsmokers.
Vitamin E	15 mg from food (equivalent to 22 IU natural sources or 33 IU synthetic form vitamin E)	15 mg from food (equivalent to 22 IU natural sources or 33 IU synthetic form vitamin E)	30 IU	1,000 mg alpha-tocopherol (equivalent to 1,500 IU natural source vitamin E or 1,100 IU synthetic form vitamin E)	
Selenium	55 mcg	55 mcg	70 mcg	400 mcg	
Beta carotene and other carotenoids	Due to conflicting evidence, no recommended level	Due to conflicting evidence, no recommended level	None identified	Due to conflicting evidence, no UL recommended	

Source: National Academy of Sciences. *Dietary Reference Intakes.* Washington, D.C.: National Academy Press, 2000. Reprinted with permission in *A Healthcare Professional's Guide for Evaluating Dietary Supplements.* Chicago: American Dietetic Association, American Pharmaceutical Association, 2000.

VITAMIN AND MINERAL SUPPLEMENTS (SELECTED): CLAIMS, BENEFITS, RISKS

Here's what the symbols mean:

↑ — Evidence comes from several controlled human studies.

?↑ — Preliminary evidence comes from only a few controlled human studies or from laboratory studies with cell or tissue samples.

↔ — Evidence is uncertain and based on conflicting, controlled human research.

↓ — Research doesn't support the claim.

NR — Not enough human research has been done yet, or the research quality is poor.

NUTRIENT SUPPLEMENT	MEDIA OR MARKETING CLAIMS	EFFECTIVENESS	SAFETY/RISKS See chapter 4 for the risks of taking excessive amounts of vitamins and minerals. These abbreviations refer to the Dietary Reference Intakes, explained in chapter 1: AI—Adequate Intake RDA—Recommended Dietary Allowance UL—Tolerable Upper Intake Level
Boron	● Prevents osteoporosis	NR	● UL—20 mg per day
	● Prevents/treats arthritis	NR	● Doses above 50 mg associated with toxicity
	● Increases muscle mass	NR	
	● Improves memory	NR	
	● Reduces hot flashes	NR	
	● Improves sex drive	NR	
Calcium	● Prevents osteoporosis	↑	● Usually safe in doses below the UL—2,500 mg daily
	● Reduces blood pressure	?↑	● May interfere with absorption of drugs and other nutrients— for example, iron, fluoride, tetracycline, biphosphate (used to treat osteoporosis), salicylates, atenolol
	● Reduces risk of colon cancer	↔	
	● Helps symptoms of PMS	↔	● Avoid taking a calcium supplement if you have been diagnosed with hyperthroidism, hypercalciuria (too much urinary calcium), or sarcoidosis
Chromium	● Helpful for people with diabetes	?↑	● AI is 25 to 35 mcg daily for adults age 19–50; over age 50, AI is 30 mcg for men and 20 for women
	● Lowers cholesterol levels	↔	● Long-term effects of high doses unknown*
	● Reduces body fat	↓	
	● Promotes muscle building	↓	
	● Prevents osteoporosis	NR	
Folate/folic acid	● Prevents birth defects	↑	● Usually safe below the UL—1,000 mcg a day for adults
	● Helps prevent heart disease	?↑	● Doses above 400 mcg daily may mask pernicious anemia in individuals with a vitamin B_{12} deficiency
	● Anticancer (colon)	NR	
	● Anticancer (cervical)	↔	● More than 5,000 mcg a day interferes with anticonvulsant medications
	● Antidepression	NR	
Magnesium	● Reduces cardiovasculardisease	↔	● Usually safe in supplemental doses below the UL—350 mg per day
	● Lowers blood pressure	↔	● Caution for people with kidney disease
	● Diabetics often are deficient	?↑	
	● Alleviates migraine headaches	↔	
	● Good for PMS	↔	
	● Enhances exercise performance	↓	
Pantothenic acid	● Lowers cholesterol	NR	● No reported adverse effects*
	● Increases energy, improves sport performance	↓	● UL not established
	● Good for rheumatoid arthritis	NR	
	● Antistress vitamin	NR	
Potassium	● Lowers blood pressure	?↑	● High doses of potassium-chloride prescriptions (6,000 to 12,000 mg daily) are linked to serious side effects: gastrointestinal lesions, hemorrhage, intestinal obstruction
			● Caution for people with kidney disease

Nutrient Supplement	Media or Marketing Claims	Effectiveness	Safety/Risks
Selenium	• Anticancer	?↑	• UL—400 mg daily for adults
	• Important for a healthy heart	↔	• Doses of 750 mcg or more daily are associated with
	• Enhances immunity	NR	toxic effects
	• Important for athletes	↓	
Beta carotene	• Anticancer	↔	• For beta carotene, but not vitamin A, may increase risk of lung
	• Prevents cardiovascular disease	↓	cancer and fatal heart disease in middle-aged male smokers
	• Enhances immunity	NR	• Vitamin A, but not beta carotene, can be toxic in doses that are ten
	• Improves vision and reduces cataract formation	NR	times the RDA
			• UL—3,000 mcg of RAE** daily; for supplements, that equals 10,000 IU
	• Reverses aging of skin	NR	• If you're pregnant, doses higher than 3,000 RAE of vitamin A can be dangerous!
			**This abbreviation is explained in "Vitamin A and Carotenoids: Good Picks" in chapter 4: RAE—Retinol Activity Equivalents*
Vitamin A	• Enhances immunity	?↑	
	• Improves vision (if deficient)	↑	
	• Fights skin disorders (only as prescription vitamin A analogs)	↑	
	• Reverses aging of skin	NR	
Vitamin B₁ (thiamin)	• Increases energy, prevents fatigue	NR	• No reported adverse effects*
	• Good for the elderly, especially for those with Alzheimer's disease	↔	• No UL established
	• Needed during stress	NR	
	• Prevents canker sores	NR	
Vitamin B₂ (riboflavin)	• Helpful for migraines	NR	• No reported adverse effects*
	• Increases energy	NR	• No UL established
Vitamin B₃ (niacin, nicotinic acid, nicotinamide)	• Lowers cholesterol levels (nicotinic acid)	↑	• Usually safe in doses below the UL—35 mg niacin equivalents per day for adults
	• May prevent development of diabetes (nicotinamide)	↔	• Use higher doses (pharmacological doses) of nicotinic acid only under the care of a physician, due to their serious adverse effects
	• Improves arthritis symptoms	NR	
Vitamin B₆ (pyridoxine)	• Improves carpal tunnel syndrome symptoms	↔	• Generally regarded as safe in doses below the UL—100 mg daily for adults
	• Relieves symptoms of PMS	↔	• Long-term use of very high doses (500 to 5,000 mg daily) linked to nerve damage
	• Important for a healthy heart	?↑	
	• Beneficial for asthmatics	↓	
	• Helpful in autistic disorder	↔	
Vitamin B₁₂ (cobalamin)	• Elderly are often deficient	↑	• No reported adverse effects*
	• Improves dementia symptoms	NR	• No UL established
	• Improves sleep quality	NR	
	• Help for people with diabetes	NR	
	• Improves neurological function in AIDS	NR	
	• Important for heart health	NR	
	• Increases energy	NR	
Vitamin C	• Treats the common cold	↔	• Avoid taking vitamin C if you have been diagnosed with hemochromatosis
	• Helpful for asthma	↔	• If you have recurring kidney stones, keep your intake to less than 100 mg of vitamin C daily
	• Needed for immunity	?↑	
	• Enhances exercise by reducing oxidative damage	↓	• May interfere with blood and diagnostic tests
	• Reduces the risk of heart disease	NR	• UL—2,000 mg per day; diarrhea and cramping may occur with higher doses
	• Protects against cancer	?↑	
	• Reduces the risk of cataracts	?↑	

VITAMIN AND MINERAL SUPPLEMENTS (SELECTED): CLAIMS, BENEFITS, RISKS *(continued)*

NUTRIENT SUPPLEMENT	MEDIA OR MARKETING CLAIMS	EFFECTIVENESS	SAFETY/RISKS
Vitamin D	• Necessary for bone health	↑	• Usually safe in doses below the UL—2,000 IU or 50 mcg daily
	• Improves calcium absorption	↑	
	• Reduces risk of cancer (colon, breast)	↔	
Vitamin E	• Reduces risk of heart attack	↔	• May increase bleeding
	• Prevents cancer	↔	• If you're taking anticoagulant medications, make sure your doctor monitors your use of vitamin E
	• Improves immunity in the elderly	?↑	• UL—1,000 mg of alpha-tocopherol daily for adults (equal to 1,500 IU natural vitamin E, or 1,100 IU of dl-alpha-tocopherol synthetic vitamin E)
	• Helpful in neuropsychiatric disorders	?↑	
	• Improves lung function	?↑	
	• Prevents cataracts	?↑	
	• Improves diabetes	?↑	
	• Enhances exercise capacity	NR	
	• Helpful for HIV	NR	
	• Anticancer	NR	
Zinc	• Treats colds	↔	• Ongoing intake of doses above the UL daily may impair immune function, induce copper deficiency, and negatively affect cholesterol levels
	• Reduces cancer risk	NR	• High doses of zinc may cause nausea and vomiting
	• Needed by female athletes	NR	• UL—40 mg daily for adults
	• Clears skin	NR	
	• Enhances fertility	NR	
	• Improves immunity among the elderly	NR	
	• May prevent progression of age-related macular degeneration	?↑	

*Long-term studies are needed to fully evaluate its safety for humans.

Source: Adapted from Allison Sarubin Fragakis, *The Health Professional's Guide to Popular Dietary Supplements* 2nd edition (Chicago: American Dietetic Association, 2002).

• *Chaparral.* This traditional Native American medicine can cause rapid, potentially irreversible liver damage.

• *Comfrey.* Supplements with comfrey (common, prickly, or Russian) pose serious health hazards, most notably for liver damage and as a possible carcinogen.

• *Ephedrine, ma huang* (ephedra sinica), *epitonin.* Being medicinal herbs, supplements with these ephedrine alkaloids are often touted as energy enhancers. Classified as a dietary supplement, ephedrine also is a component of many weight-loss teas and other aids. It's a stimulant closely related to methamphetamine, and is especially dangerous when combined with other stimulants. Hazards range from nervousness, dizziness, rapid heartbeat, and changes in blood pressure to muscle injury, seizures, nerve damage, heart attack, hepatitis, psychosis, stroke, and even death. People with health problems already, such as high blood pressure, heart disease, or diabetes, are at special risk.

• *Lobelia.* Also called Indian tobacco, it acts similarly to nicotine in the body; among the potential dangers: breathing problems, rapid heartbeat, sweating, low blood pressure, coma, and even death. It's particularly harmful to children, pregnant women, and people with heart disease.

• *Germander.* Its use may lead to liver disease, possibly to death.

• *Magnolia-stephania preparation.* Its use may lead to kidney disease and possibly permanent kidney failure.

• *Willow bark.* Marketed as an aspirin-free product, willow bark contains an ingredient that converts to the active ingredient found in aspirin. Potential health

HERBALS AND OTHER BOTANICALS (SELECTED): CLAIMS, BENEFITS, RISKS

Here's what the symbols mean:

↑ — Evidence comes from several controlled human studies.

?↑ — Preliminary evidence comes from only a few controlled human studies or from laboratory studies with cell or tissue samples.

↔ — Evidence is uncertain and based on conflicting, controlled human research.

↓ — Research doesn't support the claim.

NR — Not enough human research has been done yet, or the research quality is poor.

HERBAL OR OTHER BOTANICAL SUPPLEMENT	MEDIA OR MARKETING CLAIMS	EFFECTIVENESS	SAFETY/RISKS
Echinacea	• Protects against the common cold/flu	↔	• Do not take ... 　• If you have a health problem with reduced immunity 　• If you take medications that stimulate the immune system, such as corticosteroids 　• If you take medications that may be toxic to the liver, such as anabolic steroids 　• Continuously, for more than eight weeks*
	• Boosts the immune system	?↑	• Potential allergic reaction in people with asthma or sensitivity to grass pollens
Garlic	• Lowers cholesterol	?↑	• May increase bleeding
	• Lowers blood pressure	?↑	• Should be monitored if you take anticoagulant medications
	• Improves circulation	?↑	• Avoid taking 7 days before surgery*
	• Anticancer	↔	• May cause stomach discomfort at high doses
	• Antibiotic, antibacterial, antiparasitic, antiviral	↔	• Raw garlic may irritate stomach lining; not for people with active gastrointestinal disease
Ginkgo biloba	• Enhances memory (in Alzheimer's disease)	↔	• May increase bleeding
	• Improves memory and concentration (in healthy individuals)	NR	• Should be monitored if you take anticoagulant medications • Avoid taking 36 hours before surgery*
	• Improves circulation (with pain while walking)	?↑	
	• Strong antioxidant	↑ (in vitro)	
Ginseng	• Enhances exercise	↓	• Avoid taking with certain medications, such as phenelzine sulfate, estrogen therapy, corticosteroids, and digoxin (digitalis)
	• Energy and mood booster	NR	• May adversely affect blood glucose levels for people with diabetes*
	• Heart tonic	↔	
	• Aphrodisiac	NR	• Avoid at least 7 days before surgery
	• Normalizes imbalances in different disease states	NR	
Goldenseal (Hydrastis canadensis)	• Herbal antibiotic; reduces mucus and soothes sore throat	NR	• No scientific data available to evaluate its safety*
	• Protects against travelers' diarrhea	NR	
	• Good for menstrual difficulties	NR	
	• Masks drug use in urine tests	NR	
Green tea extract	• Strong antioxidant	↑ (human studies) ?↑ (lab studies)	• Be aware that some supplements may contain caffeine
	• Anticancer	?↑	
	• Protects the heart	NR	
	• Antiviral, antibacterial	NR	

593

HERBALS AND OTHER BOTANICALS (SELECTED): CLAIMS, BENEFITS, RISKS (continued)

HERBAL OR OTHER BOTANICAL SUPPLEMENT	MEDIA OR MARKETING CLAIMS	EFFECTIVENESS	SAFETY/RISKS
Kava *(Piper methysticum)*	• Antianxiety, antidepression • Sleep aid	?↑ NR	• Potentially dangerous interaction when combined with antianxiety medications such as benzodiazepine, or alcohol • May affect motor reflexes; do not use while operating heavy machinery • Although controversial, concern about a link to liver toxicity • Avoid if you have liver disease • Do not use for more than three months without medical advice
Ma huang *(Ephedra)*	• Enhances weight loss, but be cautious! • Helps asthma • Nasal decongestant • "Herbal ecstasy"; produces euphoric, enhanced sexual sensations	?↑ ?↑ ?↑ NR	• Potentially dangerous! • Associated with serious adverse effects such as heart attack, stroke, insomnia, tremors, death • FDA advises that all individuals avoid ma huang products! It's even riskier for those with hypertension, cardiovascular disease, thyroid disease, diabetes, neurological disorders, and men with an enlarged prostate.
Saw palmetto *(Seronoa repens)*	• Natural remedy for enlarged prostate • Prevents prostate cancer	?↑ NR	• May be linked to gastrointestinal discomfort in rare cases • Talk to your doctor regularly if you use this herb*
St. John's wort	• Alleviates depression • Promotes emotional well-being • Lifts mood—makes you happy	?↑ NR NR	• Do not take with antidepressant medications due to the potentially dangerous combined effects • Decreases effectiveness of a variety of medications; check with your physician • May make skin sensitive to sunlight, especially for fair-skinned people

Valerian *(Valeriana officinalis)*	• Enhances sleep
	• Antistress, antianxiety
		?↑
		NR
			• Do not take . . .
			  • with barbiturates or other sleep medications
			  • if you have liver disease
			• Discontinuing its use may be associated with withdrawal symptoms; taper off slowly
			• May cause morning drowsiness with high doses (900 mg)*

Wheat grass, barley grass	• Antioxidant protection • Supports the immune system • Concentrated source of several nutrients • Lowers cholesterol	NR (in lab studies) NR (in human studies) ↓ NR	• No reported adverse effects*
Yohimbine *(yohimbe)*	• Increases sex drive • Aids in weight loss • Builds muscle	↓ NR NR	• Potentially dangerous! • Doses of 4 mg to 20 mg have been associated with serious harmful effects, such abnormal heartbeat, tremors, and low blood pressure • Toxicity may be enhanced by taking phenothazines (drug used for mental disorders) • Not for people with high or low blood pressure, bipolar disorder, or liver or kidney disease

*Long-term studies are needed to fully evaluate its safety for humans.

Source: Adapted from Allison Sarubin Fragakis, *The Health Professional's Guide to Popular Dietary Supplements* 2nd edition (Chicago: American Dietetic Association, 2002).

hazards include Reye's syndrome, a potentially fatal disease that's linked to aspirin intake in children with chicken pox or flu symptoms. Adults can have an allergic reaction to willow bark.

● *Wormwood.* This herbal ingredient may cause neurological symptoms such as numbness of legs and arms, loss of intellect, delirium, and paralysis.

● *Yohimbe.* Derived from tree bark, yohimbe has several active ingredients, including yohimbine, with potentially dangerous side effects: kidney failure, seizures, nervous system disorders, paralysis, fatigue, stomach problems, and death. Because yohimbine is a MAO (monoamine oxidase) inhibitor, it is especially harmful when taken at the same time as tyramine-containing foods such as liver, cheese, or red wine, and with over-the-counter medications with phenylpropanolamine (some nasal decongestants and diet aids).

Two other ingredients, often found in herbal supplements, have potential health hazards: germanium (a nonessential mineral) may result in kidney damage, possibly death, and L-tryptophan (an amino acid) may result in a potentially fatal blood disorder that can cause high fever, muscle and joint pain, weakness, skin rash, and swelling of the arms and the legs.

Other Supplements

As supplement categories, nutrient and herbal supplements are often the first to come to mind. However, store shelves and Internet sites are filled with other types of supplements. *Many are addressed in the chart "Selected Other Supplements: Claims, Benefits, Risks" in this chapter.*

● Enzymes and hormones—for example, coenzyme Q10, DHEA, melatonin

For up-to-date and reliable information about the safe, effective use of supplements, access these Web sites:

● Office of Dietary Supplements—*http:// dietary-supplements.info.nih.gov*

● U.S. Pharmacopoeia—*http://www.usp.org*

● University of Illinois—*http://www.uic/edu/ pharmacy/research/diet/ce.html*

For more about these dietary supplements, see these chapters:

● Amino acid supplements—chapter 19.
● Carnitine—chapter 19.
● Chromium picolinate—chapter 19.
● Creatine—chapter 19.
● Dehydroepiandrosterone (DHEA)— chapter 19.
● Ergogenic aids—chapter 19.
● Fiber pills and powders—chapter 6.
● Fish oil supplements—chapter 22.
● Garlic supplements—chapter 22.
● Glucosamine—chapter 22.
● Laetrile—chapter 22.
● Lecithin—chapter 22.
● Pangamic acid—chapter 19.
● SAM-e—chapter 22.
● Shark cartilage—chapter 22.
● Spirulina—chapter 19.
● Wheat germ and wheat germ oil—chapter 19.

● Ergogenic aids—for example, chromium picolinate, creatine

● Others—for example, acidophilus, bee pollen, carnitine, conjugated linoleic acid, fish oil, flaxseed, glucosamine, laetrile, lecithin, royal jelly, shark cartilage, spirulina

Supplements: Safe? Effective?

Even though dietary supplements are big business, manufacturing standards for their quality, potency, and effectiveness have lagged behind their phenomenal market growth. Product information is often misleading, despite limited government regulations. While scientific claims may be given, well-designed scientific studies for supplements are limited

Quality and Effectiveness: Who's in Control?

If you buy a supplement, are you getting what you think you paid for? Maybe, but maybe not, despite government regulations.

SELECTED OTHER SUPPLEMENTS: CLAIMS, BENEFITS, RISKS

Here's what the symbols mean:

↑ — Evidence comes from several controlled human studies.

?↑ — Preliminary evidence comes from only a few controlled human studies or from laboratory studies with cell or tissue samples.

↔ — Evidence is uncertain and based on conflicting, controlled human research.

↓ — Research doesn't support the claim.

NR — Not enough human research has been done yet, or the research quality is poor.

OTHER SUPPLEMENTS	MEDIA OR MARKETING CLAIMS	EFFECTIVENESS	SAFETY/RISKS
Acidophilus/ lactobacillus acidophilus (LA)	• Improves digestion of dairy products	↔	• No reports of serious adverse effects*
	• Prevents vaginal yeast infections	↔	
	• Prevents antibiotic-associated diarrhea	↔	
	• Lowers cholesterol levels	↔	
	• Protects against cancer	NR	
	• Clears up skin	NR	
Bee pollen	• Nature's perfect food	↓	• Not advised for people with asthma or allergies to honey or bee stings
	• Increases vitality, memory, well-being	NR	• *Note:* Not "magical," bee pollen is composed of the same nutrients found naturally in food: starch, sugars, protein, and a small amount of fat
	• Improves exercise performance	NR	
	• Combats respiratory tract infections, endocrine diseases, colitis, allergies	NR	
Branched chain amino acids (BCAAs)	• Improves exercise performance (physical and mental)	↔	• Doses higher than 20 g may cause gastrointestinal distress and may impair performance and induce fatigue*
Carnitine (L-carnitine)	• Good for the heart	?↑	• No serious adverse effects reported with doses ranging from 0.5 to 6 g a day*
	• Improves aerobic power	↓	• Larger doses associated with nausea and diarrhea
	• Improves neurological function	↔	
	• Improves immune function (AIDS)	NR	
	• Energy enhancer	NR	
	• Burns fat	NR	
Creatine	• Increases muscular strength	?↑	• Not to be used by people with renal disease or insufficiency
	• Delays fatigue—greater gains	NR	• Avoid exceeding a dose of 2 to 5 g a day
	• Burns fat, increases muscle mass	NR	• May cause weight gain/water retention
	• Increases strength in the elderly	NR	
	• Increases strength in people with muscular diseases	?↑	
	• Increases strength in people with heart disease	NR	
Conjugated linoleic acid (CLA)	• Reduces body fat and builds muscles	↓	• No serious adverse effects found in short-term studies.
	• Reduces appetite	↓	
	• Anticancer	NR (in humans)	
	• Good for the cardiovascular system	NR	
	• Improves glucose tolerance	NR	
Gamma-linolenic acid (evening primrose oil, black currant oil, borage seed oil)	• Helpful for PMS and other female health problems	↔	• Not to be used with tricyclic antidepressants or anticonvulsants
	• Eliminates pain of rheumatoid arthritis	↔	• Borage seed oil shouldn't be taken if drugs with potential liver-related side effects are being taken, too.
	• Beneficial for allergic skin reactions and clears up acne	↔	
	• Helpful for people with diabetes	NR	
	• Improves symptoms of heart disease	NR	
	• Prevents hair loss	NR	

OTHER SUPPLEMENTS	MEDIA OR MARKETING CLAIMS	EFFECTIVENESS	SAFETY/RISKS
Coenzyme Q10 (ubiquinone)	• Cardioprotective • Enhances exercise performance • Reduces breast cancer risk • Supports immune function/AIDS • Neurological problems • Slows aging	?↑ ↓ NR NR NR NR	• No reported serious adverse effects with 100-200 mg per day* • May cause mild gastrointestinal distress • *Note:* Coenzyme Q10 is also a body chemical, produced in body cells, that aids in energy production and works as an antioxidant. There's no agreement that ingesting additional coenzyme Q10 offers extra benefits.
DHEA (dehydro-epiandosterone)	• Offsets aging • Improves memory • Enhances sexual prowess • Enhances immunity • Improves cardiovascular function • Anticancer • Treats lupus • Helpful for those with AIDS • Weight reduction	NR NR NR ↔ ↔ ↔ ↔ NR ↓	• Self-supplementation not advised • May increase the risk of breast, endometrial, or prostate cancer • May promote masculine characteristics • May decrease HDL (good) cholesterol level

Fish oil (contains DHA, or docos-ahexanoic acid, and EPA, or eicosapentaenoic acid)	• Cardioprotective:
	  • Lowers tryglycerides
	  • Improves lipids and glucose control for people with diabetes
	  • Lowers blood pressure
	  • Improves effects of atherosclerosis
	  • Reduces risk of death from heart attack
	• Improves rheumatoid arthritis
	• Improves ulcerative colitis
	• Improves psoriasis
		
		↑
		?↑
		
		?↑
		↔
		?↑
		
		?↑
		?↑
		↓
			• May increase bleeding
			• Should be monitored if you take anticoagulant medications
			• Avoid taking before surgery*

Flaxseed	• Reduces cholesterol levels • Reduces heart disease risk • Anticancer • Alleviates rheumatoid arthritis pain • Improves symptoms of lupus, multiple sclerosis, eczema, psoriasis	↔ NR NR (in vitro) NR NR	• Doses higher than 45 g of flaxseed powder cause loose bowels • May increase bleeding if taken with another blood thinner • Flaxseed oil shouldn't be used in high-temperature cooking*
Glucosamine	• Relieves arthritis pain • Heals tendons and ligaments • Improves symptoms of tendonitis and bursitis	?↑ NR NR	• In short-term studies, no serious adverse effects* • Some controversy regarding glucosamine and blood glucose control. To be safe, people with diabetes should have glucose levels monitored.
Lecithin/choline	• Improves exercise endurance • Helps Alzheimer's patients • Improves memory • Reduces liver degeneration	↓ ↓ NR NR	• Mild side effects are linked to high doses (20 g) of choline: gastrointestinal symptoms, urinary incontinence, and diarrhea* • Ongoing use may affect the nervous system if taking high doses of choline regularly; safe in doses of 3.5 g or less choline per day
Melatonin	• Regulates sleep • Reduces jet lag • Prevents cancer • Slows aging process • Increases sex drive	↔ ↔ NR NR NR	• Not known if long-term use of melatonin supplements inhibits the body's natural melatonin production*
Royal jelly	• Antibacterial/fights infection • Improves cardiovascular system • Reduces signs of aging • Improves mental alertness • Improves stamina and fatigue • Reduces symptoms of depression	NR NR NR NR NR NR	• Not advised for people with asthma or a genetic predisposition to allergies • *Note:* Royal jelly—exotic and expensive—isn't jelly, but instead a salivary secretion produced by worker bees to nourish all young larvae and to serve as the sole food for future queen bees.

SELECTED OTHER SUPPLEMENTS: CLAIMS, BENEFITS, RISKS *(continued)*

OTHER SUPPLEMENTS	MEDIA OR MARKETING CLAIMS	EFFECTIVENESS	SAFETY/RISKS
Soy protein and isoflavones	• Lowers cholesterol levels	↑	• If you're a woman diagnosed with breast cancer or at risk for breast cancer, avoid these supplements.*
	• Reduces risk of breast and prostate cancer	NR	
	• Hormone replacement therapy	NR	
	• Reduces risk of osteoporosis	NR	
Shark cartilage	• Cures cancer	NR	• Not enough data to evaluate safety* • One report of hepatitis linked to taking shark cartilage
Spirulina/blue-green algae	• Immune booster	NR	• No reported adverse affects
	• Lowers cholesterol levels	NR	
	• Reduces cancer risk	NR	
	• Improves intestinal health	NR	
Whey protein	• Anabolic agent	NR	• No reported adverse effects* • Avoid use if you have been diagnosed with renal failure or insufficiency • Avoid if allergic to cow milk

*Long-term studies are needed to fully evaluate its safety for humans.

Source: Adapted from Allison Sarubin Fragakis, *The Health Professional's Guide to Popular Dietary Supplements* 2nd edition (Chicago: American Dietetic Association, 2002).

Although foods and drugs are highly regulated, supplements aren't. Enacted in 1994, the FDA's Dietary Supplement Health and Education Act (DSHEA) requires that supplements be safe, unadulterated, and properly labeled, be produced with good manufacturing practices, and be promoted with label information that's truthful. The FDA proposed Good Manufacturing Practices for supplements for review and targeted approval in 2002.

The responsibility for proof, however, lies with the manufacturer, not with the FDA. The manufacturer is expected to ensure that the supplement's label information (Supplement Facts and ingredient list) is accurate, that its ingredients are safe, and that the declared contents match what's inside the container.

The FDA doesn't currently require supplement testing—for safety, effectiveness, or interactions—before launching a supplement into the marketplace. It doesn't require approval before producing or selling it. If, however, an ingredient is new (marketed after October 1994), manufacturers must provide the government with evidence that the supplement is "reasonably expected to be safe" at the labeled dosage. The FDA can take action if the supplement is either unsafe or mislabeled.

For a growing list of dietary supplements, U.S. Pharmacopeia (USP), an independent, not-for-profit organization, sets quality standards: for strength, quality, and purity of supplements. If manufacturers voluntarily comply, they may display the "USP" or "NF" (National Formulary) letters along with the lot number and expiration date of the product. This is industry-reported compliance, not third-party assessment. USP's *United States Pharmacopeia—National Formulary* manual shows supplement standards for:

● *Disintegration,* or how fast it breaks down into smaller pieces.

● *Dissolution,* or how fast and how well it dissolves in a solution similar to digestive juices.

● *Purity,* whether it has an acceptable limit of impurities.

● *Strength,* or how much of the vitamin, mineral, or active ingredient it contains.

● *Expiration,* or how long it retains its quality.

While some supplements are labeled accurately and completely, many aren't, and what's stated on the label may not be what's in the container. The potency or purity may be misrepresented or inconsistent.

Have You Ever Wondered

. . . if any herbal supplement can replace or enhance medication for depression? If your doctor has prescribed medication for depression, follow the guidance; don't mix or change antidepressants. Mixing may result in harmful interactions—for example, St. John's wort interacts with antidepressants such as Prozac and amoxapine. The combination may be additive. And a herbal treatment may not yield the intended outcome. If you choose to try a herbal, talk to your physician first.

Herbs may be misidentified, indicating the wrong part or type of herb. The dosage's safety and effectiveness aren't regulated either. Bottom line: It's up to you to be a discriminating consumer!

Several independent organizations—e.g., NSF International, U.S. Pharmacopeia (USP), and ConsumerLab.com—have initiated certification programs, designed to assess whether a supplement really contains what the manufacturer declares on the label. (The "USP letters" mentioned previously have a different meaning than the "USP Verified" mark.) A fee-based service to industry, each certifying organization sets its own assessment criteria—some more in-depth than others. Some audit manufacturing practices; some do ongoing surveillance.

A step in the right direction, it's hard to discern precisely what a specific certification mark on a supplement label means and how each mark's criteria differ, however. Although a certifying mark helps you know if you're getting what you paid for, it does *not* verify a supplement's overall safety or effectiveness. No certifying mark? It could mean several things: the supplement didn't meet certification criteria, or the assessment is in progress, or perhaps the supplement hasn't been submitted for review.

What about regulations for advertising supplements? The Federal Trade Commission (FTC) regulates the advertising of supplements, including media infomercials and Internet promotion. Like the FDA, its resources for monitoring are limited.

Also note, supplement recalls are voluntary. Recalling a harmful product is no guarantee that it's been removed entirely from store shelves . . . despite good intentions by reputable manufacturers.

Supplements: Marketplace Confusion

Believe it or not, many supplement manufacturers do provide reliable product information. In fact, by law, supplement labels must bear Supplement Facts and claims that cannot mislead.

However, many companies don't abide by the supplement "rules." A regulatory environment that's less restrictive than the early 1990s has allowed more products and more misinformation to enter the marketplace, and deceptive marketing tactics are rampant throughout the supplement industry. For well-intentioned consumers—eager to take responsibility for their health—the sea of science and fiction is often confusing and misleading, and ultimately may be costly and harmful.

What misleading tactics may be used? Supplements are often promoted with pseudoscience. *See "Ten Red Flags of Junk Science" in chapter 24.*

● *Borrowed research.* Study results that may or may not apply to the product: perhaps supplements with different potencies or formulations, or derived from different parts of the plant.

● *Distorted data.* Information that's "spun" to match the product claim. Again, the formulation or dosage may differ from the supplement used in the original study. Less reputable manufacturers may present their "proof" in a format—charts and tables, cited references—that looks like a reliable research study.

● *Claims that research is under way.* In other words, no specific data are available.

● *Unreliable studies.* Poorly designed research that hasn't been published in peer-reviewed publications.

● *Testimonials.* Statements, not based in sound science, from "satisfied" customers or celebrities

Science behind Supplements: More Needed

To show the effectiveness of a supplement and its active ingredients, more good research is needed! Good research should provide data from randomized, placebo-controlled, double-blind studies—not just one study, but several that duplicate the results. In reality, current laws do not require manufacturers to conduct research, and few do. *See chapter 24 for definitions of research terms.*

To further complicate what's known and unknown, many supplements—for example, botanicals—have two or more active ingredients. Yet, all the bio-active substances haven't been identified, nor what they do. Potencies differ when the same herbal supplement derives from different parts of a plant or different varieties. Growing conditions may affect the potency of bio-active substances. Even if sound research exists for the safety and effectiveness of one active ingredient, it may not exist for all ingredients, and usually not for the combination. Typically the potency of active ingredients in combination products is less than the amount used in single ingredient studies. More unknowns: There's not enough scientific evidence to know how much of a supplement or its bio-active substitutes offer benefits, how much may be harmful, the health effects of dosages beyond the label dosage, or any interaction with food or medication.

In the future, sound research data may become available for more supplements as more funding comes from the National Institutes of Health, including the Office of Dietary Supplements (ODS) and the National Center for Complementary Medicine (NCCAM). Until sound science reveals more, the best consumer advice: a healthy skepticism.

See chapter 24 for more about judging nutrition information, scientific reports, and nutrition quackery.

Supplements: Questions to Ask an Expert

With so many supplement products and so many unknowns about them, these are questions you can explore with qualified nutrition experts—before you take a supplement:

● What are the claims? Who's making them? Why? Are the claims valid?

● Where did the product information come from? Is the manufacturer a trusted, nonbiased source?

● Is the supplement generally safe? Can it cause harm in *any* dosage?

● Does the product come from a company that's known, or highly likely, to follow safe, appropriate manufacturing practices?

● What's known about the supplement's effectiveness for its proposed benefit?

● How do the active ingredients work in the body?

● What plant or plants and part of the plant or plants do the main active ingredients come from?

● How much of the active ingredients does the supplement have? What else does it contain?

● What are the risks and benefits of using the supplement: for anyone, for you?

● What scientific evidence supports this product formula or brand?

● What side effects might result from taking this supplement?

● How much (dose), how often, and how long is it safe for you to take it?

Source: Adapted from American Dietetic Association/American Pharmaceutical Association, *A Healthcare Professional's Guide to Evaluating Dietary Supplements* (2000).

If You Take a Supplement . . .

Before you head down your store's supplement aisle, order a supplement online, or pick up a product at your fitness center, get supplement savvy. Buy and use dietary supplements with the same consumer wisdom you use when you buy a car or make any major investment. This time that major investment is you and your health—for the short term and the long term!

Guidelines for Supplement Use

Keeping up with the explosion of supplements and supplement claims can be overwhelming! If you take supplements, strive to use them with good health sense, and ask for expert guidance.

For All Supplements . . .

Before you decide to take a dietary supplement, go with the tried-and-true as your best approach for fitness. There's plenty of scientific evidence supporting the benefits of physical activity, healthful eating, and a healthful lifestyle. If you take a supplement—any supplement—keep these general tips in mind:

● Give up the notion that dietary supplements are simple, immediate solutions to your health problems. Even supplements that offer benefits take time and ongoing use to make a difference.

● Skip the lure of this myth: "Even if a supplement won't help me, at least it won't hurt me." High dosages, taken long enough or combined with other supplements, can be harmful.

● *Best practice:* Talk to your doctor *before* you take any supplement! That's especially important if you're under age eighteen, pregnant or breast-feeding, chronically ill, elderly, or taking prescription or over-the-counter medicines. *See "Warning: Supplement Interactions!" in this chapter.*

● If you're already taking a dietary supplement, tell your doctor to make sure it's safe and appropriate for you and your health status. Be prepared to discuss:

  ● Supplement name, type, and daily or weekly dose (Bring the container if you can.)

  ● How long you have taken it and plan to take it, and why

  ● How long you've had the symptoms you're treating with the supplement, and if your symptoms have improved

  ● Other medications (over-the-counter and prescription) you're taking

  ● Any health problems or illnesses
    ● Whether you're pregnant or breast-feeding
    ● Whether you drink alcohol or smoke; if so, how often and how much
    ● If you have allergies
    ● If you're on a special eating plan (self-prescribed or medically prescribed)

Supplements: If You Have an Adverse Reaction . . .

● Immediately inform your healthcare provider if you think you have suffered a serious harmful effect or illness from a dietary supplement.

● Report any serious problems to the FDA's MedWatch hotline: (1-800-FDA-1088), fax (1-800-FDA-0178), or *(http://vm.fda.gov/medwatch/report/hcp.htm)* online. Either you or your healthcare provider can do this. Be prepared to identify the probable product.

● For a general concern or complaint about any supplement, contact your nearest FDA District Office. Find the phone number on the *http://vm.fda.gov/opacom/backgrounders/complain.htm* Web site.

● If you're pregnant, planning to become pregnant, or breast-feeding, be sure to talk to your healthcare provider about supplements! Some are safe, even recommended. Others, such as some herbal and other botanical supplements, aren't.

● Unless your pediatrician prescribes them, avoid giving supplements to your child or teen. That includes herbals, which may not be as "safe" as claimed. *For more about supplements and children see "What about Nutrient Supplements?" in chapter 16 and "Caution: Herbals Not for Kids!" in this chapter.*

● Look out for supplements with fraudulent claims. Besides not doing what they say, they may be costly or harmful.

● Look for products labeled with the voluntary USP (U.S. Pharmacopeia) or NF letters, which indicates that the manufacturer self-reports voluntary standards of quality. Some reputable companies choose to pay for independent certification; often national brands from larger companies have stricter quality controls. Remember that certification marks represent differing criteria; most important, they indicate whether a label matches the contents of the supplement, not its overall safety or effectiveness.

● Remember that "natural" doesn't mean safe.

● Stick with the dosage on the label; heed all warnings. The dosage is set by the manufacturer—not by FDA regulations and likely not by scientific advice. Boosting the dosage without medical supervision can be dangerous. An insignificant substance can become harmful when a supplement is consumed beyond the label dosage.

● Follow the directions printed on the label. Some supplements are more effective taken with food; others, on an empty stomach. Ask your healthcare provider for a list of foods and drinks to avoid consuming with the supplement. Usually water is the best drink.

● Keep dietary supplements in a safe place—away from places where children may reach them! Adult iron supplements are the most common cause of poisoning deaths among children in the United States!

● Keep supplements in a cool, dry place—preferably away from the stove and not in the bathroom. Heat and moisture affect their quality and effectiveness. Keep them in their original containers (label still on).

● Check the expiration date. Supplements lose some potency as they get closer to their expiration date.

● On the same note, skip the urge to "prescribe" a supplement for someone else. Even if it works for you, it may not be safe or effective for someone else.

● Want information about the contents of supplements? Write to the manufacturer. The FDA doesn't have the resources to analyze supplements. *Tip:* Companies that provide scientific information about their products are more likely to be reliable resources; still, be wary and careful.

● Ask a registered dietitian or your healthcare provider about the effectiveness of specific supplement products—and the research behind their claims. Show the supplement container, or reveal the information you've gathered.

● Stay skeptical of supplement marketing—even with label or advertising claims. *See "Play 'Ten Questions'" in chapter 24 to help you evaluate their claims.*

For Vitamin/Mineral Supplements . . .

If your doctor or a registered dietitian recommends a supplement—either a vitamin-mineral combination or a single nutrient such as calcium—follow his or her professional guidance. *That includes the general guidelines in "For All Supplements . . ." on page 600.* Choose the product recommended for you.

If you're healthy and self-prescribe a dietary supplement, first ask yourself if you really need it. Think about the foods you typically eat and what they contain. If you're eating a healthful diet—following guidelines from the Food Guide Pyramid—you're likely getting all the nutrients you need already. *See "The Food Guide Pyramid: Your Healthful Eating Guide" in chapter 10.*

● Remember, for most healthy people: food before pills. Use supplements as supplements—not replacements—for nutrients in healthful meals and snacks. Choose food with variety, balance, and moderation in mind: plenty of fruits, vegetables and grains, especially whole grains, for their vitamins and fiber; lean meat, fish, and poultry, for their minerals; and dairy foods, for their calcium (and other nutrients).

Warning: Supplement Interactions!

● *Dealing with cancer, diabetes, heart disease, immune problems, kidney problems, thyroid problems, ulcers, or other health problems?* Talk with your doctor before using dietary supplements, and about the potential for harmful interactions.

● *Taking prescription or over-the-counter medication?* Supplements—when combined with medications or other treatments—may interfere with or boost their action, even be harmful or life-threatening. *See "Food and Medicine" in chapter 22.* For example:
  ● Folic acid can interact with anticonvulsant medications.
  ● Vitamin E, garlic, and gingko biloba may thin blood—dangerous when taken with blood-thinning medication such as Coumadin and aspirin.
  ● Garlic supplements may interact with drugs used in HIV therapy such as saquinavir, which is a protease inhibitor.
  ● The combination of foxglove (the source of digitalis, or digoxin) and cardiac medication is dangerous for those with heart disease.
  ● St. John's wort may reduce the effect of heart drugs, antidepressants, antiseizure drugs, anticancer drugs, birth control drugs, certain HIV drugs, and anti-transplant-rejection drugs.

● *Planning for any surgery?* Avoid *all* supplements two to three weeks ahead, according to guidelines from the American Society of Anesthesiologists. Although herbal supplements may seem "innocent," their use can cause complications such as bleeding, heart instability, low blood sugar, blood pressure changes, and other drug interactions. Among those linked to surgical complications are ephedra, garlic, ginkgo, ginseng, kava, St. John's wort, and valerian.

● Choose a vitamin-mineral combination. Limit the potency to 100 percent or less of the Daily Values (DV) for your age and gender; use the Supplement Facts on the label to judge the product. A supplement with 100 percent of the DV is likely more than enough, especially if you're eating a healthful diet, too. Avoid large doses!

● Choose a supplement for your unique needs. Consider your age, gender, and medical status. *Note:* If you're under stress, don't count on a stress vitamin pill to help. Stress doesn't increase nutrient needs.

● For economy, consider the generic brand. Paying more for the same product generally offers no additional benefits. You also may save by buying synthetic vitamins rather than natural ones. For the most part, their chemical makeup is the same. One exception is "natural" vitamin E (d-alpha-tocopherol on the ingredient list), which is more potent than the synthetic form (dl-tocopherol). In most cases, however, your body won't know the difference between synthetic and natural, but your wallet will because the "natural" products likely cost more.

Don't be lured by extra ingredients: choline, inositol, lecithin, PABA, herbs, and enzymes. They add to the cost but offer no proven nutritional benefits.

● Check the expiration date on the label. Over time, nutrient supplements lose some potency.

● Take the supplement in the recommended dosage. There's no need to double dose on days when you've missed a meal. Rather than popping a pill, make up for foods you missed with your food choices on the next day. Because supplements can have druglike effects, too much taken at one time can be dangerous.

● Remember, no nutrient supplement provides the full complement of vitamins, minerals, and other important nutrients found in food that you need for health. A supplement has only what's listed on its label. If you rely on supplements, you miss out on the full variety of nutrients, as well as fiber, phytonutrients, and other substances supplied by food.

● Be cautious about doubling up on certain nutrients. If you're already taking multivitamin/mineral supplements, taking a single vitamin or mineral supplement as well may be too much! Read the label.

For Herbal and Other Botanical Supplements . . .

Helpful or harmful? Even though herbal and other botanical products are sold over the counter, use them with caution and discretion. Some offer varying degrees of health benefit—perhaps backed up by tradition or by emerging scientific evidence. Yet many don't deliver on the myriad of benefits they claim, dispensing more fraud than fact. Others have harmful, even life-threatening side effects.

Besides the general guidelines in "For All Supplements . . ." presented earlier in this chapter, protect your health and increase your chances for any potential benefits by following these guidelines:

● Seek unbiased, science-based sources of information about herbals. Relying on product claims can mislead you. The poorly defined term "natural" doesn't mean safe or healthful. Ask a registered dietitian or other qualified nutrition expert for reliable information—what's known and unknown—about the supplement.

● Before you take a herbal supplement, find out about the risks and potential side effects. Then decide with your doctor if it's safe and appropriate for you—or if other known health strategies would yield safe, effective results.

● Always consult a qualified health professional. Be cautious of those who call themselves a "herbalist," "herb doctor," "health counselor," or "master herbalist." These job titles aren't regulated.

● For serious illness, avoid self-medicating with herbal or other botanical supplements. That may delay known treatment that can help you.

● Tell if you're taking herbal supplements. Talk to your doctor, since some supplements don't mix well with medications.

● Skip herbal remedies if you're taking medication—either prescription drugs or over-the-counter medications. These products may interfere with your medications. The combination could make your medication ineffective, or together they may create a harmful side effect.

● If you're pregnant (or trying to get pregnant) or breast-feeding, avoid herbal remedies unless your doctor gives them an okay. Substances in these remedies may pass to your baby. These products aren't meant for children, either.

● If you get a doctor's okay, use herbal products only as directed. Take single-herb products, not herbal mixtures, unless recommended by a qualified practitioner with expertise in herbal therapies. If you have an adverse effect, you can identify the source more easily if you're taking single-herb products.

● If a herbal product seems to cause any negative side effects, stop taking it, and contact your doctor

Caution: Herbals Not for Kids!

Even though supplement companies aggressively target kids and parents, herbal and other botanical supplements may not be as safe or effective for your child or teen as you may think! Some supplements are useless; others, potentially harmful. Consider this: In the big picture of scientific research, little evidence exists on the safety and effectiveness of botanical supplements for adults. Their use among children and teens is virtually untested. In other words, we don't know the short- or long-term benefits, or more importantly, the risks.

Warning: Despite FDA warnings against ephedra for anyone—including those under age eighteen—weight-loss products with ephedra and "energy-boosting" energy drinks are available to teens. Among the dangers: severe chest pain. *See "Herbal Ingredients: Hazardous to Health!" in this chapter.*

right away. Your doctor should contact the FDA's MedWatch hotline, which monitors adverse reactions to food and dietary supplements. *See "Supplements: If You Have an Adverse Reaction . . ." in this chapter. See "Herbal Teas: Health Benefits?" in chapter 8.*

The Supplement Label

A supplement label looks somewhat like a food label. Required by the Dietary Supplement Health and Education Act, the label must provide specific information you can use to make an informed decision:

● *Statement of identity.* Look for the product name, perhaps "ginseng." The term "dietary supplement" or a descriptive phrase, such as "vitamin and mineral supplement," also must appear. If the product is a botanical, the plant part must be identified.

● *Net quantity of the ingredients.* That might be the number of capsules, perhaps "sixty capsules," in the package or container, or the weight.

● *Disclaimer with any structure/function claim. See "Claim Check!" in this chapter.*

● *Supplement Facts.* This gives the serving (or dosage), the amount and the percent Daily Values (DVs) per serving if appropriate, and the active ingredient. *See "Check the Supplement Facts" on this page.*

● *Directions for use.* This might indicate how often to take the supplement, perhaps "Take one capsule daily"; whether the supplement is best taken with or without food; safety tips; or storage guidelines. Be aware, however: Suggested dosage is meaningless when little is known about the benefits and risks of many supplements.

● *Ingredients.* The list must be in descending order by common name or proprietary blend. *See "Ingredients Labeling, Too" in this chapter.*

● *Name and address of the manufacturer, packager, or distributor.* Use this contact information to get more product information.

As an option, supplement labels also may carry product claims: nutrient content claims, health claims, or structure/function claims.

Check the Supplement Facts

How do you know about the nutrition in a dietary supplement? Check the Supplement Facts panel, which must appear on *all* supplements. Its format is similar to the familiar Nutrition Facts you see on food products. To use the Supplement Facts panel:

● Check the serving size, or an appropriate unit, such as a capsule, packet, or teaspoonful. That's what the nutrition information is based on. Unlike Nutrition Facts for foods, serving size isn't standardized for supplements; neither is the potency, or nutrient amount, per serving. The manufacturer makes that decision.

Have You Ever Wondered

. . . if herbal supplements are safe to take if you have allergies? Remember that herbal and other botanical supplements are made from the bark, flowers, leaves, and seeds of plants. If you're prone to allergic reactions, check with your healthcare professional before taking them. *See chapter 21 for more about allergies.*

. . . if a supplement without cautionary information on the label is safe? Warnings about potential adverse effects of a supplement's use do not need to be printed on the label. To find out, you need to contact the manufacturer directly for substantiated evidence.

● Check the quantity and the percent Daily Values (DVs) for any of fourteen nutrients, including sodium, vitamin A, vitamin C, calcium, and iron, if the levels are significant. Other vitamins or minerals must be listed, too, if they are added or referred to with a nutrient content claim on the label.

On the Supplement Facts, you probably won't find a nutrient if it isn't present. For example, cod liver oil lists fat on the panel, but a calcium supplement won't because it doesn't contain fat.

If the supplement has a substance with no Daily Value, the quantity per serving must be listed—for example, "15 mg. omega-3 fatty acids."

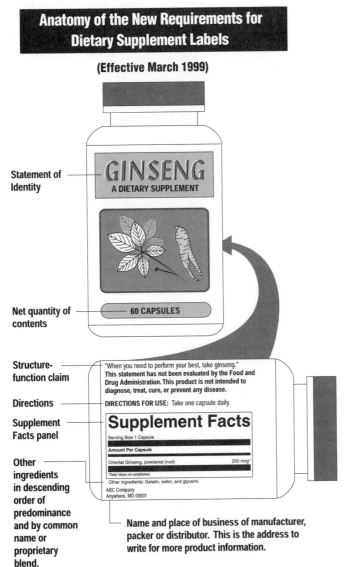

Anatomy of the New Requirements for Dietary Supplement Labels

(Effective March 1999)

Statement of Identity

Net quantity of contents

Structure-function claim

Directions

Supplement Facts panel

Other ingredients in descending order of predominance and by common name or proprietary blend.

GINSENG
A DIETARY SUPPLEMENT

60 CAPSULES

"When you need to perform your best, take ginseng." This statement has not been evaluated by the Food and Drug Administration. This product is not intended to diagnose, treat, cure, or prevent any disease.

DIRECTIONS FOR USE: Take one capsule daily.

Supplement Facts
Serving Size 1 Capsule
Amount Per Capsule
Oriental Ginseng, powdered (root)   250 mcg*
*Daily Value not established.
Other ingredients: Gelatin, water, and glycerin.
ABC Company
Anywhere, MD 00001

Name and place of business of manufacturer, packer or distributor. This is the address to write for more product information.

Claim Check!

Confused about marketing claims for supplements? Not surprising! Some label claims (nutrient content claims and health claims) are backed by scientific consensus, yet many (structure/function claims) aren't, at least not yet. Loose supplement regulations, including many product claims that push "over the edge" of credibility, leave many consumers misguided, bewildered, or both.

Some product claims are clearly illegal—for example, "cures cancer," "treats arthritis," " prevents impotence." According to FDA regulation, no dietary supplement can legally state or imply that it can help diagnose, treat, cure, or prevent disease.

Here's what marketers can claim about supplements—and how the claims are regulated—on package labels. *Since claims for food and for dietary supplements are similar, see chapter 11 for more information.*

Nutrient Content Claims. "High in calcium" … "excellent source of folate" … "iron-free" … like food packaging, dietary supplement labels can carry nutrient content claims if they contain a specific level of a nutrient in a single serving. The claims, carefully regulated by the U.S. Food and Drug Administration (FDA), are similar to nutrient content claims for food. For example, any product with at least 20 percent of the Daily Value per serving can be labeled as "high" or "excellent source" of that nutrient.

What does a nutrient content claim tell you? It's just a clue. You need to read the Supplement Facts to know the specific nutrient content of one dose, or "serving."

Wonder why a supplement would be "iron-free"? It's a product meant for the age fifty-plus market, when women's iron needs drop.

Health Claims. "Calcium can reduce the risk of osteoporosis." "Folic acid protects against neural tube defects." Health claims that describe the link between nutrients or substances in food, and health, can be used on supplements. These FDA-regulated statements are based on scientific consensus—you can trust these claims, too. *For a list of approved health claims for food and supplement labeling, see the Appendices.* Two health claims have been approved for supplements but not for food products: (1) omega-3 fatty acids and their role in reducing the risk for heart disease and (2) B vitamins (folic acid, vitamin B_6 and vitamin B_{12}) and reduced risk for vascular disease.

Structure/Function Claims. Echinacea: "boosts the immune system." Zinc: "helps treat the common cold." Garlic: "helps maintain cardiovascular health." Lutein: "helps maintain healthy eyes."

Structure/function claims like these may appear on

dietary supplements as well as on food labels. These claims describe what the dietary ingredient is intended to do to in the body or to promote health. However, research to support these claims is often limited, with no scientific consensus.

By regulation, the manufacturer, not the FDA, must substantiate that the statements are truthful and not misleading. Because the FDA does not approve them, supplement labels with these claims must carry an FDA disclaimer: "This statement has not been evaluated by the Food and Drug Administration. This product is not intended to diagnose, treat, cure, or prevent any disease."

Ingredients Labeling, Too

The label shows ingredients, given their common name or proprietary blend, in descending order by weight. If an ingredient isn't listed in the Supplement Facts, it must be in the ingredients statement—for example, rose hips as the vitamin C source. Besides the active ingredients, other substances—fillers, colorings or flavors, sweeteners—must be listed.

For herbal and other botanical supplements, potency often differs when different parts of a plant are used. If the supplement contains these ingredients, the label must identify what part of the plant it comes from—for example, ginseng may come from a root. The ingredient source may appear on an ingredients statement or near the product's statement of identity.

Have You Ever Wondered ?

. . . if the same supplement can be sold by several names? Yes; that adds to consumer confusion. However, the ingredient list must list the common name.

Botanical supplements may have a common name and a botanical name—for example, St. John's wort, often promoted to treat mild to moderate depression, also is known as *Hypericum perforatum.*

In other cases, the common name may refer to a category. Ginseng may refer to *Panax ginseng* or *Panax japonicus* (Asian ginsengs) or to *Panax quinquefolius L.* (American ginseng), each with different effects. Siberian ginseng *(E. senticosus)* isn't botanically related to either one!

. . . what the term "high potency" on a dietary supplement label means? According to recent government regulations, "high potency" means that a nutrient in a food product, including a dietary supplement, provides 100 percent or more of the Daily Value (DV) for that vitamin or mineral. The term also can refer to a product with several ingredients if two-thirds of its nutrients contribute more than 100 percent of the DVs. *See chapter 10 for more about DVs.*

. . . if chelated mineral supplements are any better? Chelation binds minerals to other substances, supposedly making minerals easier for the body to absorb. While that may be true, many minerals found naturally in food aren't very bioavailable; that's considered when their Dietary Reference Intakes are established. In the overall picture, chelation isn't important—if you're meeting your day's mineral recommendation.

Need more strategies for appropriate use of dietary supplements? Check here for "how-tos":

- Find out about *safe* supplement use for children—see chapter 16.
- Get savvy about ergogenic supplements for athletic performance—see chapter 19.
- Sort through misleading information about supplements—see chapter 24.
- Talk to a qualified nutrition expert about safe and appropriate supplements for you and your family—see chapter 24.

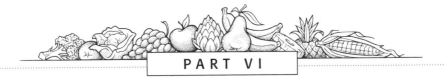

PART VI

Resources

More about
Healthful Eating

Well Informed?

Are you well informed . . . or often confused about conflicting nutrition information? Can you easily find reliable nutrition information . . . or do you feel frustrated sorting through a maze of scientific news about healthy eating? For that matter, how do you stay up-to-date?

Probably, popular media—television, magazines, newspapers, and perhaps the Internet—are part of your health education "mix," alerting you to up-to-date food and nutrition issues, concerns, and advice. In fact, many consumers rely on media more than health professionals. For your own good health, you're wise to find credible sources and learn to judge the value of nutrition advice before using it to make your eating, lifestyle, and health decisions.

Where do teens and children learn about healthful eating? First and foremost, from you. So being well informed yourself ultimately teaches them. As kids get older, they learn from school, friends, and media, too. For kids already computer-savvy, Web sites are fast becoming an easy and private health information resource. Your challenge as a parent, caregiver, or teacher? Knowing enough to provide accurate information . . . and to direct those in your care to sources of sound eating and lifestyle guidance!

Need Nutrition Advice?

When do you need smart eating advice? Every day! Sometimes you may need to know a little more . . .

- If you're pregnant—or trying to get pregnant
- If you need guidance *and confidence* for breast-feeding
- If you're trying to deal with the "ups and downs" of infant or child feeding
- If you're trying to steer your teen toward healthier eating
- If you want to put in your peak performance for sports
- If you're struggling with your weight—or just trying to gain or lose a few pounds
- If you need to change your eating habits to prevent or manage a health problem—yours, or a family member's
- If you're caring for an aging parent or friend
- If you simply want to eat smarter to stay fit

When you need nutrition advice, ask a qualified expert. Your health—and that of your family—depend on it!

The Real Expert . . . Please Stand Up

Just who is a qualified nutrition expert? Sometimes it's hard to tell. Qualified nutrition experts, with specific academic and training credentials, know the science of nutrition. Their degrees in nutrition, dietetics, public health, or related fields (such as biochemistry, medicine, or a nutrition specialty in family and consumer sciences) come from well-respected colleges and

Who Is a Registered Dietitian?

The initials "RD" after someone's name mean "registered dietitian." A registered dietitian is a food and nutrition authority who has met academic and training requirements to earn the RD credential—and so provide credible nutrition guidance to the public.

As an important member of the healthcare team, an RD may have specialized expertise, perhaps in pediatric, maternal, or sports nutrition; oncology, cardiovascular, or renal nutrition; weight counseling; or diabetes education. Besides being in healthcare, education, and research, registered dietitians also provide nutrition and food expertise in business (marketing, sales), government (public policy, government programs), food service (restaurant, institutions) management, fitness (education, training), communications (media, public relations, writing), and in private practice counseling and consulting.

To earn the RD credential, an individual first must complete at least four years of education in nutrition or a related field from an accredited college or university program that's approved by the American Dietetic Association. He or she also is required to complete nine hundred hours of supervised practice in nutrition and dietetics. Many dietetics professionals earn graduate degrees as well.

To become registered, candidates must pass an extensive examination, administered by the Commission on Dietetic Registration, the credentialing agency of the American Dietetic Association. All RDs are required to stay current with ongoing continuing education. Only dietitians who have passed the exam and maintain their continuing education are considered "registered."

Some registered dietitians also have specialized credentials, such as Board Certified Specialists in Pediatric Nutrition (CSP) or in Renal Nutrition (CSR), or as Certified Diabetes Educators (CDE). And some RDs pursue recognition for advanced-level practice, with the credential FADA, or Fellow of the American Dietetic Association.

universities. The title "dietitian" or "nutritionist" often describes what they do.

Letters after a name don't necessarily qualify someone to provide nutrition services. Even when that person holds other academic degrees, nutrition may not be his or her specialty. Probe further.

The initials RD for "registered dietitian" or DTR for "dietetic technician, registered" do mean the person has met specific educational requirements in nutrition and health. *See "Who Is a Registered Dietitian?" and "Who Is a Dietetic Technician, Registered?" in this chapter.* In states with licensing, dietitians may have more credentials, such as LD (licensed dietitian); terms differ from state to state. Many qualified nutrition experts also have advanced degrees, such as M.S., M.Ed., Sc.D., M.D., or Ph.D.

In many states the titles "nutritionist" and "diet counselor" aren't regulated, so terms like these may be used by those not properly qualified to give accurate nutrition information or sound advice. For example, salespeople for dietary supplements, so-called health advisers, and some authors may call themselves "nutritionists." In reality, they instead may be self-proclaimed experts, perhaps with just a little nutrition training or with only mail-order credentials.

Mail-order, diploma-mill credentials may appear impressive—but don't be fooled. The U.S. Department of Education defines a "diploma mill" as an organization awarding degrees without requiring its students to meet the established educational standards followed by reputable institutions. To see if an institution is accredited, not simply a diploma mill, check in your library for a list of accredited educational institutions.

Licensing qualified nutrition experts in many states helps ensure credible nutrition guidance and quality healthcare. Although qualifications for licensing differ from state to state, they often reflect the same education and training required to become an RD.

How to Find Nutrition Help . . .

Need personal nutrition counseling? Food assistance for a friend or a family member? Answers to nutrition questions? Check with health, education, and social service organizations in your community, as well as dietitians in private practice for direct services.

Who Is a Dietetic Technician, Registered?

The initials "DTR" after a person's name stand for "dietetic technician, registered." It signifies that the individual is qualified to be part of the nutrition care or food service management team. DTRs often are considered partners in practice with registered dietitians. Job responsibilities may include teaching nutrition classes, offering diet counseling, performing diet histories, assessing a person's nutritional status, or managing aspects of a food-service operation. DTRs typically work in hospitals or extended care facilities; many also work in businesses, government agencies, education, retail sales and marketing, academic institutions, or fitness centers.

Currently there are two ways to attain the DTR credential. First is by completing requirements for an associate degree from an ADA-accredited/approved dietetic technician program. Second is completing a baccalaureate degree, didactic program in dietetics from an ADA-accredited/approved college or university. Either way, 450 hours of supervised field experience in healthcare facilities, food-service operations, or community nutrition programs must be completed. Many DTRs earn additional degrees that complement their food and nutrition background. DTRs also must successfully complete a comprehensive registration exam administered by the Commission on Dietetic Registration, the credentialing agency of the American Dietetic Association.

Once they earn their credential, dietetic technicians, registered must stay current with ongoing continuing education. Only individuals who pass the exam and maintain their status through continuing education are considered *registered*. People with job titles that include "dietetic technician," "diet tech," or "diet clerk"—without being a DTR—or who are "RD-eligible" are not generally recognized as qualified to provide reliable food and nutrition services.

To Find a Qualified Nutrition Expert

Start with these sources:

- Your doctor, health maintenance organization (HMO), or local hospital for a referral

- Your local dietetic association, public health department, Cooperative Extension Service, or the nutrition department of an area college or university

- The American Dietetic Association at *www. eatright.org* (go to "Find a Dietitian"). Or call 800/366-1655 for a referral to a registered dietitian in your area.

See "The Real Expert . . . Please Stand Up" in this chapter to help you choose a qualified nutrition expert.

To Find Food and Nutrition Services

Agencies, institutions, and businesses—often staffed with qualified nutrition experts—provide direct food or nutrition services. Whether for you and for someone you know who might benefit, consider these resources:

Child Nutrition Programs. Schools, as well as early childhood centers, after-school programs, and summer camps, may provide nutritious breakfasts and lunches for children. Often local programs get support partly through the USDA's Child Nutrition Program. By regulation, school meals and snacks must meet strict nutrition guidelines. The program also provides nutrition education for children. *See "For Kids Only—Today's School Meals" in chapter 16.*

Extension Service. Each state's Extension program provides consumer information on various topics, including food, nutrition, and food safety. State land-grant universities employ nutrition experts as part of the Extension staff. Look for food and nutrition information online from Extension offices across the nation. Or check your local newspaper for a regular feature written by Extension nutrition staff.

Food Stamp Program. The food stamp program, administered by state agencies and funded by the U.S. Department of Agriculture (USDA), provides food assistance to needy families and individuals. Food stamps are used like cash in food stores and some farmers' markets. For the nearest food stamp office, check your county public health department or government pages of your phone book.

Health Organizations. For help with specific health issues, check health organizations such as the American Heart Association, the American Diabetes Association, and the Food Allergy and Anaphylaxis Network—as well as the American Dietetic Association. *Also check "Resources You Can Use," at the end of this book.* Their Web sites offer a wealth of information, and perhaps a gateway to other credible food, nutrition, and health Web sites.

Home-Delivered Meals. People who can't leave their homes or who can't prepare food independently may seek services for home-delivered meals. For those who qualify, government or community agencies provide meals at low cost. Check with a social worker, religious group, or state or area Agency on Aging.

Senior Citizens' Meal Programs. Community agencies may serve low-cost meals and offer social contact for senior citizens. To find services, check with a social worker, health department, religious group, or state or area Agency on Aging.

Soup Kitchens and Food Pantries. For those who are homeless or have limited resources for food, private and religious groups may provide food at no cost. Often social workers, social agencies, and religious groups offer referrals.

Women, Infants, and Children (WIC) Program. This federal government program offers food assistance and nutrition education to pregnant women, infants, and preschoolers. Again, the county or other local public health department can help, or check the government pages in your phone book.

For More about Food Products

Food Industry Groups. Food companies and food industry groups provide information about the nutrients and ingredients in their products. Many also offer healthful eating and lifestyle information on their Web sites, package labels and print materials, or through their toll-free phone numbers (often printed on food packages). Through their consumer response services—staffed by dietitians or other qualified food and nutrition professionals—you also may find answers to individual consumer questions.

When You Consult an Expert . . .

Whether you seek nutrition counseling on your own or follow up from a doctor's referral, here's how you can make the most of your time with a qualified nutrition professional. For an office visit . . .

● *Have a medical checkup first.* A qualified nutrition professional needs to know your health status before providing dietary guidance. Your healthcare provider can share your blood pressure and information from blood tests, such as blood cholesterol, triglycerides, blood glucose (sugar), hemoglobin, and hematocrit levels, among others.

Some health problems are managed in part or completely by diet and perhaps physical activity. If so, your doctor may refer you to a dietitian for appropriate diet therapy. In many states, private health insurance and managed care plans cover nutrition counseling (also known as medical nutrition therapy) with a registered dietitian for some health conditions, such as diabetes. Ask for a referral if you qualify.

● *Share your goals.* If you seek nutrition advice on your own, know what you want to accomplish. Do you want to lose weight? Gain weight? Have more energy for sports? Lower your blood cholesterol level? Live a healthier lifestyle? Think about your goals ahead . . . and make them realistic.

● *Forget miracles and magic bullets.* A qualified nutrition professional will focus on changes in your lifestyle and food choices, not on quick results, miracle cures, or costly dietary supplements.

● *Tell about dietary supplements you're taking.* That includes herbal remedies and botanicals. Some supplements interact with medications (even over-the-counter types), rendering them ineffective or causing harmful side effects. *See "Food and Medicine" in chapter 22.* Dietary supplements taken in very large doses also may cause adverse health reactions. *See chapter 23, "Supplements: Use and Abuse."*

● *Be prepared to answer questions.* Expect to talk about your eating habits, any adverse reactions to food, dietary supplements, your weight history, food preferences, general medical history, family history of health problems, medications, special diets, any nutrition instruction you've had, and your lifestyle habits. With those insights, a dietitian can customize food and nutrition advice to match your lifestyle and health needs.

● *For weight counseling or sports nutrition, expect to have your weight and body composition checked—* usually height, weight, and a skinfold measurement in several spots on your body (or other techniques to measure body composition).

● *Ask for clarification.* If you don't understand the

terms used in the counseling session, ask! Terms such as "blood glucose level," "HDLs," "triglycerides," "anaphylactic reaction," "fortified," "saturated fat," "trans fatty acids," and "Nutrition Facts" are nutrition-related lingo. You need to know what they mean.

● *Be specific with your questions.* You're the most important person on your healthcare team. You can only comply with dietary recommendations if you have a clear understanding of the advice offered.

● *Be open to professional health advice.* For example, if your healthcare provider talks about your weight, it's for your own health benefit.

● *Keep careful eating records*—if you're asked. Record everything you eat and drink, including snacks, perhaps for several days. Write down the amounts (in cups, ounces, tablespoons, or the like) and how the foods were prepared, such as "fried" or "baked." *For a few other tips see "Dear Diary . . ." in chapter 2.*

● *Involve your family.* If you take a nutrition class or seminar or have a one-on-one meeting with a nutrition professional, bring your support along. The support of family and friends helps ensure success.

● *Follow up, as advised,* so your progress can be monitored and your questions answered. Follow-up visits are great moral support, too!

● *Stick with it!* A change in body weight, blood cholesterol levels, and other physical conditions may take time. With your healthcare provider and support team, plan for gradual results.

Be Your Own Judge!

Do you rely on popular media—magazines, newspapers, TV, the Internet—for nutrition updates? Fortunately, there's plenty of reliable nutrition information available today—shared in a context that can apply to you. Yet, the airwaves, print, and the Web are also full of nutrition hype, misleading reports, and quackery. How can you be a nutrition-savvy media consumer—and sort fact from fiction?

You Can't Judge a Book by Its Cover

Although magazine racks, bookstore shelves, newspaper columns, and the Internet bombard you with healthful eating advice, being a best-seller or a highly visible source doesn't necessarily make the advice reliable. Despite many threads of truth, the messages may be laced with misinformation or offer advice in a context that doesn't apply to you. Before you accept what you read or hear, give it a reliability check.

Who Wrote It?

Check the author's qualifications. A reputable nutrition author usually is educated in the field of nutrition, medicine, or a related specialty, with a degree or degrees from an accredited college or university. He or she usually is a credentialed member of a credible nutrition organization—for example, an RD or a DTR. Today you can find many books, magazine articles, newspaper columns, and online information written by qualified nutrition experts. *See "The Real Expert . . . Please Stand Up" in this chapter.*

Many credible writers are affiliated with an accredited university or medical center that offers nutrition or related health research, programs, or courses. An "accredited" institution generally is certified by an agency recognized by the U.S. Department of Education. Check the reference department of your local library for an institution's accreditation.

Why Was It Published?

For healthful eating advice, find resources with a balanced nutrition message meant to inform you, not advertise products to buy. As a consumer, try to analyze what's being said or implied. If it's not clear, ask a qualified nutrition expert.

Is the Nutrition Advice Credible?

Check the sources cited. Reliable advice about nutrition and active living is backed up with credible sources such as:

● *Government entities.* For example, the National Academy of Sciences/Office of Medicine, the U.S. Department of Health and Human Services (DHHS), the U.S. Department of Agriculture (USDA), and Centers for Disease Control and Prevention (CDC) base healthful eating and lifestyle guidelines on the most current research and consensus from scientific experts. Among the guidelines often cited: Dietary Reference Intakes, the Food Guide Pyramid, and the

CDC's body mass index and physical activity guidelines.

● *Credible professional nutrition and health organizations.* They, too, base their advice on sound science and government guidelines.

● *Peer-reviewed scientific journals.* Research reported in peer-reviewed journals goes through the scrutiny of several experts before it can be printed, so in medical news stories, look for the journal citing. If you choose, you can read the original research. Among the peer-reviewed journals: *New England Journal of Medicine, Lancet, Journal of the American Medical Association, and Journal of the American Dietetic Association.*

As you read, note that credible nutrition experts don't claim to have all the answers. If scientific evidence isn't conclusive or if the issues are controversial, they say so.

Check "Resources You Can Use" at the back of this book for many—but not all—government and health agencies, professional organizations, and food industry groups that provide credible information.

Have You Ever Wondered

. . . how to access credible scientific journals? University, medical school, and large urban libraries have them. With Internet access you can check online through MEDLINE, a database managed by the National Library of Medicine, a division of the U.S. National Institutes of Health. MEDLINE*plus (http://www.nlm.nih.gov/medlineplus/)* is especially designed for consumer ease; the site can link you to the National Library of Medicine's PubMed Web site *(www.ncbi.nlm.nih.gov/pubmed/)* with access to scientific journal abstracts and articles. Some journals have their own online presence, perhaps available at no charge.

. . . how to judge today's alternative-nutrition approaches? New stories about dietary supplements, herbal remedies, and holistic therapies need to stand up to the same scrutiny as any scientific research report—and the study itself needs the same rigor and precision. Testimonials and anecdotes aren't enough.

What Do Credible Experts Say?

Look for reviews by credible experts. For a book, start inside or on the cover itself, where you may find a list of reviewers. Like those of the author, reviewers' credentials or affiliations help you judge the reliability of nutrition information. *See "Nutrition in Cyberspace" in this chapter for ways to evaluate nutrition Web sites.*

Words to the Wise

"May"	Does not mean "will"
"Contributes to," "is linked to," or "is associated with"	Does not mean "causes"
"Proves"	Scientific studies gather evidence in a systematic way, but one study, taken alone, seldom proves anything.
"Breakthrough"	This happens only now and then—for example, the discovery of penicillin or polio vaccine. But today this word is so overworked as to be meaningless.
"Doubles the risk," "triples the risk"	May or may not be meaningful. Do you know what the risk was in the first place? If the risk was one in a million, and you double it, that's still only 1 in 500,000. If the risk was 1 in 100 and doubles, that's a big increase.
"Significant"	A result is "statistically significant" when the association between two factors has been found to be greater than what might occur at random (this is worked out by a mathematical formula). But people often take "significant" to mean "major" or "important."

Source: © Health Letter Associates, 1996, *www.WellnessLetter.com.*

For an expert judgment, contact a registered dietitian or other qualified nutritionist connected with a local college, university, hospital, Extension program, public health department, or in private practice.

Read between the Headlines

Every day, nutrition and health news make headlines. In this age of instant communication, research often hits the media before nutrition experts can review and interpret the findings. Today's report may appear to contradict what you heard last week. Adding to the challenge, general reporters assigned to medical stories usually need to report complex medical news quickly, in a short, simple way. The result? Consumer confusion.

Legitimate scientists aren't out to mislead you. Responsible journalists aren't, either. Uncovering the mysteries of nutrition and the human body is a complex process. As new findings emerge, research may seem to contradict itself. But differences in two or more reports reflect how scientists continue to learn—sharing research results and questioning each step along the way. Scientific debate leads to more studies. Eventually—perhaps after years of study—recommendations based on sound science (repeated, conclusive evidence) can be shared with the public. In today's popular media, you can listen to the debate.

As science unravels more about the links among nutrition, health, and chronic disease, reports heard today will eventually prove to be both true and false. You can't expect to dissect every research report. But you can use caution and common sense before jumping to conclusions and changing your food and lifestyle choices:

● *Go beyond headlines.* An attention-grabbing headline may leave a different impression than the full newspaper article or news brief itself. Read or listen to the whole story. Often response from other experts or "bottom line" advice appears at the story's end.

● *Remember—once isn't enough!* The results of one study aren't enough to change your food choices. They're just one piece of a bigger scientific puzzle. True nutrition breakthroughs take years of study and the support of repeated findings from many scientific studies. That's why health organizations, government agencies, and health experts may appear conservative; their guidance reflects consistent, well-researched findings.

● *Check the report.* Do other studies support the evidence? And does it build on what scientists know already? Responsible scientists and careful journalists report research within the context of other studies. And one study rarely changes their nutrition advice.

● *Recognize preliminary findings for what they are—preliminary!* Read them with interest. But wait for more evidence before you make major changes.

● *Look for the human dimension.* Animal studies may be among the first steps in researching a hypothesis. But the results don't always apply to humans.

● *Learn to be research-savvy.* Read more about the study itself before applying its conclusions to you. Ask yourself: Are the people studied like you—perhaps in age, gender, health, ethnicity, geographic location, and lifestyle? Did the study include a large group of people? Was the study long-range? Longer studies, with more people, more likely produce valid results. Even by asking these questions, it's hard for consumers to assess research methods. *See "Scientific Studies: Coming to Terms" in this chapter.*

● *Consider its context in the real world of healthful eating.* Does the study tell how the findings relate to overall food choices, lifestyle, and other research? A responsible report tells how research fits within the broader context of what is already known.

● *Know what the words mean.* Credible nutrition reports are careful with what they say so they won't mislead you. Research results may "suggest," but that isn't the same as "prove." And "linked to" doesn't mean "causes." *Don't jump to conclusions—get to know "Words to the Wise" on page 614.*

● *Check out the source.* Ask a qualified nutrition expert to help. Credible research comes from credible institutions and scientists, and it's reported in credible, peer-reviewed scientific and professional journals. Before nutrition research is published in reputable journals, it must meet well-established standards of nutrition research. If research is attributed simply to "they" or to some other elusive source, be wary of its results.

● *Watch for follow-up reports.* Breaking scientific news is often followed up by review and advice from nutrition experts. For example, registered dietitians often appear in media, helping to interpret news reports on nutrition issues.

Even when the research has been well conducted, different scientists may view the results differently. And it may take time for nutrition experts to study the research methods and findings. So don't always expect an immediate response. For the best news stories about health, look for those that report a full perspective, not one study.

● *Keep a healthy skepticism.* That's especially true when evaluating news about fantastic nutrition "discoveries," "ground-breaking procedures," and "revolutionary therapy." *See "Case against Health Fraud" in this chapter.*

● *Watch out for absolutes!* Responsible scientists don't claim "proof" or "cause" until repeated studies show that the findings are conclusive.

● *Seek a qualified opinion.* Take the article with you! Before you change your eating style, consult a registered dietitian, other qualified nutrition expert, or doctor. Even promising research may not apply to you. For example, a report may suggest a heart healthy benefit from red wine, but if you're taking an MAO inhibitor (an antidepressant), the combination may raise your blood pressure. So emerging science about wine may not benefit you—and drinking wine may be harmful in your case!

Nutrition in Cyberspace

Browsing the Web, you've probably noticed that food and nutrition information is proliferating in cyberspace, with thousands of health-related sites debuting each year. Search engines can quickly direct you to breaking nutrition news, sound eating advice, healthful recipes, government agencies, other credible nutrition resources, food product information, and even the chance to "chat" with a registered dietitian. However, like other media, the Internet also is littered with nutrition misinformation.

Clearing Up the Web of Confusion

How do you determine if a Web site provides information you can trust, or instead, if credible sources are quoted to "spin" a sense of legitimacy into unreliable sources? Use the same healthy skepticism with online information that you use to evaluate other nutrition information. Also ask yourself: Does it . . .

● Identify the sponsor or the owner of the site? That's your clue to the site's perspective and potential bias. The three-letter suffix on a Web site address is your first clue. Those that end in *.edu* (educational institution), *.gov* (government agencies), and perhaps *.org* (organizations, often nonprofit) tend to be the most credible. Those ending in *.com* are commercial sites and in *.net* are networks, Internet service providers, or organizations. Many *.com* sites have responsible consumer information; just be a savvy consumer.

Several new suffixes, approved for use, might be used for Web sites with nutrition and health information: *.biz* (businesses), *.coop* (business cooperatives), *.info* (general use), *.museum* (museums), *.name* (individuals), and *.pro* (professionals).

● Name contributors or perhaps an editorial board, with their credentials and perhaps an affiliation? No matter what the media, credible information comes from qualified nutrition experts. Look for a contact address or phone number if you want to talk or write directly.

Today many registered dietitians who work in consulting or private practice have personal Web sites. You can verify their RD credential by contacting the Commission on Dietetic Registration of the American Dietetic Association. *See "Resources You Can Use" at the back of this book for contact information.*

● Provide facts with cited sources, not just opinions? Look for information supported by established scientific findings.

● Link to credible online sites? Other Web sites may have supporting data or guidelines. Be aware, however, that an unreputable site may hyperlink to a credible site—perhaps a government nutrition site—to give a trustworthy perception.

● Have an educational purpose, or only a hidden guise of sound nutrition advice? If it's promotional (selling something), the information is likely biased. Since there's no peer review for online nutrition, many charlatans are selling products and "cures" with unfounded benefits or perhaps dangerous side effects.

Scientific Studies: Coming to Terms

You've read news reports of nutrition studies. But what do all the terms mean?

Bias. Problems in the study design that affect the reliability of the results; perhaps the subjects weren't chosen right.

Blind (single or double) study. Study (*single blind*) where the subjects don't know if they're in the experimental or placebo group until after the study's over; study (*double blind*) where the researchers don't know either, so they can't influence the outcome.

Clinical trial. Studies done to directly show the effectiveness and the safety of a supplement, medication, or treatment with a selected group of people.

Confounding variable. A "hidden" and related variable (perhaps an unknown phytonutrient) that the researcher attributes to something different.

Control group. The study group that doesn't have the treatment. A control group is used to know if a treatment has an effect.

Correlation. An association between two research variables, such as eating lycopene and reduced risk for prostate cancer. A correlation does not prove cause and effect, but may suggest further study.

Epidemiological study. Study of the incidence and prevalence of a health condition among a specific group of people, such as neural tube defects among newborns.

Generalizability. Describes how much research results apply to the general population of people who are like the studies' subjects.

Incidence. How many new cases of a disease or health condition as of a specific date, for a defined population.

In vitro study. Laboratory study with cells or tissue samples, usually done before an *in vivo* study.

In vivo study. Study with living subjects, either animal or human research.

Meta-analysis. A way to pool quantitative data from many studies to see what overall conclusions can be drawn, such as the pooling of more than forty studies on oats and more than twenty-five studies on soy protein to show their links to cholesterol-lowering.

Morbidity. Number of deaths in relation to a population.

Mortality. Number of people with an illness in relation to a population.

Observational study. Study that identifies a link between a health condition and behavior, such as overweight and TV-watching, but doesn't prove cause and effect.

Placebo. A "fake" treatment, perhaps a sugar pill, that appears to be the same as the treatment under study. It's used to remove bias when study subjects don't know which treatment they have.

Placebo effect. Positive results among subjects who think they're getting the real treatment.

Prevalence. How many *existing cases* of a disease or a health condition as of a specific date, for a defined population.

Prospective study. Study that poses the research questions, then follows groups of people, often for decades.

Random sample. A way to choose study subjects whereby anyone from a target population has an equal chance to be picked. In that way the results can be more easily generalized to a larger group.

Reliability. Describes research that is carefully controlled so the data can be reproduced. In other words, the researcher would get the same result with the same study subject several times.

Retrospective study. Study that uses recorded data or recall of the past. Because the study relies on memory or some variables that can't be easily controlled, this type of research has limitations.

Risk. The probability that something (perhaps a heart attack, stroke, cancer, diabetes, osteoporosis) will happen. "Risk" doesn't necessarily mean something will happen.

Risk factor. A factor that's statistically linked to the incidence of disease, such as a high BMI as a risk factor for heart disease. Again, it doesn't necessarily mean cause and effect.

Validity. The accuracy or truthfulness of the study's conclusion, and if the study measured what it meant to study.

Variable. A factor such as age, gender, or food choices in a study that differs among the people being studied. An *independent variable* is the one being studied; a *dependent variable,* perhaps lower blood sugar level or LDL cholesterol level, happens as a result of the treatment.

Adapted from source: Reprinted with permission of the International Food Information Council Foundation, Washington, D.C.

● Indicate regular updates and postings? Credible Web sites are updated often to offer the most current advice. **Caution:** Being current doesn't necessarily make it accurate.

● Provide sound information, not just "bells and whistles"?

● Pass other credibility tests? *See "Read between the Headlines" in this chapter.* Anyone can launch a site. Like any media report, being on the Internet doesn't ensure reliability.

● Have a nutrition expert as a host for forums and chatrooms? Many unsponsored bulletin boards bring interested people together, with chat from undisclosed sources who often aren't experts. Be wary!

"Well" Connected Links

Search engines list legitimate and less reliable Web sites side-by-side; you need skills to sort them out. That's why it's wise to tap health-related resources that indicate high standards:

● Use gateway sites that link to responsible organizations—for example, the U.S. Department of Health and Human Services' Healthfinder (*http://www. healthfinder.gov*) hyperlinks to hundreds of responsible sites, as does the gateway in the American Dietetic Association's site (*www.eatright.org*).

● Check with a reputable Web site that rates other sites, such as Tufts Nutrition Navigator (*http://www. navigator.tufts.edu*).

● Review more than one Web site for information on the same nutrition topic; use several search engines. With information often in "sound bites," usually one site isn't complete enough.

● Look for sites with the HON-code symbol, showing they adhere to the HONcode (Health On the Net Foundation) principles. An example: the WebMD Web site, which provides online, consumer-focused health information (*www.webmd.com*). These sites voluntarily comply with a code of conduct for health and medical Web sites. HON is an honor symbol and system, so still be a careful consumer of the Web site's information.

Have You Ever Wondered

. . . how to judge food scares that circulate through e-mail? Being 100 percent sure about these food scares takes research. What appears in your e-mail is likely a hoax (1) if it wasn't written by the e-mail sender, (2) if you're asked to forward the e-mail, (3) if it claims not to be a hoax or an urban legend, (4) if it appeals to your emotions, and (5) if it doesn't cite a legitimate source or a credible Web site. Read critically for obvious false claims, poor logic, and lack of common sense. If you're still not sure, you might check Web sites such as *http://www.quackwatch.com* or *http://www. urbanlegends.com* that debunk food myths.

● Ask a nutrition expert, such as an RD or a DTR, who has a quick ability to see nuances of Web site bias and inaccuracy. If you find news of interest on the Internet, such as about a phytonutrient link to health, or a dietary supplement, print the information with the name and address of the Web site; take it to your healthcare provider or a nutrition expert for a perspective.

To find reliable nutrition and health Web sites, see "Resources You Can Use" at the back of this book.

E-Nutrition Advice: Just for You

With a few mouse clicks, you can calculate your BMI, assess your day's food choices, even tie in to online weight control counseling and support. Before using a search engine, consider this:

● If you wish, use quick, online assessments to become aware of your own food choices and perhaps health issues, but not to replace your healthcare provider. For a reliable diagnosis and prescribed eating plan, see a qualified healthcare provider in person, who also can review your medical history. You can't easily check credentials for a Web site healthcare provider.

● For the same reasons, get advice or a prescription for a dietary supplement from your doctor. As an aside, buying supplements online may, or may not, cost less, and the quality is uneven.

● Even on trustworthy healthcare sites that do online

nutrition assessments and counseling, there's a wrinkle: *privacy.* To protect the privacy of your records and avoid a Pandora's box of e-marketing, provide personal data on encrypted, or secured, sites only. If a "closed padlock" appears on the Web page, the data you provide are encrypted and secure. And pay attention to "alarms" on the site that warn that you're moving from secure to insecure parts of the Web site.

Case against Health Fraud

Can you "lose weight while you sleep"? Can a dietary supplement assure "no more arthritic pain" or "cure for AIDS"? Can a device guarantee "a bigger bustline" or "spot reduction"?

Americans spend billions of dollars annually on products and services that make such claims. Health quackery is the most common type of fraud aimed at the elderly and others. Easy remedies are hard to resist! Yet many are simply useless; others, potentially harmful. Either way, it's health fraud.

Nutrition quackery thrives among people who are uninformed or already misinformed, desperate for help, overconfident about possible risks, or alienated from traditional healthcare. And quacks can more easily manipulate those people who are already leaning in their direction, perhaps with ploys that seem reasonable: "We really care about you," "What have you got to lose?," "Science doesn't have all the answers," or "We treat medicine's failures."

Health fraud means promoting, for financial gain, a health remedy that doesn't work—or hasn't yet been proven to work. The remedy may be a device, treatment, service, plan, special foods, or other product. Although fraud is rampant in many areas of health, often it's linked to nutrition—perhaps to a dietary supplement, a herbal product, a weight-loss device, or a new diet program.

So what is quackery? The term comes from the term "quacksalver," referring to medieval peddlers of salves who sounded like quacking ducks when they used their voices to promote their wares. That's why they were called "quacks."

Quacks promote health fraud. Their motivation may be strictly financial gain. But often, quacks sincerely believe in the value of their product, treatment,

or service. They don't mean to deceive you. Instead, they lack scientific understanding.

Health fraud and quackery have grown dramatically in the past several decades. Why such growth? Among the reasons, there's an unprecedented interest in personal healthcare. In general, people today take more personal responsibility for staying healthy. That interest has created a huge demand for products and services that promote health. Legitimate business uses this opportunity to provide products, treatments, and services that do have scientifically proven benefits. But this same wave of interest also has spawned a fanfare of health fraud and quackery, leaving people more vulnerable than ever.

With looser government regulation, the misuse of dietary supplements—and quackery surrounding them—have grown dramatically. Today supplement manufacturers need to prove harm, not safety. That allows claims for supplements to appear more credible than they really are. *For more about the use and abuse of supplements, see chapter 23.*

There's another common reason for the growth of health fraud. Some people expect a quick or easy "health fix." They may count on today's "medicine" to undo the results of an unhealthful lifestyle. However, it's not that simple—even if quacks lead you to believe otherwise.

What Are the Consequences?

Nutrition quackery exploits consumers, and it carries significant health and economic risks along the way. Among them:

● *False hopes.* Dream on! Quacks may promise—but unsound nutrition advice, products, or services won't prevent or cure disease.

● *A substitute for reliable healthcare.* False hopes, created through quackery, may delay or replace proper health promotion, medical care, or follow-up treatment. If you follow the advice of quackery, you may lose something you can't retrieve: time for effective treatment!

● *Interference with sound eating and lifestyle habits.* That happens when quackery replaces proven guidance.

● *Unneeded expense.* In the best-case scenario, some

products and services touted by quacks simply don't work—and cause no harm, either. Why waste your hard-earned money on devices, products, and services that have no effect?

● *Potential harm.* Nutrition quackery also can put your health at risk. Taking very large doses of some vitamins and minerals, in the form of dietary supplements, can have toxic side effects. For example, excessive amounts of vitamin A during pregnancy increase the chances of birth defects. Inappropriate supplement use can lead to harmful drug-nutrient interactions. For example, taking vitamin K can be risky if you take blood-thinning drugs. *For more about specific vitamins and minerals see chapter 4.*

Over-the-counter herbal products, marketed as dietary supplements, are sources of potent drugs. Yet, unlike medications, herbal products aren't well regulated. *See "Herbals and Other Botanicals: Help or Harm?" in chapter 23.*

Quackery: What You Can Do

No one has to be the victim of nutrition fraud. To protect yourself, you just need to know how to identify fraud and quackery, and where to find sound nutrition information.

● Retain a healthy skepticism as your best defense against a "quack attack." And take time to be well informed before you invest in a nutrition product, treatment, or service. *Give it the "Ten Questions" test on page 621 before you buy.*

● Seek advice from reliable sources. If you're suspicious about a statement, product, or service, contact a credible nutrition source—for example, a registered dietitian, your public health department, the medical or nutrition department of a nearby college or university, or your county Extension office. *See "Need Nutrition Advice?" in this chapter.*

● Report nutrition fraud. If you suspect that a statement, product, or service is fraudulent or false, inquire with the appropriate government agency or file a complaint.

To the Postal Service. Contact your postmaster or someone else in the Postal Service if you've been the victim—or target—of nutrition fraud through the mail. It's illegal to use the Postal Service to make false claims about or to sell fraudulent products or services.

To the FDA. Make inquiries or file complaints about false claims for dietary supplements with the U.S. Food and Drug Administration (FDA). That includes concerns about inadequate information on package labels.

To the FTC. For questions or concerns about false or misleading claims in advertising, contact the Federal Trade Commission (FTC).

Have You Ever Wondered

. . . how to check out diet scams? Besides talking with a nutrition expert, check the Federal Trade Commission (*http://www.ftc.gov*), which may list diet scams it's prosecuted.

Ten Red Flags of Junk Science

A new health or nutrition report? Before you jump to conclusions, check it out. Any combination of these signs should send up a red flag of suspicion.

1. Recommendations that promise a quick fix.
2. Dire warnings of danger from a single product or regimen.
3. Claims that sound too good to be true.
4. Simplistic conclusions drawn from a complex study.
5. Recommendations based on a single study.
6. Dramatic statements that are refuted by reputable scientific organizations.
7. Lists of "good" and "bad" foods.
8. Recommendations made to help sell a product.
9. Recommendations based on studies published without peer review.
10. Recommendations from studies that ignore differences among individuals or groups.

Source: Developed by the Food and Nutrition Science Alliance (FANSA).

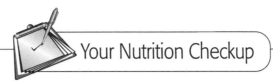

Play "Ten Questions"

Suspicious when something sounds too good to be true? To avoid the lure, arm yourself with these questions—even when you aren't suspicious!

Ask: Does the promotion of a nutrition product, regimen, service, treatment, or device . . .

Yes	No	
☐	☐	**1.** Try to lure you with scare tactics, emotional appeals, or perhaps with a "money-back guarantee" rather than proven results?
☐	☐	**2.** Promise to "revitalize," "detoxify," or "balance your body with nature"? Or does it claim to increase your stamina, stimulate your body's healing power, or boost your energy level?
☐	☐	**3.** Offer "proof" based on personal anecdotes or testimonials rather than sound science?
☐	☐	**4.** Advise supplements as "insurance" for everyone? Or recommend very large doses of nutrients? "Very large" means significantly more than 100 percent of the Daily Values (DVs). *See the Appendices for DV levels.*
☐	☐	**5.** Claim it can "treat," "cure," or "prevent" diverse health problems . . . from arthritis to cancer to sexual impotence?
☐	☐	**6.** Make unrealistic claims such as "reverse the aging process" or "cure disease" or "quick, easy approach"?
☐	☐	**7.** Blame the food supply as the source of health or behavior problems? Belittle government regulations? Or discredit the advice of recognized medical authorities?
☐	☐	**8.** Claim that its "natural" benefits surpass those of "synthetic" products?
☐	☐	**9.** Mention a "secret formula"? Or fail to list ingredients on its product label or to state any possible side effects?
☐	☐	**10.** Come from a "nutrition expert" without accepted credentials? Does that person also sell the product?

Now score yourself:

In this game of "Ten Questions," you might spot quackery with just one "yes" answer! Here's why.

1. *Fact:* Playing on emotion, misinformation, or even fear is common among nonscientific pseudo-experts. Emotional words used to promote a product can be an instant tip-off to quackery: "guaranteed," "breakthrough," and "miraculous" are used for emotional appeal. *For a list of commonly used terms, see "Spotting a Fraud" in chapter 2.* So are false claims that most Americans are poorly nourished or that foods or additives are "deadly poisons."

2. *Fact:* Pseudo-medical jargon such as "detoxify," "rejuvenate," or "balance your body chemistry" suggests misinformation. These terms have no meaning in physiology. To sort valid medical terms from hype, ask a credible expert to decipher any confusing terms or phrases. A supplement can't increase

your strength, immunity, stamina, or energy level, either. *For more about supplements promoted to athletes see "Ergogenic Aids—No Substitute for Training" in chapter 19.* "Ergogenic" means the potential to increase work output; a supplement can't do that!

3. *Fact:* Nutrition is a science based on fact, not emotion or belief. Be skeptical of case histories and testimonials from satisfied users—if that's the only proof that a product works. Instead look for medical evidence from a reputable institution or a qualified health expert. Without scientific evidence, a reported "cure" may have other causes. Sometimes the ailment disappears on its own. The "cure" actually may have a placebo effect; its benefit may be psychological, not physical. The person may have been misdiagnosed in the first place. And even chronic ailments don't always have symptoms all the time.

4. *Fact:* Everyone does *not* need a vitamin supplement! Most healthy people can get enough nutrients by following a varied, balanced eating plan with enough servings from the Food Guide Pyramid. Quacks rarely say who does *not* need a supplement. *See "The Food Guide Pyramid: Your Healthful Eating Guide" in chapter 10.*

For most people, there's no added benefit from taking more than 100 percent of the DVs for vitamins and minerals. Except for a nutrition deficiency, there's no proof that nutrients alone prevent or cure anything. So ignore the hype! On the contrary, taking too much may be harmful. *See chapter 23, "Supplements: Use and Abuse."*

5. *Fact:* No nutrition regimen, device, or product can treat all that ails you. And they can't cure many health conditions, including arthritis, cancer, and sexual impotence. Even when they're part of credible treatment or prevention strategies, nutrition factors are typically just one part of overall healthcare.

6. *Fact:* Most health-promoting approaches take some effort. Claims that sound too good to be true probably are. But quacks know that's what people want to hear. Quackery thrives because people want simple cures and magic ways to change what's imperfect.

7. *Fact:* Quacks often belittle the regular food supply, government regulation, and the established medical community. They even claim that the traditional health community is suppressing their work. Instead they call for "freedom of choice". . . and describe unproved methods as alternatives to current, proven methods. However, alternatives promoted through quackery are typically untested and may be ineffective or even unsafe. Among well-researched methods, you'll find choices.

By discrediting traditional approaches, quacks are attempting to funnel your healthcare dollars toward their own financial gain.

8. *Fact:* There's nothing magical about products promoted as "natural." From the standpoint of science, the chemical structure of natural and synthetic dietary supplements is essentially the same. And the body uses them in the same manner. (There's one exception: "natural" vitamin E is more potent than its synthetic form.) Herbal products aren't necessarily safe just because they're "natural." Even substances found in nature can have natural toxins, with potent, druglike effects.

9. *Fact:* By law, a medication must carry product information on its packaging. That includes the product's ingredients, use, dosage, warnings, precautions, and what to do if adverse reactions occur. However, products or regimens sold through quackery may not report all this information, including potential side effects or dangers.

10. *Fact:* Quacks are typically salespeople. Rather than offering accurate advice, their bottom line is to sell you something. Be wary when someone tries to diagnose your health status, then offers to sell you a remedy, such as a routine dietary supplement.

Be wary of the methods used to assess your health or need for supplements. Many invalid tests may be hard to distinguish from legitimate clinical assessments. Those often used by quacks include hair analysis, iridology, and herbal crystallization analysis, among others. Computerized questionnaires can't supply enough information either to determine your need for a supplement. Get an opinion from a qualified health professional before getting these assessments or making changes based on the results.

Quackery underlies many regimens focused on weight loss or gain, too. *To judge programs for their effectiveness and safety see "Questions to Ask . . . About Diet Programs" in chapter 2.*

Resources You Can Use

Looking for sound nutrition information? You have many reliable resources: professional associations, health agencies, government agencies, and credible nutrition newsletters. Besides brochures, booklets, and consumer hotlines, many provide reliable on-line nutrition information. Your local hospital, public health, extension service, and many food industry groups are other reliable resources you might tap.

General Nutrition

American Dietetic Association
216 West Jackson Boulevard
Chicago, IL 60606-6995
Online: *http://www.eatright.org*
Consumer Nutrition Hotline:
800/366-1655 for recorded messages in English or Spanish, or to obtain a referral to a registered dietitian in your area

Center for Nutrition Policy and Promotion
U.S. Department of Agriculture
1120 20th Street, NW, North Lobby, Suite 200
Washington, DC 20036
202/418-2312
Online: *http://www.cnpp.usda.com*

Cooperative Extension Service
(Contact your state's land-grant university.)

Food and Nutrition Information Center
National Agricultural Library
U.S. Department of Agriculture, Room 304
10301 Baltimore Avenue
Beltsville, MD 20705-2351
301/504-5719
Online: *http://www.usda.gov/fnic*

International Food Information Council (IFIC)
1100 Connecticut Avenue, NW, Suite 430
Washington, DC 20036
202/296-6540
Online: *http://ific.org*

National Academy of Sciences/Food and Nutrition Board
2101 Constitution Avenue, NW
Washington, DC 20418
202/334-1732
Online: *http://www.nas.edu*

Nutrition, Health, and Food Management Division
American Association of Family and Consumer Sciences
1555 King Street
Alexandria, VA 22314
703/706-4600
Online: *http://www.aafcs.org*

Society for Nutrition Education
9202 North Meridian Street, Suite 200
Indianapolis, IN 76260
317/571-5618

U.S. Government (gateway to nutrition sites)
Online: *http://www.nutrition.gov*
Online: *http://www.heathfinder.gov*

Dietary Supplements

Food and Drug Administration
Online: *http://www.cfsan.fda.gov/~dms/supplmnt.html*

National Center for Alternative and Complementary Care
NCCAM Clearinghouse
P.O. Box 7923
Gaithersburg, MD 20898
888/644-6226
Online: *http://nccam.nih.gov/fcp/*

U.S. Pharmacopoeia
12601 Twinbrook Parkway
Rockville, MD 20852
800/822-8772
Online: *http://www.usp.org/frameset.htm*

Food Safety, Labeling, and Advertising

American Association of Poision Control Centers
National hotline to local centers:
1-800-222-1222

CDC's National Prevention Information Network
Clearinghouse for HIV/AIDs, STDs, and TB Material
P.O. Box 6003
Rockville, MD 20849-6003
800/458-5231
Online: *http://www.cdcpin.org*

Center for Food Safety and Applied Nutrition
CFSAN Outreach and Information Center
200 C Street, SW (HFS-555)
Washington, DC 20204
888-723-3366 or 888/SAFE-FOOD
Online: *http://www.vm.cfsan.fda.gov*

FDA's Food Information and Seafood Hotline
888-723-3366
FDA's MEDWatch Program
800/FDA-1088

Federal Trade Commission (FTC)
600 Pennsylvania Avenue, NW, Room 130
Washington, DC 20580
Online: *http://www.ftc.gov*
Consumer number: 877/FTC-HELP
(Or contact your regional FTC office.)

Food and Drug Administration (FDA)
Consumer Information Office
5600 Fishers Lane, HFI-40 or HF-12
Rockville, MD 20857
301/827-7130
(Or contact your regional FDA office.)
Online: *http://www.fda.gov*

Food Safety and Inspection Service
U.S. Department of Agriculture
14th Street and Independence Avenue, SW
Washington, D.C. 20250
202/720-2791

Food Safety and Inspection *(continued)*
USDA's Meat and Poultry Hotline
800/535-4555
Online: *http://fsis.usda.gov/OA/
   programs/mphotlin.htm*

National Lead Information Center
1019 19th Street, NW, Suite 401
Washington, DC 20036
800/532-3394
Online: *http://epa.gov/lead*

U.S. Environmental Protection Agency
Areil Rios Building
1200 Pennsylvania Avenue, NW
Washington, DC 20490
Online: *http://www.epa.gov*
Drinking Water Hotline
800/426-4791

**U.S. Government (gateway to food
   safety sites)**
Online: *http://www.foodsafety.gov*

Food Sensitivities

**American Academy of Allergy, Asthma,
   and Immunology**
611 East Wells Street
Milwaukee, WI 53202
414/272-6071
Online: *http://www.aaaai.org*

American Celiac Society
59 Crystal Avenue
West Orange, NJ 07052-3570
973/325-8837

Celiac Sprue Association/USA
P.O. Box 31700
Omaha, NE 68131-0700
402/558-0600
Online: *http://www.csaceliacs.org*

Children's P.K.U. Network
3970 Via de la Valle, Suite 116E
Del Mar, CA 92014
858/509-0767
Online: *http://www.rarediseases.org*

Food Allergy and Anaphylaxis Network
10400 Eaton Place, Suite 107
Fairfax, VA 22030-2208
703/691-3179
Online: *http://www.foodallergy.org*

**Gluten Intolerance Group of North
   America**
15110 10th Avenue, Suite A
Seattle, WA 98166-1820
206/246-6531
Online: *http://www.gluten.net*

P.K.U. Parents
8 Myrtle Lane
San Anselmo, CA 94960
415/457-4632

Maternal, Infant, Child, and Adolescent Nutrition

American Academy of Pediatrics
141 Northwest Point Boulevard
Elk Grove Village, IL 60007-1098
847/434-4000
Online: *http://www.aap.org*

**American Foundation for Maternal
   and Child Health**
439 East 51st Street, 4th Floor
New York, NY 10022
212/759-5510

**American School Food Service
   Association**
700 South Washington Street, Suite 200
Alexandria, VA 22314
703/739-3900
Online: *http://www.asfsa.org*

La Leche League International
P.O. Box 4079
Schaumburg, IL 60173-4079
800/LALECHE (800/525-3243) or
   847/519-7730
Online: *http://www.lalecheleague.org*

Nutrition and Aging

**American Association of Retired
   Persons**
601 E Street, NW
Washington, DC 20049
202/434-2277
Online: *http://www.aarp.org*

Elder Care Locator
927 15th Street, NW, 6th Floor
Washington, DC 20005
800/677-1116
Online: *http://www.n4a.org*

**National Association of Area Agencies
   on Aging**
927 15th Street, NW, 6th Floor
Washington, DC 20005
202/296-8130
Online: *http://www.n4a.org*

**National Institute on Aging
   Information Office**
Building 31, Room 5C-27
31 Center Drive, MSC 2292

Bethesda, MD 20892
301/496-1752
Online: *http://www.nih.gov/nia*

General Health and Disease Prevention/Treatment

General

**American Academy of Family
   Physicians**
11400 Tomahawk Creek Parkway
Leawood, KS 66211-2672
800-274-2237 or 913-906-6000
Online: *http://www.aafp.org*

American Health Foundation
1 Dana Road
Valhalla, NY 10595
914/592-2600
Online: *http://www.ahf.org*

American Medical Association
515 North State Street
Chicago, IL 60610-4377
312/464-5000
Online: *http://www.ama-assn.org*

American Public Health Association
800 I Street, NW
Washington, DC 20001
202/777-2752
Online: *http://www.apha.org*

**Centers for Disease Control and
   Prevention**
1600 Clifton Road Northeast
Atlanta, GA 30333
404/639-3311 or 800/311-3435
Online: *http://www.cdc.gov*

Congress for National Health
National Wellness Institute
P.O. Box 827
Stevens Point, WI 54481-0827
715/342-2969
Online: *http://www.nationalwellness.org*

Minority Health Resource Center
P.O. Box 37337
Washington, DC 20013-7337
800/444-6472
Online: *http://www.omhrc.org*

National Center for Health Statistics
U.S. Department of Health and Human
   Services
6525 Belcrest Road, Room 1064
Hyattsville, MD 20782-2003
301/458-4636
Online: *http://www.cdc.gov/nchs*

National Health Information Center
P.O. Box 1133
Washington, DC 20013-1133
301/565-4167 or 800/336-4797
Online: *http://www.health.gov/nhic*
Toll-free health information:
http://www.health.gov/NHIC/Pubs/tollfree.htm
Federal health information and clearinghouses: *http://www.health.gov/NHIC/Pubs/clearinghouses.htm*

National Institutes of Health
9000 Rockville Pike
Bethesda, MD 20892
301/496-4000
Online: *http://www.nih.gov/health*

U.S. Department of Health and Human Services
200 Independence Avenue, SW
Washington, DC 20201
202/619-0257
Online: *http://www.hhs.gov*
Online: *http://www.healthfinder.gov*

Alcoholism

National Clearinghouse for Alcohol and Drug Information
11426 Rockville Pike, Suite 200
Rockville, MD 20852
301/468-2600 or 800-729-6686
Online: *http://www.health.org/nhic*

National Council on Alcoholism and Drug Dependence
20 Exchange Place, Suite 2902
New York, NY 10005
212/269-7797
Online: *http://www.ncadd.org*

Cancer

American Cancer Society
1599 Clifton Road, NE
Atlanta, GA 30329-4251
404/320-3333 or 800/227-2345
Online: *http://www.cancer.org*

American Institute for Cancer Research
1759 R Street, NW
Washington, DC 20009
202/328-7744
Online: *http://www.aicr.org*

National Cancer Institute
NCI Inquiries Office
Building 31, Room 10A0331, Center Drive, MSC 2580

Bethesda, MD 20892-2580
800/4-CANCER (800/422-6237) or 301/435-3848
Online: *http://www.nci.nih.gov*
Online: *http://www.5aday.gov*

Cardiovascular (Heart) Disease

American Heart Association
7272 Greenville Avenue
Dallas, TX 75231-4596
214/706-1173 or 800/AHA-USA1 (800/242-8721)
Online: *http://www.americanheart.org*

National Cholesterol Education Program and National Heart, Lung, and Blood Institute
P.O. Box 30105
Bethesda, MD 20824-0105
301/592-8573
Online: *http://www.nhlbi.nih.gov/*

Diabetes

American Diabetes Association
Attn.: Customer Service
1701 North Beauregard Street
Alexandria, VA 22314
800/342-2383
Online: *http://www.diabetes.org*

Joslin Diabetes Center
Nutrition Services
Joslin Clinic
1 Joslin Place
Boston, MA 02215
617/732-2400
Online: *http://www.joslin.org*

Juvenile Diabetes Foundation International
120 Wall Street
New York, NY 10005
212/785-9500
800/JDF-CURE (800/533-2873)
Online: *http://www.jdf.org*

National Diabetes Information Clearinghouse
1 Information Way
Bethesda, MD 20892-3560
301/654-3327 or 800/860-8747
Online: *http://www.niddk.nih.gov/health/diabetes*

Digestive Disease

Digestive Disease National Coalition
507 Capitol Court NE, Suite 200

Washington, DC 20002
202/544-7497
Online: *http://www.ddnc.org*

National Digestive Diseases Information Clearinghouse
2 Information Way
Bethesda, MD 20892-3570
301/654-3810 or 800/891-5389
Online: *http://www.niddk.nih.gov/health/digest*

Eating Disorders

National Association of Anorexia Nervosa and Associated Disorders
P.O. Box 7
Highland Park, IL 60035
847/831-3438

National Eating Disorders Organization
6655 South Yale Avenue
Tulsa, OK 74136
918/481-4044
Online: *http://www.kidsource.com/nedo*

Oral Health

American Dental Association
211 East Chicago Avenue
Chicago, IL 60611
312/440-2500
Online: *http://www.ada.org*

Osteoporosis

National Osteoporosis Foundation
1232 22nd Street, NW
Washington, DC 20037-1292
202/223-2226 or 800/223-9994
Online: *http://www.nof.org*

Weight

Healthy Weight Network
402 South 14th Street
Hettinger, ND 58639
701/567-2646 – fax
Online: *www.healthyweight.net*

Overeaters Anonymous
6075 Zenith Court, NE
Rio Rancho, NM 87124
505/891-2664
Online: *http://www.overeatersanonymous.org*

Shape Up America
6707 Democracy Boulevard, Suite 306
Bethesda, MD 20817
Online: *http://www.shapeup.org*

Sports Nutrition and Physical Activity

American Alliance for Health, Physical Education, Recreation, and Dance
1900 Association Drive
Reston, VA 20191-1598
703/476-3400
Online: *http://www.aahperd.org*

American College of Sports Medicine
401 West Michigan Street
Indianapolis, IN 46202-3233
317/637-9200
Online: *http://www.acsm.org*

American Council on Exercise
5820 Oberlin Drive, Suite 102
San Diego, CA 92121-3787
Consumer Fitness Hotline
800/529-8227 or 800/825-3626

American Running and Fitness Association
4405 East-West Highway, Suite 405
Bethesda, MD 20814
301/913-9517 or 800/776-ARFA (-2732)
Online: *http://www.americanrunning.org*

Fifty-Plus Fitness Association
P.O. Box 20230
Stanford, CA 94309
415/323-6160
Online: *http://www.50plus.org*

International Center for Sports Nutrition
502 South 44th Street, Suite 3012
Omaha, NE 68105-1065
402/559-5505

National Fitness and Wellness Coalition
1800 Silas Deane Highway
Rocky Hill, CT 06067
203/721-1055

President's Council on Physical Fitness and Sports
Hubert H. Humphrey Building
200 Independence Avenue, SW
Washington, DC 20201
202/690-9000
Online: *http://www.surgeongeneral. gov/ophs/pcpfs.htm*

Women's Sports Foundation
Eisenhower Park
East Meadow, NY 11554
800/227-3988

YMCA of the USA
101 North Wacker Drive
Chicago, IL 60606
800/USA-YMCA (800/872-9622) or 312/977-0031

Vegetarian Eating

North American Vegetarian Society
P.O. Box 72
Dolgeville, NY 13329
518/568-7970
Online: *http://www.navs-online.org*

Vegetarian Resource Group
P.O. Box 1463
Baltimore, MD 21203
410/366-VEGE (8343)
Online: *http://www.vrg.org*

Food Technology/Biotechnology

Functional Foods for Health
University of Illinois at Urbana-Champaign, Chicago
1302 West Pennsylvania Avenue
Urbana, IL 61801
217/333-6364
Online: *http://www.ag.uiuc.edu/ffh*

International Food Additives Council
5775 Peachtree-Dunwoody Road, Suite 500-G
Atlanta, GA 30342
404/252-3663

International Food Biotechnology Council
1126 16th Street, NW
Washington, DC 20036
202/659-0074

Office of Biotechnology
Food and Drug Administration
200 C Street, SW
Washington, DC 20204
202/205-4144

Health Fraud

Consumer Health Research Institute
300 East Pink Hill Road
Independence, MO 64057
816/228-4595
Online: *http://www.ncahf.org*

National Council against Health Fraud, Inc.
P.O. Box 141
Fort Lee, NJ 07024
201/723-2955
Online: *http://www.cahf.org*

Quackwatch, Inc.
Online: *http://www.quackwatch.com*

Food Industry Associations

Almond Board of California
1150 Ninth Street, Suite 1500
Modesto, CA 95354
209/549-8262
Online: *http://www.AlmondsAreIn.com http://www.GetYourE.org*

American Dry Bean Board
115 Railway Street
Scottsbluff, NE 69361
Online: *http://www.americanbean.org*

American Egg Board
1460 Renaissance Drive
Park Ridge, IL 60068
847/296-7043
Online: *http://www.aeb.org*

California Olive Oil Council
PO Box 7520
Berkeley, CA 94707
888/718-9830
Online: *http://www.cooc.com/home.html*

Calorie Control Council
5775 Peachtree-Dunwoody Road, Suite 500-G
Atlanta, GA 30342
404/252-3663
Online: *http://www.caloriecontrol.org*

Canned Food Alliance
6 PPG Place 14th Floor
Pittsburgh, PA 15222
412/456-3596
Online: *http://www.mealtime.org*

Distilled Spirits Council of the United States
1250 Eye Street NW, Suite 400
Washington, DC 20005
202/682-8837
Online: *http://www.discus.org*

Flax Council of Canada
465-176 Lombard Avenue
Winnipeg, MB
Canada R3B 0T6
(204) 982-2115
Online: *http://www.flaxcouncil.ca*

Food Marketing Institute
655 15th Street, NW
Washington, DC 20005
202/452-8444
Online: *http://www.fmi.org*

Glutamate Association
555 13th N Street, NW
Atlanta, GA 30342
202/783-6135
Online: *http://www.msgfacts.com*

Infant Formula Council
5775 Peachtree-Dunwoody Road,
    Suite 500-G
Atlanta, GA 30342
404/252-3663

International Bottled Water
    Association
1700 Diagonal Road, Suite 650
Alexandria, VA 22314
703/683-5213 or 800/WATER11
Online: *http://www.bottledwater.org*

National Cattlemen's Beef Association
5420 South Quebec Street
Greenwood Village, CO 80111
303/694-0305
Online: *http://www.beef.org*

National Chicken Council
1055 15th Street, NW, Suite 930
Washington, DC 20005
202/296-2622
Online: *http://www.eatchicken.com*

National Coffee Association
15 Maiden Lane, Suite 1405
New York, NY 10038
212/766-4007
Online: *http://www.ncausa.org*

National Dairy Council (Dairy
    Management, Inc.)
O'Hare International Center
10255 West Higgins Road, Suite 900
Rosemont, IL 60018-5616
847/803-2000 or 800/426-8271
Online: *http://www.dairyinfo.com*

National Fisheries Institute, Inc.
1901 North Fort Myer Drive, Suite 700
Arlington, VA 22209
703/524-8880

National Pasta Association
2102 Wilson Boulevard, Suite 920
Arlington, VA 22201
202/637-5888
Online: *http://ilovepasta.org*

National Potato Promotion Board
1050 Battery Street
San Francisco, CA 94111
415/984-6143
Online: *http://www.potatohelp.com*

National Pork Producers Council
P.O. Box 10383
Des Moines, IA 50306
515/223-2600
Online: *http://www.nppc.org*

National Restaurant Association
1200 17th Street, NW
Washington, DC 20036-3097
202/331-5900 or 800/424-5156
Online: *http://www.restaurant.org*

The Peanut Institute
2336 Lake Park Drive
Albany, GA 31707
888/8PEANUT
Online: *http://www.peanut-institute.org*

National Turkey Federation
1225 New York Ave., NW, Suite 400
Washington, DC 20005
202/898-0100
Online: *http://www.turkeyfed.org*

Produce for Better Health Foundation
5-A-Day Program
5301 Limestone Road, Suite 101
Wilmington, DE 19808-1249
302/738-7100
Online: *http://www.5aday.com*

Produce Marketing Association
1500 Casho Mill Road
P.O. Box 6036
Newark, DE 19714-6036
302/738-7100
Online: *http://www.pma.com*

Rice Council of the USA
6699 Rookin Street
Houston, TX 77074
713/270-6699
Online: *http://www.USArice.com*

Snack Food Association
1711 King Street, Suite One
Alexandria, VA 22314
703/836-4500 or 800/628-1334
Online: *http://www.sfa.org*

The Sugar Association, Inc.
1101 15th Street, NW, Suite 600
Washington, DC 20005
202/785-1122
Online: *http://www.sugar.org*

The Tea Council of the U.S.A.
420 Lexington Avenue, Suite 825
New York, NY 10170
212/986-6998
Online: *http://www.teausa.com*

United Fresh Fruit & Vegetable
    Association
727 North Washington Street
Alexandria, VA 22314
703/836-3410
Online: *http://www.uffva.org*

United Soybean Board
16640 Chesterfield Grove Road,
    Suite 130
Chesterfield, MO 63005
800/989-8721
Online: *http://www.soybean.org*

Wheat Foods Council
19841 Crossroads Drive, Suite 105
Parker, CO 80138
303/840-8787
Online: *http://www.wheatfoods.org*

Nutrition Newsletters

Consumer Reports on Health
101 Truman Avenue
Yonkers, NY 10708
914/378-2300
Online: *http://www.consumerreports.org*

Environmental Nutrition
52 Riverside Drive, Suite 15-A
New York, NY 10024-6599
Online: *http://www.
    environmentalnutrition.com*

FDA Consumer
Superintendent of Documents
U.S. Government Printing Office
Washington, DC 20401
202/512-1800
Online: *http://www.bookstore.gpo.gov/*

Food & Fitness Advisor
The Center for Women's Health
Weill Medical College of Cornell
    University
P.O. Box 420235
Palm Coast, FL 32142-0235
800/829-2505

Mayo Clinic Health Letter
Subscription Services
P.O. Box 53889
Boulder, CO 80321
800/333-9037
Online: *http://www.mayohealth.org*

Tufts University Health and
    Nutrition Letter
10 High Street, Suite 706
Boston, MA 01220
Online: *http://www.healthletter.tufts.edu*

University of California, Berkeley
    Wellness Letter
Health Letter Associates
P.O. Box 420148
Palm Coast, FL 32142
800/829-9080

Appendices

1997–2001 Dietary Reference Intakes

Recommended Dietary Allowances and Adequate Intakes

The Dietary Reference Intakes—established by the Food and Nutrition Board of the National Academy of Sciences—include Recommended Dietary Allowances (RDAs) and Adequate Intakes (AIs). RDA levels meet the nutrient needs for most healthy people; AIs have been established for nutrients without enough scientific evidence for an RDA. Still, they're goals to strive for.

As always, the best way to consume enough of these nutrients is to follow guidance from the Food Guide Pyramid. *See "Nutrients: How Much?" in chapter 1 for more about the DRIs.*

Tolerable Upper Intake Levels

Tolerable Upper Intake Levels (ULs), also part of the DRIs, represent the maximum intake that probably won't pose risks for health problems for most people. With so many fortified foods and nutrient supplements, be aware of excessive levels!

Protein: 1989 Recommended Dietary Allowances

Recommended Dietary Allowances also are set for protein. New recommendations for macronutrients, including protein, as well as fiber, are scheduled for release in 2002.

AGE		PROTEIN (GRAMS)
Infants	0–6 months	13
	6–12 months	14
Children	1–3 years	16
	4–6	24
	7–10	28
Males	11–14 years	45
	15–18	59
	19–24	58
	25–50	63
	51+	63
Females	11–14 years	46
	15–18	44
	19–24	46
	25-50	50
	51+	50
Pregnant		60
Lactating	1st 6 months	65
	2nd 6 months	62

Source: Adapted with permission from National Academy of Sciences, *Recommended Dietary Allowances,* 10th ed. (Washington, D.C.: National Academy Press, 1989).

Dietary Reference Intakes: Recommended Intakes for Individuals, Vitamins
Food and Nutrition Board, The Institute of Medicine, National Academies

Life Stage Group	Vitamin A (µg/d)[a]	Vitamin C (mg/d)	Vitamin D (µg/d)[b,c]	Vitamin E (mg/d)[d]	Vitamin K (µg/d)	Thiamin (mg/d)	Riboflavin (mg/d)	Niacin (mg/d)[e]	Vitamin B$_6$ (mg/d)	Folate (µg/d)[f]	Vitamin B$_{12}$ (µg/d)	Pantothenic Acid (mg/d)	Biotin (µg/d)	Choline[g] (mg/d)
Infants														
0-6 mo	400*	40*	5*	4*	2.0*	0.2*	0.3*	2*	0.1*	65*	0.4*	1.7*	5*	125*
7-12 mo	500*	50*	5*	5*	2.5*	0.3*	0.4*	4*	0.3*	80*	0.5*	1.8*	6*	150*
Children														
1-3 y	**300**	**15**	5*	**6**	30*	**0.5**	**0.5**	**6**	**0.5**	**150**	**0.9**	2*	8*	200*
4-8 y	**400**	**25**	5*	**7**	55*	**0.6**	**0.6**	**8**	**0.6**	**200**	**1.2**	3*	12*	250*
Males														
9-13 y	**600**	**45**	5*	**11**	60*	**0.9**	**0.9**	**12**	**1.0**	**300**	**1.8**	4*	20*	375*
14-18 y	**900**	**75**	5*	**15**	75*	**1.2**	**1.3**	**16**	**1.3**	**400**	**2.4**	5*	25*	550*
19-30 y	**900**	**90**	5*	**15**	120*	**1.2**	**1.3**	**16**	**1.3**	**400**	**2.4**	5*	30*	550*
31-50 y	**900**	**90**	5*	**15**	120*	**1.2**	**1.3**	**16**	**1.3**	**400**	**2.4**	5*	30*	550*
51-70 y	**900**	**90**	10*	**15**	120*	**1.2**	**1.3**	**16**	**1.7**	**400**	**2.4**[h]	5*	30*	550*
>70 y	**900**	**90**	15*	**15**	120*	**1.2**	**1.3**	**16**	**1.7**	**400**	**2.4**[h]	5*	30*	550*
Females														
9-13 y	**600**	**45**	5*	**11**	60*	**0.9**	**0.9**	**12**	**1.0**	**300**	**1.8**	4*	20*	375*
14-18 y	**700**	**65**	5*	**15**	75*	**1.0**	**1.0**	**14**	**1.2**	**400**[i]	**2.4**	5*	25*	400*
19-30 y	**700**	**75**	5*	**15**	90*	**1.1**	**1.1**	**14**	**1.3**	**400**[i]	**2.4**	5*	30*	425*
31-50 y	**700**	**75**	5*	**15**	90*	**1.1**	**1.1**	**14**	**1.3**	**400**[i]	**2.4**	5*	30*	425*
51-70 y	**700**	**75**	10*	**15**	90*	**1.1**	**1.1**	**14**	**1.5**	**400**	**2.4**[h]	5*	30*	425*
>70 y	**700**	**75**	15*	**15**	90*	**1.1**	**1.1**	**14**	**1.5**	**400**	**2.4**[h]	5*	30*	425*
Pregnancy														
≤18 y	**750**	**80**	5*	**15**	75*	**1.4**	**1.4**	**18**	**1.9**	**600**[j]	**2.6**	6*	30*	450*
10-30 y	**770**	**85**	5*	**15**	90*	**1.4**	**1.4**	**18**	**1.9**	**600**[j]	**2.6**	6*	30*	450*
31-50 y	**770**	**85**	5*	**15**	90*	**1.4**	**1.4**	**18**	**1.9**	**600**[j]	**2.6**	6*	30*	450*
Lactation														
≤18 y	**1,200**	**115**	5*	**19**	75*	**1.4**	**1.6**	**17**	**2.0**	**500**	**2.8**	7*	35*	550*
19-30 y	**1,300**	**120**	5*	**19**	90*	**1.4**	**1.6**	**17**	**2.0**	**500**	**2.8**	7*	35*	550*
31-50 y	**1,300**	**120**	5*	**19**	90*	**1.4**	**1.6**	**17**	**2.0**	**500**	**2.8**	7*	35*	550*

NOTE: This table (taken from the DRI reports, see www.nap.edu) presents Recommended Dietary Allowances (RDAs) in **bold type** and Adequate Intakes (AIs) in ordinary type followed by an asterisk (*). RDAs and AIs may both be used as goals for individual intake. RDAs are set to meet the needs of almost all (97 to 98 percent) individuals in a group. For healthy breastfed infants, the AI is the mean intake. The AI for other life stage and gender groups is believed to cover needs of all individuals in the group, but lack of data or uncertainty in the data prevent being able to specify with confidence the percentage of individuals covered by this intake.

[a] As retinol activity equivalents (RAEs). 1 RAE=1 µg retinol, 12 µg β-carotene, 24 µg α-carotene, or 24 µg β-cryptoxanthin in foods. To calculate RAEs from REs of provitamin A carotenoids in foods, divide the REs by 2. For preformed vitamin A in foods or supplements and for provitamin A carotenoids in supplements, 1 RE=1 RAE.

[b] Cholecalciferol. 1 µg cholecalciferol=40 IU vitamin D.

[c] In the absence of adequate exposure to sunlight.

[d] As α-tocopherol. α-Tocopherol includes RRR-α-tocopherol, the only form of α-tocopherol that occurs naturally in foods, and the 2R-stereoisomeric forms of α-tocopherol (RRR-, RSR-, RRS-, and RSS-α-tocopherol) that occur in fortified foods and supplements. It does not include the 2S-stereoisomeric forms of α-tocopherol (SRR-, SSR-, SRS-, and SSS-α-tocopherol), also found in fortified foods and supplements.

[e] As niacin equivalents (NE). 1 mg of niacin=60 mg of tryptophan; 0-6 months=preformed niacin (not NE).

[f] As dietary folate equivalents (DFE). 1 DFE=1 µg food folate=0.6 µg of folic acid from fortified food or as a supplement consumed with food=0.5 µg of a supplement taken on an empty stomach.

[g] Although AIs have been set for choline, there are few data to assess whether a dietary supply of choline is needed at all stages of the life style, and it may be that the choline requirement can be met by endogenous synthesis at some of these stages.

[h] Because 10 to 30 percent of older people may malabsorb food-bound B$_{12}$, it is advisable for those older than 50 years to meet their RDA mainly by consuming foods fortified with B$_{12}$ or a supplement containing B$_{12}$.

[i] In view of evidence linking folate intake with neural tube defects in the fetus, it is recommended that all women capable of becoming pregnant consume 400 µg from supplements or fortified foods in addition to intake of food folate from a varied diet.

[j] It is assumed that women will continue consuming 400 µg from supplements or fortified food until their pregnancy is confirmed and they enter prenatal care, which ordinarily occurs after the end of the periconceptional period—the critical time for formation of the neural tube.

Dietary Reference Intakes: Recommended Intakes for Individuals, Minerals
Food and Nutrition Board, The Institute of Medicine, National Academies

Life Stage Group	Calcium (mg/d)	Chromium (µg/d)	Copper (µg/d)	Fluoride (mg/d)	Iodine (µg/d)	Iron (mg/d)	Magnesium (mg/d)	Manganese (mg/d)	Molybdenum (µg/d)	Phosphorus (mg/d)	Selenium (µg/d)	Zinc (mg/d)
Infants												
0-6 mo	210*	0.2*	200*	0.01*	110*	0.27*	30*	0.003*	2*	100*	15*	2*
7-12 mo	270*	5.5*	220*	0.5*	130*	11	75*	0.6*	3*	275*	20*	3
Children												
1-3 y	500*	11*	340	0.7*	90	7	80	1.2*	17	460	20	3
4-8 y	800*	15*	440	1*	90	10	130	1.5*	22	500	30	5
Males												
9-13 y	1,300*	25*	700	2*	120	8	240	1.9*	34	1,250	40	8
14-18 y	1,300*	35*	890	3*	150	11	410	2.2*	43	1,250	55	11
19-30 y	1,000*	35*	900	4*	150	8	400	2.3*	45	700	55	11
31-50 y	1,000*	35*	900	4*	150	8	420	2.3*	45	700	55	11
51-70 y	1,200*	30*	900	4*	150	8	420	2.3*	45	700	55	11
>70 y	1,200*	30*	900	4*	150	8	420	2.3*	45	700	55	11
Females												
9-13 y	1,300*	21*	700	2*	120	8	240	1.6*	34	1,250	40	8
14-18 y	1,300*	24*	890	3*	150	15	360	1.6*	43	1,250	55	9
19-30 y	1,000*	25*	900	3*	150	18	310	1.8*	45	700	55	8
31-50 y	1,000*	25*	900	3*	150	18	320	1.8*	45	700	55	8
51-70 y	1,200*	20*	900	3*	150	8	320	1.8*	45	700	55	8
>70 y	1,200*	20*	900	3*	150	8	320	1.8*	45	700	55	8
Pregnancy												
≤18 y	1,300*	29*	1,000	3*	220	27	400	2.0*	50	1,250	60	13
10-30 y	1,000*	30*	1,000	3*	220	27	350	2.0*	50	700	60	11
31-50 y	1,000*	30*	1,000	3*	220	27	360	2.0*	50	700	60	11
Lactation												
≤18 y	1,300*	44*	1,300	3*	290	10	360	2.6*	50	1,250	70	14
19-30 y	1,000*	45*	1,300	3*	290	9	310	2.6*	50	700	70	12
31-50 y	1,000*	45*	1,300	3*	290	9	320	2.6*	50	700	70	12

NOTE: This table presents Recommended Dietary Allowances (RDAs) in **bold type** and Adequate Intakes (AIs) in ordinary type followed by an asterisk (*). RDAs and AIs may both be used as goals for individual intake. RDAs are set to meet the needs of almost all (97 to 98 percent) individuals in a group. For healthy breastfed infants, the AI is the mean intake. The AI for other life stage and gender groups is believed to cover needs of all individuals in the group, but lack of data or uncertainty in the data prevent being able to specify with confidence the percentage of individuals covered by this intake.

SOURCES: Dietary Reference Intakes for Calcium, Phosphorus, Magnesium, Vitamin D, and Fluoride (1997); Dietary Reference Intakes for Thiamin, Riboflavin, Niacin, Vitamin B$_6$, Folate, Vitamin B$_{12}$, Pantothenic Acid, Biotin, and Choline (1998); Dietary Reference Intakes for Vitamin C, Vitamin E, Selenium, and Carotenoids (2000); and Dietary Reference Intakes for Vitamin A, Vitamin K, Arsenic, Boron, Chromium, Copper, Iodine, Iron, Manganese, Molybdenum, Nickel, Silicon, Vanadium, and Zinc (2001). These reports may be accessed via www.nap.edu.

Source: Reprinted with permission from the National Academy of Sciences, *Dietary Reference Intakes* (Washington, D.C.: National Academy Press, 1997–2001).

Dietary Reference Intakes (DRIs): Tolerable Upper Intake Levels (UL*), Vitamins
Food and Nutrition Board, The Institute of Medicine, National Academies

Life Stage Group	Vitamin A (μg/d)[b]	Vitamin C (mg/d)	Vitamin D (μg/d)	Vitamin E (mg/d)[c,d]	Vitamin K	Thiamin	Riboflavin	Niacin (mg/d)[d]	Vitamin B6 (mg/d)	Folate (μg/d)[d]	Vitamin B12	Pantothenic Acid	Biotin	Choline (g/d)	Carotenoids[e]
Infants															
0-6 mo	600	ND[f]	25	ND	ND	ND	ND	ND	ND	ND	ND	ND	ND	ND	ND
7-12 mo	600	ND	25	ND	ND	ND	ND	ND	ND	ND	ND	ND	ND	ND	ND
Children															
1-3 y	600	400	50	200	ND	ND	ND	10	30	300	ND	ND	ND	1.0	ND
4-8,y	900	650	50	300	ND	ND	ND	15	40	400	ND	ND	ND	1.0	ND
Males, Females															
9-13 y	1,700	1,200	50	600	ND	ND	ND	20	60	600	ND	ND	ND	2.0	ND
14-18 y	2,800	1,800	50	800	ND	ND	ND	30	80	800	ND	ND	ND	3.0	ND
19-70 y	3,000	2,000	50	1,000	ND	ND	ND	35	100	1,000	ND	ND	ND	3.5	ND
>70 y	3,000	2,000	50	1,000	ND	ND	ND	35	100	1,000	ND	ND	ND	3.5	ND
Pregnancy															
≤18 y	2,800	1,800	50	800	ND	ND	ND	30	80	800	ND	ND	ND	3.0	ND
19-50 y	3,000	2,000	50	1,000	ND	ND	ND	35	100	1,000	ND	ND	ND	3.5	ND
Lactation															
≤18 y	2,800	1,800	50	800	ND	ND	ND	30	80	800	ND	ND	ND	3.0	ND
19-50 y	3,000	2,000	50	1,000	ND	ND	ND	35	100	1,000	ND	ND	ND	3.5	ND

[a] UL = The maximum level of daily nutrient intake that is likely to pose no risk of adverse effects. Unless otherwise specified, the UL represents total intake from food, water, and supplements. Due to lack of suitable data, ULs could not be established for vitamin K, thiamin, riboflavin, vitamin B12, pantothenic acid, biotin, or carotenoids. In the absence of ULs, extra caution may be warranted in consuming levels above recommended intakes.

[b] As preformed vitamin A only.

[c] As α-tocopherol; applies to any form of supplemental α-tocopherol.

[d] The ULs for vitamin E, niacin, and folate apply to synthetic forms obtained from supplements, fortified foods, or a combination of the two.

[e] β-Carotene supplements are advised only to serve as a provitamin A source for individuals at risk of vitamin A deficiency.

[f] ND = Not determinable due to lack of data of adverse effects in this age group and concern with regard to lack of ability to handle excess amounts. Source of intake should be from food only to prevent high levels of intake.

SOURCES: Dietary Reference Intakes for Calcium, Phosphorus, Magnesium, Vitamin D, and Fluoride (1997); Dietary Reference Intakes for Thiamin, Riboflavin, Niacin, Vitamin B6, Folate, Vitamin B12, Pantothenic Acid, Biotin, and Choline (1998); Dietary Reference Intakes for Vitamin C, Vitamin E, Selenium, and Carotenoids (2000); and Dietary Reference Intakes for Vitamin A, Vitamin K, Arsenic, Boron, Chromium, Copper, Iodine, Iron, Manganese, Molybdenum, Nickel, Silicon, Vanadium, and Zinc (2001). These reports may be accessed via www.nap.edu.

Dietary Reference Intakes (DRIs): Tolerable Intake Levels (UL[a]), Elements
Food and Nutrition Board, The Institute of Medicine, National Academies

Life Stage Group	Arsenic[b]	Boron (mg/d)	Calcium (g/d)	Chromium	Copper (μg/d)	Fluoride (mg/d)	Iodine (μg/d)	Iron (mg/d)	Magnesium (mg/d)[c]	Manganese (mg/d)	Molybdenum (μg/d)	Nickel (mg/d)	Phosphorus (g/d)	Selenium (μg/d)	Silicon[d]	Vanadium (mg/d)[e]	Zinc (mg/d)
Infants																	
0-6 mo	ND[f]	ND	ND	ND	ND	0.7	ND	40	ND	ND	ND	ND	ND	45	ND	ND	4
7-12 mo	ND	ND	ND	ND	ND	0.9	ND	40	ND	ND	ND	ND	ND	60	ND	ND	5
Children																	
1-3 y	ND	3	2.5	ND	1,000	1.3	200	40	65	2	300	0.2	3	90	ND	ND	7
4-8 y	ND	6	2.5	ND	3,000	2.2	300	40	110	3	600	0.3	3	150	ND	ND	12
Males, Females																	
9-13 y	ND	11	2.5	ND	5,000	10	600	40	350	6	1,100	0.6	4	280	ND	ND	23
14-18 y	ND	17	2.5	ND	8,000	10	900	45	350	9	1,700	1.0	4	400	ND	ND	34
19-70 y	ND	20	2.5	ND	10,000	10	1,100	45	350	11	2,000	1.0	4	400	ND	1.8	40
>70 y	ND	20	2.5	ND	10,000	10	1,100	45	350	11	2,000	1.0	3	400	ND	1.8	40
Pregnancy																	
≤18 y	ND	17	2.5	ND	8,000	10	900	45	350	9	1,700	1.0	3.5	400	ND	ND	34
19-50 y	ND	20	2.5	ND	10,000	10	1,100	45	350	11	2,000	1.0	3.5	400	ND	ND	40
Lactation																	
≤18 y	ND	17	2.5	ND	8,000	10	900	45	350	9	1,700	1.0	4	400	ND	ND	34
19-50 y	ND	20	2.5	ND	10,000	10	1,100	45	350	11	2,000	1.0	4	400	ND	ND	40

[a]UL=The maximum level of daily nutrient intake that is likely to pose no risk of adverse effects. Unless otherwise specified, the UL represents total intake from food, water, and supplements. Due to lack of suitable data, ULs could not be established for arsenic, chromium, and silicon. In the absence of ULs, extra caution may be warranted in consuming levels above recommended intakes.

[b]Although the UL was not determined for arsenic, there is no justification for adding arsenic to food or supplements.

[c]The ULs for magnesium represent intake from a pharmacological agent only and do not include intake from food and water.

[d]Although silicon has not been shown to cause adverse effects in humans, there is no justification for adding silicon to supplements.

[e]Although vanadium in food has not been shown to cause adverse effects in humans, there is no justification for adding vanadium to food and vanadium supplements should be used with caution. The UL is based on adverse effects in laboratory animals and this data could be used to set a UL for adults but not children and adolescents.

[f]ND=Not determinable due to lack of data of adverse effects in this age group and concern with regard to lack of ability to handle excess amounts. Source of intake should be from food only to prevent high levels of intake.

SOURCES: Dietary Reference Intakes for Calcium, Phosphorus, Magnesium, Vitamin D, and Fluoride (1997); Dietary Reference Intakes for Thiamin, Riboflavin, Niacin, Vitamin B₆, Folate, Vitamin B₁₂, Pantothenic Acid, Biotin, and Choline (1998); Dietary Reference Intakes for Vitamin C, Vitamin E, Selenium, and Carotenoids (2000); and Dietary Reference Intakes for Vitamin A, Vitamin K, Arsenic, Boron, Chromium, Copper, Iodine, Iron, Manganese, Molybdenum, Nickel, Silicon, Vanadium, and Zinc (2001). These reports may be accessed via www.nap.edu.

Source: Reprinted with permission from the National Academy of Sciences, *Dietary Reference Intakes* (Washington, D.C.: National Academy Press, 1997–2001).

Growth Charts: Body Mass Index for Children and Teens

Body Mass Index (BMI) charts for adults are *not* meant for children and teens. For that reason, separate charts, using percentiles, were developed by the Centers for Disease Control and Prevention for girls and boys ages two to twenty, to track their growth based on BMI (see page 634).

BMI/growth charts *are not* meant to diagnose a child's or a teen's weight status but may suggest whether a child or a teen is at risk for being overweight or underweight. A child or a teen whose BMI is at the 5 percent or less percentile *may* be underweight; at the 85 to 95 percent percentile *may* be at risk of overweight; or at the 95 percent or more percentile *may* be overweight. Healthcare professionals use these charts to track a child's or a teen's growth over time; your healthcare professional should determine if your child has a weight problem and what action to take, if any.

Body Mass Index for Adults

This table allows you to determine your body mass index without having to perform calculations. Locate your height in the left-hand column. Scanning across that row, find the number closest to your weight. At the top of that column is your BMI. If your height or weight isn't listed in the table, here's a shortcut method for calculating BMI: multiply your weight (in pounds) by 703 and then divide this number by your height (in inches) squared (i.e., height × height). *For more information on what your BMI number means, refer to chapter 2.*

BODY MASS INDEX

HEIGHT	19	20	21	22	23	24	25	26	27	28	29	30	35	40
4'10"	91	96	100	105	110	115	119	124	129	134	138	143	167	191
4'11"	94	99	104	109	114	119	124	128	133	138	143	148	173	198
5'0"	97	102	107	112	118	123	128	133	138	143	148	153	179	204
5'1"	100	106	111	116	122	127	132	137	143	148	153	158	185	211
5'2"	104	109	115	120	126	131	136	142	147	153	158	164	191	218
5'3"	107	113	118	124	130	135	141	146	152	158	163	169	197	225
5'4"	110	116	122	128	134	140	145	151	157	163	169	174	204	232
5'5"	114	120	126	132	138	144	150	156	162	168	174	180	210	240
5'6"	118	124	130	136	142	148	155	161	167	173	179	186	216	247
5'7"	121	127	134	140	146	153	159	166	172	178	185	191	223	255
5'8"	125	131	138	144	151	158	164	171	177	184	190	197	230	262
5'9"	128	135	142	149	155	162	169	176	182	189	196	203	236	270
5'10"	132	139	146	153	160	167	174	181	188	195	202	207	243	278
5'11"	136	143	150	157	165	172	179	186	193	200	208	215	250	286
6'0"	140	147	154	162	169	177	184	191	199	206	213	221	258	294
6'1"	144	151	159	166	174	182	189	197	204	212	219	227	265	302
6'2"	148	155	163	171	179	186	194	202	210	218	225	233	272	311
6'3"	152	160	168	176	184	192	200	208	216	224	232	240	279	319
6'4"	156	164	172	180	189	197	205	213	221	230	238	246	287	328

WEIGHT (LBS)

OVERWEIGHT | OBESE

Source: World Health Organization

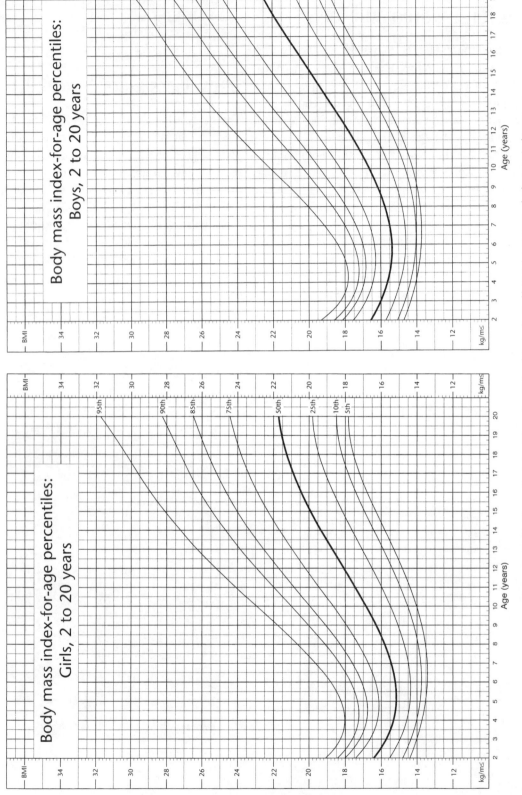

Body mass index-for-age percentiles: Boys, 2 to 20 years

Body mass index-for-age percentiles: Girls, 2 to 20 years

Source: Centers for Disease Control and Prevention, National Center for Health Statistics, CDC Growth Charts: United States. *http://www.cdc.gov/nchs/about/major/nhanes/growthcharts/charts.htm.* May 30, 2000.

Carbohydrates in Common Foods

"CARBO" FOODS

	SERVING	ENERGY (CALORIES)	CARBOHYDRATES (GRAMS)
BREAD, CEREAL, RICE, AND PASTA These foods provide a higher percentage of complex carbohydrates.			
Bagel	½	85	15
Biscuit (2" across)	1	105	15
Blueberry muffin	1	110	15
Bread (white, whole-wheat)	1 slice	60	10
Bread sticks	2 sticks	75	15
Bun (hot dog, hamburger)	½	60	10
Cereal	1 oz. (1 cup)	110	25
Cereal (cooked Cream of Wheat)	½ cup	65	15
Corn bread (2" square)	½ piece	90	15
English muffin	½	75	15
Graham crackers	2 squares	60	10
Noodles (spaghetti)	½ cup cooked	80	15
Oatmeal (cooked)	½ cup	75	15
Oatmeal (flav. instant)	1 packet	110	25
Pancakes (4" across)	1	55	10
Popcorn (plain)	1 cup popped	25	5
Pretzels	1 oz.	105	20
Rice (brown)	½ cup cooked	115	25
Rice (white)	½ cup cooked	110	25
Saltines	5 crackers	60	10
Tortilla (flour)	1	85	15
Waffles (3½" across)	1	60	10
OTHER BAKED GOODS These foods provide both complex and simple carbohydrates.			
Angel food cake	1 piece	140	30
Animal crackers	5	55	10
Chocolate cake	1 piece	235	40
Fig bar	1	50	10
Granola bar	1	110	15
Oatmeal raisin cookie	1	60	10
COMBINATION FOODS These foods provide a higher percentage of complex carbohydrates.			
Bean burrito	1	395	30
Pizza (cheese)	1 slice	290	40

For the carbohydrate content of specific foods, check the Nutrition Facts panel on food labels.

"CARBO" FOODS *(continued)*

	SERVING	ENERGY (CALORIES)	CARBOHYDRATES (GRAMS)
FRUITS These foods provide a higher percentage of simple carbohydrates.			
Apple	1 medium	80	20
Apple juice	¾ cup	85	20
Applesauce	½ cup	115	30
Banana	1	105	25
Cantaloupe	½ cup	30	5
Cherries (raw)	10	50	10
Dates (dried)	5	115	30
Fruit cocktail (packed in own juice)	½ cup	55	15
Grape juice	¾ cup	70	15
Grapes	½ cup	75	20
Orange	1 med.	65	15
Orange juice	¾ cup	85	20
Pear	1	75	20
Pineapple	½ cup	40	10
Dried plums (prunes)	5	100	25
Raisins (seedless)	⅓ cup	150	40
Raspberries	½ cup	30	5
Strawberries	½ cup	25	5
Watermelon	½ cup	25	5
VEGETABLES These foods provide a higher percentage of complex carbohydrates.			
Carrot	1 med.	30	10
Corn	½ cup	90	20
Lima beans	½ cup cooked	110	20
Peas (green)	½ cup	65	10
Potato (baked, plain)	1 large	220	50
Sweet potato	1 large	120	30
MILK, YOGURT, AND CHEESE These foods provide a higher percentage of simple carbohydrates.			
Frozen yogurt (low-fat)	1 cup	220	35
Fruit flavored yogurt	1 cup	225	40
Milk (1%)	1 cup	120	10
Milk (fat-free)	1 cup	85	10
Pudding	½ cup	160	30

Source: Debbi Sowell Jennings and Suzanne Nelson Steen. *Play Hard, Eat Right (*Minneapolis: Chronimed Publishing, 1995).

% Daily Values: What Are They Based On?

The % Daily Values (% DV) on food and supplement labels are considered average nutrient levels, not necessarily your specific nutrient needs. You may need more or less.

For daily nutrient recommendations specific to your age and gender, see the Dietary Reference Intakes (DRIs)—*shown elsewhere in the Appendices and explained in chapter 1.*

The following values are for adults and children ages four and older. Protein levels are different for infants under a year (14 grams); children one to four years (16 grams); pregnant women (60 grams); and nursing mothers (65 grams).

NUTRIENT/FOOD COMPONENT	100% DV IS EQUAL TO THIS AMOUNT
Total fat	65 g*
Saturated fat	20 g*
Cholesterol	300 milligrams
Sodium	2,400 milligrams
Potassium	3,500 milligrams
Total carbohydrate	300 g*
Dietary fiber	25 g†
Protein	50 g*
Vitamin A	5,000 IU
Vitamin C	60 mg
Calcium	1,000 mg
Iron	18 mg
Thiamin	1.5 mg
Riboflavin	1.7 mg
Niacin	20 mg
Vitamin D	400 IU
Vitamin E	30 IU
Vitamin B_6	2 mg
Folate	400 mcg
Vitamin B_{12}	6 mcg
Biotin	300 mcg
Pantothenic acid	10 mg
Phosphorus	1,000 mg
Iodine	150 mcg
Magnesium	400 mg
Zinc	15 mg
Copper	2 mg

*Based on a 2,000-calorie reference diet.
†Based on 11.5 grams per 1,100 calories.

Health Claims on Food Labels

WHAT DO HEALTH CLAIMS ON FOOD LABELS TELL YOU?

HEALTH CLAIMS ON FOOD LABELS	HOW IT MIGHT APPEAR ON THE LABEL
Calcium and osteoporosis	Regular exercise and a healthy diet with enough calcium help teens and young adult white and Asian women maintain good bone health and may reduce their high risk of osteoporosis later in life.
Sodium and hypertension	Diets low in sodium may reduce the risk of high blood pressure, a disease associated with many factors.
Dietary fat and cancer	Development of cancer depends on many factors. A diet low in total fat may reduce the risk of some cancers.
Saturated fat and cholesterol and the risk of coronary heart disease	While many factors affect heart disease, diets low in saturated fat and cholesterol may reduce the risk of this disease.
Fiber-containing grain products, fruits, and vegetables, and cancer	Low-fat diets rich in fiber-containing grain products, fruits, and vegetables may reduce the risk of some types of cancer, a disease associated with many factors.
Fruits, vegetables, and grain products that contain fiber, particularly soluble fiber, and their risk of coronary heart disease	Diets low in saturated fat and cholesterol and rich in fruits, vegetables, and grain products that contain some types of dietary fiber, particularly soluble fiber, may reduce the risk of heart disease, a disease associated with many factors.

WHAT DO HEALTH CLAIMS ON FOOD LABELS TELL YOU? *(continued)*

HEALTH CLAIMS ON FOOD LABELS	HOW IT MIGHT APPEAR ON THE LABEL
Fruits and vegetables and cancer	Low-fat diets rich in fruits and vegetables (foods that are low in fat and may contain dietary fiber, vitamin A, or vitamin C) may reduce the risk of some types of cancer, a disease associated with many factors. Broccoli is high in vitamin A and C, and it is a good source of dietary fiber.
Folate and neural tube defects	Healthful diets with adequate folate may reduce a woman's risk of having a child with a brain or spinal cord defect.
Sugar alcohol and dental caries	*Full claim:* Frequent between-meal consumption of foods high in sugars and starches promotes tooth decay. The sugar alcohols in [name of food] do not promote tooth decay. *Shortened claim* (on small packages): Does not promote tooth decay.
Soluble fiber from certain foods and the risk of coronary heart disease	Soluble fiber from foods such as [name of soluble fiber source], as part of a diet low in saturated fat and cholesterol, may reduce the risk of heart disease. A serving of [food name] supplies _____ grams of the [necessary daily dietary intake for the benefit] soluble fiber from [name of soluble-fiber source] necessary per day to have this effect.
Soy protein and risk of coronary heart disease	25 grams of soy protein a day, as part of a diet low in saturated fat and cholesterol, may reduce the risk of heart disease. A serving of [food name] supplies _____ grams of soy protein.
Plant sterol/stanol esters and risk of coronary heart disease (interim health claim)	1. Foods containing at least 0.65 gram per serving of vegetable oil sterol esters, eaten twice a day with meals for a daily total intake of at least 1.3 grams as part of a diet low in saturated fat and cholesterol, may reduce the risk of heart disease. A serving of [food name] supplies ___ grams of vegetable oil sterol esters. 2. Foods containing at least 1.7 gram per serving of vegetable oil stanol esters, eaten twice a day with meals for a daily total intake of at least 3.4 grams as part of a diet low in saturated fat and cholesterol, may reduce the risk of heart disease. A serving of [food name] supplies _____ grams of plant stanol esters.
Whole-grain foods and risk of heart disease and certain cancers	*Required wording:* Diets rich in whole grain foods and other plant foods and low in total fat, saturated fat, and cholesterol may reduce the risk of heart disease and some cancers.
Potassium and the risk of high blood pressure and stroke	*Required wording:* Diets containing foods that are a good source of potassium and that are low in sodium may reduce the risk of high blood pressure and stroke.

For definitions of terms such as "low," "rich," and "high," see "Label Lingo" in chapters 2, 3, 4, 5, 6, 7, and 11.

Sources: *Code of Federal Regulations,* Title 21, Parts 101.72-101.83 (Washington, D.C.: U.S. Food and Drug Administration, April 2001); *A Food Labeling Guide.* (Washington, D.C.: U.S. Food and Drug Administration, November 2000).

Functions of Selected Additives

A CLOSE-UP LOOK AT ADDITIVES

	Improves or Maintains Nutritional Value	Prevents Spoilage	Prevents Rancidity and Discoloration	Distributes Particles Evenly	Prevents Lumping	Retains Moisture	Makes Food Rise	Controls pH	Gives Smooth, Thick or Uniform Texture	Improves Baking Quality	Gives Color	Gives or Enhances Flavor	Sweetens
Acetic acid								X					
Acidulants or acidifiers			X					X				X	
Agar									X				
Alginate									X				
Annatto											X		
Aspartame													X
Baking powder (sodium bicarbonate and acid salts)							X						
Baking soda (sodium bicarbonate)							X						
BHA/BHT			X										
B vitamins	X												
Caffeine												X	
Calcium	X												
Calcium bromate	X									X			
Calcium proprionate	X	X											
Calcium silicate	X				X								
Calcium sulfate	X								X				
Caramel color											X		
Carob gum				X					X				
Carotene	X										X		
Carrageenan				X					X				
Cellulose						X			X				
Citric acid			X					X				X	
Corn syrup												X	X
Dextrin						X			X				
Disodium gyanylate or inosinate												X	
EDTA			X										
Gelatin									X				
Glycerine						X							
Glycerol monostearate						X							
Guar gum									X				
Herbs												X	
Hydrolyzed vegetable protein												X	
Iodine	X												

A Close-Up Look at Additives (continued)

	Improves or Maintains Nutritional Value	Prevents Spoilage	Prevents Rancidity and Discoloration	Distributes Particles Evenly	Prevents Lumping	Retains Moisture	Makes Food Rise	Controls pH	Gives Smooth, Thick, or Uniform Texture	Improves Baking Quality	Gives Color	Gives or Enhances Flavor	Sweetens
Iron	X												
Iron ammonium					X								
Lactic acid		X						X					
Lecithin				X	X								
Modified food starch					X	X			X				
Mono- and diglycerides				X									
Monosodium glutamate (MSG)												X	
Paprika											X		
Pectin				X					X				
Phosphoric acid								X					
Polysorbate				X									
Potassium sorbate		X											
Proprionic acid		X											
Propyl gallate			X										
Saffron											X	X	
Salt												X	
Silicon dioxide					X								
Sodium benzoate		X											
Sodium citrate				X									
Sodium nitrate/nitrite		X											
Sorbitan monostearate				X									
Sorbitol						X						X	X
Spices												X	
Sugar		X										X	X
Turmeric											X	X	
Vanilla												X	
Vitamin A	X												
Vitamin C	X		X										
Vitamin D	X												
Vitamin E (tocopherols)	X		X										
Xanthan gum									X				
Yeast							X						

Index